ACUTE & CHRONIC WOUNDS

CURRENT MANAGEMENT CONCEPTS

Ruth A. Bryant, PhD(candidate), MS, RN, CWOCN
Nurse Scholar in Residence
Washington State University and Providence Health Care
WOC Nursing
Sacred Heart Medical Center and Children's Hospital
Spokane, Washington

Denise P. Nix, MS, RN, CWOCN
Nix Consulting, Inc.
WOC Nursing Consultant
Minnesota Hospital Association
Minneapolis, Minnesota

FIFTH EDITION

ELSEVIER

ELSEVIER

3251 Riverport Lane
St. Louis, Missouri 63043

ACUTE & CHRONIC WOUNDS: CURRENT MANAGEMENT CONCEPTS,
FIFTH EDITION

ISBN: 978-0-323-31621-7

Notices

Library of Congress Cataloging-in-Publication Data

Acute & chronic wounds.
  Acute and chronic wounds : current management concepts / [edited by] Ruth A. Bryant, Denise P. Nix. —
Fifth edition.
    p. ; cm.
  Preceded by Acute & chronic wounds / [edited by] Ruth A. Bryant, Denise P. Nix. c2012.
  Includes bibliographical references and index.
  ISBN 978-0-323-31621-7 (hardcover : alk. paper)
  I. Bryant, Ruth A., editor. II. Nix, Denise P., editor. III. Title.
  [DNLM: 1. Wounds and Injuries—nursing. 2. Wounds and Injuries—therapy. 3. Patient Care Planning. 4. Skin Ulcer—complications. 5. Wound Healing—physiology. WY 161]
  RD98.3
  617.9'195—dc23

2015016845

Senior Content Strategist: Sandra Clark
Content Development Manager: Laurie Gower
Senior Content Development Specialist: Karen Turner
Publishing Services Manager: Jeff Patterson
Senior Project Manager: Tracey Schriefer
Design Direction: Julia Dummitt

Working together
to grow libraries in
developing countries

www.elsevier.com • www.bookaid.org

Printed in the United States of America

Last digit is the print number: 9 8 7 6 5 4 3 2 1

This book is dedicated to all those strong, amazing women out there who, due to unforeseen circumstances, find they need to redefine their future and purpose. It is dedicated to all the people who support and understand the vulnerabilities these women experience during this transition and provide the unconditional, nonjudgmental support they need to survive and ultimately prosper. I will be eternally grateful to my mother, Marilyn Elizabeth Cullivan Bryant, my WOC nursing circle of friends at Sacred Heart Medical Center (Michelle, Teresa, Becca, Beth, Robin, and Tonia) who made it very safe for me to find self-confidence, my WSU faculty friends, my sister Dorna, and my friend for life, DeeDee.

Ruth Ann Bryant

I dedicate this book to my family for all the gifts they have given me over my lifetime. To the men in my life who show me endless kindness and love: my husband Johnny, and my sons, Ian and Adam Nix.
You are my greatest blessings.
For my mom, Barbara Henry who continues to inspire and amaze me.
In loving memory of my father, Allan Henry who passed away during the writing of this book. I miss you so much Dad, every single day.

Denise (Dee Dee) Henry Nix

CONTRIBUTORS

Latricia Allen, DPM, MPH
Attending Podiatric Surgeon
Clinical Research Fellow
Veterans Affairs New England Health Care Division
Department of Surgery
Providence, Rhode Island

Michelle Best, BSN, RN, CWOCN
Sacred Heart Medical Center & Children's Hospital
Wound Care and Ostomy Department
Spokane, Washington

Jonathan S. Black, MD
Assistant Professor, Department of Plastic Surgery
University of Virginia Medical Center
Charlottesville, Virginia

Joyce M. Black, PhD, RN, CWCN, FAAN
Associate Professor
University of Nebraska Medical Center
College of Nursing
Omaha, Nebraska

Craig L. Broussard, PhD, RN, ANP-C, GNP-BC, CNS, CWS, CWCN, FAPWCS, FACCWS
President
Clinical Consultants
Port Arthur, Texas

Ruth A. Bryant, PhD(candidate), MS, RN, CWOCN
Nurse Scholar in Residence
Washington State University and Providence Health Care
WOC Nursing
Sacred Heart Medical Center and Children's Hospital
Spokane, Washington

Jane E. Carmel, MSN, RN, CWOCN
Program Co-director
Harrisburg Area Wound Ostomy Continence Nursing
    Education Program
Mechanicsburg, Pennsylvania

Renee Cordrey, PT, PhD(c), MSPT, MPH, CWS
Assistant Professor
Department of Physical Therapy and Health Care Sciences
The George Washington University
Washington, District of Columbia

David R. Crumbley, RN, MSN, CWCN
Assistant Clinical Professor
Auburn University School of Nursing
Auburn, Alabama

Dorothy B. Doughty, MN, RN, CWOCN, CFCN, FAAN
WOC Nurse Clinician
Emory University Hospital
Atlanta, Georgia

Vickie R. Driver, DPM, MS, FACFAS, FAPWCA
Professor of Orthopedic Surgery
The Warren Alpert Medical School of Brown University
Providence, Rhode Island

Eric Elster, MD, FACS, CAPT, MC, USN
Professor and Chairman
Norman M. Rich Department of Surgery
Uniformed Services University
Bethesda, Maryland

JoAnn Ermer-Seltun, RN, MS, ARNP, FNP-BC, CWOCN, CFCN
Family Nurse Practitioner, Certified Wound Ostomy and
    Continence Nurse, Certified Foot Care Nurse
Mercy Advance Wound Center & Continence Clinic
Mercy Medical Center–North Iowa
Mason City, Iowa;
Program Co-director and Faculty, webWOC Nursing
    Education Program
Minneapolis, Minnesota

Jill Evans, RN, MSN
Coordinator, Pediatric Burn Services
Medical University of South Carolina Children's Hospital
Charleston, South Carolina

Rita A. Frantz, PhD, RN, FAAN
Kelting Dean and Professor
College of Nursing
The University of Iowa
Iowa City, Iowa

Susan Gallagher, PhD, RN
Founder and Senior Clinical Advisor
Celebration Institute, Inc.
Sierra Madre, California

Daniel J. Gibson, PhD
Research Assistant Professor
University of Florida
Gainesville, Florida

Vicki Haugen, RN, MPH, CWOCN, OCN
Ostomy Wound Consultant
Chans Home Health Care
Brunswick, Maine

Ann B. Heintzelman, RN, MS, ANP-BC, CWCN
Faculty
Eastern Kansas Health Care System
Wound Management Academy
Leavenworth, Kansas

Harriet W. Hopf, MD
Professor and Vice Chair
Department of Anesthesiology
University of Utah
Salt Lake City, Utah

**Sheila Howes-Trammel, MSN, CFNP, CLNC, CCCN,
    CWCN, CFCN**
Family Nurse Practitioner
Hennepin County Medical Center
Faculty, webWOC Nursing Education Program
Minneapolis, Minnesota

Scott Junkins, MD
Associate Professor
Vice Chair, Pain Medicine
Department of Anesthesiology
School of Medicine
Medical Director, Pain Management Center
University of Utah
Salt Lake City, Utah

**Diane L. Krasner, PhD, RN, CWCN, CWS, MAPWCA,
    FAAN**
Wound and Skin Care Consultant
York, Pennsylvania

Jonathan M. LeBretton, RN, BSN
Clinical Research Nurse Coordinator
Clinical Research, Foot Care
Endovascular and Vascular Services
Department of Surgery
Boston Medical Center and Boston University School of
    Medicine
Boston, Massachusetts

Dianne M. Mackey, RN, BSN, CWOCN
Staff Educator
Home Health, Hospice, and Palliative Care
Kaiser Permanente
San Diego, California

Vincente S. Nelson, MD
Resident Surgeon
General Surgery
Walter Reed National Military Medical Center
Bethesda, Maryland

Debra S. Netsch, DNP, APRN, FNP-BC, CWOCN
Family Nurse Practitioner/Advanced Practice WOC Nurse
Ridgeview Medical Center
Waconia, Minnesota;
Co-director and Faculty
webWOC Nurse Education Program
Metropolitan State University
Minneapolis, Minnesota

Denise P. Nix, MS, RN, CWOCN
Nix Consulting, Inc.
WOC Nursing Consultant
Minnesota Hospital Association
Minneapolis, Minnesota

Daniel K. O'Neill, MD
Associate Director, Adult Offsite Anesthesiology Services
Assistant Professor of Anesthesiology
Department of Anesthesiology, Perioperative Care, and Pain
    Medicine
New York University Langone Medical Center
New York, New York

Nanjin J. Park, DPM
Clinician
Outside In Clinic
Portland, Oregon

Ben Peirce, RN, CWOCN
Vice President of Quality Management and Utilization
Woundtech
Hollywood, Florida

Priscilla L. Phillips, PhD
Department of Microbiology and Immunology
A. T. Still University
Kirksville, Missouri

Barbara Pieper, PhD, RN, ACNS-BC, CWOCN, FAAN
Professor/Nurse Practitioner
College of Nursing
Wayne State University
Detroit, Michigan

Janet M. Ramundo, MSN, RN, CWOCN, CFCN
Instructor
Emory University WOCNEC
Nell Woodruff School of Nursing
Atlanta, Georgia

Catherine R. Ratliff, PhD, GNP-BC, CWOCN, CFCN
Nurse Practitioner/Associate Professor
University of Virginia Health System
Charlottesville, Virginia

Sharon Saim, DNP, ANP-BC, CWCN
Director of the Wound Management Academy
Eastern Kansas Health Care System
Leavenworth, Kansas

Gregory Schultz, PhD
Professor
Obstetrics and Gynecology
Director
Institute for Wound Research
University of Florida
Gainesville, Florida

Dag Shapshak, MD
Associate Professor
Co-medical Director UAB Wound Care and Hyperbaric
    Medicine Clinic
Department of Emergency Medicine
University of Alabama at Birmingham
Birmingham, Alabama

Bonnie Sparks, MSN, APRN, ANP-BC, CWOCN, CWS
WOC Nurse
Atlanta Medical Center
East Point, Georgia

Nancy A. Stotts, RN, EdD, FAAN
Professor Emeritus
School of Nursing
University of California, San Francisco
San Francisco, California

**Deanna Vargo, RN, BSN, CWS, FACCWS, DAPWCA,
    CWOCN**
Clinical Resource Specialist
ConvaTec
Cuyahoga Falls, Ohio;
Wound Care Specialist
Acute/Outpatient Services
Summa Barberton Hospital
Barberton, Ohio

JoAnne D. Whitney, PhD, RN, CWCN, FAAN
Professor and Associate Dean for Research
Harborview Medical Center Endowed Professor in
Critical Care Nursing
University of Washington, School of Nursing
Nurse Scientist
Harborview Medical Center
Seattle, Washington

Annette B. Wysocki, PhD, RN, FAAN
Associate Dean for Research and Professor
College of Nursing
University of Massachusetts Amherst
Amherst, Massachusetts

Carrie Carls, RN, BSN, CWOCN, CHRN
Nursing Director
Advanced Wound Healing and Hyperbaric Medicine
Passavant Area Hospital
Jacksonville, Illinois

Lea R. Crestodina, MSN, ARNP, CWOCN, CDE
Clinical Manager Wound Care
Past Assistant Program Director
Wound Care
Emory University Wound Ostomy Continence Nursing
    Education Center
Memorial Regional Hospital/Joe DiMaggio Children's
    Hospital
Hollywood, Florida

Marilu Dixon, RN, MSN, CWOCN
Wound Ostomy Team
Sentara Virginia Beach General Hospital
Virginia Beach, Virginia

Kevin R. Emmons, DrNP, CRNO, AGPCNP-BC, CWCN
Clinical Assistant Professor
Wound Faculty–WOCNEP
School of Nursing–Camden
Rutgers, The State University of New Jersey
New Brunswick, New Jersey

Elaine Churchwell Harris, RN, MS, CCRN
Clinical Associate Professor of Adult Nursing
College of Nursing
Georgia Baptist College of Nursing of Mercer University
Atlanta, Georgia

Isabelle Reeves, RN, PhD
Associate Professor
School of Nursing
Sherbrooke University
Longueuil, Quebec

Bonnie Sue Rolstad, RN, MS, CWOCN
Program Administrator
webWOC Nursing Education Program
College of Nursing and Health Sciences
Metropolitan State University
Minneapolis, Minnesota

Mary Walden, DNP, RN, CWOCN
Professor
Itawamba Community College
Tupelo, Mississippi;
Consultant
Nursing Services
Aberdeen Pioneer Hospital
Aberdeen, Mississippi

PREFACE

Invariably, when a new edition of a textbook is released, the question from readers is, "Why should I buy this edition when I already have a previous edition?" Granted there are many resources available on wound care today unlike even 5 years ago. What this textbook and this edition bring to your library is a compilation of evidence to substantiate every aspect of the care of patients who have breaks in skin integrity. This textbook is not about dictating to the reader a recipe to follow for wound care. Rather, this textbook is about giving you, the reader, the knowledge and insight you need to discern quality, evidence-based care from arbitrary, unsubstantiated, or antiquated skin and wound care. It is about imparting to you the essential pieces of information you need to differentiate types of wounds and skin lesions so that you can derive the correct diagnosis and treatment plan. It is about outlining the normal process of wound repair in conjunction with identifying wound manifestations and needs so that you are empowered to develop the most appropriate plan of care tailored in partnership with the patient and family to reinforce the success of the treatment plan.

In addition to updating the content within each chapter, including references, there are some unique features in this fifth edition. One of those unique features is the addition of Clinical Consults at the end of every chapter. These are real-life clinical vignettes conveyed via a clinical documentation progress note using the ADPIE* or in some cases, the SBAR** scheme. It is our hope that this addition will model how to apply the new knowledge gained from that chapter into practice. Another unique feature of this edition is positioning the discussion of noncompliance (Chapter 29) within the Health Belief Model theoretical framework. By doing so, the discussion becomes positive and empowering as a means of engaging patients and family members in their self-care and risk-reduction efforts. A third unique feature of this edition is the revision of Chapter 19 to incorporate the current terminology of culture and tissue-based products (CTPs), rather than skin substitutes, in keeping with the Centers for Medicare & Medicaid Services (CMS) 2014 Hospital Outpatient Prospective Payment System (HOPPS) rule. The very popular self-assessment questions (Appendix B) have been edited and revised and continue to be extremely valuable to readers who are preparing for one of the wound certification exams. Chapter 2 (Billing, Reimbursement, and Setting Up a Clinic) has been updated to address the new ICD-10 codes. Chapter 16 (Wound Infection: Diagnosis and Management) now has a section devoted to biofilm. Finally, in an effort to reduce redundancy, we have removed many of the resources that are now readily available on the Internet.

We trust you will find this fifth edition of *Acute & Chronic Wounds: Current Management Concepts* beneficial to you personally as well as professionally. We are confident it will be an essential foundation guiding your everyday clinical practice. We appreciate your commitment to providing quality and evidence-based care to our patients.

ACKNOWLEDGMENTS

We would like to acknowledge the staff at Elsevier—Karen Turner, Tracey Schriefer, and Laura Bayless—and the many proofreaders, artists, and editors who contributed their talents. We are very grateful for their hard work, patience, and diligence.

Ruth and DeeDee

*Assessment, Diagnosis, Plan, Intervention, Evaluation
**Situation Background Assessment Recommendation

TABLE OF CONTENTS

SECTION I: Foundations

1 Principles for Practice Development to Facilitate Outcomes and Productivity, 1
Ruth A. Bryant and Denise P. Nix
Educational Preparation of the Wound Specialist, 1
National Certification: Value and Routes, 2
Roles, Functions, and Responsibilities of a Wound Specialist, 2
Prevalence/Incidence Studies, 13
Marketing, Justifying, and Securing the Wound Specialist Role: Benefits and Outcomes, 15

2 Billing, Reimbursement, and Setting Up a Clinic, 21
Deanna Vargo and Ruth A. Bryant
Creating the Business Plan, 21
Clinic Management, 21
Clinic Structure, 22
Clinic Operations, 24
Affordable Care Act and Payment Systems, 30
Factors that Influence Provider Reimbursement, 33
Coding and Billing for Services and Supplies, 36

3 Anatomy and Physiology of Skin and Soft Tissue, 40
Annette B. Wysocki
Skin Layers, 40
Skin Functions, 46
Factors Altering Skin Characteristics, 51

4 Wound-Healing Physiology and Factors That Affect the Repair Process, 63
Dorothy B. Doughty and Bonnie Sparks
Mechanism of Wound Healing, 63
Wound-Healing Process, 64
What Makes a Chronic Wound Chronic?, 73
Mediators of Wound Healing, 74
Extremes of Repair: Scarless Healing Versus Excessive Scarring, 75
Factors Affecting the Repair Process, 76

5 Types of Skin Damage and Differential Diagnosis, 82
Ruth A. Bryant
Assessment, 82
Mechanical Forces, 82
Moisture-Associated Skin Damage, 87
Medical Adhesive–Related Skin Injury, 93
Vascular Damage, 94
Infectious Agents, 95
Allergic Factors, 101
Radiation, 102

6 Skin and Wound Inspection and Assessment, 109
Denise P. Nix
Significance, 109
Assessment, 109
Reassessment and Evaluation of Healing, 119

SECTION II: Pressure Ulcers

7 Pressure Ulcers: Impact, Etiology, and Classification, 124
Barbara Pieper
Scope of the Problem, 124
Vulnerable Patient Populations, 126
Terminology, 127
Causative Factors, 127
Pathophysiologic Changes, 132
Classification of Pressure Ulcers, 135

8 Developing and Maintaining a Pressure Ulcer Prevention Program, 140
Ruth A. Bryant and Denise P. Nix
PUPP Justification, 140
Components of a PUPP, 143
Establishing a Best-Practice Bundle, 143
Creating Infrastructure to Sustain the PUPP, 155

9 Support Surfaces, 162
Denise P. Nix and Dianne M. Mackey
Interface Tissue Pressures: Past and Present, 162
Physical Concepts and Therapeutic Functions, 162
Components, 164
Categories and Features, 166
Support Surface Selection Criteria, 171

SECTION III: Lower Extremity Wounds

10 Lower Extremity Assessment, 177
JoAnn Ermer-Seltun
General Appearance of the Limb, 177
Functional–Sensory Status, 179
Perfusion, 181
Diagnostic Testing, 182

11 Arterial Ulcers, 186
Dorothy B. Doughty
Epidemiology, 186
Etiology, 187
Risk Factors for Lead, 188
Pathology of Arterial Ulceration, 191
Assessment, 191
Noninvasive Testing for Lead, 193
Invasive Testing for Lead, 196
Management of the Patient with Arterial Ulceration, 197
Patient Education, 200

12 Venous Ulcers, 204
Jane E. Carmel and Ruth A. Bryant
    Epidemiology, 204
    Venous Structure and Function, 205
    Chronic Venous Disease, 205
    Assessment, 209
    Management, 212
    Compression Therapy, 213
    Compression Wraps, 216
    Compression Garments, 218
    Intermittent Pneumatic Compression, 219
    Local Wound Care, 220
    Adjunct Therapies, 221
    Surgical Interventions, 221
    Follow-Up and Lifelong Maintenance, 223

13 Lymphedema, 227
Catherine R. Ratliff
    Epidemiology, 227
    Pathophysiology, 227
    Types of Lymphedema, 228
    Stages of Lymphedema, 230
    Lipedema, 230
    Diagnostic Tests, 231
    Assessment, 232
    Prevention, 233
    Management, 234
    Complications, 236

14 Neuropathic Wounds: The Diabetic Wound, 239
Vickie R. Driver, Jonathan M. LeBretton, Latricia Allen,
and Nanjin J. Park
    Epidemiology, 239
    Pathogenesis, 240
    Assessment, 244
    Management, 252

15 Foot and Nail Care, 263
Sheila Howes-Trammel and Ruth A. Bryant
    Quality of Life, 263
    Structure and Function, 263
    Physical Assessment, 266
    Prevention and Routine Management, 269
    Management of Specific Conditions, 276

SECTION IV: Wound Bed Preparation

16 Wound Infection: Diagnosis and Management, 283
Nancy A. Stotts
    Continuum of Microorganism Bioburden, 284
    Management of Bioburden, 288
    Evaluation, 292

17 Wound Debridement, 295
Janet M. Ramundo
    Methods of Debridement, 296
    Selection of Debridement Method, 301

18 Principles of Wound Healing and Topical Management, 306
Ruth A. Bryant and Denise P. Nix
    Principles of Wound Management, 306
    Types of Dressings, 308
    Components of a Dressing Change, 317
    Dressing Selection, 319
    Documentation and Reimbursement, 321

SECTION V: Biophysical and Biologic Agents

19 Cellular- and/or Tissue-Based Products for Wounds, 325
Sharon Saim, Ann B. Heintzelman, and Ruth A. Bryant
    Indications for Use, 325
    Classification of Products, 326
    Bilayered CTPs, 333
    Future Directions, 334

20 Molecular and Cellular Regulators, 337
Gregory Schultz, Priscilla L. Phillips, and Daniel J. Gibson
    Biologic Roles of Cytokines and Growth Factors, 337
    Adhesion Molecules and Adhesion Receptors in Inflammation, 338
    Cytokines, 341
    Growth Factors, 342
    Major Families of Growth Factors, 343
    Integrating Growth Factors into Clinical Practice, 345

21 Negative Pressure Wound Therapy, 350
Debra S. Netsch, Denise P. Nix, and Vicki Haugen
    Mechanism of Action, 350
    Indications and Uses, 352
    Safety, Contraindications, and Precautions, 353
    Clinical Application, 354

22 Hyperbaric Oxygenation, 361
Craig L. Broussard
    History, 361
    Physiologic Effects, 361
    Indications, 362
    Contraindications, 364
    Protocols and Clinical Application, 364
    Topical Oxygen is not HBO, 366

23 Electrical Stimulation, 369
Rita A. Frantz
    Effects of Electrical Stimulation, 369
    Indications and Contraindications, 371
    Types of Electrical Stimulation, 372
    Payment Coverage, 373

24 Ultraviolet Light and Ultrasound, 377
Renee Cordrey
    Ultraviolet Light, 377
    Ultrasound, 379

SECTION VI: Critical Cofactors

25 Wound Pain: Impact and Assessment, 386
Diane L. Krasner
Perceptions About Pain, 386
Consequences of Wound Pain, 387
Pain Physiology, 388
Classifications, 388
Assessment, 390
Wound Pain Care Models, 394
Translation to Practice, 395

26 Managing Wound Pain, 399
Harriet W. Hopf, Dag Shapshak, Scott Junkins, and Daniel K. O'Neill
Nonpharmacologic Pain Control, 399
Pharmacologic Interventions, 400

27 Nutritional Assessment and Support, 408
Nancy A. Stotts
Malnutrition, 408
Screening and Assessment, 410
Nutrient Needs for Healing, 414
Nutritional Support, 416

28 Perfusion and Oxygenation, 419
JoAnne D. Whitney
Effect of Oxygen and Perfusion in Wound
    Healing, 419
Factors that Alter Perfusion and Oxygenation, 420
Interventions to Improve Perfusion and Oxygen, 422
Measuring the Response, 424

29 Eliminating Noncompliance, 428
Denise P. Nix, Ben Peirce, and Vicki Haugen
Significance, 428
Goal Setting, 429
Patient Perceptions and the Health Belief Model, 429
Informed Refusal, 437

SECTION VII: Acute and Traumatic Wounds

30 Uncommon Wounds and Manifestations of Intrinsic Disease, 441
Ruth A. Bryant
Infectious Etiology, 441
Spider Bites, 443
Pyoderma Gangrenosum, 443
Vasculitis and Connective Tissue Disorders, 446
Calciphylaxis, 448
Martorell Hypertensive Ischemic Leg Ulcer, 448
Epidermolysis Bullosa, 450
Extravasation, 452
Immune Reactions, 454
Frostbite, 456
Primary Malignancy and Malignant
    Transformation Wounds (Marjolin Ulcer), 458
Blood Dyscrasias, 458

31 Traumatic Wounds: Bullets, Blasts, and Vehicle Crashes, 462
Vincente S. Nelson, David R. Crumbley, and Eric Elster
Etiology of War Wounds, 462
Acute Management of Traumatic Wounds, 464
Subacute Management of Traumatic Wounds, 468

32 Burns, 475
Jill Evans
Epidemiology, 475
Types of Burn Injury, 475
Evaluation of Burn Injury, 477
Pathophysiology of Burn Injury on the Body, 479
Phases of Burn Care, 480
Outpatient Burn Management, 486

33 Reconstructive Surgery, 490
Joyce M. Black and Jonathan S. Black
History of Surgery for Wounds, 490
Surgical Decision Making, 490
Selection of Wound Closure Method, 491
Nonoperative Conditions, 493
Urgent Operative Conditions, 493
Preoperative Management, 494
Operative Management, 495
Postoperative Management, 497

34 Surgical Wounds and Incision Care, 499
JoAnne D. Whitney
Surgical Wound Closure, 499
Surgical Wound Assessment, 500
Topical Incision Care, 503

SECTION VIII: Special Patient Populations

35 Skin Care Needs of the Obese Patient, 507
Susan Gallagher
Defining Obesity, 508
Altered Skin Function, 508
Unique Needs, 508
The Surgical Experience, 511
Nutritional Considerations, 513
Quality Improvement, 513

36 Skin Care Needs of the Neonatal and Pediatric Patient, 516
Denise P. Nix, Michelle Best, and Ruth A. Bryant
Neonatal Terminology and Skin Characteristics, 516
Skin Inspection and Risk Assessment, 518
Pediatric Conditions that Affect the Skin, 518

37 Managing Wounds in Palliative Care, 531
Ruth A. Bryant
Definition of Terms, 531
Palliative Wound Care, 532
Nonmalignancy-Related Wounds, 532
Malignancy-Related Wounds, 534
Objectives in the Care of the Malignant
    Cutaneous Wound, 534
Evaluation, 538

38 Management of Draining Wounds and Fistulas, 541
Ruth A. Bryant and Michelle Best
   Epidemiology and Etiology, 541
   Terminology, 542
   Manifestations, 544
   Medical Management, 544
   Nursing Management, 547
39 Percutaneous Tube Management, 562
Ruth A. Bryant
   Gastrostomy and Jejunostomy Devices, 562
   Placement Approaches, 563
   Feeding Tube Features, 570
   Low-Profile Gastrostomy Device (Button), 571
   Nursing Management of Enteric Tubes, 572
   Complications, 575
   Tube Removal, 576
   Patient Education, 576
   Miscellaneous Drain Tubes, 577

Appendix A: Examples of Tools Used to Support Skin and Wound Care, 579
   American College Physicians Evidence for Pressure Ulcer Risk Assessment Tools, 579
   Policy and Procedure: Prevention of Pressure Ulcers, 580
   Policy and Procedure: Wound Assessment, Documentation, and Quality Tracking, 581
   Policy and Procedure: Wound Management, 582

Policy: Nail, 583
Policy: Antiembolism Stockings, 583
Interdepartmental Handoff, 585
Pressure Ulcer Prevention Algorithm, 586
Skin Care Instructions, 587
Alginate Dressing Change Procedure, 588
Gel/Ointment/Enzyme Dressing Change Procedure, 588
Hydrocolloid Dressing Change Procedure, 589
Hydrogel-Saturated Gauze Dressing Change Procedure, 589
Wound and Skin Care Competencies, 590
Safe Skin Gap Analysis: Operating Room, 592
Aultman Surgical/Procedural Positioning Communication Tool, 593
Safe Skin Gap Analysis: Respiratory Equipment, 594
Safe Skin Gap Analysis: Cervical Collar, 595
Safe Skin ICU Pledge, 595
Pressure Ulcer Prevention Patient and Family Education, 596
Medicare Coverage of Support Surfaces, 598
Satisfaction Survey, 599
Activity Log, 600
Appendix B: Self-Assessment Exercises, 601
   Questions, 601
   Answers, 611

Principles for Practice Development to Facilitate Outcomes and Productivity

Ruth A. Bryant and Denise P. Nix

OBJECTIVES

1. Describe the services provided by the wound specialist.
2. Identify a certification process that is legally defensible.
3. Distinguish between prevalence and incidence, addressing how each is calculated and the clinical utility of each measure.
4. Describe the data that are collected and used to drive practice and justify the wound specialist position.
5. Provide an example of two stakeholders and why they hold that position in a skin and wound care practice.
6. Cite three examples of how the wound specialist can affect cost savings within an institution.

A comprehensive wound care program is essential to any organization, agency, or health care system offering a full scope of services to its clientele. The wound specialist can provide a multitude of valuable services: state-of-the-art, evidence-based wound management; staff education; control of wound-related costs; quality improvement activities; protocol and formulary development; pressure ulcer risk reduction; and insight into efficient use of personnel and resources. The wound specialist is instrumental in bringing together many departments to more fully appreciate and manage the condition of the patient with a wound. In addition, the wound specialist can affect the quality of care in an organization or agency through administrative activities, collaboration with materials management personnel, establishment of a skin safety team, and provision of direct and indirect patient care through consultation and staff education.

Many factors contribute to a successful practice as a wound specialist. Obviously the specialist must have a strong knowledge base in wound care and the relevant pathologies. In addition, the specialist must establish credibility, which is earned by demonstrating clinical competence, critical thinking, organization, self-confidence, and an eagerness to collaborate and share information with colleagues. However, a successful practice also requires the wound specialist to integrate business skills to develop goals that reflect the organization's mission and goals, effectively define services, identify benefits of services, outline a marketing approach to potential referral sources, and draft a conservative but realistic budget. Many decision-making tools and clinical resources are needed in a wound management program. The wound specialist would be wise to assemble a business plan for new skin-related and wound-related programs. Components of a business plan are listed in Chapter 2, Box 2-1. This chapter discusses the application of business skills in terms of qualifications, role development, time management, data collection, marketing, value-added services, and outcomes measurement.

EDUCATIONAL PREPARATION OF THE WOUND SPECIALIST

When an organization is developing a skin and wound management program, it is incumbent upon the administration to demand appropriate educational preparation, qualifications, and credentialing of the health care professional who will function as the wound specialist. Appropriate education and certification should not be confused with attendance at individual seminars or continuing education courses. Upon completion of a continuing education course, the attendee receives a certificate of completion. **However, in no way** should this certificate of completion be misconstrued as an indication of the attendee's expertise, mastery, or competence. The certificate simply denotes the individual's attendance at the educational event.

NATIONAL CERTIFICATION: VALUE AND ROUTES

National certification yields many benefits to the individual, the employer, and the patient (Box 1-1) (Bonham, 2009; Cary, 2001; Fleck, 2008; Woods, 2002). National certification is the formal recognition of an individual's knowledge and expertise in a defined functional or clinical area of care. National certification is intended to protect the public and should validate an individual's specialty knowledge, experience, and clinical judgment. Not all programs are legally defensible or psychometrically sound. The following components of the organization providing the certification are important to assess: national accreditation, eligibility criteria (educational degree, formal wound care education, structured clinical practicum in wound care, prior clinical experience), and recertification requirements. Collectively, these components influence the extent to which the certification designation is legally defensible (Hess, 2005). Checklist 1-1 presents questions to ask when comparing certifying organizations and certifications.

National Accreditation and Testing Standards

Accreditation of the certifying organization by an independent national certifying body is important because accreditation denotes the certifying organization's compliance with national standards relevant to all aspects of the certification process. Additionally, accreditation ensures that the certification credential meets specific criteria consistent with a testing process that is psychometrically sound (i.e., accuracy and effectiveness of each test item). A strong psychometric foundation underlying the certifying process assures candidates of fairness and accuracy of content in the testing process.

Eligibility Criteria

A key distinction among the certification designations is the education and clinical experience criterion for eligibility. Eligible disciplines and their educational preparation differ among certifying organizations. For example, the designation CWOCN© (Certified Wound, Ostomy, Continence Nurse) is bestowed only upon eligible baccalaureate-prepared nurses, whereas other certifications are available to licensed practical nurses.

Preexamination wound-specific coursework and clinical practicum requirements vary among certifying organizations. Coursework requirements can range from 0 to 5 days to many weeks. Similarly, required clinical experience varies among certifying bodies, ranging from "experience" with care, management, or research related to wounds to a more rigorous competency-based precepted clinical practicum to facilitate integration of new knowledge into an actual patient care setting in the presence of a qualified, experienced expert.

Recertification Requirements

In the ever-changing world of wound care and the need to stay current, recertification requirements are critically important and vary among credentialing organizations. Required frequency of recertification is 5 or 10 years, depending on the organization. Methods of recertification vary significantly and include self-assessment, proof of experience, and retesting.

ROLES, FUNCTIONS, AND RESPONSIBILITIES OF A WOUND SPECIALIST

The wound specialist is not responsible for conducting every wound assessment or dressing change. Clarity in terms of

TABLE 1-1 Delineation of Roles of Wound Specialist and Staff Nurse	
Wound and Skin Specialist	**Staff Nurse**
Facilitate creation and implementation of pressure ulcer risk assessment protocol.	Conduct risk assessment per protocol.
Establish protocol for prevention guidelines to correlate with risk assessment.	Implement appropriate risk reduction interventions.
Establish protocol for management of minor skin lesions (candidiasis, skin tears, incontinence-associated dermatitis, Stage I and II pressure ulcers).	Implement appropriate care of minor skin lesions.
Formulate skin and wound care product formulary to specify indications and parameters for use of products.	Use wound products per formulary. Notify wound specialist if product performs poorly or if expected outcome is not achieved.
Conduct comprehensive assessment, establish plan of care for complex patients (e.g., leg ulcers, Stages III and IV pressure ulcers), conduct regular reevaluation of healing.	Notify wound specialist of complex patients. Conduct focused wound assessment. Implement appropriate care per wound specialist's direction and facility protocols.
Provide competency-based staff education for new employees and annual competency-based education for existing employees.	Identify and recommend topics of interest for staff education and updates.
Track outcomes and identify skin and wound care issues. Initiate quality improvement activities.	Participate in quality improvement activities.

expectations of the wound specialist, staff nurse, and physical therapist (PT) is essential to promote collaboration and deliver comprehensive and effective skin and wound care. This clear delineation of roles is important to foster an empowering environment, avoid duplication of efforts, and maximize the efficient use of resources, including personnel. Table 1-1 provides examples of role delineation of a wound specialist and a staff nurse.

Participation in staff orientation programs is a key strategy to communicate roles, functions, and responsibilities. This setting offers an opportunity to orient new staff members to their role in maintaining skin health, providing wound care, performing skin assessment and surveillance, performing risk assessment, and preventing pressure ulcers. The wound specialist should take the time to instruct personnel on when and how to access the wound specialist. Key stakeholders (e.g., physicians, information technology personnel, purchasing director, materials management, director of nursing) should be contacted and the role of the wound specialist discussed and clarified. Stakeholders, by definition, may affect or be affected by the skin and wound program; thus keeping them involved and informed can minimize or eliminate negative ramifications. As with all discussions, emphasizing the benefits of the skin and wound care program to the success of the facility or patient practice is important. The support and confidence of key stakeholders are so critical that the extra effort and time taken to nurture these relationships are well worth it. Ultimately, however, the wound specialist will need to demonstrate competence and confidence in his or her practice. Regardless of the health care setting in which the wound specialist will practice, role implementation will share common overlapping components: clinical consultant/expert, leader/coordinator, educator, change agent, and facilitator of evidence-based practice (EBP) and quality improvement to improve outcomes (Box 1-2).

Consultant

Although many wound specialists provide direct patient care for the most complex wounds, in most settings the wound specialist serves primarily as a consultant. As a consultant, the specialist can better meet the majority of patients' needs by coordinating a skin and wound care program implemented by a multidisciplinary team of health care providers. The consultant role builds on the foundations of the wound specialist's clinical expertise in wound-related pathophysiology, physical assessment, wound assessment, appropriate use of interventions, and documentation. A successful consultant must effectively communicate, collaborate, and educate. Clinical decision-making tools and resources, such as protocols, product formularies, and standardized care plans, pave the way for the specialist to adopt a consultative approach within the organization (Pasek et al, 2008).

Educator

Knowledge about skin inspection, pressure ulcer prevention, basic wound care, and comprehensive, accurate documentation is essential to maintaining and restoring skin integrity. Information about wound and skin care is increasingly available from the literature and from commercial sources. Reimbursement restrictions provide greater incentive for staff to familiarize themselves with basic skin care and pressure ulcer prevention. However, the wound specialist needs to organize the information into retrievable and clinically useful formats so that a formulary of wound and skin care products is available; the process for selecting and ordering an appropriate support surface is specified; and the documentation is comprehensive, easily accomplished, and not repetitive. As an educator, the wound specialist will develop routine orientation sessions to introduce new staff to the pressure ulcer prevention program, addressing, for example, basic wound assessment, support surface selection, and the essential nature of skin inspection and risk assessment.

BOX 1-2　Roles of the Wound Specialist

Consultant/Expert
- Evaluates patient response to treatment and the progress of wound healing, making adjustments and modifications as indicated
- Where qualified and appropriate, provides conservative sharp debridement of devitalized tissue and applies silver nitrate to epibole, granulation tissue, and areas with minor bleeding
- Provides consultation and follow-up for patients with draining or chronic wounds, fistulas, or percutaneous tubes through outpatient clinic visits and/or phone consultations; initiates appropriate referrals for medical or surgical intervention

Educator
- Provides appropriate education to patient, caregiver, and staff regarding skin care, wound management, percutaneous tubes, and draining wound/fistula management
- Assists staff to maintain current knowledge and competence in the areas of skin and wound care through orientation and regularly scheduled education
- Attends continuing education programs related to skin and wound management

Change Agent (see Tables 1-2 and 1-3)
- Identifies barriers to change
- Provides evidence that persuades staff that change will achieve desired outcome
- Considers all stakeholders when planning change
- Communicates aspects of practice changes that will positively affect key stakeholders (especially the staff expected to implement the change)

Program Coordinator/Leader
- Provides consultation and assistance to staff in developing and implementing protocols used in the identification and management of patients with potential or actual alteration in skin integrity
- Provides guidance to staff in implementation of protocols to identify, control, or eliminate etiologic factors for skin breakdown, including selection of appropriate support surface
- Establishes protocols and guidelines for appropriate and cost-effective use of therapeutic support surfaces
- Maintains records and statistics and submits reports to employer
- Analyzes inventory and recommends appropriate additions and deletions to ensure quality and cost-effectiveness of products used for skin and wound care
- Serves on agency-wide committees and participates in agency-wide projects as requested
- Coordinates wound management teams or committees

Facilitator of EBP and Quality Improvement
- Assists staff to maintain current state-of-the-art practice by reviewing and revising policies and procedures to be consistent with national guidelines and other sources of evidence-based literature
- Provides leadership with prevalence and incidence studies
- Conducts product evaluations or contributes to research studies related to skin and wound care when indicated; submits reports and recommendations based on results
- Participates in public policy through guideline development, consensus statements, advisory panel membership, etc.

By auditing chart documentation or surveying the staff's knowledge about specific areas of wound care, the specialist can identify additional needs and target follow-up educational activities to satisfy those needs (Beeckman et al, 2013). Beitz, Fey, and O'Brien (1999) warn that "professional staff who perceive little need for additional wound care education may 'tune out' opportunities for increasing their knowledge base because they consider themselves 'competent.'" This information underscores the importance of using pretests and other means of educational needs assessments; however, education does not guarantee practice change.

Change Agent

Although education is an important role and tool for the wound specialist, it can be viewed as a burden that will increase workload rather than an innovation that eventually will decrease workload and improve patient outcomes (Landrum, 1998b). The organization will need to integrate principles for innovation adaptation to increase the likelihood of success with the educational efforts. An individual's reaction to and decision about new information, ideas, or practice (i.e., innovations) develops over time and seldom is spontaneous. Rogers' *Diffusion of Innovations* (2003) provides a framework for changing practices in a group, individual, or organization (Dobbins et al, 2005; Landrum, 1998a). This theory describes how people adopt innovations using five stages: knowledge, persuasion, decision, implementation, and confirmation (Table 1-2). Whether the innovation is implementing a new product or improving upon an existing product, and whether the innovation is preventive or has immediate observable results, a failure to consider these stages can spell disaster and frustration. Table 1-2 outlines these stages, defines each stage, and discusses considerations relative to skin and wound care.

Innovation is more likely to be adopted and behaviors changed when the innovation is perceived as relevant and consistent with the individual's attitudes and the perceived attitudes of colleagues within the organization (Dobbins et al, 2005). Generally, an individual will seek like-minded peers who already have embraced the innovation to discuss the consequences of adopting the innovation, and an individual's motivation to embrace the innovation is increased when these colleagues are supportive and positive about the innovation. Five attributes of an innovation significantly influence the rate at which it is adopted: relative advantage, compatibility, complexity, trialability, and observability (Table 1-3). These attributes should be considered before the persuasion stage so that adjustments can be made to enhance the likelihood of success with the education efforts.

TABLE 1-2 Five Stages of Rogers's Innovation-Decision Process

Stage	Description
Knowledge	Individual becomes aware of an innovation and of how it functions. May occur with reading, reviewing posted flyers, attending lectures.
Persuasion	Favorable or unfavorable attitude toward an innovation forms. To form a favorable attitude, the individual must be convinced that the innovation has greater value than current practice (e.g., identify patients at risk for pressure ulcers or target appropriate interventions).
Decision	Individual receives enough information to form an opinion about innovation. Individual pursues activities that lead to adoption or rejection of the innovation.
Implementation	Once an individual makes a decision to adopt the innovation, barriers (structural, process, psychological) to implementation must be overcome (e.g., adequate number of forms is available).
Confirmation	Individual seeks to reinforce his or her decision. Observable and positive results are critical at this stage to prevent a reversal in decision. Careful monitoring is required, and information validating positive effects is important (e.g., decrease in incidence of pressure ulcers after adoption of new risk assessment tool).

Data from Landrum BJ: Marketing innovations to nurses, Part 1: How people adopt innovations, *J Wound Ostomy Continence Nurs* 25:194–199, 1998.

TABLE 1-3 Attributes that Influence Adoption of Innovation

Attributes of Innovation	Description
Relative advantage	Is this better than an existing practice (e.g., potential decrease in costs, decrease in staff time, ease of use)?
Compatibility	Is this consistent with the individual's existing values, experiences, and needs?
Complexity	Is this innovation difficult to understand or use? For example, when a protocol is developed that links risk assessment scores with nursing interventions, the decision about which preventive nursing intervention to use may be perceived as less complex than before the protocol; therefore, the protocol may be more likely to be adopted.
Trialability	Can the individual experiment with the innovation on a limited basis?
Observability	Are the results of an innovation visible to others? Subtle outcomes are harder to communicate to others, so the innovation often is slower to be adopted.

Adapted from Landrum BJ: Marketing innovations to nurses, Part 1: How people adopt innovations, *J Wound Ostomy Continence Nurs* 25:194–199, 1998.

T (timeframe). This type of narrowly defined question facilitates the search so as to obtain the most relevant and best evidence (Melynyk & Fineout-Overholt, 2011). Sample PICOT questions are provided in Box 1-3.

Evidence-Based Care. Integrating evidence into practice is a fundamental expectation of the wound specialist and a key component of an EBP. Defined as "the integration of best research evidence with clinical expertise and patient values to facilitate clinical decision making" (Sackett et al, 2000), EBP acknowledges that the care provided patients should not be based on habit, but rather supported by the best possible evidence of effectiveness. Evidence-based practice requires consideration of the following types of evidence: external evidence (i.e., research, theories, expert panel), internal evidence (i.e., clinical expertise, QI, patient data), and patient preferences and values (Melynyk & Fineout-Overholt, 2011). Providing evidence-based care requires that we *synthesize* the best available evidence from what is currently known.

Many individual and organizational barriers exist to research utilization and evidence-based care (DiCenso et al, 2005; Melynyk & Fineout-Overholt, 2011). One individual barrier is feeling inadequately prepared to evaluate the quality of research and a lack of knowledgeable colleagues with whom to discuss research. In addition, access to the literature may be a hardship because of workload and time limitations. On an organizational level, barriers may arise from a lack of

Facilitator of Evidence-Based Practice and Quality Improvement

The wound specialist serves a pivotal role in facilitating and implementing EBP and quality improvement (QI) studies within the context of skin and wound care for the facility or agency. Examples of QI activities that the wound specialist could participate in are discussed later in this chapter. Many wound specialists have a role in public policy through guideline development, consensus statements, advisory panel membership, and research. These activities have helped shape public policy by strengthening the evidence base and educating lawmakers to help improve outcomes through better access to appropriate supplies, equipment, and services.

Regardless of the type of project being planned (i.e., EBP, QI, or research), the first step in the process is to formulate and refine a question. PICOT is a common format recommended for phrasing the question. A well-designed PICOT question contains the following pieces of information: P (patient population), I (intervention or issue of interest), C (comparison intervention or group, O (outcome), and

BOX 1-3   Sample PICOT Questions

- In the home care patients with a wound (P), how does dressing change technique using clean technique by the patient in the home (I) compared with changing dressings using sterile technique by professional nursing in the outpatient clinic (C) affect outcomes (O) following a patient education program (T)?*
- In patients with advanced illness (P), how do Stage I and II pressure ulcers (I) compared with Stage III and IV pressure ulcers (C) affect the rate of complete healing (O) among patients referred to a regional palliative care program between May 2005 and June 2006 (T)?†
- In the nursing home patient population (P), how does skin inspection (I) conducted by a single nurse or by two nurses (C) affect the pressure ulcer prevalence rate (O) over a 3-year timeframe (T)?‡

*Adapted from Chan LN, Lai CKY: The effect of patient education with telephone follow-up on wound healing in adult patients with clean wounds: a randomized controlled trial, *J Wound Ostomy Continence Nurs* 41(4):345–355, 2014.
†Adapted from Maida V, Ennis M, Coban J: Wound outcomes in patients with advanced illness, *Int Wound J* 9:683–692, 2012.
‡Adapted from Kottner J, Tannen A, Halfens R, et al: Does the number of raters influence the pressure ulcer prevalence rate? *Appl Nurs Res* 22(1):68–72, 2009.

TABLE 1-4   Hierarchy of Preprocessed Information Sources

	Hierarchy Levels	Examples
(Highest-Level Resource)	Systems	Clinical practice guidelines
		Evidence-based textbook summaries
		Clinical Evidence (BMJ Publishing Group)
	Synopses of syntheses	Evidence-based abstract journals (e.g., *Evidence-Based Nursing*)
		Systematic reviews
	Syntheses	*Cochrane Reviews*
		Cochrane Library (www.cochrane.org)
		UpToDate (Resource for preappraised evidence-based clinical decisions published by Wolters Kluwer Health)
	Synopses of single studies	Evidence-based abstract journals
(Lowest-Level Resource)	Single studies	PubMed clinical queries

interest, motivation, vision, and strategy on the part of leadership. Organizational barriers also may be related to library access, the extent of library holdings, and Internet access. Recognizing and overcoming these barriers is important in order to positively impact implementation of EBP.

To embark on the path of evidence-based care, the specialist must keep abreast of relevant health care literature to "find the evidence." In the face of a constantly growing body of health care literature, remaining current in the literature may seem impossible or all consuming. However, preappraised literature is increasingly available that expedite access to evidence (Fine-Overholt et al, 2011).

Preappraised literature are products that have been developed by an individual or group that has reviewed the literature, filtered out the flawed studies, and included only the methodologically strongest studies. A hierarchy of preappraised literature with relevant examples is given in Table 1-4. Such sources include practice guidelines, clinical pathways, evidence-based abstract journals, and systematic reviews. For example, guidelines pertinent to skin and wound care are available through the Wound, Ostomy and Continence Nurses Society™ (WOCN®, 2008, 2010a, 2011a, 2012a), Wound Healing Society (Hopf et al, 2006; Robson et al, 2006; Steed et al, 2006; Whitney et al, 2006), National Guideline Clearinghouse (www.guideline.gov), Association for the Advancement of Wound Care (www.aawconline.org), the Cochrane Collaboration (www.cochrane.org), and the National Pressure Ulcer Advisory Panel/European Pressure Ulcer Advisory Panel/Pan Pacific Pressure Injury Alliance (https://international-pressure-ulcer-guidelines.myshopify.com).

When appraised literature relative to a particular clinical issue is not available, unprocessed resources are necessary.

Unprocessed resources are databases (e.g., CINAHL, MEDLINE, EMBASE) that contain millions of primarily original study citations (Table 1-5). The World Wide Web also is an unprocessed resource, although its potential for inaccurate information is substantial. Seven criteria have been developed (Table 1-6) that can be used to assess the quality of health care information obtained from the Internet (AHCPR, 1999; O'Sullivan, 2011).

Because the methodological quality of studies obtained using unprocessed sources will vary, each study or report will require a critical appraisal to differentiate misleading research reports from valid reports. Many sources that discuss the critical appraisal of research are available (Callihan, 2008; Webb, 2008). However, many providers are not comfortable with their research appraisal skills. To simplify the process, Cullum and Guyatt (2005) propose asking three discrete, sequential questions, as discussed in Table 1-7.

The value of research-based care to the organization and the patient is significant. Results of a metaanalysis of studies have demonstrated that research-based care offers patients better outcomes than does routine procedural care. However, the wound specialist not only should *apply* evidence to practice, but also should *generate* evidence from practice (Ehrenberg et al, 2004). Evidence can be generated by publishing individual case studies or by partnering with doctoral-prepared researchers to design and conduct basic research that answers clinically relevant questions.

TABLE 1-5   Unprocessed Sources of Evidence

Database	Maintained by	Unique Features	Contents
CINAHL	Information systems and updated quarterly	Largest bibliographic database specifically related to nursing, allied health disciplines, and consumer health	Full text articles Clinical practice guidelines Bibliographies of major articles Research instruments Government publications Comments Book reviews Evaluations of multimedia and computer software and systems Patient education materials
MEDLINE	United States National Library of Medicine	Readily accessible Searching effectively requires thorough knowledge of how database is structured and publications are indexed	Comprehensive coverage of health care journals
EMBASE	Elsevier Science	Comprehensive bibliographic database of worldwide literature Requires thorough knowledge of how database is structured and publications are indexed	Biomedical and pharmaceutical literature fields Indexes large proportion of European biomedical and science literature

TABLE 1-6   Criteria for Evaluating Internet Health Information

Criteria	Description
Credibility	Includes source, currency, relevance/utility, and editorial review process for the information
Content	Must be accurate, complete, and provide an appropriate disclaimer
Disclosure	Includes informing the user of the purpose of the site, as well as any profiling or collection of information associated with site use
Links	Evaluated according to selection, architecture, content, and back-linkages
Design	Encompasses accessibility, logical organization (navigability), and internal search capability
Interactivity	Includes feedback mechanisms and means for information exchange among users
Caveats	Clarifies whether site functions as marketer of products and services or as provider of primary information content

Data from Agency for Healthcare Research and Quality (AHRQ): *Assessing the quality of Internet health information: summary,* Rockville, MD, June 1999, AHRQ. http://www.ahrq.gov/research/data/infoqual.htm Accessed Jan. 22, 2014.

Historically, a gap in health care has existed between what is known and what is practiced. The wound specialist has a critical leadership role in making EBP a reality. When leaders not only expect but also promote EBP to staff, quality of care is enhanced and optimal patient outcomes are achieved. Caregivers are most effective at integrating research into practice when the leader is clinically based, has specific clinical expertise and knowledge, and expresses a positive attitude toward research (Ferguson et al, 2004).

Evidence ranking. Evidence derives from many sources, and each source has its own merits and deficiencies. Clinical observations, expert opinions, and generalizations from physiology constitute the weakest forms of evidence. Systematic studies, such as clinical trials, prospective studies, and case studies, provide a higher level of evidence. Typical classification schemes place the metaanalysis and randomized clinical trial (RCT) as the highest levels of evidence because they are designed to reduce the risk of bias and have less risk of systematic errors. However, not all clinical questions can be researched using an RCT design (e.g., rare conditions, ethical concerns). In addition, the RCT is not an appropriate design for a prognosis or diagnosis question. Therefore different specialties and organizations often adopt variations of the classification scheme to best meet the types of questions being posed, yet all share common threads with the goal of providing a consistent method for interpreting the quality of evidence. Table 1-8 provides the definition of the levels of evidence used by the WOCN® Society in their guideline development process. Tables 1-9, 1-10, and 1-11 provide the criteria used in the development of the international pressure ulcer guidelines specific to intervention studies, prognostic studies, and diagnostic studies. The Centre for Evidence-Based Medicine (CEBM) is a valuable resource for detailed information about resources and tools concerning levels of evidence (http://www.cebm.net).

Quality Improvement. Quality improvement activities incorporate elements of research and are a high priority for the wound specialist. Quality improvement initiatives often are initiated to improve processes that will decrease cost, save time, or improve patient or staff satisfaction (Orsted et al,

TABLE 1-7 Guide for Evaluating Intervention-Based Research

Steps	Description	Related Study Design Questions
1. Are the results valid?	The study must be designed and conducted in a valid manner so that the results are believable and credible. A study design that is less than rigorous and contains sources of bias will generate skewed and false conclusions. Only when the study methods are valid and rigorous should the reader continue on to further assess the study results.	Did intervention and control groups begin the study with a similar prognosis? Were patients randomized? Was randomization concealed? Were patients analyzed in the groups to which they were randomized? Were groups shown to be similar in all known determinants of outcome, or were analyses adjusted for differences? Did intervention and control groups retain a similar prognosis after the study started? Were patients aware of group allocation? Were clinicians aware of group allocation? Were outcome assessors aware of group allocation? Was follow-up complete?
2. What are the results?	Any difference between the groups in the study will be expressed in terms of a risk measure, such as risk reduction or benefit increase. The accuracy of the risk measure (the effect of the intervention) will be expressed in terms of a confidence interval or p-value. In general, a narrow confidence interval, which does not include zero, suggests more precision and, therefore, greater confidence in the results.	How large was the intervention effect? How precise was the estimate of the intervention effect?
3. How can results be applied to patient care?	The patients in the wound care specialist's practice should be similar to the patient population that participated in the study if the research results are to be applied to them.	Were the study patients similar to the patients in my clinical setting? Were all of the important outcomes considered? Are the likely intervention benefits worth the potential harm and costs?

TABLE 1-8 Rating of Research Evidence

Level I	A randomized controlled trial (RCT) that demonstrates a statistically significant difference in at least one important outcome defined by $p < .05$. Level I trials can conclude that the difference is not statistically significant if the sample size is adequate to exclude a 25% difference among study arms with 80% power.
Level II	An RCT that does not meet level I criteria.
Level III	A nonrandomized controlled trial with contemporaneous controls selected by some systematic method. A control might have been selected because of its perceived suitability as a treatment option for an individual patient.
Level IV	A before-and-after study or a case series of at least 10 patients using historical controls or controls drawn from other studies.
Level V	A case series of at least 10 patients with no controls.
Level VI	A case report of fewer than 10 patients.

From Wound, Ostomy and Continence Nurses Society™.

TABLE 1-9 Level of Evidence for Intervention Studies

Level 1	Randomized trial(s) with clear-cut results and low risk of error OR systematic literature review or metaanalysis according to the Cochrane methodology OR meeting at least 9 of 11 quality criteria according the AMSTAR appraisal tool.
Level 2	Randomized trial(s) with uncertain results and moderate to high risk of error.
Level 3	Nonrandomized trial(s) with concurrent or contemporaneous controls.
Level 4	Nonrandomized trial(s) with historical controls.
Level 5	Case series with no control. Specify number of subjects.

Reprinted with permission from National Pressure Ulcer Advisory Panel, European Pressure Ulcer Advisory Panel, and Pan Pacific Pressure Injury Alliance. Haesler E, editor: *Prevention and treatment of pressure ulcers: clinical practice guideline*, Osborne Park, Western Australia, 2014, Cambridge Media.

TABLE 1-10   Levels of Evidence for Diagnostic Studies

Level 1	Systematic review of high-quality (cross-sectional) studies according to the quality assessment tools with consistently applied reference standard and blinding.
Level 2	Individual high-quality (cross-sectional) studies according to the quality assessment tools with consistently applied reference standard and blinding among consecutive persons.
Level 3	Nonconsecutive studies, or studies without consistently applied reference standards.
Level 4	Case controls studies, or poor or nonindependent reference standard.
Level 5	Mechanism-based reasoning, study of diagnostic yield (no reference standard).

Reprinted with permission from National Pressure Ulcer Advisory Panel, European Pressure Ulcer Advisory Panel, and Pan Pacific Pressure Injury Alliance. Haesler E, editor: *Prevention and treatment of pressure ulcers: clinical practice guideline*, Osborne Park, Western Australia, 2014, Cambridge Media.

TABLE 1-11   Levels of Evidence for Prognostic Studies

Level 1	Systematic review of high-quality (longitudinal) prospective cohort studies according to the quality assessment tools.
Level 2	A prospective cohort study.
Level 3	Analysis of prognostic factors among persons in a single arm of a randomized controlled trial.
Level 4	Case series or case controls studies, or poor-quality prognostic cohort study, retrospective cohort study.
Level 5	Not applicable.

Reprinted with permission from National Pressure Ulcer Advisory Panel, European Pressure Ulcer Advisory Panel, and Pan Pacific Pressure Injury Alliance. Haesler E, editor: *Prevention and treatment of pressure ulcers: clinical practice guideline*, Osborne Park, Western Australia, 2014, Cambridge Media.

2009). Evidence demonstrates that a facility's ongoing involvement in QI initiatives (including evidence-based guideline introduction and implementation, regular prevalence surveys, and annual national surveys) is associated with significant reductions in wounds within the facility (Bales and Duvendack, 2011; Bales and Padwojski, 2009; Kelleher et al, 2012). Such activities often consist of simple chart audits designed to ascertain the adequacy of documentation of assessment parameters, interventions, and effects or outcomes. Without a QI process, delays, inefficiencies, or harmful interventions may go undetected and thus contribute to staff or patient dissatisfaction, delayed discharge, or increased costs of care. Quality improvement activities that should be central to all wound care programs are prevalence and incidence

studies (discussed later in this chapter) and pressure ulcer prevention programs (Chicano and Drolshagen, 2009; Hiser et al, 2006; Orsted et al, 2009).

Program Coordinator

A fundamental need of any practice is a skin safety program consisting of skin and wound care policies, dressing change procedures, decision support tools, skin and wound care product formularies, support surface algorithms, and treatment protocols. Decision support tools enhance the clinician's decision-making capacity (Ehrenberg et al, 2004), thus empowering caregivers to act independently and wisely in a consistent fashion. Specifically, treatment protocols guide staff to (1) address critical assessment parameters, (2) perform steps of assessment and treatment procedures in a proper sequence, (3) learn proper application and utilization of specific products, and (4) assess the effectiveness of interventions (Pasek et al, 2008).

Policies and procedures are essential for guiding the delivery of care and meeting standards required by The Joint Commission and state health departments. Relative to skin and wound care, each facility or health care organization should develop policies for skin assessment, pressure ulcer risk assessment, wound cleansing, wound assessment, treatment of wounds, documentation and staging, compression therapy, debridement, and culturing. In addition, a policy should exist to delineate appropriate interventions for different levels of pressure ulcer risk, as well as for high-risk patients. Examples of policies, procedures, and decision-making tools are given in Appendix A.

Skin and wound assessment parameters (see Chapter 6) should be incorporated into the admission database to ensure that the data are collected. Such data can also be incorporated into daily documentation flow sheets. Flow sheets that are dedicated to wound assessment and wound care interventions are particularly useful because they will best reflect changes in wound status over time at a glance. Documentation in multiple places increases the risk of errors, inconsistencies, and omissions and should be avoided. Electronic medical records are becoming more common in the health care setting, but may not necessarily facilitate appropriate documentation or effective integration of wound- and skin-related EBP guidelines (Milne et al, 2009). Therefore it is critical that the wound specialist serve as content expert when choosing or building an electronic documentation system so that wound- and skin-specific data can be aggregated into relevant clinical information (Golinko et al, 2009).

Skin Safety Committees and Teams. Wound care is a team effort. Each member of the team has an invaluable and irreplaceable contribution. A team approach to wound care is critical to the adoption of patient-centered care delivery. The members of a team focus on working together to achieve a mutually agreed upon goal, and team members are accountable for attaining the desired results. However, functioning as a team to provide integrated services is inconsistently provided and poorly understood (Moore et al, 2014). The terms *multidisciplinary*, *interdisciplinary*, and *transdisciplinary* are misunderstood and commonly used interchangeably. The distinction among these terms is provided in Table 1-12. An additional member of the interdisciplinary wound care team that has been proposed by the collaboration of international wound care organizations is the "wound navigator" (Moore et al, 2014). The role of this individual would be to facilitate the integration of the patient's perspective into a wound care plan and would be akin to the individual who assists cancer patients in their management.

TABLE 1-12	Team Model Terms
Term	**Description**
Multidisciplinary	• Utilize skills and experience of individuals from different disciplines • Each provides a specific service to the patient • Consists of separate individual consultations • Members work independently • Focus is on *issues* relevant to their specialty • May meet regularly as a group to discuss patient's care but in absence of the patient
Interdisciplinary	• Separate discipline approaches are integrated into a single consultation • History taking, assessment, diagnosis, interventions, and goals are conducted as a team together with the patient at one time • Team members represent relevant clinical disciplines • Interactions are guided by specific team functions and processes • Patient is a member of the team and empowered to form part of decision-making process and goal setting • Goal is to achieve team-defined patient outcomes • All members encouraged to question each other and explore alternative pathways to achieve best outcome
Transdisciplinary	• Most advanced level • Disciplinary lines are blurred • Members consists of stakeholders who transcend boundaries of the individual discipline • New knowledge is brought to the team

Modified from Moore A, Butcher G, Corbett LQ, et al: Exploring the concept of a team approach: managing wounds as a team, *J Wound Care* 23(Suppl 5):S1–S38, 2014; Jessup RL: Interdisciplinary versus multidisciplinary care teams: do we understand the difference? *Aust Health Rev* 31(3):330–331, 2007.

Successful skin safety programs have reported the use of multidisciplinary meetings and interdisciplinary collaboration (Ackermann, 2012; Thommas, 2008; Tippet, 2009). As a leader and program coordinator, the wound specialist will develop programs and projects that reflect the needs of the patient population; are consistent with the priorities of the corporation; and are fiscally responsible, evidence based, and educationally and professionally valuable to the staff. A skin and wound care program is basic and essential to all care settings and facilities. In the United States the gold standard for a comprehensive wound care program is a system-wide skin safety committee with unit-based skin care teams. Such programs consistently demonstrate enhanced clinical outcomes, reduced liability, increased staff satisfaction, and reduced costs (Andriessen et al, 2009; Chicano and Drolshagen, 2009; Hiser et al, 2006; Lloyd-Vossen, 2009; McIsaac, 2007; Orsted et al, 2009). Keys to the success of a skin and wound care program are dissemination of information; involvement of all stakeholders; and consistent, intuitive documentation.

From a structural aspect, the program will need a mechanism for oversight of the program and for operationalizing the program at the bedside. Program oversight is provided by a system-wide committee (e.g., skin safety committee) that is responsible for creating policies and procedures, formularies, decision-making guides, documentation tools, and educational resources. This group also facilitates transfer of knowledge and guidelines to the unit and bedside (Lloyd-Vossen, 2009). Members of the skin safety committee providing oversight of the program are representative of all stakeholders and key decision makers, including administration, pharmacy, purchasing, and utilization review/risk management.

The success of the skin safety program ultimately lies with the ability to embed the program into the facilities infrastructure and operationalize the program at the unit level and on to the bedside. Operationalizing or implementing the skin safety program will be dictated by the size of the facility or agency, the magnitude of the existing skin and wound care needs, and the available personnel. The mechanism created for operationalizing the skin safety program requires identifying who will implement the program at the bedside. Small agencies or facilities often provide operationalization of the program and oversight. Larger facilities or agencies often identify unit-based nurse champions (described in the next section) for operationalization to the bedside.

Responsibilities and membership. Responsibilities and membership will vary according to the needs of the patient population, community laws, and the regulating bodies of the various disciplines involved. Skin safety committees and teams may fulfill many functions (Boxes 1-4 and 1-5).

Certification in wound care. At least one member of the skin safety team should possess a legally defensible certification in wound care issued by an independent national certification organization that validates specialty knowledge, experience, and clinical judgment. As previously stated, this is particularly important for the delivery of quality outcomes and the ability to legally defend the validity of the

---

BOX 1-4 Skin Safety Committee Oversight Responsibilities

Protocols and Decision-Making Tools
- Decision-making tools linking risk assessment with preventive interventions
- Offloading (specialty beds, heels, chair cushions)
- Policies or guidelines for pressure ulcer prevention, assessment, and treatment
- Protocols for care of common clinical conditions (e.g., incontinence, incontinence-associated dermatitis, skin tears)

Formulary
- Skin care and continence products
- Wound care products
- Offloading products

Documentation
- Admission database to incorporate wound and skin assessment
- Ongoing documentation methods for prevention, assessment, and treatment
- Patient education

Education
- Patient education materials
- Staff educational needs assessment
- Staff orientation
- Annual education and competency
- Newsletter for just-in-time updates, announcements, learnings

Quality Management
- Review AHEs and RCA
- Implement infrastructure changes based on AHE and RCA findings
- Analyze unit-based reports for outcomes and trends

Research
- Clinical trials of products using standard evaluation protocols
- Prevalence and incidence studies
- Ongoing review of literature to maintain evidence-based practice

AHE, Adverse health event; *RCA,* root-cause analysis.

BOX 1-5 Potential Members of a Skin Safety Committee

- Medical director
- Certified wound specialist
- Certified wound care nurse (CWCN©, CWON©, CWOCN©)
- Physical therapist
- Nursing leader
- Unit-based nurse champions
- Dietician
- Occupational therapist
- Speech therapist
- Quality management representative
- Consultants/ad hoc members
  - Infection control specialist
  - Dermatologist
  - Podiatrist
  - Orthotics specialist
  - Diabetologist
  - Gerontologist
  - Plastic surgeon
  - Information technologist
  - Vascular surgeon
  - Pharmacist

CHECKLIST 1-2 Maintenance of Infrastructure

✓ Ensure time and staff are available to convert policies, procedures, and formulary with every change in contract, documentation, or technology. New initiatives (e.g., revised documentation forms, conversion to electronic medical records) require adaptations to existing processes and procedures, reorientation of staff.

✓ Network with key stakeholders and committees that can affect infrastructure; be visible and "in the loop" so that decisions that may impact the skin and wound care program are recognized and addressed.

✓ Include the patient as a key stakeholder; conduct patient satisfaction surveys, customized patient education to reflect patient demographics.

✓ Report to a director or vice president, not unit manager.

✓ Ensure program is sustainable, regardless of new technology, changes in staffing, changes in care delivery model.

✓ Position wound specialist as a high-profile change agent, not a technician.

✓ Generate data and reports that justify sufficient staffing without compromise.

✓ Utilize operation reports as tools for monitoring and driving change, not as tasks to complete (Box 1-7).

---

certification (Checklist 1-2). This member will serve as content expert specifically related to pressure ulcer prevention and wound care.

When this member is a certified wound, ostomy, and continence nurse (CWOCN©) or a certified wound care nurse (CWCN©), the committee reaps additional benefits. Wound, ostomy, and continence nursing is a specialty recognized by the American Nurses Association (WOCN®, 2010b). Wound, ostomy, and continence nurses have expertise in a full range of skin issues (e.g., incontinence-associated dermatitis, tube site care, ostomy skin issues, complex fistula care) and the nurse's multifaceted role (WOCN®, 2012b). Given the increased incidence of device-related pressureulcers

(see Chapter 8), the nurse with this broader skill set is invaluable to the skin safety committee. A productivity survey of WOC nurses showed that two-thirds are prepared at the baccalaureate level and slightly less than one-third are prepared at the master's degree or doctorate level (WOCN®, 2012b). The certified WOC nurse often serves as the skin and wound care program coordinator by (1) organizing outcomes measurement studies and prevalence and incidence studies; (2) providing individualized holistic patient assessments; (3) making recommendations for wound care products, adjunctive therapies, and specialty beds or equipment; (4) performing debridements, if within the individual's skill level and scope of practice; (5) providing ongoing assessment and evaluation of healing for patients with complex wounds; and (6) educating staff in the prevention, assessment, and treatment of skin and wound problems. Research has demonstrated faster healing when a WOC nurse is involved in the care of a patient with a wound (Arnold & Weir, 1994; Bolton et al., 2004; Harris, & Shannon, 2008; Peirce et al, 2008).

Director. The director of the skin safety team is a physician or mid-level provider. This person oversees ongoing treatment and overall management of patients with complex wounds. The director interacts as needed with primary and consulting providers to facilitate consistent and effective skin and wound management that is in alignment with overall patient goals. Responsibilities include, but are not limited to, assisting the facility in the development and implementation of policies and procedures for prevention and treatment of skin breakdown that are consistent with national guidelines. Ideally, the director of a skin safety team is a certified wound specialist. However, when supported by qualified and competent team members, a provider without certification can be highly effective.

Nursing. The registered nurse directs the development and implementation of an individualized plan of care based on the needs and goals assessed for the patient. Nursing focuses on risk assessment, early problem identification, preventive measures to promote skin integrity, and responses to treatments. The nurse documents and reports condition changes and revises the plan of care as necessary. In the United States several training pathways for nurses are available, ranging from licensed practical nurses to registered nurse to advanced practice nurses and nurses with doctoral degrees. The nurse is instrumental in providing valuable patient-centered input to the committee.

Unit-based skin champions. As previously discussed, the success of the skin safety program ultimately lies with the ability and commitment of the nurse to operationalize the program at the unit level and on to the bedside. Unit-based champions are a core group of staff nurses with a special interest and additional education in skin health and wound management. This group of nurses becomes the "eyes and ears" of the program oversight committee. In addition, these unit-based skin care members are empowered to identify and problem solve adverse clinical findings, such as Stage I pressure ulcers and incontinence-associated dermatitis. Unit-based champions must be provided the information, tools, and resources and education they need to conduct staff education and lead the initiative for skin and wound care. A wound treatment associate (WTA) continuing education program is an example of additional education that can be

provided. The WTA is a credential designated to a registered nurse (RN), licensed practical nurse/licensed vocational nurse (LPN/LVN), or military medic with a certificate of completion from a WOCN®-endorsed WTA© continuing education program that functions under the direction of a supervising advanced practice registered nurse (APRN), WOC nurse, or physician (WOCN®, 2011b). Wound treatment associate continuing education can be conducted onsite.

The process by which the unit-based skin team member functions is dictated by census, patient acuity, length of stay, and realistic staff expectations. In one scenario, the unit-based skin team members make rounds of all patients with a skin-related issue or a Braden scale rating less than 15 once or twice weekly, based on a list of patients to be seen provided by the charge nurse. Between rounds, any Stage I or II pressure ulcers would be reported immediately to a member of the unit-based skin team so that a root-cause analysis can be performed to identify the source and take corrective action. This information is taken back to the program oversight committee to further evaluate and make modifications to the infrastructure (policies, procedures, decision-making tools) as needed so that the situation does not recur.

Physical therapy. The role of the PT can differ widely among care settings and facilities. If involved in wound care, the role of the PT may appear to overlap with that of the certified wound nurse or the WOC nurse. Physical therapists may collaborate during evaluation and care planning, or they may coordinate a team. Physical therapists often are involved throughout the process of care, from preventing breakdown to facilitating healing. Physical therapy interventions address range of motion, strength training, seating and positioning, support surfaces, and functional mobility training. Physical therapists may offer therapeutic intervention for contractures, edema, motor control, muscle weakness, and pain. Other interventions, such as electrical stimulation, pulsed lavage, and sharp debridement, may be within the scope of practice for some PTs. As with nurses, PTs should function within their scope of practice, be regulated by accredited educational programs and curricula, and have certifications with sound practicum experience.

Occupational therapy. The occupational therapist (OT) plays a rehabilitative role, assessing cognitive and functional capabilities and then introducing patient-specific adaptive techniques and equipment. Patient-specific adaptive techniques and equipment promote the patient's optimal performance of activities of daily living, including the patient's ability to take an active role in wound care. The patient with a slow-healing or nonhealing wound may benefit from the expertise of the OT in promoting the patient's overall health maintenance and quality of life by incorporating skin and wound care into the patient's and family's daily routine.

Speech therapy. The speech therapist helps promote optimal nutrition by ensuring that the patient is able to safely swallow. Speech therapy may include strengthening oral and/or pharyngeal musculature, performing swallowing trials for diet advancement, and/or providing compensatory techniques with oral intake to improve the safety of the patient's swallowing and reduce aspiration risk. The speech therapist focuses on improving the patient's ability to effectively communicate to his or her maximum functional level. Cognitively, speech therapy works to improve cognitive-linguistic skills for safe and effective communication upon the patient's transition to the least restrictive environment possible.

Dietitian or nutritionist. The dietitian promotes optimal nutrition through nutritional assessment and intervention. The dietician monitors relevant laboratory values, anthropometric measurements, and food intake or nutrition support parameters. The dietitian collaborates with the team in making recommendations that optimally meet the nutritional needs and goals of the patient.

Social services. The social worker is a key member of the skin safety team. The patient with a wound often is vulnerable and requires astute assessment of the home situation, particularly as it relates to the patient's safety, support, and ability to realistically adhere to wound management goals. The social worker is knowledgeable about financial resources and the barriers to follow-up care that are unique to each individual situation. The social worker obtains prior authorization for supplies and other services needed upon discharge to prevent unexpected costs to the patient. As the key liaison between care settings, the social worker coordinates and leads discharge-planning conferences, which include the patient, skin safety team members, and the family. Representatives from facilities and agencies responsible for future care often are included in discharge-planning meetings for patients who have complex management issues. This collaboration among the patient, the family, and the health care team members from both settings helps to establish mutual goals and continuity in care.

Utilization review. In the United States the utilization review (UR) specialist functions as a critical link among the patient, the physician, and the payer (insurance company, health maintenance organization, state or federal provider). Both nurses and social workers may hold UR positions. In many care settings, UR responsibilities have become incorporated into the case management role. The UR specialist provides information to payers to ensure funding for the most appropriate and cost-effective care.

PREVALENCE/INCIDENCE STUDIES

Prevalence and incidence measures are the primary measures of how frequently a condition, such as a pressure ulcer, develops. Incidence can be reflected as cumulative incidence or incidence density. These terms are not interchangeable. Box 1-6 provides the formula for calculating each measure.

Prevalence

Prevalence is the number of individuals who have a specific condition at a particular moment in time. Expressed as a percentage or proportion (or a ratio, not a rate), prevalence is a cross-sectional measure. As a snapshot in time, prevalence reflects how many people in a target population (e.g., patients in the orthopedic unit) have a condition (e.g., a pressure ulcer) at a point in time (e.g., one particular day or during the month of July). For example, the prevalence of pressure ulcers in the orthopedic unit for the month of July may be 5 out of a unit census of 50 (5/50, or 10%). The issue of whether the condition is "new" or ongoing is irrelevant when calculating prevalence; all patients with the condition at that point in time are counted. Generally considered to be a stable measure, prevalence should not vary significantly over time unless changes in practice patterns, referral bases, or marketing have occurred or the average duration of the disease has changed. As a measure of disease frequency (or burden of disease), prevalence is a useful tool for health care planning. Because it is a reflection of the general norm, prevalence provides a means of identifying workload needs, staff needs, or resource allocation needs to satisfy the demands of a particular disease burden or volume. Prevalence should never be misconstrued as a measure of quality of care or a measure of risk. An institution or agency that specializes in wound care is expected to have a high volume or prevalence of wounds because marketing strategies are geared toward recruiting or enrolling patients with wounds.

Incidence

Incidence is the proportion of patients who *acquire* the condition over a given period of time. The term *nosocomial* refers to hospital acquired. In the case of pressure ulcers, for example, the incidence is the number of patients in a

---

BOX 1-6 Formulas for Prevalence, Cumulative Incidence, and Incidence Density

$$\text{Prevalence}^* = \frac{\text{No. of persons with a condition (e.g., pressure ulcer)}}{\text{No. of persons in the target population at a particular point in time}} \times 100$$

$$\text{Cumulative incidence}^* = \frac{\text{No. of persons who develop the condition of interest (e.g., pressure ulcer) during a specific time period}}{\text{No. of persons in the study population (e.g., hospital, unit) during a specific time period}} \times 100$$

$$\text{Incidence Density}^\dagger = \frac{\text{No. of persons developing the condition (e.g., new pressure ulcer)}}{\text{Total time (patient-days or patient-years) persons were free of the condition or observed}} \times 1000$$

*Expressed as a percentage.
†Expressed as a rate or a percentage.

defined population (e.g., patients in the intensive care unit) who initially were ulcer free but then developed a pressure ulcer within a particular time (e.g., during their hospital stay). Incidence is calculated as a cumulative incidence (expressed as a percentage) or as incidence density (expressed as a rate).

Cumulative Incidence. *Cumulative incidence* is the number of new patients in a group who develop a condition over a period of time. The denominator for cumulative incidence is the total number of people in the population being observed at the beginning of the designated time period. Cumulative incidence is a measure of risk and provides an estimate of the probability (risk) of developing a condition or disease over a specific period of time (Kelsey et al, 1996). Therefore cumulative incidence can be used to gauge the effects of risk factors and prevention efforts. Characteristics of cumulative incidence include the following (Gordis, 1996):

1. Cumulative incidence is a measure of *new* (not existing) cases of a particular condition.
2. The denominator must include only those individuals *at risk* for developing the condition.
3. Cumulative incidence always refers to a specific time period (e.g., 1 day, 1 week, 1 month, 1 year).
4. As with prevalence, cumulative incidence is a proportion (not a rate) and ranges from 0% to 100%.
5. All individuals in the group at risk (represented by the denominator) are followed or observed for the entire time period specified.

To calculate cumulative incidence, consider the following situation. The number of patients on an orthopedic unit on July 1 is 50 (the population at risk); 5 were admitted with an existing pressure ulcer, and 5 developed a pressure ulcer after admission. The cumulative incidence of pressure ulcers on the orthopedic unit is calculated as follows. A total of 50 patients are at risk (the denominator), and 5 of the 50 patients developed a pressure ulcer, so the cumulative incidence of pressure ulcers in patients on the orthopedic unit on July 1 is 5/50, or 10%.

Incidence Density. Incidence density differs from cumulative incidence in that the denominator used to calculate incidence density is the aggregate duration of exposure. Thus incidence density is a rate that can be reported as patient-days or device-days (Streed and Loehne, 2007; WOCN®, 2004). For example, when the incidence density rate of pressure ulcers on an orthopedic unit in the month of July is calculated, the length of time that each patient remains on the unit will vary. Some patients may be on the unit 3 days before being discharged, whereas others may be on the unit for 2 weeks. Consequently, these individuals will be observed (and at risk) for different periods of time. The first patient is at risk for pressure ulcer formation for only 3 days, whereas the second patient is at risk for 2 weeks. If these two patients developed a pressure ulcer during their time on the unit, the incidence density rate would be 2 per 17 patient days. A

formula for calculating incidence density per 1000 patient-days is provided in Box 1-6.

A more feasible technique for calculating incidence density uses the number of patient-days available from the agency or facility. The formula for this technique is as follows: number of pressure ulcers divided by number of patient-days, multiplied by 1000 to give a rate. For example, during 1 month, eight incident pressure ulcers are reported with 8000 patient-days. The incidence density then is 1 per 1000 patient days, or a rate of 1.0.

Benchmarks and Generalizability of Results

Cumulative incidence is commonly reported in the literature; however, using the data for benchmarking and comparisons has limitations. The groups from which the cumulative incidence is drawn must be comparable with regard to key risk factors, such as acuity and patient mix, as well as data collection methods. The National Database of Nursing Quality Indicators (NDNQI) can provide realistic benchmarks by enrolling large numbers of facilities and breaking down data according to level of risk so that similar facilities can be compared. Furthermore, NDNQI provides pressure ulcer education (available at www.nursingquality.org) to promote consistent techniques for data collection throughout participating facilities.

Reliance on cumulative incidence measure alone has limitations. Because cumulative incidence is generally obtained through a 1-day study performed annually or quarterly, it reflects adverse events discovered on 1 day. However, from a quality-of-care perspective, all adverse events need to be reported and tracked 24 hours per day, 7 days per week, so that root-cause analysis can be determined and corrective action implemented in a timely fashion. For this purpose, an incidence density process using concurrent real-time data collection is critical. The success of concurrent real-time data collection is dependent on the infrastructure in place. The reporting process must be clear (i.e., what exactly to report), simple (e.g., a 1-minute process rather than a 15-minute report), and accessible 24/7. Data should be sent to a central location for immediate analysis and action by qualified staff (Kartes, 1996).

Methodology

Prevalence and incidence studies can be an onerous undertaking, but yield considerable information if the objective is clear from the onset. *Prevalence and Incidence: A Toolkit for Clinicians* (WOCN®, 2004) and the NDNQI pressure ulcer education site (www.nursingquality.org) outline the specific steps required to prepare for and conduct a prevalence and incidence study. They also provide documentation forms generally required of such a process and education for data collectors.

A key decision in planning the study is determining the staffing mix and the numbers for data collection. Data were analyzed from pressure ulcer prevalence studies conducted in nursing homes between 2004 and 2006 on differences in observed rates when one nurse, compared with two nurses, conducted skin inspections. Results revealed that the number of raters did not influence the observed rate, leading researchers to conclude that adequate preparation and training of staff nurses for data collection were sufficient to achieve reliable data (Kottner et al, 2009).

Another important decision in planning the study is determining which population to study, or the at-risk population. The term *at risk* implies, from an epidemiologic standpoint, those individuals who have the potential for developing a condition; *at risk* does *not* refer to the pressure ulcer risk assessment score obtained by using the Braden scale, for example. With this broader interpretation of the concept of at risk, all patients in the hospital may be assumed to be at risk for pressure ulcer formation, for example. However, whether the assumption holds that all patients who are hospitalized are at risk is arguable. When studies report the incidence for hospital-wide populations, they often exclude pediatric, obstetric, or mental health patient populations. For this reason, conducting incidence and prevalence studies on targeted patient populations may be more meaningful and more feasible (Baumgarten et al, 2003; Dugaret, 2012; McLane et al, 2004; Nijs et al, 2009; Shahin, 2008). For example, a study could examine all patients undergoing an operation lasting 3 hours or longer, all patients with a specific diagnosis such as hip fracture, patients who have diabetes and are admitted to home care from Hospital Z, or all patients on a specific hospital unit. Allman et al (1995) reported a 12.9% cumulative incidence of pressure ulcers after a median of 9 days from admission to final skin examination in a specific patient population: patients were 55 years or older, had a hip fracture or were confined to a bed or chair for at least 5 days, and did not have a Stage III or greater pressure ulcer.

MARKETING, JUSTIFYING, AND SECURING THE WOUND SPECIALIST ROLE: BENEFITS AND OUTCOMES

Employing a wound specialist yields many benefits to the organization, the value of which is more dramatic in the current climate of cost constraints. Through efficient use of materials, accurate and thorough documentation, prompt reassessment and revisions to the plan of care, and adherence to a formulary, the wound specialist has the potential to positively impact staff retention, physician satisfaction, facility reimbursements, infection rates, and patient satisfaction.

A key factor to a successful skin and wound care practice is effective communication and marketing of the role and the service. Measuring productivity and outcomes and communicating benefits are critical in securing and maintaining the role. Demonstrating and communicating the impact are essential so that the specialist and the services provided remain visible and the administration can justify the budget required to fund the wound specialist's position and program. This goal is accomplished not only through

outstanding outcomes but, more importantly, by tracking and communicating outcomes through routine operations reports to key stakeholders and committees. These reports will help remind the administration that a low incidence of wound-related and skin-related problems is a result of having a qualified wound specialist; it is not an indication that staffing for the wound specialist should be reduced. This section outlines the benefits of having a wound specialist and the operations reports that are necessary to market, justify, and secure the role of the wound specialist. Checklist 1-2 provides tips for maintaining program infrastructure and securing the specialist's role. Box 1-7 provides examples of productivity and outcomes that can be communicated through an operations and outcome presentation report. Appendix A contains an example of a patient satisfaction survey.

Increased Accountability

One benefit of the services of a wound specialist is increased accountability for national guidelines and compliance with regulatory statutes. The Centers for Medicare & Medicaid Services (CMS) and The Joint Commission are clear in their intent to encourage all facilities to adopt evidenced-based pressure ulcer protocols. The surveyor community has a common language that should be used in the medical record when referring to pressure ulcers. For example, CMS recognition and definition of the *avoidable* and *unavoidable* pressure ulcer in long-term care and *present on admission* (POA) criteria (see Chapter 8) highlight the need for incorporation of regulatory updates into practice (van Rijswijk and Lyder, 2005). Wound specialists are in a position to implement the requisite pressure ulcer prevention and treatment components. In addition to performing implementation, the wound

---

BOX 1-7   Potential Items to Include in an Operations and Outcomes Report

Operations
- Number and type of patients (example in Appendix A)
- Number of visits, type of visit, time spent
- Trends (volume, issues, demographics)
- Referral sources and utilization patterns (e.g., physicians, units, facilities)
- Specific activities and scope of practice (e.g., managing patient population, quality improvement activities, committees, projects, education)

Outcomes
- Cost avoidance and cost savings with improved resource utilization processes (i.e., specialty beds and product usage before and after formularies, algorithms, and decision tools are implemented)
- Reduction in preventable skin injury (i.e., concurrent tracking for rates and P&I studies)

Patient Satisfaction Survey (example Appendix A)

specialist can facilitate documentation that is clear and appropriate and accurately reflects appropriate prevention, assessment, and treatment of pressure ulcers.

Improved Financial Outcomes

Cost-effectiveness is a significant method for acquiring the administration's support. The wound specialist has the opportunity to help prevent costly wounds, use resources more efficiently, and, in some situations, to generate revenue. Through ongoing continuing education opportunities, the wound specialist can foster state-of-the-art patient care and EBP by using products that have scientific evidence of their effectiveness. Again, not only do the patients benefit from this expertise, but the facility also benefits financially by cutting expenditures. The wound specialist can work with QI team members to identify select aspects of care that can be monitored and tracked over time and thus obtain outcomes data and clinical effectiveness information.

Reduction of Preventable Wounds. The costs of caring for a patient with a wound range widely across the world. Estimated cost of individual patient care ranges from $20,900 to $151,700 per wound (AHRQ, 2011). When a major amputation is required, the cost will increase by a factor of seven because of the need to make home improvements to accommodate a wheelchair (Apelquist et al, 1994). In addition, up to 85% of amputations can be avoided when an effective care plan for the patient with a diabetic foot ulcer is followed (International Best Practice Guidelines, 2013). When patients at risk are identified and interventions are put in place before the wound develops or progresses, morbidity and health care costs are decreased (Ortegon et al, 2004; Padula et al, 2011).

Faster Healing Rates. Studies have shown that patients who were cared for by a WOC nurse specialist had better outcomes in terms of healing rates and/or costs of care compared with patients cared for by other nurses (Arnold & Weir, 1994; Bolton et al, 2004; Harris & Shannon, 2008; Peirce et al, 2008).

Efficient Use of Resources. The wound specialist must become cognizant of the implications of the efficient use of resources (both materials and personnel). Information on the cost implications of the skin and wound care practice or the cost savings that have been generated must be gathered and specifically communicated routinely to the supervisor. Wound management is costly; in most situations, wound management is more costly than prevention (Padula et al, 2011). Effective wound management reduces costs by allowing use of fewer supplies and providing more efficient and effective use of dressings. In addition, cost savings can be realized when preventive interventions are linked to risk level (Richardson et al, 1998). This practice could result in a significant decrease in annual expenditures for materials used. Cost-effectiveness is a positive way of acquiring the support

of the nursing administration, which is essential to obtaining institutional support.

The wound specialist should become involved with the establishment of supply contracts in order to sort through the maze of different products and their indications. A successful means of proven cost-effectiveness is limiting the number of similar supplies stocked by the facility. When a formulary for skin and wound care products and support surfaces is created, use of these products can be standardized and simplified. Furthermore, the wound specialist can serve as a resource to materials management, providing clarification on product use. Collaboration with materials management can increase the success of contractual arrangements with manufacturers and increase the facility's ability to maintain compliance with contracts.

Another area with potential for cost savings is standardizing the use of support surfaces. A policy that describes patient indicators for the use of specialty beds should be developed, and compliance with contracts for these specialty beds should be supported. A procedure for "stepping down" from a specialty bed as the patient's condition warrants should be established. In addition, units with a high prevalence of at-risk patient populations might benefit from the implementation of replacement mattresses. Standardizing the products and providing indicators or patient characteristics that guide the use of these products can reduce overuse and enhance appropriate use.

Finally, by incorporating appropriate use of skin and wound care products and state-of-the-art wound care, the wound specialist affects the use of personnel. Decreased frequency of dressing changes, expedient access to the correct dressing supplies, and printed directions for dressing changes will reduce staff frustration and time required for wound care.

Revenue Generation. Depending on payer sources, the level of education of the wound specialist and whether or not the specialist is employed by the institution, the services that are provided may be billable. Working closely with the billing department and fiscal intermediaries may be productive with regard to revenues. Chapter 2 provides specific details about the development of an outpatient clinical practice and reimbursement.

The skin and wound care program, like all departments, must have a means for tracking productivity. A mechanism for documenting visits and referrals can be formulated with the assistance of the billing department. One possible method is a system of "charge codes" for skin and wound care services based on increments of time or services provided. This is an excellent way to track, document, and justify the value of a wound specialist. However, the specialist should avoid providing services that are considered basic nursing care in order to inflate the number of charges. The specialist should not focus solely on the number of patients or charges, but rather on the types of patients and services provided. This charging system also may assist with the compilation of workload and time management data for the department. Another consideration is whether the wound specialist's interventions are affecting outcomes.

Depending on payer sources, the services that are provided through the skin and wound care program might be billable, for example, if the services are classified as a therapy rather than a nursing service. The availability of skin and wound care services may enable the institution to market itself for managed care contracts. This again defines the value of a skin and wound care program. However, inpatient skin and wound care services will seldom, if ever, be revenue-producing. Working closely with the billing department and fiscal intermediaries may be instructive.

The value of a skin and wound care program is not limited to just providing care to inpatients. The wound specialist can serve as a link to community and outreach programs and provide education that draws attention and referrals to the wound care program and the facility. The wound specialist can provide education within his or her facility in collaboration with colleagues, such as PTs and OTs. Grants to conduct some of these programs may be available from manufacturers. The manufacturers often have established programs that have been approved by licensing boards for continuing education hours, and these programs may be a cost-effective way to provide continuing education to staff. Continuing medical education programs also may be attractive; for example, well-recognized speakers may be invited to conduct an educational session.

When starting the skin and wound care program, the specialist initially may conduct a series of chart audits or a prevalence and incidence study as described in the previous section of this chapter (Chicano and Drolshagen, 2009; Orsted et al, 2009). These activities may provide information that would be helpful in determining whether a certain problem (e.g., pressure ulcers, inadequate documentation) exists. From this information, the continuous improvement process can be initiated with involved departments and personnel so that problems can be discussed and possible solutions identified. As the wound specialist begins an inpatient practice, visibility is essential. Being open to new ideas and opportunities will assist the wound specialist in creating and maintaining a successful program. Maintaining visibility and an alliance with physicians and staff will reinforce the message that the skin and wound care program is an indispensable service.

Staff Retention and Satisfaction

A key role of the wound specialist is establishing decision-making tools to expedite and standardize delivery of care. These tools help the staff to develop their comfort level in skin and wound care, facilitate utilization of products, and implement appropriate preventive interventions. Recognition and rewards can be provided for program contributions or accomplishments. Establishing skill competencies in wound care can provide a professional objective that the staff can strive for, again targeting the individual's personal satisfaction.

Critical features of a successful, enduring skin and wound care program are routine and regular operations reports, analysis of clinical practice data, and sharing of these data (see Box 1-7). Clinical practice data become the tool by which workload is measured, trends are identified, outcomes are quantified, and the valuable contribution of the wound specialist is recorded and measured. Data collection should be purposeful and outcomes oriented. In fact, data collection and practice improvement are inseparable because improvement requires measurement (Nelson et al, 1998). Clinical practice data should include time management and outcomes reports.

Patient Satisfaction and Improved Quality of Life

Having a chronic wound can decrease satisfaction and quality of life by factors that impact physical, psychological, emotional, social, and occupational aspects of life (Herber et al, 2007). Specific experiences impacting quality of life include intolerable pain, fatigue, embarrassing drainage and odor, depression, shame, isolation, impaired ability to perform activities of daily living (ADL), and job loss (Fagervik-Morton and Price, 2009; Gorecki et al, 2010; Persoon, 2004; Ribu and Whal, 2004). Patients also report a decrease in satisfaction and frustration with health professionals and service due to lack of explanation, conflicting information related to treatment options, diagnostic tests, and progress reports (Beitz, 2005; Herber et al, 2007).

The wound specialist is uniquely qualified to help prevent or minimize some of these devastating experiences, with expertise in holistic assessment of the patient with a wound (see Chapter 6) and use of appropriate dressings to help manage pain, exudate, and odor with products that consider the patient's needs and lifestyle (see Chapter 18). Quality of life and strategies for improvement are discussed in Chapters 25, 29, 37, and throughout this text. Quality-of-life questionnaires and scales, as well as patient satisfaction surveys, can be used to measure outcomes (Augustin et al, 2010; Iglesias et al, 2005; Price and Harding, 2004).

Operations and Outcomes Reports

When cost containment, efficient use of resources, and managed care dominate discussions, information concerning time use is invaluable. This type of data can validate any subjective perception of an increase or change in workload and communicates a strong objective message. Data should be recorded daily and tabulated weekly, monthly, quarterly, and annually. Summary data (e.g., number of patient referrals, number of visits, average length of visits, average number of visits per patient or wound type, reason for referral, number of projects/activities, and time per project) should be submitted to the wound specialist's supervisor on a monthly basis, with trends highlighted. Plots can graphically display time or volume by month. Data collection can be maintained by hand on paper or by computer through one of the many commercially available software packages. Reports can be generated from an electronic medical record system through collaboration with the information technology department. Appendix A contains an example of a simple database created using the Microsoft Excel program.

Benefits of services to the organization become tangible and coherent when they are phrased in terms of outcomes. Outcomes should include specific patient population outcomes and organizational outcomes. Potential outcomes should be discussed relative to behaviors or physical conditions that can be affected by the wound specialist. For example, an outcome of shortened length of stay in the hospital may not be realistic because many variables impact an individual's length of stay and are not necessarily under the control of the wound specialist. However, the outcome could be rephrased to more precisely define the patient population or type of wound for which length of stay will be decreased. Another outcome could address the control of wound care products. However, in order for this outcome to be feasible, tools that will assist the staff in appropriate product use, such as protocols and a formulary, would be required.

CLINICAL CONSULT

Memorandum

To: Medical and Nursing Staff

From: Nursing Administration and Wound Care Department

S: Weekend coverage for new patient referrals for wound consultations.

B: In the past our wound care staff was not available on weekends or holidays for new patient referrals.

A: With an increasingly shorter length of stay for hospitalized patients and the growing number of referrals for wound care, we will pilot a new weekend/holiday coverage policy.

R: For nonemergent new patient consults, please initially refer to the new online wound and skin troubleshooting guidelines. If this is not sufficient, contact the house nursing supervisor and he or she will contact the oncall wound care specialist to determine if a phone call will adequately address the problem or if the wound care specialist will need to make a hospital visit. After 3 months we will ask for feedback on the process and determine our ongoing plan for better coverage of our wound care patients. Thank you all for the great care you consistently give our patients.

SUMMARY

Establishing a skin and wound care practice in any setting requires the skills of an entrepreneur and a strong foundation in pathophysiology and clinical management. The wound specialist must determine how his or her role will be implemented, how his or her relationship with colleagues will be defined, what quality management processes can be implemented, and what type of data is needed. Data should describe how time is spent and what outcomes are being achieved. The wound specialist must stay current in the art and science of wound management by adopting lifelong learning strategies, such as regularly attending continuing education programs, critically reading journals, and monitoring select websites. The time and energy spent in initial and ongoing practice development are critical to a successful, satisfying, and effective skin and wound care practice.

REFERENCES

Ackerman CL: "Not on my watch": treating and preventing pressure ulcers, *Medsurg Nurs* 20(2):86–93, 2011.

Agency for Healthcare Research and Quality (AHRQ): *Assessing the quality of Internet health information: summary*, Rockville, MD, June 1999, AHRQ. http://www.ahrq.gov/research/data/infoqual.htm. Accessed Jan 26, 2014.

Agency for Healthcare Research and Quality (AHRQ): *Are we ready for this change? Preventing pressure ulcers in hospitals: a toolkit for improving quality of care*, Rockville, MD, April 2011, AHRQ. http://www.ahrq.gov/professionals/systems/long-term-care/resources/pressure-ulcers/pressureulcertoolkit/putool1.html. Accessed Jan 26, 2014.

Allman RM, Goode PS, Patrick MM, et al: Pressure ulcer risk factors among hospitalized patients with activity limitation, *JAMA* 273(11):865–870, 1995.

Andriessen AE, Polignano R, Abel M: Development and implementation of a clinical pathway to improve venous leg ulcer treatment, *Wounds* 21(5):127–133, 2009.

Apelquist J, Ragnarson-Tennvall G, Persson U, et al: Diabetic foot ulcers in a multidisciplinary setting. An economic analysis of primary healing and healing with amputation, *J Intern Med* 235:463–471, 1994.

Arnold M, Weir D: Retrospective analysis of healing in wounds cared for by ET nurses versus staff nurses in a home setting, *J Wound Ostomy Continence Nurs* 24:456–460, 1994.

Augustin M, Herberger K, Rustenbach SJ, et al: Quality of life evaluation in wounds: validation of the Freiburg Life Quality Assessment-wound module, a disease-specific instrument, *Int Wound J* 7(6):493–501, 2010.

Bales I, Duvendack T: Reaching for the moon: achieving zero pressure ulcer prevalence, an update, *J Wound Care* 20(8):374–347, 2011.

Bales I, Padwojski A: Reaching for the moon: achieving zero pressure ulcer prevalence, *J Wound Care* 18(4):137–144, 2009.

Baumgarten M, Margolis D, Berlin JA, et al: Risk factors for pressure ulcers among elderly hip fracture patients, *Wound Repair Regen* 11:96–103, 2003.

Beeckman D, Clays E, Van Hecke A, et al: A multi-faceted tailored strategy to implement an electronic clinical decision support system for pressure ulcer prevention in nursing homes: a two-armed randomized controlled trial, *Int J Nurs Stud* 50(4):475–486, 2013.

Beitz JM, Fey J, O'Brien D: Perceived need for education vs. actual knowledge of pressure ulcer care in a hospital nursing staff, *Dermatol Nurs* 11(2):125, 1999.

Bolton L, McNees P, van Rijswijk L, et al: Wound-healing outcomes using standardized assessment and care in clinical practice, *J Wound Ostomy Continence Nurs* 31:65–71, 2004.

Bonham P: The role of wound, ostomy and continence (WOC) specialty nurses in managing complex cases, *Remington Report* 17:10, 2009.

Callihan D: Simplifying the process of research review for the novice researcher, *J Wound Ostomy Continence Nurs* 35(1): 30–33, 2008.

Cary AH: Certified registered nurses: results of the Study of the Certified Workforce, *Am J Nurs* 101(1):44–52, 2001.

Chicano SG, Drolshagen C: Reducing hospital-acquired pressure ulcers, *J Wound Ostomy Continence Nurs* 36(1):45–50, 2009.

Cullum N, Guyatt G: Health care interventions and harm: an introduction. In DiCenso A, Guyatt G, Ciliska D, editors: *Evidence-based nursing: a guide to clinical practice*, Philadelphia, 2005, Mosby.

DiCenso A, Ciliska D, Guyatt G: Introduction to evidence-based nursing. In DiCenso A, Guyatt G, Ciliska D, editors: *Evidence-based nursing: a guide to clinical practice*, Philadelphia, 2005, Mosby.

Dobbins M; Ciliska, D. Estabrooks, C et al: Changing nursing practice in an organization. In DiCenso A, Guyatt G, Ciliska D, editors: *Evidence-based nursing: a guide to clinical practice*, Philadelphia, 2005, Mosby.

Dugaret E, Videau MN, Faure I, et al: Prevalence and incidence rates of pressure ulcers in an emergency department, *Int Wound J* 11:386–391, 2012.

Ehrenberg A, Fraser KD, Gunningberg L: Can decision support improve nurses' use of knowledge? *J Wound Ostomy Continence Nurs* 31(5):256–258, 2004.

Fagervik-Morton H, Price P: Chronic ulcers and everyday living: Patients' perspective in the United Kingdom, *Wounds* 21(12):318–323.

Ferguson L, Milner M, Snelgrove-Clarke E: The role of intermediaries: getting evidence into practice, *J Wound Ostomy Continence Nurs* 31(6):325–327, 2004.

Fineout-Overholt E, Berryman DR, Hofstetter S, et al: Finding relevant evidence to answer clinical questions. In Melnyk BM, Fineout-Overholt E, editors: *Evidence-based practice in nursing & healthcare. A guide to best practice*, ed 2, Philadelphia, 2011, Lippincott Williams & Wilkins.

Fleck C: To certify or not to certify; that is the question, *Todays Wound Clin* 2(3):26, 2008.

Golinko MS, Clark S, Rennert R, et al: Wound emergencies: the importance of assessment, documentation, and early treatment using a wound electronic medical record, *Ostomy Wound Manage* 55(5):54–61, 2009.

Gordis L: *Epidemiology*, Philadelphia, 1996, Saunders.

Gorecki C, Lamping DL, Brown JM, et al: Development of a conceptual framework of health-related quality of life in pressure ulcers: a patient-focused approach. *Int Nurs Stud* 47:1525–1534, 2010.

Harris C, Shannon R: An innovative enterostomal therapy nurse model of community wound care delivery: a retrospective cost-effectiveness analysis, *J Wound Ostomy Continence Nurs* 35(2):169–183, 2008.

Herber OR, Schnepp W, Rieger MA: A systematic review on the impact of leg ulceration on patients' quality of life, *Health Qual Life Outcomes* 5:4, 2007.

Hess CT: WOC credentials: a legally defensible process, Wound, Ostomy and Continence Nursing Certification Board, 2005. http://www.wocncb.org/pdf/value_of_certification.pdf. Accessed Jan 20, 2014.

Hiser B, Rochette J, Philbin S, et al: Implementing a pressure ulcer prevention program and enhancing the role of the CWOCN© impact and outcomes, *Ostomy Wound Manage* 52(2):48–59, 2006.

Hopf HW, Ueno C, Aslam R, et al: Guidelines for the treatment of arterial insufficiency ulcers, *Wound Repair Regen* 14(6):693–710, 2006.

Iglesias CP, Birks Y, Nelson EA, et al: Quality of life of people with venous leg ulcers: a comparison of the discriminative and responsive characteristics of two generic and a disease specific instruments, *Qual Life Res* 14(7):1705–1718, 2005.

International best practice guidelines: *Wound management in diabetic foot ulcers*, Wound International, 2013. http://www.woundsinternational.com/pdf/content_10803.pdf. accessed July 13, 2015.

Kartes SK: A team approach for risk assessment, prevention, and treatment of pressure ulcers in nursing home patients, *J Nurse Care Qual* 10(3):34–45, 1996.

Kelleher AD, Moorer A, Makic MF: Peer-to-peer nursing rounds and hospital-acquired pressure ulcer prevalence in a surgical intensive care unit: a quality improvement project, *J Wound Ostomy Continence Nurs* 39(2):152–157, 2012.

Kelsey JL, Marmot MG, Stolley PD, et al, editors: *Methods in observational epidemiology*, ed 2, New York, 1996, Oxford University Press.

Kottner J, Tannen A, Halfens R, et al: Does the number of raters influence the pressure ulcer prevalence rate? *Appl Nurs Res* 22(1):68–72, 2009.

Landrum BJ: Marketing innovations to nurses, Part 1: How people adopt innovations, *J Wound Ostomy Continence Nurs* 25:194–199, 1998a.

Landrum BJ: Marketing innovations to nurses, Part 2: Marketing's role in the adoption of innovations, *J Wound Ostomy Continence Nurs* 25:227–232, 1998b.

Lloyd-Vossen J: Implementing wound care guidelines: observations and recommendations from the bedside, *Ostomy Wound Manage* 55(6):50–55, 2009.

McIsaac C: Closing the gap between evidence and action: how outcome measurement informs the implementation of evidence-based wound care practice in home care, *Wounds* 19(11):299–309, 2007.

McLane KM, Bookout K, McCord S, et al: The 2003 national pediatric pressure ulcer and skin breakdown prevalence survey: a multisite study, *J Wound Ostomy Continence Nurs* 31(4):168–178, 2004.

Melnyk BM, Fineout-Overholt E: *Evidence-based practice in nursing & healthcare. A guide to best practice*, ed 2, Philadelphia, 2011, Lippincott Williams & Wilkins.

Milne CT, Trigilia D, Houle TL, et al: Reducing pressure ulcer prevalence rates in the long-term acute care setting, *Ostomy Wound Manage* 55(4):50–59, 2009.

Moore A, Butcher G, Corbett LQ, et al: Exploring the concept of a team approach: managing wounds as a team, *J Wound Care* 23(Suppl 5):S1–S38, 2014.

Nelson EC, Splaine ME, Batalden PB, et al: Building measurement and data collection in to medical practice, *Ann Intern Med* 128:460–466, 1998.

Nijs N, Toppets A, Defloor T, et al: Incidence and risk factors for pressure ulcers in the intensive care unit, *J Clin Nurs* 18(9): 1258–1266, 2009.

Orsted HL, Rosenthal S, Woodbury MG: Pressure ulcer awareness and prevention program: a quality improvement program through the Canadian Association of Wound Care, *J Wound Ostomy Continence Nurs* 36(2):178–183, 2009.

Ortegon MM, Redekop WK, Niessen LW: Cost-effectiveness of prevention and treatment of the diabetic foot: a Markov analysis, *Diabetes Care* 27(4):901–907, 2004.

O'Sullivan M: TRUTHFUL: A method to assist patients with evaluation health information on the internet, *Online J Nurs Informatics* 15(3), 2011.

Padula WV, Mishra MK, Makic MB, et al: Improving the quality of pressure ulcer care with prevention: a cost-effectiveness analysis, *Med Care* 49(4):385–392, 2011.

Pasek TA, Geyser A, Sidoni M, et al: Skin care team in the pediatric intensive care unit: a model for excellence, *Crit Care Nurse* 28(2):125–135, 2008.

Peirce B, Tiffany M, Kinsey H, et al: Using OASIS data to quantify the impact of WOC© nursing on patient outcomes in home healthcare: a multicenter study (Abstract), *J Wound Ostomy Continence Nurs* 33(Suppl 1):532, 2006.

Persoon A, Heinen MM, Vleuten CJM, et al: Leg ulcers: a review of their impact on daily life, *J Clin Nurs* 13:341–354, 2004.

Price P, Harding K: Cardiff Wound Impact Schedule: the development of a condition-specific questionnaire to assess health-related quality of life in patients with chronic wounds of the lower limb, *Int Wound J* 1(1):10–17, 2004.

Ribu L, Wahl A: Living with diabetic foot ulcers: a life of fear, restrictions, and pain, *Ostomy Wound Manage* 50:57–67, 2004.

Richardson GM, Gardner S, Frantz RA: Nursing assessment: impact on type and cost of interventions to prevent pressure ulcer, *J Wound Ostomy Continence Nurs* 25(6):273–280, 1998.

Robson MC, Cooper DM, Aslam R, et al: Guidelines for the treatment of venous ulcers, *Wound Repair Regen* 14(6):649–662, 2006.

Rogers EM: *Diffusion of innovations,* ed 5, New York, 2003, Free Press.

Sackett DL, Straus SE, Richardson WS, et al: *Evidence-based medicine: how to practice and teach EBM,* ed 2, London, 2000, Churchill Livingstone.

Shahin ES, Dassen T, Halfens RJ: Pressure ulcer prevalence and incidence in intensive care patients: a literature review, *Nurs Crit Care* 13(2):71–79, 2008.

Steed DL, Attinger C, Colaizzi T, et al: Guidelines for the treatment of diabetic ulcers, *Wound Repair Regen* 14(6):680–692, 2006.

Streed SA, Loehne HB: Preventing infections to improve wound care outcomes: an epidemiological approach, *Wounds* 19(11):320–330, 2007.

Thomas ME: The providers' coordination of care: a model for collaboration across the continuum of care, *Prof Case Manage* 13(4):220–227, 2008.

Tippet AW: Reducing the incidence of pressure ulcers in nursing home residents: a prospective 6-year evaluation, *Ostomy Wound Manage* 55(11):52–58, 2009.

van Rijswijk L, Lyder CH: Pressure ulcer prevention and care: implementing the revised guidance to surveyors for long-term care facilities, *Ostomy Wound Manage* 51(Suppl 4):7–19, 2005.

Webb JJ: Nursing research and evidence-based practice. In Cherry B, Jacob SR, editors: *Contemporary nursing: issues, trends, & management,* ed 4, St. Louis, MO, 2008, Mosby.

Whitney J, Phillips L, Aslam R, et al: Guidelines for the treatment of pressure ulcers, *Wound Repair Regen* 14(6):663–679, 2006.

Woods DK: Realizing your marketing influence, Part 3: Professional certification as a marketing tool, *J Nurs Adm* 32(7–8):379–386, 2002.

Wound, Ostomy and Continence Nurses Society™ (WOCN®): *Prevalence and incidence: a toolkit for clinicians,* Glenview, IL, 2004, WOCN®.

Wound, Ostomy and Continence Nurses Society™ (WOCN®): *Guideline for management of patients with lower extremity arterial disease (WOCN® clinical practice guideline series #1),* Mount Laurel, NJ, 2008, WOCN®.

Wound, Ostomy and Continence Nurses Society™ (WOCN®): *Guideline for management of pressure ulcers (WOCN® clinical practice guideline series #2),* Mount Laurel, NJ, 2010a, WOCN®.

Wound, Ostomy and Continence Nurses Society™ (WOCN®): *Wound, ostomy and continence nursing scope & standards of practice,* Mount Laurel, NJ, 2010b, WOCN®.

Wound, Ostomy and Continence Nurses Society™ (WOCN®): *Guideline for management of patients with lower extremity venous disease (WOCN® clinical practice guideline series #1),* Mount Laurel, NJ, 2011a, WOCN®.

Wound, Ostomy and Continence Nurses Society™ (WOCN®): *Position statement about the role and scope of practice for wound care providers,* Mount Laurel, NJ, 2011b, WOCN®.

Wound, Ostomy and Continence Nurses Society™ (WOCN®): *Guideline for management of patients with lower extremity neuropathic disease (WOCN® clinical practice guideline series #1),* Mount Laurel, NJ, 2012a, WOCN®.

Wound, Ostomy and Continence Nurses Society™ (WOCN®): *2012 WOC Nursing Salary and Productivity Survey,* Mount Laurel, NJ, 2012b, WOCN®.

Wound, Ostomy and Continence Nursing Certification Board (WOCNCB): *Choosing Wound/Ostomy Certification?* https://www.wocncb.org/pdf/Wound%20Certification%20Comparison%20Chart.7.15.14.pdf. accessed July 13, 2015.

Billing, Reimbursement, and Setting Up a Clinic

Deanna Vargo and Ruth A. Bryant

OBJECTIVES

1. Describe how wound clinics may differ with regard to their management, location, staff, and services offered.
2. List key components of a wound clinic.
3. List documentation that must be in the medical record to meet Medicare and billing requirements.
4. Distinguish among the different Medicare and insurance programs, including how they relate to billing for clinic services and supervision requirements.

Patients come to wound care clinics expecting state-of-the-art treatments. Many patients are seeking advanced technologies and evidence-based care and are anticipating improved healing by clinicians knowledgeable about wound care. In general, the types of patients typical of an outpatient wound clinic include patients with chronic and difficult-to-heal wounds, such as pressure ulcers; venous, arterial, and diabetic wounds; and skin disorders and unusual wound types. The common goal of an outpatient wound clinic is to provide standardized, consistent, evidence-based wound care, which includes the comprehensive care of the patient, addressing underlying etiologies, addressing cofactors, and teaching self-care to prevent recurrence. This chapter outlines the essential components of the operation and structure of an outpatient wound clinic and the impact of various regulatory issues and reimbursement requirements.

CREATING THE BUSINESS PLAN

The first step in creating a new clinic is to establish a business plan (Box 2-1). The goal of a business plan is to provide a step-by-step guide to follow when creating a new program or project. A well-constructed business plan is an important tool to use when obtaining administrative support because the plan will enumerate the benefits of the service and summarize existing internal and external competitors. The business plan should include a pro forma or projected operating budget for the next 5 years. Getting started requires consideration of several topics that should be covered in the business plan: the local health care environment, referral sources, customers, competitors, regulators, and revenue sources. The business plan must emphasize the product or service being proposed, as well as the marketing plan. A key element of the business plan is often referred to as the unique service advantage, which is what this business will do that no other business currently does, or how this new business will do it better than the competition does. Completion of a business plan will reveal commitment to goals and serve as a tool to highlight focus on improved outcomes and financial advantages the new business will provide.

The benefits of a wound care clinic to a hospital or organization are numerous (Box 2-2) and should be outlined in the business plan. A completed sample business plan is available through the Wound, Ostomy and Continence Nurses Society's™ *The Wound Ostomy and Continence Nursing Educational Essentials* 5th edition, *Professional Practice Manual* (WOCN®, 2013).

CLINIC MANAGEMENT

Although wound clinics offer similar services, they differ in their management arrangements and structure. Management can be overseen externally by a managed contract or proprietor, or they may be self-directed (internal), similar to a provider private practice. Table 2-1 lists advantages of both types of management. Available resources are a key consideration in determining the type of management needed. Resources include guidelines for care, policies, and forms; materials for staff and patient education; and quality improvement processes. Another essential consideration is access to the staff with expertise in developing these resources. External management often has these resources ready for use. However, such an arrangement could conservatively commit more than half of the wound center revenue to the management contract. Decision makers should be aware of the type and extent of support that the management company can provide before choosing that company as a partner.

CLINIC STRUCTURE

Structurally, the physical space of a wound clinic can be attached to a hospital (a hospital-based clinic or hospital outpatient clinic) or freestanding (clinic without any physical attachment to a hospital). The hospital-based clinic is a portion of a hospital that provides diagnostic, therapeutic, and rehabilitation services to sick or injured persons who do not require hospitalization. When determining the physical location of the clinic, particularly of the hospital-based clinic, it is important to consider ease of patient access to the clinic and ease of parking. Within the clinic space itself, a variety of issues must be considered in the design of the individual treatment rooms, the floor plan, the location of stocked equipment, lighting, and the need for stretcher access or lounge chair space (Checklist 2-1). Consultation with the facility maintenance department or facility planning department early in the planning to assist with these unique clinic space issues may be beneficial.

Billing Differences

The billing of clinic services is one of the consistent differentiations between the hospital-based clinic and the freestanding clinic based on the Medicare billing system. At a hospital-based clinic, services billed to Medicare or Medicaid patients will be reimbursed at the Medicare facility rate (facility submits a facility rate for the overhead cost and physician submits a separate bill for professional services). At a freestanding clinic, services billed to Medicare or Medicaid patients will be reimbursed at the Medicare nonfacility rate (a higher reimbursed dollar amount compared with the facility rate because the overhead cost is not billed separately).

Additional Means of Financial Viability

The survival of any wound clinic will depend on more than desire and quality outcomes. No wound center can continue to provide care unless the costs of providing care are covered. Wound care is a volume business—that is, the center must see a certain number of patients in order to create a positive cash flow. The bottom-line number of patients who must be seen will depend on the center's overhead: salaries, rent, utilities, cost of supplies, and other expenses. Financial success is difficult to attain if professional charges are the sole source of income, such as with the freestanding clinic.

A hospital-based clinic can offer additional referrals to the hospital for laboratory, radiology, nuclear medicine, magnetic resonance imaging, arteriogram, and surgical procedures and even for admissions, all of which add to the clinic's financial viability. The clinic should record these referrals and communicate to administrators in regular reports to reinforce the financial contributions of the wound center (Treadwell, 2007). Hospital outpatient clinics have the ability

TABLE 2-1   Advantages of External versus Internal Clinic Management

External (Outside) Management	Internal (Self-directed) Management
Policy and documentation forms already developed	Able to create policy and forms that flow with current hospital tools already in place
Education and resources available via managed company	Establish and seek education via both national and local conferences based on clinic focus
Able to compare productivity and outcome numbers with other management facilities to gauge quality outcomes	Quality care program based on internal data or nationally available data
Established evidence-based pathway provided	Create clinic pathway to fit patient population and current hospital protocols using available evidence-based resources
Decisions and goals made at the corporate level and can be implemented with corporate support	Decisions and goals made at local level with flexibility to respond based on internal assessment and preferences
Audits by oversight to determine compliance, alert to national changes	Verify changes to payment rate, make local coverage determinations at least quarterly, make policy/form changes as prompted from data to fit local changes
Database system to assist with reports and documentation	If database desired, may choose from many available for reports and documentation; this option may offer benchmarking with other sites for outcome comparisons
Potential for faster startup/growth due to already created tool and knowledge	Potential to add services other than wound care if clinic desires (e.g., nail care, ostomy clinic, lymphedema, continence clinic)
Staffing needs determined by job descriptions	Less outgoing expense, increased clinic revenue potential

CHECKLIST 2-1   Clinic Space and Supply Needs

Space-Related
✓ Individual treatment rooms with sinks
✓ Adequate front office space
✓ Offices
✓ Waiting area (include bariatric-friendly furniture)
✓ Clinic workspace
✓ Dictation area
✓ Storage areas
✓ Clean and dirty utility rooms

Hyperbaric-Related (If Applicable)
✓ Patient changing rooms
✓ Oxygen supply
✓ Fire safety
✓ Floor weight loading with consideration to wax on floor and types of lights in ceiling

Nail Care-Related (If Applicable) (see Chapter 15)
Debridement-Related
✓ Forceps (toothed and/or smooth)
✓ Scalpels with blade (no. 10, 11, 15)
✓ Clamps or hemostats
✓ Curettes of several sizes
✓ Scissors or tissue nippers (various types: bandage removal, sharp for cutting tissue or dressings)

✓ Rongeurs
✓ Punch biopsy
✓ Sterile drapes
✓ Dressings

Wound Management-Related
✓ Normal saline
✓ Dressings
✓ Tube stabilizers
✓ Ostomy and wound pouches
✓ Wound measuring guides
✓ Camera
✓ Monofilaments
✓ Doppler
✓ Pulsate lavage supplies/noncontact low-frequency ultrasound (if applicable)
✓ Durable equipment that accommodates bariatric and spinal cord-injured population
✓ Transfer devices (e.g., hover mat, Hoyer lift)
✓ Examination tables and chairs
✓ Offloading overlay surface
✓ Scales
✓ Full range of blood pressure cuff sizes

Lists specify items other than routine examination room-related supplies, such as gloves, gowns, masks, and drapes.

to obtain the facility fee for services provided by charging the facility rate when procedures are performed; this will assist in capturing facility-operating expenses.

In contrast, the freestanding clinic may increase financial stability by performing some of the necessary supplementary procedures in the center. Vascular evaluations with Doppler, transcutaneous oxygen pressure ($TcPO_2$) studies, and measurements of ankle-brachial index (ABI) can generate charges for the center and enhance the bottom line. Clinics may choose to provide outpatient intravenous antibiotic therapy, ostomy care/education, lymphedema therapy, or foot and nail services, allowing patients to come to a familiar location for multiple services. In turn, these visits provide the staff with an opportunity to keep a close eye on the patient's wound while offering one-stop convenience to the patient.

CLINIC OPERATIONS

Numerous operations-related issues must be addressed: regulatory compliance, consents, infection control, national guidelines, laboratory and radiology needs, staff education, documentation, billing guidelines, and much more. Many of these issues are common to all outpatient clinics regardless of their location.

Hours of Operation and Scheduling

Hours of operation need to accommodate the population served and be compatible with staff availability and support services, such as transportation, laboratory, and radiology departments. The schedule should include time allocated for follow-up communication, staff education, meetings, quality reviews, audits, and emergency visits. Allowing for unscheduled emergency visits may avoid costly trips to the emergency department and unnecessary hospital admissions. The wound clinic has readily available focused resources to address wound care needs in an outpatient environment. This is significant in helping to prevent unplanned readmissions, which precipitate negative financial impact with recent health care changes of the Affordable Care Act (ACA).

Special scheduling considerations include a longer time slot for new patients and anticipated procedures, teaching sessions, and review of test results. As the clinic volume grows, it will be prudent to establish predetermined time slots for these types of visits. A communication process should be established so that the scheduling staff is aware of these special needs. This can be accomplished with a notation on the medical record or on the scheduling book to remind scheduling staff to consider this information before scheduling the appointment.

Another consideration for scheduling is staff and skill mix needs. For example, a plastic surgeon with many immobile individuals may require higher numbers of staff to help position and hold patients versus a podiatry clinic, where the majority of patients can self-ambulate and remove/replace their shoes.

Chart Preparation, Storage, and Electronic Medical Records

Before the appointment, the clerical staff should prepare the necessary forms and verification of insurance authorization. New patients will need to provide a history and sign consent forms, in addition to any documentation forms necessary for return visits. Locked file storage within the clinic will be necessary, with potential for offsite storage if space is limited. However, it is important to consider how accessible these records will be if a request is made to retrieve them. A master list for storage boxes should be maintained to assist with retrieval, sign-out, and replacement.

The electronic medical record (EMR) has been utilized for years in wound clinics to aid clinical documentation, financial tracking/billing, regulatory compliance, audits, and outcome tracking. A growing number of companies have a focused attention on EMR use for the wound clinic (i.e., Wound Expert, Intellicure, Indigo). Privacy and security regarding the confidentiality of all patient health information is a priority, and facility policies must be implemented and followed for all patient records.

Obtaining Consents

Preprinted consent forms (treatment, photography, surgical/biopsy) should be available and signed before the visit. Consents can be mailed or faxed to the appropriate authority before the appointment to prevent delay in treatment when the patient is unable to sign independently. A protocol for the frequency of renewing consents should be established. Some facility registration cycles require monthly consents with each new registration; others refer to this as a recurring series and require annual updates if the patient has continued uninterrupted visits during the course of treatment. All consents should be maintained in the legal patient's records.

Regulations and Compliance

With the numerous rules and regulations existing today that ultimately impact quality of care, reputation, and payment for services, most organizations have a compliance program to oversee both corporate and regulatory issues. The objective of a compliance program is to identify potential sources of risk and implement policy and process modifications to reduce risk (Hess, 2008). Corporate compliance addresses employee behaviors and ethical issues in an attempt to protect the corporation from criminal and civil liability. This is accomplished through corporate-sponsored training activities on topics such as code of conduct (e.g., sexual harassment, interaction with vendors, ethics, publication, involvement with media), grievance without retribution procedures, and disciplinary processes.

Regulatory issues are dictated by whether the clinic is freestanding or hospital based. Most hospital-based clinics are included in annual hospital audits/surveys and are required to follow standard hospital policies; freestanding clinics may not have the same requirements. During the planning process, regulatory requirements within the geographic area need to be addressed as established by The Joint Commission, the Department of Health, and the Certificate of Need (Fusaro et al, 2008). Compliance with National Patient Safety Goals (including patient identification, appropriate hand-off communication, and medication safety) and with coding and billing guidelines is essential to the financial health of a clinic. Coding experts should be used in setting up the "charge master" (clinic billing charges linking codes and dollar amounts), training staff in coding visits and procedures, and ensuring accurate documentation that reflects compliance and maximizes payment.

The clinic staff should be familiar with and in compliance with the Health Insurance Portability and Accountability Act (HIPAA) of 1996 privacy rule. The HIPAA was enacted for many reasons, including improving the portability and continuity of health insurance coverage and combating waste, fraud, and abuse in health insurance and delivery of health care (U.S. Department Health and Human Services, 2009). The HIPAA privacy rule also established national standards to protect the privacy of a patient's health information from health plans, health care clearinghouses, and most health care providers. Further information and guidance on implementing the HIPAA privacy rule are available on the websites listed in Table 2-2.

Insurance Authorization. Generally, Medicare policy requires providers to update beneficiary payer information for every admission, outpatient encounter, or start of care before submitting a bill to Medicare. The provider should retain a copy of the completed questionnaire on file or online for audit purposes. It is prudent for providers to retain these records. When a provider believes Medicare may not cover his or her services as medically reasonable and necessary, the provider should give the patient an acceptable advance beneficiary notice (ABN); otherwise, the provider generally cannot hold the patient liable if Medicare denies payment. Managed care contracts and some group health care plans may require prior

authorization for care at the wound clinic. Authorizations may come open ended or may have restricted timeframes and visit numbers. A tracking system needs to be created so that staff is alerted when reauthorization is required.

Some wound treatment orders require authorization before implementation (e.g., biologic skin grafts, negative pressure wound treatments, noncontact low-frequency ultrasound); therefore the provider and staff should be aware of these requirements to prevent loss of reimbursement. In addition, the office staff should verify that the provider is covered by the insurance plan.

Treatment Orders. In most wound clinics a physician or a nonphysician provider (advanced practice registered nurse or physician's assistant) is present to see the patient at each visit. A physician referral or a prior physician order to treat is not required by the Centers for Medicare & Medicaid Services (CMS); however, a referral may be required by the individual patient's insurance plan. The office staff should be familiar with this requirement so that they can obtain the necessary authorization. A copy of this order must remain in the patient's record.

TABLE 2-2 Website Addresses Relevant to Clinic Function, Structure, and Operations

Information Available	Website URL
Directory and information	http://www.cms.hhs.gov
Guidance on HIPAA privacy rules and teaching materials	http://www.hhs.gov/ocr/privacy/hipaa/understanding/index.html
Local information regarding coverage	http://www.cms.gov/medicare-coverage-database/overview-and-quick-search.aspx?show=all&clickon=search
Fee schedules	http://www.cms.hhs.gov/FeeScheduleGenInfo/
Hospital outpatient PPS	http://www.cms.gov/Medicare/Medicare-Fee-for-Service-Payment/HospitalOutpatientPPS/index.html
CPT codes	http://www.cms.gov/Medicare/Coding/ICD9ProviderDiagnosticCodes/codes.html, or http://www.ama-assn.org//ama/pub/physician-resources/solutions-managing-your-practice/coding-billing-insurance/cpt/about-cpt.page
Healthcare Common Procedure Coding System HCPCS	http://www.cms.gov/Medicare/Coding/MedHCPCSGenInfo/index.html
Directory of Fiscal Intermediaries and Intermediary Carriers and Medicare Contractors	http://www.cms.gov/About-CMS/Agency-Information/Aboutwebsite/contractorwebguidlines.html
Medicare Coverage Database with current NCDs and draft and final LCDs	http://www.cms.gov/mcd/overview.asp
NCCI edits	http://www.cms.gov/Medicare/Coding/NationalCorrectCodInitEd/
ICD-10 information	http://www.cms.gov/icd10
Quality initiatives link	http://www.cms.gov/Medicare/Quality-Initiatives-Patient-Assessment-Instruments/QualityInitiativesGenInfo/index.html
Prior Authorization Process for Certain Durable Medical Equipment, Prosthetic, orthotics, Supplies Items	http://www.cms.gov/Research-Statistics-Data-and-Systems/Monitoring-Programs/Medicare-FFS-Compliance-Programs/Prior-Authorization-Initiatives/Prior-Authorization-Process-for-Certain-Durable-Medical-Equipment-Prosthetic-Orthotics-Supplies-Items.html

CPT, Current Procedural Terminology; *HIPAA,* Health Insurance Portability and Accountability Act of 1996; *LCD,* local coverage determination; *NCCI,* National Correct Coding Initiative; *NCD,* national coverage determination.

When no physician or nonphysician provider is scheduled to see the patient, auxiliary staff (nursing, technicians, and therapist) must meet supervision criteria before billing the incident to the physician services. In this case the order for treatment and documentation of visit must be maintained in the medical record, including the provider's treatment plan showing his or her active involvement with prior and ongoing care. Additionally the facility should maintain a record of the supervising physician for each visit (consider documenting in the record at the encounter); auxiliary staff must also be certain to follow the scope of practice pertaining to license and state law. Incident to services are further explained later in this chapter.

Documentation. Documentation alone will not guarantee reimbursement; however, to receive payment for services, appropriate and complete documentation must be provided. This should include the following:

- Accurate diagnoses are documented by clinic staff and the physician treating the patient.
- Exact anatomic locations of all wounds treated are denoted, including specific and consistent measurements.
- Clinic and provider documentation support each other.
- Provider documentation is present, supports the necessity of treatment, and is linked to the diagnosis code (Fife and Weir, 2007).
- Treatments, including the dressing specifics, are recorded. Many treatment modalities and dressings (e.g., dermal substitutes, negative pressure wound therapy, debridement) are reimbursed based on the size of the affected area (Sullivan, 2007).

Additional documentation needed to complete the clinic chart is listed in Table 2-3. Documentation requirements are extensive. Compliance is facilitated by building prompts within the documentation system of the medical record.

Debridement. Wound debridement is an integral part of the day-to-day care provided in wound clinics. As required by Medicare, documentation of debridement must communicate exactly what was done and the rationale. Specifically documentation must include type of tissue removed, depth of removal, instrument used (type of instrument, dressing, medication), wound size, condition of wound/bleeding stopped, and how the wound was redressed after debridement (Fife, 2007). A clear picture must be presented, given the Office of the Inspector General (OIG) report revealing that 64% of claims for debridement did not meet Medicare requirements (OIG, 2007). Chapter 17 provides critical information related to debridement.

Contractor or Payer Audits. Regular audits are conducted by the CMS through their Recovery Audit Contractors (RAC) program (CMS, 2015a). Implemented in 2008, RAC's mission is to identify overpayments and underpayments to health care providers and suppliers. Contractors must comply with national coverage determinations (NCDs) and local coverage determinations (LCDs).

TABLE 2-3	Items in an Outpatient Clinic Chart
Comprehensive admission assessment	Patient's name, gender, race, ethnicity, primary language spoken, address, phone number, date of birth, height/weight, name and phone of any legally authorized representative, past and present diagnoses, wound history, reason for visit, barriers to care, allergies, current mediations, advanced directive, family history
Wound assessment, compliance/teaching record	Vital signs, any medicine changes, procedure or hospitalizations since last visit, reason for visit, complete wound description and photography (if applicable), compliance to treatment plan, pain, any teaching reviewed at visit and response to teaching, treatment applied before discharge, vascular assessment if lower extremity wounds
Physician progress notes	Reason for visit and relevant history, physician examination findings and prior diagnostic test results, assessment, clinical impression or diagnosis, plan of care, rationale for ordering any test, patient's progress and response to changes in treatment plan; codes reported on billing statement should be supported in the documentation; any consult advice provided or received acknowledged as reviewed
Discharge orders	Any new test or medications ordered, wound treatment orders, next follow-up appointment or consult appointment, compression or offloading instructions
Acuity	Used by hospital-based clinic if no procedure was completed to bill evaluation and management of services based on facility resources acuity score; all resources considered should be supported in the medical record (consider acuity form a permanent documentation form to prevent charges not documented; use as a documentation and scoring tool)
Billing form	Complete listing of any diagnosis codes or procedure codes used for billing; supporting documentation must be in the medical record
Consents, insurance information, HIPAA documents	Consent for treatment, consent for photography, insurance information or copy of insurance card, HIPAA notification

Auditors will often request specific documentation to demonstrate compliance (Checklist 2-2). Common issues reviewed by auditors include:

- Every service billed must be documented because the patient's record must contain clear evidence that the service, procedure, or supply actually was performed or supplied.
- The medical necessity for choosing the procedure, service, or medical supply must be substantiated.
- Every service must be coded correctly. Diagnoses must be coded to the highest level of specificity, and procedure codes must be current.
- Documentation must clearly indicate who performed the procedure or supplied the equipment.
- Legible documentation, which may be dictated and transcribed, is required. Existing documentation may not be embellished; however, additional documentation that supports a claim may be submitted.
- Voluntary disclosure of information by the provider is encouraged. When an error is discovered, any overpayment should be returned to Medicare (Centers for Medicare & Medicaid Services, 2004).

Clinic Composition: Staffing with an Interdisciplinary Team

Much like any wound team, the outpatient wound clinic requires the coordination and contribution of a variety of individuals and professionals and an extensive referral network. Members of the staff should have a job description and expectations that align with their educational preparation as outlined in Chapter 1. Each member of the outpatient wound clinic team will be instrumental in patient recruitment. The following describes additional roles unique to the outpatient setting.

Table 2-4 lists examples of Wound Clinic Interdisciplinary Team Members.

CHECKLIST 2-2 Typical Documentation Items Requested by Audit Contractor or Payer

✓ Office records (progress notes, current history and physical, treatment plan)
✓ Documentation of identity and professional status of clinician
✓ Laboratory and radiology reports
✓ Comprehensive problem list
✓ Current list of prescribed medications
✓ Progress notes for each visit indicating patient's response to prescribed treatment
✓ Documentation supporting time spent with patient when time-based codes are used
✓ Required referrals or prescriptions (for many nonphysician services/supplies)
✓ Required Certificates of Medical Necessity

TABLE 2-4 Wound Clinic Interdisciplinary Team Members

Position	Onsite	Available as Consultant
Medical director	X	
General surgeon		X
Peripheral vascular surgeon		X
Orthopedic surgeon		X
Dermatologist		X
Reconstructive surgeon		X
Podiatry		X
Infectious disease		X
Geriatrician		X
Occupational therapist		X
Certified wound care nurse (CWCN©, CWOCN©, CWON©)	X	
Registered nurse	X	
Physical therapist (may be certified wound specialist)	X	
Medical or surgical assistant	X	
Office staff (e.g., receptionist)	X	
Diabetes educator	X	
Dietitian	X	
Billing/coder	X	

Clinic Director. The clinic director is often a nurse and may or may not be certified in wound care. This position provides oversight of the clinic, including staffing, scheduling, materials management, staff preparation/education, regulatory compliance, and profitability. Routine and frequent contact of the clinic director with insurance, billing, and coding personnel will facilitate early identification of any problems in reimbursement or documentation so that corrective steps can be taken promptly. Educational outreach programs can be used to become acquainted with possible referral sources, such as home health care agencies, nursing homes, physician offices, urgent care centers, and emergency rooms.

Nurse Coordinator. Nurses in the clinic provide a key role in the operation of the clinic and coordination of care. Responsibilities often include checking in the patient, interviewing the patient, removing dressings, assessing the wound, and collaborating with the wound specialist and interdisciplinary team members to evaluate and implement the plan of care. Basic competencies in wound care and skin assessment are essential to optimal functioning of the nursing staff in the wound clinic (Morrison, 2007).

Insurance and Billing Coder. The value and expertise of insurance and billing coders cannot be understated. Close collaboration with the coding department will secure optimal regulatory compliance and reimbursement. In addition, insurance coordinators for the wound department may assist with preapprovals from various private insurance companies. This position may be part of the facility coding team or a person assigned to the department to obtain preapprovals and support the coders with communication to the clinic.

Ancillary Staff. Ancillary clinic staff may include schedulers, medical assistants, and surgical assistants, who may work in the clinic and assist with office duties. Expectations may include preparation of forms and consents, patient registration, placing appointment reminder calls, scheduling tests, and data entry for billing and supplies. Training ancillary staff to work in the clinical area (within their job scope and reporting significant findings to clinic nurses and physicians) and to cover the office allows for flexibility in scheduling during slow clinic times and vacation schedules.

Utilizing the ancillary staff while scrutinizing staffing ratios (nursing hours vs. ancillary hours and all hours worked vs. patient visits) will assist with monitoring worked hours per patient visit. Closely watching this ratio may show the need to bring on new staff as clinic visits increase, alter staff hours during slower days during the week, and shift staff hours to busier work days.

Referral Network

Outpatient care, in large part, requires referrals to, and use of, community services: local transportation companies, durable medical equipment (DME) companies, orthotics and prosthetics suppliers, physician offices, home care agencies, laboratories, and radiology and other hospital departments. Everyone in the clinic should be familiar with how to access these resources and the requirements that must be fulfilled in order to complete a referral. This kind of detail when providing care to the clinic patient will convey a sense of calmness and confidence to the patient and facilitate the patient's ability to follow through, which ultimately will enhance outcomes.

Hospital facilities likely have access to onsite laboratory, radiology, vascular laboratory, surgical suite, and emergency rooms. The place or site to which the patient is referred must always be the patient's choice rather than a mandate that the patient be sent to a particular facility. The insurance company often drives this decision. When referral sites are freestanding, it may be beneficial to have a list of local sites where such tests can be obtained, along with their hours of business, addresses, and contact information.

Durable medical equipment (DME) supplies will be a common need of the wound clinic patient. Most patients are unaware of where to obtain supplies and what products may be equivalent substitutes. Therefore the patient will need a list of local DME providers, as well as mail-order companies, to facilitate accessing supplies. The patient who has limited mobility cannot easily pick up supplies and will need either free home delivery or mail delivery. Providing patients with written instructions detailing their wound care supplies and the wound care procedure will facilitate continuity in their care. In many situations, wound care orders can be sent directly to the DME; however, proposed changes may require altering current processes. A proposed rule by CMS: *Medicare Program; Prior Authorization Process for Certain Durable Medical Equipment, Prosthetic, Orthotics and Supplies (DMEPOS) Items*, would establish a prior authorization process for certain DMEPOS that are frequently subject to unnecessary utilization. This is in response to the 2012 reporting period that found approximately 94% of DMEPOS improper payments were due to insufficient documentation, which could be avoided with a preapproval process. At time of this text the proposal includes items that are high cost (over $1000 and rental over $100, i.e., negative pressure wound therapy pumps, diabetic shoes and inserts, powered beds, overlay and mattress) (CMS, 2014a).

Clinic Space and Equipment

Equipment needed for the wound clinic is similar to that needed in many routine outpatient clinics; however, additional equipment items unique to the care of the patient with a wound are necessary to provide the patient with efficient care (see Checklist 2-1).

Room Equipment. At a minimum, multipatient rooms should have privacy curtains separating patients. Individual rooms are preferred to facilitate privacy. From an infection control perspective, rooms in which treatments have the potential to generate aerosolization should be separated by walls rather than curtains to prevent the spread of microorganisms. Considering how the patient will arrive may be critical to determining what equipment to place in a room. Carts and large wheelchair transports may be cumbersome when turning corners and should be considered early in the planning phase.

The type of clinic room equipment may vary depending on the type of patients expected. Spinal cord injury or reconstructive surgery clinics may require space to accommodate patients arriving on stretchers, with pneumatic treatment tables and additional staff or adaptive equipment to assist with transfers. An offloading overlay surface should be added to the examination table to reduce pressure and provide comfort; it also can be used for educational purposes when teaching positioning and hand checks. Examination chairs (e.g., podiatry chairs) are preferable for the ambulatory patient with a lower extremity ulcer. The positioning made available with this type of chair will facilitate patient comfort, allow for better visualization of lower extremity wounds, promote ergonomic movements by the staff, thus reducing their risk of musculoskeletal injury, and maintain a good distance from the floor so that the risk of cross-contamination from microorganisms on the floor is minimized.

A stand for treatment supplies with wheels that can be positioned within reach of the patient and caregiver, as well as a place for documentation, will be needed for each room.

Additional items needed include a stool for the clinician, a visitor chair, and good lighting. Basic equipment includes items such as thermometers, sphygmomanometers, needle boxes, gloves boxes, dirty linen containers, trashcans, and hazardous waste receptacles.

Wound centers may want to purchase a bariatric treatment chair. Many treatment chairs have a weight limit between 275 and 400 pounds; however, a certain patient population will require a treatment chair that can hold between 500 and 800 pounds.

Another important piece of equipment for wound centers is a scale to help monitor nutrition and fluid balance, especially when diuretics are used with compression wraps. Patient safety should be considered when purchasing a scale. A scale with handrails provides a stable base for patients to step onto. A wheelchair scale may be necessary, or one with a weight limit up to 850 pounds.

Wound Care Supplies. A formulary of wound care supplies for the wound clinic will need to be developed. The formulary should be selected with knowledge of the most common wound needs seen in the clinic and the function of the various dressings. The range of products included in the formulary should be kept narrow to reduce the potential for confusion on utilization, ordering, or storage. Due to product expiration dates, supplies used less often or for specific procedures (e.g., biologic graft) may need to be special ordered.

Pharmaceuticals (topical anesthetics and topical creams) should be kept locked and made available for minor procedures such as debridement. Medications should not be administered without a provider's order. Patients attending a clinic where medications cannot be administered should be encouraged to take a pain medication before their visit.

Many wound care visits will require conservative sharp debridement, so appropriate tools should be available. However, no package should be opened during room setup in anticipation of debridement. Rather, package materials should be opened only after the need for the tools is confirmed. Basic sharp debridement tools can be disposable or resterilized; consider patient volumes when determining the number of tools needed and the time allotment for resterilizing equipment.

Education

Education of patients and staff is a vital component of any wound care program in any setting and is addressed throughout this textbook. In the outpatient setting, documentation of the education and handouts provided and their understanding is important, not only in providing quality wound care, but also can be used to justify additional clinic visits, as well as potential referrals (e.g., psychiatrist, cognitive evaluation, home care). When setting up a clinic, planners should consider the variety of electronic media that can be used and made available to the patient, either in a separately designated "education" room or from a library, from which the patient can access the material, review it at home, and then return it (Armstrong et al, 2008).

Staff education should be mandatory and competency based for a variety of reasons, such as patient safety, appropriate use of resources, improved patient care, standardization of care, and compliance with facility policy. The Federal Register and State Operating Manuals have requirements for policies to address education when protocols are utilized (Calloway, 2012). Education time is essential for staff to keep abreast of any new developments in their field and be informed to follow proper safety procedures. Checklist 2-3 provides a list of competencies to be considered for staff education in a wound clinic.

Policies, Procedures, and Guidelines

As described in Chapter 1, the wound specialist plays a pivotal role in integrating research findings into policies, procedures, and guidelines for the clinic. Evidence-based policies, procedures, and guidelines for care must be readily available to clinic personnel. Familiarity with these documents should be addressed through competency-based staff education programs as already described. See Checklist 2-3 for a list of possible wound clinic policies.

CHECKLIST 2-3 Examples of Wound Clinic Policies and Competencies

Policies	Competencies
✓ Wound measurement	✓ Wound measurement
✓ Wound photo	✓ Wound photography
✓ Direct supervision/"incident-to" visits	✓ Wound culture
✓ Quality program	✓ Compression wraps
✓ Conservative care designation	✓ Negative pressure wound therapy
✓ Chart order	✓ Low-frequency ultrasound treatments
✓ Billing guidelines	✓ Skin inspections
✓ Form completion guidelines	✓ Room cleaning between patients
✓ Clinic scheduling	✓ Isolation/infection control
✓ Position descriptions and responsibilities	✓ Offloading techniques
✓ Insurance authorization process	✓ Ankle-brachial index
✓ HIPAA/EMR/Health information security and privacy	✓ Monofilament/sensory testing
	✓ Conservative sharp debridement
	✓ Chemical cautery with silver nitrate
	✓ Pulsate lavage

HIPAA, Health Insurance Portability and Accountability Act; *EMR*, electronic medical record.

Continuous Quality Improvement Plan

Quality outcome data are necessary to evaluate compliance with evidence-based wound care and progress of the overall treatment plan. The data may be shared with the patient to encourage continued treatment, shared with insurance companies to demonstrate medical necessity, and compared locally or nationally to display the cost benefit of treatment. Although economic factors in wound care are common measures in product evaluation, ultimately the bottom line is efficacy. An inexpensive product that makes up for its low cost with increased clinic visits due to delayed healing time quickly loses its product price advantage; additional costs will be incurred if infection develops (Jacobs and Tomazak, 2008). Healing time in relation to cost is another valuable piece of outcome data. Stratification of data by etiology, providers, and clinic days provides additional information about efficiency, effectiveness, and best practice. Further analysis includes measuring the impact of clinic-based care on the number of home care visits, use of wound care–related medications, acute care readmissions, emergency room visits, number of surgical procedures, limb salvage, and healing times. These data are useful for substantiating best practices and for marketing the clinic.

AFFORDABLE CARE ACT AND PAYMENT SYSTEMS

Successful wound management is a culmination of quality wound care practices and knowledge of coverage and payment polices. Reimbursement is based on what is done and documented at the clinic visit. Knowing the type of insurance and whether authorization is required, keeping track of visits, and knowing whether the patient has Medicare/Medicaid and how this coverage affects billing are essential.

The CMS is responsible for establishing the payment system for Medicare and Medicaid beneficiaries. It pays the majority of the health care dollars in the United States. Billing principles are similar for other insurance types using the billing codes established by the American Medical Association (AMA) known as diagnosis codes, also known as the International Classification of Diseases, 10th Revision (ICD-10) codes, to support the disease/reason for visit. Acronyms are common in the billing process, and a directory of acronyms related to the billing process is provided in Box 2-3.

Affordable Care Act

The ACA is changing the way health care is delivered and addresses coverage issues for all, the rising cost of care, and improved care delivery—including the coordination and safety of care. This means transparency of costly mistakes and readmissions, keeping patients healthy, rewarding quality instead of quantity, and building on the health information technology infrastructures. This concept is familiar to many who have worked within the outpatient wound clinic over the years where outcomes were tracked, patients were directed to return to the clinic for issues versus readmissions, and education was

---

BOX 2-3 Acronyms Related to Billing and Reimbursement Process

APC: Ambulatory Payment Classification—System used for outpatient services, attached to assigned CPT code for payment.

CPT: Current Procedural Terminology—Codes that describe the procedure performed, such as debridement.

DME: Durable Medical Equipment—Supplies ordered by physician for use in the home (item must be reusable).

DMERC: Durable Medical Equipment Regional Carrier—Contractor for CMS who provides claims processing and payment for DME.

E&M: Evaluation and Management—CPT code used to obtain the fee for the corresponding services provided.

FI: Fiscal Intermediary—Contractor for CMS who processes claims for services covered under Medicare.

HCPCS: Healthcare Common Procedure Coding System—Uniform method used by providers and suppliers to report professional services, procedures, and supplies (codes describe dressing supply) assigned and maintained by local Medicare contractors.

ICD-10: International Classification of Diseases, 10th Revision—National coding method designed to enable providers to effectively document the medical condition, symptom, or complaint that forms the basis for rendering a specific service.

LCD: Local Coverage Determination—Formal statement developed through a specifically defined process that defines the service, provides information about when the service is considered reasonable and necessary, outlines any coverage criteria and/or documentation requirements, and provides coding information.

Level II HCPCS—Method for obtaining reimbursement for products, supplies, or procedures not covered in the CPT codes.

MAC: Medicare Administrative Contractor—A single authority consisting of integrated fiscal intermediaries and carriers responsible for the receipt, processing, and payment of Medicare claims. The MAC will perform functions related to the beneficiary and provider service, appeals, provider outreach and education, financial management, program evaluation, reimbursement, payment safeguards, and information systems security.

NCCI: National Correct Coding Initiative—Developed to promote correct coding by providers and supplies (to prevent payment for noncovered and/or incorrectly coded services).

NCD: National Coverage Determination—Developed by CMS to describe the circumstances for Medicare coverage for a specific medical service procedure or device.

OPPS: Outpatient Prospective Payment System—A prospective payment system (fee schedule) that sets payments for individual services as identified by the HCPCS codes and used for hospital outpatient services, certain Part B services furnished to hospital inpatients who have no Part A coverage, and partial hospitalization services furnished by hospitals and community mental health centers.

PPS: Prospective Payment System—Method of reimbursement in which Medicare payment is made based on a predetermined, fixed amount.

provided to patients and caregivers to care for wounds at home. The outpatient areas should expect to become a growing focus of early assessment on preventing infections and readmissions by utilizing experts to avoid unnecessary readmissions via the emergency department or nonspecialist provider. These clinics may provide areas of expanded value to the hospital partner by providing care of the ostomy, lymphedema, and burn patient if not already addressed.

The ACA is a landmark health bill signed into law by President Obama in 2010. Paying for value is a focus, as the hospital will be rewarded based on the quality of care it provides to patients via the Value-Based Purchasing Program; the Hospital Readmissions Reduction Program will reduce payment to hospitals with relatively high rates of potentially preventable readmissions. Promoting better care and protecting patients are addressed via the adoption of the electronic record, as well as reporting hospital-acquired conditions, with possible payment penalties for those with high rates. Reducing health costs is addressed in the Medicare durable medical equipment, prosthetics, orthotics, and supplies (DMEPOS) competitive bidding and by fighting fraud (CMS, 2014b).

The fundamentals of traditional Medicare remain with additional incentives and penalties assigned for quality outcomes, technology use, and cost containment. These changes will modernize our health care system and fight waste, fraud, and abuse. Being aware of key provisions and how they affect care changes and financial outcomes will remain critical (i.e., reduce the number of hospital readmissions, reduce hospital-acquired conditions, bundling payments, improved quality reporting) (CMS, 2014b).

Medicare

Title XVIII of the Social Security Act, designated "Health Insurance for the Aged and Disabled," is more commonly known as Medicare. The Social Security Amendments of 1965 created a health insurance program for aged persons to complement retirement, survivor, and disability insurance benefits. When first implemented in 1966, Medicare covered most persons aged 65 years and over. In 1973 additions made to Medicare benefits included (1) persons entitled to Social Security or Railroad Retirement disability cash benefits for at least 24 months, (2) most persons with end-stage renal disease, and (3) certain otherwise noncovered aged persons who elected to pay a premium for Medicare coverage.

Medicare traditionally has consisted of two parts: Part A and Part B (Original Medicare). A third part, Part C, or the Medicare Advantage program (also known as Medicare + Choice), is available to individuals who qualify for Original Medicare. The drug coverage, known as Medicare Part D, is provided by private health plans; this coverage can be drug only or can be provided through a Medicare Advantage plan that offers comprehensive benefits.

Medicare Part A. Medicare Part A, referred to as "Hospital Insurance," helps cover services and supplies related to inpatient hospital stays. In addition, Part A covers care in a skilled nursing facility (SNF) if the care follows a Medicare Part A–covered 3-day hospital stay. Finally, Part A covers hospice and, in some situations, home health care. When the beneficiary is entitled to Part A benefits, the beneficiary's red, white, and blue Medicare identification card will indicate "Hospital (Part A)."

Medicare Part B. Medicare Part B, commonly known as "Medical Insurance," essentially helps cover doctors' services, certain medical items, and outpatient care when such services are provided under a doctor's care and are documented to be medically necessary. Specifically, clinical laboratory services, some home health care, outpatient hospital services, blood transfusions (after the first 3 pints), some preventive services, ambulance services (when other transportation would endanger health), and medical social services are provided under Part B. Physical therapy and some home health care furnished by hospitals, SNFs, and other institutional providers likewise are eligible for Part B coverage. When the beneficiary has Part B benefits, the Medicare card will stipulate "Medicare (Part B)." Part B requires payment of a monthly premium that usually is taken out of the beneficiary's Social Security, Railroad Retirement, or Office of Personnel Management Retirement payment. Otherwise, Medicare will bill for the premium every 3 months. In addition to the premium, the beneficiary must meet an annual deductible and pay all coinsurance amounts unless he or she has other supplemental insurances.

Providers who submit Part B claims should always refer to their carrier's local coverage determinations (LCDs) and other billing guidance for specific coverage and payment criteria. Box 2-4 gives a list of services and supplies covered under Part B, when medically necessary.

Medicare Advantage Plan, Part C. The Medicare Advantage program was established by the Balanced Budget Act of 1997 (BBA). This program consists of a set of options created by the BBA to provide care under contract to Medicare, to possibly reduce the beneficiary's out-of-pocket expenses, and to offer more health care and contractor choices. The Medicare Advantage plan must provide the same services a beneficiary would be eligible to receive from Medicare if he or she were in Original Medicare. However, the beneficiary technically still is "on Medicare" but has selected a different contractor and is required to receive services according to that contractor's arrangements.

Providers, suppliers, and their billing personnel must be aware that Medicare Advantage plans do not operate under the same coverage and payment policy for claims processing as Original Medicare. If a beneficiary is a member of a Medicare Advantage plan, the local Part B carrier cannot process claims for that beneficiary. When claims are submitted, the local Medicare Part B carrier will deny payment (except for dialysis services). After the denial, the carrier will automatically transfer the claim to the appropriate Medicare

---

BOX 2-4 Services and Supplies Covered under Medicare Part B, When Medically Necessary

Medical Care and Other Services
- Doctor's services
- Outpatient medical and surgical services and supplies
- Diagnostic examinations and tests
- Ambulatory surgery center facility fees for approved procedures
- DME such as wheelchairs, hospital beds, oxygen, walkers
- Second surgical opinions
- Outpatient mental health care
- Outpatient physical and occupational therapy, including speech/language therapy

Clinical Laboratory Services
- Blood tests
- Urinalysis
- Other tests requested by provider

Home Health Care
- Part-time skilled nursing care
- Physical therapy
- Occupational therapy
- Speech/language therapy
- Home health aide services
- Medical social services
- DME such as wheelchairs, hospital beds, oxygen, walkers
- Medical supplies and other services

Additional Coverage Related to Wound Care
- Ambulance services when other transportation would endanger the patient's health
- Artificial limbs that are prosthetic devices and their replacement parts
- Braces (arm, leg, back, neck)
- Emergency care
- Medical nutrition therapy services for people who have diabetes or kidney disease (unless currently on dialysis), with doctor's referral
- Medical supplies, such as ostomy pouches, surgical dressings, splints, casts, some diabetic supplies
- Second surgical opinion by a doctor (in some cases)
- Services of a practitioner, such as clinical social worker, physician's assistant, nurse practitioner
- Telemedicine services in some rural areas
- Therapeutic shoes for people with diabetes (in some cases)
- X-ray films, magnetic resonance imaging, computed tomographic scanning, electrocardiography, and some other purchased diagnostic tests

DME, Durable medical equipment.

Advantage plan. The medical managed care plan is not responsible for paying Medicare Advantage claims, except when (1) the physician or supplier is affiliated with the Medicare Advantage plan or (2) the physician or supplier furnishes emergency services, urgently needed services, or other covered services not reasonable available through the Medicare Advantage plan.

A provider may be reimbursed when filing a claim to a Medicare Advantage plan if he or she is an in-network provider. An out-of-network provider may be covered if specific criteria are met as stipulated by the Medicare Advantage plan, such as prior authorization. If the plan denies the claim, the provider has the right to appeal the claim. An out-of-plan provider may also collect the full fee directly from the patient for services provided if the patient did not receive prior authorization. Before rendering services, a provider who is an affiliate with a Medicare Advantage plan should emphasize to his or her patients what their financial liability will be if they did not receive prior authorization to see the out-of-plan provider.

Medicaid

Title XIX of the Social Security Act is a federal/state entitlement program that pays for medical assistance for certain individuals and families with low incomes and limited resources. The program, known as Medicaid, became law in 1965 as a cooperative venture jointly funded by the federal and state governments for furnishing medical assistance to eligible needy persons. Medicaid is the largest source of funding of medical and health-related services for America's poorest individuals.

Each state (1) establishes its own eligibility standards; (2) determines the type, amount, duration, and scope of services; (3) sets the rate of payment for services; and (4) administers its own program. Medicaid eligibility and/or services within a state can change during the year.

Medicare beneficiaries who have low incomes and limited resources may also receive help from the Medicaid program. For persons who are eligible for full Medicaid coverage, Medicare health care coverage is supplemented by services that are available under their state's Medicaid program, according to eligibility category. When a patient is "dual enrolled," the Medicare program pays for any services that are covered by Medicare before the Medicaid program makes any payments, as Medicaid is always the "payer of last resort."

Group Health Plans, Medicare Secondary Payer Program, and Medicare Coordination of Benefits

Until 1980 Medicare was the primary payer in all situations except those involving workers' compensation. Since 1980, changes in the Medicare law have resulted in Medicare being the secondary payer in situations. The Medicare Secondary Payer (MSP) program protects Medicare funds and ensures that Medicare does not pay for services reimbursable under private insurance plans or other government programs.

The MSP program precludes Medicare from making primary claims payment when a beneficiary has other insurance that should pay first. If a beneficiary is covered by a group health plan as a benefit of current employment, charges for medical services must first be submitted to the group health plan (CMS, 2006).

The Medicare Coordination of Benefits (COB) program works to identify health care coverage that beneficiaries may have that pays primary to Medicare and to coordinate the payment process to prevent mistaken Medicare primary payments. Although the various insurance programs may set separate guidelines, they generally follow similar guidelines as established by the Medicare and/or Medicare Advantage Programs. Monthly verification for services and specific procedures may be necessary to gather payment.

Medigap (Supplemental Insurance)

A Medigap policy is a health insurance policy sold by private insurance companies to fill "gaps" in the Original Medicare plan. The Medigap policy must clearly identify it as "Medicare Supplemental Insurance."

FACTORS THAT INFLUENCE PROVIDER REIMBURSEMENT

When implemented in 1966, Medicare was a fee-for-service insurance plan. Part B providers were paid on a reasonable charge basis for most services. Since then Congress has mandated several changes to the Medicare reimbursement models that vary depending on the care setting and services provided. Today most payments are based on federally established predetermined payments per procedure or item rather than randomly created clinic or hospital fees. Several factors influence the amount of payment the provider is reimbursed: the care setting, the payer or payment plan, and the type of provider.

Care Setting: Nonfacility/Freestanding Sites (Part B)

Part B providers include physicians, ARNPs, physical therapists in private practice, and suppliers of DMEPOS. A Part B provider will always accept assignment on claims submitted on behalf of the Medicare beneficiary. When a Part B provider accepts assignment, the Part B provider agrees to bill the beneficiary only for any coinsurance or deductible that may be applicable and accepts the Medicare payment as full payment.

Physician services are paid by the carrier based on the Medicare Physician's Fee Schedule (MPFS). A fee schedule is a complete listing of fees used by Medicare to pay doctors or other providers/suppliers. This comprehensive listing of "fee maximums" is used to reimburse a physician and/or other providers on a fee-for-service basis. The Centers for Medicare & Medicaid Services develops fee schedules for physicians, ambulance services, clinical laboratory services, and DMEPOS. These fee schedules provide listings for facility rates and nonfacility rates; the nonfacility rates are utilized when services are provided in a standard office setting/nonfacility site.

Care Setting: Hospital Outpatient Facility Settings (Part B)

Reimbursement is limited to a facility fee rate when services are performed in one of the following settings: (1) an inpatient or outpatient hospital setting, (2) a hospital emergency room, (3) a SNF, (4) a comprehensive inpatient or outpatient rehabilitation facility, (5) an inpatient psychiatric facility, or (6) an ambulatory surgical center (ASC). Medicare pays less for services provided in these settings because Medicare assumes the physician's overhead and other related expenses are lower than they would have been in a standard office setting. Physicians are not allowed to bill the beneficiary for the difference. The fee schedule is updated annually on January 1 and available online (see Table 2-2).

Care Setting: Hospital-based Clinic (Part A)

Part A providers include comprehensive outpatient rehabilitation facilities (CORFs); end-stage renal disease (ESRD) facilities; home health agencies (HHAs), including hospital subunits; hospitals (including freestanding facilities or units of a medical complex, such as critical access hospitals [CAHs]); and outpatient rehabilitation facilities (ORFs).

Today most Part A providers, including hospitals, SNFs, and HHAs, receive payments through a prospective payment system (PPS), which is designed to cover the costs of all items and services furnished to beneficiaries while they are under the care of that facility. A PPS is a method of reimbursement in which Medicare payment is made based on a predetermined, fixed amount. The payment amount for a particular service is derived based on the classification system of that service (e.g., diagnosis-related groups [DRGs] for inpatient hospital services and ambulatory payment classifications [APCs] for outpatient services).

Many items and services that once were billable now are covered under the "Consolidated Billing" provisions of the Part A PPS system. Under this coverage, many dressing supplies and services (e.g., physical therapy) must be billed by the facility even if the services were furnished by a Part B provider (in which the payment would generally fall within the PPS). Part B suppliers should contact their Medicare Administrative Contractor (MAC) to learn what "Consolidated Billing" provisions may apply to their provider type or services they furnish.

All services paid under the new PPS to the outpatient clinic are classified into APCs. Services in each APC are similar clinically in terms of the resources they require. A payment rate is established for each APC. Depending on the services provided, hospital clinics may be paid for more than one APC per encounter. The APC codes are attached to the assigned Current Procedural Terminology (CPT) code as further described in the Procedure Codes section and in Table 2-5.

Medicare Managed Care Plan

A beneficiary can select a managed care plan to provide Medicare services. Centers for Medicare & Medicaid Services will pay a fixed amount (i.e., a capitated rate) to the managed care plan selected by the beneficiary. Centers for Medicare & Medicaid Services pays the plan, which then reimburses the provider for services. However, enrollment as a Part B provider does not ensure payment from a Medicare managed care plan.

TABLE 2-5	Types of Codes Necessary for Provider Billing		
Code	Description	Caveat	Example
ICD-10-CM	The first 3 digits pertaining to category, the following digits addressing etiology, anatomic sites, and severity Primary diagnosis code followed by secondary diagnosis—example showing secondary diagnosis for pressure ulcer	Identified as 3- to 7-digit numbers	L8993 Pressure Ulcer unspecified site stage 4 L89153 Pressure Ulcer sacral region stage 3 L89154 Pressure Ulcer sacral region stage 4
CPT	Describes the procedure or service provided	Identified as a 5-digit code	11041: debride skin full-thickness 97597: active wound care/20 cm or under
HCPCS	Describes dressing, supplies, drugs, or procedures that do not have a CPT code	Identified as a letter and numbers	A6234: hydrocolloid dressing 4×4 with adhesive A6257: transparent film, 4×4 size

CPT, Current Procedural Terminology; *HCPCS,* Healthcare Common Procedure Coding System; *ICD-10,* International Classification of Diseases, 10th Revision.

Provider reimbursement in a managed care plan is based solely upon the terms of the provider's agreement with the plan, regardless of the amount Medicare pays for the services.

Nonphysician Practitioners

Medicare allows payment for services furnished by nonphysician practitioners, which includes the advanced practice registered nurse (APRNs) (e.g., NP, clinical nurse specialist, nurse anesthetist) and physician's assistant. The APRN may provide physician services and bill as the provider with the APRN's provider number. Medicare reimburses the APRN at a rate of 85% of the physician rate. Medicare will pay 80% of the patient's bill for the services, and the patient will pay 20% (Buppert, 2007). A service that does not meet Medicare's definition of a "physician service" will not be reimbursed. For example, health services that are within the realm of nursing but are not "physician services" are not covered under Medicare Part B. Medicare defines physician services as diagnosis, therapy, surgery consultation, and care plan oversight (Buppert, 2007). Box 2-5 lists Medicare rules for APRN payment. No separate payment may be made to the nonphysician practitioner if a facility or other physician payment is also made for such professional services (CMS, 2006).

In general, Medicare requires that practices bill services under the provider number of the individual clinician performing the service. However, Medicare rules allow "incident-to" billing (i.e., submitting bills under a physician's provider number for services provided by a supervised employee) reimbursed at a rate of 100% of the physician rate. For services billed as "incident to," the APN must follow the incident-to rules discussed next and use the physician's provider number on the claim. In this situation, the APRN or PA provider number is not needed.

Incident-to-Physician Services and Direct Supervision

Incident-to-physician services may be provided by auxiliary staff (any individual acting under the supervision of a physician, regardless of whether the individual is an employee,

The APRN meets Medicare qualification requirements;
The practice or facility accepts Medicare's payment, which is 85% of the physician fee schedule rate for bills submitted under the APRN's provider number;
The services performed are "physician services" or those for which a physician can bill Medicare;
The services are performed in collaboration with a physician;
The services are within the APRN's scope of practice as defined in state law; and
No facility or other provider charges are paid with respect to the furnishing of the services.

leased, or employed independent contract) or the APRN and PA. Therapeutic services and supplies that are incident to the services of the physician in the course of diagnosis or treatment of an injury or illness are referred to as incident-to-physician's professional services. To be covered as incident-to-physician's services, the services and supplies must be furnished and represent an expense to the legal entity billing for the services or supplies (clinic, physician—in a private office) and must be an integral, although incidental, part of the physician's professional service. The services must be furnished under the order of a physician and under the direct supervision of a physician. A service or supply could be considered to be incident-to when furnished during a course of treatment where the physician performs an initial service and subsequent services of a frequency reflect the physician's active participation in the management of the course of treatment, which is documented in the medical record (CMS, 2014c).

"Direct supervision" means the physician has performed the initial service and periodically is involved in care; the physician must be present and on the premises and immediately available to furnish assistance and direction throughout the performance of the procedure. It does not mean that the physician must be present in the room when the procedure is performed (Vargo, 2009). In the office setting this means the physician must be present in the office suite. In the physician-directed clinic, direct supervision may be the responsibility of several physicians as opposed to an individual attending physician; the clinic physician ordering the service need not be the physician who is supervising the service (CMS, 2014c). A hospital service or supply would not be considered incident to a physician's service if the attending physician merely wrote an order for the services or supplies and referred the patient to the hospital without being involved in the management of that course of treatment (CMS, 2009). During any course of treatment rendered by the auxiliary or nonphysician practitioner, the physician must personally see the patient periodically and sufficiently often to assess the course of treatment and the patient's progress and, where necessary, to change the treatment regimen. Clinicians must follow scope of practice and follow state laws. Centers for Medicare & Medicaid Services would expect that hospitals have credentialing procedures to ensure that services furnished are being provided by qualified practitioners in accordance with all applicable laws and regulations.

In addition to the Medicare Benefit Policy Manual, supervision criteria can be verified with the local MAC.

General Supervision

Few wound care services may be provided with general supervision which means supervision is not required during the performance of the procedure. All other hospital outpatient therapeutic services require a minimum of direct supervision. Effective January 1, 2013, Healthcare Common Procedure Coding System (HCPCS) codes G0127 (Trimming of dystrophic nails), 11719 (Trimming of nondystrophic nails), 29580 (Strapping; Unna boot), and 29581 (Application of multilayer compression system: leg [below knee], including ankle and foot) are listed as general supervision codes (CMS, 2012). Scope of practice and state law requirements will need to be met; however, the direct supervision of a physician will not be required during the service.

Fiscal Intermediaries, Carriers, and Medicare Administrative Contractors

Medicare Part A and Part B claims are processed by nongovernmental organizations or agencies that contract to serve as fiscal agents between providers and suppliers and the federal government. Historically these claims processors were known as fiscal intermediaries (FIs) and carriers. These contractors apply Medicare coverage rules to determine appropriateness of claims for Part A (claims for institutional services, including inpatient hospital claims, SNFs, HHAs, and hospice services) and Part B (claims submitted by institutional providers, including hospital outpatient services). Providers who submit claims should always refer to their local LCD policy and other billing guidance for specific coverage and payment criteria.

From October 2004 through October 2011, FIs and carriers were integrated into MACs. As a single authority, the MAC was responsible for the receipt, processing, and payment of Medicare claims. In addition to providing core claims processing operations for both Medicare Part A and Part B, MAC performed functions related to the beneficiary and provider service, appeals, provider outreach and education (also referred to as provider education and training), financial management, program evaluation, reimbursement, payment safeguards, and information systems security. To access the most current information on Medicare contractors, see the website reference listed in Table 2-2.

National Coverage Determinations and Local Coverage Determinations

National coverage determinations (NCDs) were developed by CMS to describe the circumstances for Medicare coverage for a specific medical service procedure or device. National coverage determinations outline the conditions for which a service is considered to be covered or not covered. Once published by the CMS, an NCD is binding on all Medicare contractors and providers or suppliers. A list of current NCDs available on the CMS website is provided in Table 2-2. Box 2-6 gives a list of Medicare NCDs pertaining to wound care.

The LCD is a formal statement developed through a specifically defined process that (1) defines the service, (2) provides information about when the service is considered reasonable and necessary, (3) outlines any coverage criteria and/or specific documentation requirements, (4) provides specific coding and/or modifier information, and (5) provides references upon which the policy is based. Copies of draft and final LCDs are available with the Medicare Coverage Database (see Table 2-2 for the CMS website).

Generally the LCD is an administrative and education tool used to assist providers and suppliers in completing claims for payments correctly and to guide medical reviewers. These documents specify the clinical circumstances that qualify for select service and the correct coding. The contractor shall ensure that all LCDs are consistent with all regulations and national coverage payment and coding policies. If a contractor develops an LCD, this LCD applies only within the geographic area in which that contractor services.

BOX 2-6 Medicare National Coverage Determinations Pertaining to Wound Dressings and Modalities

- Porcine skin and gradient pressure dressings
- Treatment of decubitus ulcers
- Hyperbaric oxygen therapy for hypoxic wounds and diabetic wounds of the lower extremities
- Electrical stimulation and electromagnetic therapy for treatment of wounds
- Noncontact normothermic wound therapy
- Nonautologous blood-derived products for chronic nonhealing wounds

Clinic personnel who are primarily responsible for ensuring fiscal success in the wound clinic should be aware of any NCD and LCD pertaining to the wound care services provided in the clinic and verify updates frequently throughout the year. A mechanism should be in place for this information to be shared with the practitioners, who are expected to read and know the information. In the event both an NCD and an LCD address the same procedure or service, the NCD will always take precedence. In the absence of an NCD addressing a specific procedure or service, local Medicare contractors may establish an LCD that summarizes medical necessity, criteria for coverage, codes for novel procedures or supplies, and references upon which a temporary coverage policy is based.

CODING AND BILLING FOR SERVICES AND SUPPLIES

Both prospective payment billing (for the hospital outpatient department) and fee-for-services billing (for provider services) require identifying the diagnosis and services provided via the coding methods described in the following section. Table 2-5 lists the types of codes necessary for provider billing.

Medical Condition Codes (ICD-10)

The national coding method designed to enable providers to effectively document the medical condition, symptom, or complaint that forms the basis for rendering a specific service is known as the ICD. The most current is the tenth revision, known as ICD-10. These codes have multiple parts. The new ICD-10 codes have 3 to 7 digits, with the first 3 digits pertaining to category and the following digits addressing etiology, anatomic sites, and severity; these codes now allow for much more specific detail to be captured from the documentation. ICD-10 codes are able to capture initial encounters or subsequent, acute or chronic, right or left, normal healing, or delayed healing (CMS, 2014d).

To provide more detail about the diagnosis and procedures provided, ICD-10 diagnoses codes increased from ~ 14,500 to ~ 70,000. Similarly, procedure codes increased from ~ 4,000 to ~ 72,000. The number of codes available for pressure ulcers increased from 13 to 25 codes incorporating location and stage, and venous ulcer codes increased from 4 to 50.

A template of relevant wound-specific ICD-10 codes with CPT codes should be created to facilitate the efficient and accurate capturing of charges.

Procedure Codes (CPT)

Procedures provided in the clinic are billed using CPT codes that describe the procedures performed, such as debridement, strapping, biopsy, chemical cautery, application of negative pressure, and application of biologic skin substitutes. These codes are derived from a standardized numeric coding system developed and maintained by the AMA.

It is essential to match the CPT codes to the services performed during the wound clinic visit in order to bill both CMS and private health insurance programs. A created list of all services provided should be reviewed with the billing/coding department to find the most closely related code to the service provided, with frequent reviews to incorporate any changes to the frequently used codes. The physician-reported procedure codes and the facility-reported procedure codes should match and be supported via documentation in the medical record.

When no procedure is completed and the patient receives care, the visit is billed using an evaluation and management (E&M) service code. The E&M code is also a CPT code used to obtain the fee for the corresponding services provided. Evaluation and management codes are based on the complexity of the service rendered to the patient. Unlike procedure codes, the E&M code level of the physician service and the clinic service may not always match. The physician will utilize this code to describe how the information about the patient's illness-related condition was gathered and analyzed and the course of treatment devised. The facility will base the E&M level on the acuity-scoring tool.

Evaluation and management codes 99211 through 99215 describe varying levels of complexity for an "established patient" visit. Codes 99201 through 99205 describe varying levels of complexity for the "new patient" visit. Taken collectively, when visit levels are graphed, the majority of visits would be expected to be in the middle level of complexity and present as a bell curve.

Supply Codes (HCPCS)

Medicare does not allow for reimbursement of routine dressing supplies provided during a clinic visit. Under the outpatient prospective payment system (OPPS), the cost of routine dressing supplies considered integral to the visit are bundled into the visit codes and costs of many procedures; thus, supplies are included in the payment for the service (i.e., packaged services). No separate payment is made for packaged services. Although supplies may be marked on the bill to show the cost of the visit, most insurance providers will not reimburse for wound care supplies used during an outpatient clinic visit and tend to follow the Medicare guidelines on packaged codes. For example, routine supplies, anesthesia, recovery room use, and most drugs are considered an integral part of a surgical procedure, so payment for these items is packaged into the APC payment for the surgical procedure (Centers for Medicare & Medicaid Services, Medicare Benefit Policy Manual chapter 15, 2014).

Unless a facility is also a DME provider, the ability for an outpatient clinic to provide and bill supplies for use at home is cost prohibitive. The patient may qualify for home dressing supplies per Medicare guidelines if home care is not providing the wound care. Medicaid may reimburse for supplies if home care is active, and group health plans may offer coverage at times with a possible copayment. Understanding how to assist patients in obtaining home supplies is integral to successful patient outcomes. Patients will need information about suppliers in their area, as well as those that do business by mail (electronic and postal) and by phone. The wound specialist should be aware of additional services provided by suppliers, such as billing insurance directly, offering free delivery, obtaining physician prescriptions for supplies, and making reminder phone calls for reorders. Box 2-7 lists the Medicare guidelines for DME orders.

Knowledge of coverage limits and criteria will assist with the ordering of products that are readily available in the community and reimbursed by Medicare. This valuable information on coverage can be obtained from the CMS website (see Table 2-2).

A complete list of supplies frequently used in the clinic, such as hydrocolloid, alginates, or compression wraps, should be developed and matched to the corresponding HCPCS. These codes describe the dressing supply assigned and maintained by local Medicare contractors. Level II HCPCS provides a method for obtaining reimbursement for products, supplies, or procedures not covered in CPT codes.

In the OPPS, outpatient clinics are encouraged to mark on the bill all supplies used at each visit, regardless of expected reimbursement. The total cost of the visit will help ensure future reimbursement of clinic CPT and E&M services by showing the average cost of visits over time.

National Correct Coding Initiative Edits

The CMS developed the National Correct Coding Initiative (NCCI) to promote correct coding by providers and suppliers. National Correct Coding Initiative edits apply to claims that contain more than one procedure on the same patient, on the same date, and by the same provider or supplier. Payment edits are designed and put in place to prevent payment for noncovered and/or incorrectly coded services. These edits are also used to select targeted claims for review before payment (Vargo, 2008). The NCCI edits can be located online at

---

BOX 2-7 Medicare Guidelines for DME Arrangements for the Home

1. Written orders for DME can be submitted as a photocopy, facsimile image, electronic file, or original "pen-and-ink" order.
2. For dressing supplies that will be provided on a periodic basis, the written order should include:
   - The start date of the order
   - A detailed description listing all options or additional features that will be separately billed or that will require an upgraded code
3. Medical necessity information (diagnosis code) is not considered part of the order, although it may be included within the same document.
4. Someone other than the physician may complete the detailed description of the item or service; however, the treating physician must review the detailed description and personally sign and date the order to indicate agreement.

Example: One 4×4 hydrocolloid dressing changed two times per week for 1 month, or until the ulcer is healed.
DME, Durable medical equipment.

---

the CMS website listed in Table 2-2. Wound debridement codes include the wound debridement, the dressing placed after the debridement, and the assessment and documentation of the wound; therefore, E&M would not be added to the bill along with the debridement because E&M is a necessary part of the debridement and is already captured in the debridement code.

Modifier 59: Distinct Procedural Service

Under certain circumstances, the physician may need to indicate that a procedure or service was distinct or independent from other services performed on the same day. Multiple procedures involving one wound site are almost always billed under one code. The code modifier 59, Distinct Procedural Services, applies when multiple procedures involving multiple anatomic sites or different patient encounters are performed. In this situation, it is appropriate to bill for additional procedures, adding the modifier 59 to indicate that the various procedures involved were at different wound sites even though they were performed on the same day.

Misuse of modifier 59 proceeded the introduction of four new HCPCS modifiers effective January 2015 that are more specific. Modifier 59 remains available; however, the most descriptive modifier should always be used.

The four new HCPCS referred to as X{EPSU} modifiers: (1) XE Separate Encounter—a service that is distinct because it occurred during a separate encounter, (2) XS Separate Structure—a service that is distinct because it was performed on a separate organ/structure, (3) XP Separate Practitioner—a service that is distinct because it was performed by a different practitioner, (4) XU Unusual Non-overlapping Service—the use of a service that is distinct because it does not overlap unusual component of the main service (Schaum, 2014) .

Understanding the edits for bundled services and the code modifier for multiple services is essential to comprehending expected reimbursement.

Status Indicator

Current Procedural Terminology codes are assigned a status indicator (SI). A T indicates that reimbursement will be adjusted downward to a discount for multiple procedures. An S indicates that no downward adjustment will be made, that is, no discount for multiple procedures. This adjustment reflects a situation where multiple services are provided with the understanding that resources (e.g., room setup, registration) for multiple procedures will not be duplicated for each of the additional procedures. For example, if three debridements are done to three different anatomic sites on the same patient on the same day, the first debridement is paid in full and the additional debridements are paid at a discounted rate.

Wavier of Deductible and Coinsurance

Routinely waiving the collection of deductible or coinsurance from a beneficiary constitutes a violation of the law pertaining to false claims and kickbacks. Where a physician/supplier makes a reasonable collection effort for the payment of coinsurance/deductibles, failure to collect payment is not considered a reduction in the charges. To be considered reasonable collection efforts, the efforts must be similar to those made to collect from non-Medicare patients.

This may include actions such as subsequent billings, collection letters, and telephone calls or personal contacts that constitute a genuine, rather than token, collection effort (CMS, 2015b).

CLINICAL CONSULT

S: Please see attached business plan including a list of patients and interventions provided this past year by the Wound, Ostomy and Continence Nurses Society™ after readmissions within 30 days of initial hospital stays.

B: As you are aware, in addition to the financial penalty hospitals with excess Medicare readmissions receive, Medicare Hospital Readmissions Reduction Program (HRRP) provides financial incentive to lower readmission rates.

A: An outpatient wound clinic could help the hospital with the HRRP, save money, and increase patient satisfaction.

R: We respectfully request your review of the attached proposal and permission to begin meeting with key stakeholders to further explore the possibility of providing wound care services across the continuum of care.

CHECKLIST 2-4   Establishing an Outpatient Clinic

✓ Determine services to be provided
✓ Create business plan
✓ Gain support and approval from administration and medical colleagues
✓ Decide clinic structure and staffing needs
  • Management/clinic director
  • Medical director
  • Wound specialist nationally certified as CWCN or CWS
  • Nurse
  • Physical therapist
  • Insurance and billing coders
  • Ancillary staff
✓ Determine clinic location and space needs
✓ Develop compliance program
  • HIPAA privacy rule
  • Centers for Medicare & Medicaid Services
  • The Joint Commission
  • Department of Health Certificate of Need
  • National Patient Safety Goals
  • Billing codes
  • Corporate compliance
✓ Meet with coders and create charge master
  • Establish policies

  • Documentation
  • Photography
  • Frequency of visits
  • Referrals for tests and consults
  • Infection control
  • Treatment orders
  • Obtaining consents
  • Debridement
  • Staffing
  • Staff education
  • Wound care outcomes
  • Insurance authorization
✓ Create patient and staff education and competencies
✓ Determine equipment needs and formulary of supplies
✓ Create/gather teaching documents, including list of durable medical equipment contacts
✓ Establish operations
  • Hours
  • Scheduling
  • Documentation forms
  • Chart storage and retrieval
  • Room cleaning
✓ Develop marketing plan

HIPAA, Health Insurance Portability and Accountability Act of 1996.

SUMMARY

Clinics will obtain reimbursement differently depending on the clinic structure (i.e., hospital-based clinic, freestanding clinic). The freestanding clinic will mirror the physician office in utilizing the physician fee schedule for reimbursement, whereas the hospital outpatient department will utilize the hospital outpatient prospective payment system (HOPPS). In the hospital outpatient clinic, when a physician sees a patient while utilizing the hospital staff, a bill is submitted by the physician (at a lower reimbursement rate than if the patient were seen in his or her private office) and a bill is submitted by the facility (to capture hospital resources of room, staff, and supplies based on the HOPPS). Further differences between clinics consist of determining who the practitioners will be: physician, nonphysician practitioner (reimbursed at 85% of the physician rate when billing physician services), nurse, PT, or a combination, while also considering which multidiscipline programs will be attached to the clinic. Checklist 2-4 summarizes steps to consider for establishing a successful outpatient clinic.

REFERENCES

Armstrong DG, Ayello EA, Capitulo KL, et al: New opportunities to improve pressure ulcer prevention and treatment: implications of the CMS inpatient hospital care present on admission (POA) indicators/hospital-acquired conditions (HAC) policy, *Adv Skin Wound Care* 21(10):469–478, 2008.

Buppert C: *Billing for nurse practitioners services—update 3 2007: guidelines for NPs, physicians, employers, and insurers*, 2007. http://www.medscape.com/viewprogram/7767_pnt. Accessed July 2, 2014.

Calloway SD: *CMS Requirements on order sets, protocols, preprinted orders, and standing orders* Emergency Medicine Patient Safety Foundation, 2012. http://www.tha.org/.../standing%20order%20article%20final%20rev.docx. Accessed June 5, 2014.

Centers for Medicare and Medicaid Services (CMS): Recovery audit program, April 9, 2015a. http://www.cms.gov/NewsroomMediaReleaseDatabase/Fact-Sheets/2008-Fact-Sheets-Items/2008-10-06.html. Accessed June 14, 2015.

Centers for Medicare and Medicaid Services (CMS): *Affordable Care Act update: implementing Medicare cost savings*, 2010. http://www.cms.gov/apps/docs/aca-update-implementing-medicare-costs-savings.pdf. Accessed June 15, 2015.

Centers for Medicare and Medicaid Services (CMS): Prior authorization process for certain durable medical equipment, prosthetic, orthotics, supplies items, May 23, 2014a. http://www.cms.gov/Research-Statistics-Data-and-Systems/Monitoring-Programs/Medicare-FFS-Compliance-Programs/Prior-Authorization-Initiatives/Prior-Authorization-Process-for-Certain-Durable-Medical-Equipment-Prosthetic-Orthotics-Supplies-Items.html Accessed June 15, 2015.

Centers for Medicare and Medicaid Services (CMS): *Reference guide for Medicare physicians and supplier billers*, ed 2, 2006. No.11049 - ICN006209. http://amcp.org/WorkArea/DownloadAsset.aspx?id=11778. Accessed June 15, 2015.

Centers for Medicare and Medicaid Services (CMS): *ICD-10 Basics for Medical Practice*, 2014d. http://www.cms.gov/Medicare/Coding/ICD10/Downloads/ICD10BasicsforPractices20140819.pdf. Accessed March 17, 2015.

Centers for Medicare and Medicaid Services (CMS): *Medicare benefit policy manual: Chapter 15-Covered medical and other health services. Section 60: services and supplies, Rev 202*, Dec 31, 2014c. https://www.cms.gov/Regulations-and-Guidance/Guidance/Transmittals/downloads/bp102c15.pdf. Accessed June 15, 2015.

Centers for Medicare and Medicaid Services (CMS): *Medicare benefit policy. Update of the Hospital Outpatient Prospective Payment System (OPPS), January 16, 2009. (Publication no. 100-02), CMS Manual System*, Jan 16, 2009. http://www.cms.hhs.gov/transmittals/downloads/R101BP.pdf. Accessed, June 14, 2015.

Centers for Medicare and Medicaid Services (CMS): *Supervision file – Hospital outpatient therapeutic services*, Nov 27, 2012. https://www.cms.gov/Medicare/Medicare-Fee-for-Service-Payment/HospitalOutpatientPPS/Downloads/CY2013-OPPS-General-Supervision.pdf. Accessed June 15, 2015.

Centers for Medicare and Medicaid Services (CMS): *Lower costs, better care: reforming our health care delivery system* (Fact sheet), Jan 30, 2014b. http://www.cms.gov/Newsroom/MediaReleaseDatabase/fact-sheets/2014-fact-sheets-items/2014-01-30-03.html. Accessed June 15, 2015

Centers for Medicare and Medicaid Services (CMS): *Medicare claims processing manual. Chapter 23 - Fee schedule administration and coding requirements. Section 80.8.1- Waiver of deductible and coinsurance, Rev 3190* , Feb 6, 2015b. http://www.cms.hhs.gov/manuals/downloads/clm104c23.pdf. Accessed March 17, 2015

Fife C: The debridement dilemma, *Todays Wound Clin* 1(2):24–27, Fall 2007.

Fife C, Weir D: Getting started, *Todays Wound Clin* 1(1):22–26, Spring 2007.

Fusaro ME, Brotman D, Laboda B, et al: *Principles to initiate and maintain a successful wound care center* (APWCA white paper, version 1.1), 2008. http://www.apwca.org/Resources/Documents/APWCA-Wound-Cntr-Priniciples-061508%5B1%5D.pdf. Accessed July 2, 2014.

Hess CT: Developing a wound care compliance program (part 1), *Adv Skin Wound Care* 21(10):496, 2008.

Jacobs AM, Tomczak R: Evaluation of Bensal HP for the treatment of diabetic foot ulcers, *Adv Skin Wound Care* 21:461–465, 2008.

Medicare Program: Prior Authorization Process for Certain Durable Medical Equipment, Prosthetic, Orthotics, and Supplies (DMEOPS) Items (Proposed rule), *Federal Register* 19:30511–30531, May 28, 2014. https://federalregister.gov/a/2014-12245. Accessed June 16, 2014.

Morrison CA: If you build it, they will come: marketing your wound clinic to its fullest potential, *Todays Wound Clin* 1(1):32–33, Spring 2007.

Office of Inspector General (OIG): *Medicare payments for surgical debridement services in 2004* (Report no. OEI-02-05-00390), May 2007.

Schaum K: Begin preparing for 2015 coding changes: use 4 new modifiers instead of modifier 59, *Adv Skin Wound Care* 27(11):488–489, 2014.

Sullivan V: Educating staff—what wound clinic clinicians need to know, *Todays Wound Clin* 1(1):14–17, Spring 2007.

Treadwell T: How are we doing? Evaluating your wound clinic operations, *Todays Wound Clin* :29–31, Spring 2007.

U.S. Department Health and Human Services: *Health information privacy*, 2009. http://hhs.gov/ocr/privacy/hipaa/understanding/index.html. Accessed July 2, 2014.

Vargo D: Make sense of wound care billing: turn your cents into reimbursement dollars, *J Wound Ostomy Continence Nurs* 35(2):186–198, 2008.

Vargo D: Direct supervision requirements and incident to services: a primer for the WOC nurse, *J Wound Ostomy Continence Nurs* 37(2):148–151, 2009.

Wound, Ostomy and Continence Nurses Society™ (WOCN®): *Educational essentials*, ed 5, *Professional practice manual (2011) Business plan template workbook*, Mount Laurel, NJ, 2013, WOCN®.

3

Anatomy and Physiology of Skin and Soft Tissue

Annette B. Wysocki

OBJECTIVES

1. Describe the mechanisms by which the skin is able to provide its six major functions.
2. Describe the structures, function, and cellular composition of the skin layers, including layers within the dermis and epidermis.
3. Explain the relationship between skin pigmentation and protection against ultraviolet radiation.
4. Compare and contrast the structural and cellular development of the skin in the fetus, premature infant (between

23 and 32 weeks' gestation), full-term neonate, adolescent, and adult.
5. Describe at least two effects on the skin of the following: hydration, sun, nutrition, soaps, and medications.
6. Compare and contrast the structure and function of dark and lightly pigmented skin.

The skin is the one organ of the body that is constantly exposed to a changing environment. Maintaining its integrity is a complex process, and without appropriate treatment, assaults from surgical incisions, injuries, or burns can lead to life-threatening consequences.

The skin of the average adult covers approximately 3000 in^2, or an area almost equivalent to 2 m^2. From birth to maturity the skin covering will undergo a sevenfold expansion. It weighs about 6 lb (or up to 15% of total adult body weight), is the largest organ of the body, and receives one third of the body's circulating blood volume. The skin forms a protective barrier against the external environment while maintaining a homeostatic internal environment. Epidermal appendages (nails, hair follicles, sweat or sebaceous glands) that are lined with epidermal cells are also present in the skin. During healing of partial-thickness wounds, these epidermal cells migrate to resurface the wound. This organ is capable of self-regeneration and can withstand limited mechanical and chemical assaults. The skin varies in thickness from 0.5 mm in the tympanic membrane to 6 mm in the soles of the feet and the palms of the hands. Variations are attributable to differences in the thickness of the skin layers covering underlying organs, bones, muscle, and cartilage. Diseases of the skin can result from genetic causes, so-called genodermatoses, infection, immune dysfunction, and trauma. Skin diseases can involve some or all skin layers and, in the case of various skin cancers, metastasize to other organs and/or tissues.

Population projections indicate that changing demographics will occur over the next decades and that by 2043, a majority of the U.S. population will be composed of people with skin of color, a "majority-minority" population. By 2060 the population is expected to be 31% Hispanic, 14.7% African American, 8.2% Asian, 1.5% American Indian and Native Alaskan, and 0.3% Native Hawaiian and other Pacific Islanders (U.S. Census Bureau, 2012). Unique characteristics of darker versus lighter pigmented skin (Box 3-1) are described throughout the chapter.

SKIN LAYERS

Human skin is divided into two primary layers: epidermis (outermost layer) and dermis (innermost layer) (Figure 3-1). These two layers are separated by a structure called the basement membrane. Beneath the dermis is a layer of loose connective tissue called the hypodermis, or subcutis.

Epidermis

The epidermis, the outermost skin layer, is avascular and derived from embryonic ectoderm. This layer is relatively uniform in thickness over the body, between 75 and 150 μm, except on the soles and palms, where thickness is between 0.4 and 0.6 mm. The epidermal layer is constantly being renewed, with turnover time ranging from 26 to 42 days. Complete epidermal renewal occurs over a period lasting between 45 and 75 days, or about every 2 months (Odland,

BOX 3-1 Unique Characteristics of Darker Pigmented Skin

- Higher lipid content in stratum corneum
- Increased junctional integrity
- Stratum corneum contains melanosomes (light skin has no melanosomes in stratum corneum)
- Inflammatory reactions (i.e., reddened areas) can be masked
- Inflammation may appear violet-black or black
- Vitiligo and keloids more common
- More blood vessels and dilated lymph channels
- Less abundant distribution of elastic fibers
- Greater protection against photoaging or dermatoheliosis due to no obvious signs of damage to elastic fibers upon exposure to sunlight
- Increase in hair breakage and higher prevalence of traumatic alopecia
- More prone to pseudofolliculitis due to spiral configuration and curvature of hair follicles
- Better protection against skin cancer due to increased synthesis, amount, distribution of melanin
- Can mask precancerous and cancerous tumors due to increased melanin content
- Reduced level of vitamin D

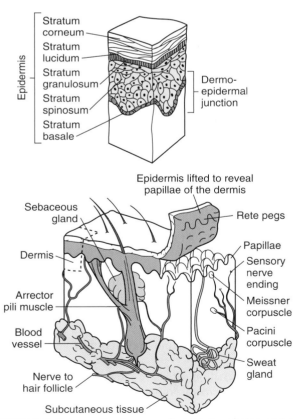

FIGURE 3-1 Schematic diagram of anatomy of skin and subcutaneous tissue. (From Hooper BJ, Goldman MP: *Primary dermatologic care*, St. Louis, MO, 1999, Mosby.)

1991). The epidermal layer is composed of stratified squamous epithelial cells, or keratinocytes, and is divided into five layers (see Figure 3-1). These layers, beginning from the outermost to the innermost, are the stratum corneum, stratum lucidum, stratum granulosum, stratum spinosum, and stratum basale (stratum germinativum or, simply, the basal layer).

Stratum Corneum. The stratum corneum, or horny layer, is the top layer and is composed of dead keratinized cells. These squames, or corneocytes, are the cells that are abraded by the daily mechanical and chemical trauma of hand washing, scratching, bathing, exercising, and changing of clothes. The stratum corneum is composed of layers of thin, stacked, pancake-appearing, anucleate cells. Approximately 80% of these cells are filled with keratin, a tough, fibrous, insoluble protein; hence, they are called keratinocytes. Keratinocytes are initially formed in the basal layer and undergo the process of differentiation. The normal stratum corneum is composed of completely differentiated keratinocytes. Keratin is resistant to changes in temperature and pH and to chemical digestion by trypsin and pepsin. This same protein is found in hair and nails; in these structures, keratin is referred to as "hard" keratin compared with the "soft" keratin of the skin (Jacob et al, 1982; Solomons, 1983). Stratum corneum thickness varies with age, gender, and disease. In the deeper layer of the stratum corneum, the stratum compactum, the keratin is more densely packed and the cells have a diminished capacity to bind water (Haake, Scott, and Holbrook, 2001). In the upper layer, the stratum dysjunctum, cells are partly shed as a result of proteolytic degradation of the desmosomes.

The stratum corneum is enriched with a lipid matrix that enhances the barrier properties of the skin. This lipid-rich matrix is composed of about 50% ceramides, 25% cholesterol, and 15% free fatty acids and has a unique lamellar organization (the mortar) seen between corneocytes (the bricks) that is first detected in the upper layer of the stratum spinosum where their assembly begins (Feingold and Elias, 2014). The composition of the lipid-rich matrix changes with aging. Although not universally agreed upon, across the skin color spectrum, differences in the stratum corneum exist as summarized by Taylor (2002). At least two studies (LaRuche and Cesarini, 1992; Rienertson and Wheatley, 1959) report that black stratum corneum has a higher lipid content and this may in part contribute to the conflicting results regarding strateum corneum thickness. The stratum corneum in darkly pigmented skin has been reported to have increased junctional integrity as evidenced by the increased number of tape strippings required to remove the stratum corneum. Whether the stratum corneum is thicker in darkly pigmented skin is unclear (Taylor, 2002).

Stratum Lucidum. The stratum lucidum is directly below the stratum corneum. This layer is found in areas where the epidermis is thicker, such as the palms of the hands and the soles of the feet, but it is absent from thinner skin, such as the eyelids. This layer can be one to five cells thick and is transparent. Cell boundaries often are difficult to identify in histologic sections under a light microscope. The stratum lucidum is a transitional layer where active lysosomal enzymes degrade the nucleus and cellular organelles before they are moved into the stratum corneum (Jacob et al, 1982; Wysocki, 1995).

Stratum Granulosum. The stratum granulosum, or granular layer, is beneath the stratum lucidum when the stratum lucidum is present; otherwise, the stratum granulosum lies beneath the stratum corneum. This layer is one to five cells thick and is so named because of the granules present in the keratinocytes of this layer. The cells of the stratum granulosum have not yet been compressed into a flattened layer and are diamond shaped. The structures contained in these cells are keratohyalin granules, which become intensely stained with the appropriate acid and basic dyes. The proteins contained in these granules (profilaggrin, intermediate keratin filaments, and loricrin) help to organize the keratin filaments in the intracellular space. Profillaggrin is cleaved to form filaggrin, which is further degraded to form urocanic acid and pyrrolidone carboxylic acid. Both urocanic acid and pyrrolidone carboxylic acid provide additional hydration to the stratum corneum and limited filtering against ultraviolet radiation (UVR). The major component of the cornified envelope is loricrin, which is cross-linked to other protein components (involucrin, cystatin A, small proline-rich proteins [SPRR1, SPRR2], elafin, envoplakin) that together form up to 70% of the molecular mass of the cells in this layer. Cells in this layer still have active nuclei (Millington and Wilkinson, 1983; Wheater et al, 1987).

Stratum Spinosum. The stratum spinosum is below the stratum granulosum. This layer often is described as the prickly layer because cytoplasmic structures in these cells take on this morphology. Generally the cells of this layer are polyhedral. A prominent feature of the prickle layer is the desmosome, a type of cell–cell junction. The desmosomes provide adhesion between cells and resistance to mechanical forces. Cells in this layer begin to synthesize involucrin, a soluble precursor of the cornified envelopes (Millington and Wilkinson, 1983). The spinous cells contain large bundles of newly synthesized keratin filaments (K1/K10) in addition to K5/K14 still present from the basal layer (Haake et al, 2001). The identification of various classes of desmosomal proteins (plakoglobin, desmoplakin, plakophilins) and transmembrane glycoproteins (desmogleins, desmocollins) has led to the identification of their roles in various epidermal pathologies, such as bullous impetigo, pemphigus vulgaris, and other genodermatoses.

Stratum Basale or Stratum Germinativum. The stratum basale, or stratum germinativum, is the innermost epidermal layer. It often is referred to simply as the basal layer (see Figure 3-1). It is a single layer of mitotically active cells called basal keratinocytes, or basal cells. These active cells respond to several factors, such as extracellular matrix, growth factors, hormones, and vitamins. Skin metabolism is mediated by glucose. Glucose utilization in the skin is comparable to that in muscle. Glucose leaving the circulation crosses the basement membrane and forms a concentration gradient that decreases as the glucose moves to the upper layers of the epidermis.

Once cells leave the basal layer they begin an upward migration, which can take 2 to 3 weeks. A cell takes approximately 14 days to move to the stratum corneum and another 14 days to move through the stratum corneum and desquamate (Haake, Scott, and Holbrook, 2001). After leaving the basal layer, the cells begin the process of differentiation. All layers of the epidermis consist of peaks and valleys, but this arrangement is more dramatic in the basal layer such that these protrusions are partly responsible for anchoring the epidermis, thus providing structural integrity. These epidermal protrusions of the basal layer point downward into the dermis and are called rete ridges, or rete pegs. The basal layer is the primary location of mitotically active cells of the epidermis and has been noted to have increased proliferative capacity compared with cells at the top of the ridges (Briggaman, 1982).

Epidermal stem cells compose about 10% of the basal cell population. These stem cells have a slow cell cycle. When labeled with a radiolabeled DNA precursor, epidermal stem cells retain the label for long periods; thus they are identified as label-retaining cells (Bickenbach, 1981). Once cell division occurs, daughter cells that will undergo differentiation as they move toward the stratum corneum are called transient amplifying cells. These transient amplifying cells make up approximately 50% of the basal keratinocyte population (Lavker and Sun, 2000). Transient amplifying cells progress to become postmitotic cells that then terminally differentiate. A portion of the stem cell population is found in the epidermal crypts of the rete pegs and in the bulge region of hair follicles. Dividing cells go through the cell cycle, and the G_1 phase is shortened in states such as wound healing. The normal keratinocyte cell cycle time is 300 hours, but may be as short as 36 hours when psoriasis is present. These stem cell compartments and the transient amplifying cells both are capable of limited or continuing cell division and thus are the cells most likely to reside long enough in the skin to undergo genetic modifications that lead to the development of skin cancers. The use of stem cells alone and in combination with tissue-engineering approaches is an area of active research and development in wound care (Griffith and Naughton, 2002).

Tissue oxygenation data have shown that the oxygen pressure in the epidermis is low compared with other tissue, at around 0.2% to 8%, compared with 10% in the dermis. These low partial pressures result in a mildly hypoxic microenvironment with a resulting expression of hypoxia inducible factor-1α (HIF-1α). HIF-1α targets a number of genes important for skin homeostasis and repair, including genes that encode proteins for cell growth and apoptosis, cell adhesion and migration, angiogenesis, melanogenesis, DNA repair, and extracellular matrix synthesis and repair and mediates glucose uptake for cell metabolism (Rezvani et al, 2011).

Melanocytes, the cells responsible for skin pigmentation as a result of melanin synthesis, also are distributed in the basal layer. Melanocytes are dendritic cells that arise from melanoblasts, which derive from the neural crest. During development, they migrate to other locations, including the bulge region of hair follicles, the choroid of the eye, the heart, and the brain (Goding, 2007). Melanocytes are also required for hearing; genetic mutations resulting in a loss of melanocytes are a major cause of deafness (Steel and Barkway, 1989). Melanin is packaged inside the cell into melanosomes, which are transported via the cytoskeletal network of microfilaments and microtubules to the dendritic processes of the melanocyte, where they are then transferred to keratinocytes. Incorporation into the keratinocytes is thought to occur via one or more of the following processes: release and endocytosis, engulfment, active transport, or passage through channels or pores between the melanocyte and neighboring keratinocytes (Boissy, 2003). Melanocytes can be detected by 50 days' gestation in fetal development (Holbrook, 1998). Under normal conditions, melanocytes rarely divide. In normal skin, the number of melanocytes present is nearly the same, regardless of skin color. There is approximately one melanocyte for every 36 basal cells. Dendritic melanocyte structures are responsible for the transfer of pigment to a large number of keratinocytes. The primary difference between light- and dark-skinned individuals is the size, number, and distribution of melanosomes, the structures containing the melanin pigment, and the activity of the melanocytes. Carotene or carotenoids are responsible for imparting the yellow hue to the skin of some individuals (Jacob et al, 1982; Sams, 1990; Solomons, 1983).

Melanin pigment is a complex polymer that is synthesized from tyrosine by activity of the tyrosinase gene pathway. Melanin is difficult to study because it is relatively insoluble (Boissy, 2003). The two primary types of melanin are brown/black eumelanin and red/yellow pheomelanin (Lin and Fisher, 2007). Pheomelanin is more photolabile, and damage leads to release of oxygen radicals such as hydrogen peroxide, superoxide, and hydroxyl radicals, resulting in oxidative stress and DNA damage (Lin and Fisher, 2007). Constitutive synthesis, or the synthesis that occurs at basal levels, results primarily from genetic regulation. Facultative synthesis is the additional up-regulation or down-regulation of melanin synthesis in response to UVR, hormones, cytokines, immune regulation, chemical exposure, or other agents (Boissy, 2003). Interestingly, once delivered to the keratinocytes, melanosomes are preferentially, although not exclusively, clustered around the apical side of the nucleus, where they can more effectively provide protection from UVR to prevent DNA damage leading to mutations (Boissy, 2003). In addition to its photoprotective effect, melanin is thought to act as a sink for

highly reactive oxygen species that can also lead to DNA damage (Goding, 2007). Pathologies associated with melanocytes or pigmentation are melanoma, dyschromias such as vitiligo and melasma, xeroderma pigmentosa, and albinism.

As a result of genetics, genetic recombination, and selective environmental pressures (e.g., UVR intensity and exposure, age, hormonal influences), skin pigmentation demonstrates considerable variation across the human population. Presently more than 150 genes have been identified that either directly or indirectly affect skin color (Yamaguchi and Hearing, 2009). Key proteins and receptors identified with the synthesis and transport of melanin or melanosomes include melanocyte-stimulating hormone, melanocortin-1 receptor (MC1R), keratinocyte growth factor, and protease-activated receptor-2. The red hair/light skin phenotype is associated with mutations found in the residues of MC1R, which lead to increased risk for skin cancer (Miyamura et al, 2006). Thus the skin color spectrum ranges from dense black, with the highest level and distribution of melanosomes, to various shades of brown to white and finally to albino, or the complete absence of pigment (but not an absence of melanocytes). In general, Caucasian and Asian skin has smaller melanosomes that form small clusters or aggregates, whereas dense African skin has larger melanosomes that are distributed primarily as single units (Montagna et al, 1993; Szabo et al, 1969; Szabo et al, 1972). In darkly pigmented skin, despite the hydrolytic degradation that occurs with keratinocyte differentiation, some melanosomes can still be seen in the stratum corneum, whereas in light skin no melanosomes are seen in the stratum corneum (Boissy, 2003). Various shades of brown skin occur across African, African American, Hispanic, Asian, Caucasian, and Native American peoples; these shades are influenced by the number, size, and distribution of melanosomes. The range of variation can even occur in the same individual, depending on skin location and sun exposure (Szabo, 1954). In general, the density of melanocytes is slightly higher in skin covering the upper dorsal surfaces compared with skin on the lower dorsal surfaces, and the amount of melanin present in the skin correlates well with visible skin pigmentation seen on physical examination (Miyamura et al, 2006).

Intensely pigmented skin can mask the detection of skin inflammatory reactions, which is seen as reddened areas in light-skinned individuals that may appear in response to conditions such as contact dermatitis, pressure, or folliculitis. Inflammation may appear as darker areas in black skin, violet-black in intensely black skin, or black in brown skin. Other signs of inflammation may include the detection of heat or warmth to touch or induration detected as skin tightening or hardening over areas where there is skin damage. Dermatologic disorders accompanied by inflammation can result in postinflammatory hypopigmentation or hyperpigmentation that can be especially distressing to individuals with more darkly pigmented skin in which the color contrast can be dramatically evident. Other dermatologic disorders more commonly associated with darkly pigmented skin include vitiligo and keloids. Keloids occur 3 to 18 times more frequently in darkly pigmented skin, and the incidence has been reported as between 4.5% and 16% in Chinese, Hispanic, and African American individuals (Oluwasanmi, 1974; Robles and Berg, 2007; Taylor, 2002; Taylor, 2003).

Universal agreement concerning comparative differences, if any, across the skin color spectrum for transepidermal water loss (TEWL), strateum corneum structure, epidermal thickness, and sweat and sebaceous gland number or distribution is fraught with numerous points of criticism that include low numbers of subjects, variation in age, gender, circadian rhythms, use of emollients, relative temperature and humidity, geographic location, location of skin sample, sun-exposed versus sun-protected areas, nutrition, validity and reliability of instrumentation, and accurate indexing to skin color (McDonald, 1988; Taylor, 2002). It has been noted that there are 31 climate zones around the globe subject to the adaptation, lifestyle, and conditions of people with various customs and resources, and climate can influence birth weight, body shape, and cranial morphology (Lambert et al, 2008). Thus, definitive studies of skin biology across the range of the skin color spectrum relative to age and gender await more exhaustive and comprehensive research studies and may require more precise instrumentation for some measures.

Basement Membrane Zone

The basement membrane zone (BMZ), or dermal–epidermal junction, is the area that separates the epidermis from the dermis. Closer examination of the BMZ in the past decade has revealed the BMZ to be more complex than previously believed. Basal keratinocytes use hemidesmosomes to structurally and functionally attach to the BMZ. The BMZ is subdivided into two distinct zones: the lamina lucida and the lamina densa. The lamina lucida is so named because it is an electron-translucent zone compared with the electron-dense zone of the lamina densa. The major proteins found in the BMZ are fibronectin, an adhesive glycoprotein; laminin, a glycoprotein; type IV collagen, a non–fiber-forming collagen; and heparin sulfate proteoglycan, a glycosaminoglycan. A lesser amount of type VII collagen has also been detected. The BMZ anchors the epidermis to the dermis and is the layer that is affected in blister formation associated with dermatologic diseases, second-degree burns, full-thickness wounds, and mechanical trauma. During wound healing the BMZ is disrupted and must be reformed (Sams, 1990).

Dermis

The dermis, or corium, is the thickest tissue layer of the skin. Compared with the cellular epidermal layer, the dermis is sparsely populated (primarily by fibroblast cells) and is vascularized and innervated. The dermal layer is derived from the middle embryonic germ layer, the mesoderm. Dermal thickness ranges from 2 to 4 mm, but on average is 2 mm. Variations in dermal thickness account for differences in total skin thickness that have been measured throughout the body.

The dermis of the back is thicker than the dermis covering the scalp, forehead, abdomen, thigh, wrist, and palm.

The dermal vasculature consists of a network of papillary loops, supported by a deep horizontal plexus. The vasculature functions to provide nutritional support, immune surveillance, wound healing, thermal regulation, hemostasis, and the inflammatory response. Formation of the vascular system involves vasculogenesis and angiogenesis. Vasculogenesis is the process that occurs de novo during embryonic development and is mediated by angioblasts derived from the mesoderm. Angiogenesis is the process whereby new vessels are formed from preexisting vessels. It is involved in wound healing, tumor growth and metastasis, hemangiomas, telangiectasia, psoriasis, and scleroderma. Vascular endothelial growth factor (VEGF), or vascular permeability factor, is secreted by keratinocytes in response to hypoxia. It is increased in wound healing and is responsible for stimulating angiogenesis. Other factors that stimulate angiogenesis include acidic and basic fibroblast growth factor, interleukin-8, platelet-derived endothelial growth factor, placental growth factor, transforming growth factor-α and transforming growth factor-β, oncostatin M, angiogenin, and heparin-binding epidermal growth factor. Inhibitors of angiogenesis include angiostatin, thrombospondin, endostatin, interferon-γ, interleukin-12, and platelet factor-4.

The major proteins found in the dermis are collagen and elastin. The other category of proteins found occupying the space between collagen and elastin fibers is referred to as the ground substance. The ground substance in black skin is distinctly more abundant in both the papillary and reticular layers than in white skin (Montagna and Carlisle, 1991). This category of proteins is largely composed of proteoglycans and glycosaminoglycans. Included in this category of proteins are chondroitin sulfates and dermatan sulfate (versican, decorin, biglycan), heparan and heparan sulfate proteoglycans (syndecan, perlecan), and chondroitin-6 sulfate proteoglycans. Although these proteins account for only approximately 0.2% of the dry weight of the dermis, these large molecules are capable of binding up to 1000 times their volume. Thus, proteoglycans and glycosaminoglycans play a role in regulating the water-binding capacity of the dermis, which can determine dermal volume and compressibility. Hyaluronan is also found in the dermis and in higher abundance in fetal skin, where it forms a watery, less stable matrix that allows greater cell movement; it also is a critical factor in scarless healing (Longaker, Adzick, et al, 1990). Hyaluronan can bind growth factors and provide cellular linkages with other matrix materials that together function to regulate cell migration, adhesion, proliferation, differentiation, morphogenesis, and tissue repair (Haake and Holbrook, 1999). Other glycoproteins found in the dermis include fibronectin, thrombospondin, laminin, vitronectin, and tenascin. These glycoproteins are synthesized and secreted by fibroblasts in the dermis.

Data indicate that skin fibroblasts from different anatomic locations contain different transcriptional patterns that can indicate position and can be differentiated from fibroblasts in other locations using microarray analysis (Chang et al, 2002). Fibroblasts present in the dermis range in size and number. It has been reported that fibroblasts in black facial skin were larger, occurred in greater numbers, and were more likely to be binucleated or multinucleated compared with white skin. Overall, the dermis in black skin was thick and compact compared with thinner and less compact in white skin (Montagna and Carlisle, 1991). In this same study, collagen fiber bundles were observed to be smaller, more tightly packed and were oriented parallel to the epidermis in black skin, and had more fiber fragments. Somewhat in contrast, white skin was noted to have larger collagen fiber bundles with some degraded collagen fragments, which may have resulted from sun exposure, but had greater variability in the number of fibroblasts. No differences in mast cells were observed. However, black skin did have more binucleated and multinucleated macrophages in the papillary dermis, and the accompanying melanophages in black skin contained melanosomes both singly and in complexes, whereas in white skin the melanophages were almost exclusively in complexes (Montagna and Carlisle, 1991). Again, these findings should be viewed with caution given the lack of comprehensive studies across the skin color spectrum. The dermis is a matrix that supports the epidermis. It can be divided into two areas: papillary dermis and reticular dermis (see Figure 3-1). The papillary and reticular layers appear more distinct in white skin and less distinct in black skin (Montagna and Carlisle, 1991).

Papillary Dermis. The papillary dermis lies immediately below the BMZ and forms interdigitating structures with the rete ridges of the epidermis called dermal papillae. The dermal papillae contain papillary loops (Figure 3-2), which supply the necessary oxygen and nutrients to the overlying epidermis via the BMZ. The collagen fibers contained in the papillary dermis are much smaller in diameter and form smaller, wavy, cablelike structures compared with the reticular dermis. This portion of the dermis also contains small elastic fibers and has a greater proportion of ground substance than the reticular dermis. The superficial subepidermis in darkly pigmented skin contains more numerous blood vessels, along with many more dilated lymph channels (Montagna and Carlisle, 1991). The papillary dermis also contains lymphatic vessels that play a role in controlling interstitial fluid pressure by resorption of fluid and assist in clearing the tissues of cells, lipids, bacteria, proteins, and other degraded substances. The papillary lymph vessels drain into the horizontal plexus of larger lymph vessels located in the deep subpapillary venous plexus. This system is further connected to the lymph system in the reticular dermis. Fluid flow through this system is partially controlled through arterial pulsations, muscle contractions, and body movement. Renewed interest in the skin lymphatic system has resulted from the identification of markers such as VEGF-C, VEGFR-3, and lymphatic vessel endothelial receptor-1 (LYVE-1) and the findings of the role of these lymphatic vessels in tumor promotion (Chu, 2008).

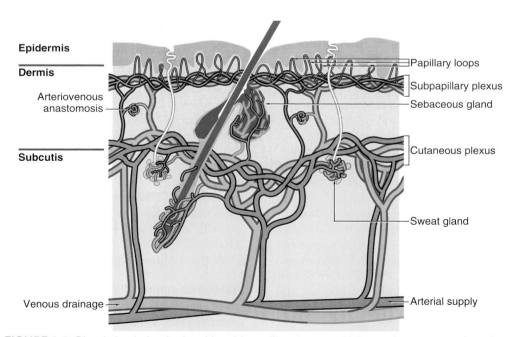

FIGURE 3-2 Blood circulation in the skin with papillary loops, which supply oxygen and nutrients to the epidermis, and dermal cutaneous plexuses, which arise from the deeper blood supply located in the hypodermis. (From Young B, O'Dowd G, Woodford P: *Wheater's functional histology: a text and colour atlas*, ed 5, Edinburgh, 2006, Churchill Livingstone.)

Reticular Dermis. The reticular dermis (the area below the papillary dermis) forms the base of the dermis. The collagen fibers in the reticular dermis are thicker in diameter and form larger cablelike structures than in the papillary dermis. There is no clear separation of papillary and reticular dermis because the collagen fibers change in size gradually between the two layers. Thicker elastic fibers are found in the reticular dermis, but substantially less ground substance is present. A complex of cutaneous blood vessels is found in this part of the dermis.

Dermal Proteins. Collagen, the protein that gives the skin its tensile strength, is the major structural protein found in the dermis and accounts for 25% of the skin's total weight (Stryer, 1995). The primary constituents of collagen are proline, glycine, hydroxyproline, and hydroxylysine. Collagen is secreted by dermal fibroblasts as tropocollagen, which undergoes additional extracellular processing so that mature collagen fibers are formed. Normal human dermis is primarily composed of type I collagen, a fiber-forming collagen. Type I collagen represents 77% to 85% of the collagen present; type III collagen, also a fiber-forming collagen, represents the remaining 15% to 23% (Gay and Miller, 1978; Wysocki et al, 2005). Very small amounts of type V collagen (less than 5%) and type VI collagen also are present.

Elastin, another protein found in the dermis, provides the skin's elastic recoil, a feature that prevents the skin from being permanently reshaped. It is a fiber-forming protein, like collagen. Elastin has a high amount of proline and glycine. However, unlike collagen, elastin lacks large amounts of hydroxyproline. Elastin fibers form structures, similar to coils, that allow this protein to be stretched and, when released, to return to its inherent configuration. Elastin accounts for less than 2% of the skin's dry weight (Millington and Wilkinson, 1983; Sams, 1990; Wysocki, 1995). Elastin is distributed with collagen but in smaller amounts. Large concentrations of elastin are found in blood vessels (especially the aortic arch near the heart) and lymphatic vessels. The distribution of elastic fibers ranges from less abundant in darkly pigmented skin to more abundant in light skin. Upon exposure to sunlight, elastic fibers in darkly pigmented skin show no obvious signs of damage, whereas elastic fibers in light skin show obvious signs of elastosis (Montagna et al, 1993). The lower distribution of elastic fibers in darkly pigmented skin also extends to the anchorage of hair follicles, leading to an increase in hair breakage and a higher prevalence of traumatic alopecia in both men and women (Taylor, 2002). Furthermore, the curvature of hair follicles and the spiral configuration seen in Africans and African Americans lead to pseudofolliculitis, especially in men who shave.

Other cells found in the dermis are mast cells, macrophages, and lymphocytes. All of these cells are involved with immune surveillance of the skin, often referred to as the skin immune system. The dermis also contains dermal appendages that include hair follicles, sebaceous glands, and eccrine and apocrine sweat glands.

Hypodermis

Hypodermis, or superficial fascia, forms a subcutaneous layer below the dermis. It is an adipose layer containing a subdermal plexus of blood vessels giving rise to the cutaneous plexus in the dermis, which in turn gives rise to the papillary plexus and loops of the papillary dermis (see Figure 3-2). The hypodermis attaches the dermis to underlying structures. This layer provides insulation for the body, a ready reserve of energy, and additional cushioning; it also adds to the mobility of the skin over underlying structures (Haake and Holbrook, 1999). Growing hair follicles and apocrine and eccrine sweat glands can extend into this layer. The hypodermis is largely absent in certain pathologic disease states, such as Werner syndrome and scleroderma. Adipocytes form the primary cells in this tissue layer, and their activity is regulated by leptin.

SKIN FUNCTIONS

The skin provides several functions: protection, immunity, thermoregulation, sensation, metabolism, and communication (Jacob et al, 1982; Millington and Wilkinson, 1983; Woodburne and Burkel, 1988).

Protection

The skin protects the body against aqueous, chemical, and mechanical assaults; bacterial and viral pathogens; and UVR. It also prevents excessive loss of fluids and electrolytes in order to maintain the homeostatic environment. The effectiveness of the skin in preventing excessive fluid loss can be seen in patients with burns. Patients with burns involving 30% of their body can lose up to 4.1 L of fluid compared with 710 ml for normal adults (Rudowski, 1976). The skin maintains the internal milieu, and a progressive decrease in water content across the epidermal layers helps to prevent excessive transepidermal water loss under basal conditions. Water constitutes 65% to 70% of the basal layer, and decreases to 40% in the granular layer and 15% in the stratum corneum (Warner et al, 1988). The skin's barrier function is so effective that percutaneous drug delivery is limited except in premature babies and in newborns. In general, compounds are restricted to those with a molecular mass of 500 daltons or less with a daily dose of 10 mg or less. Protection against mechanical assaults is mainly provided by the tough fibroelastic tissue of the dermis, collagen, and elastin.

Protection against Pathogens. Protection against aqueous, chemical, bacterial, and viral pathogens is provided by the stratum corneum, secretions from the sebaceous glands, and the skin immune system. Epithelial cells have pattern recognition receptors as part of the skin immune system that are capable of recognizing microbes via their cell wall components, nucleic acids, and flagella and have the ability to recruit immune cells. The primary line of defense against all of these agents is an intact stratum corneum (Roth and James, 1988). The insoluble protein keratin, found in the horny layer, provides good resistance. In addition, the constant shedding of squames from the stratum corneum prevents the entrenchment of microorganisms.

Sebum, a lipid-rich, oily substance secreted by the sebaceous glands onto the skin surface, usually via hair follicles and shafts, provides an acidic coating with a pH ranging from 4 to 6.8 (Spince and Mason, 1987) and a mean pH of 5.5 (Roth and James, 1988; Wysocki et al, 2005). Salt and electrolytes from eccrine sweat provide additional acidification. This acidity, together with natural antibacterial substances found in sebum, retards the growth of microorganisms. These glands are stimulated by sex hormones (androgens) and become very active during adolescence. Sebum, along with keratin, provides resistance to aqueous and chemical solutions. When sebaceous glands occur in association with hair follicles, they are called a pilosebaceous unit. Sebaceous glands are not found on palms or soles; they occur in areas that lack hair, such as lips. These glands are largest when they are located on the face and when associated with hair follicles. Sebaceous glands may increase in size by 100 to 150 times as sebum accumulates. Maximum secretion occurs in persons in their late teens to early twenties. Rates of secretion are higher in men and decline 32% per decade in females compared with 23% per decade in males.

Resistance to pathogenic microorganisms is also provided by normal skin flora through bacterial interference (Noble, 2004; Weinberg and Swartz, 1987). Conceptually, the two categories of skin flora are (1) resident (bacteria normally found on a person) and (2) transient (bacteria not normally found on a person and usually shed by daily hygienic practices, such as bathing and hand washing). Resident bacteria are found on exposed skin; moist areas such as the axillae, perineum, and toe webs; and covered skin. Bacterial microcolonies are found in hair follicles and at the edges of squames as halos in the upper loose surface layers. It has been estimated that in healthy skin a 1-cm^2 area is covered with 1 million or more bacteria, including those in appendages such as the hair follicle and sebaceous glands (Grice et al, 2008). The skin microbiome has been examined using 16S rRNA, a highly conserved gene across different species of bacteria, in combination with polymerase chain reaction (PCR) to provide a more comprehensive topographic map that demonstrates the regional diversity across air-exposed and covered skin surfaces where creases and moisture can shift the bacterial populations (Grice et al, 2009). It is estimated that only 1% of bacterial species are identified using standard laboratory methods using bacterial culture media. The most predominant phyla represented are Actinobacteria (51.8%), represented by the genera and *Propionibacteria;* Firmicutes (24.4%), represented by the genera *Staphylococci;* Proteobacteria (16.5%); and Bacteroidetes (6.3%) (Grice et al, 2009). A noteworthy finding is that gram-negative

bacteria are abundant on dry surfaces, having previously thought to be rare skin colonizers. Furthermore, sequence data using the 16S approach indicate that swab, scrape, or punch biopsy are each sufficient to obtain a representative sample of the community membership of the bacteria present (Grice et al, 2008). Generally, the following species of bacteria are routinely found on human skin: Staphylococcus, Micrococcus, Peptococcus, Corynebacterium, Brevibacterium, Propionibacterium, Streptococcus, Neisseria, and Acinetobacter. The yeast Pityrosporum, the fungi Malassezia, and the mite Demodex are also found. Not all species are found on any one individual, but most individuals have at least five of these genera. Normal viral florae are not known to exist (Noble, 2004). However, viruses have been detected in compromised skin and in individuals who are not immunocompetent.

An association exists between skin pH and bacteria. For example, Propionibacterium acnes grow well at pH values of 6 and 6.5, but its growth is markedly decreased at pH 5.5 (Korting and Braun-Falco, 1996). However, this association can vary depending on the specific bacterial species involved and the body location. The formation of bacterial biofilms has been scrutinized (Wysocki, 2002), and the role of normal skin flora in the formation of these biofilms is an area of active investigation. Biofilms are essentially an extracellular polysaccharide matrix, or glycocalyx, in which microorganisms are embedded. Biofilms are composed of mixed bacterial species living in their own microniche in a complex, metabolically cooperative microbial community that maintains its own form of homeostasis and rudimentary circulatory system (Costerton et al, 1995). Biofilms are resistant to host immune responses and are markedly more resistant to antibiotic and topical bactericidals (Xu et al, 2000). Reports indicate that biofilm cells can be at least 500 times more resistant to antibacterial agents (Costerton et al, 1995). Biofilm formation is familiar to clinicians and can be identified on endotracheal tubes, Hickman catheters, central venous catheters, contact lenses, and orthopedic devices. Pseudomonas aeruginosa forms biofilms in conjunction with other bacterial species. Quorum sensing by bacteria is a feature in biofilm formation. These biofilms complicate the eradication of infections because they give rise to sessile and planktonic bacteria. Planktonic bacteria can be cleared by phagocytosis, antibodies, and antibiotics (Costerton et al, 1999). Sessile bacteria in biofilms can evade antibiotics by giving rise to planktonic bacteria, which respond to antibiotics and host immune responses, but the sessile bacteria remain. Cycles of antibiotic treatment often are administered without success, and the symptoms of infection recur. In these situations, biofilm formation should be suspected, and surgical removal of the sessile population most likely will be required to eliminate the pathogenic bacteria. Moist skin areas, such as the axillae, perineum, toe webs, hair follicles, nail beds, and sweat glands, are especially prone to an increased presence of bacteria. Protection from bacterial invasion is mediated in part by antimicrobial peptides (AMPs), proteins called defensins

(Hoffmann et al, 1999), cathelicidins, and protegrins and RNases (Simanski et al, 2012). More than 1,200 AMPs have been identified, and in the skin they are found in keratinocytes, mast cells, neutrophils, sebocytes, and eccrine epithelial cells (Nakatsuji and Gallo, 2012). Findings show that β-defensin is abundant in skin and may be important for wound healing. Defensins act in conjunction with phagocytosing neutrophils and the membrane attack complex of complement. Thus, optimal skin and wound care is a cornerstone of clinical practice in preventing the progression from bacterial colonization to infection (Wysocki, 2002).

Protection against Ultraviolet Radiation. Protection against UVR is provided by skin pigmentation, which results from synthesis of the pigment melanin. Harmful effects are primarily attributable to UVA, the long-wave form of UVR, which ranges spectrally from 320 to 400 nm, and UVB, the short-wave ultraviolet form, which ranges from 290 to 320 nm (Council on Scientific Affairs, 1989). Approximately 90% to 99% of UVA reaches the planet's surface compared with only 1% to 10% of UVB. The shorter the waves, the more dangerous they are. UVC is effectively blocked by an intact ozone layer. Holes appearing in the ozone layer have raised concern over the effects of UVR in causing skin diseases. Because darker-skinned individuals have increased synthesis, amount, and distribution of melanin, they are better protected against skin cancer. More melanin is distributed in all layers of the epidermis in dark skin than in light skin (Spince and Mason, 1987).

Darkly pigmented black skin provides more efficient protection from both UVB and UVA. The mean transmission of UVB is approximately 7.4% and that of UVA is 17.5% in darkly pigmented skin compared with 29.4% and 55.5%, respectively, in white skin. The mechanism for the more efficient absorption and scattering of UVB and UVA in darkly pigmented skin is attributed to the larger size and number of melanosomes in black skin. The superior UVB/UVA efficiency in black skin can provide a skin protection factor of approximately 13.4 compared with 3.4 for white skin (Montagna et al, 1993), with a range from 10- to 15-fold that is seen in the absence of melanin when the minimal erythematous dose is used as a measure (Lin and Fisher, 2007). However, in terms of protection against various types of skin cancer, highly pigmented skin affords a 500 to 1000 times reduction in risk (Lin and Fisher, 2007). An inverse relationship exists between melanin levels and DNA damage, with darker skin having less DNA damage. Higher melanin levels also decrease damage to basal stem cells and melanocytes in the deep epidermis. Thus, DNA damage in darkly pigmented skin is largely restricted to the upper layers of the epidermis, whereas DNA damage in lightly pigmented skin occurs throughout all layers of the epidermis (Miyamura et al, 2006). Melanocytes in darkly pigmented skin are more efficient than melanocytes in lighter skin in their response to the same UVR challenge (Miyamura et al, 2006). The immediate response in darkly pigmented skin leads to a more efficient

distribution and trafficking of melanosomes to the upper epidermis. An actual increase in melanin synthesis is largely a delayed response (Tadokoro et al, 2005). Finally, UV-induced apoptosis leading to removal of damaged cells is higher in darkly pigmented skin, resulting in an overall lower incidence of skin carcinogenesis (Yamaguchi et al, 2008). However, even individuals with darkly pigmented skin can develop skin cancers, and the increased melanin content often can mask precancerous and cancerous lesions, leading to poorer outcomes when the lesions eventually are detected and treated.

Clinically, the skin phototype (SPT) system was developed as a valid and practical tool to characterize the reactivity of human skin to ultraviolet radiation UVR based on the minimal erythematous dose and the ability to tan upon sun exposure (Fitzpatrick, 1988; Pathak, Nghiem, and Fitzpatrick et al, 1999). It is one of the most widely used systems to classify skin pigmentation by dermatologists and the Food and Drug Administration (Fitzpatrick, 1988; Taylor, 2002). Originally this system was developed to guide the exposure of individuals receiving psoralen ultraviolet A (PUVA) for psoriasis when it was found that hair and eye color were not sufficient to determine the level of exposure (Fitzpatrick, 1988). Over time the system was expanded from primarily one that defined various light-skinned individuals to include darkly pigmented skin. The SPT system ranges from I (ivory, white) to VI (dark brown or black) and is now defined based on (1) constitutive or unexposed skin color, (2) minimal erythematous dose and minimal melanogenic dose for UVB and UVA, (3) reactivity to ultraviolet light, (4) sunburn and tanning history, (5) immediate pigment darkening, (6) delayed tanning, (7) extent of photoaging, and (8) susceptibility to skin cancer (Pathak et al, 1999).

Exposure to UVR can lead to skin cancer, sunburn (first- or second-degree burns), compromised immunity, and long-term skin damage. Sun-exposed epidermal skin is thicker and rougher than unexposed skin, is more prone to benign and malignant growths, and tends to have a greater decrease in Langerhans cells (which seems to occur independent of skin color) (Scheibner et al, 1986). And the increase in skin pigmentation that occurs in sun-exposed skin also leads to an increase in pigmentation in sun-protected skin (Stierner et al, 1989). Infrequent sun exposure may be more harmful than regular exposure (Miyamura et al, 2006). Sun-exposed dermis has increased elastogenesis and a greater decrease in mature collagen with fragmented collagen fibrils compared with unexposed dermis.

Skin Immune System. The skin immune system also provides protection against invading microorganisms and antigens. The cells of the skin that provide immune protection are the Langerhans cells, which are antigen-presenting cells found in the epidermis; interstitial dendritic cells in the dermis; tissue macrophages, which ingest and digest bacteria and other substances; mast cells, which contain histamine (released in inflammatory reactions); and dendrocytes. Immune cells (dendritic cells, monocytes, macrophages, B cells, T cells) and some nonimmune cells (fibroblasts, epithelial cells, endothelial cells) found in the skin have pattern recognition receptors, most notably toll-like receptors that can initiate an immune response especially against microbial molecules. Both macrophages and mast cells are found in the dermis (Auger, 1989; Benyon, 1989; Wolff and Stingl, 1983). Using a standard panel of 41 allergens, allergic contact dermatitis and irritant contact dermatitis overall do not appear to be different in white compared with black individuals, although their response to specific allergens is different (DeLeo et al, 2002).

Langerhans cells are responsible for the recognition, uptake, processing, and presentation of soluble antigens and haptens to sensitized T lymphocytes. This occurs through binding of T cells to Langerhans cells. Exposure to UVB light decreases the functional capability of Langerhans cells (Bergstresser et al, 1980). Dermal dendritic cells are now recognized as having a more prominent role in antigen presentation, with Langerhans cells remaining important for activation of regulatory cells.

Tissue macrophages are derived from monocytes, which arise from bone marrow precursor cells. Macrophages are among the most important cells of the skin's immune system because they are versatile. Once monocytes migrate into the tissue, they differentiate and become macrophages. Cells in the dermis that are not completely differentiated are difficult to distinguish, and much effort has been made in the past decade to recognize the various cells in the dermis. Macrophages, in addition to their antibacterial activity, can process and present antigens to immunocompetent lymphoid cells; are tumoricidal; and can secrete growth factors, cytokines, and other immunomodulatory molecules. Macrophages are involved in coagulation, atherogenesis, wound healing, and tissue remodeling (Haake and Holbrook, 1999).

Mast cells are usually distributed in the papillary dermis, around epidermal appendages, blood vessels and nerves in the subpapillary plexus, and in subcutaneous fat. These cells are distributed in connective tissue throughout the body in places where organs interface with the environment. Mast cells contain or secrete a host of proteins on demand. Thus mast cells are the primary effector cells in allergic reactions. They also are involved in conditions of subacute and chronic inflammatory disease. Increased numbers of mast cells have been detected in tissues affected by chronic eczema, psoriasis, scleroderma, porphyria cutanea tarda, lichen simplex chronicus, lichen planus, and in healing wounds. As a part of the skin immune system, mast cells play a role in protecting against parasites, stimulating chemotaxis, and promoting phagocytosis; are involved in the activation and proliferation of eosinophils; are capable of altering vasotension and vascular permeability; and can promote connective tissue repair and angiogenesis (Haake and Holbrook, 1999).

Dermal dendrocytes are highly phagocytic cells found in the papillary and upper reticular dermis. They also are distributed near vessels in the subpapillary plexus, reticular dermis, and subcutaneous fat. These immunologically competent cells are highly phagocytic and can be recognized as melanophages. Their numbers are increased in fetal, infant, and photoaged skin and in pathologic skin conditions such as psoriasis and eczema (Headington, 1986). Their numbers are decreased in malignant fibrotic tumors and fibroproliferative lesions, such as keloids, scars, and scleroderma (Headington and Cerio, 1990).

Thermoregulation

Thermoregulation of the body is provided by the skin forming a barrier between the outside and inside environments, thus maintaining the body's temperature. The two primary thermoregulatory mechanisms are circulation and sweating. Blood vessels can either dilate to dissipate heat or constrict to shunt heat to underlying body organs. When dilated, these vessels have increased blood flow and release heat by conduction, convection, radiation, and evaporation. Vasoconstriction is often accompanied by the action of arrector pili muscle attached to hair follicles. This action results in the hair standing vertically. In mammals that depend on hair for warmth, this action fluffs up the fur to increase thermal capacity. The resulting visible bulge around hair shafts is commonly referred to as goose bumps. In humans, shivering is more important than the vertical orientation of hair for maintaining body temperature when the outside environment is cold (Jacob et al, 1982; Sams, 1990). In cold weather the "core" body temperature encompasses a smaller zone, whereas in warm weather the "core" is expanded. Sensations of cold and warm are generally detected below 30°C and above 37°C, respectively. Clinically it has been estimated that for each 1°C (1.8°F) increase in fever, a patient's fluid and calorie needs increase by 13%. At rest, the trunk, viscera, and brain account for 70% of heat production but compose only 36% of body mass. However, during exercise, muscle and skin account for 90% of heat production but represent 56% of body mass (Wenger, 1999).

Unlike other skin structures, hair follicles have a repeated cycle of growth and regression. Follicle development begins in month 4 of gestation. The hair growth cycle consists of anagen (growth phase), catagen (follicle involution), and telogen (dormant or resting phase) phases. In addition, a population of epidermal stem cells in the bulge region of the hair follicle contributes to reepithelialization in partial-thickness wounds. Hair shape varies depending on ethnicity and location. Asians have the largest diameter scalp hair and Caucasians the smallest. In the scalp, approximately 85% of hair is in anagen phase and 15% in telogen phase. The anagen phase lasts from 2 to 5 years. On the extremities, anagen lasts from 22 to 28 days (Freinkel, 2001).

Sweating occurs when the activity of the sweat glands is increased. It has been estimated that the human body has from two to five million sweat glands ranging in size from 0.05 to 0.1 mm. Sweat glands are of two types—eccrine and apocrine. Eccrine glands arise from epidermal invagination and are found abundantly on the palms of the hands and the soles of the feet. These glands are largely under the control of the nervous system, responding to temperature differences and emotional stimulation. Their secretory activity also is influenced by muscular activity. These sweat glands, located in the dermis as a coil, secrete fluid that is 99% to 99.5% water; the remainder consists of sodium chloride, urea, sulfates, and phosphates (Solomons, 1983; Spince and Mason, 1987). The pH is slightly acidic. Thermoregulatory control occurs as a result of cooling when fluid evaporates from the skin surface, since evaporation requires heat. The odor associated with sweat is largely a result of bacterial action. Eccrine sweat glands are capable of producing 1 to 4 L of sweat per hour, resulting in a 75% to 90% reduction in body heat. Man is capable of losing heat more rapidly and for longer periods than is any other animal (Quinton, 1983).

Apocrine sweat glands usually are found in association with hair follicles; they do not play a significant role in thermoregulation. These coiled, tubular glands are present in the axillae and in the anogenital area; modifications of these glands are found in the ear and secrete ear wax, or cerumen (Spince and Mason, 1987). There are approximately 100,000 apocrine glands, each 2 to 3 mm in diameter. Apocrine glands produce secretions in small amounts. The secretions are turbid, and they contain iron, carbohydrates, and lipids.

In general, no differences in the quantity, structure, or function of eccrine or apocrine sweat glands between individuals have been identified (Badreshia-Bansal and Taylor, 2009). However, scant data on functional activity indicate that white individuals have a higher degree of sweating with physical labor than do black Africans or Asian Indians and that eccrine gland activity for Hispanic individuals falls between that of white and black individuals (Badreshia-Bansal and Taylor, 2009). Other data indicate that the sodium content in sweat is lower in Africans, indicating the existence of a more efficient electrolyte conservation system in Africans (Badreshia-Bansal and Taylor, 2009). It has been reported that apocrine glands, sweat glands that are a combination of exocrine and eccrine glands, are more abundant in the facial skin of blacks compared with whites (Montagna and Carlisle, 1991). The significance of these findings, if any, awaits more comprehensive study.

Sensation

Nerve receptors located in the skin are sensitive to pain, touch, temperature, and pressure. Nerve fibers are located in the dermis and throughout the epidermis. Nerve structures in the skin originate from the neural crest and are detectable in the developing embryo at approximately 5 weeks' gestation. When stimulated, these receptors transmit impulses to the cerebral cortex, where they are interpreted. Combinations of the four basic types of sensations result in burning, tickling, and itching (Jacob et al, 1982). These sensations are propagated by unmyelinated free nerve endings, Merkel cells, Meissner corpuscles, Krause end bulbs, Ruffini terminals, and pacinian corpuscles. Identification of particular responses with specific nerve structures has not been successful, in part because some receptors seem to respond to a variety of stimuli. However, Meissner corpuscles are involved in touch reception; pacinian corpuscles (see Figure 3-1) respond to pressure, coarse touch, vibration, and tension; and free nerve endings respond to touch, pain, and temperature (Wheater et al, 1987). Merkel cells are instrumental in propagating light sensory touch in the skin (Maricich et al, 2009) and are distributed in the rete ridges among basal keratinocytes. They can be identified in association with hair follicles, digits, lips, and regions of the oral cavity.

Skin sensation is a part of the body's integrative response to protect itself from the surrounding environment. Sensation assists with the skin's regulatory function and can signal sweating, shivering, weight shifts (Parish et al, 2007), laughter, and scratching.

Merkel cells function as mechanoreceptors. In the epidermis these cells produce nerve growth factor, whereas in the dermis, Merkel cells express receptors for nerve growth factor (Narasawa et al, 1992). Merkel cells are found around the arrector pili muscle in the bulge region of hair follicles and contribute to the development of eccrine sweat glands, nails, and nerves of the skin (Boulais and Misery, 2008; Kim and Holbrook, 1995; Narasawa et al, 1996).

Sensation also moderates the psychobiologic phenomena made famous by Harlow (Harlow and Zimmermann, 1959; van der Horst et al, 2008), who demonstrated the preference of young animals for objects that were warm and those that provided better tactile sensitivity. In addition, early studies by Spitz (1947) point to the importance of touch in mediating social interactions with children and infants. Deprivation of touch can lead to psychomotor retardation and increased risk of death (Ottenbacher et al, 1987). Stroking, handling, talking, and playing resulted in a 60% decrease in aortic atherosclerotic lesions (Nerem et al, 1980), even though study groups had the same cholesterol-containing diet, blood pressures, heart rates, and serum cholesterol levels.

In healing wounds, sensory nerves sprout abundantly for about the first 3 weeks, then return to their normal density. The role of neuropeptides in stimulating growth of connective tissue is increasingly being recognized. This includes a role for these neuropeptides in modulating matrix production by fibroblasts and in acting as growth factors for keratinocytes (Baraniuk, 1997; Kiss et al, 1995; Metze and Luger, 2001).

Metabolism

Synthesis of vitamin D in the skin occurs in the presence of sunlight. Ultraviolet radiation converts a sterol (7-dehydrocholesterol) to cholecalciferol (vitamin D). Vitamin D participates in calcium and phosphate metabolism and is important in the mineralization of bone. Because vitamin D is synthesized in the skin but then transmitted to other parts of the body, it is considered an active hormone when converted to calcitriol (1,25-dihydroxycholecalciferol) (Lehninger, 1982; Stryer, 1995). Synthesis of vitamin D is higher in lightly pigmented skin and lower in darkly pigmented skin (Badreshia-Bansal and Taylor, 2009; Wilkins et al, 2009), a condition that may have implications for mood and cognitive status (Wilkins et al, 2009) and for protection against cardiovascular disease, diabetes, and some cancers (Harris, 2006). On the other hand, the reduced level of vitamin D in darkly pigmented skin does not seem to be associated with a higher level of osteoporotic fractures (Harris, 2006). Consequently, clinicians are being encouraged to promote an increased level of vitamin D intake, especially among individuals with darkly pigmented skin (Harris, 2006; Wilkins et al, 2009).

Communication

In addition to its biologic, structural, functional, and physiologic functions, human skin functions as an organ of communication and identification. The skin over the face is especially important for identification of a person and plays a role in internal and external assessments of beauty. Injury to the skin can result not only in functional and physiologic consequences, but also in changes in body image. Scarring from trauma, surgery, or incisions can lead to changes in clothing choices, avoidance of public exposure, and decreased self-esteem. Research (Koblenzer, 2005; Shuster et al, 1978) indicates that self-image is progressively reduced with increased scarring from facial acne. Adolescents are especially sensitive to physical appearance (Bernstein, 1976; Van Loey and Van Son, 2003). As an organ of communication, facial skin, along with underlying muscles, is capable of expressions such as smiling, frowning, and pouting. The sensation of touching can convey feelings of comfort, concern, friendship, and love.

FACTORS ALTERING SKIN CHARACTERISTICS

Many factors alter the normal characteristics of the skin. Predominate factors include age, sun, hydration, soaps, nutrition, smoking, obesity, medications, and allergens and irritants. Although normal age-related changes in the skin cannot yet be changed, the effects of the other variables that affect the skin can be modified or prevented.

Age

The aging process is associated with numerous morphologic and functional changes in the skin (Tables 3-1 and 3-2). Distinctive differences exist in fetuses, premature infants (23 to 32 weeks' gestation), full-term newborns, adults, and older adults. By the midcentury of 2060, approximately one in five Americans will be 65 years or older (U.S. Census Bureau, 2012); therefore, understanding age-related changes in the skin is important for all health care providers in any health care setting so that complications can be averted.

A key feature of fetal tissue that has come under more intense investigation is its ability for scarless healing (Longaker, Whitby, et al, 1990; Siebert et al, 1990). Until 120 days' gestation, wounds in the fetal lamb heal without scarring. Differences in chemical composition and growth factor concentrations of fetal skin contribute to its capacity for scarless healing and are summarized in Box 3-2 (Bullard et al,

2003; Longaker, Adzick, et al, 1990). An understanding of the factors that contribute to the phenomenon may lead to the achievement of scarless healing in adults. For example, in the laboratory setting, topical application of hyaluronic acid has been associated with a reduction in scar formation in postnatal wounds.

At birth, the skin and nails are thinner than those in an adult, but with aging they will gradually increase in thickness. Formation of the epidermal and dermal layers occurs within the first 2 weeks of embryonic development. Epidermal development is complete by the end of the second trimester, and at birth, epidermal thickness is almost that of adult skin, although newborn skin is not as effective as adult skin in providing a barrier to transcutaneous water loss. On the other hand, development of the dermis lags behind and does not take on the characteristics of adult dermis until after birth. Until about 6 months of age, the ratio of type I to type III collagen is similar to that in the fetus; soluble collagen is approximately 24%, compared with 1% in the adult.

Immature skin, or skin from premature infants between 23 and 24 weeks' and up to 32 weeks' gestation, requires special attention compared with that of infants beyond 32 weeks' gestation. In particular, before 28 weeks' gestation the skin is thin and poorly keratinized and functions weakly as a barrier. An article appearing in *Lancet* (Immature skin, 1989) has characterized the skin of infants born at the limits of viability as more suitable to an "aquatic environment" than to atmospheric conditions. Transepidermal water loss is high, and application of adhesives to the outer immature epidermal layer can leave behind raw, damaged skin prone to infection and occasional scarring. At 24 weeks' gestation, TEWL can be 10 times greater per unit area compared with an infant born at term (Rutter, 1996). Infants born between 22 and 25 weeks' gestation may require up to 4 weeks to develop a functional stratum corneum (Evans and Rutter, 1986; Harpin and Rutter, 1983; Kalia et al, 1998; Rutter, 1996). In addition, premature infants have high evaporative heat losses that result in increased risk for hypothermia.

Because premature infants have a greater surface-area-to-volume ratio compared with full-term infants, they are at an increased risk for skin complications and systemic toxicity from topically applied agents. These infants may also have alterations in metabolism, excretion, distribution, and protein binding of chemical agents, placing them at increased risk for local or systemic toxicity from soaps, lotions, or other topical agents (Weston and Lane, 1999). Other dangers are percutaneous absorption of topical agents, including antiseptics. Hemorrhagic necrosis of the dermis from alcohol absorption has been reported if the alcohol does not quickly evaporate, and is sometimes mistaken for bruising. The use of topical antibiotic sprays containing neomycin should be avoided, since it is an ototoxic aminoglycoside. Thus water-based topical antiseptics are preferred but should be used sparingly. Cleaning should be done with care, using normal saline or water. Chlorhexidine, a commonly used antiseptic, is not known to have any adverse effects, but it is probably

TABLE 3-1 Morphologic Differences in Skin at Various Ages

	Premature Newborn	Term Newborn	Adult	Aged
Skin thickness (total)	Approximately 50% of adult Higher surface-to-weight ratio Approximately 13% of body weight	Approximately 70% of adult Higher surface-to-weight ratio	Full thickness Approximately 3% of body weight	Approximately 65%–70% of adult
Periderm	Present up to approximately 120 days	Absent	Absent	Absent
Epidermis	Thinner (2–3 cells thick) Stratum corneum absent until 2–4 weeks after air exposure Melanin production absent/low Immature junctional integrity Fewer desmosomes Immature keratin filament bundles	Equivalent to smaller adult, more uniform cell size Reduced melanin production Vernix caseosa present Immature melanin granule formation	Mature stratum corneum Junctional integrity Immune cells and melanin production relative to skin phototype	Epidermal thinning is minimal (10%–50%) Increased corneocyte surface area Decreased number of active melanocytes by 10%–20% each decade Increased time for epidermal turnover Loss of epidermal stem cell population Progressive reduction in moles from 15–40 in the 30s to 4 at 60–80 years Increase in apoptosis below granular layer
Dermal–epidermal junction	Flat Absent to few rete pegs/dermal papillae before 34 weeks with immature hemidesmosomes	Rete ridges only weakly developed at birth	Mature with full junctional integrity	Flat with loss of rete pegs/dermal papillae
Dermis	Thin Higher type I-to-type III collagen ratio Approximately 24% soluble collagen compared with 1% in the adult Smaller, more uniform collagen fibers/fiber bundles in both papillary and reticular dermis High amount of hyaluronic acid Higher water content More immature elastin fiber bundles Fibroblasts more abundant in reticular dermis	Thinner (approximately 60% of adult) Much higher cellular component compared with mature adult skin Higher type I-to-type III collagen ratio persists Collagen development continues up to 3–6 months postnatally Smaller, finer collagen fiber bundles Some immature elastin fiber bundles become mature at approximately 3 years Fibroblasts more abundant in reticular dermis	Mature array of collagen and elastin fibers Larger, denser collagen fiber bundles in reticular dermis 1% of collagen is soluble Elastin fibers mature in size, distribution Fibroblasts more abundant in papillary dermis Level of advanced glycation end-products begins to increase around age 35 years	Approximately 20% loss of dermal thickness (1% reduction each year) Increase in size, number, diameter of elastic fibers Decrease in elastin synthesis Decrease in number of fibroblasts Decrease in synthesis and turnover of collagen types I and III Increase in collagen cross-linking Slight decrease in levels of hyaluronic acid, glycosaminoglycans, proteoglycans Increased matrix metalloproteinase expression Increase in advanced glycation end-products
Subcutaneous	No/little subcutaneous tissue	Thinner subcutaneous tissue	Mature subcutaneous tissue	Contraction of septae in subcutaneous fat Loss of subcutaneous fat Changes more dramatic in papillary than reticular dermis

TABLE 3-1 Morphologic Differences in Skin at Various Ages—cont'd

	Premature Newborn	Term Newborn	Adult	Aged
Vasculature	Capillary beds not organized Poor/reduced vasoconstriction/vasodilation of cutaneous vessels	Capillary beds not completely organized, continues up to 14–17 weeks postnatally	Mature organization of cutaneous vessels in papillary and reticular dermis	Approximately 30% reduction in venular cross-sections Approximately 60% reduction in peak cutaneous blood circulation Reduced vascular response Up to 50% reduction in vascular wall thickness at age 80 years Decreased vasoconstriction/vasodilation arteriole response Decrease in vascular endothelial growth factor Decreased endothelial cell permeability response
Innervation/sensation	Meissner corpuscles not fully developed Nervous network not as organized Axon flare response attenuated	Meissner corpuscles not fully developed Axon reflex muted	Mature complement of Meissner and pacinian corpuscles	Reduced number of pacinian and Meissner corpuscles to one third that in adult Pain threshold increases up to 20%
Apocrine glands	Present	Present	Present and active	Reduction in gland size, function
Immune cells	Decreased immune function	Reduced immune function	Mature immune function	Langerhans cells reduced by 20%–50% Up to 50% reduction in mast cells Increase in autoantibodies (bullous pemphigoid, antinuclear antibodies, antithyroglobulin, rheumatoid factor)
Eccrine glands	Structure present by 24–29 weeks but not responsive until 36 weeks, with cells more undifferentiated	Structure present but not responsive for one to several days after birth, with complete neural control by age 2–3 years		15% reduction in number of glands, with 70% reduction in sweating
Sebaceous glands	Large and active	Large and active but decreased in size, activity Sebum composition different from adult	Increased estrogen and androgens at puberty Increase activity of pilosebaceous glands	Decreased sebum production by approximately 65%, but number and size remain similar to adult
Hair	Lanugo hair may be present	Vellus and terminal hair present	Axillary and pubic hair appear at puberty	Reduced hair follicle density Reduced/absent hair follicle melanocyte activity Increased time for hair growth Up to approximately 50% gray/white hair by age 50 years 20% decrease in number of hair follicles by 60 years Reduction in hair diameter Bitemporal hair line recession in both genders Increased baldness in at-risk individuals

Data for this table compiled from the following resources; complete references provided at end of chapter.
Braverman, 1986; Bullard et al, 2003; Chang and Orlow, 2008; Evans and Rutter, 1986; Gilchrest, 1989; Gilchrest, 1991; Gilchrest et al, 1982; Harpin and Rutter, 1983; Holbrook, 1991; Kalia et al, 1998; Lavker et al, 1986; Lin and Carter, 1986; Longaker et al, 1990; Metze and Luger, 2001; Nordlund, 1986; Rutter, 1988; Sauder, 1986; Silverberg and Silverberg, 1989; Varani et al, 2006; Yaar and Gilchrest, 2007; Yanagishita, 1994

TABLE 3-2 Functional Differences in Skin among Premature Newborn, Term Newborn, Adult, and Aged

	Premature Newborn	Newborn	Adult	Aged
Protection	Highly permeable TEWL 10 times higher at 24 weeks of prematurity TEWL up to 100 g/m²/hr Skin maturation may require up to 5–7 weeks Higher surface-to-body weight ratio leading to greater absorption and toxicity from topical agents Excessive fluid loss and risk of hypernatremia Low melanin production leading to increased sunburn risk Increased risk of bacterial invasion Increased risk of trauma up to 15% or more of body surface area from monitor probes, rubbing, tape stripping Higher pH becomes more acidic over time (up to 8 days or more) Stratum corneum hydration higher than newborn or adult	Somewhat permeable leading to increased risk of toxicity from topical agents TEWL 6–8 g/m²/hr More readily sunburns Active sebaceous glands due to maternal hormone exposure Sebum secretion higher at birth than at 6 months Slightly higher pH compared with adult that stabilizes over 2 days Reduced stratum corneum hydration initially	Mature barrier function with good resistance to penetration Protection from UV radiation related to skin phototype	Decreased barrier function Delayed barrier recovery of stratum corneum Dry, flaky stratum corneum Higher pH (<5.0 vs. 4.5) at 80+ years (increased risk of infection) Decline in lipid content Decline in sebum production Loss of UV protection due to decrease in melanocyte activity Delayed wound healing Increased risk of mechanical injury (i.e., skin tears) Decrease in skin turgor Higher risk of premalignant and malignant lesions
Immune	Antimicrobial peptides (dermcidin, LL-37) in sweat absent Decreased IgG, IgM Reduced neutrophil chemotaxis and neutrophil phagocytosis Decreased T lymphocytes			Muted allergic and contact reactions Decreased inflammatory reaction Sun-protected skin more reactive than sun-exposed skin Impaired humoral/cell-mediated immunity Decreased DNA repair capacity Increased oncogene activation
Sensation	Sensory nerve endings present and functioning			Decreased/delayed sensory perception Increased risk of burn injury 20% increase in radiant pain threshold
Metabolism	Immature metabolism Oxygen absorption and carbon dioxide excretion 6–11 times higher before 30 weeks but upon air exposure for 2–3 weeks approaches that of adult		Vitamin D production peaks with decreased synthesis depending on skin phototype	Decreased metabolism Reduced vitamin D production contributing to osteoporosis, diabetes, hypertension, tumor formation Decreased clearance of transepidermal substances Increased UV-induced reactive oxygen species damage
Thermoregulation	High risk of hypothermia Reduced/no sweating for up to 24 days Compromised ability to regulate body temperature requires humidified thermal incubator Evaporative heat loss can exceed resting heat production	Reduced sweating for up to 5 days	Full sweating capability	Loss of ability to control/maintain body temperature when exposed to cold or excessive heat by vasoconstriction, vasodilation, shunting

IgG, Immunoglobulin G; *IgM,* immunoglobulin M; *TEWL,* transepidermal water loss; *UV,* ultraviolet.

BOX 3-2   Unique Characteristics of Fetal Skin

- Collagen deposition occurs more rapidly (Longaker et al, 1990)
- Collagen deposition follows normal dermal pattern (Longaker et al, 1990)
- Approximately 30% to 60% of collagen is type III (10% to 15% in adult skin) (Bullard et al, 2003)
- Higher concentrations of hyaluronic acid than in adult (Siebert et al, 1990)
- Less TGF-β1 in fetal wounds (Roberts and Sporn, 1996)
- Differential patterns of expression of various isoforms of TGF-β in fetal wounds
- Difference in cell responses
  - Decrease in inflammatory cells, particularly polymorphonuclear leukocytes and macrophage
  - Platelets do not aggregate in response to collagen
  - Platelets do not release same amount of TGF-β1 and platelet-derived endothelial growth factor-AB as adult cells
  - Fibroblasts can migrate at faster rate
  - Fibroblasts synthesize more total collagen
- Differences in protease and inhibitor activity, level of growth factors, and expression of homeobox genes detected (Bullard et al, 2003)

TGF, Transforming growth factor.

absorbed from the skin and should be used judiciously. Likewise iodine has been reported to be absorbed, leading to goiter and hypothyroidism (Rutter, 1988). If required, moisturizing creams or ointments may be applied to dry, flaking, or fissured skin, and the best agents appear to be those with few or no preservatives, since these offer the greatest benefit with decreased risk (Weston and Lane, 1999). Other topical agents that can place the premature or neonate at risk are aniline dyes (methemoglobinemia), hexachlorophene (neurotoxicity), corticosteroids (adrenal suppression), lidocaine-prilocaine cream or EMLA (methemoglobinemia, seizures, petechiae), N,N-dimethyl-meta-toluamide or DEET (neurotoxicity), salicylates (salicylism, metabolic acidosis, encephalopathy), and silver sulfadiazine (kernicterus, agranulocytosis) (Mancini, 2004).

The next period of change occurs in adolescence, when hormonal stimulation results in increased activity of sebaceous glands and hair follicles. Sebaceous glands increase their secretory rate, and hair follicles become activated, giving rise to secondary sexual characteristics. From adolescence to adulthood there is a gradual change in skin characteristics. By the time the skin reaches mature adulthood, several changes become apparent. The dermis decreases in thickness by about 20%, whereas the epidermis remains relatively unchanged. Epidermal turnover time is increased; this means that wound healing may take longer. For instance, in young adults, epidermal turnover takes about 21 days, but by 35 years of age this turnover time is doubled. Barrier function is reduced, and such reduction may increase the risk of irritation. The number of active melanocytes per unit body surface

area decreases with aging, which means that protection against UVR is diminished. However, across the lifespan, darker skin offers greater protection against photoaging or dermatoheliosis (Miyamura et al, 2006). Skin dryness is also associated with aging and an increase in wrinkles. Sensory receptors are diminished in capacity, meaning that the skin is more likely to be burned or traumatized without perception. Vitamin D production is decreased and may be a factor in osteomalacia.

With aging there is a decrease in the number of Langerhans cells, which affects the immunocompetence of the skin and can lead to an increased risk of skin cancer and infection by invading microorganisms. The density of Langerhans cells changes from 10 per 3 mm cross-section of unexposed skin in 22- to 26-year-old persons to 5.8 per 3 mm cross-section in 62- to 68-year-old persons (Gilchrest et al, 1982). There is also a decrease in the number of mast cells and melanocytes. The inflammatory response is decreased, and such a decrease may alter allergic reactions and healing. A decrease in the number of sweat glands, diminished vascularity, and a reduction in the amount of subcutaneous fat compromise the thermoregulatory capacity of the skin. Epidermal-dermal junction changes, such as the flattening of the prominent dermal papillae and of the rete ridges, alter junctional integrity. Consequently, the skin is more easily torn in response to mechanical trauma, especially shearing forces. Because the epidermal rete pegs flatten, the unique microenvironment of the basal keratinocytes changes; it is thought that this explains the decrease in epidermal proliferative capacity that occurs with aging (Lavker et al, 1986).

Skin elasticity decreases with age and is related to a combination of aging and solar damage. Microscopic analysis of collagen and elastin fibers reveals that these are more compact, with a loss of ground substance from the spaces between these cable-like structures. Collagen fibers appear to be unwinding, whereas elastin fibers appear to be lysing. The degradation of elastin can be detected at about 30 years of age, but becomes marked at 70 years of age (Braverman, 1986). Changes in dermal proteoglycans usually occur after 40 years of age (Yanagishita, 1994). By 70 years of age, most of the elastin network is affected. Changes in collagen content and structure are mediated by an underexpression of procollagen; an overexpression of collagenase (MMP-1), stromelysin (MMP-3), and gelatinase A (MMP-2); and a decreased expression of tissue inhibitors of matrix metalloproteinase-1 (TIMP-1). Fibroblasts in aged skin have a reduced ability to synthesize collagen type I and type III, and collagen fragments further reduce the ability of fibroblasts to synthesize new collagen. In addition, fibroblasts in young adult skin have a higher amount of their cell surface in contact with collagen and exhibit more extensive cell spreading compared with fibroblasts in old skin (Varani et al, 2006). There is also a marked reduction in vascular beds in the vertical capillary loops in the dermal papillae. There is an approximately 35% decrease in the cross-sectional area of these loops in aged skin. It is thought that this leads to atrophy of the hair bulbs, the sweat glands, and the sebaceous glands. Because the hypodermis also becomes thinner, mature individuals are more prone to pressure necrosis (Gilchrest, 1989). With aging, a progressive loss of mechanoreceptors to one third of their average density occurs from the second to the ninth decades (Metze and Luger, 2001).

The density of skin melanocytes is relatively constant until about 40 years of age. By about 45 years of age, skin melanocytes have decreased in density to approximately half that seen between 30 and 39 years of age (Nordlund, 1986). Melanocytes decrease 6% to 8% each decade after age 30. It is thought that the loss of skin melanocytes contributes to an increase in the formation of skin cancers. Other overt changes are wrinkling and sagging, which occur as a result of the loss of underlying tissue, in addition to changes seen in collagen and elastin.

Changes in hair color and hair follicles also accompany aging. Age-related changes in active melanocytes result in gray hair. About 50% of the body's hair will be gray by the age of 50 in about 50% of the population. This change is accompanied by a reduction in the number of hair follicles and a decrease in the diameter of the hair. The rate of hair growth is also decreased (Silverberg and Silverberg, 1989). Nail growth rates also decrease by 40% to 50%.

Changes in thermoregulatory capacity occur with age, and older individuals are more prone to hypothermia and heat stroke. This has been attributed to changes in blood capillaries and eccrine sweat glands. In healthy older individuals, sweating may be decreased by up to 70% (Gilchrest, 1991). Sebum secretion also declines with age. Barrier function decreases with aging due to the decreased level of all the major lipid species, especially ceramides. In addition, corneocytes are larger and less cohesive. In addition to these changes, pain perception is dulled, and there is reduced skin reactivity upon exposure to irritants. Cutaneous immune function also changes with aging, as seen by a reduction in Langerhans cell density. Skin damaged by sun exposure, or actinically damaged skin, has been found to have a 50% reduction of Langerhans cell density compared with sun-protected skin (Sauder, 1986). Reduced immunocompetence of the skin is thought to contribute in part to skin cancer in the elderly.

Other factors that may contribute to the development of skin cancer in aged individuals are cumulative exposure to carcinogens, diminished DNA repair capacity, decreased melanocyte density, and alterations in dermal matrix (Lin and Carter, 1986). Not surprisingly, wound healing in older individuals is delayed compared with that of younger individuals.

Menopausal changes appear to somewhat accelerate skin changes in women where the decrease in circulating levels of estrogen result in a reduction in dermal collagen and elasticity. Other changes include a reduction in dermal hydration, increased dryness, dermal thinning, reduced vascularity, an altered response to oxidative stress, and wrinkling. Surface lipids are also reduced due to changes in sebaceous gland function. Changes in estrogen and progesterone affect

inflammatory response, keratinocyte proliferation, collagen and hyaluronic acid synthesis, and matrix metalloproteinase (MMP) activity (Yaar and Gilchrest, 2007).

Sun

Excessive exposure to UVR can have harmful effects that accelerate aging of the skin. For this reason the condition associated with UVR-damaged skin is referred to as photoaging. Dermatologically, the condition is called dermatoheliosis. Across the lifespan, darker skin offers greater protection against photoaging and dermatoheliosis (Miyamura et al, 2006). Obvious clinical signs of photodamaged skin are dryness, tough and leathery texture, wrinkling as a result of collagen and elastin degeneration, and irregular pigmentation from changes in melanin distribution (Box 3-3) (Silverberg and Silverberg, 1989; Young and Walker, 2008). Excessive exposure to UVR increases the risk of developing skin cancers such as basal or squamous cell carcinoma and malignant melanoma, especially in white or lightly pigmented skin. Damage to the DNA of skin cells leads to transformation of cells and cancer (Council on Scientific Affairs, 1989). Changes also occur in epidermal and dermal cells. Epidermal cells become thickened (Varani et al, 2006) and more numerous, and dermal vessels become dilated and tortuous. Langerhans cells are reduced in number by approximately 50%, thereby diminishing the immunocompetence of the skin (Lober and Fenske, 1990).

Exposure to excessive UVR results in the production of reactive oxygen species that lead to activation of several cell

---

BOX 3-3 Photoaging Effects on Skin Characteristics

- Hyperkeratosis
- Atrophy
- Leathery appearance, especially in lighter skin phototypes
- Melanosomes may be increased with increase in dopa-positive melanocytes up to twofold
- Telangiectasia
- Further elastogenesis/degeneration accompanied by mass accumulations
- Increased lysozyme deposition on elastic fibers
- Decreased amounts of mature collagen
- Further increased matrix metalloproteinase activity
- Presence of hyperplastic fibroblasts
- Perivascular infiltrate of lymphocytes, histiocytes, mononuclear cells, mast cells
- Prominent grenz zone (a zone of normal-appearing dermis just below the epidermis, but below this normal-appearing zone is abnormal dermis)
- Glycosaminoglycans and proteoglycans increase
- Reduction in vascular circulation
- Venule wall thickening
- Further reduction in number of Langerhans cells
- More infiltrating mononuclear cells present
- Increased CD4[+] T cells

surface receptors such as interleukin-1, epidermal growth factor, and keratinocyte growth factor, which signal the induction of the nuclear transcription complex AP-1. The AP-1 complex blocks synthesis of collagen types I and III by suppressing expression of transforming growth factor-β. These same reactive oxygen species lead to damage of the lipid cell membrane, which results in release of prostaglandins that are responsible for mediating inflammatory reactions (Yaar and Gilchrest, 2007). Together these processes can create a pattern of heightened inflammation that is responsible for the net degradation of collagen tissue by the activation and overexpression of MMPs, particularly MMP-1, MMP-3, MMP-8, and MMP-9. Other cell-mediated damage results from damage to mitochondrial DNA, protein oxidation (especially in the upper dermis), and telomere shortening (Yaar and Gilchrest, 2007).

The effects of reactive oxygen species in aged skin are not effectively countered by the presence of the naturally occurring antioxidant enzymes, such as catalase, superoxide dismutase, and glutathione peroxidase, and nonenzymatic molecules, such as coenzyme Q10, ascorbate or vitamin C, tocopherol or vitamin E, and carotenoids, which are present at higher levels in young adult skin. Over the past decade, the study of the reactive oxygen species system and its role in skin damage has resulted in the use of various antioxidants in topical sunscreens and cosmetics. Among the antioxidants used are tocopherol acetate, stable forms of vitamin C, vitamin E, polyphenolic molecules such as procyanidin and flavonoids, curcumin, genistein (found in soybeans), and resveratrol (found in red wine, nuts, and grapefruit) (Yaar and Gilchrist, 2007). Other agents that have been investigated or are being used to reverse the effects of photodamaged skin include dietary lipids such as omega-3 fatty acids and eicosapentaenoic acid, osmolytes, and α-hydroxy acids derived from fruit, sugarcane, and dairy products. Retinoids have been used since the 1980s to abrogate the effects of sun damage that can be seen visually and histologically. More recently, retinoids have been used as a pretreatment approach (Yaar and Gilchrest, 2007).

Exposure to UVR can lead to sunburn. Sunburn is partly the result of a vasodilatory response that increases blood volume. Whether an individual will become sunburned depends on the extent of skin pigmentation. Naturally, those with the least pigmentation are more prone to sunburn and the harmful, long-term effects of UVR. Severe short-term exposure of unprotected, lightly pigmented skin can lead to blistering (a second-degree burn).

There is an association between melanoma and sunburn. An individual who has sustained more than six serious sunburns is at increased risk for melanoma (Green et al, 1985). Exposure to UVR and the rise of malignant melanomas have led to the development of more effective sun-blocking agents. Over time the lifetime risk of malignant melanoma has increased from 1:1500 people in 1930 to 1:250 in 1980 to 1:62 in 2005, and as of 2015, it is expected to be 1:50 (Potts, 1990; Rigel et al, 2010). It is estimated that 65% to 90% of all melanomas result from UVR exposure. And while melanomas account for 3% of all skin cancers, they are responsible for 75% of all deaths from skin cancer, with basal cell carcinoma accounting for 80% to 85% and the remaining 15% to 20% accounted for by squamous cell carcinoma. Sunscreens should be used on a regular basis, applied at least 30 minutes before sun exposure, and have a sun protection factor (SPF) ranging from 15 to 30 (Pathak et al, 1999). Individuals with moderately pigmented skin require about three to five times more exposure to UVR to induce sunburn inflammation compared with Caucasians; individuals with darker skin require 10 times more exposure (McGregor and Hawk, 1999; Young and Walker, 2008). The age-adjusted incidence rates for melanoma have been reported as 1.0 per 100,000 for blacks versus 4.5 for Hispanics and 21.6 for white non-Hispanics (Rouhani et al, 2008).

Hydration

Adequate skin hydration is normally provided by sebum secretion and an intact stratum corneum with its keratinized cells. Several factors can affect skin hydration, including relative humidity, removal of sebum, and age. Each of these factors increases water loss from the skin, leading to dryness and scaling. Application of emollients to the skin replaces the barrier function of lost sebum or decreased evaporative water loss when the relative humidity is low. Retention of water in the epidermal layers after application of a lotion leads to swelling of the skin, which is perceived as smoothness and softness.

Various products often are promoted with claims of superiority over other products without adequate in vitro, in vivo, or clinical data. The superiority of oil baths over water baths was found to be only marginal (Stender et al, 1990). Twenty minutes after both kinds of baths, skin hydration was increased when measured by water evaporation and electrical conductance and capacitance. A small but significantly greater amount of water was bound in the skin after the oil bath, but no change was seen in evaporation, conductance, or capacitance. Thus, increases in water-holding capacity of the skin after an oil bath may not be of importance. However, a difference in skin-surface lipids was found, and the difference lasted at least 3 hours. This effect is comparable to that seen with application of a traditional moisturizing lotion. The authors of the study concluded that because daily use of bath oil is not practical, application of moisturizing lotions may be more advantageous, and the beneficial effects of bath oils are related to lipidization of the skin surface (Stender et al, 1990).

Soaps

Washing or bathing with an alkaline soap reduces the thickness and number of cell layers in the stratum corneum (White et al, 1987). Generally, soap emulsifies the lipid coating of the skin and removes it, along with resident and transient bacteria. Excessive use of soap or detergents can interfere with the water-holding capacity of the skin and may impair bacterial resistance. Use of alkaline soaps increases skin pH, which may change bacterial resistance. The time for recovery to normal skin pH of 5.5 depends on the length of exposure. Ordinary washing requires 45 minutes to restore skin pH, whereas prolonged exposure can require 19 hours (Bettley, 1960). Other agents that can lead to delipidization or dehydration of skin are alcohol and acetone. Currently, acidic skin cleansers appear to be less irritating than neutral or alkaline cleansers, and some evidence suggests that acidic cleansers decrease the number of acne lesions on the face (Korting and Braun-Falco, 1996).

Nutrition

Normal, healthy skin integrity can be maintained by adequate dietary intake of protein, carbohydrate, fats, vitamins, and minerals. Under normal conditions in healthy persons, supplementary nutrition is not beneficial if dietary intake is adequate. If the skin is damaged, increased dietary intake of some substances, such as vitamin C for collagen formation, may be beneficial. A healthy diet of protein supplies the necessary amino acids for protein synthesis. Fats are broken down into essential fatty acids, which cells can use to form their lipid bilayer. Carbohydrates are digested to supply energy for cell metabolism. Maintenance of normal, healthy skin requires ingestion of the following: vitamins C, D, and A; the B vitamins pyridoxine and riboflavin; the mineral elements iron, zinc, and copper; and many others. Adequate dietary intake can be ensured by ingestion of amounts consistent with the recommended daily allowances (RDAs) (Boelsma et al, 2001; Roe, 1986).

Smoking

Smoking decreases capillary blood flow and changes the oxygen gradient in skin via its vasoconstrictive effects. Data indicate that the dermis in smokers has a reduced level of collagen and elastin fibers, leading to tissue that is less elastic and hardened as a result of an increase in reactive oxygen species and MMPs. Epidermal effects include keratinocyte dysplasia, telangiectasias, roughness, and excessive wrinkling (Kennedy et al, 2003; Leow and Maibach, 1998). Furthermore, a dose–response effect of smoking and wrinkle formation has been identified, leading to premature skin aging (Kennedy et al, 2003). Yellow discolored nails and mustaches are frequently seen in heavy users of tobacco products, including cigarettes and pipes. Tobacco smoke contains a number of mutagens and carcinogens, including polycyclic aromatic hydrocarbons, heterocyclic amines, and nitrosamines. Premature graying of hair can be seen in both men and women, and frequently accelerated hair loss can be seen in men (Ortiz and Grando, 2012).

Obesity

Obesity (body mass index >30 kg/m^2) is now a recognized risk factor for a number of skin diseases. These include an increased risk of melanoma and nonmelanoma skin cancers (Tobin et al, 2013). High circulating levels of leptin, detected in obesity, have been found to confer a 1.56-times increase in risk for melanoma. Obese individuals exhibit changes in immune capacity as measured by lower levels of cytotoxic T lymphocytes and natural killer cells. Both of these cell populations are important to defend the body against cancer (Tobin et al, 2013). Obesity is also associated with increased inflammation and the presence of psoriasis, an inflammatory dermatoses. Other skin conditions associated with obesity are lymphedema and cellulitis, hidradenitis suppurativa, intertrigo with candida infection, observation of acanthosis nigricans, and various cutaneous infections. Obese individuals are more likely to become diabetic, and uninjured diabetic skin has been found to be mechanically compromised (Bermudez et al, 2011).

Medications

Various medications affect the skin, and the prevalence rate of skin reactions to medications in hospitalized individuals is 2% to 3% (Gerson et al, 2008; Ramdial and Naidoo, 2009). Some of the best-studied medications are the corticosteroids, which interfere with epidermal regeneration and collagen synthesis (Ehrlich and Hunt, 1968; Pollack, 1982; Ramdial and Naidoo, 2009; Wicke et al, 2000). Medications also cause photosensitive and phototoxic reactions. Some categories of medications that can affect the skin are antibacterials, antihypertensives, analgesics, tricyclic antidepressants, antihistamines, antineoplastic agents, antipsychotic drugs, diuretics, hypoglycemic agents, sunscreens, and oral contraceptives (Potts, 1990; Ramdial and Naidoo, 2009). Skin eruptions have been more frequently reported for antibiotics, antiepileptics, antiarrhythmic, and anticoagulants (Gerson et al, 2008). Skin flora can be changed by the use of antibacterials, orally administered steroids, and hormones. Analgesics, antihistamines, and nonsteroidal antiinflammatory drugs can alter inflammatory reactions. Thus, whenever drugs are prescribed and skin reactions occur, medications should always be checked to determine whether they are responsible.

Allergens and Irritants

Additionally, metals such as nickel, cobalt, gold, and chromate; plants such as poison ivy and poison oak; and foods such as chamomile, tomatoes, mango, citrus, garlic, and shiitake mushrooms can lead to inflammatory skin changes resulting in contact dermatitis with exposure. Nickel is recognized as one of the most common allergens, with an increasing prevalence as high as 28% in females and 5% in males (Schram et al, 2010). Other sources of skin reactions are associated with cosmetics, including personal care products that contain fragrances, preservatives, antioxidants, botanicals, and cosmetic vehicles. Reactions to these personal care products have been reported in up to 23% of women and 17.8% in men (Alani et al, 2013).

CLINICAL CONSULT

A: Referral received from primary provider for an 88-year-old woman with persistent diffuse fine macular–papular rash over lower back, buttocks, and both legs. Rash has become bothersome and increasingly pruritic. Significant macular-papular rash with satellite lesions under both breasts; slight erythema. Pruritus more intense under both breasts. Patient well dressed, independent, and physically active. Describes self as 30 pounds overweight. Recently developed UTI and is finishing 10-day course of antibiotic. Patient describes hands as very sore. Denies any medication allergies. Acknowledges she recently changed both laundry detergent and bath soap. Reports daughter recently bought her new bath soap and laundry detergent that had a fragrant smell. Lower extremities thin, no discoloration in skin tone, no edema, dry flaking skin apparent. Macular-papular rash present under pendulous breasts; skin intact.

Hands very dry with cracks apparent in fingertips. Applies lotion occasionally to her hands
D: Dry skin and candidiasis under pendulous breasts.
P: Treat candidiasis, moisturize skin, reduce exposure to possible irritants.
I: (1) Antifungal powder to apply under breasts twice daily. (2) Apply an over-the-counter, high-grade moisturizing cream daily to her dry skin on legs and hands. (3) Increase water intake to 8 glasses daily. (4) Provided with education about loss of emollients, elasticity, and moisture with aging skin. (5) Discontinue new bath soap and evaluate for improvement in overall skin condition, especially on back. Discontinue laundry detergent if condition has not improved.
E: Return to wound clinic in 4 weeks; if condition worsens, call wound clinic for referral to dermatologist.

SUMMARY

As the body's largest organ, the skin serves several complex functions: protection, thermoregulation, sensation, metabolism, and communication. Numerous factors that influence the skin's ability to adequately provide these functions are age, UVR exposure, hydration, medications, nutrition, obesity, irritants, and soaps. The skin's integrity also can be jeopardized by many of these factors.

Wound management and skin care must be grounded in a comprehensive knowledge base of the structure and function of the skin. After reviewing this chapter, the care provider should closely scrutinize many of the skin care practices and bathing routines that are subconsciously engrained in day-to-day patient care activities and that may compromise the function and integrity of the skin.

REFERENCES

Alani JI, Davis MDP, Yiannias JA: Allergy to cosmetics: a literature review, *Dermatitis* 24:283–290, 2013.

Auger MJ: Mononuclear phagocytes, *BMJ* 298:546–548, 1989.

Badreshia-Bansal S, Taylor SC: The structure and function of skin of color. In Kelly AP, Taylor SC, editors: *Dermatology for skin of color*, New York, 2009, McGraw-Hill.

Baraniuk JN: Neuropeptides in the skin. In Bos JD, editor: *Cutaneou immunology and clinical immunodermatology*. ed 2, Boca Raton, 1997, CRC Press, pp 311–323.

Benyon RC: The human skin mast cell, *Clin Exp Allergy* 19:375–387, 1989.

Bergstresser PR, Toews GB, Streilein JW: Natural and perturbed distributions of Langerhans cells: responses to ultraviolet light, heterotopic skin grafting, and dinitrofluorobenzene sensitization, *J Invest Dermatol* 75:73–77, 1980.

Bermudez DM, Herdrich BJ, Xu J, et al: Impaired biomechanical properties of diabetic skin, *Am J Pathol* 178:2215–2223, 2011.

Bernstein NR: Appearance: concepts of perception and disfigurement (Chapter 1), *Emotional care of the facially burned and disfigured*, Boston, 1976, Little, Brown, pp 13–22.

Bernstein NR: Body and face images: personality and self-representation (Chapter 2), *Emotional care of the facially burned and disfigured*, Boston, 1976, Little, Brown, pp 23–40.

Bernstein NR: Disfigurement and personality development, (Chapter 3), *Emotional care of the facially burned and disfigured*, Boston, 1976, Little, Brown, pp 41–75.

Bettley FR: Some effects of soap on the skin, *BMJ* 1:1675–1679, 1960.

Bickenbach JR: Identification and behavior of label-retaining cells in oral mucosa and skin, *J Dent Res* 60:1611–1620, 1981.

Boelsma E, Hendriks HF, Roza L: Nutritional skin care: health effects of micronutrients and fatty acids, *Am J Clin Nutr* 73(5):853–864, 2001.

Boissy RE: Melanosome transfer to and translocation in the keratinocyte, *Exp Dermatol* 12(Suppl 2):5–12, 2003.

Boulais N, Misery L: The epidermis: a sensory tissue, *Eur J Dermatol* 18:119–127, 2008.

Braverman IM: Elastic fiber and microvascular abnormalities in aging skin, *Dermatol Clin* 4:391–405, 1986.

Briggaman RA: Epidermal-dermal interactions in adult skin, *J Invest Dermatol* 79(Suppl 1):21–24, 1982.

Bullard KM, Longaker MT, Lorenz HP: Fetal wound healing: current biology, *World J Surg* 27:54–61, 2003.

Chang HY, Chi JT, Dudoit S, et al: Diversity, topographic differentiation, and positional memory in human fibroblasts, *Proc Natl Acad Sci USA* 99(20):12877–12882, 2002.

Chang MW, Orlow SJ: Neonatal, pediatric and adolescent dermatology. In Wolff K, Gilchrest B, Katz S, et al (eds): et al, editors: *Fitzpatrick's dermatology in general medicine*, ed 7, New York, 2008, McGraw-Hill.

Chu DH: Development and structure of skin. In Wolff K, Gilchrest B, Katz S, et al (eds): et al, editors: *Fitzpatrick's dermatology in general medicine*, ed 7, New York, 2008, McGraw-Hill pp 57–73.

Costerton JW, Lewandowski Z, Caldwell DE, et al: Microbial biofilms, *Annu Rev Microbiol* 49:711–745, 1995.

Costerton JW, Stewart PS, Greenberg EP: Bacterial biofilms: a common cause of persistent infections, *Science* 284:1318–1322, 1999.

Council on Scientific Affairs: Harmful effects of ultraviolet radiation, *JAMA* 262:380–384, 1989.

DeLeo VA, Taylor SC, Belsito DV, et al: The effect of race and ethnicity on patch test results, *J Am Acad Dermatol* 46:S107–S112, 2002.

Ehrlich HP, Hunt TK: Effects of cortisone and vitamin A on wound healing, *Ann Surg* 167:324–328, 1968.

Evans NJ, Rutter N: Development of the epidermis in the newborn, *Biol Neonate* 49:74–80, 1986.

Feingold KR, Elias PM: Role of lipids in the formation and maintenance of the cutaneous permeability barrier, *Biochim Biophys Acta* 1841:280–294, 2014.

Fitzpatrick TB: The validity and practicality of sun-reactive skin types I through IV, *Arch Dermatol* 124:869–871, 1988.

Freinkel RK: Hair. In Freinkel RK, Woodley DT, editors: *The biology of the skin*, New York, 2001, Parthenon, pp 77–86.

Gay S, Miller S: *Collagen in the physiology and pathology of connective tissue*, Stuttgart, Germany, 1978, Gustav Fischer Verlag.

Gerson D, Sriganeshan V, Alexis JB: Cutaneous drug eruptions: a 5-year experience, *J Am Acad Dermatol* 59:995–999, 2008.

Gilchrest BA: Skin aging and photoaging: an overview, *J Am Acad Dermatol* 21:610–613, 1989.

Gilchrest BA: Physiology and pathophysiology of aging skin. In Goldsmith LA, editor: *Physiology, biochemistry, and molecular biology of the skin*, ed 2, New York, 1991, Oxford University Press pp 1425–1444.

Gilchrest BA, Murphy GF, Soter NA: Effect of chronologic aging and the ultraviolet irradiation on Langerhans cells in human epidermis, *J Invest Dermatol* 79:85–88, 1982.

Goding CR: Melanocytes: the new black, *Int J Biochem Cell Biol* 39(2):275–279, 2007.

Green A, Siskind V, Bain C, et al: Sunburn and malignant melanoma, *Br J Cancer* 51:393–397, 1985.

Grice EA, Kong HH, Conlan S, et al: Topographical and temporal diversity of the human skin microbiome, *Science* 324:1190–1192, 2009.

Grice EA, Kong HH, Renaud G, et al: A diversity profile of the human skin microbiota, *Genome Res* 18:1043–1050, 2008.

Griffith LG, Naughton G: Tissue engineering—current challenges and expanding opportunities, *Science* 295:1009–1014, 2002.

Haake AR, Holbrook K: The structure and development of skin. In Freedberg IM, et al, editors: *Fitzpatrick's dermatology in general medicine*, ed 5, New York, 1999, McGraw-Hill pp 70–114.

Haake A, Scott GA, Holbrook KA: Structure and function of the skin: overview of the epidermis and dermis. In Freinkel RK, Woodley DT, editors: *The biology of the skin*, New York, 2001, Parthenon, pp 19–46.

Harlow HF, Zimmermann RR: Affectional responses in the infant monkey, *Science* 130:421–432, 1959.

Harpin VA, Rutter N: Barrier properties of the newborn infant's skin, *J Pediatr* 102:419–425, 1983.

Harris SS: Vitamin D and African Americans, *J Nutr* 136(4):1126–1129, 2006.

Headington JT: The dermal dendrocyte, *Adv Dermatol* 1:159–171, 1986.

Headington JT, Cerio R: Dendritic cells and the dermis, *Am J Dermatopathol* 12:217–220, 1990.

Hoffmann JA, Kafatos FC, Janeway CA, et al: Phylogenetic perspectives in innate immunity, *Science* 284:1313–1318, 1999.

Holbrook KA: Structure and function of the developing human skin. In Goldsmith LA, editor: *Physiology, biochemistry, and molecular biology of the skin*, ed 2, New York, 1991, Oxford University Press pp 64–101.

Holbrook KA, Vogel AM, Underwood RA, et al: Melanocytes in human embryonic and fetal skin: a review and new findings, *Pigment Cell Res* 1(Suppl):6–17, 1998.

Immature skin, *Lancet* 334(8672):1138, 1989 DOI: http://dx.doi.org/10.1016/S0140-6736(89)91497-9.

Jacob SW, Francone CA, Lossow WJ: *Structure and function in man*, ed 5, Philadelphia, 1982, Saunders.

Kalia VN, Nonato LB, Lund CH, et al: Development of skin barrier function in premature infants, *J Invest Dermatol* 111:320–326, 1998.

Kennedy C, Bastiaens MT, Bajdik CD, et al: Effect of smoking and sun on aging skin, *J Invest Dermatol* 120:548–554, 2003.

Kim DK, Holbrook KA: The appearance, density and distribution of Merkel cells in human embryonic and fetal skin: their relation to sweat glands, and hair follicle development, *J Invest Dermatol* 104:411–416, 1995.

Kiss M, Wlaschek M, Brenneisen P, et al: Alpha-melanocyte stimulating hormone induces collagenase/matrix metalloproteinase-1 in human dermal fibroblasts, *Biol Chem Hoppe Seyler* 376:425–430, 1995.

Koblenzer CS: The emotional impact of chronic and disabling skin disease: a psychoanalytic perspective, *Dermatol Clin* 23(4):619–627, 2005.

Korting HC, Braun-Falco O: The effect of detergents on skin pH and its consequences, *Clin Dermatol* 14(1):23–27, 1996.

La Ruche G, Cesarini JP: Histology and physiology of black skin, *Ann Dermatol Venereol* 119(8):567–574, 1992.

Lambert MI, Mann T, Dugas JP: Ethnicity and temperature regulation, *Med Sport Sci* 53:104–120, 2008.

Lavker RM, Sun TT: Epidermal stem cells: properties, markers, and location, *Proc Natl Acad Sci USA* 97(25):13473–13475, 2000.

Lavker RM, Zheng PS, Dong G: Morphology of aged skin, *Dermatol Clin* 4:379–389, 1986.

Lehninger AL: *Principles of biochemistry*, New York, 1982, Worth.

Leow YH, Maibach HI: Cigarette smoking, cutaneous vasculature, and tissue oxygen, *Clin Dermatol* 16:579–584, 1998.

Lin AN, Carter DM: Skin cancer in the elderly, *Dermatol Clin* 4(3):467–471, 1986.

Lin JY, Fisher DE: Melanocyte biology and skin pigmentation, *Nature* 445:843–850, 2007.

Lober CW, Fenske NA: Photoaging and the skin: differentiation and clinical response, *Geriatrics* 45:36–40, 42, 1990.

Longaker MT, Adzick NS, Hall JL, et al: Studies in fetal wound healing, VII. Fetal wound healing may be modulated by hyaluronic acid and stimulating activity in amniotic fluid, *J Pediatr Surg* 25:430–433, 1990.

Longaker MT, Whitby DJ, Adzick NS, et al: Studies in fetal wound healing, VI. Second and early third trimester fetal wounds demonstrate rapid collagen deposition without scar formation, *J Pediatr Surg* 25:63–68, 1990.

Mancini AJ: Skin, *Pediatrics* 113:1114–1119, 2004.

Maricich SM, Wellnitz SA, Nelson AM, et al: Merkel cells are essential for light-touch responses, *Science* 324:1580–1582, 2009.

McDonald CJ: Structure and function of the skin. Are there differences between black and white skin?, *Dermatol Clin* 6(3):343–347, 1988.

McGregor JM, Hawk JLM: Acute effects of ultraviolet radiation on the skin. In Freedberg IM, et al, editors: *Fitzpatrick's dermatology in general medicine*, ed 5, New York, 1999, McGraw-Hill pp 1555–1561.

Metze D, Luger T: Nervous system in the skin. In Freinkel RK, Woodley DT, editors: *The biology of the skin*, New York, 2001, Parthenon, pp 153–176.

Millington PF, Wilkinson R: *Skin*, Cambridge, 1983, Cambridge University Press.

Miyamura Y, Coelho SG, Wolber R, et al: Regulation of human skin pigmentation and responses to ultraviolet radiation, *Pigment Cell Res* 20(1):2–13, 2006.

Montagna W, Carlisle K: The architecture of black and white facial skin, *J Am Acad Dermatol* 24:929–937, 1991.

Montagna W, Prota G, Kenney JA: *Black skin: Structure and function*, San Diego, 1993, CA Academic Press.

Nakatsuji T, Gallo RL: Antimicrobial peptides: old molecules with new ideas, *J Invest Dermatol* 132:887–895, 2012.

Narasawa Y, Hashimoto K, Kohda H: Merkel cells participate in the induction and alignment of epidermal ends of arrector pili muscles of human fetal skin, *Br J Dermatol* 134:494–498, 1996.

Narasawa Y, Hashimoto K, Nihei Y, et al: Biological significance of dermal Merkel cells in development of cutaneous nevus in human fetal skin, *J Histochem Cytochem* 40:65–71, 1992.

Nerem RM, Levesque MJ, Cornhill JF: Social environment as a factor in diet-induced atherosclerosis, *Science* 208:1475–1476, 1980.

Noble WC, editor: *The skin microflora and microbial skin disease*, Cambridge, 2004, Cambridge University Press.

Nordlund JJ: The lives of pigment cells, *Dermatol Clin* 4:407–418, 1986.

Odland GF: Structure of the skin. In Goldsmith LA, editor: *Physiology, biochemistry, and molecular biology of the skin*, ed 2, New York, 1991, Oxford University Press.

Oluwasanmi JO: Keloids in the African, *Clin Plast Surg* 1:179–195, 1974.

Ortiz A, Grando SA: Smoking and the skin, *Int J Dermatol* 51:250–262, 2012.

Ottenbacher KJ, Muller L, Brandt D, et al: The effectiveness of tactile stimulation as a form of early intervention: a quantitative evaluation, *J Dev Behav Pediatr* 8:68–76, 1987.

Parish LC, Lowthian P, Witkowski JA: The decubitus ulcer: many questions but few definitive answers, *Clin Dermatol* 25(1):101–108, 2007.

Pathak MA, Fitzpatrick TB, Nghiem P, et al: Sun-protective agents: formulations, effects, and side effects. In Freedberg IM, et al, editors: *Fitzpatrick's dermatology in general medicine*, ed 5, New York, 1999, McGraw-Hill.

Pathak MA, Nghiem P, Fitzpatrick TB: Acute and chronic effects of the sun. In Freedberg IM, et al, editors: *Fitzpatrick's dermatology in general medicine*, ed 5, New York, 1999, McGraw-Hill pp 1598–1607.

Pollack SV: Systemic medications and wound healing, *Int J Dermatol* 21:489–496, 1982.

Potts JF: Sunlight, sunburn, and sunscreens, *Postgrad Med* 87:52–55, 59–60, 63, 1990.

Quinton PM: Sweating and its disorders, *Annu Rev Med* 34:429–452, 1983.

Ramdial PK, Naidoo DK: Drug-induced cutaneous pathology, *J Clin Pathol* 62(6):493–504, 2009.

Rezvani HR, Ali N, Nissen LJ, et al: HIF-1α in epidermis: oxygen sensing, cutaneous angiogenesis, cancer, and non-cancer disorders, *J Invest Dermatol* 131:1793–1805, 2011.

Rienertson RP, Wheatley VR: Studies on the chemical composition of human epidermal lipids, *J Invest Dermatol* 32:49–59, 1959.

Rigel DS, Russak J, Friedman R: The evolution of melanoma diagnosis: 25 years beyond the ABCDs, *CA Cancer J Clin* 60:301–316, 2010.

Roberts AB, Sporn MB: Transforming growth factor-B. In Clark RAF, editor: *The molecular and cellular biology of wound repair*, ed 2, New York, 1996, Plenum Press pp 275–308.

Robles DT, Berg D: Abnormal wound healing: keloids, *Clin Dermatol* 25(1):26–32, 2007.

Roe DA: *Nutrition and the skin*, New York, 1986, Liss.

Roth RR, James WD: Microbial ecology of the skin, *Annu Rev Microbiol* 42:441–464, 1988.

Rouhani P, Hu S, Kirsner RS: Melanoma in Hispanic and black Americans, *Cancer Control* 15:248–253, 2008.

Rudowski W: *Burn therapy and research*, Baltimore, 1976, Johns Hopkins University Press.

Rutter N: The immature skin, *Eur J Pediatr* 155:S18–S20, 1996.

Rutter N: The immature skin, *Br Med Bull* 44: 957–970, 1988.

Sams WM: Structure and function of the skin. In Sams WM, Lynch PJ, editors: *Principles and practice of dermatology*, New York, 1990, Churchill Livingstone.

Sauder DN: Effect of age on epidermal immune function, *Dermatol Clin* 4:447–454, 1986.

Scheibner A, Hollis DE, McCarthy WH, et al: Effects of sunlight exposure on Langerhans cells and melanocytes in human epidermis, *Photodermatology* 3:15–25, 1986.

Schram SE, Warshaw EM, Laumann A: Nickel hypersensitivity: a clinical review and call to action, *Int J Dermatol* 49:115–125, 2010.

Shuster S, Fisher GH, Harris E, et al: The effect of skin disease on self image, *Br J Dermatol* 90(Suppl 16):18–19, 1978.

Siebert JW, Burd AR, McCarthy JG, et al: Fetal wound healing: a biochemical study of scarless healing, *Plast Reconstr Surg* 85:495–502, 1990.

Silverberg N, Silverberg L: Aging and the skin, *Postgrad Med* 86:131–136, 1989.

Simanski M, Köten B, Schröder JM, et al: Antimicrobial RNases in cutaneous defense, *J Innate Immun* 4:241–247, 2012.

Solomons B: *Lecture notes on dermatology*, ed 5, Oxford, 1983, Blackwell Scientific.

Spince AP, Mason EB: *Human anatomy and physiology*, Menlo Park, CA, 1987, Benjamin/Cummings.

Spitz R: An inquiry into the genesis of psychiatric conditions in early childhood. In Nagera H, editor: *Psychoanalytical studies of the child*, vol 2, London, 1947, International.

Steel KP, Barkway C: Another role for melanocytes: their importance for stria vascularis development in the mammalian inner ear, *Development* 107:453–463, 1989.

Stender IM, Blichmann C, Serup J: Effects of oil and water baths on the hydration state of the epidermis, *Clin Exp Dermatol* 15:206–209, 1990.

Stierner U, Rosdahl I, Augustsson A, et al: UVB irradiation induces melanocyte increase in both exposed and shielded human skin, *J Invest Dermatol* 92:561–564, 1989.

Stryer L: *Biochemistry*, ed 4, New York, 1995, Freeman.

Szabo G: The number of melanocytes in human epidermis, *Br Med J* 1:1016–1017, 1954.

Szabo G, Gerald AB, Pathak MA, et al: Racial differences in the fate of melanosomes in human epidermis, *Nature* 222:1081–1082, 1969.

Szabo G, Gerald AB, Pathak MA 7 Fitzpatrick TB, et al: The ultrastructure of racial color differences in man. In Riley V, editor: *Pigmentation: its genesis and biological control*, New York, 1972, Appleton-Century-Crofts pp 23–41.

Tadokoro T, Yamaguchi Y, Batzer J, et al: Mechanisms of skin tanning in different racial/ethnic groups in response to ultraviolet radiation, *J Invest Dermatol* 124:1326–1331, 2005.

Taylor SC: Skin of color: biology, structure, function, and implications for dermatologic disease, *J Am Acad Dermatol* 46(2 Suppl Understanding):S41–S62, 2002.

Taylor SC: Epidemiology of skin diseases in people of color, *Cutis* 71:271–272, 2003.

Tobin A-M, Ahern T, Rogers S, et al: The dermatological consequences of obesity, *Int J Dermatol* 52:927–932, 2013.

U.S. Census Bureau: An older and more diverse nation by midcentury. (n.d.) The Free Library. (2014). Retrieved July 17, 2015 from http://www.thefreelibrary.com/An+Older+and+More+Diverse+Nation+by+Midcentury.-a0182890016.

van der Horst FCP, Leroy HA, van der Veer R: "When strangers meet": John Bowlby and Harry Harlow on attachment behavior, *Integr Psych Behav* 42:370–388, 2008.

Van Loey NE, Van Son MJ: Psychopathology and psychological problems in patients with burn scars: epidemiology and management, *Am J Clin Dermatol* 4(4):245–272, 2003.

Varani J, Dame MK, Rittie L, et al: Decreased collagen production in chronologically aged skin: roles of age-dependent alteration in fibroblast function and defective mechanical stimulation, *Am J Pathol* 168:1861–1868, 2006.

Warner RR, Myers MC, Taylor DA: Electron probe analysis of human skin: determination of the water concentration profile, *J Invest Dermatol* 90(2):218–224, 1988.

Weinberg AN, Swartz MN: General considerations of bacterial diseases. In Fitzpatrick TB, *Dermatology in general medicine: textbook and atlas*, New York, 1987, McGraw-Hill.

Wenger CB: Thermoregulation. In Freedberg IM, et al, editors: *Fitzpatrick's dermatology in general medicine*, ed 5, New York, 1999, McGraw-Hill.

Weston WL, Lane AT: Neonatal dermatology. In Freedberg IM, et al, editors: *Fitzpatrick's dermatology in general medicine*, ed 5, New York, 1999, McGraw-Hill.

Wheater PR, Burkitt HG. *Functional histology: a text and colour atlas*. ed 2, Edinburgh, 1987, Churchill Livingstone.

White MI, Jenkinson DM, Lloyd DH: The effect of washing on the thickness of the stratum corneum in normal and atopic individuals, *Br J Dermatol* 116:525–530, 1987.

Wicke C, Halliday B, Allen D, et al: Effects of steroids and retinoids on wound healing, *Arch Surg* 135(11):1265–1270, 2000.

Wilkins CH, Birge SJ, Sheline YI, et al: Vitamin D deficiency is associated with worse cognitive performance and lower bone density in older African Americans, *J Natl Med Assoc* 101(4): 349–354, 2009.

Wolff K, Stingl G: The Langerhans cell, *J Invest Dermatol* 80:17S–21S, 1983.

Woodburne RT, Burkel WE: *Essentials of human anatomy*, New York, 1988, Oxford University Press.

Wysocki AB: A review of the skin and its appendages, *Adv Wound Care* 8(2 Pt 1):53–54, 56–62, 1995.

Wysocki AB: Evaluating and managing open skin wounds: colonization versus infection, *AACN Clin Issues* 13(3): 382–397, 2002.

Wysocki AB, et al: Skin, molecular cell biology of. In Meyers RA, editor: *Encyclopedia of molecular cell biology and molecular medicine*, ed 2, vol 13, Weinheim, Germany, 2005, Wiley-VCH Verlag GmbH & Co. KgaA, pp 217–250.

Xu KD, McFeters GA, Stewart PS: Biofilm resistance to antimicrobial agents, *Microbiol* 146:547–549, 2000.

Yaar M, Gilchrest FA: Photoageing: mechanism, prevention and therapy, *Br J Dermatol* 157:874–887, 2007.

Yamaguchi Y, Hearing VJ: Physiological factors that regulate skin pigmentation, *Biofactors* 35(2):193–199, 2009.

Yamaguchi Y, Beer JZ, Hearing VJ: Melanin mediated apoptosis of epidermal cells damaged by ultraviolet radiation: factors influencing the incidence of skin cancer, *Arch Dermatol Res* 300(Suppl 1):S43–S50, 2008.

Yanagishita M: A brief history of proteoglycans, *EXS* 70:3–7, 1994.

Young AR, Walker SL: Acute and chronic effects of ultraviolet radiation on the skin. In Wolff K, et al, editors: *Fitzpatrick's dermatology in general medicine*, ed 7, New York, 2008, McGraw-Hill.

4

Wound-Healing Physiology and Factors that Affect the Repair Process

Dorothy B. Doughty and Bonnie Sparks

OBJECTIVES

1. Compare and contrast wound-healing processes for each type of closure: primary intention, secondary intention, and tertiary intention.
2. Distinguish between partial-thickness wound repair and full-thickness wound repair, addressing the key components, phases, usual timeframes, and wound appearance.
3. Explain the difference between acute and chronic full-thickness wounds.
4. Describe four characteristics of a chronic wound.
5. Describe the role of the following cells in the wound repair process: platelets, polymorphonuclear leukocytes,

macrophages, fibroblasts, endothelial cells, and keratinocytes.
6. Explain how bioactive agents (e.g., growth factors and cytokines) and extracellular matrix proteins (e.g., matrix metalloproteinases and tissue inhibitors of metalloproteinases) help to regulate the repair process.
7. Describe features and characteristics of scarless healing.
8. Distinguish between keloid and hypertrophic scarring and the treatment of each.
9. Identify conditions and comorbidities that affect the wound-healing process.

For centuries, wound healing was regarded as a mysterious process, with wound management based on practitioner preference as opposed to scientific principles. Research over the past 3 decades has contributed much information regarding the wound-healing process and the factors that facilitate it. We now know that repair is an extremely complex process involving hundreds, possibly thousands, of overlapping and "linked" processes (Goldman, 2004). It is critical for all wound care clinicians to base their interventions and recommendations on current data and to remain abreast of new findings and their implications for care. This chapter reviews the process of wound healing and discusses the implications for wound management.

MECHANISM OF WOUND HEALING

The ability to repair tissue damage is an important survival tool for any living organism. Regardless of the type or severity of injury, repair occurs by only two mechanisms—regeneration, or replacement of the damaged or lost tissue with more of the same, and scar formation, replacement of damaged or lost tissue with connective tissue that lacks some of the functions of the original tissue. Regeneration is the preferred mechanism of repair because normal function and appearance are maintained. Scar formation is a less

satisfactory alternative and occurs when the tissues involved are incapable of regeneration. Many invertebrate and amphibian species have the ability to regenerate entire limbs. Humans have only limited capacity for regeneration, and most wounds heal by scar formation (Calvin, 1998; Mast and Schultz, 1996; Wilgus, 2007).

In humans, the mechanism of repair for any specific wound is determined by the tissue layers involved and their capacity for regeneration. Wounds that are confined to the epidermal and superficial dermal layers heal by regeneration because epithelial, endothelial, and connective tissue can be reproduced. In contrast, deep dermal structures (e.g., hair follicles, sebaceous glands, sweat glands), subcutaneous tissue, muscle, tendons, ligaments, and bone lack the capacity to regenerate; therefore loss of these structures is permanent, and wounds involving these structures must heal by scar formation (Martin, 1997; Mast and Schultz, 1996).

The standard repair mechanism for human soft tissue wounds is connective tissue (scar) formation; however, an exception to this rule is the early-gestation fetus. Intrauterine surgical procedures performed during the second trimester result in scarless healing, a phenomenon that has been consistently reproduced in laboratory studies. Interestingly, the fetus loses the ability to heal without scarring at approximately 22 to 24 weeks' gestation. Repair during the third trimester and the postnatal period follows the "usual" rules for repair and results in scar formation. A number of differences in the molecular environment for repair in the early-gestation fetus are thought to contribute to scarless repair and are discussed throughout this chapter (Bullard et al, 2002; Dang et al, 2003; Wilgus, 2007; Yang et al, 2003).

The mechanism of healing for a specific wound depends on the tissue layers involved (partial-thickness vs. full-thickness), onset and duration (acute vs. chronic), and type of wound closure (primary, secondary, or tertiary intention).

Partial Thickness/Full Thickness

Partial-thickness wounds involve only partial loss of the skin layers; that is, they are confined to the epidermal and superficial dermal layers. Full-thickness wounds involve total loss of the skin layers (epidermis and dermis) and frequently involve loss of the deeper tissue layers as well (subcutaneous tissue, muscle, and bone) (see Figure 3-1). The timeframe for repair and the repair process itself differ significantly for partial-thickness and full-thickness wounds.

Acute/Chronic

Acute wounds typically are traumatic or surgical in origin. Acute wounds occur suddenly, and in most individuals, move rapidly and predictably through the repair process and result in durable closure. In contrast, chronic wounds fail to proceed normally through the repair process. Chronic wounds frequently are caused by vascular compromise, chronic inflammation, or repetitive insults to the tissue, and they either fail to close in a timely manner or fail to result in durable closure (Brissett and Hom, 2003; Pradhan et al, 2009).

Primary, Secondary, Tertiary

Classification of repair as primary-, secondary-, or tertiary-intention healing is based on the ideal of primary surgical closure for all wounds. Primary closure minimizes the volume of connective tissue deposition required for wound repair and restores the epithelial barrier to infection (Figure 4-1, A). Approximated surgical incisions are said to heal by primary intention; they usually heal quickly, with minimal scar formation, as long as infection and secondary breakdown are prevented. Wounds that are left open and allowed to heal by scar formation are classified as healing by secondary intention (Figure 4-1, B). These wounds heal more slowly because of the volume of connective tissue required to fill the defect. They are vulnerable to infection because they lack the epidermal barrier to microorganisms until late in the repair process. These wounds are characterized by prolongation of the inflammatory and proliferative phases of healing. Chronic wounds such as pressure ulcers and dehisced incisions typically heal by secondary intention. Wounds managed with delayed closure are classified as healing by tertiary intention, or delayed primary closure (Figure 4-1, C). This approach is sometimes required for abdominal incisions complicated by significant infection (Gabriel et al, 2010). Closure and/or

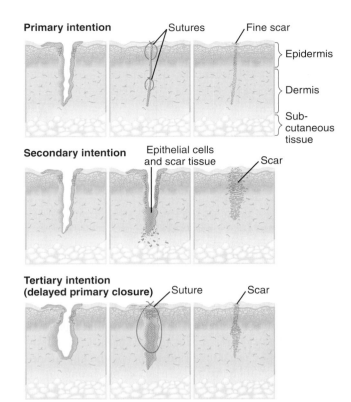

FIGURE 4-1 A, Wound healing by primary intention, such as with a surgical incision. Wound edges are approximated and secured with sutures, staples, or adhesive tapes, and healing occurs by epithelialization and connective tissue deposition. **B,** Wound healing by secondary intention. Wound edges are not approximated, and healing occurs by granulation tissue formation, contraction of the wound edges, and epithelialization. **C,** Wound healing by tertiary (delayed primary) intention. Wound is kept open for several days. The superficial wound edges then are approximated, and the center of the wound heals by granulation tissue formation. (From Black JM, Hawks JH: *Medical surgical nursing, clinical management for positive outcomes*, ed 7, St. Louis, MO, 2005, Saunders.)

approximation of the wound is delayed until the risk of infection is resolved and the wound is free of debris.

WOUND-HEALING PROCESS

Wound healing is best understood as a cascade of events. Injury sets into motion a series of physiologic responses that are coordinated and sequenced and that, under normal circumstances, result in durable repair. Critical factors in the repair process include the cells that establish a clean wound bed and generate the tissue to fill the defect, the bioactive molecules that control cellular activity (growth factors and cytokines), and the wound-healing environment (extracellular matrix [ECM]). The wound-healing environment (matrix) provides a scaffold that promotes cell migration, and it contains a number of substances that regulate the activity of growth factors and cytokines and promote cell migration (e.g., matrix metalloproteinases) (Cheresh and Stupack, 2008; Gill and Parks, 2008; Macri and Clark, 2009).

Our current understanding of wound repair is based primarily on acute wound-healing models. Therefore the processes for partial-thickness wound healing and full-thickness wound healing by primary intention are presented first, followed by a discussion of the repair process for wounds that heal by secondary intention.

Partial-Thickness Wound Repair

Partial-thickness wounds are shallow wounds involving epidermal loss and possibly partial loss of the dermal layer (see Plate 1). Partial-thickness wounds typically are less than 0.2 cm in depth. These wounds are moist and painful because of the loss of the epidermal covering and the resultant exposure of nerve endings. When the wound involves loss of the epidermis with exposure of the basement membrane, the wound base appears bright pink or red. In the presence of partial dermal loss, the wound base usually appears pale pink with distinct red "islets." These "islets" represent the basement membrane of the epidermis, which projects deep into the dermis to line the epidermal appendages. These islands of epidermal basement membrane are important in partial-thickness wound healing because all epidermal cells are capable of regeneration, and each islet will serve as a source of new epithelium (Hunt and Van Winkle, 1997; Winter, 1979).

The major components of partial-thickness repair include an initial inflammatory response to injury, epithelial proliferation and migration (resurfacing), and reestablishment and differentiation of the epidermal layers to restore the barrier function of the skin (Monaco and Lawrence, 2003; Winter, 1979). If the wound involves dermal loss, connective tissue repair (granulation tissue formation) will proceed concurrently with epithelial repair (Table 4-1) (Jahoda and Reynolds, 2001).

Epidermal Repair. Tissue trauma triggers the processes that result in epidermal repair: an acute inflammatory response followed by epidermal mitosis and migration

(Harrison et al, 2006). The inflammatory response produces erythema, edema, and a serous exudate containing leukocytes. When this exudate is allowed to dry on the wound surface, a dry crust, commonly referred to as a "scab," is formed. In partial-thickness wounds, the inflammatory response is limited, typically subsiding in less than 24 hours (Winter, 1979).

Epidermal resurfacing begins as the inflammatory phase subsides and is dependent on two processes: proliferation of epidermal cells throughout the wound bed and lateral migration of the epidermal cells at the leading edge. In order to migrate laterally, the keratinocytes at the wound edge must undergo several changes. First they must acquire a migratory phenotype. This involves breakdown of their attachments to adjacent cells, the basement membrane, and the underlying dermis. These attachments normally prevent lateral migration and provide epithelial stability. The keratinocytes then must undergo cytoskeletal alterations that support lateral movement. These alterations include flattening of the cells at the advancing edge of the epithelium and formation of protrusions known as lamellipodia, which attach to binding sites in the wound bed. The migratory keratinocytes then move across the wound bed by alternately attaching to the ECM and then detaching and reattaching at a more distal point (Harrison et al, 2006; Monaco and Lawrence, 2003).

The epithelial cells within the wound bed continue this pattern of lateral migration until they contact epithelial cells migrating from the opposite direction. Once the epithelial cells meet, lateral migration ceases; this phenomenon is known as contact inhibition (Hunt and Van Winkle, 1997; Monaco and Lawrence, 2003).

Epithelial resurfacing is supported by increased production of basal cells just behind the advancing edge and throughout the wound bed. The process typically peaks between 24 and 72 hours after injury. The rate of reepithelialization is affected by a number of factors of clinical significance. For example, resurfacing is promoted by maintenance of a moist wound surface. Winter (1979) found that partial-thickness wounds left open to air required 6 to 7 days to resurface, whereas moist wounds reepithelialized in 4 days. This is because cells can migrate much more rapidly in a moist environment (Figure 4-2). In contrast, when the surface of the wound is covered with a scab, migration is delayed while the epithelial cells secrete enzymes known as matrix metalloproteinases (MMPs). The MMPs lift the scab by cleaving the bonds that attach it to the wound bed, creating a moist pathway that supports keratinocyte migration (Harrison et al, 2006; Monaco and Lawrence, 2003; Winter, 1979). Interestingly, hypoxic conditions in the wound bed also serve to stimulate keratinocyte migration, probably through increased production of the MMPs that promote lateral migration. This positive response to wound bed hypoxia is lost in the elderly, which may be one factor contributing to slower rates of reepithelialization in the aged (O'Toole et al, 2008). In contrast, high bacteria levels may serve as an impediment to reepithelialization. Data indicate that keratinocyte migration

TABLE 4-1	**Partial-Thickness Repair**	
Level of Injury (Tissue Layers Involved)	**Primary Phases of Repair**	**Outcomes**
Epidermal loss	Inflammation (brief) Epithelial resurfacing Restoration of normal epithelial thickness/ repigmentation	No loss of function No scar No change in skin appearance or color
Possible partial dermal loss	Dermal repair (if dermal loss involved)	Restoration of rete ridges/ dermal papillae when dermis involved

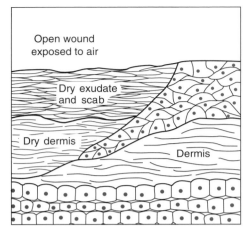

FIGURE 4-2 Migration of epidermal cells in moist environment and dry environment.

is inhibited by bacterial byproducts such as lipopolysaccharide (Loryman and Mansbridge, 2008). In vivo evidence strongly suggests that elevated glucose levels are another major impediment to epidermal proliferation and migration. This may be one factor contributing to delayed healing of superficial wounds in diabetic patients with poorly controlled glucose levels (Lan et al, 2008).

The newly resurfaced epithelium appears pale, pink, and dry in people of all races (see Plate 1). Because it is only a few cell layers thick, the new epithelium is very fragile and requires protection against mechanical forces such as superficial shear and friction.

Once epithelial resurfacing is complete, the epithelial cells resume vertical migration and epidermal differentiation so that normal epidermal thickness and function are restored. The normal anchors to adjacent epidermal cells and to the basement membrane are reestablished (Harrison et al, 2006). The "new" epidermis gradually repigments, matching the individual's normal skin tone (see Plate 1). This is clinically relevant, as the wound is not completely healed until repigmentation has occurred (Monaco and Lawrence, 2003).

Regulatory factors. The processes of epithelial proliferation and migration are regulated by a complex interplay between various MMPs and selected growth factors. Specifically, lateral migration is dependent on normal levels and function of multiple MMPs, which serve to break the attachments that bind the edge keratinocytes to adjacent cells and the underlying wound bed. In addition to playing a key role in establishment of a migratory phenotype, MMPs facilitate continued resurfacing by assisting the migrating keratinocytes to detach from the wound bed. Repetitive detachment and distal reattachment are critical to the resurfacing process (Gill and Parks, 2008). Epithelial proliferation is dependent in part on keratinocyte attachment to the ECM and in part on exposure to growth factors. Keratinocyte attachment is required for the cell to exit from the G_0 phase of mitosis, and growth factors are required to stimulate cellular reproduction. A number of growth factors promote keratinocyte proliferation includeing transforming growth factor-α (TGF-α), keratinocyte growth factor, platelet-derived growth factor (PDGF), and epidermal growth factor (EGF). See Chapter 20 for a detailed discussion of the molecular factors regulating wound repair.

Dermal Repair. In wounds involving both dermal and epidermal loss, dermal repair proceeds concurrently with reepithelialization. By the fifth day after injury, a layer of fluid separates the epidermis from the dermal tissue. New blood vessels begin to sprout, and fibroblasts become plentiful by about the seventh day. Collagen fibers are visible in the wound bed by the ninth day. Collagen synthesis continues to produce new connective tissue until about 10 to 15 days after injury. This new connective tissue grows upward into the fluid layer. At the same time, the flat epidermis falls down around the new vessels and collagen fibers, re-creating ridges at the dermal–epidermal junction. As the new connective tissue gradually contracts, the epidermis is drawn close to the dermis (Winter, 1979). Insulin and insulin-like growth factor may contribute to reformation of the dermal–epidermal junction.

Full-Thickness Wound Repair: Wounds Healing by Primary Intention

Full-thickness wounds, by definition, extend at least to the subcutaneous tissue layer and possibly as deep as the fascia–muscle layer or bone (see Plate 2). Full-thickness wounds may be either acute or chronic. This section addresses acute wound healing by primary intention, such as a surgical incision.

Many steps are involved in full-thickness repair, but they are commonly conceptualized as four major phases: hemostasis, inflammation, proliferation, and remodeling. Considerable overlap exists among the phases, and the cells involved in one phase produce the chemical stimuli and substances that serve to move the wound into the next phase. Thus normal repair is a complex and well-orchestrated series of events (Figure 4-3) and is affected by a number of systemic and local factors, including the wound environment.

Hemostasis. Any acute injury extending beyond the epidermis causes bleeding, which activates a series of overlapping events designed to control blood loss, establish bacterial control, and seal the defect. Immediately upon injury, disruption of blood vessels exposes the subendothelial collagen to platelets, which trigger platelet activation and aggregation. Simultaneously, injured cells in the wound area release clotting factors that activate both the intrinsic and extrinsic coagulation pathways. As part of the coagulation pathway, circulating prothrombin is converted to thrombin, which is used to convert fibrinogen to fibrin. The end result is formation of a clot composed of fibrin, aggregated platelets, and blood cells. Hemostasis is further accomplished by a brief period of vasoconstriction mediated by thromboxane A_2 and prostaglandin 2-α, substances released by the damaged cells and activated platelets. Clot formation seals the disrupted vessels so that blood loss is controlled. The clot also provides a temporary bacterial barrier, a reservoir of growth factors, and an interim matrix that serves as scaffolding for migrating cells (Brissett and Hom, 2003; Monaco and Lawrence, 2003; Phillips, 2000).

Clot formation, followed by fibrinolysis (clot breakdown), is a critical event in the sequence of wound healing (Figure 4-4). The activation and degranulation of platelets cause the α-granules and dense bodies of the platelets to rupture, releasing a potent "cocktail" of energy-producing compounds and cytokines/growth factors (including complement factor C5a). These substances attract the cells needed to begin the repair process. They also provide fuel for the energy-intensive process of wound healing. The platelet-derived substances thought to be most critical to repair include PDGF, TGF-β, and fibroblast growth factor-2. Thus

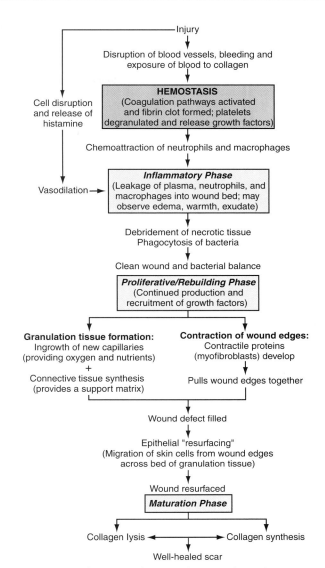

FIGURE 4-4 Cascade of events in wound repair process.

hemostasis, which is the body's normal response to tissue injury, actually initiates the entire wound-healing cascade. The importance of hemostasis to wound healing is underscored by the finding that inadequate clot formation is associated with impaired wound healing and that the extrinsic coagulation pathway is critical to repair (Brissett and Hom, 2003; Monaco and Lawrence, 2003).

Inflammation. Once the bleeding is controlled, the focus becomes control of infection and establishment of a clean wound bed. This process can be compared with the repair of a damaged home or building. Before rebuilding can begin, the damaged components must be removed. Wound "cleanup" involves breakdown of any devitalized tissue and elimination of excess bacteria by a team of white blood cells. Acute wounds, such as sutured lacerations or incisions, typically have limited devitalized tissue and low bacterial loads, so the cleanup phase usually is brief, lasting only hours to a few days (Braiman-Wiksman et al, 2007; Pradhan et al, 2009).

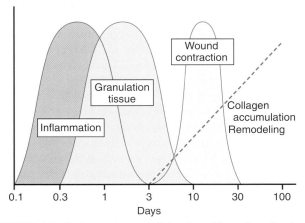

FIGURE 4-3 Orderly phases of healing. Time line (in days) reflects healing trajectory of acute wound healing model. (Modified from Clark RA: Cutaneous wound repair. In Goldsmith LA, editor: *Physiology, biochemistry and molecular biology of the skin*, ed 2, vol 1, New York, 1991, Oxford University Press. Found in Kumar V, Cotran RS, Robbins ST: *Robbins basic pathology*, ed 7, Philadelphia, 2003, Saunders.)

Within 10 to 15 minutes after injury, vasoconstriction subsides, followed by vasodilation and increased capillary permeability. Vasoactive substances released by damaged cells and by clot breakdown (histamine, prostaglandins, complement factor, thrombin) mediate this response. The dilated capillaries permit plasma and blood cells to leak into the wound bed. Clinically, this process is observed as edema, erythema, and exudate. At the same time, the damaged cells and platelets produce cytokines and growth factors that attract leukocytes (neutrophils, macrophages, lymphocytes) to the wound bed. The twin processes of chemoattraction and vasodilation result in the delivery of multiple phagocytic cells to the wound site within minutes of injury (Gill and Parks, 2008; Pradhan et al, 2009; Rodriguez et al, 2008).

Leukocyte migration out of the vessels and into the wound bed occurs via margination and diapedesis. Margination involves adherence of the leukocytes to the endothelial cells lining the capillaries in the wound bed. Integrins on the surface of the leukocytes attach to cell adhesion molecules on the surface of the endothelial cells, causing the leukocytes to "line up" against the vessel wall. Through a process known as diapedesis, the leukocytes migrate through the dilated capillaries into the wound bed (Cross and Mustoe, 2003; Monaco and Lawrence, 2003; Wilgus, 2007).

The first leukocytes to arrive in the wound space, the neutrophils, are present in the wound bed within minutes after injury and dominate the scene for the first 2 to 3 days. The primary function of neutrophils is phagocytosis of bacteria and foreign debris. Neutrophils first bind to the damaged tissue or target bacteria via cell adhesion molecules and then engulf and destroy the target molecules via intracellular enzymes and free oxygen radicals. In addition, growth factors released by the neutrophils attract additional leukocytes to the area (Cross and Mustoe, 2003).

By days 3 to 4 after injury, the neutrophils begin to spontaneously disappear as a result of apoptosis and are replaced by macrophages (activated monocytes). The macrophages continue to phagocytize bacteria and break down damaged tissues as already described. In addition, the macrophages release a large number of potent growth factors that stimulate angiogenesis, fibroblast migration and proliferation, and connective tissue synthesis.

T lymphocytes are present in the wound tissue in peak quantities between days 5 and 7 after injury. T lymphocytes contribute to the inflammatory phase of wound healing by secreting additional wound-healing cytokines and by destroying viral organisms and foreign cells. Thus significant deficiencies of T lymphocytes can delay or compromise the repair process (Monaco and Lawrence, 2003).

Although all leukocytes contribute to elimination of bacteria and establishment of a clean wound bed, macrophages contribute the most significantly to the repair process. Studies indicate that wounds can heal without neutrophils, especially if no bacterial contamination is present. However, elimination of macrophages severely compromises wound repair (Cross and Mustoe, 2003; Gabriel et al, 2010).

The result of the inflammatory phase of wound healing is a clean wound bed. In acute wounds healing by primary intention, the inflammatory phase lasts approximately 3 days. At this point, bacterial levels usually are controlled, and any devitalized tissue has been removed. Elimination of these noxious stimuli allows the wound to transition to the "rebuilding" phase. This transition involves apoptosis of the inflammatory cells, possibly due in part to the effects of antiinflammatory cytokines and increased production of growth factors that promote proliferation as opposed to inflammation (Demidova-Rice et al, 2012; Goldman, 2004). However, in wounds complicated by necrosis and/or infection, the inflammatory phase is prolonged and wound healing is delayed (Burns et al, 2003). A prolonged inflammatory phase increases the risk for wound dehiscence because approximation of the incision is totally dependent on the closure material (sutures, staples, fibrin glue) until sufficient connective tissue has been synthesized to provide tensile strength to the incision. (Tensile strength during the inflammatory phase is 0%.)

Factors affecting the duration and intensity of inflammation. The intensity and duration of the inflammatory phase appear to be critical factors in the amount of scar tissue produced. Numerous studies support a strong link between prolonged inflammation and hyperproliferative scarring (Dubay and Franz, 2003; Pradhan et al, 2009; Rahban and Garner, 2003; Robson, 2003). Thus the clinician needs to have a clear understanding of both proinflammatory and antiinflammatory factors and the implications for wound management. As noted, local factors such as bacterial load and presence of devitalized tissue are major proinflammatory factors that should be aggressively managed through debridement and appropriate use of topical dressings and antimicrobial agents (Demidova-Rice et al, 2012). Necrotic tissue and infection trigger production of cytokines that attract excessive numbers of inflammatory cells to the wound bed; these inflammatory cells produce reactive oxygen species (ROS) that, in conjunction with proinflammatory cytokines, cause degradation of the growth factors needed for normal function of proliferative cells such as fibroblasts. Thus necrosis and infection are major impediments to wound healing.

The ECM is another important determinant; it can either promote or inhibit inflammation, depending on the types of MMPs produced and their functions. Some MMPs promote inflammation by releasing proinflammatory cytokines from the cells in the wound bed; proinflammatory cytokines attract inflammatory cells to the wound bed (Pradhan et al, 2009). Other MMPs inhibit inflammation by degrading proinflammatory cytokines or inhibiting their release. For example, tumor necrosis factor-α (TNF-α) is a proinflammatory cytokine that normally is present at high levels during the early inflammatory phase, and levels of TNF-α are controlled by two ECM proteins. One protein, a disintegrin and metalloproteinase (ADAM-17), promotes release of TNF-α. Another protein, a tissue inhibitor of metalloproteinase-3 (TIMP-3), controls ADAM-17, thereby reducing production of TNF-α. Research is ongoing into factors that determine the combination and concentration of ECM proteins and into strategies for measuring and controlling levels of various MMPs to achieve therapeutic outcomes (Gill and Parks, 2008; Macri and Clark, 2009).

Diabetes is a clinical condition associated with prolonged inflammation. Some data suggest that leukocyte migration may be impaired in people with this condition; in addition, the leukocytes that do migrate to the wound bed frequently are dysfunctional, especially in the presence of hyperglycemia. The end result of diminished leukocyte migration and impaired leukocyte function is failure to effectively control bacterial loads. This situation results in a persistent stimulus for proinflammatory cytokines, chronic inflammation, and delayed healing (Pradhan et al, 2009). Conditions resulting in ischemia/hypoxia also produce prolonged inflammation, because oxygen and ROS are required for oxidative killing of bacteria. The inability to control bacteria that accompanies hypoxia results in chronic inflammation and failure to heal. Hyperbaric oxygen therapy can improve tissue oxygen levels, contribute to bacterial control, and reduce the production of proinflammatory cytokines, thus promoting the repair process (Rodriguez et al, 2008; Thom, 2009).

Conditions and medications that affect the function of autonomic and sensory nerves and their receptors may also affect inflammation. For example, diabetes is associated with diminished production of substance P, a neuropeptide that normally contributes to a healthy inflammatory response by supporting vasodilation and leukocyte migration. Diminished production of substance P may be one factor leading to compromised inflammation and impaired healing in the diabetic population (Pradhan et al, 2009). Preliminary research suggests β-adrenergic agents may reduce inflammation by reducing neutrophil recruitment and production of inflammatory cytokines (Pullar et al, 2008).

Proliferation. The third phase of acute full-thickness wound healing is the proliferative phase. During this phase, the wound surface is covered with new epithelium that restores the bacterial barrier, vascular integrity is restored, and the incisional defect is mended with new connective tissue. The key components of the proliferative phase are epithelialization, neoangiogenesis, and matrix deposition/collagen synthesis. Limited contraction of the newly formed ECM also may occur.

Epithelialization. Epithelialization of a full-thickness wound healing by primary intention begins within hours after injury and typically is complete within 24 to 48 hours. This "neoepithelium" is only a few cells thick but is sufficient to provide a closed wound surface and a bacterial barrier. This process is the basis for the Centers for Disease Control and Prevention's recommendation that new surgical incisions be covered with a sterile dressing for the first 24 to 48 hours postoperatively. Until reepithelialization is complete, the potential for bacterial invasion exists, and the wound should be managed with sterile wound care and a cover dressing that

provides a bacterial barrier (Mangram et al, 1999; Yamamoto et al, 2014). As with partial-thickness wound repair, the processes of lateral migration, vertical migration, and differentiation continue throughout the proliferative phase and gradually reestablish epidermal thickness and function (Braiman-Wiksman et al, 2007; Myers et al, 2007). In full-thickness wounds, the new epidermis is slightly thinner than the original epidermis. Because the neoepidermis is covering scar tissue rather than normal dermis, the rete pegs that normally dip into the dermis are lacking (Monaco and Lawrence, 2003).

Granulation tissue formation. A hallmark outcome of the proliferative phase is the formation of granulation tissue, which begins as the inflammatory phase subsides, at 3 to 4 days postinjury (Braiman-Wiksman et al, 2007). Granulation tissue is composed primarily of capillary loops and newly synthesized connective tissue proteins and is often referred to as the ECM. Fibroblasts and inflammatory cells also are present in this new matrix. Neoangiogenesis and connective tissue synthesis occur simultaneously in a codependent fashion to form the new ECM that will fill the wound defect. Through angiogenesis, new capillaries are formed and joined with existing severed capillaries, thus restoring the delivery of oxygen and nutrients to the wound bed. At the same time, a new "provisional" ECM is formed through the synthesis of connective tissue proteins such as type III collagen (Figure 4-5) (Pradhan et al, 2009).

Neoangiogenesis. Endothelial cells typically are quiescent. Neoangiogenesis requires stimulation by growth factors, which convert the quiescent cells to actively proliferating cells. Molecules in the ECM also play a critical role by influencing the response of endothelial cells to angiogenic growth factors (Cheresh and Stupack, 2008). Neoangiogenesis occurs by two mechanisms: production of new vessels by local endothelial cells and recruitment of circulating stem progenitor cells to form new vessels de novo (Thom, 2009).

The growth factors that stimulate production of new vessels are produced by the cells in the wound bed (injured endothelial cells, macrophages, fibroblasts, keratinocytes) and include vascular endothelial growth factor (VEGF), basic fibroblast growth factor, and possibly PDGF. The most important angiogenic growth factor is VEGF; in addition to stimulating local endothelial cells to proliferate and migrate, VEGF attracts stem progenitor cells to the wound bed and stimulates them to differentiate into endothelial cells (Braiman-Wiksman et al, 2007; Gill and Parks, 2008; Thom, 2009). A number of ECM factors also affect neoangiogenesis. One is the provisional matrix itself, which affects the migration of endothelial cells (Gill and Parks, 2008). Another is the level of TIMP-3, which has a very negative effect on angiogenesis. TIMP-3 binds to the receptor sites for VEGF and blocks its angiogenic effects (Gill and Parks, 2008). A third factor is the level of nitric oxide, which promotes angiogenesis by activating MMP-13 (Lizarbe et al, 2008).

Clinical factors affecting neoangiogenesis include oxygen levels within the wound bed, patient age, gender, diabetes,

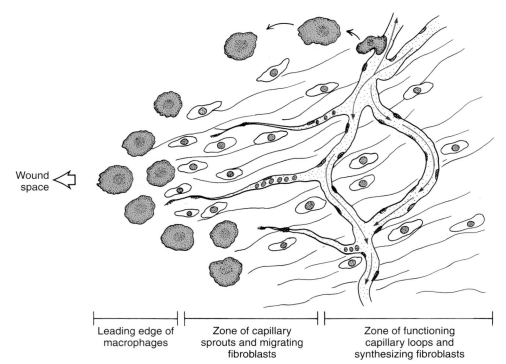

Wound
space

| Leading edge of macrophages | Zone of capillary sprouts and migrating fibroblasts | Zone of functioning capillary loops and synthesizing fibroblasts |

FIGURE 4-5 Advancing module of reparative tissue during proliferative and remodeling phases. (From Whalen GF, Zetter BR: Angiogenesis. In Cohen IK, Dieglemann RF, Lindbald WJ, editors: *Wound healing: biochemical and clinical aspects*, Philadelphia, 1992, Saunders.)

coronary artery disease, radiation therapy, and chemotherapy. Hypoxia acts as an initial stimulus to angiogenesis, but persistent hypoxia interferes with endothelial cell proliferation and new vessel formation. Hyperglycemia and glycolysis are associated with production of substances that are toxic to endothelial cells. Diabetes, aging, female gender, coronary artery disease, radiation therapy, and chemotherapy all interfere with angiogenesis by reducing mobilization of stem progenitor cells, thus compromising the potential for de novo development of new vessels. Aging is also associated with dysfunction and impaired mobilization of local endothelial cells, partly due to impaired expression of VEGF and other angiogenic stimuli. Of interest, some data suggest that exercise can partially reverse these age-related changes (Hoenig et al, 2008; Rodriguez et al, 2008; Thom, 2009). Therapeutic modalities that may promote angiogenesis include exogenous application of basic fibroblast growth factor and topical or systemic administration of erythropoietin (EPO). Animal studies and limited human case reports indicate potent stimulation of angiogenesis and granulation tissue formation with each of these therapies; EPO has also been associated with inhibition of excessive inflammation (Hamed et al, 2014; O'Goshi and Tagami, 2007).

Matrix deposition/collagen synthesis. Fibroblasts are responsible for synthesis of the connective tissue proteins that compose the provisional ECM; therefore fibroblasts are critical to the repair process. Fibroblasts migrate into the wound bed from the surrounding tissues in response to growth factors

and interleukins released by degranulating platelets, activated leukocytes (neutrophils and macrophages), and keratinocytes. Migration requires up-regulation of binding sites (integrin receptors) on the cell wall, which is mediated by PDGF and TGF-β. This up-regulation of binding sites is essential because fibroblasts migrate by maintaining attachment to one binding site while extending lamellipodia in search of another site. Once the fibroblast is able to bind to a new site, it releases the original attachment and "moves" in the direction of the wound bed (Monaco and Lawrence, 2003; Myers et al, 2007).

Fibroblasts begin to appear in the wound bed toward the end of the inflammatory phase, 2 to 3 days after injury. By day 4, fibroblasts are the predominant cells in the wound matrix (Dubay and Franz, 2003). Once fibroblasts arrive at the wound site, growth factors bind to fibroblast receptor sites and trigger intracellular processes that move the fibroblasts into the reproductive phase of the cell cycle, thus stimulating proliferation of the fibroblast. Finally, the fibroblasts are converted into "wound fibroblasts" by TGF-β, a growth factor secreted by macrophages. These wound fibroblasts differ from typical dermal fibroblasts in that they exhibit decreased proliferative behavior but increased synthesis of connective tissue proteins such as collagen (Frank et al, 2002).

Collagen synthesis follows the established process for synthesis of any protein. The collagen molecule is characterized by a glycine-X-Y repeating sequence. The collagen molecule must undergo a series of intracellular modifications before the molecule is secreted into the extracellular environment and becomes part of the ECM. One of the most critical modifications is "cross-linking" of the proline and lysine molecules, a process known as hydroxylation. These cross-links are essential for the development of tensile strength. A number of factors are required for normal hydroxylation, including oxygen, ascorbic acid, iron, copper, and selected enzymes. Thus hypoxia, vitamin C deficiency, copper deficiency, and iron deficiency all can compromise hydroxylation and the development of tensile strength. High-dose corticosteroids also can impair tensile strength because corticosteroids suppress the enzymes needed for hydroxylation. Following intracellular modifications, the collagen molecule is secreted into the extracellular environment as the triple helix procollagen. It then undergoes additional steps that culminate in the formation of cross-linked fibrils. The enzyme lysyl oxidase is essential to these processes and to the development of stable collagen fibers (Monaco and Lawrence, 2003).

The early granulation tissue is a provisional matrix characterized by unstructured collagen and high levels of fibronectin. This provisional matrix also includes vibronectin, laminin, and proteoglycans such as hyaluronic acid (Braiman-Wiksman et al, 2007; Gill and Parks, 2008; Schneider et al, 2008). As the ECM matures, collagen becomes the predominant protein, representing a little over 50% of the new ECM. Proteoglycans such as hyaluronic acid are present in small amounts but serve critical functions. For example, hyaluronic acid facilitates cell migration, protects cells against free-radical and proteolytic damage, and contributes viscoelastic properties to the new matrix (Chen and Abatangelo, 1999; Monaco and Lawrence, 2003).

Wounds healing by primary intention, such as sutured incisions, require a limited amount of connective tissue to mend the defect. In these wounds, ECM production is essentially complete within 14 to 21 days (Hunt and Van Winkle, 1997; Monaco and Lawrence, 2003). Although the granulation tissue is not visible in these wounds, a "healing ridge" can be palpated just under the intact suture line by days 5 to 9. The healing ridge is produced by the newly formed connective tissue proteins. Absence of this healing ridge indicates impaired healing and increased risk for dehiscence (Hunt and Van Winkle, 1997).

Factors affecting granulation tissue formation. Factors affecting granulation tissue formation include perfusion status, oxygen levels, nutritional status, and glucose levels/diabetes. Granulation tissue formation is very much an oxygen-dependent process. Hypoxia can act as a stimulus to fibroblast proliferation and initial collagen synthesis, but adequate levels of oxygen (30–40 mm Hg) are absolutely essential for the latter steps in collagen synthesis and for the cross-linking that provides tensile strength. Adequate oxygen levels are also required for prevention of infection. Infection rates in surgical wounds are inversely proportional to oxygen levels (Rodriguez et al, 2008). Tissue oxygenation of acute wounds is discussed in more detail in Chapters 28 and 34. Nutritional status affects granulation because granulation tissue formation requires adequate

levels of protein and micronutrients such as ascorbic acid, iron, and copper. Diabetes is associated with delayed deposition of granulation tissue and insufficient production of collagen to establish a mature matrix (Braiman-Wiksman et al, 2007).

Contraction. Contraction occurs when specialized fibroblasts known as myofibroblasts exert tractional forces on the ECM, reducing the size of the wound. Wounds healing by primary intention have limited or no contraction because the wound edges have been surgically approximated (Monaco and Lawrence, 2003).

Maturation/Remodeling. The final phase in full-thickness wound healing is the maturation, or remodeling, phase, which begins around day 21 after wounding and continues beyond 1 year. The early collagen is characterized by poorly organized fibers having limited tensile strength. At 3 weeks after injury, the healing wound exhibits only 20% of the strength of intact dermis. The provisional matrix is gradually converted to a mature and relatively acellular scar, a process that involves replacement of the type III collagen in the provisional matrix with type I collagen, the type normally found in dermal tissue. However, even the final form of collagen does not exhibit the normal basket-weave pattern of the collagen in unwounded dermis. Rather, the fibers of "repair collagen" are aligned parallel to the stress lines of the wound. The new ECM also lacks elastin, which provides the uninjured skin with elasticity; thus scar tissue is "stiff" compared with normal tissue (Monaco and Lawrence, 2003; Rodriguez et al, 2008).

Remodeling involves the dual processes of synthesis and degradation of the ECM and is regulated by fibroblasts and ECM proteins (MMPs). The new collagen that is formed is more orderly and provides more tensile strength to the wound; tensile strength improves steadily during the 2 to 3 months following initial injury and repair. However, the tensile strength of the remodeled ECM (scar tissue) is never more than 80% of the tensile strength in nonwounded tissue (Hunt and Van Winkle, 1997).

An imbalance between the dual processes of matrix synthesis and matrix breakdown can complicate wound healing. For example, hypertrophic scarring and keloid formation are believed to be caused in part by an excess of matrix synthesis compared with matrix degradation (Rahban and Garner, 2003; Wilgus, 2007). In contrast, hypoxia, malnutrition, or excess levels of MMPs can interfere with synthesis and deposition of new matrix proteins, resulting in wound breakdown (Monaco and Lawrence, 2003).

Full-Thickness Wound Repair: Wounds Healing by Secondary Intention

Although full-thickness wounds healing by secondary intention (e.g., pressure ulcers) proceed through the same phases as full-thickness wounds healing by primary intention, key differences do exist within each phase. These differences are summarized in Table 4-2 and discussed here.

TABLE 4-2 Full-Thickness Repair Process

	Primary Intention	Secondary Intention
Examples	Laceration Surgical incision	Chronic wound (e.g., pressure ulcer, venous ulcer) Wound dehiscence
Hemostasis	Bleeding Platelets rupture and release growth factors Coagulation pathways (intrinsic and extrinsic) activated	No bleeding No coagulation Hemostasis absent
Inflammatory phase	Any necrotic tissue removed Bacterial balance restored Duration usually limited to 1–3 days unless complicated by infection	Necrotic tissue removed Bacterial balance restored Duration prolonged until nonviable tissue eliminated and bacteria controlled; also prolonged by presence of excess proinflammatory cells
Proliferative phase	Epithelialization (first event in proliferative phase) Synthesis of connective tissue Duration typically 14–21 days	Granulation tissue formation • Neoangiogenesis • Synthesis of connective tissue proteins Contraction of wound edges Epithelialization (last event in proliferative phase) Duration is dependent on size and depth of wound and host's ability to synthesize new extracellular matrix
Maturation (remodeling phase)	Collagen synthesis and lysis Tensile strength partially reestablished	Collagen synthesis and lysis Tensile strength partially reestablished

Absence of Hemostasis. The absence of hemostasis has a tremendous impact on the healing trajectory of wounds. Bleeding and hemostasis do not occur in wounds healing by secondary intention. Failure to bleed and clot compromises the repair process because the wound-healing sequence of events is normally initiated by clot breakdown and the subsequent release of growth factors. One theorized benefit of surgical debridement of chronic wounds is to trigger clot formation and the release of growth factors so that the repair process is reactivated.

Prolonged Inflammatory Phase. The inflammatory phase frequently is prolonged. Because the goal of this phase is to establish a clean wound bed and to obtain bacterial balance, the wound will remain in this phase until necrotic tissue has been eliminated and bacterial loads have been controlled. Wounds healing by secondary intention frequently are characterized by large amounts of devitalized tissue and heavy bacterial loads. Thus the inflammatory phase generally lasts considerably longer than the 3 days that are typical in the approximated incision.

Prolonged Proliferative Phase. The proliferative phase is prolonged, and the sequence of events is different. In wounds healing by primary intention, epithelialization occurs first, followed by angiogenesis and formation of a limited volume of connective tissue proteins (ECM); contraction does not occur or is very limited. These processes usually are complete within 14 to 21 days. In secondary-intention wound healing, the proliferative phase begins with granulation tissue formation (to fill in the soft tissue defect), followed by contraction (to minimize the defect); epithelialization is the final phase.

The volume of granulation tissue required to fill the defect (and the time required for this phase of repair) is determined by the size of the wound and the degree to which contraction is able to reduce the size of the defect. Because the wound bed is visible, the clinician is able to assess progress in healing. Healthy granulation tissue presents as a red, vascular, granular wound bed as a result of the numerous capillary loops in combination with the newly synthesized ECM proteins (see Plate 3).

Increased Amount of Contraction. Contraction is much more important in secondary-intention wound healing than in closed wounds because contraction reduces the size of the soft tissue defect and thus reduces the amount of granulation tissue required. The rate of contraction for open wounds averages 0.6 to 0.7 mm/day (Gabbiani, 2003; Monaco and Lawrence, 2003). The degree to which a specific wound will contract is determined partly by the mobility of the surrounding tissue. For example, the tissue surrounding sacral and abdominal wounds is quite mobile and can contract easily. In contrast, the tissue surrounding a wound on the extremity or overlying a bony prominence has limited potential for contraction. Contraction is considered undesirable in some wounds because it can cause cosmetic deformities or flexion contractures of joints.

Contraction is mediated by myofibroblasts, modified fibroblasts that contain actin and myosin monofilaments and smooth muscle proteins. Differentiation of fibroblasts into myofibroblasts is stimulated by growth factors such as TGF-β1 and PDGF. Substances within the ECM itself are also thought to contribute to the development of myofibroblasts. Intracellular actin filaments and extracellular fibronectin work jointly to establish a contractile force that compresses and "shrinks" the ECM, thus pulling the wound edges toward each other (Demidova-Rice et al, 2012; Gabbiani 2003).

Delayed Epithelialization. Because full-thickness wounds involve loss of the deep dermis and epidermal appendages (along with their epithelial lining), epithelialization in these wounds proceeds from the periphery of the wound inward in a centripetal fashion. Epithelial migration requires an open, proliferative wound edge. Closed, nonproliferative wound edges, also known as epibole, are sometimes seen in open wounds healing by secondary intention, probably due to premature keratinization of the wound edges (Figure 4-6 and Plate 4). In these wounds, an open edge must be reestablished, by either surgical excision or chemical cauterization, before epithelial migration can occur (Schultz, Sibbald, Falanga, 2003).

Prolonged Remodeling. The remodeling process for wounds healing by secondary intention is essentially the same as that for wounds healing by primary intention. Clinicians and caregivers must remain acutely aware that newly "healed" wounds initially lack tensile strength, and measures should be initiated to minimize stress on the remodeling wound until tensile strength has developed, which occurs 2 to 3 months after closure. For example, the patient with a newly healed pressure ulcer should remain on a therapeutic support surface and should minimize time spent lying on the involved surface.

WHAT MAKES A CHRONIC WOUND CHRONIC?

An acute wound in a relatively healthy host will heal fairly quickly because of a cascade of growth factors, cytokines, and matrix proteins that tend to keep the acute wound on the "healing track." In clinical practice, however, chronic wounds such as pressure ulcers, vascular ulcers, and neuropathic wounds behave much differently and may be extremely slow to heal. In order to intervene effectively, the clinician must be knowledgeable regarding the various factors contributing to delayed healing.

Over the past decade, extensive research analyzing the cellular, biochemical, and molecular components of acute and chronic wounds has significantly expanded the understanding of the detailed complexities of normal wound healing and the pathophysiologic mechanisms of chronic wounds. Box 4-1 summarizes the characteristics of a chronic wound.

Underlying Pathology

The nature of the injury differs between acute and chronic wounds. Acute wounds usually begin with a sudden, solitary insult and proceed to heal in an orderly manner. In contrast, chronic wounds are commonly caused by an underlying pathologic process, such as vascular insufficiency, that produces repeated and prolonged insults to the tissues. Failure to correct or control the underlying pathology can result in a persistent cycle of injury that causes repetitive tissue damage. In contrast, correction of the underlying pathology frequently can shift the wound to a healing pathway (Goldman, 2004).

Increased Levels of Inflammatory Substances

Chronic wounds frequently are complicated by impediments to healing, such as ischemia, necrotic tissue, heavy bacterial loads, and high levels of proinflammatory MMPs. These factors prolong the inflammatory phase of wound healing by continuing to recruit macrophages and neutrophils into the wound bed. In addition, high levels of proinflammatory MMPs are associated with ongoing destruction of the ECM (Demidova-Rice et al, 2012; Gill and Parks, 2008; Goldman, 2004). Studies indicate that the levels of inflammatory substances in chronic wounds are 100 times higher than the levels in acute wounds (Berg Vande and Robson, 2003). Fortunately, this cycle can be interrupted by elimination of the noxious stimuli, that is, by debridement of necrotic tissue and control of the bacterial burden (Goldman, 2004).

BOX 4-1 **Characteristics of a Chronic Wound**
Prolonged inflammatory phase
Cellular senescence
Deficiency of growth factor receptor sites
No initial bleeding event to trigger fibrin production and release of growth factors
High level of proteases

Stratum corneum
Stratum lucidum
Stratum granulosum
Stratum spinosum
Basal cells of epidermis

FIGURE 4-6 Left, Closed wound edges in which epidermis of wound edges has rolled under so that epithelial cells cannot migrate. Right, Open wound edges from which epithelial cells can migrate.

Low Levels of Growth Factors

In addition to high levels of inflammatory proteases, low levels of growth factors commonly characterize the environment of chronic wounds. Normal levels of growth factors are critical to repair, because a "threshold level" of growth factors is required to move target cells out of the quiescent G_0 phase and into the reproductive cycle (Berg Vande and Robson, 2003). The low levels of growth factors commonly found in chronic wounds may be the result of inadequate production by the cells of the wound bed (or insufficient numbers of "producer" cells). Additional potential causes include rapid breakdown of growth factors by the high levels of MMPs or "binding" of the growth factors by the ECM (Berg Vande and Robson, 2003; Steed, 2003). Although this imbalance between inflammatory and proliferative stimuli usually is thought to be the cause of impaired healing, some investigators suggest that the imbalance instead may be a result of chronicity. When the wound begins to heal, the ratio of inflammatory to proliferative stimuli normalizes (Goldman, 2004; Henry and Garner, 2003).

Cellular and ECM Abnormalities. Current evidence suggests distinct phenotypic differences in the fibroblasts and keratinocytes found in chronic wounds compared with those found in acute wounds. Specifically both fibroblasts and keratinocytes exhibit reduced proliferative behavior and reduced motility, possibly due in part to abnormalities in the ECM (Demidova-Rice et al, 2012). Additional differences noted in the fibroblasts and keratinocytes of chronic wounds include reduced numbers of growth factor receptor sites and increased cellular senescence (that is, decreased ability to proliferate) (Telgenhoff and Shroot, 2005). Because all phases of wound healing are controlled primarily by growth factors, reduced binding sites or reduced responsiveness would significantly alter the cells' ability to contribute to wound healing. Cellular senescence may occur in the elderly as a normal component of aging and may contribute to the delayed healing commonly seen in this population. In addition, the high levels of ROS common to the chronic wound environment can cause DNA damage and loss of the cells' ability to replicate normally, even in younger individuals. Fortunately, this type of cellular senescence is reversible through optimal wound management (Berg Vande and Robson, 2003; Pittman, 2007; Telgenhoff and Shroot, 2005).

Miscellaneous Host Conditions

Additional "host factors" that trigger chronicity in a wound include ischemia, malnutrition, and comorbidities such as diabetes (Steed, 2003). Malnutrition is a particularly common contributor to wound chronicity. Fibroblasts that lack the requisite raw ingredients cannot synthesize connective tissue proteins. The importance of nutritional status is reflected in studies documenting consistently impaired wound healing in patients whose albumin levels were lower than 2.0 g/L (Burns et al, 2003). In addition, a study on wound fluid as a predictor of healing found the only constituents to reliably predict healing were total protein and albumin, that is, albumin levels greater than 2.0 g/L (James et al, 2000; Schultz et al, 2003).

Pale, pink tissue that is smooth rather than granular is indicative of delayed healing and a compromised ability to synthesize collagen and other connective tissue proteins (see Plate 5).

Denervation

Denervation is another potential cause of failure to heal. Sensory nerves secrete neuropeptides (e.g., substance P) that are highly chemotactic for inflammatory cells. Therefore denervated wounds are subject to impaired inflammation and compromised healing. Denervation may be one of the factors contributing to chronicity of pressure ulcers in patients with spinal cord injury and neuropathic ulcers in diabetic patients (Macri and Clark, 2009; Richards et al, 1997).

In summary, differences in the healing trajectory for acute and chronic wounds stem from the nature of the injury, the cellular events that follow injury, and miscellaneous host factors. In general, healing wounds are characterized by high mitotic activity, therapeutic levels of inflammatory cytokines, low levels of proteases, and mitotically competent cells. In contrast, chronic wounds exhibit low mitotic activity, excessive levels of inflammatory cytokines, high levels of proteases, and senescent or mitotically incompetent cells.

MEDIATORS OF WOUND HEALING

In order for healing to occur normally, the critical cells must be recruited to the wound bed (at the appropriate time), stimulated to reproduce, and then directed to carry out essential functions, such as neoangiogenesis, connective tissue synthesis, and reepithelialization. This complex process is controlled and coordinated by an equally complex array of regulatory substances; key elements include bioactive molecules, matrix proteins, and the matrix itself. The effect of these regulatory factors is further influenced by "host" factors, such as cell receptor sites, cellular senescence, availability of nutrients, and cofactors required for phagocytosis and collagen synthesis, and comorbid conditions, such as hypoxia and diabetes. This section provides a brief overview of regulatory factors, which are discussed further in Chapter 20.

Bioactive Molecules

Bioactive molecules include growth factors and cytokines. They are produced by the cells in the wound bed (e.g., platelets, neutrophils, macrophages, and fibroblasts) and act as "directors" of cell function and thus of the repair process. They do so by attracting the needed cells to the wound bed, stimulating them to proliferate, and then directing the cells to carry out specific aspects of repair. For example, TNF-α is a proinflammatory cytokine that attracts neutrophils and macrophages to the wound bed and is present in high concentrations during the inflammatory phase, whereas VEGF is a growth factor that supports proliferation and migration of endothelial cells and therefore is important during angiogenesis (Gill and Parks, 2008; Macri and Clark, 2009; Thom, 2009).

Matrix Proteins

Growth factors and cytokines act as "controllers" for the cells critical to the repair process. However, it is increasingly apparent that proteins within the ECM control the levels and function of growth factors and cytokines. Key categories of matrix proteins include MMPs, ADAMs, and tissue inhibitors of metalloproteinase (TIMPs). Matrix metalloproteinases and ADAMs can "up-regulate" the levels of growth factors and cytokines by cleaving them from the cell and thus activating them; however, they also can "down-regulate" the levels of growth factors and cytokines by degrading them or by inhibiting their release. Tissue inhibitors of metalloproteinase control the activity of MMPs by binding to them, thus blocking their effects (Gill and Parks, 2008).

Extracellular Matrix

The ECM serves as a scaffold for migrating cells and as a repository for growth factors. It also influences the response of the cells to growth factors. For example, keratinocyte proliferation requires both attachment to the ECM and stimulation by growth factors. Cell migration is another aspect of repair that is dependent on both matrix proteins and integrins within the matrix itself. Matrix proteins promote migration by degrading the bonds between the migrating cells and the underlying wound bed, and the matrix promotes reattachment through the expression of binding sites (integrins) within the matrix. The matrix also supports cell-to-cell communication. The ECM needs to be porous and pliable in order to support the movement of cells, nutrients, and growth factors through the wound environment (Cheresh and Stupack, 2008; Schultz and Wysocki, 2009). Dermal matrix dressings (see Chapter 19) may be beneficial to support cell migration and granulation tissue formation, in select wounds (Nataraj et al, 2007).

Host Factors

A number of host factors influence cells' response to growth factors, cytokines, and matrix proteins. One of these factors is the type of receptors on the cell wall. This is an important factor because all cells within the wound bed are exposed to the same mix of regulatory substances, but only select cells respond. In addition, different cells may exhibit different responses to the same regulatory substance because regulatory substances exert their effects primarily through binding with cell receptors. Therefore only cells with the specific receptor sites respond to the regulatory substance, and the effects of receptor binding vary based on cell type. For example, PDGF stimulates migration of some cells and mitosis in others, but it has no effect on other cells (Martin, 1997; Witte and Barbul, 1997). Furthermore, fibroblasts and keratinocytes in elderly individuals have a decreased number of receptor sites, which may explain why elderly patients tend to exhibit a diminished response to some regulatory substances (Ashcroft et al, 2002).

Other factors that impact an individual's ability to heal normally are systemic factors such as nutritional status, perfusion, oxygenation, and comorbidities such as diabetes. These factors are addressed briefly in this chapter and in greater depth in other chapters in this text.

EXTREMES OF REPAIR: SCARLESS HEALING VERSUS EXCESSIVE SCARRING

This chapter has focused on what is currently considered "normal" repair for full-thickness wounds, that is, formation of granulation tissue (scar) to mend the defect, with a covering of new epithelium. This form of repair represents an intermediate point between "ideal" repair, also referred to as scarless healing, and "abnormal" repair. Hypertrophic and keloid scars are examples of abnormal repair or excessive scarring. As we learn more about the factors that lead to "normal" and excessive scarring, we hope to be able to optimize repair and minimize scarring for all patients.

Scarless Healing

As mentioned earlier in this chapter, the early-gestation fetus typically heals without scarring, an ability that is lost at 22 to 24 weeks of gestation (Samuels and Tan, 1999). Features and characteristics of early-gestation healing are listed in Box 4-2. One significant difference is a markedly diminished inflammatory response. Multiple studies using various models have demonstrated that inflammation is minimal or essentially absent in early-gestation (scarless) healing. This finding is consistent with other studies showing a strong link between the intensity and duration of the inflammatory response and the subsequent development of scar tissue (Wilgus, 2007). The specific factors thought to contribute to this very minimal inflammatory response include the following: (1) Fetal platelets release much lower levels of proinflammatory growth factors and cytokines, most specifically the profibrotic isoforms of TGF-β. TGF-β is responsible for attracting inflammatory cells to the wound bed, for promoting angiogenesis and fibroblast activity, and for remodeling

---

BOX 4-2   Characteristics of Scarless Healing

Decreased amount of platelet-derived growth factor
Decreased amount of proinflammatory proteases and growth factors
Increased levels of fibronectin and hyaluronic acid
Balance of TIMP and MMP
New collagen structure and function indistinguishable from native collagen

MMP, Matrix metalloprotease; *TIMP*, tissue inhibitor of matrix metalloprotease.

of the ECM; (2) Marked reduction in migration of inflammatory cells (neutrophils, macrophages, and T cells); this is partially due to the lower levels of proinflammatory growth factors and partially due to the fact that the fetal immune system is poorly developed; (3) Marked reduction in angiogenic stimuli linked to scar formation (VEGF, TGF-β1, PDGF, and prostaglandin E2) (Walraven et al, 2014; Wilgus, 2007).

Another difference in early-gestation healing is the rate at which epithelial resurfacing occurs. Rapid up-regulation of the adhesion molecules within the ECM allows cells to move laterally, which promotes early keratinocyte migration (Wilgus, 2007).

Most importantly, a number of differences in fetal healing contribute to production of a new ECM that retains the characteristics of unwounded tissue. One contributing factor may be the high levels of hyaluronic acid and hyaluronic-acid-stimulating activity factor. This factor is significant because hyaluronic acid supports rapid cell migration. In addition, high levels of MMPs compared with TIMPs favor degradation of the ECM, which is thought to help prevent overproduction of collagen. Finally, fetal fibroblasts retain the ability to produce new matrix proteins that retain the basket-weave configuration characteristic of normal dermis (Wilgus, 2007).

In summary, early-gestation fetal repair is characterized by a significantly reduced inflammatory response and a rapid and balanced proliferative phase that restores the dermal architecture without scarring (see Box 4-2).

Excessive Scarring

Excessive or hyperproliferative scarring is a complication of acute full-thickness wound healing that presently is not well understood. The two types of hyperproliferative scarring are hypertrophic scars and keloid scars (see Plate 7, C and D). Both types appear raised, are red or pink, and are pruritic. Hypertrophic scars are confined to the original incisional or scar area, whereas keloids expand beyond the incision into the surrounding tissue. This expansion, sometimes described as a mushroom effect, is the result of continued proliferation of connective tissue proteins that may continue indefinitely (Atiyeh, 2005; Slemp and Kirschner, 2006).

Hypertrophic scars are characterized by increased vasculature, increased numbers of white blood cells and fibroblasts, and a thickened epidermal layer (Atiyeh, 2005). The collagen fibers in hypertrophic scars are organized and oriented parallel to the epidermal layer; however, they contain an abundance of myofibroblasts, which leads to contracture formation. One positive feature of hypertrophic scars (compared with keloids) is their potential to eventually regress during the remodeling phase (Slemp and Kirschner, 2006).

Keloids are a much more serious problem than hypertrophic scars. Keloids may continue to expand, creating both functional and cosmetic deficits. In addition, scars that initially appear to be "normal" may deviate into a pattern of keloid growth over time. Biochemical analysis of keloid scars reveals increased numbers of receptor sites for growth factors and major abnormalities in the behavior of fibroblasts and keratinocytes, which may partially explain the excessive production of ECM. Most importantly, the balance between synthesis and degradation of connective tissue proteins is lost. This loss of balance is theorized to result from abnormalities in cell-to-cell communication and immune function, failure of apoptosis (spontaneous cell death), and the effects of hypoxia and oxygen free radicals. Keloid scars are characterized by disorganized collagen bundles; however, these scars do not contain myofibroblasts and are not associated with contracture formation (Atiyeh, 2005; Hahn et al, 2013; Slemp and Kirschner, 2006).

Risk factors for hyperproliferative scarring include a strong family history (particularly important with keloid formation), age 10 to 30 years, and darkly pigmented skin. In the United States, individuals of African American descent have a 5% to 15% increased risk compared with Caucasians (Atiyeh, 2005; Slemp and Kirschner, 2006). Exposure to mechanical stretch may be a trigger for keloid production (Ogawa et al, 2012).

Strategies designed to prevent or correct hyperproliferative scarring have provided inconsistent and often suboptimal results. Surgical excision, intralesional steroids (either single or combination steroids), and topical silicone sheeting are the most commonly prescribed therapies. Table 4-3 lists current treatment options. Research is ongoing, with the goals of accurately identifying the cellular and biochemical abnormalities that produce these scars and designing therapies to prevent and correct them (Kieran et al, 2013; Sayed and Bayat, 2013; Yamamoto and Kiyosawa, 2012).

FACTORS AFFECTING THE REPAIR PROCESS

By observing a number of similar wounds and tracking their time to healing, it is possible to construct a curve that represents the healing "trajectory" for that type of wound. For example, epithelialization of a surgical wound healing by primary intention typically is complete by 48 hours, although difficult to palpate; a healing ridge develops by days 5 to 9; and initial collagen deposition should be complete by postoperative day 21. Interestingly, it also is possible to plot a "healing trajectory" for neuropathic ulcers, venous ulcers, and pressure ulcers. As described in Chapter 6, studies indicate that the usual "time to healing" is similar for all patients with a particular type of wound (Steed, 2003). Multiple factors affect the time to healing for a specific wound; it is critical for the clinician to identify and correct factors that are known to delay healing. Factors that can delay the healing process and shift the trajectory to the right are outlined in Table 4-4.

TABLE 4-3   Therapy Options for Hyperproliferative Scarring

Treatment	Indications	Considerations
Surgical excision	Hypertrophic scars Keloid scars	Recurrence rare with hypertrophic Recurrence common (45%–100%) with keloid if surgical excision is done without adjunctive therapies
Radiation (as adjunct to surgical excision)	Hypertrophic scars Keloid scars	Promotion of fibroblast apoptosis (death) Low recurrence rates (1%–35%) Theoretical risk of radiation-induced malignancy (no data)
Corticosteroid therapy (systemic), intralesional injections (single or combined agents)	Hypertrophic scars Keloid scars	Reduces scar overgrowth, pruritus, contractures Pain of repeated injections may limit patient adherence Adverse effects: skin atrophy, depigmentation, telangiectasias
Silicone gel, sheeting	Hypertrophic scars Keloid scars	Increases wound hydration Decreases fibroblast activity Down-regulates fibrogenic isoforms of TGF-β Worn 12–24 hr/day for at least 2–3 months Risk of maceration and skin breakdown with gel (gel use limited to areas where sheeting will not conform)
Laser (CDL, PDL)	Hypertrophic scars Keloid scars	Stimulates regression of keloid Reduces pruritus with hypertrophic (PDL) Variable results if used independently; best if used in conjunction with steroids or silicone gel CDL: recurrence rate as high as 50% PDL: Works best with steroids + silicone No comparative studies of laser, surgery, and adjunctive therapy
Retinoids (topical)	Hypertrophic scars Keloid scars	Suppresses collagen synthesis Increases epithelial cell turnover May be applied topically both preoperatively/postoperatively 80% of lesions have favorable short-term outcomes
Intralesional cryotherapy	Hypertrophic scars Keloid scars	Scar regression through reduction of hyperproliferative response
Compression garments	Hypertrophic scars (primary indication) Keloid scars	Hypoxic and thermal effects in compressed areas reduce fibroblast activity Must be worn 8–24 hr/day for first 6 months Must fit correctly
Antiproliferative agents (5-fluorouracil, bleomycin)	Hypertrophic scars Keloid scars	Induce scar regression 5-Fluorouracil more effective with hypertrophic Provide short-term suppression of small keloids Few small studies support use of bleomycin topically Side effects: pulmonary fibrosis, fever, rash, hyperpigmentation
Intralesional injections of verapamil	Keloid scars	Inhibit inflammation Stimulate production of collagenase and other enzymes to degrade excess extracellular matrix Used for both prevention and treatment
Immunotherapy (immunomodulators, immunosuppressants, antibody therapy [e.g., imiquimod, tacrolimus, sirolimus, tumor necrosis factor-α, interferons, interleukins])	Keloid scars	Suppress fibroblast activity Promote fibroblast apoptosis Help reduce inflammation and regulate cellular activity Significant side effects depending on agent and dose
Suture ligature	Keloid scars	Deprives tissue of nutrients and oxygen, thus promoting tissue death Keloid must be amenable to suture ligature Requires weekly office visits and daily maintenance of local wounds

Data from Al-Attar et al, 2006; Berman, 2007; D'Andrea, 2002; Franz et al, 2007; Funayama et al, 2003; Gupta and Kumar, 2001; Har-Shai, 2003; Kieran et al, 2013; Parikh, 2008; Stashower, 2006; Syed and Bayat, 2013; Xia et al, 2004.
CDL, Carbon dioxide laser; *PDL,* pulsed dye laser; *TGF,* transforming growth factor.

TABLE 4-4   Factors Affecting Wound Healing

Factor	Effects on Repair Process	Clinical Implications
Perfusion/ oxygenation Hypoxia Adequate oxygen levels	Initiates new vessel development, promoting fibroblast proliferation Critical for cellular production of ATP, bacterial killing, collagen synthesis, development of tensile strength Critical oxygen levels ≥30–40 mm Hg (higher for bacterial killing)	Hypovolemia, hypotension, vasoconstriction, vascular impairment, edema, hypoxia all deleterious to repair Intervene to promote perfusion and oxygenation: warmth, hydration, pain control, management of edema, maintenance or restoration of blood flow Supplemental oxygen may be beneficial See Chapter 28
Excessive bioburden	Causes direct tissue damage and breakdown of growth factors; inhibits keratinocyte migration, collagen synthesis, and development of tensile strength Bacteria compete with fibroblasts for oxygen and nutrients, thus delaying repair Inflammatory response to high bacterial loads keeps wound "stuck" in inflammatory phase and prevents progression to proliferative phase of repair	Debride necrotic tissue to eliminate environment favorable to bacterial growth Monitor wound for signs and symptoms of invasive infection (cellulitis or osteomyelitis); treat any invasive infection with systemic antibiotics Monitor for signs and symptoms of critical colonization or biofilm formation; remove biofilm mechanically and treat critical colonization topically (with antimicrobial agents)
Smoking/ tobacco use	Byproducts (nicotine, carbon monoxide, hydrogen cyanide) reduce oxygenation, impair immune response, reduce fibroblast activity, increase platelet adhesion and thrombus formation Smoking associated with significantly higher infection rates	Counsel patients on negative effects of tobacco use Offer comprehensive program for smoking cessation: support groups, nicotine replacement, medications (No increase in wound infection with nicotine patch) See Chapter 28
Nutritional status	Adequate nutritional status critical for collagen synthesis, tensile strength, immune function Critical nutrients include micronutrients (vitamins, minerals), key amino acids (glutamine, L-arginine), adequate protein	Nutritional assessment and support are critical aspects of effective wound care program and must include attention to micronutrients and calorie and protein intake See Chapter 27
Diabetes mellitus	Associated with • Abnormal and prolonged inflammation • Reduced collagen synthesis • Decreased tensile strength • Impaired epithelial migration • Compromised vasculature • Hyperglycemia associated with compromised neutrophil function, impaired epithelial migration	Tight Glycemic control (glucose levels <150 mg/dl) associated with a reduced incidence of postoperative wound infections See Chapter 14
Obesity	Adipose tissue poorly vascularized Large volumes of adipose tissue put additional stress on incisional lines, increasing risk of dehiscence Associated with higher incidence of infection, seroma formation, wound dehiscence	Monitor intake to ensure adequate intake of protein and micronutrients and appropriate caloric intake Incisional support (binders) beneficial in reducing risk of dehiscence See Chapter 35
Medications	Chemotherapeutic agents impair production of white blood cells and fibroblasts, interfering with both inflammatory and proliferative phases of repair and increasing risk of infection Corticosteroids suppress inflammation and reduce proliferation of keratinocytes and fibroblasts, thereby impairing both granulation and epithelial resurfacing; impact is time and dose dependent, with impairment limited primarily to patients receiving steroids in doses >40 mg/day and for at least 30 days before wounding High doses of NSAIDs may impair healing	Delay chemotherapy when possible to permit healing (delay in healing most significant when chemotherapy given within first weeks following surgery/injury) Limited data suggest that topical vitamin A may partially reverse negative effects of corticosteroids (applied to clean wound bed before dressing application). Systemic administration is not recommended at present due to concerns that this could block the intended effects of the steroids Recommended dose range is 25,000–100,000 international units per day (note this recommendation based on limited and anecdotal data) For patient with impaired healing taking high-dose NSAIDs, collaborate with prescribing provider to reduce dose if possible

TABLE 4-4   Factors Affecting Wound Healing—cont'd

Factor	Effects on Repair Process	Clinical Implications
Advanced age	Diminished proliferation of cells critical to repair Hormonal changes Increased number of senescent cells Diminished production of growth factors and possible reduction in receptor sites for growth factors Multiple existing comorbidities	Correct any reversible comorbidities Optimize nutritional status Provide evidence-based wound care
Immunosuppression	Increased susceptibility to infection Compromises body's ability to manifest signs of infection	Provide meticulous wound care to minimize risk of infection Monitor wound closely for muted signs of infection (faint erythema, mild increase in exudate, pain) and treat appropriately
Stress	Increased production of corticosteroids	Implement strategies to minimize stress: pain control, environmental management, patient education and counseling
Cellular senescence	Impairs healing due to reduced ability of cells involved in repair to replicate normally Associated with aging and with chronic wound environment, specifically high levels of ROS	Control bioburden and inflammation/levels of ROS to avoid damage to cellular DNA and "induced senescence"
Other	Malignancy Multisystem failure Failure to maintain clean, moist wound bed	Provide holistic wound management that addresses comorbidities Implement topical therapy to eliminate necrotic tissue and heavy bacterial loads Keep wound surface clean and moist

Data from Anstead, 1998; Burns et al, 2003; Ehrlich and Hunt, 1968; Ehrlich and Hunt, 1969; Greenhalgh, 2003; Hardman and Ashcroft, 2008; Howard et al, 2013; Manassa et al, 2003; Pittman, 2007; Sorensen et al, 2003; Telgenhoff and Shroot, 2005; Wang et al, 2013; Whitney, 2003; Wicke et al, 2009; Wientjes, 2002; Williams and Barbul, 2003; Wilson and Clark, 2003.
ATP, Adenosine triphosphate; *NSAID*, nonsteroidal antiinflammatory drug; *ROS*, reactive oxygen species.

CLINICAL CONSULT

A: Referral received for management of dehisced abdominal surgical incision; patient is 62-year-old African American female who underwent abdominal hysterectomy and bilateral salpingooophorectomy 6 days ago for endometrial cancer. Medical history includes type 2 diabetes mellitus (last HbA1c 8.2), obesity (height 5'5"; weight 250 lbs), gastroesophageal reflux disease (GERD), cigarette smoking (one pack per day for 42 years; stopped smoking 3 months ago), hypertension, and chronic obstructive lung disease. Upon assessment, patient is alert, oriented × 3, and very concerned about her open wound. She is mobile in bed and able to turn independently; she gets out of bed with assistance. She is coughing at intervals and states that she has moderately severe pain with coughing. Dehisced incisional wound measures 12 cm (L) × 6 cm (W) × 3 cm (D). The wound base is 60% red and smooth; 40% of the wound bed is covered with mixed yellow-tan adherent nonviable tissue. There is a moderate amount of serosanguineous drainage. The periwound skin is intact with mild erythema extending 2 cm from wound edge and slight induration. Currently on day 3 of antibiotic therapy for a surgical site infection (SSI).

D: Dehisced abdominal incision in inflammatory phase of repair. Mild erythema and slight induration indicative of resolving surgical site infection. Obesity, diabetes, and lung disease contributed to risk for SSI.
P: Optimize systemic factors to enhance wound repair; provide external support to reduce strain on wound with decreased tensile strength. Initiate measures to eliminate slough from wound bed and to promote transition to proliferative phase of repair.
I: (1) Nutritional consult to ensure macronutrients and micronutrients sufficient for repair. (2) Consult with provider to monitor blood sugars with goal of <180. (3) Abdominal binder to support incision since patient is obese and is coughing. (4) Fill wound bed with methylene blue/gentian violet foam dressing to reduce bacterial burden and provide moist environment that will enhance autolysis; cover with nonadherent superabsorbent pad and change in 2 days.
E: Will follow to evaluate/monitor effectiveness and will adapt plan as indicated. Reassess and consider negative pressure wound therapy once nonviable tissue removed.

SUMMARY

Wound healing is a complex series of events. Normally wound healing is initiated by an injury that leads to clot formation and platelet degranulation, is controlled by a myriad of cytokines and growth factors, and is affected significantly by systemic factors such as perfusion, nutritional status, and steroid levels. Effective management of any wound requires an understanding of the normal repair process and the factors that may interfere with normal repair. This understanding provides the foundation for comprehensive assessment of the wound and of the patient and for selection of interventions designed to optimize healing.

REFERENCES

Al-Attar A, Mess S, Thomassen JM, et al: Keloid pathogenesis and treatment, *Plastic Reconstr Surg* 117:286–300, 2006.

Anstead G: Steroids, retinoids, and wound healing, *Adv Wound Care* 11:277–285, 1998.

Ashcroft GS, Mills SJ, Ashworth JJ: Aging and wound healing, *Biogerontology* 3(6):337–345, 2002.

Atiyeh B: Keloid or hypertrophic scar: the controversy. Review of the literature, *Ann Plast Surg* 54(6):676–680, 2005.

Barendse-Hofmann MG, Steenvoorde P, van Doorn L, et al: Extracellular wound matrix (OASIS): exploring the contraindications and results of 32 consecutive outpatient clinic cases, *Wounds* 19(10):258–263, 2007.

Berg Vande JS, Robson MC: Arresting cell cycles and the effect on wound healing, *Surg Clin North Am* 83:509–520, 2003.

Berman B: A review of the biologic effects, clinical efficacy, and safety of silicone elastomer sheeting for hypertrophic and keloid scar treatment and management, *Dermatol Surg* 33(11):1291–1302, 2007.

Braiman-Wiksman L, Solomonik I, Spira R, et al: Novel insights into wound healing sequence of events, *Toxicol Pathol* 35:767–779, 2007.

Brissett AE, Hom DB: The effects of tissue sealants, platelet gels, and growth factors on wound healing, *Curr Opin Otolaryngol Head Neck Surg* 11(4):245–250, 2003.

Bullard KM, Longaker MT, Lorenz HP: Fetal wound healing: current biology, *World J Surg* 27:54–61, 2002.

Burns JL, Mancoll JS, Phillips LG: Impairments to wound healing, *Clin Plast Surg* 30:47–56, 2003.

Calvin M: Cutaneous wound repair, *Wounds* 10(1):12–32, 1998.

Chen WYJ, Abatangelo G: Functions of hyaluronan in wound repair, *Wound Repair Regen* 7:79–89, 1999.

Cheresh D, Stupack D: Regulation of angiogenesis: apoptotic cues from the ECM, *Oncogene* 27:6285–6298, 2008.

Cross KJ, Mustoe TA: Growth factors in wound healing, *Surg Clin North Am* 83:531–545, 2003.

D'Andrea F: Prevention and treatment of keloids with intralesional verapamil, *Dermatology* 204(1):60–62, 2002.

Dang C, Ting K, Soo C, et al: Fetal wound healing: current perspectives, *Clin Plast Surg* 30:13–23, 2003.

Demidova-Rice T, Hamblin M, Herman I: Acute and impaired wound healing: pathophysiology and current methods for drug delivery, part 1: normal and chronic wounds: biology, causes, and approaches to care, *Adv Skin Wound Care* 25(7):304–314, 2012.

Dubay KA, Franz MG: Acute wound healing: the biology of acute wound failure, *Surg Clin North Am* 83:463–481, 2003.

Ehrlich P, Hunt T: Effects of cortisone and vitamin A on wound healing, *Ann Surg* 167(3):324–328, 1968.

Ehrlich P, Hunt T: The effects of cortisone and anabolic steroids on the tensile strength of healing wounds, *Ann Surg* 170(2):203–206, 1969.

Frank S, Kämpfer H, Wetzler C, et al: Nitric oxide drives skin repair: novel functions of an established mediator, *Kidney Int* 61:882–888, 2002.

Franz M, Steed DL, Robson MC: Optimizing healing of the acute wound by minimizing complications, *Curr Probl Surg* 44(11):691–763, 2007.

Funayama E, Chodon T, Oyama A, et al: Keratinocytes promote proliferation and inhibit apoptosis of the underlying fibroblasts: an important role in the pathogenesis of keloid, *J Invest Dermatol* 121(6):1326–1331, 2003.

Gabbiani G: The myofibroblast in wound healing and fibrocontractive diseases, *J Pathol* 200:500–503, 2003.

Gabriel A, Mussman J, Rosenberg LZ, et al: *Wound healing, growth factors*, http://emedicine.medscape.com/article/1298196-overview. Accessed December 29, 2014.

Gill S, Parks W: Metalloproteinases and their inhibitors: regulators of wound healing, *Int J Biochem Cell Biol* 40:1334–1347, 2008.

Goldman R: Growth factors and chronic wound healing: past, present, and future, *Adv Skin Wound Care* 17(1):24–35, 2004.

Greenhalgh DG: Wound healing and diabetes mellitus, *Clin Plast Surg* 30:37–45, 2003.

Gupta S, Kumar B: Intralesional cryosurgery using lumbar puncture and/or hypodermic needles for large, bulky, recalcitrant keloids, *Int J Dermatol* 40(5):349–353, 2001.

Hahn J, Glaser K, McFarland K, et al: Keloid derived keratinocytes exhibit an abnormal gene expression profile consistent with a distinct causal mechanism in keloid pathology, *Wound Repair Regen* 21(4):530–544, 2013.

Hamed S, Bennett C, Demiot C, et al: Erythropoietin, a novel repurposed drug: an innovative treatment for wound healing in patients with diabetes mellitus, *Wound Repair Regen* 22(1):23–33, 2014.

Howard M, ASMI R, Evans K, et al: Oxygen and wound care: a review of current therapeutic modalities and future direction, *Wound Repair Regen* 21(4):503–511, 2013.

Hardman M, Ashcroft G: Estrogen, not intrinsic aging, is the major regulator of delayed human wound healing in the elderly, *Genome Biol* 9(5):R80, 2008.

Harrison C, Heaton MJ, Layton CM and Neil SM: et al: Use of an in vitro model of tissue-engineered human skin to study keratinocyte attachment and migration in the process of reepithelialization, *Wound Repair Regen* 14:203–209, 2006.

Har-Shai Y: Intralesional cryotherapy for enhancing the involution of hypertrophic scars and keloids, *Plast Reconstr Surg* 111(6):1841–1852, 2003.

Henry G, Garner WL: Inflammatory mediators in wound healing, *Surg Clin North Am* 83:483–507, 2003.

Hoenig M, Bianchi C, Rosenzweig A, and Sellke FW: et al: Decreased vascular repair and neovascularization with ageing: mechanisms and clinical relevance with an emphasis on hypoxia-inducible factor, *Curr Mol Med* 8(8):754–767, 2008.

Hunt TK, Van Winkle W Jr: Normal repair. In Hunt TK, Dunphy JE, editors: *Fundamentals of wound management*, New York, 1997, Appleton-Century-Crofts.

Jahoda CAB, Reynolds AJ: Hair follicle dermal sheath cells: unsung participants in wound healing, *Lancet* 358(9291):1445–1448, 2001.

James TJ, Hughes MA, Cherry GW, et al: Simple biochemical markers to assess chronic wounds, *Wound Repair Regen* 8:264–269, 2000.

Kieran I, Knock A, Bush J, et al: Interleukin-10 reduces scar formation in both animal and cutaneous wounds: results of two preclinical and phase II randomized controlled trials, *Wound Repair Regen* 21(3):428–436, 2013.

Lan CC, Liu IH, Fang AH, et al: Hyperglycaemic conditions decrease cultured keratinocyte mobility: implications for impaired wound healing in patients with diabetes, *Br J Dermatol* 159:1103–1115, 2008.

Lizarbe T, García-Rama C, Tarín C, et al: Nitric oxide elicits functional MMP-13 protein-tyrosine nitration during wound repair, *FASEB J* 22:3207–3215, 2008.

Loryman C, Mansbridge J: Inhibition of keratinocyte migration by lipopolysaccharide, *Wound Repair Regen* 16:45–51, 2008.

Macri L, Clark R: Tissue engineering for cutaneous wounds: selecting the proper time and space for growth factors, cells, and extracellular matrix, *Skin Pharmacol Physiol* 22(2):83–93, 2009.

Manassa EH, Hertl CH, Olbrisch RR: Wound healing problems in smokers and nonsmokers after 132 abdominoplasties, *Plast Reconstr Surg* 111(6):2082–2087, 2003.

Mangram AJ, Horan TC, Pearson ML, et al: Guideline for prevention of surgical site infection, *Infect Control Hosp Epidemiol* 20(1):250–278, 1999.

Martin P: Wound healing: aiming for perfect skin regeneration, *Science* 276:75–81, 1997.

Mast BA, Schultz G: Interactions of cytokines, growth factors, and proteases in acute and chronic wounds, *Wound Repair Regen* 4:411–420, 1996.

Monaco JL, Lawrence WT: Acute wound healing: an overview, *Clin Plast Surg* 30:1–12, 2003.

Myers S, Leigh IM, Navsaria H: Epidermal repair results from activation of follicular and epidermal progenitor keratinocytes mediated by a growth factor cascade, *Wound Repair Regen* 15:693–701, 2007.

Nataraj C, Ritter G, Dumas S, et al: Extracellular wound matrices: novel stabilization and sterilization method for collagen-based biologic wound dressings, *Wounds* 19(6):148–156, 2007.

Ogawa R, Okai K, Tokumura F, et al: The relationship between skin stretching/contraction and pathologic scarring: the important role of mechanical forces in keloid generation. *Wound Repair Regen* 20(2):149–157, 2012.

O'Goshi K-I, Tagami H: Basic fibroblast growth factor treatment for various types of recalcitrant skin ulcers: reports of nine cases, *J Dermatol Treat* 18:375–381, 2007.

O'Toole E, van Koningsveld R, Chen M, et al: Hypoxia induces epidermal keratinocyte matrix metalloproteinase-9 secretion via the protein kinase C pathway, *J Cell Physiol* 214:47–55, 2008.

Parikh D: Keloid banding using suture ligature: a novel technique and review of literature, *Laryngoscope* 118(11):1960–1965, 2008.

Phillips SJ: Physiology of wound healing and surgical wound care, *ASAIO J* 46(6):S2–S5, 2000.

Pittman J: Effect of aging on wound healing: current concepts, *J Wound Ostomy Continence Nurs* 34(4):412–417, 2007.

Pradhan L, Nabzdyk C, Andersen ND, et al: Inflammation and neuropeptides: the connection in diabetic wound healing, *Expert Rev Mol Med* 11:e2, 2009.

Pullar C, Manabat-Hidalgo CG, Bolaji RS, et al: β-adrenergic receptor modulation of repair, *Pharmacol Res* 58(2):158–164, 2008.

Rahban SR, Garner WL: Fibroproliferative scars, *Clin Plast Surg* 30:77–89, 2003.

Richards AM, Mitsou J, Floyd DC, et al: Neural innervation and healing, *Lancet* 350(9074):339–340, 1997.

Robson MC: Proliferative scarring, *Surg Clin North Am* 33:557–569, 2003.

Rodriguez P, Felix FN, Woodley DT, et al: The role of oxygen in wound healing: a review of the literature, *Dermatol Surg* 34:1159–1169, 2008.

Samuels P, Tan AKW: Fetal scarless wound healing, *J Otolaryngol* 28(5):296–302, 1999.

Syed F, Bayat A: Superior effect of combination vs single steroid therapy in keloid disease: a comparative in vitro analysis of glucocorticoids, *Wound Repair Regen* 21(1):88–102, 2013.

Schneider A, Garlick AJ, Egles C: Self-assembling peptide nanofiber scaffolds accelerate wound healing, *PLoS One* 3(1):e1410, 2008.

Schultz GS, Sibbald RG, Falanga V, et al: Wound bed preparation: a systematic approach to wound management, *Wound Repair Regen* 11(Suppl 1):S1–S28, 2003.

Schultz G, Wysocki A: Interactions between extracellular matrix and growth factors in wound healing, *Wound Repair Regen* 17(2):153–162, 2009.

Slemp A, Kirschner R: Keloids and scars: a review of keloids and scars, their pathogenesis, risk factors, and management, *Curr Opin Pediatr* 18(4):396–402, 2006.

Sorensen LT, Karlsmark T, Gottrup F: Abstinence from smoking reduces incisional wound infection: a randomized controlled trial, *Ann Surg* 238(1):1–5, 2003.

Stashower M: Successful treatment of earlobe keloids with imiquimod after tangential shave excision, *Dermatol Surg* 32(3):380–386, 2006.

Steed DL: Wound-healing trajectories, *Surg Clin North Am* 83:547–555, 2003.

Telgenhoff D, Shroot B: Cellular senescence mechanisms in chronic wound healing, *Cell Death Differ* 12:695–698, 2005.

Thom S: Oxidative stress is fundamental to hyperbaric oxygen therapy, *J Appl Physiol* 106:988–995, 2009.

Walraven M, Gouverneur M, Middelkoop E, et al: Altered TGF-β signaling in fetal fibroblasts: what is known about the underlying mechanism? *Wound Repair Regen* 22(1):3–13, 2014.

Wang A, Armstrong E, Armstrong A: Corticosteroids and wound healing: clinical considerations in the perioperative period, *Am J Surg* 206(3):410–417, 2013.

Whitney JD: Supplemental perioperative oxygen and fluids to improve surgical wound outcomes: translating evidence into practice, *Wound Repair Regen* 11(6):462–467, 2003.

Wicke C, Bachinger A, Coerper S, et al: Aging influences wound healing in patients with chronic lower extremity wounds treated in a specialized wound care center, *Wound Repair Regen* 17(1):25–33, 2009.

Wientjes KA: Mind-body techniques in wound healing, *Ostomy Wound Manage* 48(11):62–67, 2002.

Wilgus T: Regenerative healing in fetal skin: a review of the literature, *Ostomy Wound Manage* 53(6):16–31, 2007.

Williams JZ, Barbul A: Nutrition and wound healing, *Surg Clin North Am* 83:571–596, 2003.

Wilson JA, Clark JJ: Obesity: impediment to wound healing, *Crit Care Nurs Q* 26(2):119–132, 2003.

Winter G: Epidermal regeneration studied in the domestic pig. In Hunt T, Dunphy J, editors: *Fundamentals of wound management*, New York, 1979, Appleton-Century-Crofts.

Witte M, Barbul A: General principles of wound healing, *Surg Clin North Am* 77(3):509–528, 1997.

Xia W, Phan TT, Lim IJ, et al: Complex epithelial-mesenchymal interactions modulate transforming growth factor-beta expression in keloid-derived cells, *Wound Repair Regen* 12(5):546–556, 2004.

Yamamoto N, Kiyosawa T: Histological effects of occlusive dressings on healing of incisional skin wounds, *Int Wound J* 11(6):616–621, 2014.

Yang GP, Lim IJ, Phan TT, et al: From scarless fetal wounds to keloids: molecular studies in wound healing, *Wound Repair Regen* 11(6):411–418, 2003.

Types of Skin Damage and Differential Diagnosis

Ruth A. Bryant

OBJECTIVES

1. Describe the process of at least five factors that contribute to skin damage.
2. Distinguish among the following terms: macule, papule, plaque, nodule, wheal, pustule, vesicle, and bulla.
3. Describe the extent of tissue damage and skin manifestations associated with the four types of mechanical trauma, moisture associated skin damage (MASD), medical adhesive related skin injury (MARSI), and skin irradiation.
4. Discuss at least three interventions for the prevention and treatment of each type of mechanical trauma, MASD, MARSI, candidiasis, and radiation skin damage.
5. Distinguish between an irritant contact dermatitis and an allergic contact dermatitis.
6. Identify factors that predispose a patient to candidiasis.
7. Describe the types of lesions and distribution common to candidiasis, folliculitis, impetigo, and herpes.
8. Discriminate among incontinence-associated dermatitis (IAD), candidiasis intertrigo, Stage I or Stage II pressure ulcer, suspected deep tissue injury (sDTI), perianal herpes, tinea cruris, and inverse psoriasis.

Skin integrity can be jeopardized or compromised by a multitude of factors: mechanical, moisture, chemical, vascular, infectious, allergy, inflammatory, intrinsic disease, burn, radiation, and miscellaneous assaults. Each type of injury creates a complex set of skin responses, such as erythema, macules, papules, pustules, vesicles/bullae, erosion, and ulcers. Primary lesions of the skin are the first recognizable lesions in the skin. Plate 6 shows the definition and appearance of common primary lesions. Secondary skin lesions evolve from primary lesions due to the natural history of the disease or as a result of scratching/infection. Common secondary lesions are depicted and defined in Plate 7. Because periwound skin can develop skin complications and because many of these conditions provide clues to the etiology of the skin alteration, the health care provider for patients in acute care, home care, outpatient, and long-term care facilities must be familiar with these terms.

Before a treatment plan for any skin lesion or wound can be initiated, the underlying cause of that condition must be determined. Clues to the cause are derived from the patient's history and physical assessment and specifically by an assessment of the following parameters: location, characteristics, and distribution. These clues can be used to direct subsequent tests that may be necessary to develop a definitive diagnosis. Once the cause of the wound or skin lesion is identified, realistic goals for care can be established and a comprehensive, interdisciplinary treatment plan devised. This chapter introduces a classification system for types of skin damage, briefly describes the pathophysiologic process, and discusses the prevention and treatment of the most common types of skin damage (Box 5-1). The more uncommon skin lesions, particularly those associated with intrinsic disease, are addressed in Chapter 30.

ASSESSMENT

A systematic skin assessment and an accurate description of any lesions are essential to obtain a reasonable list of differential diagnoses. Additional assessments and diagnostic tests then can be used to derive the most likely diagnosis. Lesions should be described by five morphologic parameters: distribution, shape or arrangement, border and margins, associated changes within the lesion(s), and pigmentation. These parameters, including options for descriptive terminology, are listed in Table 5-1.

MECHANICAL FORCES

The forces that are applied externally to the skin, such as pressure, shear, friction, and skin stripping (skin tears), create mechanical skin damage. Each may occur in isolation or in combination with other mechanical insults, such as pressure and shear. This chapter presents shear, friction, and skin stripping. Pressure damage is discussed in detail in Chapter 7. Preventive interventions for pressure are discussed in Chapters 8 and 9.

TABLE 5-1   Morphologic Characteristics of Skin Lesions

Characteristic	Description	Examples
Distribution		
Localized	Lesion appears in one small area	Impetigo, herpes simplex (e.g., labialis), tinea corporis ("ringworm")
Regional	Lesions involve a specific region of the body	Acne vulgaris (pilosebaceous gland distribution), herpes zoster (nerve dermatomal distribution), psoriasis (flexural surfaces and skin folds)
Generalized	Lesions appear widely distributed or in numerous areas simultaneously	Urticaria, disseminated drug eruptions
Shape/Arrangement		
Round/discoid	Coin or fine shaped (no central clearing)	Nummular eczema
Oval	Ovoid shape	Pityriasis rosea
Annular	Round, active margins with central clearing	Tinea corporis, sarcoidosis
Zosteriform (dermatomal)	Following a nerve or segment of the body	Herpes zoster
Polycyclic	Interlocking or coalesced circles (formed by enlargement of annular lesions)	Psoriasis, urticaria
Linear	In a line	Contact dermatitis
Iris/target lesion	Pink macules with purple central papules	Erythema multiforme
Stellate	Star shaped	Meningococcal septicemia
Serpiginous	Snake-like or wavy line track	Cutanea larva migrans
Reticulate	Net-like or lacy	Polyarteritis nodosa, lichen planus lesions of erythema infectiosum
Morbilliform	Measles-like: maculopapular lesions that become confluent on the face and body	Measles, roseola
Border/Margin		
Discrete	Well demarcated or defined, able to draw a line around it with confidence	Psoriasis
Indistinct	Poorly defined, have borders that merge into normal skin or outlying ill-defined papules	Nummular eczema
Active	Margin of lesion shows greater activity than center	*Tinea* spp. eruptions
Irregular	Nonsmooth or notched margin	Malignant melanoma
Border raised above center	Center of lesion is depressed compared with the edge	Basal cell carcinoma
Advancing	Expanding at margins	Cellulitis
Associated Changes within Lesions		
Central clearing	An erythematous border surrounds lighter skin	Tinea eruptions
Desquamation	Peeling or sloughing of skin	Rash of toxic shock syndrome
Keratotic	Hypertrophic stratum corneum	Calluses, warts
Punctation	Central umbilication or dimpling	Basal cell carcinoma
Telangiectasias	Dilated blood vessels within lesion blanch completely, may be markers of systematic disease	Basal cell carcinoma, actinic keratosis
Pigmentation		
Flesh	Same tone as the surrounding skin	Neurofibroma, some nevi
Pink	Light red undertones	Eczema, pityriasis rosea
Erythematous	Dark pink to red	Tinea eruptions, psoriasis
Salmon	Orange-pink	Psoriasis
Tan-brown	Light to dark brown	Most nevi, pityriasis versicolor
Black	Black or blue-black	Malignant melanoma
Pearly	Shiny white, almost iridescent	Basal cell carcinoma
Purple	Dark red-blue-violet	Purpura, Kaposi sarcoma
Violaceous	Light violet	Erysipelas
Yellow	Waxy	Lipoma
White	Absent of color	Lichen planus

From Seidel HM, Ball JW, Dains JE, et al: *Mosby's guide to physical examination*, ed 6, St. Louis, MO, 2006, Mosby.

BOX 5-1   Classification of Skin Damage Based on Source and Irritant*

Mechanical
Pressure
Shear
Friction
Skin stripping
- Skin tears
- Medical adhesives

Moisture
Moisture-donating wound dressing
Urinary incontinence
Perspiration
Medical adhesives

Chemical
Feces
Gastrointestinal contents
Drainage from percutaneous tubes
Povidone-iodine complex (Betadine)
Alkaline soaps
Alcohol

Vascular/Neuropathic
Venous
Arterial
Neuropathic

Infectious
Fungal
Candidiasis
Dermatophyte (tinea)

Bacterial
Cellulitis
Erysipelas
Erythrasma
Folliculitis
Impetigo
Bullous impetigo
Nonbullous impetigo

Viral
Herpes simplex
Varicella-zoster virus

Allergic
Medical adhesive

Radiation

*See Chapter 30 for atypical types of skin damage.

Shear

Shear is trauma caused by tissue layers sliding against each other and results in disruption or angulation of blood vessels. Shearing force is the sliding movement of the top superficial layers of the skin over a support surface and/or subcutaneous soft tissue over muscle layers and sliding of the muscle layers over bony prominences while the underlying muscle and bone are stationary (AORN, 2008; Gefen, 2007). Skin damage is created by the interaction of tangential shear forces on the internal tissue and frictional forces (resistance) against the surface of the skin. Thus friction is always present when shearing force is present. Shear occurs when transferring a patient laterally onto the operating room table or onto a stretcher. The classic example of a shear injury occurs when the patient is in a semi-Fowler position. Because of the pull of gravity, anytime the head is higher than the foot, even when the head of bed is elevated as little as 30 degrees, shear can still occur (Gefen et al, 2013) (Figure 5-1). Ultimately, the skin is held in place while the skeletal structures pull the body (by gravity) toward the foot of the bed. Consequently, blood vessels in the area are stretched and angulated, the vasculature is disrupted, and small-vessel thrombosis and tissue death may develop (Wright and O'Connor, 2007).

Shear may cause shallow or deep ulcers and extends the tissue damage of pressure ulcers. This extension is manifested in the pressure ulcer by the presence of undermining (dissection or separation of tissue parallel to the skin surface; see Figures 5-1, 6-5). Shear injury is predominantly localized at the sacrum or coccyx and is commonly a consequence of elevating the head of the bed or improper transfer technique. However, it may also occur in other locations such as under contact casts. Prevention requires an awareness of those situations in which the skin is subjected to shearing force. For example, the patient with pulmonary distress requires the head of the bed to be elevated to facilitate adequate ventilation; however, the patient is at great risk for shear injury. Likewise, the patient with a cerebrovascular accident may experience shear injury when being transferred from the bed to the wheelchair. In the operating room, shear may be present with lateral transfers of the patient from the stretcher to the operating table (AORN, 2008).

Most strategies for prevention of shear have derived from expert opinion and have been incorporated into safe patient handling guidelines by the Centers for Disease Control and Prevention (CDC), American Nurses Association (ANA), and National Institute for Occupational Safety and Health (NIOSH) (CDC, 2014; Waters and Rockefeller, 2010; Waters et al, 2011). Because shear is an important contributing factor to pressure ulcer development, strategies to simultaneously prevent shear and pressure are warranted (see Chapter 8). The primary intervention for reducing shear is the use of lift sheets when repositioning the patient; this eliminates drag on the sacral skin because the two opposing surfaces are the bed surface and the lift sheet rather than the patient's skin. The

FIGURE 5-1 Shearing force. (Adapted from Loeper JM: *Therapeutic positioning and skin care*, Minneapolis, MN, 1986, Sister Kenny Institute.)

head of the bed should be maintained at less than 30 degrees; elevations higher than 30 degrees may be needed for meals, but should be limited to short periods of time. Also, the knee gatch can be used to interrupt gravity's pull on the body toward the foot of the bed. Many support surfaces have a slick fabric covering, which anecdotally and intuitively seems to reduce shear. A standardized method for measuring the ability of a support surface to reduce shear is not currently available.

Fontaine et al (1998) proposed a calculated pressure/shear factor (PSF), which would quantify support surface efficiency for the combined effect of pressure and shear reduction. Pressure/shear factor is calculated by adding the rounded average interface pressure (in millimeters of mercury) to the rounded average gross shearing force (g) multiplied by the impact factor of 4. The equation is as follows:

$$\text{Pressure} + (4 \times \text{shearing force}) = \text{PSF}$$

or

$$\text{mm Hg} + (4\,g) = \text{PSF}$$

A pressure sensor and a shear sensor are required to obtain the values to put into the PSF equation. Potentially, PSF could become a tangible support surface measurement. In this way, PSF would provide additional objective information on the potential for the support surface to prevent ulceration. For example, Fontaine et al (1998) studied PSF for three support surfaces classified as group 2 devices according to the Medicare Part B policy (described in Chapter 9). Pressure/shear factor was calculated for a powered, alternating-pressure mattress overlay; a powered, zoned, air-filled mattress replacement device; and a nonpowered fluid overlay. The resulting PSFs were 939, 1043, and 331, respectively. The implication of this finding is that the nonpowered fluid overlay was more effective in reducing the PSF. However, because PSF is a newly defined variable, further research is required to establish the validity of the variable, as well as its predictive value and clinical effectiveness.

Friction

The National Pressure Ulcer Advisory Panel (NPUAP) defines friction as the resistance to motion in a parallel direction relative to the common boundary between two surfaces (NPUAP, 2007). Skin injury by friction initially appears as erythema and progresses to an abrasion. As stated previously, shearing force is created by the interaction of tangential forces and friction (resistance) against the surface of the skin. Friction is frequently seen on elbows or heels because the patient easily abrades these surfaces against sheets when repositioning. Injury is characteristically very shallow and limited to the epidermis. Friction primarily affects superficial layers, and thus does not result in tissue necrosis, whereas shearing forces mainly affect deeper tissue layers (WOCN®, 2010).

Interventions to prevent friction and superficial shear involve the use of protective padding over the elbows or heels and moisturizers applied to vulnerable areas to maintain proper hydration of the epidermis. Both maneuvers decrease friction and thereby decrease shear. Transparent adhesive dressings, thin hydrocolloids, low-adhesion foam dressings, and skin sealants are effective at reducing friction. Adhesive dressings are contraindicated if the shear is sufficient to loosen the dressing. Braces, splints, prosthetic devices, and shoes should be assessed frequently for evidence of shear, and modifications (e.g., reshaping, molding, extra padding) should be implemented as needed.

Skin Stripping and Lacerations (Epidermal and Dermal)

Skin stripping is the inadvertent removal of the epidermis, with or without the dermis, by mechanical means. The International Skin Tear Advisory Panel (ISTAP) defines a skin tear as a partial thickness or full thickness wound caused by shear, friction, and/or blunt force resulting in separation of skin layers (LeBlanc et al, 2013). For most patients, skin tears do not extend hospital stay, but they are painful and distressing in appearance and can be interpreted as being the result of poor care (Ratliff and Fletcher, 2007). In the neonate or premature infant, however, skin tears are a significant portal of entry that can lead to septicemia (Furdon, 2003). Unique considerations concerning skin tears in the neonate or premature infant are addressed in Chapter 36. Data suggest that skin tears heal in 7 to 21 days, depending on the extent of tissue damage (Meuleneire, 2002; Milne and Corbett, 2005).

The ISTAP classification system for skin tears is a simple classification tool developed through consensus by LaBlanc and colleagues (2013) (Table 5-2). Type I skin tears are distinguished by a resulting skin flap or avulsed skin that can cover the exposed wound (see Plate 8). Type II skin tears (see Plates 9-11) are distinguished by partial flap loss that cannot be repositioned to cover the wound bed. Type III skin tears (see Plate 12) have total flap loss. The frequency of various locations of skin-stripping injuries is as follows: upper extremities (73% to 80%), legs and feet (20%), head (3% to 4%), and torso (3%) (Malone et al, 1991; McGough-Csarny

TABLE 5-2   Skin Tears: ISTAP Skin Tear Classification System

Type	Description
I: No skin loss	Linear or flap tear that can be re-positioned to cover the wound bed (see Plate 8)
II: Partial flap loss	Partial flap loss that cannot be repositioned to cover the wound bed (see Plates 9-11)
III: Total flap	Total flap loss exposing entire wound bed (see Plate 12)

LeBlanc et al, 2013.

and Kopac, 1998; Payne and Martin, 1990). In 2006 the Pennsylvania Patient Safety Reporting System (PA-PSRS) reported similar results and further specified the involved sites on the upper extremities (Pennsylvania Patient Safety Authority, 2006). The PA-PSRS reports the most frequent site of injury is the forearm, followed by the arm, hand, and lower extremities (Pennsylvania Patient Safety Authority, 2006).

Risk factors for a skin tear include advanced age, sensory loss, dehydration and malnutrition, history of previous skin tears, cognitive impairment, dependency, poor locomotion, and presence of ecchymosis (LeBlanc et al, 2008; McGough-Csarny and Kopac, 1998). A descriptive, cross-sectional, online survey of 1127 health care workers from 16 countries ranked equipment injury, patient transfers, falls, and dressing- or treatment-related injuries as the top causes of skin tears, respectively (LaBlanc et al, 2013).

Elderly skin and immature skin both are vulnerable to skin tears because the dermal–epidermal junction is not optimally functional. The interlocking dermal papillae and epidermal rete pegs at the dermal–epidermal junction are critical to providing resiliency and the ability to withstand mechanical forces. In the premature infant's skin, the dermal–epidermal junction is undeveloped and weak. As the skin ages, the epidermis thins, the dermal–epidermal junction flattens, and cohesion is diminished. In addition, the amounts of collagen and elastin present in the aging skin decrease so that the skin becomes wrinkled, thin, and less compliant. Furthermore, similar connective tissue changes around blood vessels increase the fragility of capillaries. Therefore mechanical stresses can trigger a subcutaneous hemorrhage (e.g., senile purpura) between the skin layers, which results in further separation of the dermis and epidermis. Disease management regimens also can alter the skin's vitality. For example, corticosteroids reduce tissue collagen strength and elasticity and thereby increase the patient's risk of skin tears. Long-term consequences of radiation therapy are epidermal atrophy, microvascular occlusions, reduced fibroblast proliferation, and tissue fibrosis.

Skin tears cannot be prevented by one individual. Because the typical individual at risk for skin tears is dependent on caregivers for many aspects of care, preventive interventions must be embraced by all staff members. Therefore staff education is a critical component of a skin tear prevention and treatment program. By using a web-based educational program, McTigue et al (2009) found that acute care registered nurses from two affiliated hospitals ($N = 416$) had significantly improved their ability to identify, assess, classify, and treat skin tears ($p < .001$) after they had completed the program.

A standardized care plan for patients at high risk for skin tears is shown in Box 5-2 (Ayello, 2003; LeBlanc et al,

---

BOX 5-2   Standardized Care Plan for Patients at High Risk for Skin Tears

1. Provide a safe environment.
   - Free room of obstacles that obstruct pathway around bed and bathroom.
   - Provide adequate lighting in resident's room.
   - Leave on nightlight in bathroom and leave door open.
   - Leave side rails down at night.
   - Make hourly rounds.
   - Provide safe area for wandering.
   - Implement bed or ankle alarm.
   - Provide well-fitting supportive shoes with skid-free soles.
   - Use protective garments for arms, legs, areas of purpura (e.g., fleece-lined jogging suits, knee-length athletic socks, stockinette doubled, skin sleeves).
   - Pad rough edges of furniture.
   - Relocate or loosen ID band when determined to be cause of skin tears.
2. Maintain nutrition and hydration.
   - Obtain dietary consult.
   - Obtain physician's order for double portions or high-protein snacks between meals.
   - Keep intake and output records.
   - Offer fluids between meals twice every shift.
   - Encourage fluids at every meal.
   - Inspect and moisturize arms and legs twice daily.
3. Protect from self-inflicted injury or injury incurred during routine cares.
   - Keep nails clipped.
   - Use wheelchair for transport only.
   - Use sling around chair legs to prevent feet from falling off footrests.
   - Position with pillows and folded blankets to prevent head and arms from dangling over side of chair.
   - Use palm of hands and lift sheet instead of fingers to position patient.
   - Use mechanical lift for transfers.
   - Obtain occupational or physical therapy consultation if needed for safe positioning.
   - Avoid adhesives when possible.
   - Use appropriate methods to avoid medical adhesive related skin injury (MARSI) (see Box 5-3).

Modified from White MW, Karam S, Cowell B: Skin tears in frail elders: a practical approach to prevention, *Ger Nurs* 15(2):95–99, 1994.

2008; White et al, 1994). Recognizing "at-risk" individuals and implementing key preventive strategies has been shown to decrease the incidence of skin tears (Bank and Nix, 2006; Brillhart, 2005). Extreme care and a gentle touch are critical when touching the patient or performing patient care, because most skin tears occur during the course of providing routine patient care activities (e.g., bathing, dressing, transferring) (Malone et al, 1991; McGough-Csarny and Kopac, 1998; White et al, 1994). Because harsh soaps and frequent bathing can reduce the skin's natural lubrication and lead to dry skin, gentle skin cleansers and frequent moisturizing are important components of skin tear prevention (Bank and Nix, 2006; Birch and Coggins, 2003; Brillhart, 2005; Hunter et al, 2002; Ratliff and Fletcher, 2007). It may be necessary to decrease bathing schedules and use humidifiers to increase environmental moisture (LeBlanc and Baranoski, 2009; LeBlanc et al, 2008). Rooms should be adequately lit to reduce the risk of bumping into furniture and equipment (Nazarko, 2005; Ratliff and Fletcher, 2007). Beyond these measures, the current focus of prevention is on the application of products and garments that serve as barriers between the skin and potential trauma; such products include commercially available skin sleeves, roll gauze, pants, and long-sleeve shirts (Bank and Nix, 2006).

If adhesives must be used, skin sealants can be placed on the skin before the tape is applied to provide protection from skin tears. Only alcohol-free skin sealants should be used when the skin is denuded or when contact with wound edges is likely because alcohol can cause intense stinging. It is important to allow the skin sealant to dry completely before applying tape. Many central-line dressing kits are prepackaged with a skin sealant.

When frequent tape removal is needed for dressing changes, application of an adhesive barrier (e.g., solid-wafer skin barrier or thin hydrocolloid) can be used on periwound skin to anchor tape and prevent skin stripping. The protocol should clearly indicate that the barrier is not changed routinely. The barrier should be left undisturbed and allowed to fall off. Loose edges should be clipped rather than removing the old barrier and applying a new one. Used in this way, the skin barrier or hydrocolloid dressing can remain in place for several days while caregivers easily apply and reapply the tape without traumatizing the epidermis. Box 5-3 summarizes interventions for preventing skin tears in conjunction with the use of medical adhesives.

Goals for topical care of skin tears include: maintain an approximated residual skin flap if applicable (gently reposition the flap over the wound surface) and maintain a physiologic wound environment; atraumatic dressing removal is critical (Baranoski, 2003; Fleck, 2007; LeBlanc et al, 2008; Roberts, 2007). Hydrocolloids, transparent films and closure strips are contraindicated. Rather silicones, foams, alginates, hydrofibers, and hydrogel dressings are favored and selected to maintain a moist wound environment while managing exudate and bacteria (LaBlanc et al, 2013; Meuleneire, 2002; Milne and Corbett, 2005; Roberts, 2007; Thomas et al, 1999). Approximated edges also may be secured with careful use of 2-octyl-cyanoacrylate (also referred to as topical skin bandage or skin glue) (Baranoski, 2003; Fleck, 2007; LaBlanc et al, 2008; LaBlanc et al, 2013; Roberts, 2007).

MOISTURE-ASSOCIATED SKIN DAMAGE

When the skin is exposed to moisture, such as body fluids, perspiration, or cleansers, for extended periods of time or repeatedly (i.e., frequent cleansing), the normal barrier function of the stratum corneum is diminished (Warner et al, 2003). As a result, skin pH rises and the risk of bacterial colonization increases, predisposing the patient to development of cutaneous infections. The two most common organisms are *Candida albicans* (from the gastrointestinal tract) and *Staphylococcus* (from the perineal skin).

The nomenclature used to describe and classify skin damage caused by these conditions is extensive and confusing. For example, dermatitis caused by chemical irritants has been referred to as irritant contact dermatitis. The term *diaper dermatitis*, familiar to most health care providers, specifically refers to inflammation of the skin in the diaper area (perineal

---

BOX 5-3   Prevention of Medical Adhesive Related Skin Injury (MARSI)*

1. Secure dressings with roll gauze, tubular stockinette, or self-adhering tape (avoids unnecessary tape on skin).
2. Apply tape without tension (prevents blistering of skin under tape).
3. Use porous tapes (allows moisture to evaporate).
4. Use skin sealants, thin hydrocolloids, or solid-wafer skin barriers under adhesives (provides protective layer over skin for adhering tapes).
5. Secure dressings with Montgomery straps (prevents repeated tape applications).
6. Remove tape slowly, peel away from anchored skin, or pull one corner of tape at an angle parallel with skin. Solvents can be used to break bond with skin, although solvents have drying effect on skin. Plain tap water can often serve this purpose effectively (decreases trauma to epidermis and dermal–epidermal junction).

Neonates (See also Chapter 36)
- Solvents and adhesive removers should not be used with the neonate due to reports of skin toxicity.
- Skin sealants should not be used with neonates less than 30 days old. Alcohol-free skin sealants may be used for the neonate greater than 30 days old.

*Rationale for intervention is given in parentheses.

or perigenital areas) of the infant (Zulkowski, 2008). However, when the same condition develops in the perineal area in the adult, it is often called *perineal dermatitis*. The dilemma with both terms is that they do not adequately address the irritant, and the terms exclude locations outside of the diaper or perineum, such as the inner thighs or buttocks.

Recognizing the multiplicity of terms and their limitations, the term *moisture-associated skin damage* (MASD) has been adopted to capture the "inflammation and erosion of the skin caused by prolonged exposure to various sources of moisture, including urine or stool, perspiration, wound exudate, mucus or saliva" (Gray et al, 2011). Sources of moisture that contain chemicals or enzymes (e.g., gastrointestinal secretions, stool, harsh cleansing solutions and solvents) are harmful to the skin due to their acidic pH, or high volume of enzymes, and will erode the top layers of the epidermis. In addition, when the presence of moisture is accompanied by mechanical factors such as friction and/or the presence of potentially pathogenic microorganisms, skin damage is accentuated. Coexisting infections that occur with MASD most often include candidiasis. Additional infections that can arise include herpes zoster or herpes simplex virus (HSV), tinea cruris (a dermatophyte infection of the squamous cells and trapped in a skin fold), and inverse psoriasis (Visscher, 2009).

There are four common conditions captured by the category of MASD: incontinence-associated dermatitis (IAD), periwound dermatitis, peristomal dermatitis, and intertrigo dermatitis (ITD). Incontinence-associated dermatitis is defined as a reactive response of the skin to chronic exposure to urine and fecal material, which could be observed as inflammation and erythema, with or without erosion or denudation (Gray et al, 2007a) (see Plate 13).

Pathophysiologic Process

The prolonged presence of moisture (more than 2 hours) on the skin places the skin at risk for overhydration and maceration of the epidermis. Although maceration is a seemingly innocent and common experience for anyone who soaks in the hot tub or washes dishes by hand, the corresponding weakening of the collagen fibers can reduce the skin's resiliency or ability to remain intact in the presence of mechanical action (e.g., friction, tape removal, pressure) or chemical exposure (e.g., gastrointestinal contents). In addition to urine, wound exudate, and perspiration, moisture-donating wound dressings such as hydrogel and saline-saturated gauze can be a source of moisture. Moisture can be trapped against the skin by clothing, diapers, gauze, wound dressings, and skin folds.

Maceration compromises protective skin mechanisms such as pH and normal flora. Increased skin pH can be triggered by exposure to ammonia in urine and to alkaline soaps; it has also been reported in the skin of persons with diabetes. As moisture penetrates the epidermis, it interacts with keratinocytes and fibroblasts, stimulating the release of cytokines, which act on the vasculature of the dermis to trigger inflammation. Consequently, the lipid bilayer structure of the stratum corneum is damaged, which may allow microorganisms to enter the epidermis (Visscher, 2009). Prolonged moisture also reduces the ability of the skin to resist additional stresses, such as shear, friction, and pressure, because of a higher frictional coefficient (Visscher, 2009), leading to secondary skin breakdown. The increased permeability of the skin and decreased barrier function contribute to bacterial overgrowth on the skin and cutaneous infection (Beeckman et al, 2011). Thus clinical manifestations of skin macerated by the presence of excess or prolonged moisture include pale skin color and a wrinkling, swollen appearance of the exposed skin surface (see Plate 14). As the length of exposure continues, the skin may become erythematous. Fissures may eventually develop from exposure to friction and shear. For example, linear shallow fissures may develop in the cleft between the buttocks, in skin folds, and between the toes.

Chemical Irritants and Moisture-Associated Skin Damage

Moisture-associated skin damage precipitated by exposure to harsh solutions or effluent can occur in the perineum, periwound, peritube, and peristomal area. When the epidermis is exposed to moisture that contains caustic or enzymatic contents, the skin will be further damaged by the chemical exposure. Fluids containing chemicals include, but are not limited to, povidone-iodine complex (Betadine), alkaline soaps, alcohol, gastrointestinal contents, and drainage from percutaneous tubes. Exposure to fecal incontinence (especially liquid to loose consistency) results in MASD because of the chemical composition of the fecal material (e.g., enzymes) combined with moisture and mechanical factors of shear and friction. Skin damage may be evident within only a few hours in the presence of a strong irritant (e.g., small bowel discharge). In fact, infants may develop a chemical-related skin injury as soon as they pass a loose stool into the diaper. In other situations, skin breakdown may occur only after repeated or prolonged exposure over several days, such as with soft or formed stool.

Moisture-associated skin damage triggered by chemical irritants can be distinguished from maceration by examining the exposure sites. Initially, irritants extract water-binding chemicals and lipids from the stratum corneum, and the skin decompensates so that it becomes dry and erythematous or develops an erythematous macular rash (Habif et al, 2011) (see Plate 13). With continued exposure to chemical irritants, the protective layer of the stratum corneum becomes damaged, resulting in a loss of epidermis in the area of exposure, which is described as superficial erosion or moist denudement. Moisture-associated skin damage resulting from exposure to chemicals is uncomfortable for the patient because the chemicals stimulate neurocutaneous pain receptors. In differentiating IAD from the various possible skin conditions in the perineal, perianal, or buttocks region, it is also important to recognize that chemical-induced IAD will only appear in the area that is directly in contact with the irritant. To facilitate further distinctions, Table 5-3 lists the typical assessment features of a variety of perineal-perianal skin conditions, including IAD, candidiasis, HSV, herpes zoster, and pressure ulcers.

Conditions Associated with IAD

Acute fecal incontinence is a common instigator of IAD. The etiology of acute fecal incontinence can be the result of a number of factors: nutritional (hyperosmolar enteric solutions, rapid rate of administration of enteric solutions, hypoalbuminemia), medications (antibiotics, cathartics), gastrointestinal function (short bowel syndrome, fat malabsorption, antibiotic-associated diarrhea, incomplete bowel obstruction, fecal impaction), and gastrointestinal disease (inflammatory bowel disease,

infection, radiation enteritis). The patient's medical history is helpful in identifying the most likely etiology; additional laboratory tests or radiologic examinations may be indicated for confirmation. A digital rectal examination should be conducted to rule out a fecal impaction causing an incomplete bowel obstruction. When a fecal impaction is present, the stool will be dry and hard, and the patient will not be able to pass the stool unassisted; diarrheal stool will be passed around the impaction (Abeloff et al, 2008). When an impaction is present, a sodium phosphate enema (i.e., Fleet enema) and oral cathartics may be indicated. A colonoscopy is beneficial to rule out other potential etiologies for diarrhea, including cytomegalovirus (CMV) in immunocompromised patients, graft versus host disease, inflammatory bowel disease (IBD), and ischemic colitis.

TABLE 5-3 Differential Diagnosis of Perineal/Perianal Skin Conditions

	Incontinence-Associated Dermatitis	Candidiasis	Herpes Zoster	Pressure
Location	Perineum Buttocks Inner thighs Groin Low abdominal skin folds	Perineum Buttocks Inner thighs Groin Low abdominal skin folds	Perianal Buttocks Genitals	Near bony prominences Coccyx, sacrum, ischium Under device/tube
Confirmed risk factors	Urinary and/or fecal incontinence	Moisture Antibiotics Immunosuppression	Immunosuppression Elderly Stress	Limited mobility or activity Dependent on others for repositioning, transferring, etc.
Blisters	Yes	No	Initially vesicles then pustules	Sometimes (Stage II)
Distribution pattern	Confluent or patchy Irregular edges with erythema Shallow denudement, and/or maceration Fleshy part of buttocks	Confluent or patchy rash Small round pustules, plaques, and/or satellite lesions	Grouped unilateral distribution of rash or ulcerations along dermatome Pustules erode into ulcerations Clusters or isolated individual shallow lesions or blisters	Isolated individual lesions on or near bony prominence or pressure-causing device Damage ranges from intact discoloration to partial- or full-thickness wounds
Color	Pink/red	Pink/red	Initial: Pink/red Ulcer may have yellow slough Later: Crust Severe cases: Necrosis	Pink, red, yellow, tan, gray, brown, black
Discomfort	Pain may be mild to severe	Itching, burning	Tingling sometimes noted initially Often very painful	Pain may be absent to severe
Diagnostic tests	None	Potassium hydroxide preparation scraping (KOH)	DNA polymerase chain reaction assay and direct immunofluorescent stain of skin scraping for VZV antigen Tzanck preparation Tissue culture	None

Antibiotic-associated diarrhea is an increasingly frequent cause of fecal incontinence. Broad-spectrum antibiotics, such as fluoroquinolones, ampicillin, amoxicillin, clindamycin, and cephalosporins, are the most common culprits (Higa and Kelly, 2013; Imhoff and Karpa, 2009). Antibiotics alter the gastrointestinal microflora, thus increasing the concentration of pathogenic organisms within the bowel. *Clostridium difficile* is the primary pathogen for antibiotic-associated colitis (Cohen et al, 2010). Although other pathogens may be responsible for diarrhea, *C. difficile* is the most common pathogen and more severe than *Escherichia coli* and *Salmonella* (Rohde et al, 2009). *C. difficile*, an opportunistic spore-forming, gram-positive anaerobic bacillus, is transmitted via the fecal–oral route, and the spores remain on surfaces for extended periods of time. Only bleach is effective at killing *C. difficile* on surfaces. *C. difficile* infection (CDI) has become the most common nosocomial diarrheal pathogen in hospitalized patients, identified as the culprit for 15% to 25% of cases (Cohen et al, 2010; Higa and Kelly, 2013; Stanley et al, 2013).

C. difficile infection ranges from being an asymptomatic carrier, to mild or moderate diarrhea, to fulminant pseudomembranous colitis. Diarrhea usually begins within 1 to 3 days after colonization; colonization can occur anywhere from 14 days to 3 months after antibiotic exposure (Higa and Kelly, 2013). Symptoms include foul-smelling, nonbloody, watery diarrhea (defined as the passage of three or more unformed stools in 24 or fewer consecutive hours), a stool test positive for toxigenic *C. difficile* or its toxins, or colonoscopic or histopathology findings demonstrating pseudomembranous colitis. Half of the patients will experience abdominal cramping and tenderness, abdominal distention, fever, leukocytosis, nausea, and dehydration (Stanley et al, 2010).

Three primary risk factors for CDI are hospitalization, recent history of antibiotic use, and over the age of 65 (Stanley et al, 2013). Modifiable secondary risk factors include post-pyloric tube feedings, gastric-acid-reducing therapy, and double-occupancy rooms. Significant inflammation of the colonic mucosa develops when *C. difficile* strains adhere to colonic cells and produce toxins. Both secretory diarrhea and osmotic diarrhea occur with *C. difficile*–associated diarrhea (CDAD) (Eddins and Gray, 2008). As the mucosal surface is damaged, liquid accumulates in the bowel lumen, resulting in secretory diarrhea. Toxins attract proinflammatory cytokines, binding to the colonic epithelium, which further damage the bowel wall and impair its ability to absorb water, electrolytes, and nutrients, thus precipitating osmotic diarrhea (Eddins and Gray, 2008).

C. difficile infection is confirmed by clinical presentation of symptoms (usually diarrhea), exclusion of other causes of diarrhea, and a stool culture or positive toxin assay (McFarland, 2009). An anaerobic stool culture for *C. difficile* is the most sensitive test, but not clinically practical due to its slow turnaround time; results are not available for 3 days (Cohen et al, 2010; Stanley et al, 2013). Although results from the enzyme immunoassay (EIA) testing are available within

2 to 3 hours, the 2010 Society for Healthcare Epidemiology of America (SHEA) guidelines describe it as suboptimal for diagnosis because it is less sensitive than the cell cytotoxin assay (Cohen et al, 2010). The more sensitive tissue culture assay also can be done to detect cytotoxin or toxin B, but results take longer. These guidelines recommend a two-step approach with an initial screening using the EIA detection of glutamate dehydrogenase (GDH) and then the cell cytotoxicity assay or toxigenic culture as the confirmatory test for GDH-positive stool specimens. A direct stool polymerase chain reaction assay provides quick results and reports fewer false-negative results than the EIA (McFarland, 2009); however, more research is needed on utility (Cohen et al, 2010). Nucleic acid amplification tests (NAATs) have been approved by the Food and Drug Administration (FDA) and are currently preferred by many laboratories (Schutze et al, 2013). These tests have quick turnaround time and do not require a two- or three-step approach, but more research is needed. Before *C. difficile* toxin assays were available, colonoscopic examinations were common; a colonic biopsy positive for pseudomembranes in the presence of diarrhea is diagnostic of CDAD (Bartlett, 2008).

Standard treatment of CDAD is (1) prompt discontinuation of the antibiotic, (2) stool toxin assay, (3) oral metronidazole for initial episode of mild to moderate CDI (500 mg three times per day for 10 to 14 days), (4) correction of fluid and electrolyte imbalance, and (5) discontinuation of antiperistalsis medications. Metronidazole should be started even before the stool culture results are available when the systemic symptoms present create a high level of suspicion of CDAD. Oral vancomycin is the drug of choice for initial episodes of severe CDI (125 mg four times per day for 10 to 14 days) (Cohen et al, 2010). This can also be given rectally when an ileus is present (500 mg in approximately 100 ml normal saline every 6 hours as retention enema). After initial antibiotic therapy, almost one fourth of patients with CDAD relapse within 2 months because spores can prevent peristalsis and delay exposure to antibiotics by "hiding" in the mucosal folds (Rohde et al, 2009). A more virulent strain has been discovered and is associated with increased disease severity and death (Cohen et al, 2010; Stanley et al, 2013). *C. difficile* infection prevention measures emphasize infection control (gowns, gloves, isolation), hand hygiene with soap and water by all people in contact with the patient (including family and visitors), environmental disinfection (chlorine-containing compounds or vaporized hydrogen peroxide on areas of potential contamination), and antibiotic stewardship (minimal use of antibiotics for the shortest duration possible and narrow-spectrum antibiotics) (Stanley et al, 2013).

Intertrigo Dermatitis

Intertrigo dermatitis is defined as inflammation resulting from moisture trapped in skin folds subjected to friction (Sibbald et al, 2013). Risk factors for ITD are hyperhidrosis, obesity, pendulous breasts, deep skin folds, immobility, and diabetes. Intertrigo dermatitis is diagnosed based on clinical findings and supplemented with laboratory tests when a secondary infection is suspected. The distribution of ITD is a mirror image with erythema, inflammation, and/or erosion (often linear) in the skin fold. Symptoms may include pruritus, pain, and odor.

Moisture-Associated Skin Damage Prevention and Treatment

The plan of care to prevent and treat MASD begins with identification of the moisture source (Zulkowski, 2012). At that point one can implement steps to reduce the presence of moisture. For example, when the source of moisture is urine, steps should be implemented to facilitate bladder control, such as with behavioral interventions, diet, and fluids.

In a systematic review of the literature, a structured skin care protocol was demonstrated to reduce the incidence of IAD (Beeckman et al, 2009). A structured skin care protocol is a three-step process: gentle skin cleansing, moisturization, and the application of a skin protectant; the type of fluid on the skin and frequency of exposure will dictate the type of skin protectant used. Box 5-4 lists interventions and products that can be used to prevent and treat MASD. Table 5-4 lists a formulary of products used to prevent and manage MASD. Unique considerations concerning the prevention and management of MASD, and specifically IAD in the neonate or premature infant, are addressed in Chapter 36.

Skin cleansers with a pH near the skin's pH are more effective than soap and water at preventing IAD (Beeckman et al, 2009). Moisturizers are an important second step in the perineal skin care regimen and often are incorporated into commercially prepared skin cleansers. The three categories of skin protectants are skin sealant, moisture barrier ointment, and moisture barrier paste. Skin sealants provide a polymer film to protect the skin from maceration but may have limited effectiveness at protecting the skin from enzymes. Moisture barrier ointments protect the skin from effluent with enzymes, but may be inadequate with high-volume output or excessively frequent effluent production or diarrhea. In these situations, a moisture barrier paste should be used. Proper use of an ointment or paste consists of applying the product and, when the surface becomes soiled, using a soft pad to gently wipe off the stained surface of the product. The skin should not be scrubbed in an attempt to completely remove the product. When the product must be completely removed, mineral oil can be used to facilitate removal. Commercially available incontinence cleansers also can be used to remove a barrier paste.

Containment devices include external pouches and indwelling catheters. Containment devices may be indicated for containment of contaminated stool for infection control purposes and/or when the frequency or volume of stool overwhelms the moisture barrier ointment or paste. Rectal pouches are adhesive ostomy pouches specifically designed

---

BOX 5-4 MASD: Types and Interventions*

Periwound
- Routine hygiene to keep skin clean and dry using skin cleanser and moisturizer.
- Use skin sealant, skin barrier ointment, skin barrier paste, or solid-wafer skin barrier to protect periwound skin.
- Use dressing with adequate absorptive capacity (see also Chapter 18).
- Change dressings before saturation occurs.
- Use low air loss support surface for moisture control of large surface areas that cannot be adequately protected with dressings, absorptive pads, or skin barrier.

Peritube or Drain (see also Chapter 39)
- Collaborate with appropriate service (i.e., intervention radiology) to determine cause of leakage, confirm proper placement, and optimal stabilization.
- Routine mild cleansing with skin cleanser and moisturizer.
- Use skin sealant, skin barrier ointment, skin barrier paste, or solid-wafer skin barrier to protect peritube skin.
- Use dressing with adequate absorptive capacity.
- Change dressings before saturation occurs.

Between Skin Folds (ITD)
- Routine hygiene to keep skin clean and dry.
- Dust intertriginous skin surfaces with absorbent skin barrier powder.

- Separate intertriginous skin surfaces with skin sealant, barrier, and/or soft cotton material (i.e., t-shirt).
- Place commercially available textile in skin fold (do not use emollients with this product).

Incontinence
- Determine and treat etiology.
- Identify patients at risk for skin damage.
- Use absorptive padding (without plastic back) as needed; change after incontinent episodes.
- Cleanse with mild incontinence skin cleanser; repeat after each incontinent episode.
- Apply moisturizer to skin.
- Apply appropriate skin barrier to keep urine and feces off epidermis.
- Apply condom catheter or external pouch.
- Use indwelling catheters *only* with clear indication, assessment of contraindications, and order; change per manufacturer's instructions.
- *Low risk* of skin breakdown (urine and/or formed, soft stools): Apply skin sealant or moisture barrier ointment; reapply skin sealant per manufacturer's instructions; reapply moisture barrier ointment with each incontinent episode.
- *High risk* of skin breakdown (impaired skin integrity apparent, actual or anticipated loose stools): Apply skin barrier *paste* and repeat per manufacturer's instructions.

*See Table 5-4 for product examples.

TABLE 5-4 Formulary of Products* Used to Prevent and Manage MASD**

Product	Purpose	Examples*	Additional Information
Perineal cleanser	Perineal skin cleansing	Coloplast CarraFoam or CarraWash, Medline Soothe & Cool, Smith & Nephew Secura	Liquid, foam, or impregnated cloth products available in rinse or no rinse.
Perineal cleanser and protectant	Combination product for cleansing and protecting perineal skin	Coloplast Baza Cleanse and Protect, Sage Comfort Shield, Medline Remedy	Skin cleanser that does not have to be rinsed off and simultaneously applies a skin protectant. Available in liquid, foam, or impregnated cloth products.
Moisture barrier ointment	Perineal skin protection	Calmoseptine ointment, Lantiseptic skin protectant, Proshield Plus skin protectant, Critic-Aide clear hydrophilic ointment	May impair adhesion if used in combination with perianal pouches.
Moisture barrier paste	Periwound, perifistula, peritube, high-risk perineal skin protection	Critic-Aide skin paste, Ilex skin protectant paste, Remedy Calazime protectant paste	More durable than moisture barrier ointment. Appropriate for open, denuded skin. Only need to remove top soiled layer of ointment before reapplication. Do not use force to remove. Mineral oil and selected perineal cleansers. May impair adhesion if used in combination with adhesive dressings and pouches. Some wound care treatments cannot be used with zinc-based pastes.
Solid skin barrier	Peristomal, perifistula, peritube, periwound skin protection	Stomahesive, Eakin, premium skin barrier	More durable than moisture barrier ointments and pastes. Available in multiple sizes and shapes (e.g., wafer, rings, strips). Waterproof; can be worn for several days.
Skin sealant	Perineal, peristomal, perifistula, peritube, periwound skin protection	No Sting Skin Prep protective dressing, Cavilon No Sting barrier film, skin gel wipe Butyl and octyl cyanoacrylate blend (e.g., Marathon)	Liquid transparent cyanoacrylate delivered by a wipe, wand, or spray. Provides a copolymer film. Some products contain isopropyl alcohol. Non–alcohol-based products should be used when skin is compromised. Butyl and octyl cyanoacrylates are wound closure adhesives intended for closure of full thickness wounds.
Skin barrier powder	Absorbs and dries weepy denuded skin to improve adherence of ointments, pastes, adhesive barriers	Stomahesive protective powder, Karaya powder, premium powder	Will impair adhesion if used on intact skin or if used in excess. Discontinue when the skin is no longer denuded.
External perianal pouch	Perianal, peristomal skin protection, containment of stool	Hollister fecal incontinence collector, ConvaTec fecal collector	Combines pouch with solid skin barrier for non-ambulatory patients. Comes with spout for use with bedside drain; spout can be cut off and replaced with provided tail closure. Odorproof and waterproof with gas filter option.
External urinary catheter	Perineal skin protection, containment of urine	Mentor-Coloplast Freedom Hollister extended wear, Hollister retracted penis pouch, Kendall Uri-Drain	Products made in variety of sizes and must be properly fit. Available in latex and nonlatex. Application involves self-adhesives or added adhesive strips.
Indwelling fecal containment device	Perianal skin protection, containment of loose stool	Hollister ActiFlo indwelling bowel catheter, ConvaTec Flexi-Seal fecal management system, Bard Digni-Care stool management system	Do not use without physician's order. Critical to read manufacturer's instruction for contraindications and safe use. May need additional perianal protection with moisture barrier paste.
Textile	Skin fold protection	InterDry Ag textile with antimicrobial silver complex	Wicks away moisture from skin-to-skin contact areas to manage moisture, odor, and inflammation. Comes in rolls; cut amount needed.

*Examples of product names are not inclusive or intended as an endorsement.
**Some of these products may not be appropriate for neonates; please see Chapter 36 and Table 36-2 specifically for important considerations in selecting skin care products for neonates.

to fit the perianal contours and contain the incontinent stool. By protecting the skin from chemicals and moisture buildup, these products can be extremely cost-effective by reducing linen changes and freeing up nursing time for other types of care. Rectal pouches also preserve the patient's dignity by containing odor and feces. Acceptable wear time for the rectal pouch is 24 hours. Extra care should be used when repositioning the patient to prevent excess shear on the pouch and the surrounding skin. Step-by-step directions for application are provided by the manufacturer and should be followed closely.

Historically, large indwelling urinary catheters or devices called rectal or colon tubes designed for enema and medication administration have been inserted into the rectum and left in place. This practice is not safe because it has the potential to damage the anal sphincter and/or perforate the bowel. Only indwelling bowel and fecal management systems approved by the FDA are designed to safely divert, collect, and contain potentially harmful and contaminated gastrointestinal waste without damaging the anal sphincter. It is important to review the manufacturer's instructions for each product to understand differences in features, indications, and contraindications. Researchers have reported efficient evacuation with minimal leakage or anorectal mucosal injury, reduction of perineal skin breakdown and pressure ulcers, and no anorectal mucosal injury (Kim et al, 2001; Kowal-Vern et al, 2009). Reduction of perineal skin injury and pressure ulcers, as well as decreased rates of urinary tract, soft tissue, skin, and bloodstream infections, also have been reported (Benoit and Watts, 2007; Kowal-Vern et al, 2009). These studies highlight the potential of these devices beyond the scope of skin protection and into the realm of managing infection and cross-contamination.

Drainage around catheters and tubes should be managed such that the drainage is eliminated, when possible, or the skin is not directly exposed to the drainage. For example, when leakage occurs around a gastrostomy tube, the first step is to ascertain proper placement and stabilization of the tube. If drainage persists once this is accomplished, appropriate use of skin barriers (particularly moisture barrier ointments, solid-wafer skin barriers, thin hydrocolloids, or foam dressings) is indicated. A solid-wafer skin barrier, hydrocolloid, or foam dressing can be trimmed to fit around a tube site; it can remain in place for several days and changed only when it loosens at the tube site. When ointment is the selected treatment, it should be reapplied periodically throughout the day to ensure adequate skin protection. However, ointments can never be used under an adhesive dressing. Regardless of the type of skin protection selected, gauze dressings are applied over the barrier to absorb drainage and are changed when damp.

Improper use of skin care products, particularly solvents, adhesives, and skin sealants, can contribute to chemical skin damage. Only pH-neutral skin cleansers should be used. Adhesive solvents must be thoroughly rinsed from the skin to prevent buildup of harmful substances. Soaps should be avoided to prevent disruption of the skin's normal acid pH. Skin sealants and adhesives, such as cements, must be allowed to dry adequately so that solvents evaporate before other products are applied.

The prevention and treatment of ITD are based on minimizing skin-to-skin contact and friction, removing irritants and moisture from the skin fold, and wicking moisture away from the vulnerable area (Sibbald et al, 2013). Prevention measures include (1) skin cleansing with pH-balanced product; (2) gentle cleansing, no scrubbing; (3) soft cloth, no washcloths; and (4) pat dry. Talc, cornstarch, antiperspirants in the skin fold, and placing bed or bath linens in the skin fold are contraindicated. Many people with obesity will offer that they routinely use a natural fiber type of material such as a cotton "t-shirt" in their skin fold to prevent moisture entrapment. A moisture-wicking textile with silver is recommended; if a secondary infection is present, appropriate systemic or topical antimicrobials will be needed.

Medical Adhesive–Related Skin Injury

Medical adhesives precipitate several forms of skin damage and are broadly labeled medical adhesive–related skin injury, or MARSI. These are extremely common complications that are often erroneously dismissed as unavoidable. Damage to the skin from medical adhesives is also a significant source of pain and discomfort for the patient. The definition of MARSI is "an occurrence in which erythema and/or other manifestation of cutaneous abnormality (including, but not limited to, vesicle, bulla, erosion, or tear) persists 30 minutes of more after removal of the adhesive" (McNichol et al, 2013). Types of MARSI include epidermal stripping, skin tears, tension blisters, maceration, folliculitis, irritant contact dermatitis, and allergic contact dermatitis. Factors that contribute to tape trauma include product-related factors (peel force, tape occlusiveness, rigidity of backing, rheology of adhesive), user technique (process of application and removal), and patient factors (age, general health, application of solvents, preps, cleansers, and anatomic site). Of these factors, the least familiar issues to most health care providers pertain to tape-related factors.

Medical adhesives contain several layers. The two key layers that affect the adhesive's properties and performance are the adhesive layer and the backing. The adhesive layer contacts with the skin and may be an acrylate, silicone, hydrogel, hydrocolloid, polyurethane, or latex. The backing of the adhesive is the more commonly used descriptor: paper, plastic, silk, cloth, foam, elastic. This backing provides the properties of stretch, conformability, occlusion, and rigidity, which are important criteria to consider in selecting an adhesive product.

Medical adhesives are both pressure sensitive and time sensitive. When the adhesive contacts the skin, firm pressure activates the adhesive to conform to the microscopic uneven surfaces of the epidermis. Over time the adhesive also warms and begins to flow to fill in the gaps in the irregular skin surface, further increasing the strength of the bond. Acrylate adhesives fill the skin gaps slowly, thus taking more time to adhere. In contrast, silicone adhesives are considered a "softer adhesive" that fills the skin gaps more quickly and provides a constant level of adherence rather than becoming more adherent over time. Box 5-5 provides a list of consensus statements for the assessment, prevention, and treatment of MARSI.

VASCULAR DAMAGE

Ulcerations, particularly on the legs or feet, can occur as a result of venous hypertension, arterial insufficiency, neuropathy, or a combination of these factors. Although these types of lesions commonly develop incidental to benign trauma (i.e., by bumping against the leg of a chair), each ulcer has distinct distinguishing features, pathologic processes, and treatment regimens. Arterial ulcers, venous ulcers, and

---

BOX 5-5 MARSI: Consensus Statement for Assessment, Prevention, Treatment

Assessment
1. During use of adhesive-containing products, the skin should be assessed for evidence of damage on a daily basis or with adhesive device changes; this is especially important for those patients deemed to be at high risk for adhesive-related injury.
2. For all medical adhesive-related skin injuries, a comprehensive assessment should be performed to determine severity and guide management.
3. Obtain a history of patient's known or suspected allergies and sensitivities to minimize the risk of medical adhesive-related skin injury.
4. The incidence of true allergic contact dermatitis related to adhesives is not known; suspected allergic contact dermatitis should be considered for referral and/or appropriate investigation (such as patch or scratch tests).

Prevention
General
1. Identification of patients at high risk for medical adhesive-related skin injury is a key component of prevention.
2. Care of the skin, including prevention of adhesive-related injury, should be a standard of care for all health care providers.
3. Prevention of medical adhesive-related skin injuries is facilitated by good nutrition and hydration.

Selection, Application, and Removal
1. Select the most appropriate adhesive product based on its intended purpose, the anatomic location the adhesive will be applied to, and the ambient conditions present at application site.
2. Appropriate product selection entails consideration of properties of adhesive-containing products such as adhesive gentleness, breathability, stretch, conformability, and flexibility.
3. Consider the potential adverse consequences of insufficient adhesion and/or adhesive failure when selecting medical adhesive products for use in securing a critical device.
4. Exercise caution when using silicone adhesives to secure some devices, as this may result in suboptimal adherence or adhesion failure.

Selection and Application
1. Anticipate changes in skin and/or joint movement following surgery and operative or other procedures when selecting and applying medical adhesive products.

2. Anticipate skin movement with edema when selecting and applying medical adhesives.

Application
1. Consider the role of skin tension (Langer's lines) and the effects of medical adhesive products when applied with the lines or against/across the lines.
2. Consider application of a skin barrier before applying an adhesive product.
3. Limit or avoid substances that increase the stickiness of adhesives, such as compound tincture of benzoin.

Application and Removal
1. Use proper application and removal techniques for adhesive-containing products.
2. Consider use of medical adhesive removers to minimize discomfort and skin damage associated with removal of adhesive products.

Electrodes
1. To prevent electrochemical burns under adhesive electrodes, powered (battery and line voltage) equipment should be maintained and monitored for dangerous leakage currents.

Infection Prevention
1. Adhesives may promote overgrowth of microorganisms. Monitor sites exposed to adhesive materials for manifestations of infection.
2. Store and use adhesive-containing products in a manner that prevents contamination.
3. Single-patient-use adhesive products are preferred.

Treatment
1. Apply evidence-based wound care principles when treating medical adhesive-related skin injuries.
2. Consult an appropriate skin or wound care specialist if a medical adhesive-related skin injury does not respond to conservative management within 7 days or if the wound deteriorates despite conservative care.

Future Research
1. Further research is needed to expand the scientific knowledge of adhesive performance and use, including mechanisms of medical adhesive-related skin injury, prediction, prevention, assessment and documentation, and treatment.

lymphedema wounds are discussed in detail in Chapters 11 through 13. Neuropathic ulcers, such as diabetic ulcers, are discussed in Chapter 14.

INFECTIOUS AGENTS

Many skin rashes or ulcers are indicative of an infectious process and can occur around wounds or be misinterpreted as a pressure, shear, or chemical injury. Infections can be categorized according to infecting organism: fungus, bacteria, virus, or arthropod. The wound care specialist may be the first person to observe some of these infections. In many cases, the wound specialist will be responsible for identifying and managing the infections. The common skin infections are discussed here; the more unusual skin infections are addressed in Chapter 30.

Fungal

Candidiasis. Candidiasis is the most common opportunistic fungal infection (Kauffman, 2008). *Candida* spp., which are yeast-like organisms that reproduce by budding, normally colonize the skin, gastrointestinal tract, genitourinary tract, and vagina. When immunologic defenses are compromised or the normal flora is altered, *Candida* spp. become opportunistic pathogens.

Cutaneous candidiasis is an epidermal infection with *Candida* spp. Although more than 150 species of *Candida* exist, the most common is *C. albicans* (see Plates 15 and 16). The primary lesion of candidiasis is a pustule or erythematous papules or plaques that may have associated scaling or crusting or a cheesy white exudate. Maceration is common. Lesions typically are beefy red, with satellite erythematous papules and pustules. Satellite lesions (outside the advancing edge of candidiasis) are an important diagnostic feature of candidiasis (Habif et al, 2011). Intact pustules are not always visible because opposing skin and clothing will unroof the pustule so that the lesion appears to be a macule or papule. Pruritus is the key indicator of candidiasis and may be severe.

A common location for development of candidiasis is in skin folds; *intertrigo* is the term used for an inflammatory condition of skin folds (see Plate 17). Intertrigo can be induced by heat, moisture, maceration, and friction. In addition to *Candida* spp., intertrigo can be complicated by other fungal infections (tinea) and by bacterial infection (erythrasma). *Candida* intertrigo is located in the skin folds (intertriginous areas) and is characterized by an intensely red, macerated, glistening, confluent macular papular rash. The half-moon-shaped edge of the rash or plaque often extends just beyond the limits of the opposing skin folds. Satellite lesions usually are present (Brannon, 2009).

Predisposing factors to candidiasis include the presence of a moist environment, a hot and humid environment, tight underclothing, diabetes, and antibiotic therapy. Skin under damp surgical dressings, the perineum, the perineal area, and intertriginous areas (beneath pendulous breasts, overhanging abdominal folds, and inguinal skin folds) are typical moist areas that provide an excellent medium for yeast growth. Diabetes predisposes the patient to development of candidiasis because the associated increase in the amount of glucose in the saliva, sweat, and urine in patients with diabetes prevents bacteria from inhibiting yeast growth (Carpenter and de Sanctis, 2008). Antibiotics predispose the patient to development of candidiasis by removing the competing organisms. An altered skin pH also increases susceptibility to yeast infection. Immunosuppressed patients and patients with irritant contact dermatitis are vulnerable to candidiasis.

Folliculitis and contact dermatitis can be confused with candidiasis. Furthermore, candidiasis can be disguised by being superimposed on irritant contact dermatitis. The distribution and types of lesions are important to identifying the underlying problem. Folliculitis, the inflammation of a hair follicle, is characterized by the presence of pustules pierced in the center by a hair (see Plate 18), whereas candidiasis causes nonfollicular pustules. Manifestations of contact dermatitis include erythema with papules, whereas pustules are unusual and warrant culture to rule out superimposed infection. Distribution can help distinguish contact dermatitis from candidiasis because a contact dermatitis conforms to the specific shape of the irritant and therefore has well-defined borders, does not have satellite lesions, and does not have pruritus.

Intertrigo candidiasis is also easily confused with tinea cruris, erythrasma (both discussed later), and inverse psoriasis. Psoriasis is a chronic inflammatory papular skin disease characterized by scaly plaques that may affect skin, nails, and joints. It is attributed to abnormal T-lymphocyte function rather than an infection (Habif et al, 2011). One of the many unique clinical forms is intertriginous psoriasis (also known as *inverse psoriasis*). It is uncommon but can occur in the groin or under the breasts. The skin appears macerated with smooth, red, sharply defined plaques. Satellite lesions will not be present unless a candidal infection is superimposed on the psoriasis. The application of a topical steroid is associated with contributing to the added complication of candidiasis.

Candidiasis is most often determined clinically by signs, symptoms, and predisposing factors. Pruritus and burning at the site are common. The most relevant laboratory test for confirming candidiasis is a potassium hydroxide preparation scraping. Scrapings from an intact pustule and the contents are needed to yield the best results. Budding spores and elongated pseudohyphae are observed. Because the skin can be colonized with *C. albicans* but not infected, swab cultures for *Candida* are not informative, as such cultures cannot distinguish between infection and colonization (Carpenter and de Sanctis, 2008).

Nonpharmacologic treatment includes reduction of predisposing factors, such as humidity, moisture, antibiotics, hyperglycemia, and tight-fitting clothes. Body powders (e.g., Zeasorb-AF) or wide-mesh gauze can be placed in intertriginous areas to absorb moisture. Prevention of moisture buildup is the most important intervention to prevent candidiasis. Box 5-4 lists additional strategies to protect the skin from moisture-related complication. Table 5-4 lists a formulary of products used to prevent moisture- or chemical-related skin damage.

Burow's solution soaks followed by air drying are soothing when maceration or severe pruritus is present. Topical antifungal creams can be applied twice daily for limited involvement, and antifungal powders can be used in less severe cases. When creams are used, they should be applied sparingly to reduce moisture entrapment. Recalcitrant or severe fungal infections require orally administered therapy.

Dermatophyte (Tinea). The dermatophyte is a type of fungus that is responsible for the majority of fungal infections on the skin, nails, and hair (Habif et al, 2011). Known as *tinea*, a dermatophyte infection infects only dead keratin, so the stratum corneum on the skin is vulnerable. A tinea infection cannot survive in the mouth or vagina because these sites do not have a keratin layer. As a pruritic superficial fungal infection, tinea can be challenging to diagnose and treat (Wiederkehr and Schwartz, 2008). The manifestations of tinea infections vary according to body site. Box 5-6 lists the types of tinea based on body location. Tinea pedis occurs on the feet and is more familiar as *athlete's foot*. Tinea cruris occurs in the groin skin folds and is more commonly known as *jock itch*. Tinea corporis is present on the body and is also known as *ringworm*, although no worm is involved with this infection.

Fungi live on damp surfaces, and most tinea infections develop on moist surfaces (e.g., skin folds, web between toes, soles of the feet). Dermatophytes can be picked up from the floor of public showers or lockers, from a pet that is infected, or from loaning or borrowing clothing items from other individuals. Some individuals may be genetically predisposed to tinea infections (Habif et al, 2011). The active border of tinea will be scaly, red, and slightly elevated. When inflammation is significant, vesicles may be present along this active border.

Tinea can be diagnosed by directly visualizing the branches of keratinized strands under the microscope. This is done with a potassium hydroxide wet mount preparation where a scale is removed from the active edge of the infection with a no. 15 surgical blade, placed on the microscope slide, and prepared for viewing (Habif et al, 2011). Dermatophytes will appear as translucent, branching, rod-shaped strands (hyphae) with uniform width. A Wood's light examination of hair will fluoresce blue to green when infected with *Microsporum* spp. of the dermatophyte fungi. Fungal infections of the skin do not fluoresce.

Box 5-7 lists the interventions for prevention of tinea infections. Treatment varies slightly by body site, but primarily consists of topical antifungal medications such as butenafine (Lotrimin Ultra), terbinafine (Lamisil), or sertaconazole (Ertaczo) applied twice daily for 2 to 4 weeks. When interdigital web spaces are severely macerated, the antifungal medication econazole nitrate (Spectazole) also provides an antibacterial effect that addresses common secondary bacterial infections (Habif et al, 2011; Noble et al, 1998; Wiederkehr and Schwartz, 2009). Moist lesions also can be treated with a Burow's solution dressing for 20 to 30 minutes two to six times daily until the skin is dry.

Topical corticosteroid creams are commonly prescribed for inflammatory skin lesions, particularly in the groin; however, corticosteroids must be avoided when a dermatophyte infection is suspected. Use of these products can alter the clinical presentation of a dermatophyte infection, creating a condition called *tinea incognito*. When topical steroids are applied, they decrease the inflammation, which is interpreted as improvement. However, the dermatophyte fungus will flourish in the localized steroid-induced immunosuppression. When the corticosteroid is discontinued because the inflammation is resolving, the rash will return, but then the appearance will be different (absent scaling at the margins, diffuse erythema, scattered pustules or papules, and brown hyperpigmentation) and the area of involvement greatly expanded. Treatment remains topical antifungal agents; oral antifungal medications may be needed for extensive lesions (red papules and pustules).

BOX 5-6   Tinea Patterns

- Tinea pedis (foot)
- Tinea cruris (jock itch) (groin)
- Tinea corporis (ringworm) (body)
- Tinea faciei (face)
- Tinea manuum (hand)
- Tinea capitis (scalp)
- Tinea of barbae (beard)
- Tinea of onychomycosis (nails)

BOX 5-7   Preventing Tinea Infections

- Expose feet to air whenever home.
- Change socks and underwear daily, especially in warm weather.
- Dry feet carefully (especially between toes) after using locker room or public shower.
- Avoid walking barefoot in public areas; wear flip-flops, sandals, or water shoes.
- Do not wear thick clothing for long periods of time in warm weather; heavy clothes will cause increased sweating, which can encourage growth of fungal infections.
- Discard worn exercise shoes. Never borrow other people's shoes.
- Do not borrow or lend personal towels or clothing to other people.
- Check pets for areas of hair loss and ask veterinarian to check pets as well. Determine whether pets are causing patient's fungal infection; otherwise, patient may become infected again, even after treatment.
- Make sure shared exercise equipment (e.g., treadmill at gym) is clean before using it.

Bacterial

Folliculitis, impetigo, and erysipelas are bacterial skin infections caused by coagulase-positive *Staphylococcus (aureus)*, coagulase-negative *Staphylococcus (epidermidis)*, or beta-hemolytic streptococcus (Bradley, 2008; File and Stevens, 2008). Although *S. aureus* can be recovered from normal intact skin, especially in the nares, axillae, and groin, it is rarely a true member of resident bacterial flora and is considered a highly invasive pathogen. Staphylococci are able to quickly develop resistance to antibiotics; all staphylococci should be considered resistant to penicillins. Methicillin-resistant *Staphylococcus aureus* (MRSA) and methicillin-resistant *Staphylococcus epidermidis* (MRSE) account for up to 50% of *S. aureus*–identified nosocomial infections in some medical centers (Bradley, 2008). Community-associated methicillin-resistant *Staphylococcus aureus* (CA-MRSA) strains also have been reported. Vancomycin-resistant *Staphylococcus aureus* (VRSA) has developed as a consequence of prolonged use of vancomycin as the primary treatment of serious MRSA infections. First-generation cephalosporins and penicillinase-resistant penicillins are the most effective drugs for treating mild to moderate infections.

Cellulitis. Cellulitis is an infection of the dermis and subcutaneous tissue that is most commonly caused by *S. aureus*, *Staphylococcus pyogenes*, and group A streptococcus (Sachdeva and Tomecki, 2008). Cellulitis is preceded by some type of break in the skin, such as an ulcer, laceration, surgical incision, bite, burn, or body piercing, which becomes the portal of entry for the infecting organism (File and Stevens, 2008). The most frequent sites on the body for occurrence of cellulitis are the posterior legs and hands. The head, abdomen, back, neck, buttocks, perigenital and perineal areas, and inner thighs are uncommon to rare sites for cellulitis (Habif et al, 2011).

Cellulitis should be differentiated from the erythema associated with venous dermatitis (see Table 12-3) or contact allergic dermatitis (distribution has very precise edges and shape is consistent with outline of offending agent). In the perineal and perigenital areas, cellulitis can be distinguished from the erythema associated with a Stage I pressure ulcer based on the location of the lesion (a Stage I pressure ulcer is most often limited to skin overlying a bony prominence). Relative to IAD, cellulitis should be distinguished from intertrigo, erythrasma, chemical denudation, and psoriasis.

Assessment findings characteristic of cellulitis include localized erythema with diffuse borders, tenderness upon palpation, warmth, and edema. Crepitus (palpation of gas in the subcutaneous tissue), however, is pathologic for aerobic infections, such as *Clostridia*, most often *Clostridia perfringens*. An elevated white blood cell count and erythrocyte sedimentation rate may be present. Recurrent cellulitis will impair lymphatic drainage and lead to lymphedema, dermal fibrosis, and epidermal thickening. A culture is required to discern the invading organism and the appropriate antibiotic initiated. Empiric treatment may begin before the culture results are obtained, but should be effective for both staphylococcal and streptococcal organisms (Habif et al, 2011). Most patients respond to oral antibiotic therapy; reevaluation and consideration of intravenous antibiotics should be considered if the patient does not respond. Clostridial infections will require high-dose intravenous penicillin in addition to prompt debridement and surgical exploration of the cellulitis site (Sachdeva and Tomecki, 2008).

Erysipelas. Erysipelas is an acute inflammatory form of cellulitis that occurs as a complication of a break in skin integrity, which occurs with abrasions or dry skin. Erysipelas differs from other types of cellulitis because it involves the cutaneous lymphatics, in the form of "streaking." This disease has a very high morbidity rate if left undiagnosed (up to 80% in infants and 75% in the elderly) (File and Stevens, 2008).

Erysipelas most commonly occurs in infants, young children, and older adults. Additional risk factors include malnutrition, alcoholism, recent infections, stasis dermatitis, lymphedema, nephrotic syndrome, and diabetes mellitus. Small, seemingly insignificant breaks in the skin can serve as a portal of entry for infection. The extremities and the face are the most common sites (Sachdeva and Tomecki, 2008).

Erysipelas means "red skin," and the involved body part is characterized by well-defined erythema. (In contrast, cellulitis is less demarcated.) The classic primary lesion is a plaque. Prodromal symptoms, such as malaise, myalgias, chills, and high fever, may occur within 4 to 48 hours of infection. The surrounding skin rapidly progresses to become erythematous, edematous, and intensely painful. Secondary lesions are vesicles, bullae, and cutaneous hemorrhage. Within 5 to 10 days of onset, desquamation of the affected area occurs (Stevens et al, 2008). Associated lymphangitis is demonstrated by the presence of erythematous streaking over lymphatics draining the area of infection.

Erysipelas usually is diagnosed by clinical findings of sharply defined erythema, edema, and/or streaking. Accompanying systemic complaints of fever, chills, malaise, and localized pain also raise suspicion for the presence of the condition. Although cultures (via needle aspiration) of any drainage from the advancing edge and skin biopsies are appropriate, the organism is difficult to culture, leaving the test uninformative. When septicemia is suspected, a white blood cell count and blood cultures are warranted.

Nonpharmacologic interventions include bed rest, elevation of the affected extremity, and hot packs. Uncomplicated cases of erysipelas can be treated with oral antibiotics. Toxic, debilitated, and elderly patients or children with extensive facial involvement or any patients with rapidly evolving erythema, pain, and swelling require intravenous antibiotics; penicillin, a cephalosporin, or nafcillin is warranted. Symptoms should diminish within 24 hours of treatment. Pain control measures are essential.

Erythrasma. A bacterial infection (corynebacterium) can develop in skin folds (e.g., axilla, groin), resulting in the condition known as *erythrasma*. This chronic condition is mildly pruritic, with a reddish-brown pigmentation, well-defined borders, and little scaling. Overweight patients, those with diabetes, and people living in warmer climates are at increased risk for developing erythrasma. This infection can be diagnosed by microscopy or culture. Erythrasma is often confused with candidiasis intertrigo based on clinical presentation, but is easily distinguished because the erythrasma rash, when exposed to long-wave ultraviolet radiation, will fluoresce to a coral pink color due to the action of the corynebacterium. The absence of satellite lesions should also help distinguish erythrasma from candidiasis. Treatment of erythrasma consists of washing the area vigorously with antibacterial soap and either applying clotrimazole lotion three times per day for 7 days, administering erythromycin tablets (500 mg) four times per day for 7 to 10 days, or applying erythromycin gel to the affected area. As with tinea infections, erythrasma can be prevented by keeping the skin dry, wearing absorbent clean clothing, and practicing good hygiene (Habif et al, 2011).

Folliculitis. Folliculitis is an inflammation of the hair follicle (see Plate 18). It can be mechanical, bacterial, or fungal in origin. Mechanical folliculitis is the result of tight clothing or persistent trauma. Bacterial folliculitis is most commonly caused by *S. aureus*. Fungal folliculitis is associated with tinea (dermatophyte infection) of the skin where hair is present (e.g., beard, head). Fungal folliculitis also can develop in the presence of untreated tinea corporis (Habif et al, 2011). Occlusion of the skin from occlusive ointment or the prolonged presence of oil or grease on the skin also will cause development of folliculitis (occlusion folliculitis). Improperly cleaned hot tubs are also responsible for causing *Pseudomonas folliculitis*. Steroids will trigger steroid folliculitis characterized by multiple small pustules and papules, resulting in a neutrophilic inflammation of the hair follicle.

The primary lesions in folliculitis are dome-shaped, 2- to 5-mm erythematous papules that surround the hair follicle and may manifest central pustules; secondary lesions are crusts and erythema (File and Stevens, 2008). Folliculitis may be limited to the superficial area of the hair follicle or progress deeper into the follicle. Although most common on the scalp or the extremities, folliculitis may develop on any hairy body location, particularly under adhesive wound dressings. Folliculitis also may develop as a secondary infection in the presence of excoriations from scratching that accompanies scabies and insect bites.

Risk factors for developing folliculitis are diabetes mellitus, obesity, malnutrition, immunodeficiency, and chronic staphylococcal infections. When treating folliculitis, avoid or reduce heat, friction, and occlusion. Antibacterial soaps should be used and hygiene improved. Potassium hydroxide examination of the hair and surrounding skin is warranted to exclude a dermatophyte infection (i.e., tinea) so that the appropriate oral antifungal medications, such as Lamisil, can be used. When folliculitis is limited and superficial, topical mupirocin is effective (Habif et al, 2011).

Impetigo. Impetigo, most commonly seen in children, is a highly contagious, superficial, vesiculopustular skin infection that is caused primarily by the gram-positive bacterium *S. aureus*. Streptococcus pyrogenes occasionally may be the offending pathogen, causing a more significant infection. Poor hygiene or malnutrition is typical of patients with impetigo. Lesions develop within 10 to 14 days (Stevens et al, 2008). The initial onset is a vesicle involving the superficial layer of the stratum corneum. The patient may experience itching and mild soreness; systemic symptoms are uncommon. Impetigo most often develops on seemingly intact skin, although it also may develop with minor breaks in the skin, such as insect bites and minor abrasions.

It is important to distinguish impetigo from HSV. Herpes simplex virus can be distinguished from impetigo by culture and by early manifestations. Herpes simplex virus begins with grouped, clear vesicles that are uniform in size, and it recurs at the same site.

Impetigo is often self-limited and resolves spontaneously, although it may also become chronic and/or recurrent. The treatment of choice for impetigo is topically administered 2% mupirocin cream (Bactroban). It has been shown to be as effective as oral erythromycin without the side effects (Habif, 2011). The cream should be applied three times daily until the lesions clear. Oral penicillin is indicated when streptococci are present. Impetigo may present clinically as bullous or nonbullous.

Bullous impetigo. Bullous impetigo is a primarily staphylococcal disease that develops when certain strains of *S. aureus* produce a specific epidermolytic toxin (File and Stevens, 2008). They may occur anywhere on the body, but the most common location is the face. One or more vesicles enlarge, creating a superficial, fragile, clear fluid-filled bulla that gradually becomes filled with cloudy fluid. When the center of the bulla collapses, a rim of the bulla roof often remains, encircling the lesion. The center of the lesion then develops a thin, honey-colored crust. When this is removed, a red, inflamed, moist base is revealed that is exudative with serous fluid. Eventually the outer edges of the bulla become dry and flaky, and a crust forms. Bullous impetigo lesions have little, if any, surrounding erythema; they can range in size from 2 to 8 cm and remain for several months. Infants must be monitored for signs and symptoms of serious secondary infections, such as septic arthritis and pneumonia (Habif et al, 2011).

Nonbullous impetigo. The lesions associated with nonbullous impetigo are asymptomatic, with minimal surrounding erythema. Lesions begin as small vesicles or pustules but soon rupture, exposing a moist, red base that becomes crusted over. The most common sites affected are around the mouth, the nose, and the extremities. In the usual sequence of events, the infectious agent is present on intact skin and, after minor trauma such as scratching, the skin is broken and an infection develops (Habif, 2011). During the early development of the lesions, group A beta-hemolytic streptococci may be isolated; however, the lesions quickly become contaminated with staphylococci. Predisposing factors for streptococcal impetigo are warm, moist climates and poor hygiene.

Viral

Viral infections, particularly HSV and varicella-zoster virus (VZV), are commonly triggered by stress and illness. It is important to recognize these highly contagious infections to facilitate prompt appropriate treatment and prevent spread to other individuals.

Herpes Simplex Virus. Herpes simplex virus infections of the epidermis are highly contagious and can be spread when a susceptible, noninfected person comes into direct contact (via mucous membrane or broken skin) with a person shedding the virus. Viral shedding occurs even in the absence of symptoms. Most transmission of HSV occurs during periods of asymptomatic shedding (Kimberlin and Whitley, 2008). Consequently, HSV infection should be considered a chronic process rather than an intermittent process, and all HSV-infected people should be treated as potentially contagious. Furthermore, because the primary infection often is subclinical, a negative history of vesicles or blisters does not rule out previous HSV infection.

Herpes simplex virus has been divided into two types: HSV-1 (oral herpes) and HSV-2 (genital herpes). HSV-1 is associated with cold sores (fever blisters); HSV-2 causes genital and perianal herpes. However, genital lesions from HSV-1 and oral lesions from HSV-2 are becoming more common, a trend that may be a consequence of sexual freedom and the ease of transmission. Ultimately, HSV lesions are not limited to the lips and genital area and may occur anywhere on the skin.

Herpes simplex virus infections have two phases: primary infection and secondary phase. During the primary infection, the virus becomes established in a nerve ganglion. HSV-1 most often occurs during childhood, whereas HSV-2 commonly occurs after sexual contact in sexually active individuals. Symptoms of the primary infection range from being undetectable to localized pain, headache, generalized aching, malaise, and tender regional adenopathy. A significant inflammatory response develops that extends from the base of the lesions down into the dermis, which results in the classic presentation of uniform, grouped vesicles on an erythematous base; the vesicles contain large numbers of infective viral particles. As more inflammatory cells are recruited to the site, vesicles become pustules that erode, drain, and crust (see Plates 19 and 20). Primary lesions last for 2 to 6 weeks and heal without scarring. As the lesion heals, the virus enters the

skin nerve endings and ascends through peripheral nerves to the dorsal root ganglia, where it remains in a latent stage.

Reactivation of the virus can occur in response to local trauma (abrasion, ultraviolet light) or systemic changes (e.g., stress, illness, fatigue, fever, compromised immune system). The virus then travels back down the peripheral nerve to the site, or in the vicinity, of the initial infection to trigger a recurrence. Prodromal symptoms of burning at the site may precede the recurrence. The reactivated virus presents as vesicles on an erythematous base, or ulcers. Crusts cover the eruptions within 24 to 48 hours and are shed in approximately 12 days, exposing a reepithelialized surface (Hunter et al, 2002).

Clinical presentation of grouped vesicles on an erythematous base is a key indicator of HSV and can be confirmed with a Tzanck smear. However, the Tzanck smear is most reliable when the lesion sampled is a vesicle; the smear becomes less reliable with pustules, crusts, and ulcers.

Primary HSV-1 infections are generally asymptomatic. When symptoms are present, the lesions include painful vesicles or shallow ulcers on the lips or lower face or in the oral cavity, and they last for 2 to 3 weeks. Recurrent HSV-1 infections are foreshadowed by pain and tingling or a burning sensation 2 to 24 hours before the eruption of vesicles (Kimberlin and Whitley, 2008). Recurrent HSV-1 lasts about 2 days as vesicles, which progress to pustules, ulcers, and eventually crusts. Complete healing occurs in 8 to 10 days.

Primary genital herpes (typically HSV-2 infection) lesions initially are macules and papules, followed by vesicles, pustules, and ulcerations. Lesions may occur on the genitalia, the perineum, and the buttocks. The lesions are extremely painful and persist for 2 to 3 weeks. Spontaneous resolution of the primary infection is common. Recurrent genital herpes is less pronounced and lasts for 8 to 10 days. Ulcers are shallow and may or may not be painful.

Herpes lesions may occur on the buttocks and are commonly misinterpreted as pressure, chemical IAD, or scabies (see Plate 20). Therefore the differential diagnosis for ulcers located in the perianal area or on the buttocks must include HSV. HSV lesions in this location will be extremely painful and have a "punched out" appearance with a pale pink wound bed and surrounding erythema. Herpes lesions can be distinguished from pressure sores in that the lesions are not limited to a bony prominence and are more typical over the fleshy part of the buttocks. These can also be distinguished from chemical irritation (such as occurs with diarrhea) by the presence of several isolated ulcers rather than the confluence of superficial denudement or erythema that impinges on the anal opening.

The clinical presentation of grouped vesicles on an erythematous base is highly suggestive of HSV, regardless of body site. The most definitive method for confirming the infection is to unroof the intact vesicle so that the vesicular fluid can be cultured. Rapid testing (within a few hours) also can be done with direct fluorescent antibody examination.

Commercially available kits can distinguish among HSV-1, HSV-2, and VZV.

Antiviral medications are effective in treating HSV infection and are available for topical, oral, and intravenous administration. Early initiation of oral acyclovir for genital herpes decreases healing time, viral shedding, and duration of pain.

Nursing care should be directed at absorbing excess moisture, avoiding trauma, and providing comfort. Alginate dressings with a secondary dressing, such as a transparent dressing or foam, can be used to absorb exudate (Chacon and Ferreira, 2009). When the lesions are relatively dry yet painful, Burrow's solution (aluminum acetate) soaks and refrigerated hydrogel dressings can relieve the topical pain. When shedding HSV lesions are present, skin cleansing should be done cautiously to prevent spreading of the virus, particularly when the lesions are present on the buttocks.

Varicella-Zoster Virus. Varicella-zoster virus causes varicella (chickenpox) and herpes zoster (shingles). Varicella-zoster virus is highly contagious and is transmitted by direct contact with either vesicular fluid or airborne droplets from the infected host's respiratory tract. Airborne transmission

as a mode for spreading VZV is very serious. Spread of varicella with no direct contact has been reported; the sole exposure was to air that flowed from the room of the infected individual to another room. Herpes zoster is contagious to patients who have never had VZV (they will get VZV not HSV) but not to individuals who have already had VZV.

Herpes zoster is an infection within the epidermis that is characteristically unilateral and occurs along one or two adjacent dermatome distributions (Figure 5-2). Eruptions result from the reactivation of VZV in cranial or spinal nerve ganglia that then spread to cutaneous nerves. Reactivation, which can occur as a result of immunosuppression, fatigue, radiation therapy, and emotional trauma, occurs in 15% of people (American Academy of Dermatology, 2008; Habif, 2011). The elderly may be predisposed to herpes zoster as a consequence of a potential decline in immunologic function. Individuals who are immunocompromised are at risk for developing VZV and experience more severe infections. These patients are more likely to develop disseminated disease with extensive skin lesions, pneumonia, hepatitis, or encephalitis (Zaia, 2008). Diagnosis is most often based on history and clinical appearance. The DNA polymerase chain

FIGURE 5-2 Segmental dermatome distribution of spinal nerves to the front, back, and side of the body. Dermatomes are specific skin surface areas innervated by a single spinal nerve or group of spinal nerves. *C,* Cervical segments; *CX,* coccygeal segment; *L,* lumbar segments; *S,* sacral segments; *T,* thoracic segments. (From Patton KT, Thibodeau GA: *Anatomy and physiology,* ed 7, St. Louis, MO, 2010, Mosby.)

reaction assay and direct immunofluorescent stain of a skin scraping for VZV antigen are accurate and rapid diagnostic tests for chickenpox and zoster and are preferred over the Tzanck preparation or tissue culture (Zaia, 2008).

Herpes zoster has characteristic manifestations that begin with a burning pain, followed by erythema and red, swollen plaques of various sizes and across part or all of a dermatome (Habif, 2011). Variously sized vesicles erupt in clusters and become purulent. This is in contrast to the uniformly sized vesicles typical of herpes simplex. These pustules then rupture and crust over (Habif, 2001). In some debilitated patients, the eruptions become more extensive and inflammatory, with blisters, necrosis, or secondary infections developing. Varicella-zoster virus in the immunocompromised patient may last from weeks to months, and the resulting ulcer may develop a black, adherent eschar (see Plate 21). Postherpetic neuralgia (pain that persists beyond 1 month after healing) is a major complication of shingles; thus aggressive analgesia is an essential component of treatment.

Treatment of herpes zoster requires acyclovir (Zovirax) 800 mg five times daily for 7 to 10 days, valacyclovir (Valtrex) 1000 mg three times per day, or famciclovir (Famvir) 500 mg three times per day (Habif, 2011). Early intervention with systemic antiviral medications lessens postherpetic neuralgia and decreases healing time and viral shedding. Topical antivirals are not recommended in the management of herpes zoster. Burrow's solution can be applied to act as an astringent on the lesions. Daily soaks with salt solutions may minimize bacterial infection (Zaia, 2008). Anecdotally, dressings that reduce moisture in the zoster lesion, such as foam, can be used to protect the lesion from trauma and friction and reduce pain at the site. Moisture-donating dressings such as hydrocolloids or transparent dressings, however, should be avoided.

ALLERGIC FACTORS

Numerous allergic responses, both local and systemic, can be manifested on the skin. Because the wound specialist is in a likely position to observe such reactions, it is important to be able to describe the manifestations accurately and to report the assessment to the physician in a timely fashion. This section focuses on those allergic responses that are localized reactions to items such as adhesives, wound care products, and solutions. These types of skin damage are commonly referred to as *allergic contact dermatitis*.

Allergic contact dermatitis is an immunologic response to an allergen. Contact dermatitis occurs more readily in the presence of a preexisting skin disorder in which the cutaneous barrier is disrupted.

A true allergic dermatitis requires exposure to an allergen and has two phases:

1. The sensitization phase (the skin of a nonsensitized individual is exposed to a substance or chemical) transpires over a 7- to 10-day period. Small molecules from the allergen pass through the epidermis and attach to an epidermal protein found on the surface of the Langerhans cell. From here these cells migrate through the dermis to the lymph nodes, where they present the allergen to T lymphocytes. Subsequently, effector and memory T lymphocytes proliferate in the lymph node, are released to circulate in the blood, and ultimately return to the skin. Here the body develops the ability to recognize the antigen when it reappears on the skin, and the T lymphocytes are now "primed" (Hunter et al, 2002).

2. When the individual is reexposed to the allergen, the elicitation phase occurs within 48 to 72 hours. Once the Langerhans cell delivers the antigen to memory T cells in the skin, effector T cells begin to produce lymphokines. Inflammatory cells are summoned by the lymphokines, and allergic manifestations can be observed. Suppressor T cells are believed to end the inflammatory reaction.

An acute inflammatory response occurs within 48 hours of reexposure to an allergen. Clinical manifestations begin with erythema, followed by pruritus. Primary lesions are vesicles, bullae, papules, plaques, and wheals. Secondary lesions include moist desquamation (see Plate 22), edema, fissure, excoriation, and crust. An acute reaction usually resolves in days to weeks, after the allergen has been removed.

The cause or source of the allergen may be obvious, or it may be obscured by other concurrent processes. A careful, detailed assessment and interview are imperative to identify the skin reaction as an allergic response. Common allergic sensitizers include poison ivy, nickel (used in jewelry), rosins, rubber compounds (used in elastic, gloves), benzocaine (used in antipruritic creams), paraphenylenediamine (dye used to color hair), and preservatives. Topical preparations with one of the following ingredients are other common allergic offenders: aloe vera, fragrances, parabens, quaternium 15, diphenhydramine (Benadryl spray or Caladryl lotion), neomycin (Neosporin), and para-aminobenzoic acid (PABA) (Habif, 2011). Overuse of soaps, cleansers, moisturizers, and cosmetics can produce reactions. Many chemicals with similar structures cross-react, so a person who is sensitive to one product may be sensitive to several other products.

The location and distribution of the skin inflammation are important clues in identifying the causative agent. Allergic contact dermatitis is localized to the skin where the product is applied, and involved areas typically have sharp margins. For example, an allergic reaction to an adhesive will be in the shape of the adhesive and will have well-defined borders. Allergic contact dermatitis can spread from the original site of application through inadvertent transfer of the allergen by the hands or, as the disease progresses, by the circulating T lymphocytes. However, the skin reaction begins and remains most severe in the area in which contact with the antigen occurred (Hunter et al, 2002).

Patch tests can be conducted to confirm the suspected agent that is causing the allergic reaction; however, these tests must be properly conducted and interpreted. Suspected allergens are applied to the skin and secured with tape. The patient's back usually is the preferred site for patch testing.

After 48 hours, the patches are removed and the test site assessed for skin damage, which is graded using a standard scale as listed in Box 5-8. Although the patch test seems simple to apply and read, it is a complicated procedure that requires training and experience to obtain valid results (Rietschel and Fowler, 2001).

Simply avoiding contact with allergens can prevent allergic contact dermatitis. However, recognizing or identifying potential allergens is the key to prevention and may not be an easy task.

When an allergic response is suspected, use of the offending product or chemical should be discontinued. Often a substitute can be used. Use of antiinflammatory medications may be warranted topically or systemically and usually is determined based on the severity of the allergic reaction.

RADIATION

Radiation therapy is an established, common treatment of cancer. It is estimated that as many as half of all patients with cancer will receive radiation therapy as a primary, adjunctive, or palliative intervention (Bolderston et al, 2006). Although the techniques and technologies for radiotherapy have improved, skin reactions and complications continue to be problematic for patients (Wells and MacBride, 2003), and the evidence for the optimal treatments for prevention and management remain inconclusive (Olascoaga et al, 2008; Wickline, 2004).

Etiology

Ionizing radiation exerts direct tissue injury to curtail the growth of neoplastic cells; however, it also generates free radicals and reactive oxygen intermediates that further damage cellular components, including DNA, proteins, and cellular membranes. In response to the free radicals, the damaged keratinocytes recruit inflammatory cytokines, specifically interleukin-1 and interleukin-6, tumor necrosis factor-α, and transforming growth factor-β (Bernier et al, 2008). Unfortunately, the effects of radiation therapy are not restricted to malignant cells. Rapidly proliferating tissues, such as intestinal mucosa, bone marrow, and skin, are more susceptible to radiation. In addition, radiosensitization techniques may be used to enhance the effect of radiation on normal and malignant tissues (Camidge and Price, 2001).

The skin is particularly vulnerable to the effects of radiation because it is in a continuous state of cellular renewal. Damage is incurred by rapidly dividing cells, such as keratinocytes, hair follicles, sebaceous glands, epidermal basal cells, endothelial cells, and vascular components. A reduction of Langerhans cells also occurs (Bernier et al, 2008). Because radiation damages the mitotic ability of stem cells in the basal layer, regrowth of new cells is slowed and skin integrity becomes impaired (Maki and Clarey-Sanford, 2007).

Pathophysiologic Characteristics

The onset of radiation dermatitis depends on dose intensity and the individual's normal tissue sensitivity. The spectrum of skin reactions that can occur with radiation therapy (radiation dermatitis) as categorized by the National Cancer Institute is listed in Table 5-5. Treatment effects will be confined to the treatment area. Early effects will generally manifest within 2 to 3 weeks after beginning therapy. Because acute radiation effects are cumulative, the greatest reactions occur toward the end of therapy. However, side effects usually are self-limiting, and most subside 1 to 3 months after therapy has ended (Bernier et al, 2008).

Initially the skin in the treatment field will develop faint, transient erythema, which may become more brisk and persistent. Erythema will appear as a red, macular rash on warm-appearing skin that may feel sensitive and tight. It is an inflammatory response thought to be caused by dilation of the capillaries and increased vascular permeability; therefore edema may accompany erythema.

TABLE 5-5   Grading of Radiation Dermatitis

Grade 1	Grade 2	Grade 3	Grade 4
Faint erythema or dry desquamation	Moderate to brisk erythema; patchy moist desquamation, mostly confined to skin folds and creases; moderate edema	Moist desquamation other than skin folds and creases; bleeding induced by minor trauma or abrasion	Skin necrosis or ulceration of full-thickness dermis; spontaneous bleeding from involved site

Adapted from National Cancer Institute: *Common terminology criteria for adverse events* version 3.0 (CTCAE), August 9, 2006. http://ctep.cancer.gov/protocolDevelopment/electronic_applications/ctc.htm. Accessed March 21, 2015.

Dry desquamation may follow and will appear as red or tan pigmented skin that is dry, itchy, and peeling or flaky. This reaction is a result of the decreased ability of the basal cells of the epidermis to replace the surface layer cells and the decreased ability of the sweat and sebaceous glands to produce sweat. As the cumulative dose of radiation increases, the erythema and dry desquamation may evolve into moist desquamation, which is characterized by exposure of the dermis as a result of blisters, peeling, and sloughing. Moist desquamation could occur by the third week of treatment and increases the risk of infection, discomfort, and pain, possibly requiring interruption of the treatment plan to allow for healing (Bernier et al, 2008; Olascoaga et al, 2008). A combination of erythema and dry and moist desquamation may be seen within a single treatment field (Wells and MacBride, 2003).

Long-term, irradiated skin will have epidermal atrophy, so the epidermis is thin, dry, and more translucent. Sweat and sebaceous glands and hair follicles usually are absent. Telangiectasias and blood vessels are easily visible. Subendothelial connective tissue in small arteries proliferates, causing narrowing and thrombosis of the microvasculature (i.e., progressive obliterative endarteritis), and loss of elasticity due to damage to the elastic fibers in the dermis causes fibrosis (Olascoaga et al, 2008). Late effects develop gradually over several months or years and are a function of the total dose, volume of the area irradiated, energy and particles used, interval between fractions, and concomitant chemotherapy or biologic modifier (Olascoaga et al, 2008). Late effects are more likely to be significant when acute reactions are significant. Late radiation damage can be further complicated by several conditions: secondary ulceration, impaired joint mobility, shedding or deformity of the nails, malignancies (basal and squamous cell), and lymphedema (caused by fibrosis of the lymph glands). When ulceration and necrosis occur years after radiation therapy, they usually occur in conjunction with trauma or infection. These lesions can become very painful and difficult to manage.

Another reaction to radiation is termed *radiation recall*, which is defined as the "recalling" by skin of previous radiation exposure following the administration of certain chemotherapeutic agents. The medications most commonly associated with radiation recall are docetaxel, doxorubicin, gemcitabine, and paclitaxel (Hird et al, 2008). Most recall reactions occur when less than 2 months separates completion of radiation therapy and resumption of chemotherapy (Azria et al, 2005; Hird et al, 2008). Once recall dermatitis is detected, chemotherapy is withheld until the dermatitis resolves; when it is resumed, premedication with corticosteroids is indicated.

Risk Factors

Substantial variations in the degree of acute and late normal tissue reactions exist even in patients who have received identical treatments. Thus identifying patients at risk for severe radiation-induced skin reactions is difficult. Treatment schedule and total dose in radiation therapy are based on the tumoricidal doses and the tolerance dose of the perifocal normal tissue.

The quality of the irradiation and its modalities, including total dose, fractionation, and interfractional interval, appear to affect functional and cosmetic outcome the most. Risk factors that appear to influence the severity, onset, and duration of radiation skin reaction include age, general skin condition, and nutritional status. At risk for the highest stages of reaction are body areas within the treatment field, including bony prominences and moist areas on the body, such as skin folds, under the breast, the axillae, neck, perineum, and groin (Wells and MacBride, 2003). Patients who are receiving combination therapy also are at risk because concomitant use of chemotherapy may sensitize the basal cells to radiation (Bernier et al, 2008).

Care of Irradiated Skin

Skin care before, during, and after radiation is aimed at minimizing the undesirable physiologic effects of radiation. Patients and caregivers are included in planning care and selection of goals and objectives. Intervention choices should be based on the available evidence of effectiveness, the ability to soothe the skin and promote patient comfort, and compatibility with ionizing radiation.

Patient education on skin care is critical when preparing the patient for radiation and during the course of the therapy. Patients should be instructed on the typical effects of radiation on the skin (dry desquamation), measures to promote moisture retention in the treatment area, the potential for radiation recall (when applicable), to protect the area from trauma and potential irritants (i.e., alcohol, perfumes, products containing α-hydroxy acid), and to only use products in the treatment field that have been approved by the health care team.

Several literature reviews on radiation skin care (prevention and management of dermatitis) have been published in the past few years (Aistars, 2006; Bernier et al, 2008; Bolderston et al, 2006; McQuestion, 2006; Nystedt et al, 2005; Olascoaga et al, 2008; Wickline, 2004). The findings from these reviews are quite similar and have been summarized in Table 5-6. A practice guideline for skin care and prevention of acute skin reactions based on these reports is given in Checklist 5-1. Most interventions have extremely limited evidence due to the absence of randomization, lack of controls, small sample size, or inconsistent outcome measures. Most recommended skin care interventions are related to bathing, hygiene, and use of topical preparations and creams. Of particular interest are the following findings:

1. Products containing aluminum, magnesium, or zinc do not cause a "bolus effect" (i.e., increased dose and skin reaction) as previously considered (McQuestion, 2006).
2. There is insufficient evidence to support or refute most topical preparations (see Table 5-6) for the prevention of acute skin reactions (Bolderston et al, 2006; McQuestion, 2006).

TABLE 5-6   Skin Care Products and Radiation Therapy: Summary of Evidence

Product	Description	Findings
Evidence for Use or FDA Approved		
Hydrophilic lotions and creams	Moisturizers: Lubriderm, Glaxal base, Eucerin, Keri lotion, Aquaphor	• May be helpful in preventing radiation skin reactions • Product should be unscented, lanolin free • Gently apply (do not rub) twice per day
Calendula ointment	Pot marigold believed to have antiviral and antiinflammatory effects Has been used to treat acne, control bleeding, soothe irritated tissue	• May decrease occurrence of radiation dermatitis (limited evidence) • Compared with Biafine, reported to provide statistically significant reduction in skin reaction, pain, and need for treatment interruption
Hyaluronic acid cream	Lubricating agent found in the body	• May be radioprotective (limited evidence) • Used to treat very dry, scaly skin
Aloe vera gel	Extracted from pulp of aloe vera leaves	• May be used to soothe, cool radiated skin for comfort • Lack of evidence supporting or refuting use for prevention or treatment of radiation dermatitis • Product does not moisturize and should be discontinued if skin becomes dry
Miaderm cream (Aiden Industries)	Formulated with aloe vera, calendula, hyaluronic acid	• FDA approved for prevention or treatment of radiation dermatitis of skin (limited evidence)
Biafine emulsion (OrthoNeutrogena)	Water-based emulsion paraffin and avocado oil are among the many ingredients	• FDA approved for treatment of radiation dermatitis, burns, other superficial wounds (limited evidence) • Contraindicated for use on bleeding wounds • Temporary tingling sensation may occur 10–15 minutes after application • Apply three times per day but not within 4 hours of radiation treatment
Topical corticosteroid creams	Used to decrease erythema and pruritus (itching)	• Radioprotective effect may be present with use of mometasone furoate or Bepanthen cream (limited evidence) • Use only temporarily with caution in collaboration with physician's order • Induces vasoconstriction, atrophy of dermal collagen, resulting in thinning of skin • Increases susceptibility to infection, masks superficial infection, delays wound healing
Contraindicated, Off Label, or Lack of Evidence for Use		
α-Hydroxy acid (AHA) cream	Glycolic acid and lactic acid most common AHAs Exfoliates and soothes dry, scaly skin (xerosis)	• Can increase radiation skin reaction • Stinging, burning may occur when applied to irritated skin
Skin sealant wipes, wands, sprays	Protective transparent film containing plasticizing agents such as copolymer Some products contain isopropyl alcohol	• Lack of evidence supporting or refuting use for prevention or treatment of radiation dermatitis • See Table 5-4 for examples of skin sealants • Do not use products with alcohol on radiated skin
Chamomile cream	Extracted from chamomile plant	• Lack of evidence supporting or refuting use for prevention or treatment of radiation dermatitis
Almond ointment	Made with almond oil	• Lack of evidence supporting or refuting use for prevention or treatment of radiation dermatitis
Petrolatum jelly–based products	Hydrophobic/water repelling	• Do not use for prevention or treatment of radiation dermatitis
Aqueous cream	Paraffin-based emulsion containing petroleum jelly, phenoxy ethanol, and purified water	• No evidence supporting use for prevention of radiation skin reactions • Contains petroleum, which is not recommended for prevention or treatment of radiation dermatitis of skin
Sucralfate/sulcralfate derivatives	Antiulcer drug for many years Protects mucous membranes during radiotherapy and chemotherapy Recently demonstrated in animal model to stimulate regeneration of the skin and accelerate wound healing	• Not FDA approved for topical use for prevention or treatment of radiation dermatitis of skin • Small studies in radiation therapy reported that cream significantly prevented acute skin reactions and damaged skin healed significantly faster (findings not consistent in subsequent studies)

FDA, Food and Drug Administration.

Information compiled from the following sources: Aistars, 2006; Bernier et al, 2008; Bolderston et al, 2006; McQuestion, 2006; Nystedt et al, 2005; Olascoaga et al, 2008; Wickline, 2004.

CHECKLIST 5-1 Prevention and Management of Radiation Skin Reactions

Promote (Do Not Limit) Personal Hygiene Practices
✓ Continue showers and baths.
✓ Use lukewarm water and mild nonalkaline soap (e.g., baby soap, Dove, Ivory, Basis).
✓ Use mild nonmedicated shampoo (i.e., baby shampoo) for scalp in patients receiving radiation therapy to the head.
✓ Use electric razor for shaving.
✓ Apply deodorant as usual to intact skin throughout treatment.

Promote Comfort
✓ Gently apply (do not rub) unscented, lanolin-free hydrophilic moisturizer twice per day (see Table 5-6 for product examples).
✓ Do not use petrolatum-based products; products with irritants such as alcohol, perfumes, or additives; or products containing α-hydroxy acids.
✓ May use aloe vera to soothe and cool the skin (does not moisturize, so discontinue if skin becomes dry).
✓ For burning and itching, apply normal saline compresses as needed or hydrocortisone cream (if ordered).

✓ Wear loose, soft, breathable, nonbinding clothing that protects skin from sun and wind.
✓ Use cool-mist humidifier if humidity is needed.

Prevent Trauma
✓ Avoid swimming in chlorinated pools, hot tubs, and lakes to minimize exposure to chemicals and bacteria.
✓ Avoid heating pads and ice packs to prevent thermal injury.
✓ Avoid adhesives and tapes to prevent skin tears.

Manage Radiation Dermatitis
✓ Normal saline soaks to provide cooling sensation and loosen crusting in treatment field.
✓ Plain, nonscented, lanolin-free hydrophilic cream for dry desquamation, but discontinue when skin breakdown occurs.
✓ Nonadherent dressings may be used for moist desquamation when it occurs during the course of radiation therapy, but should be removed during the treatment.
✓ Dressings may be used based on the wound/skin care needs (i.e., absorb moisture) once radiation therapy has concluded.

---

3. There is insufficient evidence to support or refute corticosteroids or sucralfate cream for the management of acute skin reaction (Bolderston et al, 2006; McQuestion, 2006; Olascoaga et al, 2008).
4. Calendula ointment may decrease radiation dermatitis in breast cancer patients (Bolderston et al, 2006; McQuestion, 2006).

Dressings. Numerous topical dressings have been used to treat acute radiation dermatitis, including transparent film dressings, hydrogels, foams, alginates, slow-released silver hydrofiber dressing, silver sulfadiazine (SSD) cream, and hydrocolloid dressings (Maki and Clarey-Sanford, 2007; McQuestion, 2006; Olascoaga et al, 2008). When a topical dressing is needed to manage a radiation skin injury, the type of dressing selected must be compatible with the priority needs of the skin condition. For example, transparent film dressings absorb little exudate and would be inappropriate for moist desquamation. In contrast, hydrocolloids can be used with minimal to moderate amounts of exudate, such as what occurs with moist desquamation. Given that irradiated skin is characterized by a loss of elasticity, atrophy, and fibrosis, nonadhesive wound dressings are generally preferred to minimize trauma to irradiated skin, avoid skin tears, and prevent pain upon dressing removal (see Chapter 18 for further information about wound care dressings).

Adjunctive Interventions. Hyperbaric oxygen, growth factors, biologic skin substitutes, pentoxifylline, interferon-γ therapy, and surgery have been used for treatment of radiation-induced necrotic wounds (Olascoaga et al, 2008).

Hyperbaric oxygen improves collagen formation, neovascularization, epithelialization, and leukocyte bactericidal activity to improve acute radiation injury by reducing tissue hypoxia and edema (see Chapter 22 for further discussion of hyperbaric oxygen therapy).

Growth factors can be used to manipulate the wound environment to stimulate healing of radiation ulcers. Platelet-derived growth factor, epidermal growth factor, and transforming growth factor-β stimulate tissue regeneration, remodeling, and proliferation of capillary endothelial cells, and they chemoattract neutrophils, monocytes, and fibroblasts to the wound site (see Chapter 20 for a discussion of growth factors).

Pentoxifylline, used to treat peripheral vascular disease and improve peripheral microcirculation by increasing the flexibility of red blood cells, may reduce the severity of late radiation injury when administered preventively or in the postirradiation period (Aygenc et al, 2004). In addition, time to heal of existing radiation-induced ulcers appears to be decreased (Olascoaga et al, 2008). A few studies have used interferon-γ therapy with radiation-induced ulcers to reduce fibrosis because it inhibits collagen production in normal dermal fibroblasts (Gottlöber et al, 2001). Additional studies using comparison groups and larger samples are needed to replicate these findings.

Surgical interventions may be used for treatment of some radiation-induced wounds. These procedures involve extensive surgical debridement and removal of all poor-quality tissue and timely reconstruction with well-vascularized soft tissue flaps (see Chapter 33 for further discussion of surgical interventions for wound closure).

CLINICAL CONSULT

A: Referral received for home-visit consult to a 25-year-old paraplegic who lives with his parents and has developed a nonhealing pressure ulcer on his left ischial tuberosity. His mother provides most of his care, and they live in a very clean and organized home. Other than the presenting wound, the patient is well groomed and his overall health and skin condition appear good. No other skin lesion noted following head-to-toe skin inspection. Wound 4 cm × 3 cm × 2 cm; wound bed beefy red; no granulation tissue; periwound skin with normal skin tone and intact. Moderate serous wound exudate. Afebrile. Has a reclining wheelchair and interconnected multi-cell cushion in chair. The mother expresses concern that the wound is being "scraped" when the patient is naked and needs to use his sliding board for transfer to wheelchair. She also expresses concern that on the days of his bowel program that stool may get under the dressing and into the wound. Patient reports recent 8-hour drive in friend's truck to attend concert and did not use support surface during drive.

D: Pressure ulcer; no signs of infection. Pressure precipitated by prolonged truck ride without support surface cushion and shear/friction during transfers.

P: Topical dressings to provide moist wound environment, fill wound bed, and protect from stool. Encourage protein and vitamins to meet wound healing needs. The wound will be washed with normal saline and packed with a silver hydrofiber due to the risk for infection, as it is near the rectum. The cover dressing will be occlusive adhesive foam.

I: (1) Review/reinforce measures to reduce shear/friction. (2) Must offload from sitting position (via reclining) every hour. (3) Utilize disposable underpad during shower transfers to provide a contact layer against the buttocks and a more slippery layer against the sliding board to minimize shear with transfer. (4) Refer to PT to reassess wheelchair cushion. (5) Maintain food diary for the next week. (6) Cleanse wound with NS; fill with hydrofiber and cover with occlusive silicone border adhesive foam dressing. Change twice weekly.

E: Follow-up home visit in 2 weeks to evaluate dressing effectiveness, dietary intake, PT assessment of support surface, and ability to reduce shear in transfers.

SUMMARY

The intact skin provides the first line of defense against microbial invasion and trauma. Different factors can jeopardize the skin's integrity. It is important to be able to recognize the skin-related signs of these factors so that the factors can be eliminated or their intensity reduced substantially. Most often, the type of skin damage that the wound specialist will encounter is mechanical or vascular. Only with an in-depth skin assessment and history of the skin eruption can the etiology of the skin damage be identified and the negative sequelae arrested through appropriate prevention and treatment interventions.

Because the more rare inflammatory, infectious, or disease-related skin lesions often require prompt treatment to be effective, the wound specialist should also be familiar with these types of lesions. Although the underlying disease is the critical determinant for wound healing in these situations, the wound specialist is an important partner and interdisciplinary team member because he or she can provide valuable recommendations for wound management that will best address the requirements of the wound and the needs of the patient.

REFERENCES

Abeloff MD, Armitage JO, Niederhuber JE, et al: *Abeloff's clinical oncology*, ed 4, Philadelphia, 2008, Elsevier.

Aistars J: The validity of skin care protocols followed by women with breast cancer receiving external radiation, *Clin J Oncol Nurs* 10:487–492, 2006.

Association of periOperative Registered Nurses (AORN): *AORN recommended practices for positioning the patient in the perioperative practice setting. AORN standards, recommended practices, and guidelines*, Denver, 2008, AORN.

Ayello EA and Sibbald RG: Preventing pressure ulcers and skin tears. In Boltz M, Capezuti E, Fulmer T, and Zwicker D: editors: *Evidence-based geriatric nursing protocols for best practice*, ed 4, New York, 2012, Springer, pp 298–323.

Aygenc E, Celikkanat S, Kaymakci M, et al: Prophylactic effect of pentoxifylline on radiotherapy complications: a clinical study, *Otolaryngol Head Neck Surg* 130(3):351–356, 2004.

Azria D, Magné N, Zouhair A, et al: Radiation recall: a well recognized but neglected phenomenon, *Cancer Treat Rev* 31:555–570, 2005.

Bank D, Nix D: Preventing skin tears in a nursing and rehabilitation center: an interdisciplinary effort, *Ostomy Wound Manage* 52(9):38–46, 2006.

Baranoski S: How to prevent and manage skin tears, *Adv Skin Wound Care* 16(5):268–270, 2003.

Bartlett JG: Antibiotic-associated diarrhea. In Schlossberg D, editor: *Clinical infectious disease*, New York, 2008, Cambridge University Press.

Beeckman D, Schoonhoven L, Verhaeghe S, et al: Prevention and treatment of incontinence-associated dermatitis: literature review, *J Adv Nurs* 65(6):1141–1154, 2009.

Beeckman D, Woodward S, Gray M: Incontinence-associated dermatitis: step-by-step prevention and treatment, *Br J Community Nurs* 16(8):382–389, 2011.

Benoit RA Jr, Watts C: The effect of a pressure ulcer prevention program and the bowel management system in reducing pressure ulcer prevalence in an ICU setting, *J Wound Ostomy Continence Nurs* 34(2):163–175, 2007.

Bernier J, Bonner J, Vermorken JB, et al: Consensus guidelines for the management of radiation dermatitis and coexisting acne-like rash in patients receiving radiotherapy plus EGFR inhibitors for the treatment of squamous cell carcinoma, *Ann Oncol* 19(1):142–149, 2008.

Birch S, Coggins T: No-rinse, one-step bed bath: the effects on the occurrence of skin tears in a long-term care setting, *Ostomy Wound Manage* 49(1):64–67, 2003.

Bolderston A, Lloyd NS, Wong RK, et al: The prevention and management of acute skin reactions related to radiation therapy: a systematic review and practice guideline, *Support Care Cancer* 14:802–817, 2006.

Bradley SF: Staphylococcus. In Schlossberg D, editor: *Clinical infectious disease*, New York, 2008, Cambridge University Press.

Brannon J: Intertrigo. *Yeast infection in skin folds.* About.com: dermatology, updated November 13, 2004. http://dermatology.about.com/od/fungalinfections/a/intertrigo.htm Accessed September 15, 2009.

Brillhart B: Pressure sore and skin tear prevention and treatment during a 10-month program, *Rehabil Nurs* 30(3):85–91, 2005.

Camidge R, Price A: Characterizing the phenomenon of radiation recall dermatitis, *Radiother Oncol* 59:237–245, 2001.

Carpenter CF, de Sanctis J: Candidiasis. In Schlossberg D, editor: *Clinical infectious disease*, New York, 2008, Cambridge University Press.

Centers for Disease Control and Prevention: *Workplace safety and health topics: Safe patient handling*, 2014. http://www.cdc.gov/niosh/topics/safepatient/Accessed March 21, 2015.

Chacon J, Ferreira L: Hemicellulose dressing for skin lesions caused by herpes zoster in a patient with leukemia—an alternative dressing, *Wounds* 21(1):10–14, 2009.

Cohen SH, Gerding DN, Johnson S, et al: Clinical practice guidelines for Clostridium difficile infections in adults: 2010 update by the Society for Healthcare Epidemiology of America (SHEA) and the Infectious Diseases Society of America (IDSA), *Infect Control Hosp Epidemiol* 31(5):431–455, 2010.

Eddins C, Gray M: Are probiotic or symbiotic preparations effective for the management of clostridium difficile-associated or radiation-induced diarrhea? *J Wound Ostomy Continence Nurs* 35(1):50–58, 2008.

File TM, Stevens DL: Superficial skin infections (pyodermas). In Tan JS, Tan MJ, Salata RA, File TM, Jr: et al, editors: *Expert guide to infectious diseases*, ed 2, Philadelphia, 2008, ACP Press pp 629–642.

Fleck CA: Preventing and treating skin tears, *Adv Skin Wound Care* 20(6):315–320, 2007.

Fontaine R, Risley S, Castellino R: A quantitative analysis of pressure and shear in the effectiveness of support surfaces, *J Wound Ostomy Continence Nurs* 25:233–239, 1998.

Furdon SA: *Challenges in neonatal nursing: providing evidence-based skin care*, Medscape Nurses, 2003. http://cme.medscape.com/viewarticle/465017 Accessed August 24, 2009.

Gefen A: Risk factors for pressure-related deep tissue injury: a theoretical model, *Med Biol Eng Comput* 45(6):563–573, 2007.

Gefen A, Farid KJ. Shaywitz I: A review of deep tissue injury development, detection, and prevention: shear savvy, *Ostomy Wound Manage* 59(2):26–35, 2013.

Gottlöber P, Steinert M, Bähren W, et al: Interferon-gamma in 5 patients with cutaneous radiation syndrome after radiation therapy, *Int J Radiat Oncol Biol Phys* 50:159–166, 2001.

Gray M, Black JM, Baharestani MM, et al: Moisture-associated skin damage: overview and pathophysiology, *J Wound Ostomy Continence Nurs* 38(3):233–241, 2011.

Gray M, Bliss DZ, Doughty DB, et al: Incontinence associated dermatitis: a consensus, *J Wound Ostomy Continence Nurs* 34(1):45–54, 2007.

Habif TP: *Clinical dermatology: a color guide to diagnosis and therapy*, ed 4, St. Louis, MO, 2004, Mosby.

Habif TP, Campbell JL, Chapman MS, et al: *Skin disease: diagnosis and treatment*, ed 3, Philadelphia, 2011, Elsevier.

Higa JT, Kelly, CP: New drugs and strategies for management of Clostridium difficile colitis, *J Intensive Care Med* 29:190–199, 2013.

Hird AE, Wilson J, Symons S, et al: Radiation recall dermatitis: case report and review of the literature, *Curr Oncol* 15(1):53–62, 2008.

Hunter JAA, Savin JA, Dahl MV: *Clinical dermatology*, ed 3, Oxford, 2002, Blackwell Science.

Hunter S, Anderson J, Hanson D, et al: Clinical trial of a prevention and treatment protocol for skin breakdown in two nursing homes, *J Wound Ostomy Continence Nurs* 30(5):250–258, 2003.

Imhoff A, Karpa K: Is there a future for probiotics in preventing Clostridium difficile-associated disease and treatment of recurrent episodes? *Nutr Clin Pract* 4(1):15–32, 2009.

Kauffman CA: Candidiasis. In Tan JS, Tan MJ, Salata RA, File TM, Jr: et al, editors: *Expert guide to infectious diseases*, ed 2, Philadelphia, 2008, ACP Press pp 527–540.

Kim J, Shim MC, Choi BY, et al: Clinical application of continent anal plug in bedridden patients with intractable diarrhea, *Dis Colon Rectum* 44:1162–1167, 2001.

Kimberlin DW, Whitley RJ: Herpes simplex viruses 1 and 2. In Schlossberg D, editor: *Clinical infectious disease*, New York, 2008, Cambridge University Press.

Kowal-Vern A, Poulakidas S, Barnett B, et al: Fecal containment in bedridden patients: economic impact of 2 commercial bowel catheter systems, *Am J Crit Care* 18:2–14, 2009.

LeBlanc K, Baranoski S: Prevention and management of skin tears, *Adv Skin Wound Care* 22:325–332, 2009.

LeBlanc, K., Baranowski, S: Skin tears: state of the science: consensus statements for the prevention, prediction, assessment, and treatment of skin tears, *Adv Skin Wound Care* 24(9):(Suppl 1):2–15, 2011.

LeBlanc K, Baranoski S, Christensen D, et al: International Skin Tear Advisory Panel: a tool kit to aid in the prevention, assessment, and treatment of skin tears using a Simplified Classification System ©, *Adv Skin Wound Care* Oct 26(10):459–476, 2013.

LeBlanc K, Christensen D, Orstead HL, et al: Best practice recommendations for the prevention and treatment of skin tears, *Wound Care Canada* 6(1):14–32, 2008.

Maki L, Clarey-Sanford C: Using slow-released silver hydrofiber dressings on a neck radiation burn, *J Wound Ostomy Continence Nurs* 34(5):542–545, 2007.

Malone ML, Rozario N, Gavinski M, et al: The epidemiology of skin tears in the institutionalized elderly, *J Am Geriatr Soc* 39(6):591–595, 1991.

McFarland LV: Renewed interest in a difficult disease: Clostridium difficile infections—epidemiology and current treatment strategies, *Curr Opinion Gastroenterol* 25(1):24–35, 2009.

McGough-Csarny J, Kopac CA: Skin tears in institutionalized elderly: an epidemiological study, *Ostomy Wound Manage* 44(Suppl 3A):14S–24S, 1998.

McNichol L, Lund C, Rosen T, et al: Medical adhesives and patient safety: state of the science: consensus statements for the assessment, prevention, and treatment of adhesive-related skin injuries, *J Wound Ostomy Continence Nurs* 40(4):365–380.

McQuestion M: Evidence-based skin care management in radiation therapy, *Semin Oncol Nurs* 22(3):163–173, 2006.

McTigue T, D'Andrea S, Doyle-Munoz J, et al: Efficacy of a skin tear education program: improving the knowledge of nurses practicing in acute care settings, *J Wound Ostomy Continence Nurs* 36(5):486–492, 2009.

Meuleneire F: Using a soft silicone-coated net dressing to manage skin tears, *J Wound Care* 11(10):365–369, 2002.

Milne CT, Corbett LQ: A new option in the treatment of skin tears for the institutionalized resident: formulated 2-octylcyanoacrylate topical bandage, *Geriatr Nurs* 26(5):321–325, 2005.

National Pressure Ulcer Advisory Panel (NPUAP): *Terms and definitions related to support surfaces*, 2007. http://www.npuap.org/NPUAP_S3I_TD.pdf. Accessed September 22, 2009.

Nazarko L: Preventing and treating skin tears, *Nurs Residential Care* 7(12):549–550, 2005.

Noble SL, Forbes RC, Stamm PL: *Diagnosis and management of common tinea infections, Am Fam Physician* 58(1):163–174, 177–178, 1998. http://www.aafp.org/afp/980700ap/noble.html. Accessed October 9, 2009.

Nystedt KE, Hill JE, Mitchell AM, et al: The standardization of radiation skin care in British Columbia: a collaborative approach, *Oncol Nurs Forum* 32(6):1199–1205, 2005.

Olascoaga AJ, Vilar-Compte D, Poitevin-Chacón A, et al: Wound healing in radiated skin: pathophysiology and treatment options, *Int Wound J* 5:246–257, 2008.

Patton KT, Thibodeau GA: *Anatomy and physiology*, ed 7, St. Louis, MO, 2010, Mosby.

Payne RL, Martin ML: The epidemiology and management of skin tears in older adults, *Ostomy Wound Manage* 26:26–37, 1990.

Payne RL, Martin ML: Defining and classifying skin tears: need for a common language, *Ostomy Wound Manage* 39(5):16–20, 1993.

Pennsylvania Patient Safety Authority: Skin tears: the clinical challenge, *Patient Safety Advisory* 3(3):1, 5–10, 2006. http://www.patientsafetyauthority.org. Accessed October 3, 2009.

Ratliff CR, Fletcher KR: Skin tears: a review of the evidence to support prevention and treatment, *Ostomy Wound Manage* 53(3):32–34, 2007.

Rietschel RL, Fowler JF Jr: *Fisher's contact dermatitis*, ed 5, Philadelphia, 2001, Lippincott Williams & Wilkins.

Roberts MJ: Preventing and managing skin tears: a review, *J Wound Ostomy Continence Nurs* 34(3):256–259, 2007.

Rohde CL, Bartolini V, Jones N: The use of probiotics in the prevention and treatment of antibiotic-associated diarrhea with special interest in Clostridium difficile-associated diarrhea, *Nutr Clin Pract* 24(1):33–40, 2009.

Sachdeva MP, Tomecki KJ: Cellulitis and erysipelas. In Schlossberg D, editor: *Clinical infectious disease*, New York, 2008, Cambridge University Press.

Schutze GE, Willougby RE, Committee on Infectious Diseases, et al: Clostridium difficile infections in infants and children (Policy statement), *Pediatrics* 131(1):196–200, 2013.

Sibbald RG, Kelley J, Kennedy-Evans KL, et al: A practical approach to the prevention and management of intertrigo, or moisture-associated skin damage, due to perspiration: expert consensus on best practice, *Wound Care Canada* 11(Suppl 2):4–21, 2013.

Stanley JD, Bartlett JG, Dart BW 4th, Ashcraft JH: Clostridium difficile infection, *Curr Prob Surg* 50(7):302–337, 2013.

Stevens DL, Mebane JA, and Madaras-Kelly K: Streptococcus groups A, B, C, D, G. In Schlossberg D, editor: *Clinical infectious disease*, 2nd ed New York, 2015, Cambridge University Press.

Thomas DR, Goode PS, LaMaster K, et al: A comparison of an opaque foam dressing versus a transparent film dressing in the management of skin tears in institutionalized subjects, *Ostomy Wound Manage* 45(6):22–28, 1999.

Visscher ML: Recent advances in diaper dermatitis: etiology and treatment, *Pediatric Health* 3(1):81–89, 2009.

Warner RR, Stone KJ, Boissy YL: Hydration disrupts human stratum corneum ultrastructure, *J Invest Dermatol* 120(2):275–284, 2003.

Waters TR, Rockefeller K: Safe patient handling for rehabilitation professionals, *Rehabil Nurs* 35(5):216–222, 2010.

Waters TR, Short M, Lloyd J, et al: AORN ergonomic tool 2: positioning and repositioning the supine patient in the OR bed, *AORN J* 93(4):445–449, 2011.

Wells M, MacBride S: Radiation skin reactions. In Faithfull S, Wells M, editors: *Supportive care in radiotherapy*, New York, 2003, Churchill Livingstone.

White MW, Karam S, Cowell B: Skin tears in frail elders: a practical approach to prevention, *Geriatr Nurs* 15(2):95–99, 1994.

Wickline MM: Prevention and treatment of acute radiation dermatitis: a literature review, *Oncol Nurs Forum* 31(2):237–247, 2004.

Wiederkehr M, Schwartz RA: *Tinea cruris: treatment and medication*, updated May 20, 2008. http://emedicine.medscape.com/article/1091806-overview. Accessed September 15, 2009.

Wound, Ostomy and Continence Nurses Society™ (WOCN®): *Guideline for management of pressure ulcers (WOCN® clinical practice guideline series no. 2)*, Glenview, IL, 2010, WOCN®.

Wright K, O'Connor AD: Causes and risks of pressure sores, *Nurs Resident Care* 9(11):516–523, 2007.

Zaia JA: Varicella-zoster virus. In Schlossberg D, editor: *Clinical infectious disease*, New York, 2008, Cambridge University Press.

Zulkowski K: Perineal dermatitis versus pressure ulcer: distinguishing characteristics, *Adv Skin Wound Care* 21(8):382–388, 2008.

Zulkowski K: Diagnosing and treating moisture-associated skin damage, *Adv Skin Wound Care* 25(5):231–236, 2012.

6

Skin and Wound Inspection and Assessment

Denise P. Nix

OBJECTIVES

1. Differentiate between skin inspection and skin assessment.
2. List six factors to consider when assessing darkly pigmented skin.
3. Distinguish between wound assessment and evaluation of healing.
4. Define partial-thickness and full-thickness tissue loss.
5. Compare and contrast a normal and an abnormal finding for each wound assessment parameter.
6. Describe how to measure the length, width, depth, tunneling, and undermining of a wound.

An initial skin and wound assessment provides the foundation for developing a patient's plan of care. However, ongoing skin and wound assessments also are critical because they provide the mechanism for monitoring the effectiveness of that plan, thus allowing determination of progress or deterioration of the wound. Documentation of assessment findings facilitates communication among caregivers. Because of the myriad of etiologic, systemic, and local factors commonly involved in the pathogenesis of a wound, a comprehensive patient assessment is essential to identify cofactors that may impair wound healing and jeopardize skin integrity. Whereas all patients, with or without a wound, require a skin assessment upon admission, the patient with a wound requires additional assessments, including underlying causes for the wound and healing impediments.

SIGNIFICANCE

In order to adequately convey the condition of a wound or a skin lesion, wound and skin assessment requires access to a unique vocabulary. As with monitoring blood pressure, temperature, and pulse rate, those attending to a wound need to use specific parameters to reflect its present status. The state of the science is such that both subjective and objective measures are required to adequately capture the condition of the wound. Because subjective measures by definition can vary in interpretation from one user to another, it is essential that accurate use of wound assessment terminology be emphasized in staff education and that competencies for wound and skin assessment be used (Young et al, 2014). Appendix A contains examples of competencies related to skin and wound management.

The economics of health care impose additional motivation for conducting and documenting a systematic measurement of wound healing. Without objective criteria of the status or progress of repair, it is difficult to justify treatments or assign appropriate reimbursement for services. The standard of care is to provide accurate and routine skin and wound assessments. Failure to assess the patient systematically also carries a great legal liability risk (Croke, 2003; Reising and Allan, 2009). Without accurate, consistent, and retrievable documentation, it is difficult to retrospectively create a clear picture of the patient's condition and of the care that actually was provided.

ASSESSMENT

Assessment is a two-step process that requires inspection and collection of data and then interpretation of that data so that a plan of care can be derived. During the initial encounter, an assessment provides the baseline data to which comparisons can be made to determine changes; this is the process of *monitoring*.

The word *assessment* alone as it relates to the prevention and management of wounds can be confusing because a number of assessments are required: risk assessment (see Chapter 8), skin assessment, wound assessment, and physical assessment. For clarity and safety, findings from each type of assessment must be documented using appropriate terms to describe the patient's skin or wound condition. Staff education and competencies should include how to conduct the assessments and how to link appropriate interventions to the findings (Pieper and Ratliff, 2010).

Skin Inspection and Monitoring

Skin *inspection* involves data collection related to skin changes based on visual and palpable observation, along with the patient's reports of changes in sensation/discomfort. A complete skin inspection must be completed by trained staff upon admission (for baseline data) and daily. It is important to inspect all of the skin from head to toe (WOCN®, 2010). An adequate skin inspection requires the removal of garments (including shoes and stockings) and effective positioning for optimal visualization. Staff conducting the inspection will need to gently spread skin folds (including the buttocks), check between the toes, and remove or reposition medical devices to inspect for pressure-related skin damage from devices such as oxygen tubing, nasogastric tubes, urinary tubing, drainage tubing, therapeutic stockings, and splints (Apold and Rydrych, 2012). Staff performing the skin inspection should be expected to report the overall skin condition, such as change in skin condition (e.g., intact, broken, denuded), skin color (e.g., red, dusky), texture (e.g., pinpoint macular–papular rash, dry skin), and wounds. These findings then are communicated to a registered nurse or a provider for interpretation, and additional information is collected as needed to further describe and understand the present condition.

The skin and wound condition should be monitored on a routine and regular basis as defined by the facility policy and the severity of the condition. *Monitoring* allows the staff to keep track or "watch" for changes that deviate from the baseline data. For example, 3 days after admission, a reddened area is identified through routine monitoring, whereas the baseline assessment and documentation indicated no redness upon admission. The new finding should prompt further assessment to identify etiology so that modifications to the plan of care can be implemented. Part of the plan of care will include continued monitoring and perhaps more frequent repositioning.

Frequency of wound assessment is discussed later in this chapter. However, when dressings are in place and do not require changing, the dressing should be monitored for intactness and the surrounding skin inspected for the presence or absence of discoloration (erythema, bruising), rash, break in skin integrity, and pain (van Rijswijk and Lyder, 2005). Narrative documentation can be as simple as "dressing dry and intact, surrounding skin within defined limits," or a flow chart can be used.

Therefore monitoring can occur independently of dressing change. However, if the dressing is leaking or new observations are made (swelling, pain, erythema), the dressing should be removed and a thorough wound assessment obtained. Monitoring usually occurs more frequently than an assessment or head-to-toe skin inspection, such as every 8 hours in the acute care setting or every day in the long-term care setting. To conserve staff time and patient energy, monitoring and skin inspection can be conducted at the same time that other routine cares are provided (Table 6-1).

TABLE 6-1   Routine Activities Coordinated with Skin Inspection

Routine Activity	Skin Inspection Site
Oral care and medications	Back of ears, bridge of nose, nares, and lips
Listening to lung sounds	Occiput, spinous process, neck, scapula, coccyx, and sacrum
Perineal skin care/bath	Between and under skin folds of pannus and groin
Application or removal of antiembolism stockings or splints	Feet, heels, toes
Transferring in or out of chair	Coccyx, sacrum, and ischial
Repositioning side to side	Feet, heels, toes, coccyx, sacrum, occiput, scapula, spinous process, trochanter

Skin Assessment

The standard of care is to conduct a routine and systematic skin assessment on all patients upon admission. Skin assessment parameters and deviations from normal are listed in Table 6-2. Examples and descriptions of lesions are presented in Chapter 5 (see Table 5-1 and Plates 6 and 7).

Subsequent skin assessments should be performed routinely. Frequency of reassessment is based on baseline data, care setting, and risk for skin breakdown. For example, patients require daily skin assessments when they (1) are at increased risk for skin breakdown, (2) have impaired skin integrity, or (3) are in an acute care or long-term acute care setting. Twice-daily skin assessments are recommended under and around medical devices. For individuals at risk for fluid shifts and edema formation, more often daily inspections under and around medical devices are indicated (Apold and Rydrych, 2012; NPUAP, EPUAP, PPPIA, 2014).

Skin palpation should be used to assess skin temperature, edema, and tissue consistency/texture in all patients and is of particular importance when assessing darkly pigmented skin. Skin with deviations from normal (e.g., firm to touch, boggy, warmth, coolness) should be compared with the adjacent skin or contralateral body part and documented. Since there has been some indication that localized skin pain is a precursor to skin breakdown, pain should be evaluated with each skin assessment (NPUAP, EPUAP, PPPIA, 2014).

Skin assessments require good lighting for optimal visualization. Alterations including edema, dry skin or xerosis, and color changes such as erythema and dark discoloration should be noted. As discussed in Chapters 7 and 8, erythema in individuals at risk for developing pressure ulcers can indicate early signs of skin damage. If erythema is identified, it is important to differentiate whether it is blanchable or nonblanchable. Blanchable erythema turns white when brief pressure is applied, then red when pressure is relieved, indicating reactive hyperemia or inflammatory erythema with an intact capillary bed. Nonblanchable erythema is redness that persists after

TABLE 6-2   Skin Assessment Parameters: Findings and Interpretation

Parameter	Technique and Tips	Findings	Interpretation
Color	Conduct inspection in good light; artificial light often distorts colors and masks jaundice Ask patients/family if they have noticed any skin color changes	Pallor	Anemia, decreased blood flow, or arterial insufficiency Advanced lung disease Congestive heart failure Anemia
		Central cyanosis (lips, oral mucosa, or tongue)	Venous obstruction
		Yellow	Jaundice in sclera and skin with liver disease or excessive hemolysis of red blood cells
		Brown discoloration in lower extremities	Hemosiderin staining from venous insufficiency
		Redness	Erythema, an inflammatory response, or pressure ulcer
Moisture	Visual inspection in good light	Dry skin	Xerosis Hypothyroidism
		Dermatitis or macular-papular rash in skin folds, perineum, thighs, groin	Intertrigo, tinea, or psoriasis
Temperature	Palpate using the back of fingers Infrared thermography	Generalized increased warmth	Fever Hyperthyroidism
		Local increased warmth	Inflammation
		Coolness	Hypothyroidism or poor vascularization
Olfaction	Note odor	Present	Bacteria, metabolic acidosis, hygiene issues
Texture	Palpate using back of fingers	Roughness	Hypothyroidism
Turgor	Pinch fold of skin and note speed with which it returns (normally, skin returns quickly to baseline state)	Decreased turgor	Dehydration
Lesions	Observe any lesions of the skin, noting characteristics such as type, location, color, distribution, arrangement	Primary or secondary skin lesions (macule, papule, pustule)	See Plates 6 and 7 and Chapter 5
Skin injury	Skin should be intact If skin is open, assess for type of injury	Denuded	Chemical damage, fecal incontinence
		Ulcerated	Unrelieved pressure
		Excoriated	Pruritus, xerosis
Nails (see Chapter 15 for nail abnormalities)	Inspect and palpate fingernails and toenails Note color, shape, and presence of lesions	Clubbing of the fingers	Lung problems
		Onycholysis	Painless separation of nails from nail bed beginning distally
Hair	Inspect and palpate Note quantity, distribution, texture	Alopecia	Hair loss (diffuse)
		Hirsutism	Excessive body hair (may be patchy or total)

pressure is applied and released, indicating capillary damage, which is an independent predictor of epidermal skin damage (Nixon et al, 2007; Sterner et al, 2011). Two methods of applying pressure to assess for nonblanchable versus blanchable erythema have been reported in the literature: (1) pressing a finger on the erythema for 3 seconds and then assessing for blanching immediately upon removal and (2) applying pressure with a transparent disk, watching for blanching underneath the disk. Both methods have been investigated for

reliability with mixed results; however, training and increased education and experience appear to improve reliability of both methods (Kottner et al, 2009; NPUAP, EPUAP, PPPIA, 2014; Sterner et al, 2011; Vanderwee et al, 2006).

Darker Skin Tones. Health care in the United States and Europe has experienced a shift in racial and ethnic demographics. According to the estimates of the U.S. Census Bureau, Hispanic and black people will comprise the majority of the population in America by the year 2043 (U.S. Census Bureau, 2012). Therefore accurate assessment of patients with darker skin pigmentation is an essential skill for all health care providers, and particularly wound care providers. The unique characteristics of darker versus lighter pigmented skin are summarized in Box 3-1. Teaching points and unique considerations when assessing darkly pigmented skin are provided in Checklist 6-1 (Bennett, 1995).

Unfortunately, detection and accurate identification of erythema and Stage I pressure ulcers with standard visual inspection are unreliable in persons with darkly pigmented skin (Bates-Jensen et al, 2009; NPUAP, EPUAP, PPPIA, 2014; Rosen et al, 2006; WOCN®, 2010). This inability to detect and diagnose erythema in people with darkly pigmented skin is evidenced by two studies in long-term care settings. Baumgarten and colleagues (2004) revealed an incongruity between the prevalence of Stage I pressure ulcers in Caucasians (48%) versus African Americans (20%). Later, Rosen and colleagues (2006) found that 32% of pressure ulcers detected in Caucasian residents were Stage I, whereas no Stage I pressure ulcers were detected in African American residents. The poor reliability to detect pressure-related erythema in darkly pigmented skin underscores the importance of assessing skin temperature, edema, and changes in the consistency and texture of the skin, not just the presence of erythema.

Preliminary research has been conducted on enhanced methods for detecting erythema and soft tissue edema (through increased levels of subdermal moisture) as possible methods of predicting early inflammatory signs of pressure ulcer development. In one small laboratory study with 56 healthy subjects (28 with darkly pigmented skin), researchers were able to show an enhanced ability to detect induced erythema in a variety of skin tones using a multispectral imaging system (Sprigle et al, 2009). In long-term care and spinal cord–injured patient populations, subepidermal moisture has been associated with early pressure ulcer damage before any visual indication of skin damage (Bates-Jensen et al, 2009; Guihan et al, 2012). A noninvasive, handheld dermal phase meter is used to measure subepidermal moisture. If these findings can be replicated in larger studies with additional controls for confounding variable, these modalities may emerge as useful clinical tools for detecting early damage in persons with darker skin tones.

Focused Physical Assessment

Healing is a phenomenon composed of multiple processes (see Chapter 4), each of which must function properly and sequentially. Whereas all patients require a physical assessment, the patient with a wound requires particular attention to systemic, psychosocial, and local factors that affect wound healing. A wound specialist is specifically educated to conduct this type of focused physical assessment and to interpret the results (WOCN®, 2011). The focused physical assessment should be obtained upon admission and with a change of condition. Components of a wound-focused physical assessment are listed in Checklist 6-2.

Etiology and Differential Diagnosis. Based on the wound-focused physical assessment, a differential diagnosis and likely etiology of the wound will be determined, which will drive intervention choices and treatment strategies. The completed physical assessment should help to exclude many possible etiologies for the wound, but also will exclude treatment options. For example, compression is a critical intervention for successful management of the patient with venous insufficiency; however, compression may be contraindicated for many patients with arterial disease (see Chapter 11). Offloading is needed for management of a pressure ulcer (see Chapters 8 and 9), and glucose must be managed when the patient has diabetes (see Chapter 14). Wound etiology will also provide clues regarding the type of

---

CHECKLIST 6-1 Assessing Pressure Ulcers on Darkly Pigmented Skin

✓ Color remains unchanged when pressure is applied.
✓ Color changes occur at site of pressure, which differ from the patient's usual skin color.
✓ Circumscribed area of intact skin may be warm to touch. As tissue changes color, intact skin will feel cool to touch. Note gloves may diminish sensitivity to changes in skin temperature.
✓ If patient previously had a pressure ulcer, that area of skin may be lighter than original color.
✓ Localized area of skin may be purple/blue or violet (eggplant) instead of red.
✓ Localized heat (inflammation) is detected by making comparisons to surrounding skin. Localized area of warmth eventually will be replaced by area of coolness, which is a sign of tissue devitalization.
✓ Edema (nonpitting swelling) may occur with induration and may appear taut and shiny.
✓ Patient complains of discomfort at a site that is predisposed to pressure ulcer development.

CHECKLIST 6-2 Wound-Focused Physical Assessment Parameters

✓ Wound etiology and differential diagnosis
✓ Duration of wound
✓ Cofactors that impede healing:
  • Comorbid conditions (malignancy, diabetes, cardiac, respiratory, renal issues)
  • Medications (corticosteroids, cancer medications, immunosuppressants)
  • Host infection
  • Pressure ulcer risk factors
  • Decreased oxygenation and tissue perfusion
  • Alteration in nutrition and hydration
  • Psychosocial barriers, family support, impaired access to appropriate resources, financial limitations
  • Past therapies (e.g., radiation near the site of the wound)

healing to anticipate. For example, a venous ulcer generally has little depth, so it often heals by epithelialization rather than wound contraction, which is in contrast to the deeper Stage III or IV pressure ulcer, which requires contraction for healing to occur. Measuring wound depth in the pressure ulcer clearly is an important piece of information, but may be of little relevance in venous ulcers. Various types of skin damage are discussed in Chapter 5 and throughout this text. Interpretation of the data gathered through the focused physical assessment will guide the plan of care so that wound etiology and existing cofactors can be addressed.

Duration of Wound and Critical Cofactors that Impair Healing. A 2-week-old pressure ulcer that has not improved suggests the presence of cofactors that have not been adequately addressed, such as unresolved pressure, malnutrition, osteomyelitis, critical colonization, squamous cell cancer, or infection. Guidelines for pressure ulcers and arterial wounds recommend consideration of referral and biopsy for wounds that are unresponsive following 2 to 4 weeks of appropriate topical therapies (WOCN® 2008, 2010). A biopsy is important in the "stagnant" wound to rule out less common conditions such as pyoderma gangrenosum or the conversion of the wound to a malignancy such as squamous cell carcinoma (i.e., Marjolin ulcer). Techniques for obtaining a biopsy are described later in this chapter.

Given a clear understanding of healing, these wounds must be considered out of synchronization and require re-evaluation to identify factors that impede healing. Factors that impede healing are described in chapters throughout the text and listed in Checklist 6-2. Approaches used to assess systemic cofactors that affect wound healing, along with the chapters that describe them in detail, are listed in Table 6-3.

Wound Assessment

Wound assessment is the collection of subjective data that characterize the status of the wound specifically, as well as the periwound skin (see Plate 23). Parameters that compose a wound assessment are listed in Checklist 6-3 and

CHECKLIST 6-3 **Wound Assessment Parameters**
✓ Anatomic location of wound
✓ Extent of tissue loss (i.e., stage)
✓ Characteristics of wound base
✓ Type of tissue
✓ Percentage of wound containing each type of tissue observed
✓ Dimensions of wound in centimeters (length, width, depth, tunneling, undermining)
✓ Exudate (amount, type)
✓ Odor
✓ Wound edges
✓ Periwound skin
✓ Presence or absence of local signs of infection
✓ Wound pain

described in this section. Conducting a wound assessment is a skill and requires precision and appropriate use of unique terms; use of appropriate terms is critically important. Therefore competency-based education for wound assessment is essential (Pieper and Ratliff, 2010). Before assessment, the wound must be cleansed of loose debris, particulate matter, and dressing residue so that the normal architecture and color of the wound bed and surrounding skin can be fully appreciated.

Anatomic Location. The anatomic location of the wound is important to record using proper terminology that will also provide clues about the etiology. Anatomic locations such as the sacrum and the coccyx must be clearly delineated (Figure 6-1). The location of a wound on the plantar surface of the foot can be accurately specified by terms such as *metatarsal head*. Anatomic location will also convey plan-of-care needs. For example, a wound on the ischial tuberosity should prompt caregivers to explore the patient's sitting surface. A typical venous ulcer commonly appears on the medial aspect of the lower leg and will require compression. A patient with diabetes and a plantar surface foot ulcer typically has neuropathy and will need adequate blood glucose control and offloading.

Extent of Tissue Involvement. The extent of tissue damage guides the selection of appropriate interventions to restore tissue integrity; it also provides some information about the length of time required for the healing process. Extent of tissue involvement can be described as partial thickness or full thickness, or "staged" if indicated. Numerous staging and classification systems exist that are primarily based on wound etiology and therefore are precise and descriptive for that type of wound.

Partial thickness and full thickness. A partial-thickness wound is confined to the skin layers; damage does not penetrate below the dermis and may be limited to the epidermal layers only. These wounds heal primarily by reepithelialization (see Table 4-1 and Plate 1). A full-thickness wound indicates that the epidermis and dermis have been damaged into

TABLE 6-3 **Assessment of Cofactors**		
Cofactor	**Chapter**	**Diagnostic Test**
Tissue oxygenation	28	Transcutaneous oxygen
Bacterial load	16	Culture
		Biopsy
Circulation	14	Ankle-brachial index
		Toe-brachial index
Nutrition	27	Weight
		Body mass index
		Albumin
		Total lymphocyte count
Glycemic control	14	Blood glucose, HbA1c

FIGURE 6-1 Bony structures of human body; note delineation of sacrum and coccyx. (From Patton KT, Thibodeau GA: *Anatomy and physiology*, ed 7, St Louis 2010, Mosby.)

the subcutaneous tissue or beyond; tissue loss extends below the dermis (see Table 4-2 and Plates 2–5). Wound repair will occur by neovascularization, fibroplasia, contraction, and then epithelial migration from the wound edges. Partial thickness and full thickness can be used to describe most wounds, but are not precise terms for specific types of tissue loss and depths of the wound. For example, a full-thickness wound can expose subcutaneous tissue, or it may extend to bone.

Classification systems. Accurate classification requires knowledge of the anatomy of skin and deeper tissue layers, the ability to recognize these tissues, and the ability to differentiate between them. Classification systems for vascular

and diabetic wounds assign a "grade" to the wound based on levels of tissue involvement, history of previous ulceration, presence of bony deformity, presence and severity of ischemia, and presence and severity of infection (WOCN®, 2012a; 2014). Careful evaluation of the wound bed facilitates accurate classification, a complex skill that can take time to develop. Additional classification systems include skin tears (see Chapter 5), pressure ulcers (see Chapter 7), vascular wounds (see Chapter 11), diabetic wounds (see Chapter 14), and burns (see Chapter 32). However, as with all classification systems, they tell only a small part of the story and therefore should be used in conjunction with additional wound descriptors.

Type of Tissue in Wound Base. The amount and type of tissue in the wound bed provide insight into the severity and duration of the wound, the extent to which the wound is progressing toward healing, and the effectiveness of current interventions. Healing wounds are characterized by increasing amounts of viable tissue (e.g., granulation tissue) and decreasing amounts of nonviable tissue (e.g., eschar or slough). When the wound bed contains a combination of tissue types, each type of tissue should be described in percentages—for example, "50% of the wound bed contains eschar and 50% contains granulation tissue." Terms used to describe tissue and the wound bed, as well as other descriptions used for wound assessment, are listed in Table 6-4.

Viable tissue. Viable tissue is healthy tissue, such as granulation, epithelialization, or subcutaneous tissue. Healthy granulation tissue is characteristically described as beefy, red, moist, and cobblestone-like or berry-like in appearance (see Plate 3). New epithelial tissue is light pink and dry (see Plate 1). Deviations from an optimal state should be described carefully and correlated with conditions that may account for the abnormality, such as the patient's fluid status, serum hemoglobin level, nutrition, or colonization.

Nonviable tissue. Color, texture, moisture, and adherence of necrotic tissue to the wound bed should be noted. As with viable tissue, nonviable tissue can provide information related to wound status. The presence of nonviable tissue (or necrotic tissue) in the wound often is associated with altered tissue oxygenation, wound desiccation, or increased bacterial burden. In addition, a wound initially described as dry adherent

eschar (see Plate 24) will progress to moist, softening, brown, necrotic tissue that is lifting, loosening, or demarcating from the wound base (see Plate 25). It then progresses to yellow slough, which can be firm and adherent or moist and stringy. This transformation in the color, moisture, and texture of nonviable tissue is evidence that the natural autolysis process is occurring as desired. This process of autolysis is facilitated by appropriate topical care and a moist wound environment. Chapters 17 and 18 provide details of the significance and process for debridement and moist wound healing.

Tissue color. A myriad of colors are often found in the wound bed (e.g., red, pink, yellow, tan, black, green). It is helpful to record the color of the tissue in the wound bed because the color gives a general indication of healing status. For example, if the wound bed is red and granulation tissue is present, these are considered a positive sign that conditions for healing are right. Eschar is black (see Plate 24); as it softens (thus moving closer to being debrided through autolysis), the color will transition to yellow (see Plate 25) or yellow tan; then small red islets develop in the wound bed among the nonviable yellow slough. More granulation tissue is revealed as the wound progresses (see Plates 26A and 26B).

Color can be used to differentiate normal structures from the wound bed. However, color alone does not sufficiently describe viable or nonviable tissue and trivializes the complexities of the healing process. For example, nonviable tissue could be yellow; however, viable tendon is also yellow. A wound base may be red but with an unhealthy smooth surface (lacking the cobblestone or berry-like appearance) in which case the wound should be described as "clean, nongranulating" (see Plate 5A). In contrast, healthy granulation tissue will have a red color with a cobblestone appearance (as shown in Plate 5B). A pale red color can be indicative of anemia or hypoxia. Hypergranulation tissue is also red or pink in color but is not considered healthy. Hypergranulation tissue is the overproduction of granulation tissue generally caused by excess moisture or friction (see Plate 27).

Wound Size. Several approaches to wound measurement are described in the literature, each with their own advantages and disadvantages and some more appropriate for research than the clinical setting. These techniques have been summarized in Table 6-5. For massive tissue loss, calculation of the percentage of body surface area wounded using the Lund-Browder chart is the most common and realistic measure (see Chapter 32, Figure 32-2).

Linear two-dimensional (length and width) and three-dimensional (length, width, and depth) measurement techniques using disposable plastic/acetate or paper rulers are most common in the clinical setting. Three-dimensional measurements are required with full-thickness wounds because, by definition, full-thickness wounds are below the dermis and therefore should have depth; however, shallow full-thickness wound depth may not be measurable (<1 mm). Measurements should be recorded in centimeters

TABLE 6-4	**Wound Bed Descriptors**
Necrotic, nonviable, or devitalized	Tissue that has died and therefore has lost its physical properties and biologic activity
Eschar	Black or brown necrotic, devitalized tissue; tissue can be loose or firmly adherent; hard, soft, or boggy
Slough	Soft, moist, avascular (necrotic/devitalized) tissue; may be white, yellow, tan, or green; may be loose or firmly adherent
Scab	Crust of hardened blood and serum over the wound
Granulation tissue	Pink/red moist tissue composed of new blood vessels, connective tissue, fibroblasts, and inflammatory cells fills an open wound when it starts to heal; typically appears deep pink or red; surface is granular, berry-like, or cobblestone
Clean, nongranulating	Absence of granulation wound; surface appears smooth and red but not granular and berry-like or cobblestone
Epithelial	Regenerated epidermis across the wound surface; pink and dry

TABLE 6-5   Methods of Wound Measurement

Measurement Methods	Description
Ruler-based linear method	Disposable, three-dimensional. Should include length, width, and depth and extent and location of undermining and tunneling with consistent approach. Estimated wound area = length × width × depth (see Figures 6-2 and 6-3).
Kundin wound gauge	Disposable, three-dimensional, plastic-coated paper wound gauge. Rarely used in clinical practice.
Computerized wound measurement through digital photography	Two-dimensional, noncontact method requires uploading to computer software program.
Planimetry	Two-dimensional technique where wound is traced onto a transparency and a metric grid is used to count the number of square centimeters within the wound perimeter. High reliability except when estimating partial squares.
Wound tracings	Two-dimensional technique where wound is traced, providing a pattern against which subsequent tracings can be compared.
Stereophotogrammetry	Two-dimensional. Combines video camera and software to videotape, download onto computer, and trace with a mouse; software calculates measurement. High reliability.
Wound molds	Three-dimensional. Foam or alginate substance placed into wound and retained for serial reviews. Impractical in clinical settings.
Fluid instillation	Fluid instilled into the wound, extracted, and measured. Difficult to fill wound completely. Impractical in clinical settings.
Structured light	Three-dimensional. Wound is illuminated with set of parallel lights via projector. Image is picked up by camera connected to computer. Not applicable for very large or undermining wounds. Impractical in clinical settings.

or millimeters and include the extent and location of undermining and tunneling when present. From these dimensions, the area of the wound can be estimated by multiplying length by width by depth. To strengthen the accuracy of wound measurement, a uniform approach among staff should be used. This can be facilitated by consistent patient positioning and identifying specific wound landmarks from which to align the measuring instrument (NPUAP, EPUAP, PPPIA, 2014). Documentation requirements for consistency should be described in policies, procedures, and flow sheets (examples in Appendix A).

Unfortunately, numerous potential reliability problems exist when measuring a wound. Because the perimeter of open wounds often is irregular, it can be difficult to determine the best position on the wound surface from which to obtain the measurements. Even defining the edge of the wound from which measurements should be taken will vary among providers and will introduce inconsistencies in dimensions. In addition, the rigor with which the measurement is obtained influences the results (Langemo et al, 2008). However, serial measurements repeated over time can at least be used to reveal a trend in the presence or absence of healing in the wound.

As with each wound assessment parameter, wound size should be interpreted within the context of the other parameters enumerated in Checklist 6-3. For example, as an eschar-covered ulcer undergoes autolysis, the percentage of eschar will decrease, and consequently wound dimensions will predictably increase. Looking only at wound dimensions as an assessment parameter may lead to misinterpretation of the increase as an indication of delayed or absent wound healing. However, because wound dimensions are changing at the same time that the type and volume of tissue in the wound bed are evolving from eschar to slough to granulation tissue, the increase in size that accompanies the removal of nonviable tissue is considered desirable and indicative of a positive trend in the wound-healing process.

Measuring length, width, and depth. Length and width are measured with a head-to-toe orientation, with the longest length head to toe and the widest width perpendicular to length. Researchers have found that if the width is not measured perpendicular to the longest length, the wound area can be overestimated by 70% on some wound shapes (Keast, 2004; Langemo et al, 2008; NPUAP, EPUAP, PPPIA, 2014) (Figure 6-2). The most common method of obtaining wound depth is by inserting a moist cotton-tipped applicator into the wound bed at the greatest depth and placing a mark on the applicator at the level of the skin (Figure 6-3). This mark may simply be the examiner's thumb and index finger, but an ink mark applied to the applicator at skin level should provide more accuracy in the measurement. The cotton-tipped applicator then is held against a metric ruler to determine the depth of the wound (Doughty, 2004; NPUAP, EPUAP, PPPIA, 2014). This procedure can be made simpler by using a commercially available measuring guide integrated into a cotton-tipped applicator. Unfortunately, this technique is inherently imprecise (particularly with an irregularly shaped wound bed), but it does provide a method of at least detecting a trend.

Measuring tunneling and undermining. The terms *tunnel* and *sinus tract* are often used interchangeably. A *tunnel* is a channel that extends from any part of the wound through subcutaneous tissue or muscle (Figure 6-4). *Undermining* is tissue destruction that occurs under intact skin around the

PLATE 1 A, Partial-thickness venous ulcer healing by epithelialization. **B,** Resurfaced venous ulcer lacks normal dark pigmentation because of depth of damage (below basement membrane).

PLATE 2 Stage IV pressure ulcer with exposed muscle.

PLATE 3 Full-thickness abdominal wound healing by secondary intention with healthy (red, cobblestone) granulation tissue and attached wound edges.

PLATE 4 Stage IV sacral pressure ulcer wound edges are rolled (epibole), which is an impediment to wound healing.

PLATE 5 A, Wound clean, not granulating (note lack of red cobblestone appearance), suggesting heavy bacterial load or other impediment to wound healing. **B,** Same wound after 1 week of topical antimicrobial use (note healthy red cobblestone appearance).

PLATE 6   Primary Skin Lesions

Description	Examples		
A. Macule Flat, circumscribed area that is a change in the color of the skin less than 1 cm in diameter	Freckle, flat mole (nevus), petechia, measles, scarlet fever		Measles. (From Hockenberry MJ, Wilson D: *Wong's nursing care of infants and children*, ed 8, St Louis, 2007, Mosby.)
B. Papule Elevated, firm, circumscribed area less than 1 cm in diameter	Wart (verruca), elevated mole, lichen planus		Lichen planus. (From Weston W et al: *Color textbook of pediatric dermatology*, ed 4, Edinburgh, 1996, Mosby.)
C. Patch Flat, nonpalpable, irregular-shaped macule greater than 1 cm in diameter	Vitiligo, port-wine stain, Mongolian spot, café au lait spot		Vitiligo. (From Weston W et al: *Color textbook of pediatric dermatology*, ed 4, Edinburgh, 1991, Mosby.)
D. Plaque Elevated, firm, rough lesion with flat top surface greater than 1 cm in diameter	Psoriasis, seborrheic keratosis, actinic keratosis		Plaque. (From James WD, Berger TG, Elston DM: Andrew's diseases of the skin: *Clinical dermatology*, ed 10, London, 2000, Saunders.)

PLATE 6   **Primary Skin Lesions—cont'd**

Description	Examples		
E. Wheal Elevated, irregular-shaped area of cutaneous edema; solid, transient, variable diameter	Insect bite, urticaria, allergic reaction		 Wheal. (From Farrar WE et al: *Slide atlas of infectious diseases,* St. Louis, 1992, Mosby.)
F. Nodule Elevated, firm, circumscribed lesion; deeper in dermis than a papule; 1 to 2 cm in diameter	Erythema nodosum, lipoma		 Hypertrophic nodule. (From Goldman MP: *Cutaneous and cosmetic laser surgery,* Edinburgh, 1994, Mosby.)
G. Tumor Elevated and solid lesion; may or may not be clearly demarcated; deeper in dermis; greater than 2 cm in diameter	Neoplasm, benign tumor, lipoma, hemangioma		 Lipoma. (From Lemmi FO, Lemmi CAE: *Physical assessment findings CD-ROM,* St. Louis, 2000, Saunders.)
H. Vesicle Elevated, circumscribed, superficial, not into dermis; filled with serous fluid; less than 1 cm in diameter	Varicella (chicken pox), herpes zoster (shingles)		 Vesicles caused by varicella. (From Farrar WE et al: *Slide atlas of infectious diseases,* St. Louis, 1992, Mosby.)

Continued

PLATE 6 Primary Skin Lesions—cont'd

Description	Examples
I. Bulla Vesicle greater than 1 cm in diameter	Blister, pemphigus vulgaris

Blister. (From White DE, Fenner FJ: *Medical virology*, ed 4, San Diego, Calif., 1994, Academic Press.)

| **J. Pustule**
Elevated, superficial lesion; similar to vesicle but filled with purulent fluid | Impetigo, acne |

Acne. (From Weston W et al: *Color textbook of pediatric dermatology*, ed 4, Edinburgh, 1996, Mosby.)

| **K. Cyst**
Elevated, circumscribed, encapsulated lesion; in dermis or subcutaneous layer; filled with liquid or semisolid material | Sebaceous cyst, cystic acne |

Sebaceous cyst. (From Weston W et al: *Color textbook of pediatric dermatology*, ed 4, Edinburgh, 1996, Mosby.)

| **L. Telangiectasia**
Fine, irregular red lines produced by capillary dilation | Telangiectasia in rosacea |

Telangiectasia. (From Lemmi FO, Lemmi CAE: *Physical assessment findings CD-ROM*, St. Louis, 2000, Saunders.)

(Modified from Ball JW et al, editors: *Seidel's guide to physical examination*, ed 8, Philadelphia, 2015, Mosby/Elsevier).

PLATE 7 Secondary Skin Lesions

Description	Examples		

A. Scale
Heaped-up, keratinized cells; flaky skin; irregular; thick or thin; dry or oily; varies in size

Flaking of skin with seborrheic dermatitis following scarlet fever or flaking of skin following drug reaction, dry skin

Fine scaling. (From Baran R et al: *Color atlas of the hair, scalp, and nails,* St. Louis, 1991, Mosby.)

B. Lichenification
Rough, thickened epidermis secondary to persistent rubbing; itching, or skin irritation; often involves flexor surface of extremity

Chronic dermatitis

Lichenification. (From Lemmi FO, Lemmi CAE: *Physical assessment findings CD-ROM,* St. Louis, 2000, Saunders.)

C. Keloid
Irregular-shaped, elevated progressively enlarging scar; grows beyond boundaries of wound; caused by excessive collagen formation during healing

Keloid formation following surgery

Keloid. (From Weston W et al: *Color textbook of pediatric dermatology,* ed 4, Edinburgh, 1996, Mosby.)

D. Hypertrophic scar
Overproduction of collagen, causing the scar to be raised above skin level but not outside the boundaries of the wound.

Healed wound or surgical incision

Hypertrophic scar. (From Eisele D, Smith R: *Complications in head and neck surgery,* ed 2, Philadelphia, 2009, Mosby/Elsevier.)

E. Excoriation
Loss of epidermis; linear hollowed-out, crusted area

Abrasion or scratch

Excoriation from a tree branch. (From Lemmi FO, Lemmi CAE: *Physical assessment findings CD-ROM,* St. Louis, 2000, Saunders.)

Continued

PLATE 7 **Secondary Skin Lesions—cont'd**

Description	Examples		
F. Fissure Linear crack of break from epidermis; may be moist or dry	Athlete's foot, crack at corner of mouth		 Scaling and fissures of tinea pedis. (From Lemmi FO, Lemmi CAE: *Physical assessment findings CD-ROM*, St. Louis, 2000, Saunders.)
G. Erosion Loss of part of epidermis; depressed, moist, glistening; follows rupture of vesicle or bulla	Varicella, variola after rupture		 Erosion. (From Cohen IK et al: *Wound healing*, Philadelphia, 1993, Saunders.)
H. Ulcer Loss of epidermis and dermis; concave; varies in size	Neuropathic wound ulcer		 Neuropathic foot ulcer. (Courtesy of J. Lebretton and V. Driver.)
I. Crust Dried serum, blood, or purulent exudates; slightly elevated; varies in size; brown, red, black, tan, or straw color	Scab on abrasion, eczema		 Scab.
J. Atrophy Thinning of skin surface and loss of skin markings; skin translucent and paper-like	Striae, aged skin		 Striae. (Courtesy of Antoinette Hood, MD, Department of Dermatology, School of Medicine, University of Indiana, Indianapolis, IN.)

(Modified from Wilson SF, Giddens JF: *Health assessment for nursing practice*, ed 4, St Louis, 2009, Mosby/Elsevier. In Ball JW et al, editors: *Seidel's guide to physical examination*, ed 8, Philadelphia, 2015, Mosby/Elsevier).

PLATE 8 Type I skin tear without tissue loss: linear type (full thickness). (From LeBlanc K, Christensen D, Orsted HL et al: Best practice recommendations for the prevention and treatment of skin tears, *Wound Care Canada* 6(1):22, 2008. Image courtesy of K. LeBlanc.)

PLATE 9 Type I skin tear without tissue loss: flap type (full thickness). (From LeBlanc K, Christensen D, Orsted HL et al: Best practice recommendations for the prevention and treatment of skin tears, *Wound Care Canada* 6(1):22, 2008. Image courtesy of K. LeBlanc.)

PLATE 10 Type II skin tear with less than 25% partial tissue loss. (From LeBlanc K, Christensen D, Orsted HL et al: Best practice recommendations for the prevention and treatment of skin tears, *Wound Care Canada* 6(1):22, 2008. Image courtesy of K. LeBlanc.)

PLATE 11 Type II skin tear with greater than 25% partial tissue loss. (From LeBlanc K, Christensen D, Orsted HL et al: Best practice recommendations for the prevention and treatment of skin tears, *Wound Care Canada* 6(1):22, 2008. Image courtesy of K. LeBlanc.)

PLATE 12 Type III skin tear with complete tissue loss. (From LeBlanc K, Christensen D, Orsted HL et al: Best practice recommendations for the prevention and treatment of skin tears, *Wound Care Canada* 6(1):22, 2008. Image courtesy of K. LeBlanc.)

PLATE 13 **A,** Incontinence-associated dermatitis (IAD) on perianal skin, sacral area, and buttocks. **B,** Incontinence-associated dermatitis (IAD) with superficial epidermal erosion involving the scrotum and inner thighs.

PLATE 14 Unstageable right heel pressure ulcer with peri-wound maceration.

PLATE 15 Candidiasis in moist diaper area with characteristic satellite lesions. (From Habif TP: *Clinical dermatology*, ed 5, London, 2009, Mosby/Elsevier.)

PLATE 16 Patient with an ileostomy who developed peristomal abscess that was incised. Chemical dermatitis present along inferior aspect of incision because of inadequate protection of skin from drainage. Candidiasis also presents as papular satellite lesions and solid plaquelike rash advancing into groin and over suprapubic area.

PLATE 17 **A,** Intertrigo or intertriginous dermatitis (ITD). **B,** ITD in patient with darkly pigmented skin (A, From Habif TP: *Clinical dermatology,* ed 5, London, 2009, Mosby/Elsevier.)

PLATE 18 Folliculitis, an infection of hair follicles resulting from inappropriate hair removal technique. (From Jarvis C: *Physical examination & health assessment,* ed 4, St Louis, 2004, Saunders.)

PLATE 19 Herpes simplex virus (HSV) infection. Vesicles become pustules that erode, drain, and crust.

PLATE 20 A, Peristomal herpes lesions initially suspected to be pyoderma gangrenosum. Islands of thick, soft adherent black and tan necrosis with moist denudation; abdominal skin extremely painful. **B,** Same patient with perianal herpes simplex ulcers initially misclassified as pressure ulcers. Note proliferative edges and "punched-out" appearance that is characteristic of herpes lesions. **C,** Peristomal herpes simplex after initiation of antiviral medication. Note decreased erythema and fewer islands of necrosis; also experienced less pain in abdominal skin. **D,** Same patient after 1 week of antiviral medication. Necrosis has resolved. Epithelization and granulation have occurred. Pain significantly diminished.

PLATE 21 Herpes zoster involving simple thoracic dermatome. Vesicles are clustered and erythematous.

PLATE 22 Moist desquamation after an allergic reaction in response to the second application of benzoin to a percutaneous nephrostomy site.

Wound Assessment: Anatomy of a Wound

Wound Type: Surgical

Stage: Full Thickness
Stage of Healing: Proliferative

Measurement: L, W, D in cm.

Tunneling/Sinus: None

Wound Base: 100% red, granular

Exudate Type and Level: Moderate, serosanguinous

Periwound Skin: Resolving areas of candidiasis

Wound Edges: Epithelializing

Odor: None
Pain: 4 out of 10
Signs of Infection: No local signs present

PLATE 23 Anatomy of a wound. (Courtesy of BS Rolstad).

PLATE 24 Arterial ulcer with dry, stable eschar covering. Note dry condition of leg.

PLATE 25 Arterial ulcer with loose and adherent yellow slough present in wound bed. Mild erythema present along left lateral edge.

PLATE 26 **A,** Moderately exudative venous ulcer with slough present in wound bed and eschar present along superior aspect. **B,** After 1 week of hydrocolloids and compression therapy, autolysis has occurred, and venous ulcer has presence of granulation tissue. Amount of slough and eschar is reduced; remaining eschar is softened.

PLATE 27 Stage III pressure ulcer with excess granulation tissue.

PLATE 28 Right trochanter Stage I pressure ulcer at surgical flap site.

PLATE 29 Sacral–coccygeal ulcers of mixed etiology: pressure and IAD (fecal incontinence). Note multiple degrees of tissue loss surrounding erythema.

PLATE 30 **A,** Deep Stage III pressure ulcer. **B,** Shallow Stage III pressure ulcer on the right upper chest from a medical device. **C,** Mucosal medical device–related pressure ulcer from ET tube on the inner surface of the upper lip. **D,** Mucosal pressure ulcer on the glans penis from an indwelling urinary catheter. (A, From Cain JE: *Mosby's PDQ for wound care,* St. Louis, 2009, Mosby/Elsevier.)

PLATE 31 Left ischial tuberosity, Stage IV pressure ulcer.

PLATE 32 **A,** Unstageable sacral pressure ulcer with yellow, adherent, nonviable wound base. Periwound skin shows signs of suspected deep tissue injury (sDTI). **B,** sDTI on left buttock following surgical procedure. **C,** Right trochanter unstageable eschar covered pressure ulcer with herpes lesions on the surrounding skin secondary to significant malnutrition. Cotton-tipped applicator demonstrates dead space under eschar and need for debridement to prevent abscess and massive infection.

PLATE 33 Stage II pressure ulcer (partial thickness) from a poorly fitting compression stocking. (From Morison M et al: *Chronic wound care: a problem-based learning approach*, London, 2004, Mosby, Ltd.)

PLATE 34 Typical appearance and location of venous ulcer. Surrounding skin has been moisturized to eliminate dry skin. Note hemosiderin staining of surrounding skin and ruddy red color of wound bed.

PLATE 35 **A** and **B** Atrophie blanche dermal sclerosis with dilated abnormal vasculature and ivory white plaques on the lower extremity and hemosiderin borders. (B, Courtesy JoAnn Ermer-Seltun at Mercy Medical Center-North Iowa.)

PLATE 36 Senile purpura. Red-purple discoloration greater than 0.5 cm in diameter. Note these are not caused by pressure and may be confused as sDTI.

PLATE 37 Petechiae on dorsal surface of feet and ankles. (Ball JW et al, editors: *Seidel's guide to physical examination*, ed 8, Philadelphia, 2015, Mosby/Elsevier.)

PLATE 38 Arterial ulcer with necrotic base and halo of periwound erythema.

PLATE 39 Venous dermatitis bilateral lower legs. Note extensive hemosiderin staining and lipodermatosclerosis. Venous ulceration present with densely adherent yellow slough.

PLATE 40 Diabetic foot ulcer. Charcot foot with neuropathic plantar ulcer on the first metatarsal head. Note callus and foot and toe deformities. (Courtesy of J. Lebretton and V. Driver.)

PLATE 41 Callus removal. **A,** Hyperkeratotic callus causing increased plantar pressure. **B,** After rotary debridement, the surface is smooth and conducive to pressure redistribution. (Courtesy of J. Lebretton and V. Driver.)

PLATE 42 Lymphedema. **A** and **B,** Pattern of edema associated with lymphedema does not resolve with leg elevation and usually encompasses the entire leg. (Courtesy of JoAnn Ermer-Seltun at Mercy Medical Center-North Iowa.)

PLATE 43 Antimicrobial dressings are available in a variety of formulations. (Courtesy of Bonnie Sue Rolstad.)

PLATE 44 Epithelialized venous insufficiency ulcer. Note dark periwound staining secondary to overlapping nanocrystalline silver dressing onto intact skin. (Courtesy of Julie Freyberg.)

PLATE 45 Variety of alginate dressings. (Courtesy of Bonnie Sue Rolstad.)

PLATE 46 **A,** Alginate dressing applied to fill dead space and absorb exudate in a full-thickness abdominal wound. **B,** Alginate dressing secured with a secondary transparent dressing. Note that 2 days later at the scheduled dressing change, the alginate had formed an expected gellike appearance as the wound fluid was absorbed. The periwound skin has been protected with a liquid skin barrier.

PLATE 47 Variety of foam dressings. (Courtesy of Bonnie Sue Rolstad.)

PLATE 48 **A,** Application of nonadhesive foam dressing to venous ulcer by family member. **B,** Nonadhesive foam dressing secured with stretch-net secondary dressing.

PLATE 49 Variety of sizes and shapes of hydrocolloid dressings. (Courtesy of Bonnie Sue Rolstad.)

PLATE 50 Hydrocolloid dressing prior to removal. Note the gel developing under the dressing, which is expected as the wound exudate is absorbed by the hydrocolloid.

PLATE 51 Hydrocolloid dressing after removal from a venous ulcer. Purulent-appearing exudate is present on the dressing and wound. This is expected with autolysis under a hydrocolloid dressing and should not be misinterpreted as evidence of infection. Upon cleansing, the wound bed is clean and granular.

PLATE 52 Variety of hydrogel dressings. (Courtesy of Bonnie Sue Rolstad.)

PLATE 53 Hydrogel-impregnated gauze used to maintain a moist wound bed and fill dead space in this deep abdominal wound with undermining present.

PLATE 54 This illustrates inappropriate use of a hydrogel sheet dressing because (1) it overlaps onto intact periwound skin and (2) hydrogel will facilitate autolysis, which is not recommended on a stable eschar covered heel ulcer.

PLATE 55 Liquid skin protectant formulated as wipes, sprays, wands (i.e., skin sealant). (Courtesy of Bonnie Sue Rolstad.)

PLATE 56 Variety of transparent film dressings. (Courtesy of Bonnie Sue Rolstad.)

PLATE 57 Application of a transparent dressing by a family member in the home setting.

PLATE 58 Transparent dressing prior to removal. Note collection of fluid under the dressing, which is to be expected as autolysis occurs.

PLATE 59 Necrotizing fasciitis affecting left lower arm and extending distally onto dorsal surface of hand. Note significant amount of eschar distributed over entire surface of lower arm and edema in dorsal surface of hand. (From Bolognia JL et al: *Dermatology*, ed 2, Edinburgh, 2008, Mosby/Elsevier.)

PLATE 60 Damage to periwound closed surgical incision managed with negative pressure wound therapy without appropriate protection between black foam and periwound skin.

PLATE 61 A, Circumferential left upper thigh debrided wound with dermal wound bed on 75-pound, middle-aged adult female. **B,** Epidermal CPT (Apligraf) applied along perimeter of wound to stimulate epidermal resurfacing. Note this is an off-label use of this product and is untested in this type of wound due to rarity of the condition. **C,** One week post application with epithelial advancement along wound edges apparent.

PLATE 62 A, Brown recluse spider bite. Note central necrosis surrounded by purplish area and blisters. **B,** Another example of brown recluse spider bite following debridement 7 days after the bite initially presented with ischemia that progressed to eschar. Note persistent edema in the entire hand and fingertips. (A, From Hockenberry M, Wilson D: *Wong's essentials of pediatric nursing*, ed 8, St. Louis, 2009, Mosby/Elsevier.)

PLATE 63 Classical ulceration form of pyoderma gangreno-sum. Note violaceous (purple) color of skin surrounding ulceration.

PLATE 64 Vasculitis-related ulcer that developed in patient with rheumatoid arthritis. Wound bed has attached dry, yellow slough present, and surrounding skin is slightly erythematous.

PLATE 65 A, Calciphylaxis (CUA) in young patient with end-stage renal disease. Initial appearance can be similar to bruising or sDTI but accompanied by severe pain and erythematous margins. **B,** Calciphylaxis (CUA) has a range of manifestations in this patient and is eschar covered in this wound with continued periwound erythema and extreme pain.

PLATE 66 Untreated doxorubicin (Adriamycin) extravasation of the dorsum of the hand, with tissue damage extending throughout his forearm. **A,** Swelling, redness, and blistering apparent 3 days after the extravasation occurred. **B,** Early stages of tissue necrosis appearing 1 month later. (Copyright © 2008 by Lisa Schulmeister. Reprinted with permission.)

PLATE 67 Fasciotomy incision performed to address compartment syndrome following numerous fractures and placement of a fixation device in the lower left leg. Note viable exposed muscle and ligaments apparent in the wound bed.

PLATE 68 Clinical features of toxic epidermal necrosis (TEN) with detachment of large sheets of epidermis (more than 30% of body surface area), leading to extensive areas of denudement. A few intact bullae are still present. Wrinkling and lateral sliding of skin near blisters (positive Nikolsky sign) are apparent. (From Bolognia JL et al: *Dermatology*, ed 2, Edinburgh, 2008, Mosby/Elsevier.)

PLATE 69 Graft-versus-host disease (GVHD) in a patient after allogenic bone marrow transplantation. Note macular–papular rash is barely distinguishable and has become confluent. Edema, erythema, and bulla formation are present.

PLATE 70 Edges of incision approximated with sutures and significant pooling of subcutaneous bleeding that evolved into eschar. This photograph illustrates the importance of documenting not only the condition of the incision but also the condition of the periwound skin.

PLATE 71 **A,** Abdomen of obese patient with skin breakdown under pannus due to pressure and moisture. **B,** Skin folds in patient with obesity; textile garment in place to protect from moisture entrapment. **C,** Linear ITD fissure present in skin folds. (A, Courtesy of Judith L. Gates.)

PLATE 72 Complications at the site of the gastrostomy button. **A,** Hyperplasia/hypergranulation. **B,** Cellulitis. **C,** Dehiscence. (Courtesy of Teri Crawley Coha.)

PLATE 73 Basal cell carcinoma may be a primary lesion anywhere on the body. Existing chronic wounds of various etiologies may convert to malignant cutaneous wounds also known as *Marjolin's ulcer.* (From Habif T, Campbell M, Chapman S et al: *Skin disease: diagnosis and treatment,* ed 3, London, 2011, Mosby.)

PLATE 74 **A,** Squamous cell carcinoma on buttock. **B,** Cutaneous malignant wound (fungating wound) involving the right side of the face and neck. (B, From Morison M et al: *Chronic wound care: a problem-based learning approach,* London, 2004, Mosby, Ltd.)

PLATE 75 Patient with enterocutaneous fistula with irregular surrounding skin surfaces and depression along fistula–skin junction at interior aspect and upper left aspect.

PLATE 76 Tapered layers of solid-wafer skin barrier used to help level skin depression at inferior aspect. Skin barrier paste has been applied to surrounding wound margins and in all three depressions (over skin barrier wafer wedges) to level and protect the skin from effluent. Cement has been painted onto adhesive field (over paste and wedges) to increase adhesion.

PLATE 77 A, EAF within granular wound bed. **B,** Skin barrier powder dusted over wound bed where skin barrier ring will contact. Convex oval skin barrier ring applied with flat side down to wound bed, encircling fistula orifice. **C,** Black NPWT foam trimmed to fit remaining exposed wound bed contacting with skin barrier ring. Drape applied over inverted skin barrier ring and foam and sealed to skin barrier with stoma opening cut out. Second oval convex skin barrier ring inverted and applied (creating flat surface). **D,** Create slit in foam/drape all allow for track pad. **E,** Foam applied to lead away from wound area. **F,** Drape applied over foam (only) and track pad applied. Attached to negative pressure to confirm seal. **G,** Pouch opening created to size of skin barrier ring over EAF and attached. **H,** Separation of wound bed via NPWT from EAF and pouch apparent because pouch does not tract or suck down into fistula orifice.

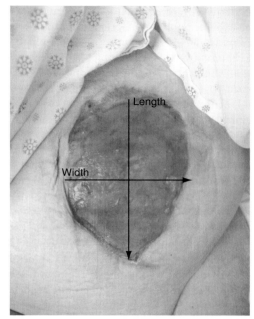

FIGURE 6-2 Measuring wound length and width.

FIGURE 6-3 Measuring wound depth.

FIGURE 6-4 Wound tunneling. Tunneling is present in this abdominal wound at the 7 o'clock position and measures 2 cm in length. Tunnel and sinus tract are often used interchangeably.

FIGURE 6-5 Undermining extends 2 cm from 7 to 11 o'clock.

wound perimeter. Pressure ulcers that have been subjected to shear often are first seen with undermining. Undermining and tunneling can be documented by measuring depth and noting the location using the face of the clock as a model. The superior aspect of the wound (12 o'clock position) points toward the patient's head, whereas the inferior aspect of the wound (6 o'clock position) points toward the patient's feet. Examples are shown in Figures 6-4 and 6-5.

Wound Shape. Terms used to describe the shape of the wound include adjectives such as round, oval, triangular, irregular, and butterfly shaped. Documenting the shape of the wound provides not only a more accurate clinical description, but also clues to wound etiology. For example, device-related pressure ulcers will be apparent because they will replicate the shape of the device, such as tubing, telemetry cable, or needle cap. Similarly, acute onset of a butterfly-shaped area of erythema over the upper buttocks and coccyx is consistent with unrelieved pressure while the patient is in the supine position.

Wound Exudate. The characteristics of wound exudate should be assessed in terms of volume (none, light, moderate, or heavy) and type (clear, serosanguineous, sanguineous,

purulent). Exudate quantity generally varies with the type of wound. For example, a venous ulcer is more exudative than an arterial ulcer. An increase in wound exudate may coincide with hyperplasia, critical colonization, biofilm, edema, or wound infection. Subjective indicators used to quantify the volume of wound exudate include frequency of dressing change and persistent presence of periwound maceration. The type of dressing used will also provide an indication of the volume of exudate, as hydrofiber and alginate dressings are much more absorbent than hydrocolloid dressings. Sodium-impregnated gauze also can be expected to contain more exudate than plain gauze. Objective measurement of the volume of wound exudate can be obtained by using a wound containment system, such as a wound pouch or closed suction.

Odor. Odor can be described as absent, faint, moderate, or strong and often varies according to wound moisture, the type and density of microorganisms present, and the amount of nonviable tissue present. Extremely odorous, purulent exudate is suggestive of an infection. However, it is important to note that most wounds have a slight odor. The type of dressing used, as well as personal and wound-related hygiene, also can affect wound odor (Keast et al, 2004).

Wound Edge. The rim of the wound or wound edge provides information regarding epithelialization, chronicity, and even etiology. Ideally, the wound edges should be attached, moist, and flush with the wound base so that epithelial cells can migrate from the wound edges across the surface of the wound bed. Unattached wound edges are those in which undermining is present between the dermis and subcutaneous tissue. Closed wound edges are characterized as dry with a loss of the intervening moist, red reproductive epithelium. In some situations, closed wound edges are also thickened and "rolled." This premature closure of the wound edge is a common complication of chronic wounds and is referred to as *epibole* (Doughty, 2004). Epibole results when squamous cells migrate along the base, wall, and edge of the wound, thus preventing migration of epithelial cells and wound closure (see Plate 4). Cautery or surgical debridement of epibole is needed to "open" the wound edges.

Periwound Skin. The periwound skin should be described in terms of color (erythema, pale, white, blue), texture (moist, dry, indurated, boggy, macerated), skin temperature (warm, cool), integrity (denudement, maceration, excoriation, stripping, erosion, papules, pustules), and presence or absence of lesions.

The periwound assessment can give clues to the effectiveness of the treatment plan and the technique used for dressing application or removal. For example, maceration (see Plate 14), dermatitis, or denudement of periwound skin occurs when exudate pools on intact skin for prolonged periods or when a moist dressing is inappropriately applied, is left on too long, and/or overlaps onto intact skin. Periwound skin stripping may indicate inappropriate adhesive removal.

Venous/arterial insufficiency, infection, pressure damage, peripheral neuropathy, pyoderma gangrenosum, vasculitis, and calciphylaxis may be present with distinct periwound features. Table 6-6 lists some pathologies that may be revealed through a careful periwound skin inspection.

Bacterial Burden. All wounds have some degree of bioburden. The extent and significance of that bioburden are conveyed with the terms *contamination*, *colonization*, *critical colonization*, *biofilm*, and *infection*. The presence or absence of local signs of infection should be documented as part of the assessment. However, it's important to remember that many chronic wounds with significant bioburden may not exhibit the classic signs of infection due to factors such as immunosuppression or the presence of biofilm. Indicators of a subclinical infection or overwhelming bioburden include delayed healing despite optimal care, discolored or friable granulation tissue, pocketing or breakdown at the wound base, and/or foul odor. A "stagnant" wound despite optimal care may indicate critical colonization or biofilm and will progress to infection without appropriate intervention. Chapter 16 presents a thorough discussion of the assessment and management of bacterial burden (including biofilm) and infection.

Wound Pain. As the fifth vital sign, pain has gained a much-deserved focus in today's health care environment. Yet wound pain is infrequently assessed and inadequately managed. Wound pain can indicate infection or deterioration and inappropriate or inadequate treatment choices. Pain can be directly related to patient satisfaction and has been shown to have a negative impact on wound healing progress. Pain should be measured regularly and frequently with a validated pain assessment scale (Reddy et al, 2003). Chapters 25 and 26 provide detailed discussions related to the assessment and management of wound pain.

TABLE 6-6	**Common Periwound Features by Wound Pathology**
Pathology	**Periwound Feature**
Venous insufficiency	Edema, brawny discoloration, hemosiderin-staining lipodermatosclerosis, dermatitis, scaling, weeping, scarring, varicose veins, maceration
Arterial	Elevation pallor, cool, dependent rubor, absent hair, xerosis, atrophy
Infection	Erythema, pain, heat, swelling, induration
Pressure	Hyperemia, edema, induration, discoloration
Peripheral neuropathy	Insensate, edema, cellulitis, erythema, induration, xerosis, fissures, callus
Pyoderma gangrenosum	Ragged borders, elevated borders, dusky red or purple, halo
Vasculitis	Palpable, nonblanchable purpura; may be associated with petechiae; nodules and vesicles may be present
Calciphylaxis	Dusky, purple, and palpable nodules progress to necrosis and ulceration; associated with renal disease; may include mottled, reticulated patches, plaques with focal central necrosis
Candidiasis	Pustular or macular-papular rash; erythematous satellite lesions

REASSESSMENT AND EVALUATION OF HEALING

Evaluation of healing involves wound assessment documented over time to reveal patterns and trends that indicate improvement or deterioration in the wound. In this way, assessment is linked to outcomes so that an evaluation of the plan of care can follow objective criteria.

Any clinical cause for suspicion, such as raised borders, unusual wound base, unexplained pain, changes in shape or color, previous history, or family history of skin cancer, requires referral for biopsy. Ulcers or lesions that do not respond to optimal therapy also warrant a referral for biopsy (Snyder et al, 2003). Biopsy technique is critical to cancer detection. It is recommended that wounds be biopsied from multiple sites (i.e., at 12, 6, 3, and 9 o'clock positions) and from multiple depths (e.g., 2, 4, and 6 mm). The biopsy sites should be recorded because rebiopsy is indicated if the wound does not respond as expected to treatment (Snyder, 2006).

Frequency of Reassessment

In general, the patient's overall condition, wound severity, health care setting, type of dressings used, and goals determine the appropriate frequency of wound assessment. Because frequency of reassessment is dependent on so many variables, the frequency interval commonly changes over time and across care settings. For example, a patient who is immunosuppressed and in acute care has greater risk for developing a wound infection and may warrant more frequent monitoring. Once the patient is stable in long-term care, the "at-risk" patient's skin should be monitored daily, but may require a full wound assessment only on admission and weekly. Once the patient is home, assessments are generally dependent on the frequency of home health worker or clinic visits. Family members should be instructed to make assessments between clinic visits and may be able and willing to monitor for trends.

National and international pressure ulcer guidelines (NPUAP, EPUAP, PPPIA, 2014; WOCN®, 2010) make specific recommendations on the frequency of monitoring, assessment, and evaluation of pressure ulcer healing, as summarized in Box 6-1. When topical wound therapy is being selected, the frequency with which the wound should be assessed must be considered. For example, a hydrocolloid on a stable wound should not be removed daily simply to conduct a wound assessment. Rather, the assessment should be obtained at the time the dressing is scheduled to be changed (i.e., every

4 days). Chapter 18 discusses the principles of wound management and the various features of local wound care options.

Regulatory Documentation Tools

Medicare's Outcome and Assessment Information Set (OASIS) and Continuous Assessment Record and Evaluation (CARE) are comprehensive patient assessments that contain information about wounds and wound management. However, these documents do not contain comprehensive wound assessments and should not replace comprehensive and focused assessments for patients with wounds. Medicare's payment to home health care agencies is based on the OASIS (revised to OASIS-C). In the future, the OASIS and regulatory documents for other health care settings will be replaced by the CARE tool.

The OASIS is a comprehensive patient assessment that includes several wound-related questions and some diagnoses. The OASIS is completed by the registered nurse or physical therapist on admission, at recertification, and at discharge. The most extensive OASIS assessment is done on admission and contains questions that cover the patient's clinical condition and functional status and includes several questions on services received. Because payment is directly affected by how several wound-related questions are answered, the Wound, Ostomy and Continence Nurses Society™ (WOCN®) developed an OASIS Guidance Document for clarification of how these questions could best be answered (WOCN.org).

The CARE tool is a standardized patient assessment tool and is expected to replace the OASIS and other regulatory documents in the future, including the Inpatient Rehabilitation Facility (IRF)-Patient Assessment Instrument (PAI), and Minimum Data Set (MDS). The CARE tool is web-based and intended for use in multiple settings, including acute care, long-term acute care, long-term care, home care, and rehabilitation. Development of the CARE tool began in 2006 and was first piloted in 2008. The project has gone through many phases involving multiple users, years of data collection, and reliability testing. A report describing the process and results was submitted to Congress in 2012, which The report described strong interrater reliability of the tool (Gage et al, 2012). Once implemented, the massive database generated by the CARE tool has the potential for comparing outcomes and learning more about best practices.

Predicting Wound Healing

It is generally agreed that the percentage of reduction in wound surface area during the initial weeks of treatment is the most reliable indicator for complete healing, and the

---

BOX 6-1 Guidelines for Frequency of Monitoring, Assessment, and Evaluation of Pressure Ulcer Healing

1. Patients at risk for skin breakdown should have at least daily skin inspections.
2. Twice-daily skin assessments are recommended under and around medical devices (more often in individuals experiencing or vulnerable to developing fluid shifts and edema).
3. Pressure ulcers should be assessed and monitored at each dressing change, or sooner if the wound or the patient's condition deteriorates.
4. Evaluation of pressure ulcer healing should occur within 2 weeks, or sooner if the patient or wound condition deteriorates.

initial size of the wound is a significant predictor of time to heal. van Rijswijk and the Multicenter Leg Ulcer Study Group (2003) monitored the healing of 61 patients with 72 full-thickness venous leg ulcers. They found that a greater than 30% reduction in ulcer area after 2 weeks of treatment was a significant ($p < .004$) predictor of the time required for healing. Kantor and Margolis (2000) conducted a cohort multicenter study of 104 patients and found that the percentage change in ulcer area during the first 4 weeks of treatment was the best prognostic indicator that the ulcers would eventually heal within 24 weeks. Similarly, Phillips et al (2000) found baseline ulcer area and duration of leg ulcer were important predictors of healing in a multicenter retrospective review of 165 patients with venous ulcers. Falanga and Sabolinski (2000) reported data based on randomized, controlled, clinical trials and presented reliable and specific findings for predicting complete healing. Initial healing time of 0.11 cm/wk or greater predicts healing, whereas rates of 0.06 cm/wk or less predict nonhealing. A prospective multicenter study of 203 patients with diabetic foot ulcers found that 4-week healing rates correlated significantly with healing at 12 weeks ($p < .01$) (Sheehan et al, 2003). Snyder and colleagues (2010) conducted a post hoc analysis of diabetic foot ulcer (DFU) treatment outcomes from two published, randomized, controlled studies (n = 133 and 117) to assess the relationship between percentage area reduction (PAR) during early standard wound care and ulcer closure by week 12. Findings confirmed that PAR in wound size is an early predictor of treatment outcome ($p \leq 0.001$). The author suggested that protocols for care should be reevaluated if greater than 50% PAR is not achieved by week 4.

Studies of neuropathic and ischemic ulcers suggest a linear relationship between initial wound radius or size and healing time (Robson et al, 2000; Zimny et al, 2002). During a controlled prospective trial examining 338 serial tracings of venous ulcers, Cardinal et al (2009) noted faster healing rates with wounds that maintained a linear relationship between margin size and wound surface size ($p < .001$).

Jones et al (2007) conducted a multisite retrospective review of medical records of patients from a variety of care settings to determine factors that influence wound healing within 3 months and nonhealing after 5 months. Researchers evaluated at least 3 months of data from 400 patients with pressure, venous, and diabetic wounds who received routine wound care by typical staff. Results showed a difference in wound healing by size, location, and socioeconomic status. Large and deep wounds were less likely to heal than small and shallow wounds. Lower extremity wounds were more likely to heal than wounds located on the iliac crest or trochanter. Patients who were not Caucasian and patients on Medicare had poor healing outcomes. Not surprisingly, nonhealing wounds were also associated with infection, heavy exudate, necrosis, and inappropriate use of wound care dressings. Edsberg and colleagues (2011) had similar findings related to initial size as a significant predictor of time to heal ($p < .023$), with smaller Stage III and IV pressure ulcers healing faster than larger Stage III and IV pressure ulcers.

Tools for Documentation and Evaluation of Healing

Several tools that enable the clinician to assess wounds are available and are presented throughout the text and in Box 6-2. These instruments attempt to enhance communication among clinicians, define a common language, and standardize assessment. Clinicians should be familiar with the strengths and limitations of the several methods currently available for assessing wound status. Staging and assessment tools are not designed to replace a comprehensive ongoing assessment. Ideally, tools should be reliable, valid, clinically useful, and theoretically based (Arndt and Kelechi, 2014).

Pillen and colleagues (2009) conducted a systematic literature review to examine available wound-healing instruments in terms of validity, reliability, and sensitivity measures of wound healing. Their review identified substantial gaps in the literature with regard to validation of the 10 wound healing instruments (see Box 6-2) found in their search. Authors reported the Pressure Ulcer Scale for Healing (PUSH) and Pressure Sore Status Tool (PSST) had been validated to the greatest extent, whereas those describing healing in leg ulcers and general or surgical wounds tended to lack comprehensive and quality evaluation. International guidelines advocate the combined use of clinical judgment and a valid and reliable pressure ulcer assessment scale to assess progress toward healing (NPUAP, EPUAP, PPPIA, 2014).

Pressure Ulcer Scale for Healing. The PUSH was developed by the National Pressure Ulcer Advisory Panel (NPUAP) to monitor pressure ulcer healing over time. The PUSH tool is designed to monitor three parameters that are considered the most indicative of healing: size (length and width), exudate amount, and tissue type. Each parameter has at least four sublevels. The subscore for each parameter is totaled, and the overall total score is calculated ranging from 0 to 17 (0 = healed). A comparison of total scores measured over time provides an indication of wound improvement or deterioration

---

BOX 6-2   Assessment of Wound-Healing Instruments

- Pressure Ulcer Scale for Healing (PUSH) #
- Bates-Jensen Wound Assessment Tool (BWAT)
- Sessing Scale (SS)
- Sussman Wound Healing Tool (SWHT)
- Wound Healing Scale (WHS)
- DESIGN
- Leg Ulcer Measurement Tool (LUMT) #
- ASEPSIS*
- Barber Measuring Tool (BMT)*
- Granulometer*

#Leg wounds
*General and surgical wounds
DESIGN, Depth, exudate, size, inflammation/infection, granulation tissue, necrotic tissue.
Data obtained from Pillen H, Miller M, Thomas J, et al: Assessment of wound healing: validity, reliability and sensitivity of available instruments, *Wound Pract Res* 17(4):208–217, 2009.

(Günes, 2009; WOCN® 2010). Numerous validation studies have been conducted using the PUSH tool. George-Saintilus and colleagues (2009) questioned the reliability of the PUSH tool when they discovered little agreement between traditional nursing observations and PUSH scores of patients with a wound residing in an extended care facility. However, subsequent studies found the PUSH tool to be valid and responsive for assessing healing for pressure, venous, and diabetic lower extremity ulcers (Hon et al, 2010).

Bates-Jensen Wound Assessment Tool. The Bates-Jensen Wound Assessment Tool (BWAT) was originally known as the PSST. The tool addresses 13 wound characteristics (Harris et al, 2010). Specific definitions are provided for each characteristic. Individual items are scored on a modified Likert scale (ranging from 1 for best for that characteristic to 5 for worst). Individual items are summed, and the total provides a measure of overall wound status. Total scores range from 13, which indicates tissue health, to 65, which indicates wound degeneration.

Although the tool is now intended for use with a variety of wound types, validity and reliability have been mostly obtained with pressure ulcers utilizing the original PSST. Content validity was established (CVI = 0.91) by a panel of nine nurses recognized as experts in wound care. Concurrent validity came from a comparison of the PSST total score to NPUAP ulcer stage, giving a correlation of $r = 0.606$ ($p = 0.001$). The tool has been through interrater reliability with raters of diverse education and training, strengthening the generalizability of these results. One study reported acceptable interrater reliability for general health care practitioners (kappa = 0.78) versus an expert "enterostomal" nurse (kappa = 0.82) (Pillen et al, 2009).

DESIGN and DESIGN R Tools. Developed in Japan, the DESIGN and the revised DESIGN R tools classify pressure ulcer severity and monitor progression toward healing. DESIGN interrater reliability results showed a high correlation with photos and real-life pressure ulcers ($r = 0.98$ with $r = 0.91$, respectively). For validity, a high correlation was found between DESIGN R and PSST scores. A positive change in at least one DESIGN R score significantly correlated with total healing within 30 days with good interrater reliability with BWAT scores (Lizaka et al, 2012; Sanada et al, 2004).

Photographic Wound Assessment Tool. The Photographic Wound Assessment Tool (PWAT) was developed from the PSST and was designed to examine the validity and reliability of wound photography. The intraclass correlation coefficient for intrarater reliability was excellent, varying from 0.86 to 0.96. Interrater reliability was dependent on the clinicians having experience in wound care. Clinicians with more than 5 years of experience had an intraclass correlation coefficient of 0.75, but only 0.34 for inexperienced students. Based on these findings, Houghton and colleagues (2000) concluded that when used by experienced wound clinicians, the PWAT suffices when a full bedside assessment is not possible.

Photography

Accurate photography may provide a template against which changes in wound status can be observed and compared. However, if photography is to be used, it should only be used as an *adjunct* to support written wound documentation of bedside assessment (NPUAP, EPUAP, PPPIA, 2014). The subject of wound photography often leads to a discussion of litigation. A blurred photograph or photography that does not follow facility policy can give the impression of poor work quality, supporting negative outcomes in a courtroom rather than the intended purpose of conveying progression of healing. If a photograph of the wound is not available, the jury could be shown a photograph of a different wound as an example of how bad it could be. States differ regarding their stance on the admissibility of photographs in court cases (WOCN®, 2012a). Another issue related to wound photography is film type: use of Polaroid film, which cannot be altered but may soon be unavailable, versus digital film, which can be altered (Sullivan, 2008).

The WOCN® Society neither recommends nor discourages the use of photography for pressure ulcer documentation. However, the organization provides a document to guide the use of photography in the clinical setting. The document outlines items and criteria that need to be included in order to be compliant with The Joint Commission, the American Health Information Management Association (AHIMA), and Health Insurance Portability and Accountability Act (HIPAA) guidelines (WOCN®, 2012a). When photography is used, the facility should have specific protocols or policies in place. Checklist 6-4 provides issues to be addressed in a wound photography protocol or policy.

CHECKLIST 6-4 Issues to Address in Policy or Protocol for Wound Photography

✓ Informed consent (who can obtain the consent and what is included)
✓ Timing of photographs (when or under what circumstances photographs are to be taken and repeated)
✓ Criteria about who can take the photographs
✓ Method of validating competency to photograph wounds (include frequency of competency revalidations)
✓ Type of camera being used
✓ Techniques used to ensure consistency in photographing and methods used to ensure photographs are not enhanced or altered (e.g., image size, distance from the wound, sample measure in frame, such as measuring guide)
✓ Appropriate patient identification (initials, medical record number, date and time markings)
✓ Maintenance and storage of photographs effectively (where they will be stored and who will have access to them)
✓ Method for releasing copies to patients upon request (authorization form)

Data from Wound, Ostomy and Continence Nurses Society™ (WOCN®): *Photography in wound documentation.* In Wound, Ostomy and Continence Nurses Society Professional Practice series, 2005. https://c.ymcdn.com/sites/wocn.site-ym.com/resource/resmgr/files/photography_in_wound_document.pdf. Accessed March 30, 2015.

CLINICAL CONSULT

A: Consulted for "sDTI pressure ulcer under leg brace, see photo in chart". Mr. Johnson is A&O × 3, 53-year-old gentleman, admitted yesterday for increased weakness and atrial fibrillation. Photo in chart shows defined purple round lesion. No documentation noted on wound flow sheet. PMH shows multiple sclerosis. Patient states he was up ad lib until yesterday, when he became extremely tired and weak. Nurse applied heel-offloading boots after use of pillows was ineffective due to leg spasms. Patient verbalized good understanding of pressure ulcer prevention and demonstrates ability to reposition effectively when asked. Left posterior leg lesion 3 × 3 cm, intact, round and slightly edematous, periwound skin intact, no local sign of infection. PT and pedal pulses palpable, no history or signs of venous insufficiency. Patient denies pain, states he didn't know it was there.

D: Complete wound assessment and differential diagnosis is not consistent with a suspected deep tissue injury pressure ulcer as it is not located over a bony prominence nor under the heel-offloading device. Suspect bruise from bumping into furniture. (Patient is on anticoagulants and states he commonly bumps into furniture at home).

P: Discussed importance for protecting himself from skin injury while on anticoagulants. Patient states he has just purchased new leather furniture to replace mission style wood furniture at home.

I: Recommendations: (1) Protect bruise from further injury especially during transfers and ambulation. (2) Continue interventions for pressure ulcer prevention.

E: Monitor bruise daily with skin inspection and call provider if it increases in dimensions, becomes painful, or deteriorates. No further plans for follow up. Please reconsult as needed.

SUMMARY

Few pathologic conditions are evaluated with a single instrument or parameter. The more intricate the process (e.g., congestive heart failure), the more clinicians rely on several measures (e.g., radiologic examination, physical examination, pulse characteristics, treadmill tests, hematocrit) to accurately capture a full description of the extent of the condition. Similarly, several parameters are required to best capture the condition of the wound.

Recognizing the difference between simply measuring the dimensions of a wound and the more complex process of assessing the status of the wound's multiple components and healing status is essential to successful wound management and holistic patient care. It is clear that evaluating wounds as if they exist separately from the patient not only is inadequate, but also is inconsistent with evidence-based practice.

REFERENCES

Apold J, Rydrych D: Preventing device-related pressure ulcers: using data to guide statewide change, *J Nurs Care Qual* 27(1):28–34, 2012.

Arndt JV, Kelechi TJ: An overview of instruments for wound and skin assessment and healing, *J Wound Ostomy Continence Nurs* 41(1):17–23, 2014.

Bates-Jensen BM, McCreath HE, Pongquan V: Subepidermal moisture is associated with early pressure ulcer damage in nursing home residents with dark skin tones: pilot findings, *J Wound Ostomy Continence Nurs* 36(3):277–284, 2009.

Baumgarten M, Margolis D, van Doorn C, et al: Black/white differences in pressure ulcer incidence in nursing home residents, *J Am Geriatr Soc* 52(8):1293–1298, 2004.

Bennett AM: Report of the task force on the implications for darkly pigmented intact skin in the prediction and prevention of pressure ulcers, *Adv Wound Care* 8(6):34–35, 1995.

Cardinal M, Eisenbud DE, Armstrong DG: Wound shape geometry measurements correlate to eventual wound healing, *Wound Repair Regen* 17(2):173–178, 2009.

Croke EM: Nurses, negligence, and malpractice, *Am J Nurs* 103(9):54–63, 2003.

Doughty DB: Wound assessment: tips and techniques, *Adv Skin Wound Care* 17:369–372, 2004.

Edsberg LE, Wyffels JT, Ha DS: Longitudinal study of stage III and stage IV pressure ulcer area and perimeter as healing parameters to predict wound closure, *Ostomy Wound Manage* 57(10):50–62, 2011.

Falanga V, Sabolinski ML: Prognostic factors for healing of venous ulcers, *Wounds* 12(Suppl 5A):42A–46A, 2000.

Gage B, Deutsch A, Smith L, et al: *The development and testing of the Continuity Assessment Record and Evaluation (CARE) Item Set: final report on CARE Item Set and current assessment comparisons, September 2012.* http://www.cms.gov/Medicare/Quality-Initiatives-Patient-Assessment-Instruments/Post-Acute-Care-Quality-Initiatives/Downloads/The-Development-and-Testing-of-the-Continuity-Assessment-Record-and-Evaluation-CARE-Item-Set-Final-Report-on-the-Development-of-the-CARE-Item-Set-and-Current-Assessment-Comparisons-Volume-3-of-3.pdf. Accessed December 7, 2014.

George-Saintilus E, Tommasulo B, Cal CE, et al: Pressure ulcer PUSH score and traditional nursing assessment in nursing home residents: do they correlate? *J Am Med Dir Assoc* 10(2):141–144, 2009.

Guihan M, Bates-Jenson BM, Chun S, et al: Assessing the feasibility of subepidermal moisture to predict erythema and stage 1 pressure ulcers in persons with spinal cord injury: a pilot study, *J Spinal Cord Med* 35(1):46–52, 2012.

Günes UY: A prospective study evaluating the Pressure Ulcer Scale for Healing (PUSH Tool) to assess stage II, stage III, and stage IV pressure ulcers, *Ostomy Wound Manage* 55(5):48–52, 2009.

Harris C, Bates-Jensen B, Parslow N, et al: Wound assessment tool, *J Wound Ostomy Continence Nurs* 37(3):253–259, 2010.

Hon J, Lagden K, McLaren AM, et al: Prospective, multicenter study to validate use of the PUSH in patients with diabetic, venous, and pressure ulcers, *Ostomy Wound Manage* 56(2):26–36, 2010.

Houghton P, Kincaid C, Campbell K, et al: Photographic assessment of the appearance of chronic pressure and leg ulcers, *Ostomy Wound Manage* 46(4):20–30, 2000.

Jones KR, Fennie K, Lenihan A: Chronic wounds: factors influencing healing within 3 months and nonhealing after 5-6 months of care, *Wounds* 19(3):51–63, 2007.

Kantor J, Margolis DJ: A multicentre study of percentage change in venous leg ulcer area as a prognostic index of healing at 24 weeks, *Br J Dermatol* 142(5):960–964, 2000.

Keast DH, Bowering CK, Evans AW, et al: Measure: a proposed assessment framework for developing best practice recommendations for wound assessment, *Wound Rep Regen* 5:S1–S17, 2004.

Kottner J, Dassen T, Lahmann N: Comparison of two skin examination methods for grade 1 pressure ulcers, *J Clin Nurs* 18(17):2464–2469, 2009.

Langemo DK, Anderson J, Hanson D, et al: Measuring wound length, width, and area: which technique? *Adv Skin Wound Care* 21:42–45, 2008.

Lizaka S, Sanada H, Matsui Y, et al: Scientific Education Committee of the Japanese Society of Pressure Ulcers. Predictive validity of weekly monitoring of wound status using DESIGN-R score change for pressure ulcer healing: a multicenter prospective cohort study, *Wound Repair Regen* 20(4):473–481, 2012.

National Pressure Ulcer Advisory Panel (NPUAP), European Pressure Ulcer Advisory Panel (EPUAP), Pan Pacific Pressure Injury Alliance (PPPIA): Haesler E, editor, *Prevention and treatment of pressure ulcers: clinical practice guideline*, Perth, Australia, 2014, Cambridge Media.

Nixon J, Cranny G, Bond S: Skin alterations of intact skin and risk factors associated with pressure ulcer development in surgical patients: a cohort study, *Int J Nurs Stud* 44(5):655–663, 2007.

Phillips TJ, Machado F, Trout R, et al: Prognostic indicators in venous ulcers, *J Am Acad Dermatol* 43(4):627–630, 2000.

Pieper B, Ratliff C: National Pressure Ulcer Advisory Panel (NPUAP) registered nurse competency-based curriculum: pressure ulcer prevention, 2010. http://www.npuap.org/wp-content/uploads/2012/03/Updated-NPUAP-RN-5-29-13.pdf. Accessed March 31, 2015.

Pillen H, Miller M, Thomas J, et al: Assessment of wound healing: validity, reliability and sensitivity of available instruments, *Wound Practice and Research* 17(4):208–217, 2009.

Reddy M, Kohr R, Queen D, et al: Practical treatment of wound pain and trauma: a patient centered approach, *Ostomy Wound Manage* 49(Suppl 4A):2–15, 2003.

Reising D, Allen P: Protecting yourself from malpractice claims, *Am Nurse Today* 2(2):39–44, 2007.

Robson MC, Hill DP, Woodske ME, et al: Wound healing trajectories as predictors of effectiveness of therapeutic agents, *Arch Surg* 135(7):773–777, 2000.

Rosen J, Mittal V, Degenholtz H, et al: Pressure ulcer prevention in black and white nursing home residents: a QI initiative of enhanced ability, incentives, and management feedback, *Adv Skin Wound Care* 19(5):262–268, 2006.

Sanada H, Moriguchi T, Miyachi Y, et al: Reliability and validity of DESIGN, a tool that classifies pressure ulcer severity and monitors healing, *J Wound Care* 13:13–18, 2004.

Sheehan P, Jones P, Caselli A, et al: Percent change in wound area of diabetic foot ulcers over a 4 week period is a robust predictor of complete healing in a 12 week prospective trial, *Diabetes Care* 26:1879–1882, 2003.

Snyder R: Skin cancers and chronic wounds. In Norman R, editor: *Handbook of geriatric dermatology*, New York, 2006, Cambridge University Press.

Snyder RJ, Cardinal M, Dauphinée DM, et al: A post hoc analysis of reduction in diabetic foot ulcer size at 4 weeks as a predictor of healing by 12 weeks, *Ostomy Wound Manage* 56(3):44–50, 2010.

Snyder RJ, Stillman RM, Weiss SD: Epidermoid cancers that masquerade as venous ulcer disease, *Ostomy Wound Manage* 49(4):63–66, 2003.

Sprigle S, Zhang L, Duckworth M: Detection of skin erythema in darkly pigmented skin using multispectral images, *Adv Skin Wound Care* 22(4):172–179, 2009.

Sterner E, Lindholm C, Berg E, et al: Category I pressure ulcers: how reliable is clinical assessment? *Orthopaedic Nurs* 30(3):194–205, 2011.

Sullivan V: In focus: the photography forecast, *Today's Wound Clinic* April 15, 2008. http://www.todayswoundclinic.com/in-focus-the-photography-forecast. Accessed December 6, 2014.

U.S. Census Bureau: *2012 National population projections*. http://www.census.gov/population/projections/data/national/2012/downloadablefiles.html. Accessed December 6, 2014.

Vanderwee K, Grypdonck MHF, De Bacquer D, et al: The reliability of two observation methods of nonblanchable erythema, grade 1 pressure ulcer, *Appl Nurs Res* 19(3):156–162, 2006.

van Rijswijk L, Lyder C: Pressure ulcer prevention and care: implementing the revised guidance to surveyors for long-term care facilities, *Ostomy Wound Manage* 51(Suppl 4):7–19, 2005.

van Rijswijk L: Multicenter Leg Ulcer Study Group: Full-thickness leg ulcers: patient demographics and predictors of healing, *J Fam Pract* 36(6):625–632, 2003.

Wound, Ostomy and Continence Nurses Society™ (WOCN®): *Guideline for management of patients with lower extremity arterial disease (WOCN® clinical practice guideline series no. 1)*, Mount Laurel, NJ, 2014, WOCN®.

Wound, Ostomy and Continence Nurses Society™ (WOCN®): *Guideline for prevention and management of pressure ulcers (WOCN® clinical practice guideline series no. 2)*, Mount Laurel, NJ, 2010, WOCN®.

Wound, Ostomy and Continence Nurses Society™ (WOCN®): *Position statement about the role and scope of practice for wound care providers,* Mount Laurel, NJ, 2011, WOCN®.

Wound, Ostomy and Continence Nurses Society™ (WOCN®): *Guideline for management of patients with lower extremity neuropathic disease (WOCN® clinical practice guideline series no. 1)*, Mount Laurel, NJ, 2012a, WOCN®.

Wound, Ostomy and Continence Nurses Society™ (WOCN®): *Photography in wound documentation (Fact sheet)*, Mount Laurel, NJ, 2012b, WOCN®. https://c.ymcdn.com/sites/wocn.site-ym.com/resource/resmgr/files/photography_in_wound_document.pdf. March 30, 2015

Young T, Rohwer A, Volmink J, et al: What are the effects of teaching evidence-based health care (EBHC)? Overview of systematic reviews, *PLoS One* 9(1):e86706, 2014.

Zimny S, Schatz H, Pfohl M: Determinants and estimation of healing times in diabetic foot ulcers, *J Diabetes Complications* 16:327–332, 2002.

7

Pressure Ulcers: Impact, Etiology, and Classification

Barbara Pieper

OBJECTIVES

1. Define pressure ulcer and terms associated with it.
2. Describe the incidence and prevalence of pressure ulcers.
3. Identify economic effects and quality-of-life impact of pressure ulcers.
4. Examine vulnerable populations (older adult, spinal cord injured, surgical, obese and underweight patients) in terms of pressure ulcer risk.
5. Describe the role of the causative factors (intensity of pressure, duration of pressure, and tissue tolerance [intrinsic and extrinsic]) for pressure ulcer formation.
6. Summarize the history of pressure ulcer classifications.
7. Describe the pathophysiologic consequences of pressure damage, including the changes that occur at the cellular level and the cone-shaped pressure gradient.
8. Define variables that influence the extent of tissue damage as a consequence of pressure.

A pressure ulcer is a localized injury to the skin and/or underlying tissue, usually over a bony prominence, as a result of pressure or pressure in combination with shear (NPUAP, EPUAP, PPPIA, 2014). Pressure ulcers present a significant health care threat to patients with restricted mobility or chronic disease and to older patients. Because of this threat, more documents about pressure ulcers are being published, such as the *Prevention and Treatment of Pressure Ulcers: Clinical Practice Guideline* (NPUAP, EPUAP, PPPIA, 2014), the Wound, Ostomy and Continence Nurses Society's™ (WOCN®) *Guideline for Prevention and Management of Pressure Ulcers* (WOCN®, 2010), *the Association for the Advancement of Wound Care's (AAWC) Venous and Pressure Ulcer Guidelines* (Bolton et al., 2014), the American College of Physicians' *Risk Assessment and Prevention of Pressure Ulcers: A Clinical Practice Guideline from the American College of Physicians* (Qaseem, Mir et al, 2015) and *Treatment of Pressure Ulcers: A Clinical Practice Guideline from the American College of Physicians* (Qaseem, Humphrey et al, 2015), the Registered Nurses Association of Ontario's (RNAO) *Risk Assessment and Prevention of Pressure Ulcers* (RNAO, 2011), *Guidelines for the Prevention of Pressure Ulcers* by the Wound Healing Society (Stechmiller et al, 2008), the Canadian Association of Wound Care's *Best Practice Recommendations for the Prevention and Treatment of Pressure Ulcers: Update 2006* (Keast et al, 2006), *Healthy People 2020* (U.S. Department of Health and Human Services, 2010), and *Pan Pacific Clinical Practice Guideline for the Prevention and Management of Pressure Injury* (Australian Wound Management Association, 2012). For the Institute for Healthcare Improvement, pressure ulcers remain a serious threat to patient safety and is a key focus of their efforts (Institute for Healthcare Improvement, 2015).

SCOPE OF THE PROBLEM

The scope of the pressure ulcer problem in the United States is examined in terms of the patient's age, diagnosis, and setting. Statistics about pressure ulcers vary because of how data were collected, variations in terminology about prevalence and incidence, concerns about litigation, and political and social events that changed American health care. The concepts of prevalence and incidence and the methods for calculation are discussed in Chapter 1.

Prevalence

Pressure ulcer *prevalence* is the proportion or percentage of patients in a defined population with at least one pressure ulcer at a given point in time (Berlowitz, 2012). In the United States across 15 studies, prevalence rates for acute care range from 0% to 15.8% (Goldberg, 2012). The prevalence of pressure ulcers in long-term care across 20 studies done in the United States has been reported as 8.2% to 32.2% (Pieper, 2012). The prevalence of pressure ulcers in home care ranges from 2.9% to 19.1% (Garcia, 2012). Pressure ulcer prevalence in pediatric populations ranges from 0.47% to 75%, with the highest occurrences in the spinal cord injured and outpatients with diagnoses of myelodysplasia and cerebral palsy; 44% of pressure ulcers were secondary to medical devices such as casts and orthoses (Baharestani, 2012). The discrepancies in prevalence can be attributed to the fact that some studies include intact pressure-damaged skin (suspected deep tissue injury or Stage I), whereas other studies exclude such lesions. Prevalence is lower when intact pressure-damaged skin is excluded from the sample. Pressure ulcers in dark-skinned persons may also be difficult to detect (Sieggreen, 2012a). Some skin conditions, such as candidiasis, incontinence-associated dermatitis, and herpetic lesions, may be misclassified as pressure ulcers. In infants and children, the diagnosis of a pressure ulcer is carefully considered because the most common types of skin breakdown in this group include diaper dermatitis, skin tears, and intravenous extravasation. Data collectors must accurately distinguish between pressure ulcers and other causes of erythema and skin ulcerations.

Incidence

Incidence is the number of patients in a defined population who initially were ulcer free but develop a pressure ulcer within a particular time period (Berlowitz, 2012). Incidence measures new conditions (e.g., pressure ulcers) and therefore is considered more reflective of the quality of care within that setting. It is a measure used to evaluate the effects of preventive and therapeutic interventions. Determining the incidence of pressure ulcers is inherently difficult because such studies require longitudinal observations. As with prevalence, incidence will vary by clinical setting. The incidence of pressure ulcers in acute care ranges from 2.8% to 9% (Goldberg, 2012). The incidence in long-term care ranges from 3.6% to 59% (Pieper, 2012) and in home care from 4.5% to 6.3% (Garcia, 2012).

Considerable methodological issues surround the calculation of incidence. For example, defining who is at risk (the number used in the denominator of the incidence formula) can have a significant influence on the resulting value, which actually may overestimate or underestimate the true frequency of the condition. Consequently, variation in reports of incidence may reflect a real difference in the frequency of the condition or simply different data collection techniques, definitions, and methods. Although differences in methodology make comparisons difficult, incidence remains an important measure. Consistency in data collection technique within the health care setting is essential to generate data that can be compared over time. National standards for the definition of terms and the process for conducting prevalence and incidence studies will also increase the comparability of these kinds of data. The National Database of Nursing Quality Indicators (NDNQI) includes pressure ulcer prevention and hospital-acquired pressure ulcer reports from more than 1705 facilities in the United States plus 12 hospitals outside the United States designed for comparisons between hospitals of similar sizes and practice levels (Bergquist-Beringer et al, 2012). Utilizing this large database, the NDNQI reported the 2010 prevalence of pressure ulcers in acute care was 9.1% and the incidence of hospital-acquired pressure ulcers as 3.7% (Bergquist-Beringer et al, 2012).

Economic Effects

In fiscal year 2007, a preventable pressure ulcer was listed as a secondary diagnosis for 300,000 Medicare patients; each pressure ulcer added $43,180 in costs to a hospital stay (AHRQ, 2011; Department of Health and Human Services, Centers for Medicare and Medicaid Services, 2008). In 2008 the Centers for Medicare and Medicaid Services (CMS) ceased payment for hospital complications considered reasonably preventable, including Stage III or IV pressure ulcers (see Chapter 8). The CMS, along with the Centers for Disease Control and Prevention (CDC), released new codes for pressure ulcers capturing wound severity (Krapfl, 2008).

Research on the costs incurred while a pressure ulcer is being managed must be viewed cautiously; the studies are not all comparable. Some studies account for all costs: room, nursing care, supplies, medications, physician fees, and so forth. Other studies examine only direct costs, such as the supplies or medications specifically indicated for that particular problem.

Facility-associated pressure ulcers add to the patient's length of stay, delay the patient's recuperation, and increase the patient's risk for developing complications. In addition, pressure ulcers often necessitate hospitalization (in certain patient populations such as the elderly and patients with a spinal cord injury) because of sepsis or the need for debridement or surgical repair. At a time of increasingly scarce health care dollars, pressure ulcers consume intense resources in the form of dressing changes, nursing care, physical therapy, medications, nutritional support, and clinician services.

The literature reports a range of costs for pressure ulcer management. Approximately, 2.5 million patients are treated each year in U.S. acute care facilities for pressure ulcers, and the cost of treating pressure ulcers is estimated at $9.1 to $11.6 billion annually (AHRQ, 2011). Pressure ulcers lead to loss of function, infection, and extended hospital stays, all of which can increase cost. Hospital length of stay for a principal pressure ulcer diagnosis was 14.1 days compared with 12.7 days for a secondary pressure ulcer diagnosis. Theisen et al (2012) reported that in Germany, older adults with pressure ulcers had longer hospital stays (mean 19 vs. 9.9 days). According to the Healthcare Cost and Utilization Project, the average cost per hospital day for a principal pressure ulcer diagnosis was $1200 compared with $1600 for a secondary pressure ulcer diagnosis (Russo et al, 2008). Nearly three of four hospitalizations with a pressure ulcer diagnosis were billed to Medicare; Medicaid patients accounted for an additional 12.5% of hospitalizations with a principal pressure ulcer.

More than half of patients with pressure ulcer stays were discharged to long-term care, which is more than three times the rate of hospitalizations for all other causes (Russo et al, 2008).

Impact on Quality and Duration of Life

Pressure ulcers may affect psychosocial needs and quality of life in terms of occurrence, recurrence, ulcer characteristics, and ulcer demands. Pressure ulcers may cause social isolation and add burden and frustration for the patient, the family, and care providers. Aspects of quality of life include change in body image, pain, odor and drainage, and financial impact. Quality-of-life research studies about persons with pressure ulcers tend to have small sample sizes, so additional research is needed. Important factors to assess are the patient's social networks; the patient's living space and environment; and the patient's mental status, learning needs, and personal goals. Pain is an ever-present problem with pressure ulcers and must be assessed (Bolton et al., 2014; NPUAP, EPUAP, PPPIA, 2014; Pieper et al, 2009). Pain assessment and management are discussed in detail in Chapters 25 and 26.

Pressure ulcers have been examined in terms of their effects on mortality rates. In 2006 hospital mortality among persons with a secondary diagnosis of a pressure ulcer was 11.6% and was 4.2% among those with a pressure ulcer as a principal diagnosis (Russo et al, 2008). Approximately 60,000 patients die each year from pressure ulcer complications (AHRQ, 2011). Pressure ulcers were reported as a cause of death among 114,380 persons (1990–2001), and the age-adjusted mortality rate was 3.79 per 100,000 population. Pressure ulcers deaths occurred mostly in persons at least 75 years old, and septicemia was reported in 39.7%. Mortality rates were higher in African Americans than in persons of other racial/ethnic groups (Redelings et al, 2005). In a home care project in Italy, residents with a pressure ulcer had a relative risk of dying of 1.92 after adjusting for age, gender, and all significant variables between the two groups of patients (Landi et al, 2007). Flattau and Blank (2014) reported that risk factors for 90-day and 180-day mortality in hospitalized patients with pressure ulcers were diabetes, chronic renal failure, congestive heart failure, metastatic cancer, and low serum albumin.

VULNERABLE PATIENT POPULATIONS

A variety of specific patient populations have been discussed in the literature as being at increased risk for pressure ulcer formation: older adults, persons with a spinal cord injury, surgical patients, obese patients, underweight patients, children, and patients at the end of life. These particular patient populations are introduced here and discussed in greater detail throughout the text.

Historically, older adults admitted to acute and long-term care facilities have been a vulnerable population. Nearly three of four (72%) older adult patients hospitalized with a secondary pressure ulcer diagnosis and 56.5% of adults with a principal diagnosis of a pressure ulcer were 65 years of age or older (Russo et al, 2008). Among persons admitted to long-term care, 10.3% to 18.4% had one or more pressure ulcers on admission

(Baumgarten et al, 2003; Siem et al, 2003). The presence of an existing pressure ulcer at the time of admission to acute care was 26.2% among persons admitted from a nursing home and 4.8% among those admitted from another living situation (Keelaghan et al, 2008; Pieper, 2012). For older adults with a pressure ulcer, coexisting conditions were fluid and electrolyte disorders, nutritional disorders, diabetes mellitus without complications, and dementia (Bolton et al, 2014; Russo et al, 2008).

Pressure ulcer prevalence for persons with spinal cord injuries ranges from 5.8% to 23.3% (Brienza and Karg, 2012). Paralysis and spinal cord injury were common coexisting conditions among younger adults hospitalized principally for pressure ulcers (Russo et al, 2008). Those with the greatest level of disability and mobility impairment have the highest pressure ulcer risk. Reported factors associated with increased incidence and prevalence of pressure ulcers in the spinal cord injured are history of pressure ulcers, coexisting medical conditions (such as diabetes mellitus and depression), rehospitalizations, nursing home stays, less than high school education, older adult, male, African American, single, behavior factors such as smoking, and time since injury (Brienza and Karg, 2012; Schubart et al, 2008).

The incidence of pressure ulcers in the perioperative period ranges from 5% to 53.4% (Ganos and Siddiqui, 2012). Associated factors were at least one comorbidity (i.e., diabetes mellitus, congestive heart failure, decreased preoperative albumin, acute renal insufficiency, recent significant weight loss), managed with a warming device, receipt of three or more anesthetic agents, and median operative time of 4.48 hours (Aronovitch, 2007; Ganos and Siddiqui, 2012). Perioperative pressure ulcer definition includes appearance of the injury up to 72 hours post operating room (Ganos and Siddiqui, 2012). Thus tissue damage may become apparent within hours or may be delayed for up to 3 days. Initial manifestations may be skin discoloration (e.g., bruising) that evolves into blister formation or necrosis. Because this process transpires over several days (i.e., 2 to 6 days), isolating the time of the original injury is complicated (Price et al, 2005). Because the length of surgery and other variables for the surgical patient cannot be changed, the surgical team must aim to decrease pressure and shear not only during the procedure, but also when transferring the patient into position before and after the procedure.

Both the obese and the underweight patient populations are vulnerable to pressure ulcer development. The morbidly obese are at risk for pressure ulcers due to their inability to turn themselves, underlying diseases, improper equipment, lack of adequate pressure redistribution, and inadequate staff numbers or staff not trained in how to turn and move such patients (Blackett et al, 2011; Knudsen and Gallagher, 2003; Mathison, 2003). Risk factors include increased perspiration and moisture (including incontinence) and not fitting well in chairs or beds, so there is pressure against equipment (Sieggreen, 2012b). In a study of elderly patients admitted to acute care, the odds of developing a pressure ulcer in patients who were obese and those who were severely obese were very low (odds ratio 0.7 and 0.1, respectively). In comparison, the odds of the underweight patient developing a pressure ulcer were almost doubled (odds ratio 1.8) (Compher et al, 2007). In contrast, Drake et al (2010) reported those with a body mass index of more than 40 and Braden scale score of 16 or less had an independent and statistically significant association with pressure ulcer occurrence.

Two additional vulnerable patient populations are children and patients at the end of life. Pressure ulcer prevalence, incidence, and risk factors for these two patient populations are presented in Chapters 36 and 37, respectively.

TERMINOLOGY

Over the years, several terms have been used to describe pressure ulcers: bedsore, decubitus ulcer, decubiti, and pressure sore. *Pressure ulcer* is the accepted term because it is more accurate and descriptive. The origin of the term *bedsore* is not known, but it predates the term *decubitus. Decubitus*, a Latin word referring to the reclining position (Fox and Bradley, 1803), dates from 1747 when the French used it to mean bedsore. However, this term is inaccurate because it does not convey the tissue destruction associated with these lesions and because these lesions can result from positions other than the lying position (such as sitting) (Arnold, 1983).

A *pressure ulcer* is defined as localized injury to the skin and/or underlying tissue, usually over a bony prominence, as a result of pressure, including pressure in combination with shear (NPUAP, EPUAP, PPPIA, 2014). A number of contributing or confounding factors are associated with pressure ulcers, but the significance of these factors has not yet been elucidated (NPUAP, EPUAP, PPPIA, 2014).

Pressure ulcers occur most commonly over a bony prominence, such as the sacrum, ischial tuberosity, trochanter, and calcaneus; however, they may develop anywhere on the body (e.g., medical device related, such as underneath a cast, splint, or cervical collar). Figure 7-1 shows the common sites for pressure ulcers and frequency of ulceration per site. The majority of pressure ulcers occur in the pelvis, but other more common locations are the sacrum/coccyx, buttocks, and the heels (Van Gilder et al, 2009).

Bony locations are most prone to pressure ulcer formation because a person's body weight is concentrated on these areas when resting on an unyielding surface. Those who have atrophy of the subcutaneous and muscle tissue layers are at even greater risk for the "mechanical load" of pressure and thus increased soft tissue and capillary compression. The coccyx, sacrum, and heel are particularly vulnerable because less soft tissue is present between the bone and skin.

CAUSATIVE FACTORS

Pressure is the major causative factor in pressure ulcer formation. However, several factors play a role in determining whether pressure is sufficient to create tissue ischemia proceeding to tissue death. The pathologic effect of excessive pressure on soft tissue can be attributed to (1) intensity of pressure, (2) duration of pressure, and (3) tissue tolerance (ability of skin and its supporting structures to endure pressure without adverse sequelae). Braden and Bergstrom (1987)

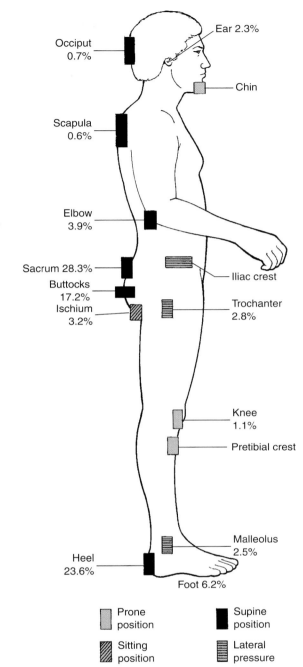

FIGURE 7-1 Sites for pressure ulcers and frequency of ulceration per site (N 5 85,838). Note: Sites for device-related pressure ulcers, which may not involve bony prominences, are not included. (Data from Van Gilder C et al: Results of the 2008–2009 International Pressure Ulcer Prevalence Survey and a 3-year, acute care, unit-specific analysis, *Ostomy Wound Manage* 55(11):39–45, 2009.)

presented a model of the factors that contribute to the intensity and duration of pressure ulcers (Figure 7-2), in combination with intrinsic and extrinsic factors that affect tissue tolerance. Defloor introduced a pressure ulcer conceptual scheme in 1999 arguing that only pressure (compressive force) and shear (shearing force) are known causative factors;

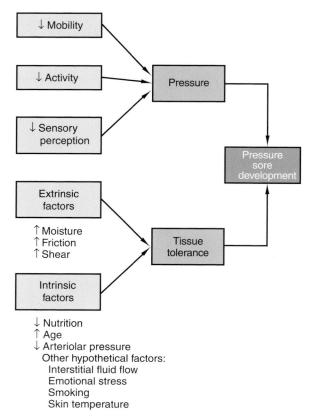

FIGURE 7-2 Factors contributing to the development of pressure ulcers. (From Braden B, Bergstrom N: A conceptual schema for the study of the etiology of pressure sores, *Rehabil Nurs* 12(1):8–12, 1987.)

therefore tissue tolerance is a modifying factor rather than a causative factor as depicted in the Braden and Bergstrom conceptual framework. Intensity and duration affect both compressive force and shearing force. Factors that affect intensity of compressive force include support, posture, body build, and medical/nursing interventions, whereas factors affecting duration of compressive force include pain reaction, pain sensitivity, mobility/activity, and medical/nursing interventions. Intensity of shearing force is determined by support, posture, maceration, and friction, whereas duration of shearing force is determined by pain reaction, pain sensitivity, mobility/activity, and medical/nursing interventions. The Defloor model also recognizes that different factors affect tissue tolerance for pressure and tissue tolerance for oxygen. Although preventive measures can be directed at pressure, shearing force, or tissue tolerance, pressure ulcer onset can only be eliminated by addressing the compressive force and the shearing force. The model consolidates known risk factors.

Intensity of Pressure

To understand the importance of intensity of pressure, it is important to review the terms *capillary pressure* and *capillary closing pressure*. *Capillary pressure* tends to move fluid outward through the capillary membrane. Exact capillary pressure is not known because of the difficulty of obtaining the measurement. Various methods have been used to estimate capillary pressure. A normal hydrostatic pressure is approximately 32 mm Hg at the arterial end of a capillary bed and 12 mm Hg at the venous end (Figure 7-3) (Kumar et al, 2005a). The mean colloidal osmotic pressure in tissue is approximately 25 mm Hg.

The term *capillary closing pressure,* or *critical closing pressure,* describes the minimal amount of pressure required to collapse a capillary (Burton and Yamada, 1951). Tissue anoxia develops when externally applied pressure causes vessels to collapse. It is believed that the amount of pressure required to collapse capillaries must exceed capillary pressure, which is considered to be 12 to 32 mm Hg, the numerical "standard" for capillary closing pressure.

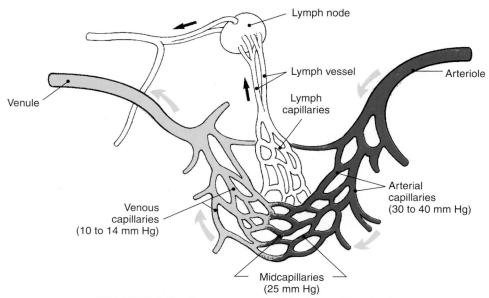

FIGURE 7-3 Capillary pressure within the capillary bed.

To quantify the intensity of pressure being applied externally to the skin, interface pressures are measured. Numerous studies measuring interface pressures have been conducted (Kosiak, 1961; Kosiak et al, 1958; Lindan, 1961). These studies showed that interface pressures attained while a person is in the sitting or supine position commonly exceed capillary pressures (Bennett et al, 1984). In 1961 Lindan used an experimental "bed" to calculate the pressure distribution over the skin of a healthy adult male in the supine, prone, side-lying, and sitting positions. Interface pressures ranged from 10 to 100 mm Hg. Interface readings as high as 300 mm Hg have been obtained over the ischial tuberosity of healthy, able-bodied male subjects when sitting in an unpadded chair (Kosiak, 1961).

Because head-of-bed elevation is important for mechanically ventilated patients in critical care and head-of-bed elevation greater than 30 degrees exposes the patient to increased shear injury and unrelieved pressure, Peterson et al (2008) examined sacral interface pressures at elevations of 0, 10, 20, 30, 45, 60, and 75 degrees in 15 healthy subjects. The elevations 30 degrees or greater had peak interface pressures significantly higher than supine. In addition, elevations 45 degrees or higher had bed interface pressures greater than 32 mm Hg.

Interface pressures in excess of capillary pressure will not routinely result in ischemia. Healthy people with normal sensation regularly shift their weight in response to the discomfort associated with capillary closure and tissue hypoxia. Unfortunately, pathologic processes such as spinal cord injury or sedation impair a person's ability to recognize or respond to this discomfort. Tissue hypoxia can then develop and progress to tissue anoxia and cellular death. Olesen et al (2010) reviewed literature on etiology of sitting-acquired deep tissue pressure ulcers. They reported (1) high interface pressure and shear forces are risk factors for wheelchair users; (2) interface pressure leads to strain and stress concentrations in the interface between bone and muscle under the buttocks; (3) ischemia experiments show pressure impinges arteries, which does not quickly lead to necrosis, but impingement of the veins does; and (4) deformation rather than hypoxia kills the cells. Gefen (2010) described a biomechanical investigation of heel pressure ulcers using a model that characterized the internal mechanical loading at the soft tissues of a supported heel. He reported a heavy-weighted foot, sharp posterior calcaneus and thin soft tissue padding, and diabetes and edema imposed risks for heel ulcers.

Duration of Pressure

Duration of pressure is an important factor that influences the detrimental effects of pressure and must be considered in tandem with intensity of pressure. An inverse relationship exists between duration and intensity of pressure in creating tissue ischemia. Specifically, low-intensity pressures over a long period can create tissue damage just as high-intensity pressure can over a short period

FIGURE 7-4 Graph demonstrating relationship between intensity and duration of pressure. (From Kosiak M: Etiology of decubitus ulcers, *Arch Phys Med Rehabil* 42:19–29, 1961.)

(Figure 7-4). Husain (1953) underscored the significance of the relationship between duration and intensity of pressure. Husain found that a pressure of 100 mm Hg applied to rat muscle for 2 hours was sufficient to produce only microscopic changes in the muscle. However, the same pressure applied for 6 hours was sufficient to produce complete muscle degeneration. The duration of time that tissues can resist periods of ischemia differs for muscle, fat, and skin; muscle tissues appear to be more susceptible to damage than skin tissue (NPUAP, EPUAP, PPPIA, 2014). Sprigle and Sonenblum (2011) noted both magnitude and duration of load must be considered; the use of different size and shape indenters, different loading parameters, and different animal models explains why a range of magnitudes and duration is linked to pressure ulcers.

Tissue Tolerance

Tissue tolerance is the third factor that determines the pathologic effect of prolonged pressure. It describes the condition or integrity of the skin and supporting structures that influence the skin's ability to redistribute the applied pressure. Compression of tissue against skeletal structures and the resulting tissue ischemia can be prevented by effective redistribution of pressure.

The concept of tissue tolerance was first discussed with the need to identify how much pressure skin could "tolerate." Later, Husain (1953) introduced the concept of sensitizing the tissue to pressure and consequently to ischemia. Rat muscle was sensitized with a pressure of 100 mm Hg applied for 2 hours. Seventy-two hours later, a mere 50 mm Hg pressure applied to the same tissue caused muscle degeneration in only 1 hour. This muscle destruction resulted during the second application of pressure, even though the intensity and duration of pressure were lower than the initial intensity and duration. This finding has significant implications for the patient population at risk for pressure ulcers. It indicates that episodes of deep tissue ischemia can occur without cutaneous manifestations and that such episodes can sensitize the patient's skin. In vitro findings show that relatively small loads cause structural changes to the dermal component of tissue. Human tissue exhibits changes visible at the surface that often are minor compared with damage seen in deeper tissue layers (Edsberg, 2007). Small increments of pressure, even if only slightly above normal capillary pressure ranges, may then result in breakdown.

Tissue tolerance is influenced by the ability of the skin and underlying structures (e.g., blood vessels, interstitial fluid, collagen) to work together as a set of parallel springs that transmit load from the surface of the tissue to the skeleton inside (Krouskop, 1983). Several intrinsic and extrinsic factors can alter the ability of the soft tissue to perform this task.

Extrinsic Factors that Affect Tissue Tolerance.

Shear. Shear is caused by the interplay of gravity and friction. It exerts a force parallel to the skin and is the result of both gravity pushing down on the body and resistance (friction) between the patient and a surface, such as the bed or chair. For example, when the head of the bed is elevated, the effect of gravity on the body is to pull the body down toward the foot of the bed. In contrast, the resistance generated by the bed surface tends to hold the body in place. However, what is actually held in place is the skin, while the weight of the skeleton continues to pull the body downward.

Because the skin does not move freely, the primary effect of shear occurs at the deeper fascial level of the tissues overlying the bony prominence. Blood vessels, which are anchored at the point of exit through the fascia, are stretched and angulated when exposed to shear. This force also dissects the tissues, resulting in undermining. High shear forces at the interface between the body and the supporting surface may exacerbate the damage caused by normal stresses alone (NPUAP, EPUAP, PPPIA, 2014).

Shear causes much of the damage often observed with pressure ulcers. In fact, some lesions that may result solely from shear are misinterpreted as pressure ulcers. Conversely, pressure ulcers may also be misinterpreted. Vascular occlusion is enhanced if shear and pressure occur together. For example, when the head of the bed is elevated more than 30 degrees, shear force occurs in the sacrococcygeal region. The sliding of the body transmits pressure to the sacrum and the deep fascia; the outer skin is fixed because of friction with the bed. The vessels in the deep superficial fascia angulate, leading to thrombosis and undermining of the dermis (see Figure 5-1). Dressings with a low-friction external surface have been reported to reduce shear force but do not significantly reduce interface pressures (Nakagami et al, 2006).

Friction. The National Pressure Ulcer Advisory Panel (NPUAP) deleted the word *friction* from the definition of a pressure ulcer (NPUAP, EPUAP, PPPIA, 2014) to reinforce that skin injuries caused by friction were not to be considered pressure ulcers (Antokal et al, 2012). Friction can cause minor to substantial skin impairment, and these lesions can occur in the same location as pressure ulcers. Friction is not a direct cause of a pressure ulcer, but is a risk factor that may contribute to or exacerbate pressure ulcer development due to the shear it creates (Antokal et al, 2012).

Alone, friction's ability to cause skin damage is confined to the epidermal and upper dermal layers and disturbs the barrier function of the stratum corneum (NPUAP, EPUAP, PPPIA, 2014). In its mildest form, friction abrades the epidermis and dermis similar to a mild burn, and sometimes is referred to as "sheet burn." This type of damage most frequently develops in patients who are restless. To prevent friction when moving up in bed, a patient who can lift independently should do so with a lift device or with use of the hands and arms. A patient who is dependent in care may need multiple caregivers to assist with moving up in bed while using a lift sheet or lift device to prevent the body from dragging.

When friction acts with gravity, the effect of the two factors is synergistic, and the outcome is shear. It is not possible to have shear without friction. However, it is possible to have friction without significant shear (such as from moving the heels repeatedly against the bed sheets).

Moisture. Moisture, specifically from incontinence, is frequently cited in the literature as a predisposing factor to pressure ulcer development. Persistent moisture alters the resiliency of the epidermis to external forces by weakening the lipid layer of the stratum corneum and collagen. Both shear and friction are increased in the presence of mild to moderate moisture, but may be decreased in the presence of profuse moisture. The high-moisture environment created by urinary incontinence can affect the skin by alkalinizing the skin's pH, thereby altering normal skin flora. Persons with fecal incontinence are more likely to develop pressure ulcers than are persons without this condition (Bergquist-Beringer and Gajewski, 2011). Clinicians need to be able to differentiate among lesions caused by moisture, moisture and friction, and pressure and shear (Doughty et al, 2012; Gray et al, 2011; Gray et al, 2012). The negative impact of prolonged moisture on the skin is discussed in greater detail in Chapter 5.

Intrinsic Factors that Affect Tissue Tolerance.

Nutritional debilitation. Although good nutrition is necessary for wound healing, the role of significant nutritional debilitation in producing pressure ulcers is often less appreciated. Poor nutritional intake and poor nutritional status correlate with the development of pressure ulcers and should be assessed (Bolton et al, 2014; Dorner et al, 2009; NPUAP, EPUAP, PPPIA, 2014). Banks et al (2009) reported malnutrition was associated with at least twice the odds ratio of having a pressure ulcer in a public health care facility. Severe protein deficiency renders soft tissue more susceptible to breakdown when exposed to local pressure because hypoproteinemia alters oncotic pressure and causes edema formation.

Oxygen diffusion and transport of nutrients in ischemic and edematous tissue are compromised. In addition, resistance to infection is decreased at low protein levels because of the effect on the immune system. Malnutrition has also been associated with altered tissue regeneration and inflammatory reaction, increased postoperative complications, increased risk of infection, sepsis, increased length of hospital stay, and death.

Certain vitamin deficiencies, particularly of vitamins A, C, and E, are a concern when assessing pressure ulcer risk. Vitamin A has a role in epithelial integrity, protein synthesis, and immune function; therefore a deficiency of vitamin A delays reepithelialization, collagen synthesis, and cellular cohesion. Vitamin C plays a role in collagen synthesis, enhanced activation of leukocytes and macrophages at a wound site, and immune function. Specific to wound healing, vitamin E aids in collagen synthesis, metabolism of fat, and stabilization of cell membranes (Posthauer, 2006). Vitamin D deficiency was not found to be an independent risk factor for pressure ulcers, but may be a marker of comorbid illnesses, which increase the risk of pressure ulcers (Kalava et al, 2011).

All nutrients have an important role in maintaining skin integrity. Cowan et al (2012) found that malnutrition, along with three other medical factors, had stronger predictive value for predicting pressure ulcers in acutely ill veterans than Braden scale total scores alone. Still, questions remain regarding how much supplementation of nutrients will positively affect outcomes. Metaanalyses of the clinical benefits of nutritional support in patients with or at risk for pressure ulcers showed an oral nutritional supplement was associated with a significantly lower incidence of pressure ulcer development in at-risk patients of 25% compared with routine care (Stratton et al, 2005). A Cochrane evaluation of enteral and parenteral nutrition on pressure ulcer prevention and treatment was not able to draw conclusions about the effect of such nutrition because of the small number of studies and methodological issues with the studies (Langer et al, 2003). However, they reported that nutritional interventions may be able to reduce the number of people who develop pressure ulcers. Researchers conclude that more research is needed about the impact of oral nutritional supplements and enteral tube feeding on prevention and treatment of pressure ulcers (Qaseem et al, 2015).

Advanced age. Several changes occur in the skin and its supporting structures with aging. The dermoepidermal junction flattens, less nutrient exchange occurs, and less resistance to shear force is present (Pittman, 2007; Reddy, 2008). With aging, gradual atrophy and greater heterogeneity of blood and lymph vessels of human skin occur (Fore, 2006; Reddy, 2008). Changes in the cutaneous nerves lead to impaired early pain warning (Fore, 2006). Skin tears occur more commonly. Loss of dermal thickness occurs; the skin appears paper thin and nearly transparent. Aging skin experiences decreased epidermal turnover, decreased surface barrier

function, decreased sensory perception, decreased delayed and immediate hypersensitivity reaction, increased vascular fragility, loss of subcutaneous fat, and clustering of melanocytes (Fore, 2006; Pittman, 2007). With these changes, the ability of the soft tissue to distribute the mechanical load without compromising blood flow is impaired. Compared with young skin, aged skin showed subepidermal separations and altered orientation of collagen fibers at an earlier time point (Stojadinovic et al, 2013). Researchers concluded that aging contributes to rapid morphologic changes and a decline in the innate inflammatory response in elderly skin, possibly contributing to pressure ulcer pathogenesis. Sopher and Gefen (2011) reported theoretically that wetness, skin aging, and/or skin wrinkling are risk factors for superficial pressure ulcers.

These changes combine with many other age-related changes that occur in other body systems to make the skin more vulnerable to pressure, shear, and friction (Pittman, 2007). For example, Wong (2011) reported for older adults who needed help turning and repositioning that repositioning from a supine to lateral position did not cause the transcutaneous oxygen to return to preload levels. She concluded the efficacy of 2-hour repositioning needs further investigation. Seating and repositioning can affect pressure even when participants are young. For example, pressure relief maneuvers and tilting can result in reductions in interface pressure and increases in buttocks blood flow (Sonenblum and Sprigle, 2011; Sonenblum et al, 2014).

Low blood pressure. Mayrovitz et al (2003) noted in a study about heels that persons with lower blood pressure require lower levels of pressure to the heels to cause breakdown. When interface pressures are near diastolic pressure, little, if any, functional pressure redistribution is realized. When perfusion is decreased by hypotension, shock, or dehydration, blood flow to the skin is likely to be compromised, thus increasing ischemia; deep tissues may be particularly vulnerable because of their extensive vascular supply (Berlowitz and Brienza, 2007). Hypotension may shunt blood flow away from the skin to more vital organs, thus decreasing the skin's tolerance for pressure by allowing capillaries to close at lower levels of interface pressure. Hypotension was a significant factor in patients with pressure ulcers in intensive care units (Terekechi et al, 2009). Man and Au-Yeung (2013) reported the odds of developing a pressure ulcer in a patient with hypotension in the acute care setting was 6.71 ($p = .001$). That said, vasopressor medications are a first-line treatment modality for hypotension (Cox, 2013). In a literature review, 7 of 10 studies reported significant associations among the broad category of vasopressors as a pressure ulcer risk factor (Cox, 2013). Research is needed to elucidate vasopressors as an independent risk factor for pressure ulcer development.

Stress. Early research identified psychosocial issues, such as emotional stress, as having an association with pressure ulcers. Cortisol may alter the mechanical properties of the skin by disproportionately increasing the rate of collagen degradation over collagen synthesis. Glucocorticoids may trigger structural changes in connective tissue and may affect cellular metabolism by interfering with the diffusion of water, salt, and nutrients between the capillary bed and the cells. Hospitalization in acute or long-term care is stressful. In examining the relationship between stress and wound healing, stress has been negatively associated with healing. Cortisol may be the trigger for lowered tissue tolerance when a person is under stress. Cortisol is the primary glucocorticoid secreted when a person is exposed to a stressor and lacks appropriate coping mechanisms to mediate the stress-related hormonal response. Higher cortisol levels were related to longer time to heal (Ebrecht et al, 2004; Gouin et al, 2008). Many factors affect cortisol: advanced age, immobility, body fat, recent surgery, stroke, and malnutrition.

Smoking. Smoking is associated with tissue hypoxia, nicotine-induced stimulation of the sympathetic nervous system resulting in epinephrine that causes peripheral vasoconstriction and decreased circulation, carbon monoxide shift of the oxygen dissociation curve, and hydrogen cyanide interference with cellular oxygen metabolism (Ahn et al, 2008). Smoking must be considered in patients at risk for pressure ulcers. Using an animal model, Tsutakawa et al (2009) reported the increased risk of pressure ulcers due to cigarette smoking is mediated, in part, by nicotine, which is elicited via an increase of inflammatory mediators in the ischemic reperfusion-treated skin. For veterans with spinal cord injury, those who smoked cigarettes had a slightly higher incidence (incidence rate ratio = 1.16) for one or more pressure ulcers during the previous year (Smith et al, 2008). In contrast, current smoking did not differ between veterans with and without pressure ulcers (Rabadi and Vincent, 2011). Bolton et al (2014) stated smoking and other substance abuse issues that affect the skin should be assessed.

Elevated body temperature. The body experiences a 10% increase in tissue metabolism with each 1° C (33.8° F) rise in skin temperature (Aronovitch, 2007). Elevated body temperatures increase metabolic rates and subsequently increase oxygen consumption rates. Elevated skin temperature exacerbates the effects of ischemia by increasing the need for oxygen (Berlowitz and Brienza, 2007). Findings on elevated body temperature are mixed. Dhandapani et al (2014) reported prolonged fever had no significant association with pressure ulcer development in patients with severe traumatic brain injury. Systemic infection or fever was associated with mortality in 90 days for hospitalized patients with pressure ulcers; it did not show a confounding effect on other variables (Flattau and Blank, 2014).

Rapp et al (2009) examined skin temperature in a small sample of nursing facility residents. Skin temperature was lowest in those who developed pressure ulcers and between low-risk and high-risk residents. They concluded the findings support skin temperature regulation as a component of tissue tolerance to pressure.

Miscellaneous factors. Other conditions, such as those that create sluggish blood flow, anemia, blood dyscrasias, or poor oxygen perfusion, may be significant intrinsic factors jeopardizing tissue tolerance. For example, greater tissue damage has been associated with increased blood viscosity and high hematocrit level. This may explain why dehydration is sometimes mentioned as a contributing factor in pressure ulcer development.

PATHOPHYSIOLOGIC CHANGES

Two primary theories explain the mechanism of pressure ulcer formation and progression (Niezgoda and Mendez-Eastman, 2006). The deep tissue injury theory holds that pressure ulcers begin from the bone and move outward. Deep tissue injury occurs first near the bone, with ischemic injury and tissue destruction continuing in an outward manner. As observed by Hussain in 1953, deep muscle tissue appears to be more susceptible to pressure damage than are skin and fat (Berlowitz and Brienza, 2007). Although it is the less favored model of pressure ulcer development, a top-to-bottom model for pressure ulcer formation proposes that skin destruction occurs at the epidermis and proceeds to deeper tissue (Niezgoda and Mendez-Eastman, 2006).

If pressure is not relieved, ischemic changes occur as a consequence of decreased perfusion; however, the occlusion also triggers a cascade of events that intensifies the extent of tissue ischemia. Hence the tissue damage typically seen with pressure is precipitated by pressure but then worsened by a series of events, such as venous thrombus formation, endothelial cell damage, redistribution of blood supply in ischemic tissue, alteration in lymphatic flow, and alterations in interstitial fluid composition.

Berlowitz and Brienza (2007) listed the four commonly hypothesized pathophysiologic explanations for pressure ulcers: (1) ischemia caused by capillary occlusion; (2) reperfusion injury; (3) impaired lymphatic function that results in accumulation of metabolic waste products, proteins, and enzymes; and (4) prolonged mechanical deformation of tissue cells. Prolonged mechanical deformation of tissue cells refers to unrelieved pressure. The remaining three hypothesized pathophysiologic explanations for pressure ulcers are described here.

Ischemia Caused by Capillary Occlusion

Obstruction of capillary blood flow by externally applied pressure creates tissue ischemia (hypoxia). If the pressure is removed in a short period, blood flow returns and the skin can be seen to flush. This phenomenon, known as *reactive hyperemia,* is a compensatory mechanism whereby blood vessels in the pressure area dilate in an attempt to overcome the ischemic episode. Reactive hyperemia, by definition, is transient and may also be described as blanching erythema. Blanching erythema is an area of erythema that becomes white (blanches) when compressed with a finger. The erythema promptly returns when the compression is removed. The site may be painful for the patient with intact sensation. Blanching erythema is an early indication of pressure and usually will resolve without tissue loss if pressure is reduced or eliminated.

When hyperemia persists, deeper tissue damage should be suspected. Nonblanching erythema is a more serious sign of impaired blood supply and suggests that tissue destruction is imminent or has already occurred; it results from damage to blood vessels and extravasation of blood into the tissues. The color of the skin can be an intense bright red to dark red or purple. Many providers misdiagnose pressure-induced nonblanching erythema as hematoma or ecchymosis. When deep tissue damage is also present, the area is often either indurated or boggy when palpated.

When pressure occludes capillaries, a complex series of events is set into motion. Surrounding tissues become deprived of oxygen, and nutrients and metabolic wastes begin to accumulate in the tissue. Damaged capillaries become more permeable and leak fluid into the interstitial space, causing edema. Because perfusion through edematous tissue is slowed, tissue hypoxia worsens. Cellular death ensues, and more metabolic wastes are released into the surrounding tissue. Tissue inflammation is exacerbated, and more cellular death occurs (Figure 7-5). Considering data from surgical patients, animal models, and in vitro cell culture models, pressure ulcers in subdermal tissue under bony prominences very likely occur approximately between the first hour and 4 to 6 hours after sustained loading (Gefen, 2008).

Muscle damage may occur with pressure ulcers and is more significant than cutaneous damage. Pressure is highest at the point of contact between the soft tissue (e.g., muscle or fascia) and the bony prominence. This cone-shaped pressure gradient indicates that deep pressure ulcers initially form at the bone–soft tissue interface, not the skin surface, and extend outward to the skin (Figure 7-6). Thus deep tissue damage may occur with relatively little initial superficial evidence of damage. The skin damage seen with pressure ulcers is often referred to as the "tip of the iceberg" because a larger area of necrosis and ischemia is assumed to be present at the tissue–bone interface. Muscle and fat tissue loading over a bony prominence is substantially higher during sitting than lying down, so pressure ulcer and deep tissue injury development are likely to occur sooner while sitting versus lying down (Gefen, 2008).

Muscle tissue is the most vascularized tissue layer between bone and skin. It is the tissue with the highest metabolic demand and the lowest tolerance to mechanical compression (Gefen, 2008). In addition, atrophied, scarred, or secondarily infected tissue has an increased susceptibility to pressure because of injured cells (Kumar et al, 2005b). An understanding of the structure of the vascular system allows formation of a rationale for this enhanced muscle damage.

The vascular circulation can be divided into three sections: segmental, perforator, and cutaneous. The segmental system is composed of the main arterial vessels arising from the aorta. The perforator system supplies the muscles, but also serves as an interchange supply to the skin. The cutaneous system consists of arteries, capillary beds, and veins draining at different levels of the skin; it serves to provide

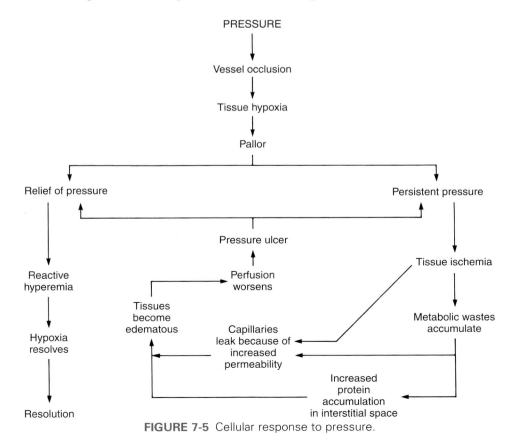

FIGURE 7-5 Cellular response to pressure.

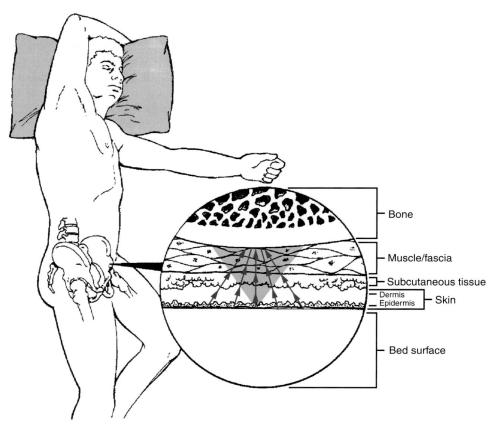

FIGURE 7-6 Amount of pressure exerted at skin level is dispersed over a large area and tapers to a point at the bone level (as indicated by the arrows), whereas the amount of tissue damage at the skin level is a pinpoint and broadens to a larger amount of tissue damage at the bone interface (indicated by the shaded area).

thermoregulation and limited nutritional support. This indicates that occlusion of the perforator system may initiate muscle damage and may also create some of the cutaneous ischemia. The significance of perforator blood flow to skin damage has been demonstrated when musculocutaneous flaps have been elevated surgically.

Reperfusion Injury

As blood returns to tissue where it was occluded, an accumulation of damaged cellular byproducts and white blood cells obstructs the capillaries, and free radicals are released. The free radicals damage cellular proteins, DNA, and cell membranes and contribute to cell death (Fowler et al, 2008). Tissue injury increases with each ischemia–reperfusion cycle, the duration of ischemia, and the frequency of ischemia–reperfusion cycles (Farid, 2007).

Externally applied high pressures, even when applied for a short duration, damage the blood vessels directly, which in turn causes tissue ischemia. The changes in larger vessels and the formation of venous thrombi impair the normal reactive hyperemia that should occur once pressure is removed. Tissue remains ischemic even after the pressure has been alleviated.

Compression of the capillary wall also damages the endothelium. Complex pathologic changes in diverse cellular systems occur with ischemia. Up to a certain point and varying among different cell types, injury is amenable to repair, but with extension of ischemic duration, cell structures continue to deteriorate (Kumar et al, 2005b). Once pressure is removed and reperfusion begins, injury can be paradoxically exacerbated and proceed at an accelerated pace, and loss of additional cells occurs. As the endothelium is shed, platelets are activated by the underlying collagen, and clot formation is triggered. Furthermore, damaged endothelial cells lose their usual anticoagulant characteristics and release thrombogenic substances that exacerbate vessel occlusion and ultimately cause increased tissue ischemia.

The redistribution of the blood supply that occurs in ischemic skin further aggravates pressure-induced tissue hypoxia. Because of the externally applied pressure, blood flow to surface capillaries is reduced, and the reduction renders these vessels more vulnerable and more permeable than before.

Impaired Lymphatic Function

The lymphatic system has a critical role in body fluid and many other functions. It must act as a conduit that directs and regulates lymph flow and as a pump that generates lymph flow (Muthuchamy and Zawieja, 2008). Thus the lymphatics are affected by pressure-induced ischemia. Lymphatic flow in pressure-damaged skin ceases. Likewise, the normal movement of interstitial fluid is inhibited by both pressure and ischemia. Consequently, protein is retained in the interstitial tissues, causing increased interstitial oncotic pressure, edema formation, dehydration of cells, and tissue irritation.

In summary, extensive or extended pressure occludes blood flow, lymphatic flow, and interstitial fluid movement. Tissues are deprived of oxygen and nutrients, and toxic metabolic products accumulate. Interstitial fluids retain proteins that dehydrate cells and irritate tissues. The ensuing tissue acidosis, capillary permeability, and edema contribute to cellular death.

CLASSIFICATION OF PRESSURE ULCERS

History and Purpose

Pressure ulcer staging has a long history (Black and Langemo, 2012). During the 1980s the International Association for Enterostomal Therapy, now known as the WOCN® Society, modified the Shea staging system, which originally was developed in 1975 (WOCN®, 2010). In 2007 the NPUAP released an updated staging system (Box 7-1). The new system improved

clarity and accuracy by adding more descriptors and creating definitions for suspected deep tissue injury and unstageable pressure ulcers (NPUAP, 2012). In 2014 the NPUAP/EPUAP international pressure ulcer classification system was released. The classification uses the same definitions, but added the term *category* (NPUAP, EPUAP, PPPIA, 2014). Some have challenged the current staging system and propose a paradigm that delineates superficial skin changes and deep pressure ulcers (Sibbald et al, 2011).

Staging of tissue layers provides increased uniformity of language and a beginning basis for evaluation of protocols. Accurate staging requires knowledge of the anatomy of skin and deeper tissue layers, the ability to recognize these tissues, and the ability to differentiate among them. Careful evaluation of the wound bed facilitates accurate staging. Staging wounds is a complex skill that can take time to develop. The staging system, which is designed for use with pressure-induced ulcers only, is based on the ability to assess the type of tissue in the wound bed. Therefore a wound bed in which the base is covered with necrotic tissue cannot be accurately staged because of the inability to visualize the normal architecture of the wound bed.

BOX 7-1   International NPUAP/EPUAP Pressure Ulcer Classification System

Pressure Ulcer Stages/Categories

Category/Stage I: Nonblanchable Erythema

Intact skin with nonblanchable redness of a localized area, usually over a bony prominence. Darkly pigmented skin may not have visible blanching; its color may differ from the surrounding area. The area may be painful, firm, soft, warmer, or cooler compared with adjacent tissue. Category I may be difficult to detect in individuals with dark skin tones. May indicate "at risk" persons.

Category/Stage II: Partial Thickness

Partial-thickness loss of dermis presenting as a shallow open ulcer with a red-pink wound bed, without slough. May also present as an intact or open/ruptured serum-filled or serosanguineous-filled blister. Presents as a shiny or dry shallow ulcer without slough or bruising.* This category should not be used to describe skin tears, tape burns, incontinence-associated dermatitis, maceration, or excoriation.

Category/Stage III: Full-Thickness Skin Loss

Full-thickness tissue loss. Subcutaneous fat may be visible, but bone, tendon, or muscle is not exposed. Slough may be present, but does not obscure the depth of tissue loss. May include undermining and tunneling. The depth of a Category/Stage III pressure ulcer varies by anatomic location. The bridge of the nose, ear, occiput, and malleolus do not have (adipose) subcutaneous tissue, and Category/Stage III ulcers can be shallow. In contrast, areas of significant adiposity can develop extremely deep Category/Stage III pressure ulcers. Bone/tendon is not visible or directly palpable.

Category/Stage IV: Full-Thickness Tissue Loss

Full-thickness tissue loss with exposed bone, tendon, or muscle. Slough or eschar may be present. Often includes undermining

and tunneling. The depth of a Category/Stage IV pressure ulcer varies by anatomic location. The bridge of the nose, ear, occiput, and malleolus do not have (adipose) subcutaneous tissue and these ulcers can be shallow. Category/Stage IV ulcers can extend into muscle and/or supporting structures (e.g., fascia, tendon, or joint capsule) making osteomyelitis or osteitis likely to occur. Exposed bone/muscle is visible or directly palpable.

Unstageable/Unclassified: Full-Thickness Skin or Tissue Loss – Depth Unknown

Full-thickness tissue loss in which actual depth of the ulcer is completely obscured by slough (yellow, tan, gray, green, or brown) and/or eschar (tan, brown, or black) in the wound bed. Until enough slough and/or eschar is removed to expose the base of the wound, the true depth cannot be determined, but it will be either a Category/Stage III or IV. Stable (dry, adherent, intact without erythema or fluctuance) eschar on the heels serves as "the body's natural (biological) cover" and should not be removed.

Suspected Deep Tissue Injury – Depth Unknown

Purple or maroon localized area of discolored intact skin or blood-filled blister due to damage of underlying soft tissue from pressure and/or shear. The area may be preceded by tissue that is painful, firm, mushy, boggy, warmer, or cooler compared with adjacent tissue. Deep tissue injury may be difficult to detect in individuals with dark skin tones. Evolution may include a thin blister over a dark wound bed. The wound may further evolve and become covered by thin eschar. Evolution may be rapid, exposing additional layers of tissue even with optimal treatment.

*Bruising indicates deep tissue injury.
National Pressure Ulcer Advisory Panel (NPUAP), European Pressure Ulcer Advisory Panel (EPUAP) and Pan Pacific Pressure Ulcer Injury Alliance (PPPUIA): Prevention and treatment of pressure ulcers: clinical practice guideline. E Haesler, editor: Cambridge Media: Osborne Park, Western Australia, 2014.

In such situations, "unstageable" should be documented. Examples of Stage I to IV pressure ulcers, suspected deep tissue injury, and unstageable pressure ulcers are provided in Plates 27 through 33. Box 7-2 gives the differential diagnoses of suspected deep tissue injury due to pressure (Ankrom et al, 2005).

Darker Skin Tones

Identifying suspected deep tissue injury and Stage I pressure ulcers in darker skin tones is difficult. Redness and other color changes are not as detectable with darker skin tones. Therefore other observable, pressure-related alterations of intact skin compared with the adjacent or opposite area on the body should be documented. Skin inspection should include assessment of changes in skin tissue consistency (firm vs. boggy when palpated), sensation (pain), edema, and warmer or cooler temperature (Bolton et al, 2014; NPUAP, EPUAP, PPPIA, 2014). Box 3-1 lists unique characteristics of darker versus lighter pigmented skin, and Checklist 6-1 gives points to consider when assessing darkly pigmented skin.

Medical Device–Related Pressure Ulcers

Pressure ulcers can develop beneath medical devices. Medical device–related (MDR) pressure ulcers have a reported incidence of 9.1%; as many as 34.5% of hospital-acquired pressure ulcers reported as MDR (Goldberg, 2012). The most common stages are I and II and common sites are ears, heels, and lower legs. Patients with a medical device are 2.4 times more likely to develop a pressure ulcer of any kind (Black et al, 2010). Although numerous risk factors have been identified, they are not unique to MDR pressure ulcers (Black et al, 2010). Medical device–related ulcers also affect children (Baharestani, 2012).

Mucosal Pressure Ulcers

Mucous tissues (i.e., lining of the gastrointestinal tract, oral cavity, nares, etc.) are also vulnerable to pressure ulcers from the presence of medical devices such as oxygen tubing, endotracheal tubes, bite blocks, nasogastric tubes, urinary catheters, and fecal containment devices. These ulcers cannot be staged using the pressure ulcer staging system or classified as partial or full thickness because the histology of mucous membrane tissue is different from skin. Therefore pressure ulcers on mucous membranes should be documented simply as mucosal pressure ulcers (NPUAP, 2009).

Reverse Staging

The practice of reverse staging, in which the wound is described as progressing from a Stage III to a Stage II to a Stage I pressure ulcer, is incorrect. Once layers of tissue and supporting structures are gone (such as with full-thickness wounds), they are not replaced. Instead, the wound is filled with granulation tissue. This staging system is to be used for describing wounds in their most severe state, and once the wounds are accurately described, these descriptor levels endure, even in the presence of healing (Black et al, 2007). Negative outcomes of reverse staging can lead to (1) denial of acute or skilled care after Stage IV ulcers have been restaged as Stage II ulcers; (2) withdrawal of pressure-reducing support surfaces when ulcers have "healed" from Stage III or Stage IV to Stage II; and (3) lower fees paid to extended care facilities for care of patients with healing Stage III and Stage IV ulcers that have been reclassified as Stage II or Stage I pressure ulcers. Therefore a Stage III pressure ulcer that appears to be granulating and resurfacing is described as a healing Stage III pressure ulcer.

> ## BOX 7-2   Differential Diagnoses of Suspected Deep Tissue Injury Due to Pressure
>
> **Bruise**: Extravasation of blood in the tissues as a result of blunt-force impact to the body. Usually about 2 weeks is required for a bruise to heal under normal conditions. History of trauma is common.
>
> **Calciphylaxis**: Vascular calcification and skin necrosis most common in patients with long-standing history of chronic renal failure and renal replacement therapy. Lesions may have a violaceous hue and be excruciatingly tender and extremely firm. Lesions are most commonly seen on the lower extremities, not over bony prominences. The incidence of these lesions is very low in general patient populations.
>
> **Fournier's gangrene**: Intensely painful necrotizing fasciitis of the perineum. May manifest initially as cellulitis.
>
> **Hematoma**: Deep-seated purple nodule from clotted blood; usually associated with trauma.
>
> **Perirectal abscess**: First sign commonly is a dull, aching, or throbbing pain in the perianal area. The pain worsens when sitting and immediately before defecation; the pain abates after defecation. A tender, fluctuant mass may be palpated at the anal verge. These abscesses can open to reveal large cavities, which can be confused with deep pressure ulcers.

> ## CLINICAL CONSULT
>
> **A:** Referral received to evaluate a large purple discolored area over left trochanter. An 87-year-old male admitted to general medicine after falling at home and lying trapped between his toilet and bathtub on the floor for between 24 and 36 hours. Trochanter painful to light palpation. No fractures per radiologic evaluation. Purple discolored area 24 cm × 12 cm, boggy upon palpation.
>
> **D:** Suspected deep tissue injury (sDTI).
>
> **P:** Pressure relief to trochanter; treat dehydration and restore fluid imbalance.
>
> **I:** (1) Initiate low air loss mattress. (2) Reposition every 2 hours in 30 degree side position to offload coccyx and trochanters. (3) Physical therapy to assess balance and safety of ambulation. (4) No topical dressing over trochanger; monitor site twice daily for changes in appearance.
>
> **E:** The definitive pressure ulcer diagnosis will be made over time, with reassessment determining if the purple tissue returns to normal color and remains intact or sloughs to reveal existing tissue damage, Stage III, IV, or unstageable pressure ulcer.

SUMMARY

Pressure ulcers present a significant economic, quality-of-life, and overall health care threat worldwide. Standards for assessment and care initially presented by the WOCN® Society have now been published by a number of dedicated disciplines and groups around the world. Once a problem considered a side effect of aging, pressure ulcers have captured the attention of payers and regulators. Although not all pressure ulcers are avoidable (see Chapter 8), pressure ulcers now are more commonly considered preventable and unacceptable (in most cases) and are considered an indicator of quality care.

REFERENCES

Ahn C, Mulligan P, Salcido RS: Smoking—the bane of wound healing: biomedical interventions and social influences, *Adv Skin Wound Care* 21(5):227–236, 2008.

Agency for Healthcare Research and Quality (AHRQ): *Preventing pressure ulcers in hospitals: a toolkit for improving quality of care*, Rockville, MD, April 2011, AHRQ. http://www.ahrq.gov/professionals/systems/long-term-care/resources/pressure-ulcers/pressureulcertoolkit/putool1.html. Accessed Feb 8, 2014.

Ankrom MA, Bennett RG, Sprigle S, et al: Pressure-related deep tissue injury under intact skin and the current pressure ulcer staging systems, *Adv Skin Wound Care* 18(1):35–42, 2005.

Antokal S, Brienza D, Bryan N, et al: *Friction induced skin injuries – are they pressure ulcers?* (National Pressure Ulcer Advisory Panel white paper), Nov 20, 2012. http://www.npuap.org/wp-content/uploads/2012/01/NPUAP-Friction-White-Paper.pdf. Accessed May 27, 2014.

Arnold HL, Decubitus: the word. In: Parish LC, Witkowski JA, Crissey JT (1983) *The decubitus ulcer*. Masson, New York, pp 1–3

Aronovitch SA: Intraoperatively acquired pressure ulcers: are there common risk factors? *Ostomy Wound Manage* 53(2):57–69, 2007.

Australian Wound Management Association: *Clinical practice guideline for the prevention and management of pressure injury*, Osborne Parke, Western Australia, 2012, Cambridge Media.

Baharestani MM: Pressure ulcers in pediatric populations. In Pieper B, editor (with the National Pressure Ulcer Advisory Panel [NPUAP]): *Pressure ulcers: prevalence, incidence, and implications for the future*, Washington, DC, 2012, NPUAP, pp 151–171.

Banks M, Bauer J, Graves N, et al: Malnutrition and pressure ulcer risk in adults in Australian health care facilities, *Nutrition* 26(9):896–901, 2010.

Baumgarten M, Margolis D, Gruber-Baldini AL, et al: Pressure ulcers and the transition to long-term care, *Adv Skin Wound Care* 16(6):299–304, 2003.

Bennett LM, Kavner D, Lee BY, et al: Skin stress and blood flow in sitting paraplegic patients, *Arch Phys Med Rehabil* 65(4): 186–190, 1984.

Bergquist-Beringer S, Gajewski BJ: Outcome and assessment information set data that predict pressure ulcer development in older adult home health patients, *Adv Skin Wound Care*, 24(9):404–414, 2011.

Bergquist-Beringer S, Gajewski BJ, Davidson J: Pressure ulcer prevalence and incidence: report from the National Database of Nursing Quality Indicators (NDNQI). In Pieper B, editor (with the National Pressure Ulcer Advisory Panel [NPUAP]): *Pressure ulcers: prevalence, incidence, and implications for the future*, Washington, DC, 2012, NPUAP, pp 175–188.

Berlowitz D: Prevalence, incidence, and facility-acquired rates. In Pieper B, editor (with the National Pressure Ulcer Advisory Panel [NPUAP]): *Pressure ulcers: prevalence, incidence, and implications for the future*, Washington, DC, 2012, NPUAP, pp 19–24.

Berlowitz DR, Brienza DM: Are all pressure ulcers the result of deep tissue injury? A review of the literature, *Ostomy Wound Manage* 53(10):34–38, 2007.

Black J, Baharestani MM, Cuddigan J, et al: National Pressure Ulcer Advisory Panel's updated pressure ulcer staging system, *Adv Skin Wound Care* 20(5):269–274, 2007.

Black J, Langemo D: Pressure ulcer staging/categorization. In Pieper B, editor (with the National Pressure Ulcer Advisory Panel [NPUAP]): *Pressure ulcers: prevalence, incidence, and implications for the future*, Washington, DC, 2012, NPUAP, pp 5–14.

Black JM, Cuddigan JE, Walko MA, et al: Medical device related pressure ulcers in hospitalized patients, *Int Wound J* 7(5):358–365, 2010.

Blackett A, Gallagher S, Dugan S, et al: Caring for persons with bariatric health care issues, *J Wound Ostomy Continence Nurs* 38(2):133–138, 2011.

Bolton ll, Girolami S, Corbett L, et al: The Association for the Advancement of Wound Care (AAWC) venous and pressure ulcer guidelines, *Ostomy Wound Manage* 60(11):24-66, 2014.

Braden BJ, Bergstrom N: A conceptual schema for the study of the etiology of pressure sores, *Rehabil Nurs* 12(1):8–12, 1987.

Brienza D, Karg P: Pressure ulcers in persons with spinal cord injury. In Pieper B, editor (with the National Pressure Ulcer Advisory Panel [NPUAP]): *Pressure ulcers: prevalence, incidence, and implications for the future*, Washington, DC, 2012, NPUAP, pp 107–112.

Burton AC, Yamada S: Relation between blood pressure and flow in the human forearm, *J Appl Physiol* 4(5):329–339, 1951.

Compher C, Kinosian BP, Ratcliffe SJ, et al: Obesity reduces the risk of pressure ulcers in elderly hospitalized patients, *J Gerontol A Biol Sci Med Sci* 62(11):1310–1312, 2007.

Cowan LJ, Stechmiller JK, Rowe M, et al: Enhancing Braden pressure ulcer risk assessment in acutely ill adult veterans, *Wound Repair Regen* 20(2):137–148, 2012.

Cox J: Pressure ulcer development and vasopressor agents in adult critical care patients: a literature review, *Ostomy Wound Manage* 59(4):50–54, 56–60, 2013.

Defloor T: The risk of pressure sores: a conceptual scheme, *J Clin Nurs* 8:206–216, 1999.

Department of Health and Human Services, Centers for Medicare and Medicaid Services: Medicare program; changes to the hospital inpatient prospective payment systems and fiscal year 2008 rates; final rule, *Federal Register* 72(162), pp 1–12, 2007 .

Dhandapani M, Dhandapani S, Agarwal M, et al: Pressure ulcer in patients with severe traumatic brain injury: significant factors and association with neurological outcome, *J Clin Nurs* 23(7–8):1114–1119, 2014.

Dorner B, Posthauer ME, Thomas D: The role of nutrition in pressure ulcer prevention and treatment: National Pressure Ulcer

Advisory Panel white paper, *Adv Skin Wound Care* 22(5): 212–221, 2009.

Doughty D, Junkin J, Kurz P, et al: Incontinence-associated dermatitis: consensus statements, evidenced-based guidelines for prevention and treatment, and current challenges, *J Wound Ostomy Continence Nurs* 39(3):303–315, 2012.

Drake DJ, Swanson M, Baker G, et al: The association of BMI and Braden Total Score on the occurrence of pressure ulcers, *J Wound Ostomy Continence Nurs* 37(4):367–371, 2010.

Ebrecht M, Hextall J, Kirtley LG, et al: Perceived stress and cortisol levels predict speed of wound healing in healthy male adults, *Psychoneuroendocrinology* 29(6):798–809, 2004.

Edsberg LE: Pressure ulcer tissue histology: an appraisal of current knowledge, *Ostomy Wound Manage* 53(10):40–49, 2007.

Farid KJ: Applying observations from forensic science to understanding the development of pressure ulcers, *Ostomy Wound Manage* 53(4):26–28, 30, 32 passim, 2007.

Flattau A, Blank AE: Risk factors for 90-day and 180-day mortality in hospitalized patients with pressure ulcers, *Int Wound J* 11(1):14–20, 2014.

Fore J: A review of skin and the effects of aging on skin structure and function, *Ostomy Wound Manage* 52(9):24–35, 2006.

Fowler E, Scott-Williams S, McGuire JB: Practice recommendations for preventing heel pressure ulcers, *Ostomy Wound Manage* 54(10):42–48, 50–52, 54–57, 2008.

Fox J, Bradley R: *A new medical dictionary*, London, 1803, Darton & Harvey.

Ganos D, Siddiqui A: Operating room. In Pieper B, editor (with the National Pressure Ulcer Advisory Panel [NPUAP]): *Pressure ulcers: prevalence, incidence, and implications for the future*, Washington, DC, 2012, NPUAP, pp 57–64.

Garcia AD: Home care. In Pieper B, editor (with the National Pressure Ulcer Advisory Panel [NPUAP]): *Pressure ulcers: prevalence, incidence, and implications for the future*, Washington, DC, 2012, NPUAP, pp 97–104.

Gefen A: Bioengineering models of deep tissue injury, *Adv Skin Wound Care* 21(1):30–36, 2008.

Gefen A: The biomechanics of heel ulcers, *J Tissue Viability* 19(4):124–131, 2010.

Goldberg M: General acute care. In Pieper B, editor (with the National Pressure Ulcer Advisory Panel [NPUAP]): *Pressure ulcers: prevalence, incidence, and implications for the future*, Washington, DC, 2012, NPUAP, pp 27–46.

Gouin JP, Kiecolt-Glaser JK, Malarkey WB, et al: The influence of anger expression on wound healing, *Brain Behav Immun* 22(5):699–708, 2008.

Gray M, Beeckman D, Bliss DZ, et al: Incontinence-associated dermatitis: a comprehensive review and update, *J Wound Ostomy Continence Nurs* 39(1):61–74, 2012.

Gray M, Black JM, Baharestani MM, et al: Moisture-associated skin damage: overview and pathophysiology, *J Wound Ostomy Continence Nurs* 38(3):233–241, 2011.

How-to Guide: *Prevent Pressure Ulcers*, Cambridge, MA, 2011, Institute for Healthcare Improvements. (Available at www.ihi. org).

Husain T: An experimental study of some pressure effects on tissues, with reference to the bedsore problem, *J Pathol Bacteriol* 66(2):347–358, 1953.

Institute for Healthcare Improvement: Pressure ulcers. http://www. ihi.org/Topics/PressureUlcers/Pages/default.aspx. Accessed July 18, 2015.

Kalava UR, Cha SS, Takahashi PY: Association between vitamin D and pressure ulcers in older ambulatory adults: results of a matched case-control study, *Clin Interv Aging* 6:213–219, 2011.

Keast DH, Parslow N, Houghton PE, et al: Best practice recommendations for the prevention and treatment of pressure ulcers: update 2006, *Adv Skin Wound Care* 20(8):337–360, 2007.

Keelaghan E, Margolis D, Zhan M, et al: Prevalence of pressure ulcers on hospital admission among nursing home residents transferred to the hospital, *Wound Repair Regen* 16(3):331–336, 2008.

Knudsen A, Gallagher S: Care of the obese patient with pressure ulcers, *J Wound Ostomy Continence Nurs* 30(2):111–118, 2003.

Kosiak M: Etiology of decubitus ulcers, *Arch Phys Med Rehabil* 42:19–29, 1961.

Kosiak M, Kubicek WG, Olson M, et al: Evaluation of pressure as a factor in the production of ischial ulcers, *Arch Phys Med Rehabil* 39(10):623–629, 1958.

Krapfl LA: Inpatient prospective payment changes: a guide for the WOC nurse, *WOC News* 3:16, 2008.

Krouskop TA: A synthesis of the factors that contribute to pressure sore formation, *Med Hypotheses* 11(2):255–267, 1983.

Kumar V, Fausto N, Abbas A: Acute and chronic inflammation. In *Robbins and Cotran pathologic basis of disease*, ed 7, Philadelphia, 2005a, Saunders.

Kumar V, Fausto N, Abbas A: Cellular adaptations, cell injury, and cell death. In *Robbins and Cotran pathologic basis of disease*, ed 7, Philadelphia, 2005b, Saunders.

Landi F, Onder G, Russo A, et al: Pressure ulcer and mortality in frail elderly people living in community, *Arch Gerontol Geriatr* 44(Suppl 1):217–223, 2007.

Langer G, Schloemer G, Knerr A, et al: Nutritional interventions for preventing and treating pressure ulcers, *Cochrane Database Syst Rev* (4):CD003216, 2003.

Lindan O: Etiology of decubitus ulcers: an experimental study, *Arch Phys Med Rehabil* 42:774–783, 1961.

Man SP, Au-Yeung TW: Hypotension is a risk factor for new pressure ulcer occurrence in older patients after admission to an acute care hospital, *J Am Med Dir Assoc* 14(8):627.e1–5, 2013.

Mathison CJ: Skin and wound care challenges in the hospitalized morbidly obese patient, *J Wound Ostomy Continence Nurs* 30(2):78–83, 2003.

Mayrovitz HN, Sims N, Taylor MC, et al: Effects of support surface relief pressures on heel skin blood perfusion, *Adv Skin Wound Care* 16(3):141–145, 2003.

Muthuchamy M, Zawieja D: Molecular regulation of lymphatic contractility, *Ann N Y Acad Sci* 1131:89–99, 2008.

Nakagami G, Sanada H, Konya C, et al: Comparison of two pressure ulcer preventive dressings for reducing shear force on the heel, *J Wound Ostomy Continence Nurs* 33(3):267–272, 2006.

National Pressure Ulcer Advisory Panel (NPUAP): *Mucosal pressure ulcers: an NPUAP position statement,* 2009. http://www.npuap. org/Mucosal_Pressure_Ulcer_Position_Statement_final.pdf. Accessed May 27, 2014.

National Pressure Ulcer Advisory Panel (NPUAP), European Pressure Ulcer Advisory Panel (EPUAP) and Pan Pacific Pressure Ulcer Injury Alliance (PPPUIA): Prevention and treatment of pressure ulcers: clinical practice guideline. In Haesler E, editor: Cambridge Media:Osborne Park, Western Australia, 2014.

Niezgoda JA, Mendez-Eastman S: The effective management of pressure ulcers, *Adv Skin Wound Care* 19(Suppl 1):3–15, 2006.

Olesen CG, de Zee M, Rasmussen J: Missing links in pressure ulcer research—an interdisciplinary overview, *J Appl Physiol* 108(6):1458–1464, 2010.

Peterson M, Schwab W, McCutcheon K, et al: Effects of elevating the head of bed on interface pressure in volunteers, *Crit Care Med* 36(11):3038–3042, 2008.

Pieper B: Long term care/nursing homes. In Pieper B, editor (with the National Pressure Ulcer Advisory Panel [NPUAP]): *Pressure ulcers: prevalence, incidence, and implications for the future*, Washington, DC, 2012, NPUAP, pp 65–88.

Pieper B, Langemo D, Cuddigan J: Pressure ulcer pain: a systematic literature review and National Pressure Ulcer Advisory Panel white paper, *Ostomy Wound Manage* 55(2):16–31, 2009.

Pittman J: Effect of aging on wound healing, *J Wound Ostomy Continence Nurs* 34(4):412–415, 2007.

Posthauer ME: The role of nutrition in wound care, *Adv Skin Wound Care* 19(1):43–52, 2006.

Price MC, Whitney JD, King CA, et al: Development of a risk assessment tool for intraoperative pressure ulcers, *J Wound Ostomy Continence Nurs* 32(1):19–30, 2005.

Qaseem A, Humphrey LL, Forciea MA, et al: Treatment of pressure ulcers: a clinical practice guideline from the American College of Physicians, *Ann Intern Med* 162:370-379, 2015.

Qaseem A, Mir TP, Starkey M, et al: Risk assessment and prevention of pressure ulcers: a clinical practice guideline from the American College of Physicians, *Ann Intern Med* 162:359–369, 2015.

Rabadi MH, Vincent AS: Do vascular risk factors contribute to the prevalence of pressure ulcer in veterans with spinal cord injury? *J Spinal Cord Med* 34(1):46–51, 2011.

Rapp MP, Bergstrom N, Padhye NS: Contribution of skin temperature regularity to the risk of developing pressure ulcers in nursing facility residents, *Adv Skin Wound Care* 22(11):506–513, 2009.

Reddy M: Skin and wound care: important considerations in the older adult, *Adv Skin Wound Care* 21(9):424–436, 2008.

Redelings MD, Lee NE, Sorvillo F: Pressure ulcers: more lethal than we thought? *Adv Skin Wound Care* 18(7):367–372, 2005.

Registered Nurses Association of Ontario (RNAO): *Risk assessment and prevention of pressure ulcers*, Toronto, ON, 2011, RNAO.

Russo CA, Steiner C, Spector W: *Hospitalizations related to pressure ulcers among adults 18 years and older*, 2006 (HCUP statistical brief no. 64), 2008. http://www.hcup-us.ahrq.gov/reports/statbriefs/sb64.pdf. Accessed Dec 20, 2013.

Schubart JR, Hilgart M, Lyder C: Pressure ulcer prevention and management in spinal cord-injured adults: analysis of educational needs, *Adv Skin Wound Care* 21(7):322–327, 2008.

Sibbald RG, Krasner DL, Woo KY: Pressure ulcer staging revisited: superficial skin changes & deep pressure ulcer framework, *Adv Skin Wound Care* 24(12):571–580, 2011.

Sieggreen M: Pressure ulcers in persons of color: race and ethnicity. In Pieper B, editor (with the National Pressure Ulcer Advisory Panel [NPUAP]): *Pressure ulcers: prevalence, incidence, and implications for the future*, Washington, DC, 2012a, NPUAP, pp 141–146.

Sieggreen M: Pressure ulcers in morbidly obese patients. In Pieper B, editor (with the National Pressure Ulcer Advisory Panel [NPUAP]): *Pressure ulcers: prevalence, incidence, and implications for the future*, Washington, DC, 2012b, NPUAP, pp 147–150.

Siem CA, Wipke-Tevis DD, Rantz MJ, et al: Skin assessment and pressure ulcer care in hospital-based skilled nursing facilities, *Ostomy Wound Manage* 49(6):42–44, 46, 48 passim, 2003.

Smith BM, Guihan M, LaVela SL, et al: Factors predicting pressure ulcers in veterans with spinal cord injuries, *Am J Phys Med Rehabil* 87(9):750–757, 2008.

Sonenblum SE, Sprigle SH: The impact of tilting on blood flow and localized tissue loading, *J Tissue Viability* 20(1):3–13, 2011.

Sonenblum SE, Vonk TE, Janssen TW, et al: Effects of wheelchair cushions and pressure relief maneuvers on ischial interface pressure and blood flow in people with spinal cord injury, *Arch Phys Med Rehabil* 2014;95(7):1350–1357.

Sopher R, Gefen A: Effects of skin wrinkles, age and wetness on mechanical loads in the stratum corneum as related to skin lesions, *Med Biol Eng Comput* 49(1):97–105, 2011.

Sprigle S, Sonenblum S: Assessing evidence supporting redistribution of pressure for pressure ulcer prevention: a review, *J Rehabil Res Dev* 48(3):203–213, 2011.

Stechmiller JK, Cowan L, Whitney JD, et al: Guidelines for the prevention of pressure ulcers, *Wound Repair Regen* 16(2):151–168, 2008.

Stojadinovic O, Minkiewicz J, Sawaya A, et al: Deep tissue injury in development of pressure ulcers: a decrease of inflammasome activation and changes in human skin morphology in response to aging and mechanical load, *PLoS One* 8(8):e69223, 2013.

Stratton RJ, Ek AC, Engfer M, et al: Enteral nutritional support in prevention and treatment of pressure ulcers: a systematic review and meta-analysis, *Ageing Res Rev* 4(3):422–450, 2005.

Terekeci H, Kucukardali Y, Top C, et al: Risk assessment study of the pressure ulcers in intensive care unit patients, *Eur J Intern Med* 20(4):394–397, 2009.

Theisen S, Drabik A, Stock S: Pressure ulcers in older hospitalized patients and its impact on length of stay: a retrospective observational study, *J Clin Nurs* 21(3–4):380–387, 2012.

Tsutakawa S, Kobayashi D, Kusama M, et al: Nicotine enhances skin necrosis and expression of inflammatory mediators in a rat pressure ulcer model, *Br J Dermatol* 161(5):1020–1027, 2009.

U.S. Department of Health and Human Services: *Healthy People, 2010*, Washington, DC, 2000, HHS.

Van Gilder C, Amlung S, Harrison P, et al: Results of the 2008-2009 International Pressure Ulcer Prevalence Survey and a 3-year, acute care, unit-specific analysis, *Ostomy Wound Manage* 55(11):39–45, 2009.

Wong V: Skin blood flow response to 2-hour repositioning in long-term care residents: a pilot study, *J Wound Ostomy Continence Nurs* 38(5):529–537, 2011.

Wound, Ostomy and Continence Nurses Society™ (WOCN®): *Guideline for prevention and management of pressure ulcers*, Glenview, IL, 2010, WOCN®.

8

Developing and Maintaining a Pressure Ulcer Prevention Program

Ruth A. Bryant and Denise P. Nix

OBJECTIVES

1. Explain three justifications for a pressure ulcer prevention program.
2. Distinguish between an avoidable and an unavoidable pressure ulcer.
3. List components of a best-practice bundle of a pressure ulcer prevention program.
4. Distinguish between a pressure ulcer risk assessment and a skin assessment.
5. Identify the risk factor subscales in the Braden scale for predicting pressure sore risk.
6. Distinguish between turning and repositioning.
7. Describe five repositioning techniques.
8. Describe why infrastructure is important to the maintenance of a successful pressure ulcer prevention program.
9. Provide examples of how an organization demonstrates skin safety as an organizational priority.

Every health care facility and health care unit needs a pressure ulcer prevention program (PUPP). When creating a PUPP, both the structure of the program (best-practice bundle) and the operations of the program (infrastructure) must be addressed. From a structural (bundle) perspective, the best-practice bundle of the PUPP has six basic components: skin inspection, risk assessment, pressure redistribution and offloading, maintaining skin health, nutrition and hydration, and patient and family education. For a PUPP to be successful, all caregivers and administration must share the belief that pressure ulcers are a negative outcome and that all health care providers play a role in their prevention. In addition, the bundle must then be integrated into the culture and infrastructure of the health care system. Evidence suggests that the infrastructure components are often the missing link to implementation and maintenance of a PUPP. Common gaps include lack of staff education, absence or insufficient involvement of physicians as well as other caregivers (i.e., nursing assistants), inadequate plan for communicating pressure ulcer risk, and deficient quality-improvement evaluations of bedside practice (Soban et al, 2011; Stechmiller, 2012). In this chapter, we define and discuss the structure of a PUPP and steps for integration into the care delivery system to ensure ongoing viability and growth of the program.

PUPP JUSTIFICATION

There are numerous reasons to justify a PUPP. Certainly economics has heightened the interest of some, but the most important reasons stem from a concern for patient safety and quality care.

Effectiveness

The most compelling argument for implementing a PUPP is that such programs have been shown to be effective in reducing the incidence of nosocomial pressure ulcers, which has become a national priority. In a systematic review of the literature on hospital-based PUPPs, Soban and colleagues (2011) reported that nearly all of the 39 studies experienced positive effects after implementing a PUPP. A number of statewide PUPPs have reported a decrease in pressure ulcers after PUPP implementation. For example, the Minnesota Department of Health (2014) reported a 33% decrease in Stage III, IV, and unstageable pressure ulcers over the course of 2 years with a statewide SAFE SKIN collaborative.

National Priority

As early as 2000, the U.S. Department of Health and Human Services (2000) document, *Healthy People 2010: Understanding and Improving Health,* listed reducing pressure ulcer incidence as an objective for all health care providers.

By fiscal year 2007, a preventable pressure ulcer was listed as a secondary diagnosis for 300,000 Medicare patients; each pressure ulcer added $43,180 in costs to a hospital stay (AHRQ, 2011). In 2008 the Centers for Medicare and Medicaid Services (CMS) ceased payment for hospital complications considered reasonably preventable, including Stage III or IV pressure ulcers, and released new codes for pressure ulcers capturing wound severity. The cost of treating pressure ulcers in the United States is estimated at $9.1 to $11.6 billion annually. Each year, about 60,000 patients die in the United States as a direct result of pressure ulcers (AHRQ, 2011). These statistics are startling when we consider the fact that people come to the hospital when they are ill, trusting that they will be taken care of and protected from adversities.

Medical errors that are clearly identifiable, preventable, and associated with serious consequences have been termed *never events* by the National Quality Forum. In its mission to "fundamentally transform health care," the National Priorities Partnership, which consists of members from 26 different national organizations and is convened by the National Quality Forum, announced six national priorities to direct health care reform to eliminate waste, harm, and inequities. Safety (the elimination of errors whenever and wherever possible) is one such priority and incorporates severe pressure ulcers, defined as Stage III or IV (National Priorities Partnership, 2008). The Institute for Healthcare Improvement (IHI) also identified the prevention of pressure ulcers as one of the 12 interventions in its 5 Million Lives campaign (Duncan, 2007).

These positions represent a dramatic shift in public policy. Pressure ulcer prevention has been in the mission of the Wound, Ostomy and Continence Nurses Society™ (WOCN®) and has been included in the curriculum for WOC nursing education programs since 1982 (Alterescu, 1991; Goode, 1991; IAET, 1987; Wright, 1991). As new technology evolved, risk assessment became more refined, and pressure ulcer prevention interventions were better understood, it was generally accepted by wound care experts that all pressure ulcers could be prevented and that their presence was a reflection on quality of care. In fact, the 5 Million Lives campaign by the IHI launched in 2007 specifically states "the goal for pressure ulcer incidence should be zero" (Duncan, 2007). Most recently, the concept of attaining a zero incidence of facility-acquired pressure ulcers is increasingly being challenged (NPUAP, EPUAP, PPPIA, 2014; WOCN®, 2010).

Reimbursement for Present on Admission Only

Once the CMS ceased payment for hospital complications considered reasonably preventable, pressure ulcers that were not present on admission (POA) became even more expensive for hospitals, adding an estimated $43,180 to a patient's hospital stay, as previously mentioned (AHRQ, 2011; Krapfl, 2008). A retrospective chart analysis of patients with Stage IV pressure ulcers calculated an average hospital cost of $129,248 to treat a hospital-acquired Stage IV pressure ulcer and related complications during just one hospital admission (Brem et al, 2010). Because patients with hospital-acquired pressure ulcers tend to have a longer length of stay (10.8 days), reimbursement for hospital care may be further compromised (Scott et al, 2006). In contrast, it has been estimated that general pressure ulcer prevention costs $54.66 per day in acute care settings (Padula et al, 2011). Checklist 8-1 provides

---

CHECKLIST 8-1 Indicators for Stage III to IV Pressure Ulcers Present on Admission

✓ Present at time the order for inpatient admission occurs. Pressure ulcer that developed during an outpatient encounter, including the emergency department, observation, or outpatient surgery, is considered POA.

✓ Pressure ulcer diagnosis documented by "provider." A provider is a physician or any qualified health care practitioner who is legally accountable for establishing the patient's diagnosis.

✓ Determination of whether the pressure ulcer was POA is based on the provider's best clinical judgment anytime during the hospital stay.

✓ Inconsistent, missing, or conflicting documentation issues are resolved by the physician.

✓ Pressure ulcer is POA when the patient is discharged with a facility-acquired pressure ulcer and later readmitted with a different diagnosis.

POA, Present on admission.
Adapted from Wound, Ostomy and Continence Nurses Society™ (WOCN®): *Inpatient prospective payment changes: a guide for the WOC nurse*, March 13, 2009. http://www.wocn.org/news/news.asp?id=67092. Accessed Feb 10, 2014.

---

the indicators for Stage III or IV pressure ulcers POA. The WOCN® Society (2009a) has published a useful guidance document to assist with interpreting the POA rule. The document clarifies the role of the WOC nurse, coder, and physician in determining whether the pressure ulcer is POA and what code to assign. For example, a suspected deep tissue injury (sDTI) is coded as an unstageable pressure ulcer. The POA rule emphasizes the importance of the PUPP component of skin inspection upon admission to any health care facility to establish a baseline for the patient so that subsequent pressure-related abnormalities in the skin can be identified.

Ability to Identify the Unavoidable Pressure Ulcer

By stating "hospital-acquired conditions (such as pressure ulcers) could be *reasonably prevented* with evidence-based guidelines," the CMS introduces the possibility that some pressure ulcers cannot be avoided (WOCN®, 2009b). Before the introduction of POA for hospitals, CMS defined the term *unavoidable pressure ulcer* (for the long-term care setting) as a pressure ulcer that develops in spite of the facility's best efforts at prevention (Checklist 8-2). However, a similar definition by the CMS for the hospital or home care setting does not exist. The WOCN® Society recognized the absence of a definition for acute care as a potential problem. To fill this gap, the WOCN® Society released a position statement (*Avoidable versus Unavoidable Pressure Ulcers*) using the CMS definition of an unavoidable pressure ulcer and refuting the assumption that all pressure ulcers are preventable (WOCN®, 2009b). There is also consensus from the National Pressure Ulcer Advisory Panel (NPUAP) that some conditions (e.g., hemodynamic instability worsened with movement) do *not* make pressure

CHECKLIST 8-2 Avoidable and Unavoidable Pressure Ulcers

Avoidable

The resident developed a pressure ulcer and the facility did *not* do one or more of the following:

✓ Evaluate the resident's clinical condition and pressure ulcer risk factors

✓ Define and implement interventions that are consistent with the resident's needs and goals and with recognized standards of practice

✓ Monitor and evaluate the impact of interventions

✓ Revise the interventions as appropriate

Unavoidable

The resident developed a pressure ulcer even though the facility *did* the following:

✓ Evaluated the resident's clinical condition and pressure ulcer risk factors

✓ Defined and implemented interventions that were consistent with the resident's needs and goals and with recognized standards of practice

✓ Monitored and evaluated the impact of interventions

✓ Revised the interventions as appropriate

CHECKLIST 8-3 Pressure Ulcer Prevention Best-Practice Audit

✓ Pressure ulcer risk assessment was documented on admission and daily.

✓ Skin inspection was documented on admission and daily.

✓ Removal of devices, such as stockings and splints, at least twice a day was documented.

✓ Devices that cannot be removed, such as indwelling tubes and drains, are stabilized and repositioned for daily skin inspection.

✓ Documented care plan linked risk assessment findings to specific preventive interventions.

✓ Patients with impaired sensory perception, mobility, and activity as defined by the risk assessment scale had the following applicable interventions documented:
  • Repositioning every 2 hours
  • Heels off bed
  • Appropriate support surfaces (mattresses, chair cushions) for pressure redistribution

✓ Patients with friction/shear risk as defined by the Braden scale had head of bed elevated ≤30 degrees documented (if medically contraindicated, physician's order and alternative plan to prevent shear injury were documented).

✓ Patients with nutritional deficits as defined by the Braden scale were followed by dietary services once the deficit was identified.

✓ Patients with incontinence have documentation that perineal cleanser and barrier were used and the underlying cause addressed.

✓ Patient/family skin safety education and patient response were documented.

✓ Standard skin safety interventions that were determined to be medically contraindicated or inconsistent with the patient's overall goals were documented or ordered by a physician and reevaluated routinely.

✓ Inability to adhere to standard skin safety interventions (i.e., noncompliance) was documented with evidence of patient/family education and ongoing efforts to reeducate or modify care plan.

ulcers inevitable, but *may* lead to unavoidable pressure ulcers. Further, consensus showed that the NPUAP continues to support the position that pressure ulcer avoidability is determined when the outcome is known and preventive interventions are evaluated (Black et al, 2011).

A PUPP is based on evidence-based guidelines or best practices and therefore provides a structure in which unavoidable pressure ulcers may be identified. Identifying a potentially unavoidable pressure ulcer may not assist with reimbursement in hospitals. However, it will help to identify whether a best practice was delivered and therefore may be useful in protecting against litigation. In addition, this definition of avoidable and unavoidable is useful in the population of patients at the end of life who may develop a pressure ulcer. Although there is support for the concept of skin failure (Black, 2011) as the end of life is near, there is no definitive confirmation that this concept is real. For now, the current definition of avoidable and unavoidable pressure ulcers allows for the possibility that a patient at the end of life could develop a pressure ulcer despite appropriate care. However, this definition also protects the patient from the assumption that pressure ulcers at the end of life are either skin failure or unavoidable. Under the current definition of "unavoidable," documentation is the only way to determine whether a pressure ulcer was or was not avoidable (Black, 2011). See Checklist 8-3 for examples of relevant audit questions for the patient's medical record.

Litigation Avoidance, Patient Trust, and Facility Reputation

Patient trust and facility reputation are other justifications for PUPP implementation as patient safety becomes transparent

through published reports on the Internet and the ability of consumers to compare facility outcomes. More than 17,000 lawsuits are related to pressure ulcers annually (AHRQ, 2011), and there is no shortage in the literature related to how patients with pressure ulcers suffer. Approximately 50% of pressure ulcers do not heal within 8 weeks (Bergstrom et al, 2005). Patients with pressure ulcers can suffer from pain, depression, infection, and sepsis. As discussed in Chapter 29, they often demonstrate significantly impaired physical and social function, self-care, and mobility. In addition, patients with pressure ulcers often require either long-term hospitalization or frequent hospital admissions.

Beyond the financial, physical, and psychological impact, errors in patient care are costly in terms of loss of trust in the system by patients, diminished satisfaction by both patients and health professionals, and loss of morale by health care professionals who are not able to provide the best care possible.

COMPONENTS OF A PUPP

A PUPP consists of a *best-practice bundle* and *infrastructure* (operations). The components of a PUPP have been widely adopted by WOC nurses for years (Bryant et al, 1992) and were included in the 1992 AHCPR Pressure Ulcer Prevention Guideline. Historically, PUPPs have been demonstrated to be effective at reducing the incidence of pressure ulcers. However, the implementation, maintenance, and survival of the PUPP were often dependent on WOC nurse involvement. Although the successful PUPP may be coordinated by the wound specialist, it should not be owned by or dependent on one individual or group. Rather, it must be adopted into the facility's overall patient safety culture, supported and protected by the administration, and therefore integrated into the facility's infrastructure. Lack of infrastructure is frequently the reason for PUPP failure. Therefore creating the infrastructure to sustain a PUPP is discussed in detail later in this chapter.

ESTABLISHING A BEST-PRACTICE BUNDLE

From a structural perspective, the best-practice bundle of the PUPP has six components: skin inspection, risk assessment, maintain skin health, pressure redistribution, nutrition and hydration, and patient education. The best-practice bundle includes research-based evidence and, when a higher level of evidence is not available, expert opinion.

Skin Inspection and Assessment

A skin inspection should be obtained for all patients upon admission. Because the admission inspection serves as a baseline for comparisons and pressure ulcers can develop quickly, this skin inspection should be obtained as soon as possible. International guidelines (NPUAP, EPUAP, PPPIA, 2014) recommend conducting a comprehensive skin inspection for those at risk as soon as possible, but within 8 hours of admission or first visit in community settings. However, physiologically a pressure ulcer can develop as early as within 1 hour (Gefen, 2008). Therefore it may be reasonable to inspect the skin within the first few hours of admission, given the need for patient repositioning and other cares that are conducive for skin inspection (see Table 6-1). Subsequent inspection and monitoring by trained staff are recommended at least daily as part of every risk assessment when patients are deemed at risk for pressure ulcers or have existing impaired skin integrity.

The frequency of skin assessment should be increased if the patient's overall condition deteriorates (NPUAP, EPUAP, PPPIA, 2014). All skin assessment findings should be documented. Skin temperature, erythema, edema, and alterations in tissue consistency should be noted by comparing adjacent skin or contralateral body part. If erythema is noted, it should be determined whether it is blanchable or nonblanchable. Optimal visualization and palpation of skin changes require adequate lighting, removal of garments, repositioning of medical devices, and the

spreading of skin folds, buttocks, and toes. Palpation of darker skin tones is particularly important, as it is not always possible to identify erythema in darkly pigmented skin. Studies report higher rates of full thickness pressure ulcers in patients with dark skin tones compared to patients with light skin tones which suggests the early indicators of pressure ulcer damage (e.g., blanching and nonblanching erythema) are not recognized in patients with dark skin tone (Baumgarten et al, 2004; Rosen et al, 2006; Van Gilder et al, 2008). Unlike inspection, skin *assessment* involves interpretation and synthesis of additional data gathered from the comprehensive holistic patient assessment, such as nutrition, perfusion, medications, and other comorbidities. Chapter 6 presents a detailed discussion related to skin assessment, inspection, and monitoring, including considerations for darkly pigmented skin (see Checklist 6-1). The concept of subepidermal moisture is also described in Chapter 6.

Risk Assessment and Screening

Chapter 7 presents a theoretical framework of pressure ulcer development and a description of intrinsic and extrinsic factors that place a patient at risk for pressure ulcer development (see Figure 7-2). As with other assessments, pressure ulcer risk assessment includes identification of subjective, objective, and psychosocial factors to determine and assess the risk and care needs of the patient (Stechmiller et al, 2008). Many of these risk factors at first glance seem intuitive. However, due to highly variable experiences and knowledge among caregivers, the accuracy of clinical judgment and intuitive sense in identifying those at risk is not reliable, as demonstrated through many studies including a recent metaanalysis (García-Fernández et al, 2014). Furthermore, the assumption that all patients are at risk and that preventive measures should be universally applied is difficult to defend due to the inefficient use of resources. Therefore, to enhance the accuracy of pressure ulcer risk assessment, experts recommend using a validated risk screening scale (Stechmiller et al, 2008; WOCN®, 2010). More recent guidelines also recommend a structured approach, but emphasize that regardless of structured method chosen, consideration of risk factors not included in most scales (e.g., perfusion, skin temperature, medical devices) and clinical judgment are essential (NPUAP, EPUAP, PPPIA, 2014).

A risk scale is a noninvasive, cost-effective method for distinguishing between patients who are at risk for developing a pressure ulcer and those who are not. Scales identify the extent to which a person exhibits a specific risk factor, thus directing the selection of interventions needed. In selecting a scale for predicting a condition such as a pressure ulcer, the scale must have demonstrated reliability and validity. *Reliability* refers to the degree to which the results obtained by the measurement procedure can be replicated. For example, if two nurses administered a pressure ulcer risk scale on the same patient at the same time and their scores were the same, the reliability of the scale would be a perfect 1.0, or 100% agreement. *Validity* refers to accuracy. A screening test such as a pressure ulcer risk scale should provide a good preliminary test of which individuals actually are at risk and which are not. Validity has two components: *sensitivity*, which correctly identifies patients at risk, and *specificity*, which correctly identifies patients not at risk. An ideal risk scale would be 100% sensitive and 100% specific, so it does not overpredict (therefore no false-positive scores) or underpredict (no false-negative scores). However, 100% is rarely achieved due to an inverse relationship between sensitivity and specificity; as the scale becomes more sensitive, specificity declines. Nevertheless, these measures of predictability are invaluable when comparing tools that attempt to predict a condition such as a pressure ulcer.

The validity and reliability of several pressure ulcer risk assessment scales have been reported in the literature and summarized in a metaanalysis (García-Fernández et al, 2014). Recommendations related to pressure ulcer risk assessment, such as frequency, who should administer it, and which patients should be assessed, are summarized in Box 8-1. These tools identify risks so they can be targeted; they logically have poor predictability rates because once a risk is identified, interventions are put in place to reduce the likelihood of pressure ulcer development. Reassessment is intuitively logical because factors known to contribute to risk clearly fluctuate

---

BOX 8-1   Pressure Ulcer Risk Assessment Scales: Summary of Recommendations

- Pressure ulcer risk assessment scales should be administered to all patients with one or more risk factors for pressure ulcer development when admitted to a hospital's medical, surgical, intensive care, orthopedic, cardiovascular, or step-down unit; home care; hospice; or extended care facility (Bolton, 2007).
- Reassessment should occur:
  - Regularly and frequently as required by the patient's condition (NPUAP and EPUAP, 2009; WOCN®, 2010)
  - When the patient's condition changes (NPUAP and EPUAP, 2009)
  - Acute care: At least every 48 hours or whenever the patient's condition changes (WOCN®, 2003, 2010)
  - Long-term care: Weekly for the first 4 weeks, monthly, then quarterly after that or when the patient's condition changes (WOCN®, 2003)
  - Home care: Every nurse visit (WOCN®, 2010)
- The Braden scale (Table 8-1), then the Norton and Waterloo scales, have the strongest body of evidence supporting validity and reliability (García-Fernández et al, 2014).
- Pressure ulcer risk assessment scales should be administered by a professional nurse (Bolton, 2007).
- Braden and Norton scales have demonstrated interrater reliability when administered by both registered nurses and licensed practical nurses (Bolton, 2007).
- Risk assessment is not valid and reliable unless those administering the assessment have access to the complete scale and subscale descriptors (Bolton, 2007).

---

with medical condition and hospital course. (See Table 8-1 and Appendix A for a list of evidence related risk assessment tools.)

Using the Braden Scale. One of the most widely used and researched pressure ulcer risk tools is the Braden Scale for the Prediction of Pressure Ulcer Risk (García-Fernández et al, 2014). Translated into many languages, numerous reports attest to the reliability (0.83 to 0.95) of the scale with adequately trained registered nurses and licensed practical nurses (Magnan and Maklebust, 2008).

The Braden scale is composed of six risk factor subscales that conceptually reflect degrees of sensory perception, skin moisture, physical activity, nutritional intake, friction and shear, and ability to change and control body position. All subscales are rated from 1 (most risk) to 4 (least risk), except the friction and shear subscale, which is rated from 1 to 3. Each rating is accompanied by a brief description of criteria for assigning the rating. Therefore the subscales identify which risk factors are present so that interventions can be targeted to reduce specific risk factors (Table 8-2) (WOCN®, 2010).

Braden scale scores are grouped according to level of risk: not at risk (>18), mild risk (15–18), moderate risk (13–14), high risk (10–12), and very high risk (≤9). When a patient has a pressure ulcer or a history of a pressure ulcer but is rated "not at risk" according to the Braden scale, it is recommended to automatically place the patient in the "at-risk" category (Maklebust et al, 2005). Likewise, the level of risk should be increased for any patient whose Braden score indicates he or she is "at risk" and who also has a fever, diastolic blood pressure less than 60, or low albumin/prealbumin (WOCN®, 2010). For example, a patient with a Braden score of 12 would be considered at moderate risk, but should be "upgraded" to the high-risk category if he or she also has a fever.

Maklebust and Magnan (2009) found that nurses who calculated scores of 13 to 18 (at risk and moderate risk) had the least amount of agreement about which interventions to implement for their patients. However, it is important to emphasize that a pressure ulcer prevention care plan is *not* based on total score alone; subscale scores, consideration of additional risk factors, and clinician judgment will serve as a more accurate guide (Gadd, 2014; NPUAP, EPUAP, PPPIA, 2014).

Accurate use of the Braden scale requires user training and retraining, even when nurses use the tool regularly and for a long period of time. A study involving more than 2500 nurses in Detroit Medical Center showed that only 75.5% of nurses correctly rated Braden scale levels (Maklebust et al, 2005). Although the two extremes of risk levels, "not at risk" and "severe risk," were most often rated correctly, the subscales "moisture" and "sensory perception" were most often misunderstood. Therefore annual competencies for risk assessment are justified (Magnan and Maklebust, 2008; Maklebust et al, 2005). Similarly, the definitions for risk factors and subscales

Patient's Name _____   Evaluator's Name _____   Date of Assessment _____

SENSORY PERCEPTION Ability to respond appropriately to pressure-related discomfort	1. Completely limited Unresponsive (does not moan, flinch, or grasp) to painful stimuli, due to diminished level of consciousness or sedation OR limited ability to feel pain over most of body.	2. Very limited Responds only to painful stimuli. Cannot communicate discomfort except by moaning or restlessness OR has a sensory impairment that limits the ability to feel pain or discomfort over half of body.	3. Slightly limited Responds to verbal commands, but cannot always communicate discomfort or the need to be turned OR has some sensory impairment that limits ability to feel pain or discomfort in one or two extremities.	4. No impairment Responds to verbal commands. Has no sensory deficit that would limit ability to feel or voice pain or discomfort.
MOISTURE Degree to which skin is exposed to moisture	1. Constantly moist Skin is kept moist almost constantly by perspiration, urine, etc. Dampness is detected every time patient is moved or turned.	2. Very moist Skin is often, but not always, moist. Linen must be changed at least once a shift.	3. Occasionally moist Skin is occasionally moist, requiring an extra linen change approximately once a day.	4. Rarely moist Skin is usually dry; linen only requires changing at routine intervals.
ACTIVITY Degree of physical activity	1. Bedfast Confined to bed.	2. Chairfast Ability to walk severely limited or nonexistent. Cannot bear own weight and/or must be assisted into chair or wheelchair.	3. Walks occasionally Walks occasionally during day, but for very short distances, with or without assistance. Spends majority of each shift in bed or chair.	4. Walks frequently Walks outside room at least twice a day and inside room at least once every 2 hours during waking hours.
MOBILITY Ability to change and control body position	1. Completely immobile Does not make even slight changes in body or extremity position without assistance.	2. Very limited Makes occasional slight changes in body or extremity position, but unable to make frequent or significant changes independently.	3. Slightly limited Makes frequent though slight changes in body or extremity position independently.	4. No limitations Makes major and frequent changes in position without assistance.
NUTRITION Usual food intake pattern	1. Very poor Never eats a complete meal. Rarely eats more than one-third of any food offered. Eats two servings or less of protein (meat or dairy products) per day. Takes fluids poorly. Does not take a liquid supplement OR is NPO and/or maintained on clear liquids or IVs for more than 5 days.	2. Probably inadequate Rarely eats a complete meal and generally eats only about half of any food offered. Protein intake includes only three servings of meat or dairy products per day. Occasionally will take a dietary supplement OR receives less-than-optimum amount of liquid diet or tube feeding.	3. Adequate Eats over half of most meals. Eats a total of four servings of protein (meat, dairy products) per day. Occasionally will refuse a meal, but will usually take a supplement when offered OR is on a tube feeding or TPN regimen, which probably meets most of nutritional needs.	4. Excellent Eats most of every meal. Never refuses a meal. Usually eats a total of four or more servings of meat and dairy products. Occasionally eats between meals. Does not require supplementation.
FRICTION & SHEAR	1. Problem Requires moderate to maximum assistance in moving. Complete lifting without sliding against sheets is impossible. Frequently slides down in bed or chair, requiring frequent repositioning with maximum assistance. Spasticity, contractures, or agitation leads to almost constant friction.	2. Potential problem Moves feebly or requires minimum assistance. During a move, skin probably slides to some extent against sheets, chair, restraints, or other devices. Maintains relatively good position in chair or bed most of the time, but occasionally slides down.	3. No apparent problem Moves in bed and in chair independently and has sufficient muscle strength to lift up completely during move. Maintains good position in bed or chair.	

Total Score _____

Risk Factor	Interventions (Skin Safety Precautions)

Impaired sensory perception, mobility, activity	1. Preventive (group 1) pressure redistribution support surface for patients with multiple intact turning surfaces and Braden score ≤18
	2. Obtain therapeutic (group 2) pressure redistribution support surface (i.e., low air loss) for patients with:
	  • Full-thickness or suspected deep tissue injury on the trunk
	  • Wounds on multiple turning surfaces
	3. Reposition every 2 hours in bed, *regardless* of bed/mattress type
	  • Avoid positioning directly on trochanter
	  • Collaborate with provider for pain control as needed to promote appropriate repositioning
	  • Use pillows to keep bony prominences from direct contact with surfaces (including keeping heels off bed)
	  • Stabilize and position tubes to prevent them from creating pressure
	4. Reposition once every hour in chair
	  • Use pressure redistribution chair cushion
	  • Return to bed after 1 hour if unable to reposition in chair
	5. Moisturize dry skin; do *not* massage reddened bony prominences
	6. Remove or reposition devices (stockings, masks, tubes) every shift for skin inspection

Moisture	1. Address cause and offer bedpan/urinal/toileting every 2 hours
	2. Notify provider and registered dietitian if patient has loose stools
	3. Use absorbent pads that wick moisture away from the body (avoid diapers/briefs with plastic backing)
	4. Skin care twice per day and after each incontinent episode to include
	  • Perineal cleanser and barrier in one
	  • Moisture barrier paste if stools are loose or perineal skin is red or open
	5. Consider containment devices for frequent loose stools (rectal pouches, Food and Drug Administration–approved indwelling fecal containment device)

Nutritional deficit	1. Consult nutritional services 2. Maintain adequate hydration
Friction and shear	1. Limit head-of-bed elevation to ≤30 degrees (unless contraindicated) 2. Use knee gatch as needed to keep patient from sliding down in bed 3. Use trapeze when indicated 4. Use lift sheet or air transfer device (HoverMatt) to move patient and prevent lateral shear 5. Protect elbows and heels with skin barriers or dressings if exposed to friction

for each risk factor are essential in both paper and electronic documentation systems. The following section discusses the Braden subscales and measurement of risk factors.

Sensory perception. With respect to pressure ulcers, *sensory perception* refers to the patient's ability to respond meaningfully to pressure-related discomfort. The extent of the deficit depends on the degree to which a patient is able to feel or communicate pressure-related discomfort. Patients without a sensory impairment move or ask to be moved if they are lying on intravenous tubing or feel pain on their tailbone. They remove or request removal of shoes, stockings, or medical devices that feel uncomfortable or too tight. Examples of patients with sensory deficits who cannot adequately communicate discomfort include those with confusion, disorientation, oversedation, or unresponsiveness. Patients who are alert and oriented may be unable to communicate discomfort (e.g., "my mask is too tight") if they are on a ventilator, speak a different language than their caregivers, or cannot feel pain due to paralysis or neuropathy.

Moisture. The more the skin is exposed to moisture, especially near a bony prominence, the more vulnerable the skin becomes to the mechanical forces of pressure, friction, and shear. Clinical examples include the patient with incontinence who is exposed to pressure, the critically ill patient with fever and diaphoresis, or the bedbound patient with poorly contained wound exudate from a perirectal abscess.

Activity. Degree of activity refers to how much a patient is in the bed or chair or is ambulating. Again, reading the subscale definitions is important. For example, "walks occasionally" means the patient spends most of the time in the chair. Therefore a few steps to the bedside commode should be scored as "walks occasionally."

Mobility. One of the problems encountered with this subscale is the tendency to confuse activity (e.g., getting up in the chair) with mobility. *Mobility* refers to the patient's ability to change or control body position. The score assigned is based on what the patient demonstrates, such as the degree to which he or she is able to change or control body position (i.e., shifting weight in the chair or turning or repositioning in bed). A patient may be able to sit in a chair (activity) but may not be able to shift his or her weight (mobility). In contrast, a patient who is agitated and moving frequently may still have a mobility deficit because the movements are not purposeful or controlled.

Nutrition. One mistake made with the Braden nutrition subscale is failure of the rater to consider "*usual* food intake pattern." For example the patient who is NPO (nil per os [nothing by mouth]) after midnight does not constitute a low nutrition score if his or her usual food intake pattern is adequate. Conversely, the patient's nutritional status may be rated "adequate" when the patient is receiving total parenteral nutrition or a tube feeding documented to "meet nutritional needs" even though the patient is malnourished. This occurs because the regimen "that meets nutritional needs" requires time to reverse the malnutrition that existed before supplementation was initiated. Therefore patients at risk for pressure ulcers with an adequate nutrition score should be placed at a higher risk level in the presence of clinical evidence of malnutrition.

Friction and shear. Friction occurs when the skin rubs against another surface. Patients who are restless or agitated commonly create friction on their elbows and heels from constant movement and rubbing against the bed surface. Friction also can occur with a brace or shoe as it slides back and forth during ambulation. *Shear* occurs when friction acts with gravity. Classic examples of actions that cause shear injury include a patient sliding down in bed after the head of the bed has been elevated for lunch or allowing the patient's buttocks to drag across the bed, stretcher, or procedure table during transfer.

Maintain Skin Health

The third component of the PUPP's best-practice bundle is preserving the protective function of the skin. Threats to the protective function of the skin include xerosis, incontinence, chemicals, friction, and shear. Interventions that minimize threats to skin integrity, including dry skin, need to be part of the routine baseline standard of care for all patients (Box 8-2). Xerosis (severe dry skin as demonstrated by pruritic, erythematous, dry, scaly, cracked, or fissured skin) is a problem for 55.6% of people 64 years and older (Paul et al, 2011). Xerosis results from loss of natural moisturizing factors, barrier abilities, and epidermal water. It is intuitive

---

BOX 8-2 Interventions to Maintain Skin Health

- Avoid alkaline soaps so that pH and normal flora of skin remain intact.
- Do not use friction when washing skin to avoid traumatizing epidermis.
- Apply moisturizer or emollient frequently to prevent xerosis.
- Encourage adequate fluid intake to prevent dehydration, which contributes to xerosis.
- Use moisture barrier ointments as needed to protect skin from chemical irritants such as fecal incontinence.
- Do *not* massage reddened areas.
- Move and transfer with lift sheet, Hoyer lift, or HoverMatt to avoid shear on buttocks due to dragging.

---

that maintaining skin integrity is important to prevent bacterial invasion and protect resilience of skin to deflect or absorb pressure, shear, or friction. Xerosis should be prevented or minimized with frequent application of moisturizers and emollients in addition to adequate water intake (Torra i Bou et al, 2005; Shannon et al, 2009).

Optimize Nutrition and Hydration

The fourth component of a PUPP's best-practice bundle is maintenance of adequate nutrition and hydration compatible with the individual's wishes and conditions (WOCN®, 2010). With weight loss and dehydration from sustained nutritional deficiencies, muscle mass is decreased so that less padding is available to distribute the patient's weight over a bony prominence (Reddy et al, 2006). Fry et al (2010) reported malnutrition and/or weight loss correlated with a fourfold higher risk of developing pressure ulcers. Although intuitively it is reasonable to conclude that malnourished patients are at risk for pressure ulcers, the data linking pressure ulcers with markers for poor nutritional status are inconsistent. While low albumin or prealbumin levels may be reported as more prevalent in or even associated with patients with a pressure ulcer compared with patients who did not develop a pressure ulcer, these relationships are not sustained when analyzed as an independent risk factor for pressure ulcer development. Key reasons for this inconsistency include that there is no widely accepted gold standard for the definition of malnutrition and typical markers for malnutrition (i.e., albumin and prealbumin) often reflect underlying or coexisting disease rather than undernutrition. However, to maintain skin resiliency (tissue tolerance) to resist the stresses known to cause pressure ulcers, patients at risk for pressure ulcers should receive adequate nutritional intake and be assisted with meals, snacks, and hydration.

Nutrition screening with a valid and reliable tool to identify the need for a comprehensive nutrition assessment can be performed by any qualified member of the health care team. Screening should be conducted on admission to the health care facility, or at first visit in community settings (NPUAP, EPUAP, PPPIA, 2014). At a minimum, if the patient has an existing pressure ulcer or the pressure ulcer risk assessment indicates the patient is nutritionally compromised, a registered dietician should be consulted for a more comprehensive nutritional assessment and specific recommendations (NPUAP, EPUAP, PPPIA, 2014; WOCN®, 2010). Depending on the patient's comorbidities, the registered dietician's recommendations may include offering fluids every 2 hours, high-protein supplements, swallowing studies, and enteral or parenteral nutrition. Fluid is a solvent and transport mechanism for nutrients and waste. Hydration status should be monitored by checking for signs of dehydration, such as changes in weight, skin turgor, urinary output (volume and concentration), elevated serum sodium, or calculated serum osmolality (NPUAP, EPUAP, PPPIA, 2014; Thomas et al, 2008). Chapter 27 discusses the details of nutritional assessment and management.

Pressure Redistribution and Offloading the Patient at Risk

Pressure redistribution and offloading are required for the at-risk patient, whether the individual is in a chair, on a transport or procedure cart, in the operating room, or in a bed. Pressure redistribution is accomplished with the use of support surfaces (see Chapter 9). Offloading is accomplished by turning and repositioning.

Repositioning Frequency. Repositioning is used to reduce the duration and intensity of pressure exerted over a bony prominence. In 1961 Kosiak recommended the frequency of repositioning to be hourly to every 2 hours, based on the interface pressure readings from healthy, able-bodied subjects. Although repositioning every 2 hours as a standard of care to prevent pressure ulcers continues to be debated, there is widespread support that a regular schedule for repositioning should continue to be the guideline for care (Black et al, 2011; Defloor et al, 2005). Most recently, international guidelines for pressure ulcer prevention and treatment recommend a reposition frequency that is determined by tissue tolerance, level of activity and mobility, general medical condition, overall treatment objectives, skin condition, and support surface. Although some of these factors are easily determined and remain constant (support surface), others cannot be measured with current technology (e.g., tissue tolerance) or may be unpredictable and labile (e.g., mobility, activity, and medical condition). Positioning regimens, including selected positions, frequency, and outcomes, should be documented (NPUAP, EPUAP, PPPIA, 2014).

Much like determining frequency for pain medications, the effectiveness of repositioning should be assessed, adjusting frequency as needed to achieve the desired outcome (e.g., no erythema). Specifically, when establishing a pressure ulcer prevention plan, positioning frequency might be determined by beginning with a schedule of every 2 hours. Persistent redness from a previous episode of pressure loading, seen when the patient is repositioned, indicates that pressure is not adequately relieved. Therefore a different support surface may be indicated or the repositioning frequency may need to be increased. Ultimately, a 4-hour repositioning schedule may be most appropriate when the patient is on an appropriate support surface, the patient's skin has remained intact and without erythema, and the patient does not have an acute illness that would precipitate a sudden change in medical condition (e.g., hemodynamic instability). Although an every-4-hour positioning schedule may be adequate in some situations for keeping the skin intact, it may be insufficient to prevent other complications associated with immobility (e.g., thromboembolism, atelectasis, aspiration).

Repositioning Techniques. Although repositioning does not reduce intensity of pressure, it does reduce the duration, which is the more critical element of pressure ulcer formation. Repositioning contributes to the patient's comfort, dignity, and functional ability (NPUAP, EPUAP, PPPIA, 2014). Repositioning techniques differ according to the patient's activity (chairbound, bedbound), location (operating room [OR], transport, emergency room, special procedures), comfort, and hemodynamic stability.

Turning. Few individuals are truly too unstable to turn (NPUAP, EPUAP, PPPIA, 2014). Turning the patient in bed is a universally accepted staple in preventing the complications associated with immobility, including pressure ulcers. The proper technique for turning to place the patient in a 30-degree side-lying position with a pillow between the knees is shown in Figure 8-1. The patient should be turned alternately from right side, to back, to left side, to back. The proper technique avoids bony prominences, nonblanchable erythema, existing wounds, and medical devices such as tubes and catheters. For example, a 90-degree side-lying position is generally undesirable because it places the patient

FIGURE 8-1 Thirty-degree lateral position.

directly on a bony prominence (trochanter) (NPUAP, EPUAP, PPPIA, 2014). When an ulcer is present on a turning surface, the turning schedule may be customized so that time spent on that turning surface is minimized.

Minor movement and slow incremental turns. Although international guidelines note that few individuals are truly too unstable to turn, slow incremental turns and minor movement (also described as miniturns, minishifts, and offloads) should be used to allow some reperfusion (NPUAP, EPUAP, PPPIA, 2014; WOCN®, 2010). For example, pillows that have been propped under the patient can be incrementally removed or placed. Ideally, the patient should also be placed on an active support surface or advanced support surface that provides more effective pressure redistribution, shear reduction, and microclimate control (see Chapter 9). The concept for weight shifting is not new—weight shifting in the chair has been a best-practice recommendation since the AHCPR Guidelines in 1992, and remains a recommendation in WOCN® Society Guidelines (2010). International guidelines for pressure ulcer prevention recommend considering incremental turns with time (e.g., 10 minutes) in between small shifts, with frequent reassessment and turning trials every 8 hours if the patient is too unstable for routine repositioning. Routine repositioning should resume as soon as the condition stabilizes (NPUAP, EPUAP, PPPIA, 2014).

There is a growing concern in the critical care literature that the term "hemodynamic instability" is being used inappropriately to describe critically ill patients, and interventions like repositioning may be withheld due to fear of affecting systemic perfusion or oxygenation. Reports of hemodynamic instability are passed on from shift to shift, without verification or inclination of when to resume or trial repositioning (Choi et al, 2008; Winkelman and Peereboom, 2010). However, experts claim that even the most critically ill patients can usually be turned (O'Connor and Walsham, 2009).

Vollman (2010) explains that research has shown that changes in the saturation of mixed venous blood (SvO_2) and heart rate following lateral turns in patients in the intensive care unit are mostly transient and return to baseline within 5 minutes. She describes the concept "gravitational equilibrium," which happens to patients who are left stationary for prolonged periods of time. Patients left supine for too long become hemodynamically "calibrated" to a supine position, creating a situation where the patient cannot adapt to changes in position. An orthostatic response can occur when the patient is rapidly moved from supine to lateral during linen changes, baths, and transfers. This is managed with *slow* incremental movements with 5- to 10-minute recovery periods in between movements. For example, slowly tilt the patient 10 degrees to one side, followed by a 5-minute recovery, then move another 10 degrees, followed by a 5-minute recovery, until attaining a 30-degree side-lying position. Vollman (2010) does not include continuous lateral rotation therapy for pulmonary care as a pressure ulcer prevention intervention, whereas others advocate lateral rotation as an opportunity to train the body to tolerate side-to-side movement (NPUAP, EPUAP, PPPIA, 2014). As described in Chapter 9, when lateral rotation is used, it is important to monitor for shear injury. Lateral rotation is not appropriate in the presence of unstable spinal fractures.

A multidisciplinary group at Virginia University Medical Center conducted a literature review and created consensus recommendations regarding the turning and repositioning of their critically ill patients. During consensus meetings, respiratory clinical experts reminded the care team that repositioning can be an actual treatment strategy for many patients with respiratory instability, citing examples like atelectasis, shunting in the context of a collapsed lung, or differences in lung compliance. The group concluded that the patient with the following conditions is too unstable to tolerate ideal repositioning for pressure ulcer prevention: active uncontrolled bleeding and a sudden desaturation or drop in blood pressure from the patient's baseline that does not recover or cannot be corrected with vasopressive agents. In these situations, the group recommended slow and cautious miniturns and weight shifts instead of 30-degree lateral turns as a temporary intervention until the patient is stabilized (Brindle, 2013).

Limiting head-of-bed elevation. Chapter 5 discusses the effects of shear injury on the skin. Shear injury is seen after the skin is dragged over a surface either laterally (during transfers) or vertically (sliding up or down in bed). Keeping the head of the bed at an angle of 30 degrees or less prevents shear (Chung et al, 2012). To minimize the pull of gravity, the knee gatch should be used to create a semi-Fowler's position (see Figure 5-1). When the head of the bed must be temporarily elevated over 30 degrees, such as when eating or drinking or during procedures, the caregiver needs to monitor the patient closely so that the head of the bed is not left in the elevated position longer than needed (e.g., 1 hour). When having the head of the bed at 30 degrees or less is medically contraindicated, the sacral region should be frequently monitored for shear injury (WOCN®, 2010), and an advanced support surface that provides more effective pressure redistribution, shear reduction, and microclimate control may be indicated (see Chapter 9). When the patient slides down in bed, a draw sheet (or alternative transfer assist device) should be used to move the patient back to a desirable position without allowing the skin to drag across the bed surface.

Transferring without lateral shear. Lateral shear results from dragging the patient across a surface or onto another surface such as an OR surface, procedure table, or cardiac chair. Traditionally, patients have been dragged with a sliding board onto another surface, or they are requested to slide (if possible) onto the new surface. Transfer assist devices are available that can safely facilitate patient movement without dragging while decreasing risk of back injury for the staff. If patients must move themselves onto the next surface, they should be asked to do so without sliding. After transfer is complete, patients should move or be moved to release any tangential forces that may have been created by the move (AORN, 2010).

Floating heels. Heels have been reported in a European study to be the second most common and severe anatomic location for pressure ulcers; the sacrum is the most common site (Vanderwee et al, 2007). A cross-sectional prevalence and incidence survey involving 85,838 hospital patients recorded an incidence of heel ulcers ranging from 23.6% to 26.1% and accounting for 41% of all sDTIs (Van Gilder et al, 2008). The plantar aspect of the heel is well constructed to resist the forces of standing and walking. However, the posterior heel has only a thin layer of fat that is bound tightly to the underlying fascia and Achilles tendon fibers and has limited ability to (1) redistribute pressure over the small area of skin overlying the posterior tubercle of the calcaneus and (2) absorb the compressive forces of shear generated during movement or transfers. Additionally, the small branches from the calcaneal and peroneal arteries and prolonged pressure on these relatively small vessels can lead to ischemia (Wong et al, 2007). Patients with diabetes and vascular disease are at increased risk for pressure ulcers on the heel, as evidenced by their diminished hyperemic response to pressure offloading (Mayrovitz and Sims, 2004). As a result, patients with vascular disease and diabetes are always at risk for pressure ulcers on the heel despite having an adequate Braden score.

Offloading products are used to "float" the heels or redistribute pressure. Options include pillows, support surfaces, and heel suspension devices. Offloading devices (fitted and used according to the manufacturer's instructions) and pillows should distribute the weight of the leg *without* putting pressure on the Achilles tendon while keeping the knees at a slight flexion. When pillows are used, they should be positioned under the calf muscle with slight knee flexion while preventing the heels from contacting the surface of the mattress. Although pillows may be readily available, they are not reliable for maintaining the offloaded heel, compress over time, and are challenging to keep in place for patients with contractures, restlessness, and spasms. Offloading via water-filled gloves, cut-out devices, and donuts are contraindicated (NPUAP, EPUAP, PPPIA, 2014; WOCN®, 2010).

A variety of pressure redistribution devices for the heel are commercially available in numerous shapes and sizes. The pressure redistribution medium used may be air, foam, or gel. In addition to pressure ulcer prevention, some devices provide functions such as safe weight bearing, insulation (beneficial to the patient with vascular conditions), and prevention and treatment of foot drop. Due to the time required to heel deeper foot wounds, the patient is at higher risk for foot drop. Therefore an offloading device that also prevents foot drop is recommended for existing full-thickness heel ulcers. Although prevention of foot drop is an important consideration for any patient with prolonged immobilization, it is also highly recommended in patients with an existing foot ulcer (such as a diabetic foot ulcer). These patients are at increased risk of foot drop because they experience prolonged reduced mobility during the significant length of time typically required to heal a foot ulcer.

Many heel offloading devices have been found effective; however, comparisons have not identified the "best" product (Cadue et al, 2008; Donnelly et al, 2011; Gilcreast et al, 2005; Walsh and Plonczynski, 2007). Product selection should address the needs of the patient. Depending on the setting, collaboration with an occupational therapist or a physical therapist may be wise to select a device that will float the heels and be compatible with ambulation or address foot drop. Use of any device, especially with patients who have a sensory perception deficit, places the patient at risk of skin damage from the device (see Plate 33); therefore, routine range of motion, repositioning, device removal, and skin inspection are critical to prevent unintended harm. This education must be provided to and reinforced for patients, families, and caregivers frequently. Routine repositioning varies by the device and manufacturer's instructions. For example, a splint could be repositioned four times per day to be consistent with a foot drop schedule, an endotracheal tube repositioned every 2 hours to be consistent with the every-2-hours standard of care for oral care of intubated patients, and antiembolism stockings removed twice daily in keeping with the manufacturer's instructions.

Seating. Moving from the bed to the chair is a position change that may decrease the patient's overall risk for pressure ulcers by making the patient more active. However, the patient in a seated position remains at risk for pressure ulcers on the coccyx and develops new pressure points on the ischial tuberosities. Patients at risk require a pressure redistribution chair cushion (further discussed in Chapter 9). Foam or rubber rings (i.e., donuts) are not indicated to relieve pressure because they concentrate the intensity of the pressure on the surrounding tissue (NPUAP, EPUAP, PPPIA, 2014; WOCN®, 2010). Patients expected to be chairbound for the long term should be evaluated and routinely reassessed by a seating specialist or team.

The type of chair the patient will be seated in affects the patient's position and posture. The posture and position prescribed should minimize pressure and shear while maximizing safety, stability, and a full range of activities (NPUAP, EPUAP, PPPIA, 2014). For example, a reclining chair will offload the ischial tuberosities but will place more pressure on the coccyx. In contrast, a commonly used straight-back chair facilitates an upright position, with most of the pressure on the ischial tuberosities, but the coccyx again becomes vulnerable to pressure damage if the patient slouches or slides.

If the patient's feet do not touch the floor while seated, the feet should be positioned on a foot rest. The foot rest should be at a height that does not raise the knees above the patient's lap, which would create more pressure under the coccyx and ischial tuberosities.

Pressure *relief* in the chair can be attained by standing up, performing pressure relief pushups, having the wheelchair tilted back 65% or more, leaning forward, or having the patient shift his or her weight from side to side every 15 minutes to 1 hour sufficiently enough to offload the ischial tuberosities and coccyx (WOCN®, 2010). Sitting should be limited (i.e., 2 hours or less at a time) if pressure relief cannot be achieved in the chair. Patients with an existing coccyx or ischial tuberosity wound should limit sitting to 1 hour or less, three times per day, on a pressure redistribution chair cushion and in a posture that minimizes pressure to the wound (e.g., erect with sacral wounds and reclined with ischial ulcers). As with all interventions, risk and benefits to skin integrity and emotional well-being with limited sitting should be regularly evaluated, with modifications as indicated (NPUAP, EPUAP, PPPIA, 2014).

Diagnostic and Procedural Hospital Settings. Little is known about the risk of pressure injury to the patient undergoing procedures in ancillary service, such as the emergency center radiology, dialysis, and special procedures. One prospective study using data from 80 patients found a 53.8% incidence of pressure ulcer development in patients undergoing lengthy radiology procedures. Patients in ancillary services are frequently subjected to high interface pressures on ancillary support surfaces and shear during patient movement and positioning during procedures. Procedures sometimes require prolonged immobilization and agents that may cause hypotension such as anesthesia and sedation (Messer, 2010). Handoff communication is critical to address continued prevention while patients are traveling on stretchers and receiving care and evaluation on special diagnostic and procedure surfaces (Haugen et al, 2011; MHA, 2013). Hospitals are beginning to address the issue with support surfaces designed for stretchers, advance notification, electronic triggers, armbands, and handoff tools that communicate pressure ulcer risk, existing skin breakdown, and positioning tips. One rapid process improvement team even found ways to shorten scan time and provide breaks as needed for offloading (Haugen et al, 2011).

Operating Room. An analysis of 15 studies conducted in the United States with perioperative patients reported a 5% to 53.4% range of incidence of pressure ulcers, with the most common sites being the sacrum, buttocks, and heels of patients who had been supine in the OR (Ganos and Siddiqui, 2012). Intraoperatively acquired pressure ulcers are not always recognized in the immediate postoperative period. Visual skin changes can appear immediately, in a few hours, or up to 72 hours following surgery. The affected area may become ecchymotic or bruised, and it may blister. Necrosis can occur within 2 to 7 days. Patients with vascular compromise and subsequent altered skin integrity may present with an area of skin that has a mottled irregular pattern that may either resolve or proceed to full-thickness skin breakdown (Aronovitch, 2007; Walton-Geer, 2009).

A validated pressure ulcer risk screening tool for the intraoperative patient population has not been developed. Patients assessed as low risk using a risk assessment scale commonly used outside of the OR have been known to develop pressure ulcers in the OR (Aronovitch, 2007). Checklist 8-4 lists pressure ulcer risk factors for intraoperative patients described in the Association of periOperative Registered Nurse's (AORN)

CHECKLIST 8-4 Pressure Ulcer Risk Factors for Intraoperative Patients

✓ Vascular, cardiac, thoracic, orthopedic surgery
✓ Impaired blood flow and hypotensive episodes
✓ Long surgeries (>3 hours)
✓ Thin stature
✓ Poor nutritional status and decreased preoperative albumin
✓ Increasing age of patient
✓ Diabetes or vascular disease
✓ Vascular procedures
✓ Lithotomy and supine positions
✓ General anesthesia
✓ Thermoregulatory devices
✓ Use of standard operating room mattresses during surgery

Standards, Recommended Practices, and Guidelines, which also include a 23-page guideline for positioning patients in the perioperative setting (AORN, 2012). International pressure ulcer prevention and treatment guidelines (NPUAP, EPUAP, PPPIA, 2014) cite many of the same risk factors, as well as low core temperature during surgery and reduced mobility on day 1 postoperatively.

Table 8-3 contains AORN (2010) recommendations for positioning and pressure ulcer prevention and the recommendations for perioperative and administrative staff-related skin safety from the international pressure ulcer prevention and treatment guideline (NPUAP, EPUAP, PPPIA, 2014). Originally created in 2008, the Minnesota Hospital Association (MHA) website contains the most recently updated preoperative pressure ulcer prevention guidance document and gap analysis used by Minnesota hospitals to embed many of these practices into the infrastructure or culture of an organization (MHA, 2014). Attention to support surfaces in the OR cannot be overemphasized, as studies have demonstrated that the standard OR mattress, defined as a 2-inch foam mattress, increases pressure ulcer risk (Aronovitch, 2007; Defloor and de Schuijmer, 2000). Appendix A contains examples of a gap analysis and a handoff tool for the perioperative environment.

Medical Devices. The incidence of device-related pressure ulcers nationwide is unknown. In 2010, 26% of full-thickness hospital-acquired pressure ulcers in Minnesota hospitals were reported to be related to medical devices (Minnesota Department of Health, 2014). Individual hospitals and organizations report medical device–related pressure ulcer incidence (all stages) ranging from 23% to 42% of all pressure ulcer stages (Black et al, 2010; Jaul, 2011; Willock et al, 2005). Researchers report that the pediatric population is particularly vulnerable, with estimates of up to 50% of pediatric pressure ulcers related to medical equipment and devices (Baharestani and Ratliff, 2007).

Examples of devices involved with pressure ulcers include cervical collars, respiratory equipment, antiembolism devices, and feeding tubes (Apold and Rydrych, 2012; Black et al, 2010;

TABLE 8-3   Perioperative Recommendations for Pressure Ulcer Prevention

	AORN (2010)	NPUAP, EPUAP, PPPIA (2014)
Before Patient Arrival to OR	• Anticipate and verify availability of appropriate positioning equipment • Select a surface that is able to reduce excessive pressure on the patient's bony prominences • Identify unique patient considerations that require additional precautions for positioning • Verify equipment is set up *before* patient arrival • Verify correct patient position and related equipment during the time-out period	• Consider high specification pressure redistribution surface prior to surgery • Position the individual in a different posture preoperatively than the posture adopted during surgery
Before transfer to OR surface	• Actively participate in monitoring the patient's tissue integrity • Remove jewelry and body piercing accessories before positioning or transferring to the procedure bed if it will cause potential injury or interfere with the surgical site • Communicate/coordinate specific patient needs to the perioperative team before initiating transfer or positioning the patient • Use a lateral transfer device for supine-to-supine patient transfer; sliding or pulling the patient can result in shearing forces and/or friction on the patient's skin	• Consider additional risk factors specific to individuals undergoing surgery, including: duration of time immobilized before surgery, length of surgery, increased hypotensive episodes during surgery, low core temperature during surgery, reduced mobility post op day 1. • Use a high specification reactive or alternating pressure support surface on the operating table for all individuals identified as being at risk of pressure ulcer development
After transfer to OR surface	• After positioning the patient, assess the patient's body alignment, tissue perfusion, and skin integrity • Elevated heels off the underlying surface when possible • For supine to Trendelenburg's or reverse Trendelenburg's, take measures to prevent patient from sliding on the procedure bed • In lateral position, ensure the ear is padded and not folded • Place hand between the safety strap and the patient to ensure the strap is not applying excessive pressure • Confirm that prep solutions have not pooled beneath the patient and check for excessive moisture (e.g., urine from incontinence) between the patient and positioning devices • Collaborate with the surgeon and anesthesiologist about positioning during long procedures	• Position the individual in such a way as to reduce the risk of pressure ulcer development during surgery • Use additional support surfaces/pads to offload pressure points on the face and body while in the prone position • Do not position the individual directly on a medical device unless it cannot be avoided • Ensure that the heels are free of the surface of the operating table • Heel suspension devices are preferable for immobilized individuals in the operating room • Offload the heel completely in such a way as to distribute the weight of the leg along the calf without placing pressure on the Achilles tendon • Position the knees in slight flexion when offloading the heels to prevent popliteal vein compression and decrease the risk of perioperative DVT
Postoperative	• Collaborate with the postoperative patient caregiver to identify patient injury due to intraoperative positioning • Evaluate the patient for signs and symptoms of physical injury related to intraoperative positioning	• Consider pressure redistribution after surgery • Position the individual in a different posture postoperatively than the posture adopted during surgery
Documentation	• Description of overall skin condition on arrival and discharge from OR • Type and location of positioning equipment • Names and titles of persons participating in positioning the patient • Patient position and new position, if repositioning becomes necessary • Postoperative assessment for injury related to position	• Document the individual's position and the anatomic areas under increased interface pressure during surgery

TABLE 8-3	**Perioperative Recommendations for Pressure Ulcer Prevention—cont'd**	
	AORN (2010)	**NPUAP, EPUAP, PPPIA (2014)**

Administrative	• Provide staff education, competency validation, and updated information on patient positioning, new positioning equipment and procedures, and ergonomic safety
	• Administrative personnel should periodically assess and document the competency of personnel in safe patient positioning and use of positioning equipment according to facility and department policy
	• Participate in developing and monitoring an organization-wide pressure ulcer prevention and management program
	• Collect and analyze information about adverse patient outcomes and "near-miss incidents" associated with positioning and use for performance improvement
	• Develop policies and procedures related to positioning; review and revise annually; keep readily available in the practice setting; include:
	  o Assessment and evaluation criteria
	  o Required documentation
	  o Safety interventions
	  o Positioning equipment care and maintenance
	  o Ergonomic safety	

Not inclusive—most recommendations specify responsibility to perioperative registered nurses.
DVT, Deep vein thrombosis; *OR*, operating room.
Association of periOperative Registered Nurses (AORN): Recommended practices for positioning the patient in the perioperative practice setting. In *Perioperative standards and recommended practices*, Denver, CO, 2010, AORN; National Pressure Ulcer Advisory Panel (NPUAP), European Pressure Ulcer Advisory Panel (EPUAP), Pan Pacific Pressure Injury Alliance (PPPIA): Prevention and treatment of pressure ulcers: clinical practice guideline, Haesler E, editor, Perth, Australia, 2014, Cambridge Media.

Jacobson et al, 2008). As shown in plate 30, device-related pressure ulcers are generally located under or near a medical device, may not be associated with a bony prominence, and often present in the shape of the device. As shown in plate 30, device-related pressure ulcers found inside the mouth (i.e., from an endotracheal tube) or other areas lined with mucosa instead of skin are not staged; instead, they are called *mucosal pressure ulcers* (NPUAP, 2009). Because many devices are near anatomic locations without fatty tissue (e.g., nares, behind ears, occiput, bridge of nose), rapid deterioration to Stage III or IV, sDTI, or unstageable pressure ulcers is often seen. Box 8-3 lists risk factors associated with medical device–related pressure ulcers. It is always important to note that failure to follow the manufacturer's application instruction can result in harm (e.g., skin damage) to the individual and can be a source of liability (NPUAP, EPUAP, PPPIA, 2014).

Similar to other types of pressure ulcers, decreasing device-related pressure ulcers involves early and frequent assessment, early identification, risk reduction, communication, collaboration, and education. The MHA website contains the most recently revised medical device–related pressure ulcer prevention guidance document used by Minnesota hospitals (MHA, 2010, 2011). Table 8-4 presents interventions and considerations for all devices and by specific devices for preventing device-related pressure ulcers. Examples of gap analysis for respiratory devices and cervical collars can be found in Appendix A.

BOX 8-3   Risk Factors Associated with Medical Device–Related Pressure Ulcers

• Sensory deficit and inability to communicate pain or "strap too tight"
• Edema near the device
• Inadequate equipment selection and/or fitting
• Inadequate positioning and stabilization of device
• Lack of routine skin inspection under and around the device
• Impaired perfusion to the area of the skin associated with the device

Compiled from Apold and Rydrych, 2012; Black et al, 2010; Boesch et al, 2012; Jaul, 2011; Mulgrew et al, 2011; NPUAP, EPUAP, PPPIA, 2014; Ong et al, 2011; Schlüer et al, 2009; Van Gilder et al, 2009.

Provide Patient and Family Education

Individuals with or at risk for pressure ulcers and their families should be given information about pressure ulcer prevention and management as part of their routine care. Yet research shows that even general education is lacking (Brace and Schubart, 2010; Hartigan et al, 2012). Formal programs for patient and family education in pressure ulcer prevention are critical to reduce the incidence of pressure ulcers in any care setting. Formal programs for patients with a spinal cord injury are common in rehabilitation centers and could serve as a model for similar educational programs for patients with any chronic

TABLE 8-4	**Prevention of Medical Device–Related Pressure Ulcers**
Device	**Preventive Interventions**
All	Consider individuals with medical devices to be at risk for pressure ulcer development
	Select medical devices that induce the least amount of skin damage
	Ensure correct size and fit to avoid excessive pressure
	Apply according to manufacturer's specifications*
	Ensure that medical devices are sufficiently secured to prevent dislodgement
	Inspect the skin under and around medical devices at least twice daily and more frequently in the presence of fluid shifts and/or signs of localized/generalized edema
	Rotate or reposition medical devices when possible
	Avoid positioning the individual directly onto medical devices
	Reposition the individual and/or the medical device to redistribute pressure and decrease shear forces
	Remove as soon as medically feasible
	Keep skin under devices clean and dry
	If indicated, choose a prophylactic dressing that isn't too thick, tight, or layered; is user friendly; manages moisture; and allows for routine skin inspection
Nasogastric tube	Consider commercial stabilizers to facilitate easier repositioning and inspection than possible with tape
	Proper application of stabilizers to keep clamp from touching skin
	Use skin sealants and commercial feeding tube stabilizer to prevent accidental dislodgment
	Change stabilizer every other day; sooner if loose or leaking
	Document skin condition with site care
Oxygen mask	Consult with respiratory therapist for proper sizing and fitting
	Refitting may be indicated as edema changes
	Consider alternative masks such as full-face masks or masks with gel borders for select patients
	Apply minimal tension to mask strap required to create adequate seal
	Add skin checks under respiratory equipment to respiratory therapist worklists or documentation
Nasal oxygen	Use commercially available nasal cannula with soft tubing
	Use commercially available foam ear protectors that are preattached or can be attached to tubing
Endotracheal tube	Combine endotracheal tube site care and inspection with oral care
	Reposition tube to different locations in mouth while ensuring depth of tube is unchanged
	Consider commercial stabilizers instead of tape to facilitate easier repositioning and inspection
	Proper application of stabilizers to keep clamp from touching mouth
Removable splint/ protector/brace	Consult physical therapist/occupational therapist for proper selection, sizing, fitting
	Keep manufacturer's application instructions accessible
	Keep schedule accessible; if not available, ask for one
	Add device removal twice per day for skin inspection to documentation
Collar	Consult with orthotics for proper sizing and fitting
	Palpate for skin changes within hairline
	Use collars that cause lower levels of mandibular and occipital pressure
Tracheostomy straps	Use commercially available foam/collar-type adjustable straps instead of ties or twill tape for comfort, pressure redistribution, and easy adjustment and to prevent inadvertent extubation

*Note: Failure to follow the manufacturer's application instruction can result in harm (e.g., skin damage) to the individual and can be a source of liability.
Compiled from Apold and Rydrych, 2012; Boesch et al, 2012; Huang, 2009; Iwai et al, 2011; NPUAP, EPUAP, PPPIA, 2014; Weng, 2008.

disease that limits mobility as the disease progresses (e.g., multiple sclerosis, terminal conditions). Such education assists the patient and caregivers to better understand why repositioning should not be delayed even when the patient "just got comfortable" or "just got to sleep." Patients and family can be empowered as advocates by reminding staff of the repositioning schedule. Patient education related to pressure ulcer prevention should include at-risk factors, skin inspection, repositioning schedule in the bed and the chair, support surfaces, and nutrition (NPUAP, EPUAP, PPPIA, 2014). Sample patient education tools are available on the NPUAP website and in the AHRQ pressure ulcer prevention tool kit.

A variety of teaching methods should be available to accommodate a variety of learning needs. Knowledge has been reported to increase with multiple methods such as printed materials, e-learning, and Internet resources (Brace and Schubart, 2010; Hartigan et al, 2012). Educational materials for patients must be at an appropriate reading level and be evaluated for design features such as organization, writing style, appeal, and appearance (Wilson and Williams, 2003; WOCN®, 2010). It may be helpful to request that caregivers come to the hospital to work with a nurse to learn techniques of care before the patient's discharge.

Both the WOCN® Society position statement and the CMS definition for unavoidable pressure ulcers emphasize the importance of preventive interventions that are consistent with the patient's needs and goals: caregivers must respect *informed* choices of individuals who decline interventions (WOCN®, 2009). For example, a patient facing the end of life may decline an intervention such as tube feeding to optimize nutrition. In this case, if a pressure ulcer developed, documentation of patient education and response could be sufficient to demonstrate *informed* refusal of care and thereby the pressure ulcer deemed to be unavoidable. Chapter 29 provides important factors to consider before documenting informed refusal of care.

CREATING INFRASTRUCTURE TO SUSTAIN THE PUPP

Creating the best-practice bundle for pressure ulcer prevention is only the first step of a PUPP. As mentioned, for a PUPP to be successful, the bundle must be integrated into the culture and infrastructure of the health care system. However, many hurdles have been identified that threaten the implementation and utilization of a PUPP. Even when a PUPP is implemented, time has shown that a PUPP is difficult to sustain. Because pressure ulcers are a complex, multifactorial problem, a holistic view of the hospital system and a change in culture are required to reduce incidence. Common gaps include lack of accountability and staff education, inadequate documentation and decision-making tools, absence of physician and other clinical care team involvement (i.e., nursing assistants, respiratory therapists, etc.), inconsistent communication of risk, and inadequate outcomes measures (Cranney et al, 2001; Krishnagopalan et al, 2002; Soban et al, 2011; Stechmiller, 2012). All caregivers and administration must share the belief that pressure ulcers are a negative outcome and that all health care providers play a role in protecting the patient from this adverse event. Implementation of a vital and enduring PUPP requires participation and oversight by management and critical scrutiny of the system's operations. The PUPP must become integrated into the day-to-day operations at the unit and systems level so that it is embedded into the infrastructure of education, documentation, decision making, and communication and handoffs (IHI, 2008). The MHA (2007) developed a roadmap for Minnesota hospitals (available on the Internet) that emphasizes these organizational components. More recently, international guidelines provided evidence for many organizational-level recommendations (NPUAP, EPUAP, PPPIA, 2014). Checklist 8-5 provides a summarized list of those recommendations, which are further described with examples in the following section. Appendix A contains examples of polices, algorithms, gap analysis, and other tools designed to assist with the process.

PUPP Team

Pressure ulcer prevention is not exclusively under the control of nurses (Jacobson et al, 2008; Padula et al, 2008). A multidisciplinary team (described in Chapter 1) is necessary to accommodate the increasing complexity of patients at risk for pressure ulcers, as well as the ever-changing amount of literature and guidelines that precipitate needed changes in policy, materials and equipment distribution, and staff education. In addition, making a sustainable change in the incidence of pressure ulcers requires a change in the culture of the organization such that the top administrators are monitoring process and outcomes data and allocating resources (e.g., staffing and time) to maintain the PUPP (Reinertsen et al, 2008). One measure of the extent of administrative support of the PUPP is the appointment of a system-wide leader or coordinator of the PUPP who has designated accountability and time for program implementation and maintenance. The PUPP coordinator should meet certain requirements for the position, primarily expertise in wound care.

Documentation

A key part of maintaining program infrastructure is providing a specific location in the medical record to document assessments and interventions relative to skin care, pressure prevention, and pressure ulcer management. To facilitate accurate documentation, flow sheets with descriptor choices should be used rather than a narrative or progress note so that staff is prompted for documentation parameters and the form is completed in its entirety. This will also provide uniformity in the use of terms so that data collection for monitoring, auditing, and trending will be expedited. The documentation forms should include risk assessment terms and definitions with subscale and total scores, skin inspection terms (intact, within defined limits, and terms to describe deviations), wound assessment parameters, offloading and positioning options, continence care, nutrition, and device removal.

Documentation should record when interventions are performed or omitted (with rationale) and when instructions are given to patients and their response. Documentation of repositioning should specify the body position in which the patient was left (back, left, or right) and the patient's tolerance (e.g., condition of offloaded bony prominence) (NPUAP, EPUAP, PPPIA, 2014). With such clarity and consistency in documentation, the risk of litigation is decreased should an adverse event occur (Brown, 2006). Frequency of documentation will vary by type of facility and the patient's overall condition. Checklist 8-6 includes items that should be documented, including those for which a designated space would facilitate ease, accuracy, and compliance.

Patient Handoffs

The frequency with which patients are harmed as a result of problematic "handoffs" is unknown, yet care plan communication lapses at the time of patient handoffs are common (Kitch et al, 2008). The Joint Commission (2008) states that an organization must define, communicate to staff, and implement a process in which information about patient care is communicated in a consistent manner. Therefore any handoff communications should include relevant information about the patient's risk of developing a pressure ulcer or the treatment and status of any existing pressure ulcers.

CHECKLIST 8-5   **Pressure Ulcer Prevention: Organizational Responsibilities**

✓ Assess knowledge and attitudes of professional staff regularly

✓ Develop an education policy for pressure ulcer prevention at an organizational level

✓ Provide regular evidence-based pressure ulcer prevention education

✓ Tailor training/education on pressure ulcer prevention to the needs of health care team members and the organization

✓ Utilize interactive/innovative learning for design/implementation of education program

✓ Evaluate learning outcomes before and after implementing education program

✓ Consider incorporating the following components:
  - Etiology and risk factors
  - NPUAP/EPUAP classification and differential diagnosis
  - Risk and skin assessment
  - Documentation of risk assessment and a preventive care plan
  - Support surfaces selection
  - Repositioning, including manual handling and use of equipment
  - Nutrition
  - Importance of an interprofessional approach
  - Patient and caregiver education

✓ Review quality, availability, ease of access, and protocols for timely implementation of equipment such as support surfaces and nutritional supplements

✓ Review/select medical devices based on ability to induce the least degree of skin damage

✓ Assess staffing characteristics (e.g., nursing care hours, qualifications of staff) and staff cohesion

✓ Use appropriate quality indicators and provide transparency:
  - Introduce an electronic system to report and track pressure ulcers
  - Conduct regular monitoring of facility-acquired pressure ulcer rates
  - Regularly inform staff members, patients, and caregivers of pressure ulcer rates

✓ Consider optimizing work procedures at a professional level:
  - Role models or designated wound care "champions"
  - Nurse-led quality improvement programs
  - Cues to perform pressure ulcer prevention

✓ Consider optimizing work procedures through the introduction of:
  - An awareness campaign
  - Standardized documentation
  - Standardized repositioning regimens (where the individual's needs will be met)
  - Multidisciplinary meetings
  - Onsite consultations
  - Computerized algorithm for selection of care strategies

CHECKLIST 8-6   **Pressure Ulcer Prevention Documentation**

✓ Pressure ulcer risk: Baseline and reassessments
✓ Skin inspection: Baseline and reassessments
✓ Routine device removal
✓ Plan of care and patient response
✓ Ongoing patient/family teaching
✓ Floating heels
✓ Repositioning frequency and position (right side, left side, etc.)
✓ Head-of-bed position
✓ Type of support surface
✓ Application of incontinent devices and barriers
✓ Nutritional supplements
✓ Tube site care
✓ Relevant consultations

A standardized process for handoffs reinforces to staff the importance of pressure ulcer prevention and facilitates consistency throughout the organization. For example, a posted turning schedule can serve as a reminder to the nurse or caregiver, as well as any other health care provider who enters the patient's room, of the time to turn a patient and the position to use (Figure 8-2).

Handoff communications between similar units for patients at high risk or with actual or potential pressure ulcers should include the following:

- Time and results of recent pressure ulcer risk assessment
- Time and results of recent skin inspection

- Location and stages of pressure ulcers
- Time of last wound assessment and dressing change
- Current offloading device(s)
- Time and position last placed
- Toleration of repositioning frequency

Handoffs from the patient care unit to another department (e.g., radiology department, OR) also necessitate communications concerning the patient's skin status and pressure ulcer risk. In particular, the staff of the receiving department should be made aware of the location and severity of any existing pressure ulcer, any positions that should be avoided, and the need for offloading (especially heels and sacrum). Appendix A provides an example of an interdepartmental handoff communication tool.

The concept of handoffs is also applicable to the transferring of the patient out of the facility at discharge. Accurate and thorough documentation is critical for continuity of care. In addition to the items listed earlier, the handoff communication should include pressure ulcer risk score, current plan of care for pressure ulcer prevention, the patient's individual response to the plan of care, and pain.

Formularies and Decision-Making Tools

A significant and valuable contribution the wound specialist can bring to any facility and any PUPP is to standardize and organize products available within his or her health care system. To bring order to the utilization of these products and

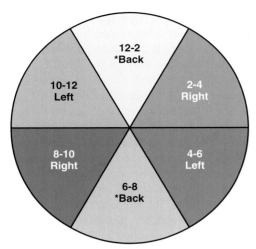

FIGURE 8-2 Example of a turning schedule. *Consider omitting from schedule for patients that are already supine during activities throughout the day.

enhance the quality of care provided, decision-making tools are used to facilitate the accuracy and efficiency of decision making, guide treatment selection, and educate the clinician concerning a particular disease entity. Annual review of these tools is recommended because changes in the pathophysiology of pressure ulcers and product research and development are ongoing and quickly paced. Decision-making tools must use language that is consistent with policies, procedures, documentation, supply order menus, and current contracts for products. If any of these factors change, revisions are necessary to keep the tools accurate and user friendly. Examples of decision-making tools include interventions based on risk factors (see Table 8-2), support surface selection (see Table 9-1), and formularies for skin care products (see Table 5-4 and throughout textbook) and wound care dressings (see Chapters 5, 16, 18, 31, and 37).

Investing in Technology

Access to, and utilization of, appropriate technology involves not only patient care items (e.g., support surfaces or devices), but also medical record documentation so that information is complete and readily available at all times. In creating the documentation system, skin care, risk assessment, nutritional assessment, and the other critical elements of a best-practice bundle must be incorporated, which requires direct input of the certified wound specialist. As technological advances in existing PUPP tools, such as support surfaces, transferring devices, and heel offloading devices, occur, the advantages of these products should be methodically reviewed by the wound specialist and presented to the PUPP team members for discussion. Similarly, the team should have a mechanism for keeping abreast of new developments in technology that may improve efficiency and reliability of interventions and the PUPP and ultimately reduce the patient's risk of pressure ulcers.

Staff Education and Competencies

All health care personnel providing care to the patient must appreciate the role they have in pressure ulcer prevention. In addition, it should not be assumed that the formal curriculum of the registered nurse, nurse practitioner, physician, physician assistant, physical therapist, and occupational therapist adequately incorporated pressure ulcer prevention and management (Magnan and Maklebust, 2008; Maklebust et al, 2005; Odierna and Zeleznik, 2003). To keep the PUPP infrastructure strong, pressure ulcer education (including how to document) should be included in new employee orientation and annual competencies for nurses and nursing assistants. The content of the education is based on the scope of practice for the position. For example, the registered nurse should minimally demonstrate competency related to pressure ulcer etiology, skin inspection, risk assessment, wound assessment, and implementation of a full range of appropriate interventions to minimize or eliminate risk factors (WOCN®, 2010). Nursing assistants may require education and competency related to monitoring the skin, reporting changes to the nurse, continence skin care, importance of nutrition, and appropriate positioning. To keep pace with the rapid changes in the science of pressure ulcer prevention and treatment, the health professional's knowledge and skills require routine and frequent updating through annual programs, at a minimum.

Staff Accountability/Ownership

Corporate culture must convey that facility-acquired pressure ulcers are no longer tolerable or "acceptable" unless documentation indicates the pressure ulcer was unavoidable. Although it is important to encourage employees to "self-report," they still must be held accountable for any errors. Just as it is unhealthy to create a punitive environment where employees are fearful of admitting errors, so, too, is it unhealthy to create an environment of toleration of less than best practices, which can lead to errors and complications such as pressure ulcers. Expectations for employees to meet this standard need to be communicated during orientation and annual education and through activities that encourage transparency and sharing of experiences (both successful and unsuccessful) and knowledge. Examples of methods for improving accountability for pressure ulcers are given in Box 8-4. Conducting good quality interdisciplinary, nonpunitive and timely root-cause analysis (RCA) is critical for staff accountability, ownership, education, and problem solving. Many facilities have found the NPUAP RCA template useful in their efforts to conduct quality RCAs (available at npuap.org).

Quality Tracking and Evaluation

Once a program as extensive and system-wide as the PUPP is implemented, feedback is needed that comes from routine measurements and quality tracking. Such feedback provides the affirmation participants need to reinforce the value of their efforts and investment in the program. Routine measurements and quality tracking will also identify areas for improvement. Once a plan for reducing or eliminating

BOX 8-4 **Improving Staff Accountability for Pressure Ulcer Prevention**

1. Implement use of NPUAP pressure ulcer root cause analysis (RCA) template available online at http://www.npuap.org
2. Arrange time for involved staff members to participate in relevant RCA
3. Create newsletters, blogs, and e-mails that share experiences and knowledge gained
4. Post commitment statements on units or in patients' rooms informing patients and families that they can expect to be repositioned and that it is okay to ask to be repositioned
5. Audit compliance with pressure ulcer preventive interventions (similar to handwashing audits)
6. Post dashboards on units sharing nosocomial rates with staff and visitors
7. Have celebrations (with treats) when facility-acquired pressure ulcer rates drop
8. Provide reviews that evaluate individual performance with pressure ulcer prevention audits, attendance and participation with relevant RCAs, unit-specific skin care initiatives, and prevalence/incidence studies

pressure is developed and the plan is implemented, the effectiveness of the intervention (turning, support surface) should be evaluated at regular intervals. Daily skin inspection should provide the information needed to determine whether the PUPP is sufficient or requires modification. As a general rule, resolution of the intensity of erythema, if present, should become apparent within 24 hours of placement upon a support surface. A patient's risk for pressure ulcer formation will vary as his or her overall condition changes; therefore routine and regular reassessment and modification of the plan of care are warranted.

Quality tracking of the PUPP should include (1) concurrent 24/7 self-reporting of nosocomial pressure ulcers, (2) process measures, and (3) outcome measures. Concurrent daily reporting of nosocomial pressure ulcers for all patients is perhaps a more important measure than are quarterly or annual incidence studies. A simple 24/7 mechanism for staff to report nosocomial pressure ulcers through quality tracking (e.g., event reports, incident reports) leads to more accurate reporting of facility-acquired pressure ulcers, more timely RCA and action plans, and early identification of weakening infrastructure. For example, a rise in the number of pressure ulcers secondary to oxygen masks may have resulted from a contract change to an inferior mask. Concurrent reporting of nosocomial pressure ulcers can uncover the problem quickly so that disciplines can unite, identify the root cause, and correct the problem quickly before more patients are injured. Conversely, a facility-wide incidence that is not reported daily cannot lead to problem resolution and pressure ulcer reduction as quickly. With an average length of stay in acute care of just a few days, countless patients are missed with such infrequent incidence studies.

Process measures capture compliance with designated components of the PUPP, for example, pressure ulcer risk assessment within 8 hours of admission, skin inspection upon admission, or daily risk assessments of "at-risk" patients. The value of process measures is heightened when correlated with concurrent self-reports. This will also be beneficial when targeting staff education.

The key outcome measure of a PUPP is the incidence of pressure ulcers and can be tabulated to reflect unit-based incidence or system-wide incidence. Pressure ulcer incidence can be obtained once yearly and compared with concurrent daily self-reporting data to essentially validate the accuracy of self-reported numbers. However, these kinds of incidence calculations cannot be considered reliable data collection for mandated public reporting. Pressure ulcer incidence can be calculated and reported in many ways, which contributes to the confusion and the wide range of data when comparisons to other facilities are attempted. To be most relevant, incidence should be reported as pressure ulcers per 100 admits or pressure ulcers per 1000 patient-days (IHI, 2008).

CLINICAL CONSULT

A: Received referral for management of a suspected deep tissue injury (sDTI) pressure ulcer on the left foot of 46-year-old Caucasian gentleman with type 2 diabetes, chronic kidney disease, and peripheral arterial disease admitted for congestive heart failure. Electronic medical record contains a photo of a dark-purple, intact lesion. Unable to discern exact location of lesion on foot by photo. Nurses consulted the dietician, placed patient on a low air loss support surface, and documented consistent repositioning and floating his heels off of the bed with use of pillows under the legs. Patient denies pain in the foot or awareness of the lesions. He is up at pleasure and walking out of the bathroom. Visibly short of breath on 2 liters of O_2 per nasal cannula; pulse oximetry 92%. Wound assessment reveals a generalized reticulate purple discoloration encompassing 4 × 4 cm on the lateral dorsal surface of the left foot. Epidermis is intact and nonblanchable. Periwound skin is intact, has no edema, and no local signs of infection. Lower extremities pulses palpable but diminished.
D: Overall assessment is not consistent with a pressure ulcer. Risk factors, patient history, distribution of lesion, and the appearance of the extremity are consistent with an arterial pathology.
P: Protect left foot from pressure and trauma to prevent break in skin integrity. Assess perfusion and circulation of lower extremity.
I: Nurse and patient understand and agree with the following plan of care: (1) Collaborate with primary care provider for further evaluation of vascular status. (2) Offloading: replace low air loss with standard pressure ulcer prevention static mattress to improve patient comfort and facilitate mobility and safety. Continue repositioning and floating heels while in bed. (3) Use appropriate footwear when up to protect from trauma. (4) Apply moisturizers daily to prevent skin dryness and maintain skin integrity. Topical dressing not indicted at this time. (5) Monitor lower extremities and lesion; notify provider for increased discoloration and size, pain, or change in temperature of extremity.
E: Will follow up to evaluate/monitor effectiveness and adapt plan as needed.

SUMMARY

Pressure ulcers are a global health concern because, for the most part, they are a costly *preventable* complication. As a consequence of unrelieved pressure, capillaries are occluded and tissue damage ensues, and the extent of tissue damage is influenced by numerous variables. Pressure ulcer prevention requires a comprehensive interdisciplinary plan that includes risk assessment; regular and routine skin assessment; reducing risk factors; patient, family, and staff education; and evaluation. Ongoing maintenance of program infrastructure is critical to sustain a low incidence of pressure ulcers. This is accomplished through (1) embedding education into patient education tools, staff orientation, and annual competencies; (2) ensuring thorough and user-friendly documentation methods and decision-making tools; (3) concurrent and reliable quality tracking; and (4) a team approach with safe handoffs and communication across settings.

REFERENCES

Agency for Healthcare Research and Quality (AHRQ): Preventing pressure ulcers in hospitals: a toolkit for improving quality of care, Rockville, MD, April 2011, AHRQ. http://www.ahrq.gov/professionals/systems/long-term-care/resources/pressure-ulcers/pressureulcertoolkit/putool1.html. Accessed Feb 8, 2014.

Alterescu V: Reflections upon the history and future of the IAET, *J ET Nurs* 18(4):126–131, 1991.

Apold J, Rydrych D: Preventing device related pressure ulcers. Using data to guide statewide change, *J Nurs Care Qual* 27(1):28–34, 2012.

Association of periOperative Registered Nurses (AORN): Recommended practices for positioning the patient in the perioperative practice setting. In *Perioperative standards and recommended practices*, Denver, CO, 2012, AORN, pp 421–444.

Aronovitch SA: Intraoperatively acquired pressure ulcers: are there common risk factors? *Ostomy Wound Manage* 53(2):57–69, 2007.

Baharestani MM, Ratliff CR: Pressure ulcers in neonates and children: an NPUAP white paper, *Adv Skin Wound Care* 20:208, 2007.

Baumgarten M, Margolis D, van Doorn C, et al: Black/white differences in pressure ulcer incidence in nursing home residents, *J Am Geriatr Soc* 52:1293–1298, 2004.

Bergquist-Beringer SB, Byron GJ, Davidson J: Pressure ulcer prevalence and incidence: report from the National Database of Nursing Quality Indicators (NDNQI). In Pieper B, editor (with the National Pressure Ulcer Advisory Panel [NPUAP]): *Pressure ulcers: prevalence, incidence, and implications for the future*, Washington, DC, 2012, NPUAP, pp 175–180.

Bergstrom N, Horn SD, Smout RJ, et al: The National Pressure Ulcer Long-Term Care Study: outcomes of pressure ulcer treatments in long-term care, *J Am Geriatr Soc* 53(10):1721–1729, 2005.

Black JM, Cuddigan JE, Walko MA, et al: Medical device related pressure ulcers in hospitalized patients, *Int Wound J* 7:358–365, 2010.

Black JM, Edsberg LE, Baharestani MM, et al: Pressure ulcers: avoidable or unavoidable? Results of the National Pressure Ulcer Advisory Panel Consensus Conference (NPUAP), *Ostomy Wound Manage* 57(2):24–37, 2011.

Boesch RP, Myers C, Garrett T, et al: Prevention of trache ostomy related pressure ulcers in children, *Pediatrics* 129(3):792–797, 2012.

Bolton L: Which pressure ulcer risk assessment scales are valid for use in the clinical setting? *J Wound Ostomy Continence Nurs* 34:368–381, 2007.

Brace JA, Schubart JR: A prospective evaluation of a pressure ulcer prevention and management e-learning program for adults with spinal cord injury, *Ostomy Wound Manage* 56(8):40–50, 2010.

Brem H, Maggi J, Nierman D, et al: High cost of stage IV pressure ulcers, *Am J Surg* 200(4):473–477, 2010.

Brindle CT: Turning and repositioning the critically ill patient with hemodynamic instability: a literature review and consensus recommendations, *J Wound Ostomy Continence Nurs* 40(3):254–267, 2013.

Brown G: Wound documentation: managing risk, *Adv Skin Wound Care* 19(3):155–165, 2006.

Bryant R, Shannon ML, Pieper B, et al: Pressure ulcer prevention and management. In Bryant R, editor: *Acute and chronic wounds: nursing management*, St. Louis, MO, 1992, Mosby, pp 105-163.

Cadue JF, Karloweicz S, Tardy C, et al: Prevention of pressure sores with a foam-body support device. A randomized control trial in a medical intensive care unit, *Presse Med* 37(1):30–36, 2008.

Choi J, Tasota FJ, Hoffman LA: Mobility interventions to improve outcomes in patients undergoing prolonged mechanical ventilation: a review of literature, *Biol Res Nurs* 10(1):21–33, 2008.

Chung CHK, Lau MCH, Leung TYC, et al: Effect of head elevation on sacral and ischial tuberosities pressure in infirmary patients, *Asian J Gerontol Geriatr* 7(2):101–106, 2012.

Cranney M, Warren E, Barton S, et al: Why do GPs not implement evidence-based guidelines? A descriptive study, *Fam Pract* 18:359–363, 2001.

Defloor T, de Schuijmer JD: Preventing pressure ulcers: an evaluation of four operating-table mattresses, *Appl Nurs Res* 13:134–141, 2000.

Defloor T, De Bacquer DD, Grypdonck MHF: The effect of various combinations of turning and pressure reducing devices on the incidence of pressure ulcers, *Int J Nurs Stud* 42:37–46, 2005.

Donnelly J, Winder J, Kernahan WG, et al: An RCT to determine the effect of a heel elevation device in pressure ulcer prevention post hip fracture, *J Wound Care* 20(7):309–318, 2011.

Duncan KD: Preventing pressure ulcers: the goal is zero, *Jt Comm J Qual Patient Saf* 33(10):605–610, 2007.

Elliott R, McKinley S, Fox V: Quality improvement program to reduce the prevalence of pressure ulcers in an intensive care unit, *Am J Crit Care* 17(4):328–334, 2008.

Fry DE, Pine M, Jones BL, et al: Patient characteristics and the occurrence of never events, *Arch Surg* 145(2):151–152, 2010.

Gadd MM: Braden scale cumulative score versus subscale scores: are we missing opportunities for pressure ulcer prevention? *J Wound Ostomy Continence Nurs* 41(1):86–89, 2014.

Ganos D, Siddiqui A: Pressure ulcers in the operating room. In Pieper B, editor (with the National Pressure Ulcer Advisory Panel [NPUAP]): *Pressure ulcers: prevalence, incidence, and implications for the future*, Washington, DC, 2012, NPUAP, pp 57–63.

García-Fernández FP, Pancorbo-Hidalgo PL, Soldevilla Agreda JJ: Predictive capacity of risk assessment scales and clinical judgment for pressure ulcers: a meta-analysis, *J Wound Ostomy Continence Nurs* 41(1):1–11, 2014.

Gefen A: How much time does it take to get a pressure ulcer? Integrated evidence from human, animal, and in vitro studies, *Ostomy Wound Manage* 54(10):26–28, 30–35, 2008.

Gilcreast DM, Warren JB, Yoder LH, et al: Research comparing three heel ulcer-prevention devices, *J Wound Ostomy Continence Nurs* 32(2):112–120, 2005.

Goode PS: Pressure ulcer prevention and early treatment, *J ET Nurs* 18(5):149–150, 1991.

Hartigan I, Murphy S, Hickey M: Older adults' knowledge of pressure ulcer prevention: a prospective quasi-experimental study, *Int J Older People Nurs* 7:208–218, 2012.

Haugen V, Pechacek J, Maher T, et al: Decreasing pressure ulcer risk during hospital procedures: a rapid process improvement workshop, *J Wound Ostomy Continence Nurs* 38(2):155–159, 2011.

Huang TT, Tseng CE, Lee TM, et al: Preventing pressure sores of the nasal ala after nasotracheal tube intubation: from animal model to clinical application, *J Oral Maxillofac Surg* 67: 543–551, 2009.

Institute for Healthcare Improvement (IHI): *5 Million Lives Campaign. Getting started kit: prevent pressure ulcers*, Cambridge, MA, 2008, IHI.

International Association for Enterostomal Therapy (IAET): *Standards of care. Dermal wounds: pressure ulcers*, Santa Ana, CA, 1987, IAET.

Iwai T, Goto T, Maegawa J, et al: Use of a hydrocolloid dressing to prevent nasal pressure sores after nasotracheal intubation, *Br J Oral Maxillofac Surg* 49:e65–e66, 2011.

Jacobson TM, Tescher AN, Miers AG, et al: Improving practice: efforts to reduce occipital pressure ulcers, *J Nurse Care Qual* 23(3):283–288, 2008.

Jaul E: A prospective pilot study of atypical pressure ulcer presentation in a skilled geriatric unit, *Ostomy Wound Manage* 57(2):49–54, 2011.

Kitch BT, Cooper JB, Zapol WM, et al: Handoffs causing patient harm: a survey of medical and surgical house staff, *Jt Comm J Qual Patient Saf* 34(10):563–570, 2008.

Kosiak M: Etiology of decubitus ulcers, *Arch Phys Med Rehabil* 42:19–29, 1961.

Krishnagopalan S, Johnson EW, Low LL, et al: Body positioning of intensive care patients: clinical practice versus standards, *Crit Care Med* 30(11):2588–2592, 2002.

Lyder CH, Ayello EA: Pressure ulcers: a patient safety issue. In Hughes RG: *Patient safety and quality: an evidence-based handbook for nurses* (Publication No. 08-0043), Rockville, MD, April 2008, Agency for Healthcare Research and Quality. http://www.ncbi.nlm.nih.gov/books/NBK2650. Accessed Feb 8, 2014.

Magnan MA, Maklebust J: The effect of web-based Braden scale training on the reliability and precision of Braden scale pressure ulcer risk assessments, *J Wound Ostomy Continence Nurs* 35(2):199–208, 2008.

Maklebust J, Magnan MA: A quasi-experimental study to assess the effect of technology-assisted training on correct endorsement of pressure ulcer preventive interventions, *Ostomy Wound Manage* 55(2):32–42, 2009.

Maklebust J, Sieggreen MY, Sidor D, et al: Computer-based testing of the Braden scale for predicting pressure sore risk, *Ostomy Wound Manage* 51(4):40–52, 2005.

Mayrovitz HN, Sims N: Effects of support surface relief pressures on heel skin blood flow in persons with and without diabetes mellitus, *Adv Skin Wound Care* 17:197–201, 2004.

Messer M: PU risk in ancillary services, *J Wound Ostomy Continence Nurs* 37(2):153–158, 2010.

Minnesota Department of Health: *Adverse health events in Minnesota 2014* (Tenth annual public report), 2014. http://www.health.state.mn.us/patientsafety/ae/2014ahereport.pdf. Accessed Feb 8, 2014.

Minnesota Hospital Association (MHA): *Device-related pressure ulcer prevention – cervical collar recommendations and guidance*, April 2010. http://www.mnhospitals.org/pressure-ulcers. Accessed Feb 8, 2014.

Minnesota Hospital Association (MHA): *Device-related pressure ulcer prevention – respiratory devices. Recommendations and guidance*, February 3, 2011. http://www.mnhospitals.org/pressure-ulcers. Accessed Feb 8, 2014.

Minnesota Hospital Association (MHA): *Roadmap SAFE SKIN*, created 2007, updated 2011. http://www.mnhospitals.org/pressure-ulcers. Accessed Nov 11, 2014.

Minnesota Hospital Association (MHA): *Pressure ulcer prevention in the O.R. Recommendations and guidance*, March 2013. http://www.mnhospitals.org/Portals/0/Documents/ptsafety/skin/OR-pressure-ulcer-recommendations.pdf. Accessed Feb 8, 2014.

Mulgrew S, Khoo A, Newton RM, et al: Pressure necrosis secondary to negative pressure dressing, *Ann R Coll Surg Engl* 93(5): e27–e28, 2011.

National Pressure Ulcer Advisory Panel (NPUAP): *Mucosal pressure ulcers: an NPUAP position statement*, 2009. http://www.npuap.org/Mucosal_Pressure_Ulcer_Position_Statement_final.pdf. Accessed April 27, 2010.

National Pressure Ulcer Advisory Panel (NPUAP), European Pressure Ulcer Advisory Panel (EPUAP): *Prevention and treatment of pressure ulcers: clinical practice guideline*, Washington, DC, 2009, NPUAP.

National Pressure Ulcer Advisory Panel (NPUAP), European Pressure Ulcer Advisory Panel (EPUAP), Pan Pacific Pressure Injury Alliance (PPPIA): Haesler E, editor: *Prevention and treatment of pressure ulcers: clinical practice guideline*, Perth, Australia, 2014, Cambridge Media.

National Priorities Partnership: *National priorities and goals for healthcare reform (Executive summary)*, 2008. http://www.nationalprioritiespartnership.org/PriorityDetails. Accessed Feb 10, 2014.

O'Connor ED, Walsham J: Should we mobilise critically ill patients? A review, *Crit Care Resusc* 11(4):290–300, 2009.

Odierna E, Zeleznik J: Pressure ulcer education: a pilot study of the knowledge and clinical confidence of geriatric fellows, *Adv Skin Wound Care* 16(1):26–30, 2003.

Ong JC, Chan FC, McCann J: Pressure ulcers of the popliteal fossae caused by thromboembolic deterrent stockings (TEDS), *Ir J Med Sci* 180(2):601–602, 2011.

Padula CA, Osborne E, Williams J: Prevention and early detection of pressure ulcers in hospitalized patients, *J Wound Ostomy Continence Nurs* 35(1):65–75, 2008.

Padula W, Mishra M, Makic M, et al: Improving quality of pressure ulcer care with prevention: a cost effective analysis, *Med Care* 49(4):385–392, 2011.

Paul C, Maumus-Robert S, Mazereeuw-Hautier J, et al: Prevalence and risk factors for xerosis in the elderly: a cross-sectional epidemiological study in primary care, *Dermatology* 223:260–265, 2011.

Powers J, Daniels D, McGuire C, et al: The incidence of skin breakdown associated with use of cervical collars, *J Trauma Nurs* 13(4):198–200, 2006.

Reddy M, Gill SS, Rochon PA: Preventing pressure ulcers: a systematic review, *JAMA* 296:974–984, 2006.

Reinertsen JL, Bisognano M, Pugh MD: *Seven leadership leverage points for organization-level improvement in health care*, ed 2 (IHI Innovation Series white paper), Cambridge, MA, 2008, Institute for Healthcare Improvement.

Rosen J, Mittal V, Degenholtz H, et al: Pressure ulcer prevention in black and white nursing home residents: a QI initiative of enhanced ability, incentives, and management feedback, *Adv Skin Wound Care* 19(5):262–268, 2006.

Schlüer AB, Cignacco E, Müller M, et al: The prevalence of pressure ulcers in four paediatric institutions, *J Clin Nurs* 18: 3244–3252, 2009.

Scott JR, Gibran NS, Engrav LH, et al: Incidence and characteristics of hospitalized patients with pressure ulcers: State of Washington, 1987 to 2000, *Plast Reconstr Surg* 117(2):630–634, 2006.

Shannon RJ, Coombs M, Chakravarthy D: Reducing hospital-acquired pressure ulcers with a silicone-based dermal nourishing emollient-associated skincare regimen, *Adv Skin Wound Care* 22(10):461–467, 2009.

Stechmiller JK: Changes in incidence and prevalence of pressure ulcers 2001-2011: innovations in prevention and treatment. In Pieper B, editor (with the National Pressure Ulcer Advisory Panel [NPUAP]): *Pressure ulcers: prevalence, incidence, and implications for the future*, Washington, DC, 2012, NPUAP, pp 227–230.

Soban LM, Hempel S, Munjas BA, et al: Preventing pressure ulcers in hospitals: a systematic review of nurse-focused quality improvement interventions, *Jt Comm J Qual Patient Saf* 37(6):245–252, 2011.

Stechmiller JK, Cowan L, Whitney JD, et al: Guidelines for the prevention of pressure ulcers, *Wound Repair Regen* 16:151–168, 2008.

The Joint Commission: *Hand-off communications*, December 9, 2008. http://www.centerfortransforminghealthcare.org/projects/detail.aspx?Project=1. Accessed Feb 10, 2014.

Thomas DR, Cote TR, Lawhorne L, et al: Understanding clinical dehydration and its treatment, *J Am Med Dir Assoc* 9(5): 292–301, 2008.

Torra i Bou JE, Segovia Gámez T, Verdú Soriano J, et al: The effectiveness of a hyperoxygenated fatty acid compound in preventing pressure ulcers, *J Wound Care* 14:117–121, 2005.

U.S. Department of Health and Human Services: *Healthy People 2010: understanding and improving health*, ed 2, Washington DC, 2000, U.S. Government Printing Office.

Vanderwee K, Clark M, Dealey C, et al: Pressure ulcer prevalence in Europe: a pilot study, *J Eval Clin Pract* 13(2):227–235, 2007.

Van Gilder C, Macfarlane GD, Meyer S: Results of nine international pressure ulcer prevalence surveys: 1989 to 2005, *Ostomy Wound Manage* 54(2):40–54, 2008.

Van Gilder C, Amlung S, Harrison P, et al: Results of the 2008-2009 International Pressure Ulcer Prevalence Survey and a 3-year, acute care, unit-specific analysis, *Ostomy Wound Manage* 55(11):39–45, 2009.

Vollman K: Introduction to progressive mobility, *Crit Care Nurse* 30:3–5, 2010.

Walton-Geer PS: Prevention of pressure ulcers in the surgical patient, *AORN J* 89(3):538–548, 2009.

Walsh J, Plonczynski D: Elevation of a protocol for prevention of facility-acquired heel pressure ulcers, *J Wound Ostomy Continence Nurs* 34(2):178–183, 2007.

Weng MH: The effect of protective treatment in reducing pressure ulcers for non-invasive ventilation patients, *Intensive Crit Care Nurs* 24(5):295–299, 2008.

Willock J, Harris C, Harrison J, et al: Identifying the characteristics of children with pressure ulcers, *Nurs Times* 101(11):40–43, 2005.

Wilson FL, Williams BN: Assessing the readability of skin care and pressure ulcer patient education materials, *J Wound Ostomy Continence Nurs* 30:224–230, 2003.

Winkelman C, Peereboom K: Staff-perceived barriers and facilitators, *Crit Care Nurse* 30:13–16, 2010.

Wong V, Stotts N, Hopf H, et al: How heel oxygenation changes under pressure, *Wound Repair Regen* 15:786–794, 2007.

Wound, Ostomy and Continence Nurses Society™ (WOCN®): *Inpatient prospective payment changes: a guide for the WOC nurse*, March 13, 2009a. http://www.wocn.org/news/news.asp?id=67092. Accessed Feb 10, 2014.

Wound, Ostomy and Continence Nurses Society™ (WOCN®): Position statement: avoidable versus unavoidable pressure ulcers, *J Wound Ostomy Continence Nurs* 36(4):378–381, 2009b.

Wound, Ostomy and Continence Nurses Society™ (WOCN®): *Guideline for prevention and management of pressure ulcers*, Glenview, IL, 2010, WOCN®.

Wright K: President's message: pressure ulcer prediction, prevention, and early treatment, *J ET Nurs* 18(4):115–116, 1991.

9

Support Surfaces

Denise P. Nix and Dianne M. Mackey

OBJECTIVES

1. List three limitations to the reliance of capillary-closing values for support surface evaluation.
2. List four factors to consider when interpreting the significance of interface tissue pressure readings.
3. Define pressure redistribution, immersion, and envelopment.

4. Explain the difference between a reactive and an active support surface.
5. Compare the advantages and disadvantages of support surface categories and features.
6. List factors to consider for appropriate selection of a support surface.

A support surface is a specialized device for pressure redistribution designed for the management of tissue loads (NPUAP, 2007). Depending on the composition of the support surface and its mechanism of action, additional therapeutic functions may include reduction of shear, friction, and moisture. Support surfaces are available in different sizes and shapes and are made for chairs and for horizontal surfaces, such as mattresses, examination and procedure tables, operating room (OR) surfaces, and, more recently, emergency and transport stretchers or gurneys.

Although there is insufficient evidence to specify a particular brand of support surface (NPUAP, EPUAP, PPPIA, 2014; Whitney et al, 2006; WOCN®, 2003, 2010), a variety of pressure-redistribution devices can help lower the incidence of pressure ulcers up to 60% (Cullum et al, 2004; Whitney et al 2006). This chapter reviews factors to consider for the (1) evaluation of support surfaces, (2) selection/evaluation of support surfaces based on individual patient assessment, and (3) creation/evaluation of a facility-wide or agency-wide support surface formulary. General guidance for the care of the patient requiring a support surface is given in Box 9-1.

INTERFACE TISSUE PRESSURES: PAST AND PRESENT

Interface tissue pressure is the force per unit area that acts perpendicularly between the body and the support surface and is measured by a sensor placed between the skin and support surface. This process is also known as *pressure mapping* (Figure 9-1). A review of 29 randomized controlled trials concluded that these measurements do not reliably predict

support surface performance (Cullum et al, 2004). However, pressure mapping continues to be used to (1) produce images for product literature that appear to show pressure redistribution, (2) compare measurements from the same patient on two different surfaces, (3) assist with adjusting inflation of a chair cushion, or (4) teach a chairbound patient what type of position change will decrease pressure over an ischial tuberosity. Box 9-2 summarizes factors to consider when reviewing literature that includes interface tissue pressures (Miller et al, 2013; Reger et al, 1988; WOCN®, 2003).

Historically, support surfaces have been categorized by comparing interface tissue pressure measurements obtained on a support surface to a standard capillary-closing value. Surfaces were then placed into categories called *pressure reduction* and *pressure relief* based on how close the interface tissue pressures were to the standard capillary-closing value; these terms are now considered invalid (NPUAP, 2007). However, because the concept of a standardized capillary-closing pressure is affected by many variables (see Box 9-2) and is unlikely to exist (Le et al, 1984), attempting to employ such a simplistic scheme to guide a process as complex as support surface selection is flawed. It is more useful to formulate a framework for support surface selection that is based on such traits as physical concepts, therapeutic functions, medium, forms, and features.

PHYSICAL CONCEPTS AND THERAPEUTIC FUNCTIONS

Physical concepts are performance-related terms used to provide standard discussions about how support surfaces perform (Christian and Lachenbruch, 2007). *Life expectancy*

BOX 9-1 General Guidance for Care of Patient Requiring a Support Surface

- Support surfaces alone neither prevent nor heal pressure ulcers and should be incorporated into a comprehensive individualized care plan.*
- Patient with or at risk* for pressure ulcers should be placed on a support surface rather than on a standard hospital mattress.
- Patient with or at risk* for pressure ulcers who sits should have a chair cushion and a sitting plan* that specifies frequency, duration, posture, and positioning needs.
- Support surfaces must be compatible with the care setting while meeting the individual needs of the patient.
- Support surfaces function best with minimal linens and pads under the patient.
- Patient must be able to assume a variety of positions on the selected surface (bed or chair) without bottoming out.
- When considering overlay use, it is important to assess risk for falls, entrapment, weight distribution, and potential for bottoming out.
- Patient should be turned and repositioned, regardless of support surface features.
- Multiple factors determine the frequency of repositioning* and must not be based solely on the features of the support surface.

- Use positioning devices and continence pads compatible with the support surface.
- A support surface that dissipates moisture (low air loss) may be indicated when moisture barriers, pouches, and dressings do not adequately protect the skin from moisture/incontinence.
- A reactive support surface with features and components such as low air loss, alternating pressure, or viscous or air fluids should be considered for patients who:
  - CANNOT be effectively positioned off their wound
  - Have pressure ulcers involving multiple turning surfaces
  - Have pressure ulcers that fail to improve despite optimal comprehensive management
- An active support surface (alternating pressure) should be considered when effective repositioning is determined by a provider to be medically contraindicated (frequent small shifts, reevaluation, and retrials at least every 8 hours should be documented).
- Always follow manufacturers' instructions for appropriate use, contraindications, and precautions (see also Checklist 9-2).

*See Chapter 8 for details.

FIGURE 9-1 Pressure-mapping device (XSensor pressure-mapping system). (Courtesy the ROHO Group, Belleville, IL.)

refers to the period of time during which a product is able to effectively fulfill its purpose. It may be affected by *fatigue* or a reduced capacity to perform due to intended or unintended use and/or prolonged exposure to chemical, thermal, or physical forces. These factors affect the ability of the support surface to redistribute pressure, control friction and shear, and manage the microclimate (temperature and humidity) of the surface (NPUAP, 2007).

Pressure Redistribution (Immersion and Envelopment)

Support surfaces are designed to prevent pressure ulcers and, through pressure redistribution, provide an environment more conducive to pressure ulcer healing. Support surfaces

---

BOX 9-2 Capillary-Closing and Interface Tissue Pressures

A *capillary-closing* pressure value should not be used to compare support surfaces for the following reasons:
- Capillary-closing values are based on measurements obtained from the fingertips of young, healthy males.
- Pressure is three to five times greater at the bone than at the surface of the skin.
- Lower capillary-closing pressures have been reported in older patients.
- Tissue interface pressures do not ensure that blood flow through the capillaries is unimpeded.

Interface tissue pressure measurements (pressure mapping) should be reported with the following disclosures:
- Population tested (healthy subjects will demonstrate lower pressure readings than debilitated subjects because normal muscle mass supports and distributes weight more effectively)
- How often equipment was recalibrated (sensors are fragile and may malfunction)
- Number of readings conducted per site (range based on multiple readings is more reliable than one single reading per site)
- Factors known to affect results:
  - Stiffness of support surface
  - Composition of body tissue
  - Transducer size and shape
  - Method of equilibrium detection
  - Uniformity of measurement technique
  - Load shape and its interaction with support material
  - Skill of person taking measurements (uniformity of technique for measuring interface tissue pressure is necessary for accuracy)

redistribute interface pressure by conforming to the contours of the body so that pressure is redistributed over a larger surface area rather than concentrated on a more circumscribed location. The therapeutic function of pressure redistribution is accomplished through immersion and envelopment. *Immersion* refers to the depth of penetration or sinking into the surface, allowing the pressure to be spread out over the surrounding area rather than directly over a bony prominence. Immersion is dependent on factors such as the stiffness and thickness of the support surface and the flexibility of the cover. *Envelopment* refers to the ability of the support surface to conform to irregularities (e.g., clothing, bedding, bony prominences) without causing a substantial increase in pressure (Brienza and Geyer, 2005; Christian and Lachenbruch, 2007; NPUAP, 2007). In contrast to the therapeutic functions of immersion and envelopment, "*bottoming out*" occurs when the depth of penetration or sinking is excessive, allowing increased pressure to concentrate over one area or bony prominence. Whitney et al (2006) define bottoming out as less than 1 inch of material between the surface and the skin when feeling under a support surface with the palm of a hand. Factors that may lead to bottoming out include (1) weight exceeds manufacturer's recommendations; (2) disproportionate weights and sizes, such as with bilateral lower extremity amputation; (3) tendency to keep the head of the bed greater than 30 degrees; and (4) inappropriate support surface settings, such as overinflation or underinflation. All support surfaces function best with minimal linen and/or plastic-backed underpads between the patient and the surface (NPUAP, 2007; NPUAP, EPUAP, PPPIA, 2014).

Friction and Shear Reduction

Friction and shear are physical concepts associated with pressure ulcer formation. *Shear stress* refers to force on the tissue; *shear strain* refers to the resulting deformation (Christian and Lachenbruch, 2007). A support surface reduces shear and friction by strategic placement of mediums and covers that allow for low-friction positioning without excessive sliding. However, the best support surface cover will not eliminate the need for additional interventions to minimize friction and shear, as described in Chapters 5 and 8.

Microclimate (Temperature and Moisture) Control

Microclimate control is a therapeutic function some support surfaces may provide. Excess moisture of the skin is a well-known factor associated with pressure ulcer development. Control of temperature at the interface surface (patient–bed boundary) helps to maintain normal skin temperature, which in turn inhibits sweating and lowers skin hydration (Mackey, 2005). A support surface should be designed to help maintain normal skin hydration and temperature (Brienza and Geyer, 2005). Porous covers help reduce moisture by allowing air to transfer between the skin and surface so that moisture and body heat can dissipate. Some mediums may be nonpermeable and prevent liquid or air from escaping, whereas others interact with the body to affect microclimate, such as with continuously pumped air flowing across the skin.

COMPONENTS

Components of a support surface are manufactured from various mediums as a means of creating pressure redistribution. Mediums are solid, fluid, and air, either used alone or in combination. The means of encapsulating the medium is considered another component of the support surface and is called the *cell* or *bladder* (NPUAP, 2007). Multiple cells can be individual or interconnected, configured in a longitudinal or latitudinal pattern (Figures 9-2 and 9-3).

Foam

Foam is available in chair cushions, overlays, mattresses for beds, transport gurneys and stretchers, and OR and procedure tables. Most foam overlays and cushions are indicated for single-patient use, whereas mattresses are intended for multiple-patient use. Both are designed for a specific weight limit and lifespan. Foam can be the sole medium or consist of hybrids that include composites of gel, air, or other more fluid materials to enhance envelopment in key areas. Benefits associated with foam support surfaces include their relatively low cost, light weight, and minimal maintenance.

Single bladder section

Latitudinal chambers section

Longitudinal chambers section

Cells section

FIGURE 9-2 Interconnected, single-bladder, longitudinal, or latitudinal cells.

FIGURE 9-3 Nonpowered static air support surface consisting of hundreds of individual air cells. (Courtesy the ROHO Group, Belleville, IL.)

A disadvantage is the limited lifespan due to fatigue caused by flexion and compression over time.

Foam can be closed cell or open cell. *Closed-cell* foam is a nonpermeable formulation in which a barrier between cells prevents gases or liquids from passing through the foam (NPUAP, 2007), potentially increasing skin temperature by preventing dissipation of body heat (Nicholson et al, 1999). *Open-cell* foam is higher-specification foam that is more effective in preventing pressure ulcers than is closed-cell foam. Examples of higher-specification foams are elastic and viscoelastic. There is no evidence that one type of high-specification foam is better than another high-specification foam (McInnes et al, 2011; NPUAP, EPUAP, PPPIA, 2014).

Elastic Foam. Elastic is high-specification foam made of porous polymer material that conforms in proportion to the applied weight. Air enters and exits the open-cell foam rapidly due to its greater density (NPUAP, 2007). The surface continues to conform until the resistance to compression exceeds the weight being applied (Christian and Lachenbruch, 2007). The combination of density and hardness determines compressibility and conformity, ultimately establishing the ability of the support surface to mechanically redistribute loading force. Density describes foam weight, reported as either pounds per cubic foot or kilograms per cubic meter. Greater density provides more durability.

Indentation force deflection (IFD), also known previously as indentation load deflection (ILD), is a measure of firmness or resistance to compression. In the United States IFD is reported as the force in pounds required to compress a prescribed size of foam by 25%. The more global foam industry tends to report the amount of force in "newtons" necessary to compress a prescribed size of foam by 40% after a process of preconditioning. Surfaces can be made with a combination of foams strategically placed to optimize pressure redistribution in targeted locations (PFA, 1994)—for example, a relatively lower-density IFD foam located closer to the surface and therefore the patient to enhance conformation, and a higher-density IFD foam located more deeply in the mattress to prevent compression or bottoming out.

A foam overlay is a single-user form of support surface placed on a mattress. If used for pressure redistribution, a foam overlay should have a base height of at least 3 inches measured from the base (or bottom) to the lower level of convolution (Figure 9-4), suitable density to ensure durability (1.3 to 1.6 lb/ft^3), IFD of 30, and ideally a ratio of 25% to 40% for compression of 2.5 or greater (Whittemore, 1998). As described later in this chapter, when considering overlay use,

it is important to assess risk for falls, weight distribution, and potential for bottoming out.

Viscoelastic (Memory) Foam. *Viscoelastic* is another high-specification open-cell foam made of porous polymer material that conforms in proportion to the applied weight. Air enters and exits the foam cells slowly, which allows the material to respond slower than elastic foam. Viscoelastic foams are a subset of urethane polymer foams that exhibit a slow recovery (memory) property. A viscoelastic foam product generally has a higher density and a lower IFD. Because of their fluid nature, when an object is placed on a viscoelastic support surface, the viscoelastic tends to displace quickly and conform to the shape of the object, with low resistance. Viscoelastic foam is available in many grades and qualities, each having properties that affect pressure redistribution and microclimate performance in unique ways. Some viscoelastic foams are engineered to change hardness within a specific temperature range. These materials tend to get softer as the material warms to body temperature, resulting in conformation similar to that of a gel. Viscoelastic support surfaces are often used in the OR (AORN, 2012) and have been shown to effectively decrease the incidence of pressure ulcers in high-risk elderly patients with fractures of the neck and femur (Cullum et al, 2001). One study of 838 patients at risk for pressure ulcers found a significantly lower pressure ulcer incidence when patients were turned every 4 hours on a viscoelastic surface compared with patients who were turned every 2 hours on a standard mattress (Defloor et al, 2005).

Gel

Gel contains a network of solid aggregates, colloidal dispersions, or polymers that may exhibit elastic properties (NPUAP, 2007). Some gel products are called *viscoelastic gel* because they respond similarly to viscoelastic foam. Gel support surfaces are intended for multiple-patient use. Because of the consistency of the medium, gels have been found to be especially effective in preventing shear. Other advantages include easy cleaning and no need for electricity. Disadvantages of gel support surfaces are that they tend to be heavy and are difficult to repair. Skin humidity can increase due to the nonporous nature of the gel and the lack of air flow. Although the gel is cool upon initial contact, skin temperature may increase after hours of constant contact. Gel must be carefully monitored, and the material must be manually moved back to the areas under bony prominences if it has migrated (Brienza and Geyer, 2005).

Fluids (Viscous Fluid, Water, Air)

Fluids are considered substances whose molecules flow freely past one another. Fluids have no fixed shape, so they take on the shape of the load with less resistance than a gel or solid component, creating a high degree of immersion. Fluid mediums include viscous fluid, water, and air. Moisture control characteristics are dependent on the ability of the medium to conduct heat and the composition of the product's cover.

Base height

Foam overlay

FIGURE 9-4 Measuring the depth of the foam overlay.

Viscous Fluid. Viscous fluid contains materials such as silicon elastomer, silicon, or polyvinyl (Brienza and Geyer, 2005). At first glance, viscous fluid can be mistaken for gel. Although many of its advantages and disadvantages are similar to those of gels, viscous fluid is free flowing and has a similar pressure redistribution response as air or water. Compared with air and water, viscous fluid is thicker, with a relatively higher resistance to flow (NPUAP, 2007).

Water. Water is a moderate-density fluid with moderate resistance to flow (NPUAP, 2007). Studies have demonstrated that water-filled support surfaces provide lower interface pressure than a standard mattress (Cullum et al, 2001). Although popular at home, water mattresses are undesirable in the hospital or long-term care setting due to multiple management concerns, including the following:
- Need for a heater to control the temperature
- Time and labor needed to drain and move the bed
- Potential for leaking
- Difficulty with repositioning and transferring and with performing cardiopulmonary resuscitation (CPR)

Air. Air is a low-density fluid with minimal resistance to flow. Air may be the sole redistribution medium, or it may be combined with other mediums (NPUAP, 2007). Support surfaces that incorporate air are available as chair cushions, overlays, mattresses, and bed systems. Most air support surfaces are easy to clean and can be reused. Air products have the potential to leak if damaged and require adequate inflation so that the body can immerse into the product. Air mattresses and overlays have the advantage of being lightweight and easy to clean.

CATEGORIES AND FEATURES

Categories of pressure redistribution support surfaces include overlays, mattress replacements, and integrated bed systems. Pressure redistribution devices may be purchased in the form of a chair cushion or transport, procedure, emergency room, or perioperative surface. All of these surfaces may be powered or nonpowered, active or reactive. Features or functional components such as low air loss, air fluidization, lateral rotation, and alternating pressure may be used alone or in combination. A variety of pressure redistribution capabilities can exist in single or multizoned surfaces. A zone is a segment with a single pressure redistribution capability. Therefore a multizoned surface has different segments with different pressure redistribution capabilities (NPUAP, 2007).

Mattress Overlays

The mattress overlay is a support surface that is placed on top of an existing mattress (Christian and Lachenbruch, 2007; NPUAP, 2007). Gel, water, and some air-filled overlays are intended for multiple-patient use and have the advantage of requiring much less storage space than mattresses and bed systems. Other overlays, such as foam and some air products, are for single-patient use and present environmental concerns

relative to disposal of the product. Overlays are thinner than mattress replacements, so there is potential for the patient to bottom out onto the mattress below. Because they are applied over an existing mattress, mattress overlays increase the height of the bed and may complicate patient transfers, alter the fit of linens, or increase the risk for patient entrapment and falls (U.S. FDA, 2006).

Mattresses

A mattress is composed of any medium or combination of mediums that is placed on an existing compatible frame. Mattresses reduce some of the high-profile–related disadvantages experienced with overlays and appear to have fewer issues with bottoming out. When first introduced, the majority of support surfaces were integrated support surfaces or overlays that were rented or purchased. When support surfaces called *replacement mattresses* entered the marketplace, many facilities realized improved skin and wound outcomes by replacing their standard mattresses with replacement mattresses (Cullum et al, 2004; Gray et al, 2001). This investment reduced lead time and labor by eliminating the need to wait for delivery of bed systems or for staff to help move the patient once risk or pressure ulcers were identified. Today, most companies no longer make mattresses that do not redistribute pressure, so their standard mattress *is* a support surface. Mattresses may include a variety of therapeutic functions such as shear and friction reduction and managing the microclimate between the patient and the support surface.

Transport, Procedure, Emergency Room, and Perioperative Support Surfaces. It stands to reason that patients who require a support surface in bed would benefit from a support surface during special procedures, surgeries, and long waits on emergency room and transport gurneys. In fact, patients on these surfaces may be more at risk for pressure ulcer development due to limited space for moving and repositioning, in addition to their potential need for sedation or anesthesia. Although limited in peer-reviewed publications, manufacturers now are creating support surface mattresses (sometimes called *pads*) with a pressure redistribution option for emergency room, transport, and procedure tables. Some companies will custom-fit their pressure redistribution products to fit surfaces other than beds.

Chapter 8 provides information related to unique risk factors specific to patients in the OR. International guidelines recommend that the at-risk individual in the OR should have a mattress with pressure-redistributing properties greater than those of the standard OR mattress (AORN, 2012; NPUAP, EPUAP, PPPIA, 2014). However, a review of the literature suggests that, due to uncontrolled variables (e.g., reaction to anesthesia, discoveries leading to longer surgery), all surgical patients should be considered at risk and placed on a mattress with pressure-redistributing properties greater than those of the standard OR mattress (Walton-Geer, 2009). A standard OR mattress is defined as a 2-inch foam surface covered with a vinyl or nylon fabric (AORN, 2012).

A number of support surface options are available for the perioperative environment including air, gel, and high-specification foam mattresses. The best OR surface for preventing pressure ulcers has not been determined. McInnes et al (2011) concluded that pressure redistribution overlays on the operating table reduce the incidence of postoperative pressure ulcers. Selection of a support surface in the OR requires careful analysis of a number of factors to ensure the product provides pressure redistribution while demonstrating compatibility with the facility's most common surgical positions, safety procedures, transfer equipment, and budget (Box 9-3).

Metaanalysis suggests that postoperative use of a pressure redistribution support surface reduces the incidence of surgery-related pressure ulcers (Huang et al, 2013; McNichol et al, 2015). Of note, the number of pads and blankets, including warming blankets placed beneath the patient and the mattress, interferes with the pressure redistribution properties of the mattress. Therefore, if a cooling blanket is placed between the patient and the OR mattress, a higher-grade surface should be considered to account for the change in pressure redistribution (AORN, 2012).

Integrated Bed Systems

An integrated bed system is a bed frame and support surface combined into a single unit. It is a rented or purchased unit whose components do not function separately (Christian and Lachenbruch, 2007; NPUAP, 2007); therefore it is used in place of an existing bed. With the integrated bed system, the features of both the frame and the support surface must be evaluated. Frames come in different widths and lengths and support a specified amount of weight. Some frames have the ability to adjust or fold for storage or transport through narrow doors and elevators. Most frames today are electric, but alternatives are available. When selecting a frame, the population to be served and the setting in which it will be used should be considered. For example, frames with built-in

---

> ### BOX 9-3 AORN Selection Recommendations for Operating Room Support Surfaces
>
> - Facilitates ability to hold patient in desired position
> - Available in variety of shapes and sizes
> - Ability to support maximum weight requirements
> - Durable material and design
> - Evidence that it can disperse skin interface pressure
> - Resistance to moisture
> - Smooth and intact surfaces
> - Low risk for moisture retention
> - Radiolucent as needed
> - Fire retardant
> - Nonallergenic
> - Promote air circulation
> - Low risk of harboring bacteria
> - Easy to use and store
> - Cost effective

---

bed exit alarms may be needed for patients who are confused and at risk for falls. Frames with built-in bed scales may be needed for the intensive care unit, where daily weights are a necessity, although many frames today include scales as standard operating equipment. Advantages and disadvantages mostly depend on whether or not the surface is rented (discussed later in this chapter).

Chair Cushions

Pressure redistribution in the chair often goes overlooked. Wounds that develop from sitting are located on the ischia during upright sitting and on the sacrum when slouching, sliding, or reclining. Pressure redistribution chair cushions should be used with seated individuals who are at risk for pressure ulcers and have reduced mobility (NPUAP, EPUAP, PPPIA, 2014). Selecting a cushion of appropriate size for the seated patient is extremely important given the potential for the patient to "bottom out," as most of the weight is applied to a relatively small body surface. Chair cushions are available in foam, air, and gel, and alternating pressure (AP) therapy and bariatric sizes.

Ring cushion (donut) devices increase venous congestion and edema and should not be used for pressure ulcer prevention and management (NPUAP, EPUAP, PPPIA, 2014; Whitney et al 2006; WOCN®, 2003, 2010).

Once implemented, chair cushions must be inspected regularly for wear and tear. Improper inflation, overcompression, or displaced gel can impair adequate pressure redistribution and lead to bottoming out.

Active (Alternating Pressure)

An *active* support surface is a powered mattress or overlay that changes its load distribution properties with or without an applied load (NPUAP, 2007). Therefore, an active support surface moves with or without a person in the bed (Christian and Lachenbruch, 2007). Active mattresses or overlays should be selected for high-risk patients when frequent repositioning is not possible (NPUAP, EPUAP, PPPIA, 2014). As of 2015, the only active support surfaces on the market are those that include the feature of alternating pressure (AP) therapy. An example of an AP therapy surface is shown in Table 9-1.

Alternating pressure is a weight-shifting feature found in overlays and mattress. Alternating pressure products have cells arranged in various patterns that are inflated and deflated with air. Rather than pressure being distributed by increasing the surface area through immersion and envelopment, pressure is periodically redistributed across the body by inflating and deflating the cells of alternating zones. *Pulsating pressure* refers to shorter-duration inflation and higher-frequency cycling for which there is less direct evidence of effectiveness (Gunther and Clark, 2000). The individual cell that composes the AP mattress or overlay must be 10 cm or greater to effectively redistribute pressure (NPUAP, EPUAP, PPPIA, 2014). Air cells can inflate and deflate in multiple stages resulting in relatively gradual transitions compared with single stage cycles. Experts agree that use of either

TABLE 9-1 Example of Support Surface Decision-Making Tool and Formulary

Criteria	Support Surface
Weight < _____ lbs AND Braden score 13 to 18 AND one of the following: • Intact skin AND can be effectively positioned • Patient CAN be effectively positioned off wound	REACTIVE SUPPORT SURFACE Example: Viscoelastic foam mattress (Visco 1) (Image courtesy of EncompassTSS)
Weight < _____ lbs AND one of the following: • Intact skin with Braden score less than 13 • Intact skin but CANNOT be effectively positioned • Patient CANNOT be effectively positioned off wound • Patient has fewer than two intact turning surfaces	REACTIVE SUPPORT SURFACE with features and components such as low air loss, viscous fluid or air fluids, OR active support surface (alternating pressure) Example: Low-air-loss mattress (Flexicair Eclipse Low Airloss Therapy Unit) (Image courtesy of Hill-Rom Services, Inc., © 2005)
Weight > _____ lbs or BMI > _____ AND Braden score 13 to 18 (at risk to moderate risk) AND one of the following: • Intact skin AND can be effectively positioned • Patient CAN be effectively positioned off wound	BARIATRIC REACTIVE SURFACE Example: Bariatric with viscoelastic foam mattress (Image courtesy of Sizewise)
Weight > _____ lbs or BMI > _____ AND one of the following: • Intact skin with Braden score less than 13 • Intact skin but CANNOT be effectively positioned • Patient CANNOT be effectively positioned off wound • Patient has fewer than two intact turning surfaces	BARIATRIC REACTIVE SUPPORT SURFACE with features and components such as low air loss, viscous fluid, or air fluids, OR active support surface (alternating pressure) Example: Bariatric with low-air-loss mattress (Image courtesy of Sizewise)

TABLE 9-1   Example of Support Surface Decision-Making Tool and Formulary—cont'd

Criteria	Support Surface
Effective repositioning is determined by a provider to be medically contraindicated (reevaluation/retrial at least every 8 hours should be documented) *Specify bariatric option for weight > _____ lbs or BMI >____*	ACTIVE SUPPORT SURFACE* Example: 'Active' Therapy Mattress Replacement (Alternating) (Image courtesy of ArjoHuntleigh)
Extensive debridement or flap surgery OR patient is on bed rest and wound(s) have deteriorated on a low-air-loss surface despite optimal wound management	AIR FLUIDIZED Example: Clinitron Air Fluidized Therapy (Image courtesy of Hill-Rom Services, Inc., © 2005)
Patient meets three of the following criteria: artificial airway, PaO_2/FiO_2 <250 with FiO_2 >0.40, requires >10 PEEP (regardless of FiO_2), desaturates with manual turning, immobile/exhibits ineffective mobility, receiving neuromuscular blockade therapy or continuous IV sedation, difficulty mobilizing secretions, ventilated with sepsis/ARDS	LATERAL ROTATION Example: TriaDyne Proventa Kinetic Therapy System (Image courtesy of KCI Licensing, Inc.)

*Refer to active support surface (alternating pressure) section of chapter for explanation.
ARDS, Acute respiratory distress syndrome; *BMI*, body mass index; *IV*, intravenous; *PaO2/FiO2*, ratio of arterial partial pressure to fractional inspired oxygen; *PEEP*, positive end expiratory pressure.

stage (single verses multiple) will assist with the prevention of partial thickness wounds. However, mattresses with the multiple stage feature are more effective in the prevention of full thickness wounds (Demarre et al, 2012; Demarre et al, 2013; McNichol et al, 2015; Vanderwee et al, 2005). Alternating pressure and pulsating pressure can be found in combination with foam and low-air-loss products.

International pressure ulcer guidelines suggest the use of an active support surface (mattress or overlay) for patients at higher risk for pressure ulcer development where frequent manual repositioning is not possible. This recommendation was derived indirectly from two studies, one of which was recognized as a poor-quality study. Iglesias and colleagues (2006) noted that pressure ulcers occurred almost 11 days sooner on an AP overlay compared with an AP mattress. However, in a study cited by International Pressure Ulcer Guidelines, no significant difference between AP mattresses and overlays was found, which led to the guidelines' statement that AP mattresses and overlays have similar efficacy in terms of pressure ulcer incidence (Nixon et al, 2006; NPUAP, EPUAP, PPPIA, 2014).

Reactive

A *reactive* support surface will move or change load distribution properties only in response to an applied load, such as the patient's body (Christian and Lachenbruch, 2007). Unlike active support surfaces that must be powered, reactive support surfaces are powered or nonpowered, with the potential to avoid the noise of a motor. Examples of reactive support surfaces include mattresses and overlays filled with foam, air, or a combination of foam and air. Gel surfaces, which may be in the form of chair cushions, overlays, mattresses and pads for stretchers, OR tables, and procedure tables, are nonpowered. Nonpowered air-filled support surfaces range from low-end prevention products that encapsulate air into a single bladder or cell to therapeutic products containing hundreds of individual interconnected cells (see Figure 9-3). All reactive support surfaces are appropriate for pressure ulcer prevention in the patient who is frequently repositioned. Some are appropriate for patients with pressure ulcers. With few exceptions, reactive support surfaces are compatible with long-term care facilities, hospitals, and home settings.

Continuous Lateral Rotation. Continuous lateral rotation is a feature that has been used for the past 30 years for the prevention and treatment of selected cardiopulmonary conditions. A continuous lateral rotation therapy bed rotates the patient in a regular pattern around a longitudinal (i.e., head to foot) axis of 40 degrees *or less* to each side. In contrast, kinetic therapy is defined as the side-to-side rotation of 40 degrees *or more* to each side. Drawing firm conclusions regarding effectiveness in the patient with cardiopulmonary disease is difficult, as these surfaces are primarily intended to facilitate pulmonary hygiene in the patient with acute respiratory conditions. Use of adult specialty beds in the rotation mode is ineffective for small children because their small

bodies are confined to one section or pillow of the surface (McCord et al, 2004).

Lateral rotation has been incorporated into some low-air-loss and air/foam mattresses, overlays, and integrated bed systems as shown in Table 9-1. One descriptive study of 30 patients on continuous lateral rotation therapy incorporated into a foam mattress replacement noted no new pressure ulcer development, with improvement of trunk and pelvis wounds (Anderson and Rappl, 2004). However, knowledge of the effects of continuous lateral rotation therapy on pressure redistribution is limited.

Therefore it is important to emphasize that continuous lateral rotation therapy does not eliminate the need for routine manual repositioning. Staff will need to take extra precautions to prevent shear, including aligning and securing the patient with bolster pads that are provided by the manufacturer and frequent turning to inspect the skin for signs of shear. Optimally, if shear injury develops, the patient would be positioned off the injured area and an alternative support surface method used. However, if the patient is still in respiratory distress, the risks and benefits of continuous lateral rotation therapy should be carefully considered before making a change (NPUAP, EPUAP, PPPIA, 2014).

Low Air Loss. One commonly misunderstood feature related to support surfaces is low air loss. The National Pressure Ulcer Advisory Panel (NPUAP) (2007) defines low air loss as a feature that provides a flow of air to assist in managing the heat and humidity (microclimate) of the skin. Low air loss consists of a series of connected pillows. A pump provides slow continuous air flow, allowing for even distribution into the porous mattress and continuous air flow across the skin (see Table 9-1). The amount of pressure in each pillow is controlled and can be calibrated according to height and weight distribution to meet the individual needs of the patient. As the patient settles down into the mattress, weight is distributed evenly for pressure redistribution. An additional component may be placed at the base of the product, such as foam or air pillows, when "bottoming out" is problematic. Low air loss can be found alone or in combination with AP, lateral rotation, and air-fluidized technology that is incorporated into overlays, mattresses, bed systems, and even a chair cushion.

The construction of a low-air-loss surface in addressing the microclimate of the skin can be achieved in two ways: with air flow under the cover or with an air-permeable cover. Most familiar to clinicians is the air-permeable cover that allows for the slow, evenly distributed release of air *through* the cover and directly to the skin. Low-air-loss surfaces with airflow *under* the cover address the skin microclimate by receiving heat, gas, and water molecules through a moisture vapor permeable cover (conducted downward from the skin) into the air stream inside the mattress, which eventually exits along the sides or ends of the mattress.

The smooth covers for low-air-loss surfaces are generally made of nylon or polytetrafluoroethylene fabric and have a low coefficient of friction. The covers are waterproof, impermeable to bacteria, and easy to clean. In order to receive the full benefits of low air loss, special underpads with a high level of moisture vapor permeability (rather than plastic-backed pads) should be used while minimizing the number and type of layers between the patient and the support surface (McNichol et al, 2015).

Low-air-loss support surfaces have been reported as an effective treatment surface and may improve healing rates of pressure ulcers (Saha et al, 2013). Because of the two aforementioned constructions (air-permeable cover vs. air flow under the cover), low air loss is associated with decreasing moisture, thereby minimizing the risk of incontinence-associated dermatitis or maceration (Cullum et al, 2004; WOCN®, 2003). Wound desiccation, however, is also possible and may be prevented by using a moisture-donating rather than absorptive dressing if the wound begins to dry.

Low-air-loss surfaces have important safety features, such as controls that instantly inflate the cushions, thus facilitating patient positioning. Fowler boost controls help prevent bottoming out by adding more air under the buttocks when the patient's head is elevated. Controls that instantly flatten the air cushions are activated before administration of CPR so that effective chest compressions are possible.

Disadvantages to this type of surface exist. Due to the lack of stability compared with a firmer mattress, low air loss may be contraindicated for patients with an unstable spine (McNichol et al, 2015). Some patients lose their ability to effectively self-position on a low-air-loss surface, again due to the lack of firmness in the surface. Additional disadvantages of low-air-loss surfaces include increased risk of bed entrapment, especially if the device is not properly adjusted. It is imperative that clinicians and involved staff are familiar with the manufacturer's recommended instructions for use. Once the proper weight setting is established, it is prudent to record the setting to ensure consistency. Low-air-loss surfaces can be costly and require electricity and special underpads that cost more than the standard underpad.

Air Fluidized. The feature of air fluidization (AF) can only be found in an integrated bed system (see Table 9-1) and was initially developed to treat patients with burns. Also known as high air loss, the surface contains silicone-coated beads that become incorporated into both air and fluid support; by pumping air through the beads, the beads behave like a liquid. The person "floats" on a sheet, with one third of the body above the surface and the rest of the body immersed in the warm, dry, fluidized beads. Body fluids flow freely through the sheet and cover, but contamination is prevented through continuous pressurization (Holzapfel, 1993). When the air-fluidized bed is turned off, it quickly becomes firm enough for repositioning or CPR.

Air-fluidized beds are most commonly used for patients with burns, myocutaneous skin flaps, and multiple Stage III or IV pressure ulcers. Using a subset of retrospectively collected National Pressure Ulcer Long-Term Care Study data, Ochs et al (2005) compared pressure ulcer outcomes of 664 residents placed on several types of support surfaces, including air fluidized, low-air-loss, powered and nonpowered overlays, and hospital mattresses. Results indicated that residents placed on air-fluidized support surfaces had larger and deeper pressure ulcers and higher illness severity scores than did residents placed on the other support surfaces. However, residents who used air-fluidized surfaces had better healing rates, fewer emergency visits, and fewer hospital admissions. Saha et al (2013) reviewed 5 studies conducted in the 1980s and 1990s and found that air-fluidized beds produced better healing in terms of reduction in ulcer size compared with several non-air-fluidized surfaces. These findings, although significant, warrant more research on variables such as initial wound size, use of dressing, debridement, nutritional status, and presence of infection and incontinence.

In the institutional environment, these products are not ideally suited to facility ownership because of the complexity and the high costs of maintenance. An air-fluidized bed system is one of the most expensive support surfaces. Air-fluidized products have a warming feature for the pressurized air, which can be comforting or harmful depending on the overall condition of the patient. Hydration issues may be more pronounced than that associated with low-air-loss surfaces. Because air-fluidized beds are heavy, they may not be safe for use in older homes. Traditional air-fluidized beds are not recommended for the patient with pulmonary disease or an unstable spine. However, air-fluidized therapy in the lower half of the bed has been combined with low air loss in the upper portion of the surface to create an adjustable bed for the patient who needs to be more upright. This bed is similar in size to a hospital bed, the head of the bed is readily adjustable, and the bed is lighter than a total air-fluidized system.

SUPPORT SURFACE SELECTION CRITERIA

Despite the lack of evidence specifying any particular brand of support surfaces, guidelines for selecting a support surface for specific patients are necessary to facilitate appropriate staff decision making and proper product use. Because multiple forms of support surfaces with a full range of features are available, it is possible to create setting-specific formularies with options compatible with the individual needs of the typical patient population for that setting .

Individual Patient Needs

Individuals with pressure ulcers or those at risk for pressure ulcers should be placed on a support surface rather than a standard hospital mattress (Cullum et al, 2004; NPUAP, EPUAP, PPPIA, 2014; Whitney et al, 2006; WOCN®, 2010). As described throughout this chapter, each support surface has disadvantages and contraindications. Therefore support surfaces must not be selected based *solely* on the patient's wound assessment, but rather on the patient's individual needs

(NPUAP, EPUAP, PPPIA, 2014). Individual needs of the patient with pressure ulcers or who is at risk for pressure ulcers are dependent on the condition and location of wounds (if applicable), activity and positioning, risk for falls and entrapment, size, weight, and patient response (McNicol et al, 2015).

For example, Rich et al (2011) reported there was little or no preventive effect of pressure-redistributing support surfaces in the at-risk but nonbedbound patient. The author concluded that the resources used to provide pressure-redistributing support surfaces to these individuals may be better allocated to other methods of pressure ulcer prevention. Critical analysis of these needs weighted with support surface indications, advantages, and disadvantages will lead to appropriate selection.

Condition and Location of Wounds. For the individual with large Stage III or IV pressure ulcers or pressure ulcers involving multiple turning surfaces, a support surface should be considered that includes features and components such as low air loss, AP, viscous fluid, or air fluids. A support surface that dissipates moisture (low air loss) may be indicated when skin barriers and dressings do not adequately protect the skin from moisture/incontinence (Cullum et al, 2004; Whitney et al, 2006; WOCN®, 2003). As discussed in the chair cushion section of this chapter, patients with sitting-surface pressure ulcers require a support surface for the chair.

Activity and Positioning. If frequent repositioning is not possible, an active support surface is indicated (NPUAP, EPUAP, PPPIA, 2014). Low-air-loss overlays may need to be changed to mattresses to prevent bottoming out if an elevated head of the bed for prolonged periods of time cannot be avoided. The patient who self-repositions, gets in and out of bed, or is attempting to increase and restore mobility and independence should use a support surface that facilitates rather than hinders activity and mobility.

Risk for Falls or Entrapment. A surface that raises the patient higher in the bed or creates more distance between the mattress and frame or side rails increases the risk for entrapment and falls. When possible, a pressure redistribution support surface that minimizes height and gaps should be selected for patients at risk for falls (U.S. FDA, 2006). Some facilities are adding fall risk assessment scores to support surface selection criteria. If the patient becomes at risk for falls or entrapment on a selected pressure redistribution support surface, additional monitoring will be necessary or an alternative pressure redistribution support surface should be selected (McNichol et al, 2015).

Size and Weight. Bed frame and mattress specifications for weight capacity must be considered. Low-air-loss products designed for adults do not provide options to accommodate the height and weight of small children (WOCN®, 2010). Children and infants can sink into and between cushions, leading to risk for entrapment and falls (McLane et al, 2004).

Many adult hospital bed frames manufactured today hold up to 500 lb. However, older frames may not be designed to hold more than 350 lb and have a width that precludes the ability of obese patients to effectively reposition for any period of time. Bariatric support surfaces are available in foam, air, gel, and water, with or without microclimate and moisture-control features. Care of the obese patient and bariatric support surface considerations are discussed in Chapter 35.

Patient Response. Once a product is selected, its effectiveness for any given patient must be reevaluated at regular intervals with the plan of care (Checklist 9-1, A). If expected outcomes are not achieved, an alternative support surface should be selected. Expected outcomes may include prevention of pressure ulcers, patient comfort, or moisture control. Wound healing may not be an expected outcome if it is not realistic or consistent with the patient's overall goals. If wound healing is an expected outcome after support surface implementation, it must be used in conjunction with documented and comprehensive pressure ulcer management.

The same factors that guided initial support surface selection should be reevaluated. Changes in patient status may guide the decision to discontinue or change a support surface. For example, the patient who once was comatose and hemodynamically unstable may require a different support surface to facilitate independence with self-positioning. Likewise, the patient on an overlay who was achieving expected outcomes may suddenly start bottoming out due to prolonged head-of-bed elevation because of respiratory distress. A patient on an overlay that previously was acceptable may be at increased risk for falling due to the onset of delirium.

Care Setting–Specific Formulary

A formulary of standardized products not only controls costs, but also is necessary to minimize confusion and mistakes related to appropriate selection and safe use (Whittemore, 1998). Considerations for compatibility with care setting include reimbursement, renting versus owning, product maintenance, safety, and facility response. Once these considerations are analyzed, a formulary can be created with a range of products intended to meet the individual needs of the patient population. Attention must then turn to creating decision-making tools and educating staff for effective product selection and safe use. Table 9-1 and Appendix A provide examples of decision-making tools to guide support surface selection. A content validated consensus and evidence-based algorithm is available (McNichol et al, 2015). Two subscale scores from the Braden Scale (mobility and moisture) have been incorporated into the tool linking clinically relevant risk factors to the decision-making process.

Reimbursement. When patients covered by Medicare Part A need a support surface, hospitals and skilled nursing facilities are financially responsible for acquiring and supplying the appropriate product. Hospitals receive a diagnosis-related group (DRG) payment based on patient diagnosis. Likewise,

CHECKLIST 9-1   Evaluating Support Surface Effectiveness

A. Individual Needs

✓ Has there been an increase in factors that place a patient at risk for pressure ulcers?
- Hemodynamic instability
- Frequent repositioning not possible
- Moisture management problems
- Increased need to keep head of the bed elevated

✓ Has the support surface caused any problems for the patient?
- Mobility impairment
- Pain or discomfort
- Sleeplessness
- Bottoming out
- Excessive dryness
- Skin breakdown

✓ Is the wound deteriorating despite appropriate care?
- Patient and caregiver education for pressure ulcer prevention and management
- Regular skin and risk assessment

- Appropriate turning and repositioning
- Appropriate wound care, including ongoing assessments and evaluation of healing
- Management of moisture and incontinence
- Nutritional support

B. Care-Setting Compatibility

✓ Does the formulary include enough options to meet the needs of the patient population?

✓ Do the formulary and selection criteria meet the fiscal needs of the setting?

✓ Is the staff competent with product procedures, such as set up, maintenance, and cleaning?

✓ Does the staff express overall satisfaction with the products?

✓ Is there an increase in entrapment, back injuries, or falls?

✓ Do the products conform to essential regulations?

✓ Are environmental concerns addressed?

✓ Does the company live up to promises for support and value-added services (see Table 9-2)?

---

skilled nursing facilities receive a per diem payment based on the resource utilization group. Therefore facilities must select the support surface that will provide the most cost-effective clinical outcome during a patient's stay.

When a patient is discharged to the home setting or converts from Medicare Part A to Medicare Part B, local coverage determination (LCD) fee schedules for support surfaces take effect. According to a report from the Office of Inspector General (Levinson, 2009), inappropriate Medicare payments for group 2 support surfaces amounted to approximately $33 million during the first half of 2007. Of the 362 claims reviewed, 86% did not meet group 2 coverage criteria, 38% were undocumented, 22% were medically unnecessary, and 17% had insufficient documentation.

When possible, selecting a support surface that matches the needs of the patient *and* meets Medicare reimbursement criteria would be ideal for patients making the challenging transition from the hospital or long-term care to home. Centers for Medicare & Medicaid Services (CMS) reimbursement criteria and product examples are listed in Appendix A. Reimbursement criteria change as technology and knowledge about support surfaces and wounds evolve. It is important to contact insurance companies, health maintenance organizations (HMOs), Medicaid, and Medicare for the most up-to-date information. Payer sources change as the patient moves through the continuum of care, and it is critical that the clinician work with the appropriate liaisons and provide documentation stating the rationale for product selections.

Renting (Leasing). For many facilities, renting support surfaces is the best option. Renting enables access to the most current technology free of any concerns about the need to update equipment. Renting support surfaces places the responsibility of maintenance and much of the liability for malfunctioning equipment with the rental company. Companies that rent equipment must provide or facilitate in-services to educate the staff on safety issues and proper use of the equipment. Rental costs may be as variable as the technology and customer service, ranging from as little as a few dollars to roughly $150 per day. Some health care agencies negotiate individual contracts with manufacturers, based on the volume of product used. However, it is important to choose a rental company that is compatible with more than just the financial needs of the facility. Table 9-2 provides a list of customer service–related items to consider during contract negotiation.

Purchasing (Owning). Advantages of owning support surface equipment include improved accessibility, decreased lead time for implementation, and potential decrease in rental expenses, particularly for critical care and bariatric surfaces. Before purchasing a product, the warranty information, guidelines for weight limit, set up, maintenance, and cleaning should be analyzed. Some frames of complete bed systems are not designed to accommodate certain mattresses. This will clearly restrict options for the facility's support surface formulary and usually more than once because frames tend to last longer than mattresses. However, many bed frame manufacturers have an "open architecture" design in which any mattress will fit the frame, allowing the clinician to choose the frame and the mattress that will best meet the needs of the patient population while opening up the possibility of mattress replacements as technology and patient needs evolve. Once the facility owns the equipment, it is responsible for storage, set up, and maintenance, which can be resource intensive for certain products or a safety/liability issue when the product is inadequately executed. Any cost analysis before purchase should consider these potential and actual financial consequences.

TABLE 9-2	**Negotiating Rental Contracts/Service Expectations**	
Company Service Provided	**Examples**
Product standardization	All low-air-loss mattresses have the CPR lever in one standard place (e.g., left side of foot of bed)
Standardized delivery and pickup times	2 to 4 hours
Safety and quality check on all units before product delivery	Flammability Product integrity (infection control/hygiene) Entrapment Labeling Biocompatibility Weight/weight capacity (maximum weight limits, safe working loads) Product expiration/lifespan
Conservation of the environment	Recycling of packaging materials Disposal and recycling of product Product is free from known harmful chemicals (PVC, DEHP, mercury, latex, etc.) Disclose all materials that compose product content/mattress core
Troubleshooting information accessible to all	Troubleshooting guides affixed to product 24-hour phone number for questions affixed to product
Daily rounds on beds by consistent and knowledgeable staff	Check whether product is in working order, appropriate labels/instructions are present and legible, patient is comfortable and is not bottoming out, timely staff education (review CPR procedures, appropriate linens and pads, etc.), interaction of surface to other products/supplies (frame, underpads, etc.)
Education	Timely in-services during daily rounds as previously described, education per 24/7 hotline calls, group in-services (orientation, yearly reviews)

CPR, Cardiopulmonary resuscitation; *DEHP,* diethylhexyl phthalate; *PVC,* polyvinyl chloride.

Product Maintenance and Safety. Keeping patients safe on a support surface is accomplished by making appropriate equipment selections; establishing proper set up, monitoring, and maintenance; facilitating optimal pressure redistribution capacity; and maintaining the barrier to environmental hazards such as fire and infectious body fluids. Maintenance requirements of support surfaces vary by design, composition, and technology. For example, support surfaces with heel zones or head zones must be placed on the bed frame in a specific orientation. Others must be turned (or flipped) regularly to maintain efficacy and checked for wear, proper inflation, and resilience. Repairing or replacing loose or broken side rails, bed controls, and CPR levers (where applicable) will help to prevent some occurrences of entrapment and falls.

Inspecting and Replacing Support Surfaces. A system should be in place to verify that the support surface is being used within its functional lifespan, as indicated by the manufacturer's recommended test method (or industry-recognized test method) *before* use of the support surface (NPUAP, EPUAP, PPPIA, 2014). Due to infection-control concerns, the expected life of a support surface cover may differ from that of the mattress itself (U.S. FDA, 2014).

Many facilities date the support surface before it is used for the first time with indelible ink and in a consistent location, so the date can be routinely checked for the manufacturer's specified lifespan. This process not only protects the patient from ineffective, damaged, or contaminated products, but it also may save money when a warranty for nonexpired

products applies. Some warranties allow for full mattress replacement as indicated over a specified timeframe. Others are prorated according to the age of the product. Some of the more complicated support surfaces may require a different process that includes accessible personnel with bioengineering expertise to maintain, repair, and troubleshoot the product.

Irrespective of manufacturer's specified lifespan, staff who have ongoing exposure to support surfaces during bedding or room changes should practice continual awareness and opportunity-based observation of support surface life expectancy. This can include, but is not limited to, nursing staff, certified nursing assistants, housekeeping, engineering, and maintenance personnel. Indicators for expired lifespan include reduced height or thickness; discoloration; altered integrity of cover, seams, zipper/zipper cover flap, or backing; degradation of internal components; or presence of odor. If any of these are observed, it is recommended that the surface be referred to engineering/maintenance for testing or evaluation for continued use (Call, 2014).

Additionally, the Food and Drug Administration (FDA) is concerned that fluid ingress from worn or damaged medical bed mattress covers may be widespread and largely underrecognized by health care providers, health care facility staff, and caregivers. From January 2011 to January 2013, the FDA received 458 reports associated with medical bed mattress covers failing to prevent blood and body fluids from leaking into the mattress (fluid ingress). Fluid ingress may occur if mattress covers become worn or damaged from small holes or rips in the fabric or from incorrect cleaning, disinfecting, and laundering procedures. The zipper on the cover may also allow fluid to penetrate the mattress. Some reports indicate that if blood and body fluids from one patient penetrate a mattress, they can later leak out from the mattress when another patient is placed on the bed. Patients are at risk for infection if they come into contact with blood and body fluids from other patients. The FDA also recommends developing an inspection plan to (1) check the expected life of the medical bed mattress and the mattress cover; (2) create an inspection plan for all medical bed mattresses in the facility; and (3) contact the medical bed mattress cover manufacturer for any additional questions (FDA, 2014). Checklist 9-2 contains items that may be used to identify reduced lifespan and infection-control concerns.

Evaluation of Outcomes. Factors to consider when evaluating a care setting–specific formulary are listed in Checklist 9-1, B. Successful implementation and ongoing use of any product will be dependent on compliance with standardization, manufacturer's customer service, effectiveness of staff education on selection criteria, and staff competency with product use, especially safety features such as CPR levers, maximum inflate mode, and other bed controls.

CHECKLIST 9-2   Inspection of Support Surfaces

Areas to inspect:
- ✓ On, around, and under support surface cover
- ✓ Mattress (over, under, and all sides)
- ✓ Seams
- ✓ Zippers
- ✓ Attached components if applicable (pumps, cords, plugs etc.)

Indicators to look for:
- ✓ Reduced mattress height or height <_____ (as specified by the manufacturer)
- ✓ Reduced thickness
- ✓ Moisture or soiling (stains, odor, wet spots)
- ✓ Altered integrity (cuts, tears, cracks, pinholes, snags)
- ✓ Degradation of internal components
- ✓ Expired lifespan of mattress or cover according to manufacturer specification*

*Failure to follow the manufacturer's instructions may result in skin damage and may be a source of liability.

CLINICAL CONSULT

A: Referral received to evaluate redness on sacrum. Patient is a 66-year-old female on the geriatric unit with 12 × 20 cm area of mixed blanching and nonblanching sacral erythema. Noted bottoming out with head of bed consistently over 30 degrees due to choking and dysphagia following a mild cerebrovascular accident.
D: Stage I pressure ulcer due to pressure and shear.
P: Implement appropriate interventions to address pressure ulcer risk factors.

I: (1) Replace current support surface with low-air-loss mattress replacement (not an overlay) to reduce shear/pressure and provide moisture management. (2) Protect heels with offloading heel boots. (3) Encourage/engage family to notify the staff and the wound team if any further skin changes occur.
E: Nurses to reassess daily and reconsult wound specialist if erythema does not decrease in dimensions.

SUMMARY

Well-designed clinical research on the effectiveness of various support surface devices is needed. The NPUAP's Support Surface Initiative (S3I) has focused efforts on the testing and reporting of criteria such as immersion, envelopment, and microclimate as they relate to support surfaces. Additional evidence-based data are still years away as the next steps bring these standardized tests into the clinical setting for evaluation of efficacy. Ideally, clinical trials should measure the effects of a particular support surface on outcomes such as incidence, comfort, cost, and satisfaction. Small sample sizes may increase the risk of false-positive results (i.e., lead to the conclu-

sion that a product makes a significant difference when it does not). In addition, sample sizes should be appropriate to allow for the most relevant and meaningful type of statistical analysis.

It is the responsibility of health care providers involved in product selection to maintain up-to-date knowledge regarding factors relevant to support surface selection. The prudent wound specialist must be familiar with the operation, indications, and contraindications of the specialty support surface products in the facility, the agency, or the patient's home.

REFERENCES

Anderson C, Rappl L: Lateral rotation mattresses for wound healing, *Ostomy Wound Manage* 50(4):50–62, 2004.

Association of periOperative Registered Nurses (AORN): Recommended practices for positioning the patient in the perioperative practice setting. In *Perioperative standards and recommended practices*, Denver, CO, 2012, AORN, pp 421–444.

Brienza DM, Geyer MJ: Using support surfaces to manage tissue integrity, *Adv Skin Wound Care* 18(3):151–157, 2005.

Christian W, Lachenbruch C: Standardizing the language of support surfaces, *Remington Rep* 15(3):11–14, 2007.

Cullum N, McInnes E, Bell-Syer SE, et al: Support surfaces for pressure ulcer prevention, *Cochrane Database Syst Rev* (3):CD001735, 2004.

Cullum N, Nelson EA, Flemming K, et al: Systematic reviews of wound care management: (5) beds; (6) compression; (7) laser therapy, therapeutic ultrasound, electrotherapy and electromagnetic therapy, *Health Technol Assess* 5(9):1–221, 2001.

Defloor T, De Bacquer D, Grypdonck MH: The effect of various combinations of turning and pressure reducing devices on the incidence of pressure ulcers, *Int J Nurs Stud* 42(1):37–46, 2005.

Demarré L, Beeckman D, Vanderwee K, et al: Multi-stage versus single-stage inflation and deflation cycle for alternating low pressure air mattresses to prevent pressure ulcers in hospitalised patients: a randomised-controlled clinical trial, *B Int J Nurs Stud* 49(4):416–426, 2012.

Demarré L, Verhaeghe S, Van Hecke A et al: The effectiveness of three types of alternating pressure air mattresses in the prevention of pressure ulcers in Belgian hospitals *Res Nurs Health* 36(5):439–452, 2013.

Gray D, Cooper PJ, Stringfellow S: Evaluating pressure-reducing foam mattresses and electric bed frames, *Br J Nurs* 10(Suppl 22):S23–S26, 2001.

Gunther RA, Clark M: The effect of dynamic pressure-redistributing bed support surface upon systemic lymph flow and composition, *J Tissue Viability* 10(3):10–15, 2000.

Holzapfel SK: Support surfaces and their use in the prevention and treatment of pressure ulcers, *J ET Nurs* 20(6):251–260, 1993.

Huang HY, Chen HL, Xu XJ: Pressure-redistribution surfaces for prevention of surgery-related pressure ulcers: a meta-analysis, *Ostomy Wound Manage* 59:36–48, 2013.

Iglesias C, Nixon J, Cranny G, et al: Pressure relieving support surfaces (PRESSURE) trial: cost effectiveness analysis, *BMJ* 332(7555):1416, 2006.

Le KM, Madsen BL, Barth PW, et al: An in-depth look at pressure sores using monolithic silicon pressure sensors, *Plast Reconstr Surg* 74(6):745–756, 1984.

Levinson D: *Inappropriate Medicare payments for pressure reducing support surfaces*, Department of Health and Human Services, Office of Inspector General (OIG), August 2009. http://www.oig.hhs.gov/oei/reports/oei-02-07-00420.pdf. Accessed Nov 6, 2009.

Mackey D: Support surfaces: beds, mattresses, overlays-oh my!, *Nurs Clin North Am* 40(2):251–265, 2005.

McCord S, McElvain V, Sachdeva R, et al: Risk factors associated with pressure ulcers in the pediatric intensive care unit, *J Wound Ostomy Continence Nurs* 31(4):179–183, 2004.

McInnes E, Jammali-Blasi A, Bell-Syer SE, et al: Support surfaces for pressure ulcer prevention, *Cochrane Database Syst Rev* (4):CD001735, 2011.

McLane KM, Bookout K, McCord S, et al: The 2003 national pediatric pressure ulcer and skin breakdown prevalence survey: a multisite study, *J Wound Ostomy Continence Nurs* 31(4):168–178, 2004.

McNichol L, Watts C, Mackey D, et al: Identifying the right surface for the right patient at the right time: generation and content validation of an algorithm for support surface selection, *J Wound Ostomy Continence Nurs* 42(1):19–37, 2015.

Miller S, Parker M, Blasiole N, et al: A prospective, in vivo evaluation of two pressure-redistribution surfaces in healthy volunteers using pressure mapping as a quality control instrument, *Ostomy Wound Manage* 59(2):44–48, 2013.

National Pressure Ulcer Advisory Panel (NPUAP): *NPUAP support surface standards initiative: terms and definitions related to support surfaces*, 2007. http://www.npuap.org/NPUAP_S3I_TD.pdf. Accessed May 11, 2009.

National Pressure Ulcer Advisory Panel (NPUAP), European Pressure Ulcer Advisory Panel (EPUAP), Pan Pacific Pressure Injury Alliance (PPPIA): In Haesler E, editor: *Prevention and treatment of pressure ulcers: quick reference guide*, Osborne Park, Western Australia, 2014, Cambridge Media.

Nicholson GP, Scales JT, Clark RP, et al: A method for determining the heat transfer and water vapour permeability of patient support systems, *Med Eng Phys* 21(10):701–712, 1999.

Nixon J, Cranny G, Iglesias C, et al: Randomised, controlled trial of alternating pressure mattresses compared with alternating pressure overlays for the prevention of pressure ulcers: PRESSURE (pressure relieving support surfaces) trial, *BMJ* 332(7555):1413, 2006.

Ochs RF, Horn SD, van Rijswijk L, et al: Comparison of air-fluidized therapy with other support surfaces used to treat pressure ulcers in nursing home residents, *Ostomy Wound Manage* 51(2):38–68, 2005.

Polyurethane Foam Association (PFA): *Joint industry foam standards and guidelines*, 1994, Indentation force deflection (IFD) standards and guidelines. http://www.pfa.org/jifsg/jifsgs4.html. Accessed Dec 15, 2014.

Reger SI, McGovern TF, Chung KC, et al: Correlation of transducer systems for monitoring tissue interface pressures, *J Clin Eng* 13(5):365–371, 1988.

Rich SE, Shardell M, Hawkes WG, et al: Pressure-redistributing support surface use and pressure ulcer incidence in elderly hip fracture patients, *J Am Geriatr Soc* 59(6):1052–1059, 2011.

Saha S, Smith MEB, Totten A, et al: *Pressure ulcer treatment strategies: comparative effectiveness* (AHRQ Publication No. 13-EHC003-EF), Rockville, MD, May 2013, Agency for Healthcare Research and Quality.

U.S. Food and Drug Administration (FDA): *Hospital bed system dimensional and assessment guidance to reduce entrapment*, March 10, 2006. http://www.fda.gov/MedicalDevices/DeviceRegulationandGuidance/GuidanceDocuments/ucm072662.htm. Accessed April 6, 2015.

U.S. Food and Drug Administration (FDA): *Damaged or worn covers for medical bed mattresses pose risk of contamination and patient infection* (FDA safety communication), April 19, 2013. http://www.fda.gov/MedicalDevices/Safety/AlertsandNotices/ucm348016.htm. Accessed April 6, 2015.

Vanderwee K, Grypdonck MH, Defloor T: Effectiveness of an alternating pressure air mattress for the prevention of pressure ulcers, *Age Ageing* 34(3):261–267, 2005

Walton-Geer P: Prevention of pressure ulcers in the surgical patient, *AORN J* 89(3):538–552, 2009.

Whitney J, Phillips L, Aslam R, et al: Guidelines for the treatment of pressure ulcers, *Wound Repair Regen* 14(6):663–679, 2006.

Whittemore R: Pressure-reduction support surfaces: a review of the literature, *J Wound Ostomy Continence Nurs* 25:6–25, 1998.

Wound, Ostomy and Continence Nurses Society™ (WOCN®): *Guideline for management of pressure ulcers* (WOCN® clinical practice guideline series no. 2), Glenview, IL, 2003, WOCN®.

Wound, Ostomy and Continence Nurses Society™ (WOCN®): *Guideline for management of pressure ulcers* (WOCN® clinical practice guideline series no. 2), Glenview, IL, 2010, WOCN®.

Lower Extremity Assessment

JoAnn Ermer-Seltun

OBJECTIVES

1. Identify critical assessment parameters of the lower extremity physical assessment.
2. For each indicator used to assess perfusion, describe the techniques and results.
3. Identify two methods for describing lower extremity edema.
4. Compare and contrast assessment parameters indicative of lower extremity venous disease (LEVD) and lower extremity arterial disease (LEAD).

In the United States chronic wounds afflict more than 6.5 million patients and cost over $25 billion to treat (Sen et al, 2009). More specifically, chronic lower extremity ulcers are thought to affect 0.18% to 1.3% of the adult population at an estimated cost of more than $1 billion annually worldwide, or $12 million in the United States (Margolis, 2013). These statistics are alarming and reflect a major threat to public health and the financial system. Most of these wounds are chronic in nature, affect the individual's quality of life, drain monetary and health care resources, and may even progress to possible limb loss if not managed appropriately. The key to successful management of any wound is an insightful assessment to determine the underlying cause so that treatment modalities address the pathologic factors. The etiologic factors of a lower extremity wound can include numerous diseases, infection, trauma, drugs, insect bites, pressure, or a combination thereof. Therefore the wound specialist must be knowledgeable regarding clinical presentation and skilled in differential assessment. Critical assessment parameters are listed in Checklists 10-1 and 10-2 and described in this chapter.

GENERAL APPEARANCE OF THE LIMB

The wound specialist must become familiar with, and proficient in, using proper descriptive dermatologic terms to describe primary or secondary lesions, the pattern of distribution, and the arrangement of lesions or other abnormalities. Careful description often leads the examiner to a specific disease state. Limb appearance should be compared with that of the contralateral limb to identify or rule out trophic changes. With the patient's shoes and socks off, the wound specialist should visually assess both extremities for varicosities, color, pigmentation, turgor, texture, dryness, fissures, hair distribution, calluses, abnormal nails, fungus, bunions, corns, bony deformities, and skin integrity (Bonham, 2003; Hirsch et al, 2006; International Best Practice Guidelines, 2013; WOCN®, 2008, 2011, 2012). The web between the toes should be assessed for hygiene issues (Bonham and Kelechi, 2008).

Trophic Changes

Trophic changes can occur when diminished blood flow can no longer support normal growth and development of the skin, hair, and nails. For example, thin and shiny epidermis, loss of hair growth, and thickened nails are often associated with, but are not diagnostic of, lower extremity arterial disease (LEAD) (WOCN®, 2008). Conversely, edema; hyperpigmentation; scaly, eczematous skin; and varicosities (dilated, swollen, torturous) may be indicative of lower extremity venous disease (LEVD) (WOCN®, 2011).

Trophic changes, however, are not definitive indicators of disease. Patterns of hair growth are affected by age, ethnicity, and perfusion status, as hair growth may be diminished or absent in the elderly and certain ethnic groups. Nail growth is also affected by factors other than perfusion, including age and fungal infections.

Appearance of Veins

The leg should be visually inspected or palpated for dilated veins, especially along the saphenous vein, beginning at the

CHECKLIST 10-1 Lower Extremity Physical Assessment

General appearance
✓ Trophic changes
✓ Hair, nail, and skin patterns
✓ Veins
✓ Skin color, shape, texture, and integrity
✓ Edema
Functional-sensory status
✓ Range of motion of ankle joint
✓ Protective sensation
✓ Vibration
✓ Deep tendon reflexes
✓ Pain
Perfusion
✓ Elevational pallor or dependent rubor
✓ Skin temperature
✓ Blood flow (bruit/thrill)
✓ Capillary refill
✓ Pulses
✓ Ankle-brachial index

CHECKLIST 10-2 Diagnostic Tests for the Lower Extremities

Noninvasive tests for LEAD
✓ Ankle-brachial index (ABI)
✓ Toe-brachial index (TBI)
✓ Transcutaneous partial pressure of oxygen (TcPO₂)
✓ Skin perfusion pressure (SPP)
✓ Pulse volume recording (PVR) and Doppler waveform study
✓ Segmental limb pressure (SLP) measurements
✓ Magnetic resonance imaging (MRI)
✓ Duplex angiography
Invasive tests for LEAD
✓ Computed tomographic angiography (CTA)
✓ Arteriography
Noninvasive test for LEVD
✓ Duplex imaging

LEAD, Lower extremity arterial disease; *LEVD,* lower extremity venous disease.

medial marginal vein on the dorsum of the foot and terminating at the femoral vein (about 3 cm below the inguinal ligament). Normally, healthy distended veins can only be visualized at the foot and ankle; the presence of dilated veins anywhere else on the leg may imply venous pathology and often is the first sign of venous insufficiency. *Dilated veins,* or *varicose veins,* are bluish, enlarged, and palpable. Often described as tortuous or rope-like, varicose veins are most often present on the back of the calf or on the inner aspect of the leg.

Small vessel changes can be detected with visual inspection. Small reddish or bluish "broken" vessels that cluster near the medial malleolus of the ankle are called *spider* or *reticular*

veins; these can also be visualized anywhere on the leg. *Ankle flare,* a larger cluster of small vessels or sunburst, occurs around the ankle. *Telangiectasias* is the presence of fine, dilated capillaries (WOCN®, 2011).

Skin Color, Shape, and Integrity

The presence of any discoloration in the skin should be noted. For example, reddish-gray-brown hyperpigmentation in the gaiter region, more specifically hemosiderin staining (see Plate 34), is another skin color change that should be noted. Hemosiderin staining is hailed as the "classic" sign of LEVD, but it also can be found if significant trauma has occurred to the lower extremity (WOCN®, 2011). This type of discoloration develops after extravasated red blood cells break down and release the pigment hemosiderin.

Atrophie blanche, also seen with LEVD, is an atrophic, thin, smooth, white plaque with a hyperpigmented border, often "speckled" with tortuous vessels, occurring near the ankle or foot. Due to its scar-like appearance, atrophie blanche is easily and often mistaken for a previously healed ulcer (see Plate 35). Its presence is considered high risk for impending ulceration.

Tiny individual reddish-purple, nonblanching discolorations on the lower extremity may be observed. When the individual discolorations are larger than 0.5 cm, they are called *purpura;* when they are smaller than 0.5 cm, they are called *petechiae.* Small blood vessels may leak under the skin and cause a blood or hemorrhagic patch that is a sign of some type of intravascular defect in individuals with normal or abnormal platelet counts. Purpura and petechiae (see Plates 36 and 37) are most often associated with LEAD (secondary to blood thinners) or vasculitis disorders such as systemic lupus erythematosus and polyarteritis nodosa. Purpura associated with vasculitis disorders is referred to as *palpable* purpura. Purpura that occurs in the elderly due to fragility of the vessels is known as *senile* purpura.

The presence of a condition known as *lipodermatosclerosis* (see Plate 39) should be noted as present or not present. Lipodermatosclerosis, a condition of the skin and soft tissues that develops in the presence of chronic swelling, is a progressive hardening or fibrosis of the soft tissues. Usually confined to the gaiter or "sock" area, lipodermatosclerosis may cause an inverted "champagne bottle" or "apple core" deformity of the lower extremity in sharp contrast to the unaffected leg.

Dermatitis (see Plate 39) manifested by scaling, crusting, weeping, excoriations (linear erosions due to scratching) from intense pruritus, erythema, or inflammation should be noted. Often these symptoms of dermatitis are misdiagnosed as cellulitis (see Table 12-3). Ulcers on the lower extremity should be noted in terms of their appearance, location, size, pain, and duration.

Edema (Extent, Pattern, Distribution)

Edema is a localized or generalized abnormal accumulation of fluid in the tissues (WOCN®, 2011). Numerous conditions can cause swelling of the lower extremity; examples include chronic venous disease, postphlebitis syndrome, iliac compression syndrome, lymphedema, and systemic disease such as chronic heart failure, pulmonary hypertension, and renal failure (Buczkowski et al, 2009). Edema causes swelling that may obscure the appearance of normal anatomy. To determine the presence of edema in the lower extremities, the appearance of one extremity should be compared with the other, noting the relative size and the prominence of veins, tendons, and bones. Edema is a significant finding in the examination of the lower extremity and should be further investigated.

Extent. Evaluating edema is challenging due to lack of objective measurement methods. One method is to have the patient sit or stand and, using a flexible tape, obtain measurements of the lower extremity at the calf and the ankle. For valid comparisons, subsequent measurements must be obtained with the patient in the same position and exact location. Calf circumference is obtained by first marking the largest part of the inner calf with a marker and then taking a measurement from the floor up to this mark (in centimeters). This is the floor-to-calf length, and all future measurements should occur at this level. Second, the calf circumference (in centimeters) at the largest portion of the calf that was previously marked is measured. The ankle circumference is measured 5 cm above the ankle. Likewise, the floor-to-ankle length is determined by placing the tape measure at 0 cm on the floor and making a dot on the skin 5 cm above the medial malleolus and then determining the circumference of the ankle (in centimeters).

The extent of edema can also be assessed by pressing firmly but gently with the index finger for several seconds on the dorsum of each foot, behind each medial malleolus, and over the shins. Edema is "pitting" when there is a visible depression that does not rapidly refill and resume its original contour (Figure 10-1). Severity of edema can be categorized by either estimating the depth of the indentation (Figure 10-1 and Box 10-1) or the length of time for the indentation to resolve. For clarity, the type of scale used should be recorded (e.g., 3+ pitting edema on a 4-point scale) (Ball et al, 2003).

The perometer, which is a computerized digital scanner, can be used to measure limb volume and is particularly useful with lymphedema and fitting compression garments. The perometer uses digital infrared technology to measure the girth and volume of an extremity (Stanton et al, 1997; Stanton et al, 2000).

Pattern and Distribution. The pattern and distribution of edema should be noted. For example, dependent edema is the accumulation of fluid in the lowest body parts, such as the feet and legs (WOCN®, 2011). With LEVD, dependent edema generally develops gradually, worsens with prolonged standing, and diminishes when the patient rests in a recumbent position with the legs elevated (WOCN®, 2011). However, the pattern of edema associated with lymphedema does not resolve with leg elevation and usually encompasses the entire leg. Another distinguishing feature of lymphedema is the presence of a positive Stemmer sign, in which a skin fold at the base of the second toe is too thick to lift. Differences in edema presentations are listed in Table 10-1. Chapter 13 provides an in-depth discussion of lymphedema.

FUNCTIONAL–SENSORY STATUS

Functional assessment includes observation for impairments in ambulation, gait, balance, use of walking aids (walker, cane), and ability to remove shoes and socks. Because loss of function may be neuropathic in origin, a focused sensory examination is an essential component of any lower extremity assessment (ADA, 2014; International Best Practice Guidelines, 2013; WOCN®, 2012). Sensory assessment (the ability to feel pain, pressure, temperature changes, vibration, and friction in the lower extremities and feet) is particularly relevant to the patient with a lower extremity wound. Failure to detect touch indicates loss of protective sensation and warrants caution if compression wraps will be applied because the patient may not sense ischemic changes in a timely manner (Bonham, 2003; WOCN®, 2011). Likewise, in patients with diabetes who also have neuropathy, motor neuropathy leads to flexion in the toes (hammer toes, claw toes), flattening of the arch, fat pad loss, and bones shifting that deteriorate into prominent plantar metatarsals (ADA, 2014). When combined with sensory (loss of sensation) and autonomic neuropathy (diminished capillary perfusion and sweat and oil gland production), a neuropathic ulcer may easily develop (ADA, 2014; International Best Practice Guidelines, 2013; WOCN®, 2012). In the case of LEAD, several studies confirmed peroneal nerve injury resulting in reduced nerve conduction velocity, poor functional outcomes, and loss of muscle strength in the lower extremities (WOCN®, 2008). These findings suggest that poor arterial

FIGURE 10-1 Pitting edema may also be categorized by depth of depression. (Ball JW, Dains JE, Flynn JA: Blood vessels. In *Seidel's guide to physical examination*, ed 8, St. Louis, MO, 2015, Mosby, pp 332–349.)

1+   2 mm
2+   4 mm
3+   6 mm
4+   8 mm

BOX 10-1 Grading Scale for Severity of Edema

1+	Slight pitting, no visible distortion Disappears rapidly
2+	Somewhat deeper pit than in grade 1, but no readily detectable distortion Disappears in 10 to 15 seconds
3+	Pit is noticeably deep and may last more than 1 minute Dependent extremity looks fuller and swollen
4+	Pit is very deep and lasts as long as 2 to 5 minutes Dependent extremity is grossly distorted

From Ball JW, Dains JE, Flynn JA: Blood vessels. In *Seidel's guide to physical examination*, ed 8, St. Louis, MO, 2015, Mosby, pp 332–349.

flow has a direct harmful effect on peroneal nerve function (McDermott et al, 2006). Signs of neuropathy include reduced sensation (detected by Semmes-Weinstein 5.07 monofilament) (HRSA, 2011), gait abnormalities caused by foot drop/drag, weakness of the ankles or feet, and loss of vibration (Boulton et al, 2008) and deep tendon reflexes (ADA, 2014; International Best Practice Guidelines, 2013).

Sensorimotor assessment is discussed in greater detail in Chapter 14.

Range of Motion of the Ankle Joint

The calf muscle pump is a critical contributor to normal venous return. Normal function of the calf muscle pump is dependent on a normally moving ankle joint. A "normal" walking motion requires flexion of the ankle joint past the 90-degree position. Therefore routine assessment of ankle range of motion should be incorporated into the physical assessment of a patient with known or suspected LEVD because elevated ankle stiffness has been associated with calf muscle pump impairment (Padberg et al, 2004). Ankle stiffness due to edema and fibrosis should be quantified according to severity: 0 = none, 1 = reduced stiffness, and 2 = nonreducible or ankylosis (Carpentier et al, 2003). A goniometer device, often used by physical therapists to measure ankle flexion/stiffness, is an objective measurement of range of motion (Bonham and Kelechi, 2008). Ankle joint equinus (the inability to dorsiflex the ankle joint less than 90 degrees) may occur with peripheral neuropathy. This loss of dorsiflexion can place extraordinary pressure on the sole of the foot, which in turn elevates the incidence of diabetic neuropathic ulceration (Caselli et al, 2002).

TABLE 10-1 Differences Between Edema, Lymphedema, and Lipedema

	Venous Edema	Lymphedema	Lipedema (Not True Edema)
Distribution	Ankle to knee May have limited foot involvement Usually unilateral	Toes to groin Usually unilateral	Ankle to groin Bilateral and symmetric
Characteristics	Pitting edema of variable severity In long-standing disease, nonpitting edema may result from tissue fibrosis	Brawny, nonpitting edema Skin and soft tissue changes common (e.g., papilloma formation, hyperkeratosis) Positive Stemmer sign (not possible to pinch fold of skin over dorsum of second toe) is early indicator Advanced disease: elephantiasis (loss of normal architecture/massive enlargement of limb)	Soft, rubbery tissue Pain on palpation common Painful bruising common Negative Stemmer sign Abnormal fat distribution from ankles to hips
Management	Elevation and compression (toes to knees) are primary approaches Intermittent pneumatic compression typically beneficial Surgery sometimes beneficial	Elevation and standard compression beneficial only in early stages Manual lymphatic drainage and inelastic compression are key elements of management Intermittent pneumatic compression frequently contraindicated	Weight loss, liposuction, but lack of evidence for long-term effect Management focus is treatment of any comorbidities, patient education, support
Risk factors	Deep vein thrombosis or thrombophlebitis Thrombophilia Obesity or multiple pregnancies Sedentary lifestyle Calf muscle pump failure	Filariasis (third world countries) Radical cancer surgery plus radiation Long-standing venous disease Vein harvesting/reconstruction	Heredity

TABLE 10-2   Pain Assessment of Patient with Leg Ulcer

Factors to be Assessed	Typical Findings		
	Venous	**Arterial**	**Neuropathic**
Characteristics	Dull Aching	Intermittent claudication Nocturnal pain Rest pain (see Box 11-3)	Burning/tingling "Shooting" "Pins and needles"
Severity	Variable Typically moderate to severe	Variable Frequently severe	Variable Commonly severe
Exacerbating factors	Dependency Increased edema Infection	Elevation Activity Infection	Variable Inactivity sometimes a precipitating factor
Relieving factors	Elevation Edema control Reduction of bacterial burden	Dependency Rest Reduction of bacterial burden	Activity such as walking

Pain

Effective pain management is a critical aspect of care for any patient with an ulcer; thus the assessment must always include determination of the type and severity of pain (both baseline and procedural), exacerbating and relieving factors, and past and present attempts to manage the pain. For the patient with a lower extremity ulcer, the pain history provides additional important etiologic clues (Table 10-2). Chapter 11 describes ischemic pain that is relieved by placing the leg in a dependent position (see Box 11-3) (Hirsch et al, 2006; WOCN®, 2008). In contrast, leg pain that is relieved by elevation is more consistent with a venous etiology (WOCN®, 2011). The patient with diabetes who is complaining of leg pain described as "pins and needles," a shooting "electrical shock," or burning sensation that is relieved by walking probably is experiencing neuropathic pain (ADA, 2014; WOCN®, 2012). Because patients with lower extremity disease may limit walking and other activities due to discomfort and comorbidities, "classic" signs of pain may not be appreciated. Extreme pain that seems out of proportion to the type of ulcer present (hyperalgesia) or pain associated with nonpainful stimuli (allodynia) should alert the clinician to further investigate for other conditions that may lead to atypical leg wounds (Alavi et al, 2012). Further discussion related to the assessment and management of pain is presented in Chapters 25 and 26.

PERFUSION

Extent of perfusion can be derived through inspection of leg temperature, position-related color changes, quality of pulses, and blood flow. Diagnostic tests used to assess perfusion include venous filling time, ankle-brachial index, and transcutaneous oxygen pressure measurements (Ball et al, 2015).

Elevational Pallor and Dependent Rubor

Presence of permanent discoloration (cyanosis, dark brown to black, pallor) of the digit and increased pain with or without ulceration may be evidence of critical digital ischemia and merits prompt investigation of the peripheral vascular system. Position-related color changes in one or both legs provide important information concerning adequacy of arterial perfusion.

Elevational Pallor. With the patient supine on the examination surface, the leg is raised to a 60-degree angle for 15 to 60 seconds. The color of the soles of the feet is observed. Normally, color should not change. When perfusion is impaired, pallor is observed in fair-skinned individuals and gray (ashen) hues in dark-skinned individuals. Box 10-2 correlates the severity of arterial occlusion with the amount of time needed for elevation pallor to occur (Gey et al, 2004).

Dependent Rubor. As for the examination for elevational pallor, the leg is raised 60 degrees while the patient is supine on the examination surface for 15 to 60 seconds. The normal leg will remain a healthy color when dependent. Initially the ischemic limb will slowly turn from white to pink and progress to a purple-red discoloration, referred to as *dependent rubor*. Color change occurs as a result of retention of deoxygenated blood in the dilated skin capillaries (Gey et al, 2004).

BOX 10-2   Assessment of Elevational Pallor

1. Raise leg to 60-degree angle for 15 to 60 seconds
2. Observe amount of time needed for pallor to appear:
   - Pallor within 25 seconds indicates severe occlusive disease
   - Pallor within 25 to 40 seconds indicates moderate occlusive disease
   - Pallor within 40 to 60 seconds indicates mild occlusive disease

From Ball JW, Dains JE, Flynn JA: Blood vessels. In *Seidel's guide to physical examination*, ed 8, St. Louis, MO, 2015, Mosby, pp 332–349.

Skin Temperature

Skin temperature of the leg is assessed by palpating lightly with the palmar surface of the fingers and hands, moving from proximal to distal, and comparing each limb to the opposite limb (e.g., right leg with left leg). Findings of unilateral coolness and a sudden marked change from proximal to distal are possible indicators of LEAD (Hopf et al, 2006). In contrast, patients with LEVD have been shown to have higher skin temperatures at the ankle (Kelechi et al, 2003; Kelechi et al, 2008; WOCN®, 2011).

When localized inflammation occurs, a slight elevation in skin temperature (2.2°C [4°F]) at that location can be detected, referred to as *infrared dermal thermometry* (IRD). Such an elevation in skin temperature was reported to be highly predictive of impending ulceration in patients with LEVD (Sayre and Kelechi, 2007) and lower extremity neuropathic disease (LEND) within 7 to 10 days (Armstrong et al, 2007). Several studies have suggested that self-monitoring of skin temperature for patients with high-risk diabetes may reduce the incidence of ulceration by modifying activity to reduce the local inflammation (Armstrong et al, 2007; Lavery et al, 2007). Although some evidence suggests IRD may also be useful to screen for pending ulceration in patients with LEVD (Kelechi et al, 2003; Sayre et al, 2007; WOCN®, 2011), more studies are needed to support the use of home thermometry for patients with LEVD (Kelechi and Bonham, 2008).

Blood Flow (Bruit/Thrill)

Blood flow through the artery should move in a laminar flow pattern. Turbulence in the flow of arterial blood occurs when some pathology, such as a clot, compression, or fatty deposit, develops within the vessel. Velocity of blood flow will slow around the source of the turbulence and cause blood cells to adhere to the vessel lining, thus forming a clot. Turbulent blood flow through an artery may be auscultated with the bell of a stethoscope and is heard as a blowing or rushing sound, which is called a *bruit* (Hirsch et al, 2006; Rumwell and McPharlin, 2004). Presence of a bruit is indicative of arterial narrowing, but because of the low-frequency sound the bruit may not always be heard (Khan et al, 2006). Turbulent blood flow may also be palpated, which is referred to as a thrill.

Capillary Refill

The capillary bed consists of small-diameter vessels that lie between the arterial and the venous systems. The time needed for the capillary bed to fill after it is occluded by pressure (capillary refill time) gives some indication of the health of the system. Delayed capillary refill (greater than 3 seconds) may indicate LEAD (WOCN®, 2008). However, the patient with LEAD may have normal capillary refill because the emptied vessels may refill in a retrograde manner from surrounding veins even if arterial inflow is markedly impaired or absent. Environmental factors such as temperature also may influence the speed of capillary refill; therefore this assessment is vulnerable to considerable subjective interpretation and should be used only to confirm a clinical

---

BOX 10-3	**Assessment of Capillary Refill Time**

- Blanch toenail bed with sustained pressure for several seconds
- Release pressure
- Observe time elapsed before nail regains full color
- In presence of arterial occlusion, refill time will be longer than 2 to 3 seconds

Caution: Decreased temperature can prolong capillary refill time. From Ball JW, Dains JE, Flynn JA: Blood vessels. In *Seidel's guide to physical examination*, ed 8, St. Louis, MO, 2015, Mosby, pp 332–349.

judgment. Box 10-3 explains how and why capillary refill time is assessed (Ball et al, 2015).

Assessment of Pulses

Pulses should be compared with the contralateral pulses and assessed in a proximal-to-distal direction. Normally pedal pulses can be palpated at both the dorsalis pedis and the posterior tibialis locations (Figure 10-2). Presence or absence of palpable pulses is not diagnostic of LEAD (Collins et al, 2006). If pulses are palpable, the patient may still have LEAD. If pulses are not palpable, a handheld Doppler probe must be used to determine the presence or absence of pulses. This assessment tool may have the highest predictive value as to whether LEAD exists (Khan et al, 2006).

The absence of Doppler pulse usually should lead to referral. However, in healthy individuals, dorsalis pedis pulse is absent in 8.1% and posterior tibialis pulse in 2.9% and both are absent in less than 2%. Therefore it is important to assess all dorsalis pedis and posterior tibialis pulses (Hopf et al, 2006).

The best way to document pulses is to use descriptive terms such as *present* or *absent*, followed by clarifying terms such as *weak* or *bounding*. Box 10-4 presents a 4-point scale that describes the amplitude of the pulse (WOCN®, 2008). Because a variety of 3- and 4-point scales are used in clinical practice, it is important to specify the type of scale used (e.g., 3+pedal pulse on a 4-point scale).

DIAGNOSTIC TESTING

When the diagnosis is unclear or wound healing fails, diagnostic studies are indicated (WOCN®, 2008, 2011, 2012).

BOX 10-4	**Assessment of Amplitude of the Pulse**

4	Bounding
3	Full, increased
2	Expected
1	Diminished, barely palpable
0	Absent, not palpable

From Ball JW, Dains JE, Flynn JA: Blood vessels. In *Seidel's guide to physical examination*, ed 8, St. Louis, MO, 2015, Mosby, pp 332–349.

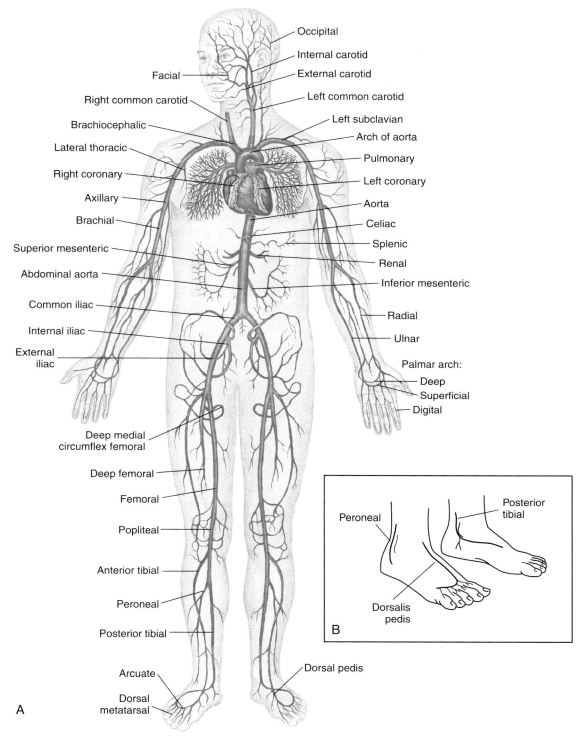

Occipital
Internal carotid
Facial
External carotid
Right common carotid
Left common carotid
Brachiocephalic
Left subclavian
Lateral thoracic
Arch of aorta
Right coronary
Pulmonary
Axillary
Left coronary
Brachial
Aorta
Superior mesenteric
Celiac
Abdominal aorta
Splenic
Common iliac
Renal
Internal iliac
Inferior mesenteric
External iliac
Radial
Ulnar
Palmar arch:
Deep
Superficial
Digital
Deep medial circumflex femoral
Deep femoral
Femoral
Popliteal
Peroneal
Posterior tibial
Anterior tibial
Dorsalis pedis
Peroneal
Posterior tibial
Dorsal pedis
Arcuate
Dorsal metatarsal

A

B

FIGURE 10-2 A, Arterial structure of lower extremity. **B,** delineates approximate location of peroneal artery, posterior tibialis, and dorsalis pedis pulses. (Ball JW, Dains JE, Flynn JA: Blood vessels. In *Seidel's guide to physical examination*, ed 8, St. Louis, MO, 2015, Mosby, pp 332–349.)

Vascular referral and studies are indicated to identify the components of the vascular system involved in the disease process, the specific pathologic process, the anatomic level of the lesions or dysfunction, and the severity of dysfunction (Hirsch et al, 2006; WOCN®, 2008). With the exception of the ankle-brachial index, these tests involve equipment that is reserved for use in a vascular laboratory by a trained technician and reviewed by a vascular radiologist or surgeon. Checklist 10-2 lists diagnostic tests used for the patient with a wound resulting from lower extremity disease. Diagnostic tests are described in detail in Chapters 11 through 15.

CLINICAL CONSULT

A: Referred to wound clinic by home care nurse for foot wound. Patient is a 58-year-old male, s/p colon resection, type 1 DM (A1c 7.8), coronary artery disease, hyperlipidemia, hypertension, retinopathy, and peripheral neuropathy. Patient was unaware of wound until nurse pointed it out. Patient reports previous callous in the same location. Right plantar aspect of the 5th metatarsal wound 2 × 2 cm punched out shape. Wound base 90% pale pink and 10% dry brown necrotic tissue, minimal exudate, calloused wound edges, periwound skin intact. No local signs of infection. Bilateral legs warm, skin thin, dry, flaky, sparse hair growth below the knee, and nail discoloration. Capillary refill is > 3 seconds. PT and DP pulses palpable but faint. No elevation pallor or dependent rubor noted. Semmes-Weinstein 5.07 monofilament test shows loss of protective sensation. Patient states legs ache at night with periodic shooting pain that is relieved with walking. Patient reports a 10 lb. weight loss since surgery.
D: Neuropathic ulceration with some level of arterial involvement. Inadequate nutrition and blood glucose management. High risk for amputation.

P: Protect feet from further pressure and trauma while minimizing potential for wound infection and ascertain level of arterial disease.
I: Home Care nurse and patient understand and agree with the following plan of care: (1) Contact provider ASAP for further evaluation of arterial perfusion; recommend toe brachial index testing due to type 1 DM causing vessel calcification. (2) Consult orthotics for custom insert and shoe to off load right 5th metatarsal; consider total contact casting if arterial perfusion is adequate. (3) Inspect feet daily, apply moisturizer to legs/feet daily, and keep toe webspaces clean and dry. (4) Conservative sharp debridement weekly to remove callous and non-viable tissue by certified wound care specialist. (5) Foam dressing for protection and exudate absorption, change three times per week. (6) Notify provider for changes in skin color, temperature, pain, or an increase size in wound size, drainage, or odor. (7) Dietary consult for assistance with blood glucose management and recent weight loss (importance of protein reviewed with patient).
E: Return to clinic in 1 week to continue callous debridement and to modify plan as needed based on consult recommendation and patient wishes.

SUMMARY

Lower extremity ulcers are an increasingly common problem and may be caused by compromised function in any component of the circulatory system (e.g., arterial, venous, lymphatic). Table 10-3 provides a brief summary of key assessment distinctions among arterial, venous, and neuropathic ulcers. However, multiple causes of lower extremity ulcers, including vasculitis, autoimmune disorders, neuropathy, and metabolic derangements, can precipitate ulcerations on the leg, with unique manifestations (Alavi et al, 2012). To further complicate the picture, many patients have ulcers of mixed etiology or comorbidities that affect management and the potential for healing. The wound specialist must utilize astute physical assessment skills and clearly and accurately document findings to facilitate an accurate differential assessment that leads to the correct diagnosis in a timely manner.

TABLE 10-3   Characteristics of Arterial, Venous, and Neuropathic Ulcers

	Arterial	Venous	Neuropathic
Location	Tips of toes (spontaneous necrosis) Pressure points (e.g., heel, lateral foot) Areas of trauma (nonhealing wounds)	Between ankles and knees; "classic" location is medial malleolus	Plantar surface over metatarsal heads Areas of foot exposed to repetitive trauma (toes, sides of feet)
Wound bed	Pale or necrotic	Dark red, "ruddy" May be covered with fibrinous slough	Typically red (if no coexisting ischemia)
Exudate	Minimal	Moderate to large amounts	Moderate to large amounts
Wound edges	Well defined	Poorly defined, irregular	Well defined Frequently associated with callous formation

TABLE 10-3   Characteristics of Arterial, Venous, and Neuropathic Ulcers—cont'd

	Arterial	Venous	Neuropathic
Other	Infection common, but signs and symptoms muted Typically painful Typically associated with other indicators (ischemia, diminished/absent pulses, elevational pallor, dependent rubor, thin fragile skin) See Plates 24, 25, and 38	Edema common Hyperpigmentation surrounding skin common Feet typically warm with good pulses (if no coexisting arterial disease) See Plates 1, 26, 34, 35, and 39	Infection common, but signs and symptoms may be muted May have coexisting ischemia See Plates 40 and 41

REFERENCES

Alavi A, Mayer D, Hafner J, et al: Martorell hypertensive ischemic leg ulcer: an underdiagnosed entity, *Adv Skin Wound Care* 25(12):563–572, 2012.

American Diabetes Association(ADA): Standards of medical care in diabetes–2014, *Diabetes Care* 37(Suppl 1):S14–S80, 2014.

Armstrong DG, Holtz-Neiderer K, Wendel C, et al: Skin temperature monitoring reduces the risk for diabetic foot ulceration in high-risk patients, *Am J Med* 120(12):1042–1046, 2007.

Ball JW, Dains, JE, Flynn JA: Blood vessels. In Seidel's guide to physical examination, ed 8, St. Louis, MO, 2015, Mosby, pp 332–349.

Bonham P: Assessment and management of patients with venous, arterial, and diabetic/neuropathic lower extremity wounds, *AACN Clin Issues* 14(4):442–456, 2003.

Bonham P, Kelechi T: Evaluation of lower extremity arterial circulation and implications for nursing practice, *J Cardiovasc Nurs* 23(2):144–152, 2008.

Boulton AJ, Armstrong DG, Albert SF, et al: Comprehensive foot examination and risk assessment. A report of the Task Force of the Foot Care Interest Group of the American Diabetes Association, with endorsement by the American Association of Clinical Endocrinologists, *Phys Ther* 88(11):1436–1443, 2008.

Buczkowski G, Munschauer C, Vasquez M: Chronic venous insufficiency, *Clin Rev* 19(3):18–24, 2009.

Carpentier PH, Cornu-Thénard A, Uhf JF, et al: Appraisal of the information content of the C classes of CEAP clinical classification of chronic venous disorders: a multicenter evaluation of 872 patients, *J Vasc Surg* 37(4):827–833, 2003.

Caselli A, Pham H, Giurini JM, et al: The forefoot-to-rearfoot plantar pressure ratio is increased in severe diabetic neuropathy and can predict foot ulceration, *Diabetes Care* 25(6):1006–1071, 2002.

Collins T, Suarez-Almazor M, Peterson NJ, et al: An absent pulse is not sensitive for the early detection of peripheral arterial disease, *Fam Med* 38(1):38–42, 2006.

Gey DC, Lesho E, Manngold J: Management of peripheral arterial disease, *Am Fam Physician* 69(3):525–532, 2004.

Hirsch A, Haskal ZJ, Hertzer NR, et al: ACC/AHA 2005 practice guidelines for the management of patients with peripheral arterial disease (lower extremity, renal, mesenteric, and abdominal aortic), *Circulation* 113(11):e463–e654, 2006.

Health Resources and Services Administration (HRSA): *Lower extremity amputation prevention (LEAP)*, 2011. http://www.hrsa.gov/hansensdisease/leap/index.html. Accessed Feb 8, 2014.

Hopf HW, Ueno C, Aslam R, et al: Guidelines for the treatment of arterial insufficiency ulcers, *Wound Repair Regen* 14(6):693–710, 2006.

International Best Practice Guidelines: *Wound management in diabetic foot ulcers*, Wounds International, 2013. http://www.woundsinternational.com/pdf/content_10803.pdf. Accessed June 1, 2014.

Kelechi TJ, Bonham PA: Lower extremity venous disorders: implications for nursing practice, *J Cardiovasc Nurs* 23(2):132–143, 2008.

Kelechi TJ, Haight BK, Herman J, et al: Skin temperature and chronic venous insufficiency, *J Wound Ostomy Continence Nurs* 30(1):17–24, 2003.

Khan N, Rahim S, Anand S, et al: A: Does the clinical examination predict lower extremity peripheral arterial disease? *JAMA* 295:536–546, 2006.

Lavery LA, Higgins KR, Lanctot DR, et al: Preventing diabetic foot ulcer recurrence in high-risk patients: the use of temperature monitoring as a self-assessment tool, *Diabetes Care* 30(1):14–20, 2007.

Margolis DJ: Epidemiology of wounds. In Mani R, Romancelli M, Shukla V, editors: *Measurements in wound healing: science and practice,* London, 2013, Springer, pp 145–153.

McDermott M, Sufit R, Nishida T, et al: Lower extremity nerve function in patients with lower extremity ischemia, *Arch Intern Med* 166(18):1986–1992, 2006.

Padberg FT, Johnston MV, Sisto SA, et al: Structured exercise improves calf muscle pump function in chronic venous insufficiency: a randomized trial, *J Vasc Surg* 39(1):79–87, 2004.

Rumwell C, McPharlin M: *Vascular technology*, ed 3, Pasadena, CA, 2004, Davies Publishing.

Sayre EK, Kelechi TJ, Neal D, et al: Sudden increase in skin temperature predicts venous ulcers: a case study, *J Vasc Nurs* 25(3): 46–50, 2007.

Sen CK, Gordillo GS, Roy S, et al: Human skin wounds: A major and snowballing threat to public health and the economy, *Wound Repair Regen* 17:673–771, 2009.

Stanton AW, Badger C, Sitzia J: Non-invasive assessment of the lymphedematous limb, *Lymphology* 33(3):122–135, 2000.

Stanton AW, Northfield JW, Holroyd B, et al: Validation of an opto-electronic limb volumeter (perometer), *Lymphology* 30(2): 77–97, 1997.

Wound, Ostomy and Continence Nurses Society™ (WOCN®): *Guideline for management of patients with lower extremity arterial disease* (WOCN ®clinical practice guideline series no. 1), Mt. Laurel, NJ, 2008, WOCN®.

Wound, Ostomy and Continence Nurses Society™ (WOCN®): *Guideline for management of patients with lower extremity venous disease* (WOCN® clinical practice guideline series no. 2), Glenview IL, 2011, WOCN®.

Wound, Ostomy and Continence Nurses Society™ (WOCN®): *Guideline for management of patients with lower extremity neuropathic disease* (WOCN® clinical practice guideline series no. 3), Glenview, IL, 2012, WOCN®.

11

Arterial Ulcers

Dorothy B. Doughty

OBJECTIVES

1. Describe etiologic factors, risk factors, pathophysiology, typical presentation, and principles of management for arterial ulcers.
2. Describe essential assessment for the patient with a suspected arterial ulcer, including history, pain assessment, physical assessment, and laboratory studies.
3. Outline a patient teaching plan for the individual with ischemic disease of the lower extremity, including lifestyle changes to maximize perfusion and measures to prevent trauma.
4. Distinguish between *critical* limb ischemia and *acute* limb ischemia, including assessment parameters and implications for management.
5. Identify indications and options for surgical revascularization and for amputation.
6. Describe pharmacologic options for management of arterial ulcers.
7. Recommend appropriate topical therapy for each of the following: ischemic ulcer covered with dry eschar and no signs of infection; ischemic ulcer covered with dry eschar and mild erythema and fluctuance of surrounding skin; open ischemic ulcer with and without signs of infection.

Arterial ulcers (also known as *ischemic ulcers*) occur as a result of severe tissue ischemia and are extremely painful. In addition, ischemic ulcers represent potential limb loss. These lesions are generally refractory to healing unless tissue perfusion can be improved, and they are prone to progress to invasive infection or gangrene, which may necessitate amputation (WOCN®, 2008). Of further concern is the likelihood of coexisting, and possibly unrecognized, cardiovascular or cerebrovascular disease. Thus any patient with an ulcer caused or complicated by arterial insufficiency requires thorough physical assessment and aggressive management. The treatment plan for these patients must be multifaceted, including measures to maximize perfusion and minimize risk of infection, evidence-based wound care, and ongoing assessment and management of ischemic pain. Effective management of ischemic disease frequently requires significant lifestyle modifications; thus patient education and counseling are essential elements of the management plan.

EPIDEMIOLOGY

Many terms are used to describe the anomalies that can affect the peripheral vascular system. *Peripheral vascular disease* describes noncardiac disease that includes numerous conditions affecting the arterial, venous, and lymphatic circulation. *Peripheral arterial disease* (PAD) specifically refers to a range of noncoronary arterial syndromes caused by an alteration in the structure and function of the arteries that supply the brain, visceral organs, and limbs; it is the preferred term for stenotic, occlusive, and aneurysmal diseases (Hirsch et al, 2006). Peripheral arterial occlusive disease describes arterial disease that is specifically occlusive in nature. Finally, *lower extremity arterial disease* (LEAD) includes only arterial disease that affects the leg arteries and excludes arterial diseases of the aorta, carotid, upper extremity, or visceral arteries (Hirsch et al, 2006; WOCN®, 2008). Most ischemic ulcers develop as a result of LEAD.

Although ischemic ulcers are much less common than those resulting from venous insufficiency or neuropathy, the underlying disease process (LEAD) is quite prevalent, especially among the elderly. It is estimated that LEAD affects one third of adults 65 and older, and similar prevalence rates are reported among younger adults who use tobacco or have diabetes mellitus. Lower extremity arterial disease is the third leading cause of morbidity related to atherosclerosis, affecting approximately 202 million people worldwide (Bonham, 2011; Fowkes et al, 2013). Unfortunately, many individuals with LEAD are undiagnosed; "silent" disease may account for almost half of cases (Aronow, 2008; Haigh et al., 2013; Sigvant et al, 2009; WOCN®, 2008).

The high prevalence of undiagnosed disease is explained by the fact that vascular disease frequently is asymptomatic until the disease process is advanced; this is true of coronary artery disease and cerebrovascular disease as well as LEAD. Unfortunately, the failure to diagnose vascular disease early results in failure to treat until the disease is advanced and the patient becomes symptomatic. Advanced (symptomatic) disease is associated with much greater risk of morbidity and mortality (e.g., myocardial infarction, cerebrovascular accident, limb loss) and is much less amenable to effective treatment; thus the focus in management of patients with any form of vascular disease (e.g., coronary artery disease, cerebrovascular disease, LEAD) must shift to routine screening to detect asymptomatic disease. Because atherosclerotic disease is the most common disease process affecting the arterial system and is a systemic phenomenon, the patient with disease in one vascular bed (e.g., coronary artery bed) is at greater risk for disease in another vascular bed (Hirsch et al, 2006). Studies indicate that patients with LEAD are very likely to have coexisting coronary artery disease or cerebrovascular disease and are at significantly greater risk for early death due to a cardiac event (Aronow, 2008; Sigvant et al, 2009; WOCN®, 2008). Ankle-brachial index (ABI) testing with a handheld Doppler is an effective bedside screening procedure. Because an abnormal ABI (<0.9 or >1.4) is an independent predictor for increased risk of cardiovascular death, individuals with an abnormal ABI should be referred for further assessment to rule out "silent but treatable" cardiac disease (Alzamora et al, 2013; Bevc et al, 2013; Jones et al, 2014).

As noted, a significant proportion of individuals with LEAD are asymptomatic. Patients who are symptomatic most commonly present with intermittent claudication (pain with walking that is relieved by rest). Others present with vague complaints of impaired mobility and leg weakness (Wennberg, 2013); the diagnosis is frequently "missed" in these individuals, whose symptoms may be attributed to aging, musculoskeletal disorders, or sedentary lifestyle.

Chronic vs. Acute Limb Ischemia

Lower extremity arterial disease results in chronic ischemia of variable severity; the disease process progresses over time and produces gradually worsening symptomatology, including the ulcers that are the focus of this chapter. In contrast, *acute limb ischemia* refers to a quickly developing or sudden decrease in limb perfusion that threatens limb viability (Hirsch et al, 2006; Norgren et al, 2007). Signs of acute limb ischemia include the six *P*s: pain, paralysis, paresthesias, pulselessness, pallor, and polar (cold extremity). Because irreversible nerve and muscle damage may occur within hours, all patients with suspected acute limb ischemia require urgent evaluation by a vascular specialist (Norgren et al, 2007).

Critical Limb Ischemia

Critical limb ischemia (CLI) is the term used to denote advanced LEAD; classic indicators of CLI include chronic ischemic rest pain, ulcerations, gangrene, and ABI less than 0.4. The goals in management of patients with CLI include healing of ulcers, limb preservation, reduced pain, and improved quality of life (Lambert and Belch, 2013; WOCN®, 2008).

ETIOLOGY

Arterial insufficiency and arterial ulcers are most common among older adults and middle-aged adults who have additional risk factors, such as diabetes, smoking, hyperlipidemia, or hypertension (Fowkes et al, 2013). The most common causative factor in these cases is atherosclerotic disease. Arterial ulcers can also occur as a result of thromboangiitis obliterans (TAO) (Buerger disease), sickle cell disease, and vasculitis (see Chapter 30); these conditions are less common but can occur among younger as well as older adults. Least common are arterial ulcers that develop as a result of entrapment syndromes, acute embolic syndromes, and arterial trauma (Hirsch et al, 2006).

Atherosclerosis

The most common cause of LEAD and arterial ulceration among older adults is atherosclerosis involving the peripheral circulation. Atherosclerotic disease can occur in any vessel in the body. In the peripheral circulation the aortic, iliac, femoral, and popliteal arteries (see Figure 10-2) are the vessels most commonly affected (Dillavou and Kahn, 2003).

Although the pathology of atherosclerotic disease is not completely understood, it is known to involve two primary processes: plaque formation and enlargement, which cause narrowing of the vessel lumen, and endothelial injury triggering an inflammatory process that ultimately results in fibrosis and hardening of the vessel wall (Hirsch et al, 2006).

Plaque formation begins with the lesion known as a "fatty streak," which is a gray or pearly white lesion that adheres to the intima (inner layer of the arterial wall). This lesion consists of a lipid core and a connective tissue covering. As further lipid accumulation occurs, the plaque enlarges, which results in progressive narrowing of the vessel lumen. Over time the plaques harden as a result of deposition of calcium salts and cholesterol crystals, causing loss of vessel elasticity, which further compromises blood flow (Hirsch et al, 2006).

The second process contributing to vessel narrowing and hardening is triggered by damage to the vessel lining. Endothelial damage results in areas where the intimal lining is denuded. Platelets aggregate over these denuded areas, causing clot formation and the subsequent release of growth factors that stimulate mitosis of the vascular smooth muscle cells and promote synthesis of connective tissue proteins such as collagen. The end result is thickening and fibrosis of the vessel wall, which further contributes to narrowing and hardening of the involved arteries. Clinically these changes result in a chronic reduction in blood flow to the tissues and a loss of the ability to respond with increased blood flow when metabolic demands are increased. In addition, acute vessel occlusion may occur as a result of sudden plaque enlargement or plaque rupture (Hirsch et al, 2006).

Lower extremity arterial disease due to atherosclerosis is a progressive disease process, ranging from asymptomatic disease to spontaneous tissue necrosis and gangrene. The severity is sometimes classified according to the Fontaine system, which designates the following levels of progression: I = asymptomatic disease, II = intermittent claudication, III = nocturnal pain, and IV = tissue necrosis/gangrene (Gardner and Afaq, 2008).

Thromboangiitis Obliterans (Buerger Disease)

Thromboangiitis obliterans, also known as Buerger disease and arteriosclerosis obliterans, is a nonatherosclerotic disease process that involves the small and medium-sized arteries in both the upper and lower extremities (Dargon and Landry, 2012). It most commonly affects young and middle-aged adults and is predominantly found in those who are heavy smokers (Dargon and Landry, 2012; Hirsch et al, 2006). The process is always bilateral and frequently involves all four limbs. The pathology of the disease remains unclear, but does not involve plaque formation. Recent studies have shown that patients with TAO have higher levels of both prothrombotic factors and inflammatory cytokines compared with healthy controls; these data suggest that inflammation or hypercoagulability may contribute to the etiology of the disease. Interestingly, inflammation can contribute to clotting by increasing the concentration of procoagulation factors, and clot formation can in turn contribute to inflammation, possibly due to the release of growth factors (Aksu et al, 2012; Dellalibera-Joviliano et al, 2012; Hus et al, 2013). Clinical indicators of TAO include cold sensitivity, rest pain, pedal claudication, digital ulceration, and gangrene. Ulceration may occur spontaneously but more commonly is precipitated by minor trauma. The most critical element of management is elimination of tobacco use, which provides consistent interruption of the disease process. In addition, selected prostacyclin analogs (e.g., iloprost) may provide improved healing and better pain relief, but only when combined with total elimination of tobacco use (Bozkurt et al, 2013). Among individuals who continue to use tobacco, digit or limb amputations are common; however, mortality is not increased (Hanly et al, 2009).

Sickle Cell Disease

Sickle cell disease is a hereditary disease that affects 90,000 to 100,000 Americans and occurs most commonly among those of African American descent (Apanah and Rizzolo, 2013). During physiologic stress in a person with sickle cell disease, the red blood cells become deformed into a crescent moon or sickle shape. These abnormal blood cells clump together and cause vascular occlusion and tissue necrosis, a phenomenon known as vasoocclusive crisis. In addition, there is increased expression of adhesion molecules on the endothelial surface during a vasoocclusive crisis; this causes the sickled cells to attach, which results in further occlusion and necrosis. One potential end result of this pathologic sequence is the development of lower extremity ulcers. Fortunately, once the crisis is resolved, blood flow typically is restored, and the ulcer slowly heals. Unfortunately, many individuals develop chronic ulcers that are very slow to heal. Many individuals with sickle cell disease also have chronic venous insufficiency, which further delays healing.

Management of sickle cell ulcers begins with measures to reduce the risk of vasoocclusive crisis, such as blood transfusions to replace the abnormal red blood cells with normal cells, and hydroxyurea, which increases the levels of fetal (normal) hemoglobin. Some studies suggest that the amino acid arginine butyrate can also increase the levels of fetal hemoglobin and may contribute to wound healing through other mechanisms. Inhaled nitric oxide is another therapy that has been shown in small studies to be of benefit, most likely due to its ability to induce vasodilation via relaxation of the vascular smooth muscle. However, at this time neither arginine nor nitric oxide is approved by the Food and Drug Administration (FDA) for treatment of sickle cell ulcers. Additional treatment measures include pain management, prompt treatment of infections, and general health promotion. Wound care is based on moist wound healing and on compression therapy to control edema (Apanah and Rizzolo, 2013; Delaney et al, 2013; Ladzinski et al, 2012). (See Table 30-7 for a list of the characteristics and treatment for sickle cell ulcers.)

Vasculitis

Another potential cause of ischemic ulceration is vasculitis, which is a general term for inflammation of vessel walls. The inflammation may produce defects in the vessel wall, allowing leakage of blood into the surrounding tissues, or it may produce vessel occlusion and tissue necrosis. The vasculitis "umbrella" comprises a large number of specific conditions that vary significantly in clinical presentation and prognosis, depending on the size and location of the inflamed vessels. The causative factors for vasculitis are not well defined, but the condition is frequently associated with either an acute allergic reaction or an autoimmune process. When the condition is associated with an autoimmune process, the patient commonly presents with systemic symptoms such as malaise, joint pain, and low-grade fever in addition to the specific symptoms produced by the inflamed vessels. Vasculitic conditions producing lower extremity ulcers typically involve midsized and small arteries and are characterized by a petechial rash, purpura, tissue necrosis, and extreme pain. Diagnosis is suggested by patient history, clinical presentation, and high serum levels of inflammatory markers and is confirmed by biopsy demonstrating vessel inflammation. Systemic management primarily involves immunosuppressive and antiinflammatory agents, as well as effective pain management. Topical therapy is based on the principles of wound bed preparation (elimination of necrotic tissue and control of bacterial burden) and moist wound healing (Aksu et al, 2012; Gaffo, 2013; Xu et al, 2009). (See Chapter 30 and Table 30-1 for further discussion of vasculitis and vasculitic ulcers.)

RISK FACTORS FOR LEAD

Risk factors for LEAD (Box 11-1) are the same as those for coronary artery disease and include both modifiable factors

BOX 11-1 Risk Factors for Lower Extremity Arterial Disease (LEAD)

Causal Modifiable (see Table 11-1)
1. Smoking
2. Diabetes
3. Dyslipidemia
4. Hypertension

Predisposing
1. Modifiable factors (obesity, inactivity, social isolation, stress)
2. Nonmodifiable factors (advanced age, male gender, post-menopausal status, family history, African American ethnicity)

Emerging
1. Elevated homocysteine levels
2. Inflammation
3. Infection
4. Renal failure

TABLE 11-1 Management of Modifiable Risk Factors

Risk Factor	Management Goals/Guidelines
Tobacco use	*Goal:* Cessation of tobacco use *Guidelines:* See Box 11–2
Diabetes mellitus	*Goal:* HbA1c 7.0% (8% for high-risk patient) *Guidelines:* • Patient education and counseling regarding diet and exercise • Oral hypoglycemics and/or insulin
Dyslipidemia	*Goals:* • LDL-C <100 mg/dl (<70 mg/dl for very-high-risk patient) • HDL-C >40 mg/dl for men, >45 mg/dl for women • Triglycerides <150 mg/dl *Guidelines:* • Patient education and counseling regarding diet and exercise • Statins
Hypertension	*Goals:* <140/90 mm Hg (nondiabetic), <130/80 mm Hg (diabetic) *Guidelines:* • Patient education and counseling regarding diet and exercise • Antihypertensive medications • Thiazide diuretics as initial drug • Angiotensin-converting enzyme inhibitor or angiotensin receptor blocker for patient with diabetic renal disease (except patient with renal artery stenosis) or congestive heart failure • β-adrenergic blocker for patient who also has coronary artery disease • Calcium channel blocker as needed for uncontrolled hypertension *Note:* Multiple agents should be used as needed to maintain blood pressure within accepted range.

HDL-C, High-density lipoprotein cholesterol; *LDL-C,* low-density lipoprotein cholesterol.

and predisposing factors. Studies have identified a number of "emerging" risk factors that appear to be associated with the development of atherosclerotic disease, but their impact is not yet well defined (Liapis et al, 2009). Although some of these risk factors, such as age, gender, and family history, are irreversible, the majority are very responsive to lifestyle modifications and pharmacologic therapy. A clear understanding of current recommendations for management of risk factors is critical because effective management of the underlying disease process is essential for wound healing, limb salvage, and long-term survival (Aronow, 2008; Liapis et al, 2009; WOCN®, 2008).

Causal Modifiable Risk Factors

The "big four" risk factors are those that appear to play a direct causal role in the development of atherosclerosis: smoking, diabetes mellitus, dyslipidemia, and hypertension. All of these risk factors are modifiable, and all contribute to cardiovascular morbidity and mortality, as well as to the progression of LEAD; thus management of these factors should be the clinician's primary focus. Table 11-1 and Box 11-2 summarize goals and guidelines for the management of modifiable risk factors (Abdulhannan et al, 2012; Fowkes, 2013; Liapis et al, 2009).

Smoking. Smoking is a highly significant risk factor for atherosclerotic disease in general and for LEAD in particular; smokers have a fourfold increased risk for LEAD. Most studies suggest a connection between pack-year history and the number and severity of vascular complications; however, the number of pack-years that constitutes a significant increased risk for vascular disease is unknown (Liapis et al, 2009; Sigvant et al, 2009; WOCN®, 2008). Smoking may be particularly harmful to women, who reportedly have a significant increase in risk with a 10-year pack history, compared with men, whose risk increases significantly with a 30-year pack history (Sigvant et al, 2009). The negative effects of tobacco on the vascular system are due to its byproducts: nicotine, carbon monoxide, and hydrogen cyanide. The most significant of these is nicotine, which is a potent vasoconstrictor and promotes platelet aggregation and clot formation. In addition to these negative effects, tobacco use potentiates the adverse effects of other risk factors for LEAD (Katsiki et al, 2013). Fortunately, smoking cessation can significantly reduce the progression of LEAD, as well as mortality rates from other vascular complications; thus smoking cessation (see Box 11-2) should be a primary target of therapy and should include patient education, patient support, nicotine replacement therapy, and pharmacologic agents when needed (Aronow, 2008; Hopf et al, 2008; Katsiki et al, 2013; Liapis et al, 2009; WOCN®, 2008).

Diabetes Mellitus. Diabetes, especially type 2, is one of the strongest predictors of LEAD, with disease most likely to involve the smaller vessels below the knee, the tibial and peroneal arteries (Gibbons and Shaw, 2012). Of great significance, patients with diabetes are at increased risk for death and limb loss caused by vascular disease; for each 1% increase in hemoglobin A1c (HbA1c) there is a 28% increase in risk of death, and patients with diabetes are 10 times more likely to progress to CLI and amputation (Hirsch et al, 2006; Liapis et al, 2009; WOCN®, 2008). Specific pathologic features associated with diabetes that contribute to LEAD include endothelial dysfunction (imbalance in production of vasoconstrictor and vasodilator substances), platelet overactivity (and, for many patients, poor response to antiplatelet therapy), and possibly increased levels of profibrotic and proinflammatory cytokines such as endothelin-1 (Ergul, 2011; Rollini et al, 2013). Clinically these pathologic processes result in vessel constriction, hypercoagulability, and overproduction of vascular smooth muscle. Insulin resistance and hyperinsulinemia may also contribute to hypertrophy of vascular smooth muscle, even in the early stages of the disease, because insulin is known to be a vascular growth factor. Fortunately, tight glycemic control (HbA1c 7.0%) can significantly reduce the risk of vascular complications and amputation; thus effective diabetes management (through diet, exercise, and pharmacologic therapy) is another key element of effective therapy for the patient with LEAD (Hopf et al, 2008). Current guidelines suggest that the "usual" goal for glycemic control is an HbA1c of around 7.0%, which correlates with a mean plasma glucose level of 126 mg/dl. For selected patients (those with newly diagnosed diabetes, long life expectancy, and no cardiovascular disease), tighter goals may be appropriate (HbA1c of

6.5%). Conversely, a less stringent goal (HbA1c < 8.0 %) may be appropriate for patients with limited life expectancy, extensive comorbidities, a history of severe hypoglycemia, or long-standing disease that is very difficult to control despite aggressive management (ADA, 2014).

Dyslipidemia. Elevated levels of cholesterol, low-density lipoprotein cholesterol (LDL-C), triglycerides, and lipoprotein(a) are independent risk factors for LEAD. Each 10 mg/dl rise in total cholesterol is associated with a 10% increase in risk (Hirsch et al, 2006; Liapis et al, 2009; WOCN®, 2008). In contrast, elevated levels of high-density lipoprotein cholesterol (HDL-C) appear to play a protective role. Recommended target levels for lipid management and strategies for maintaining normal lipid levels are provided in Table 11-1.

Hypertension. Elevated blood pressure (BP) is associated with up to a threefold increase in risk for LEAD in addition to a significant increase in risk for cardiovascular disease. Although treatment with antihypertensive medication has not been shown to improve LEAD outcomes, it is an essential element of care because of its impact on morbidity from cardiovascular and cerebrovascular disease. Current goals and guidelines for maintaining BP are listed in Table 11-1 (Aronow, 2008; Liapis et al, 2009; Mensah and Bakris, 2010; WOCN®, 2008).

Predisposing Risk Factors

Although predisposing risk factors *may* increase risk independently, they primarily act to increase the impact of primary (causative) risk factors. Predisposing risk factors include both modifiable factors (e.g., obesity, inactivity, social isolation, stress) and nonmodifiable factors (e.g., advanced age, male gender, postmenopausal status, family history, African American ethnicity). Clinicians should work with patients and other providers to eliminate or minimize modifiable factors through diet, exercise, and strategies that reduce stress and isolation. Clinicians should educate patients about the impact of nonmodifiable risk factors and the critical importance of attention to smoking cessation, glycemic control, BP control, and correction of dyslipidemia (Hopf et al, 2008; Liapis et al, 2009; WOCN®, 2008).

Emerging Risk Factors

Emerging risk factors include conditions such as elevated homocysteine levels, inflammation, infection, and indicators of renal failure.

Homocystinemia. Homocystinemia is a rare autosomal-dominant disease found in 30% to 40% of individuals with LEAD. Studies suggest that elevated homocysteine levels are associated with atherosclerosis and may increase risk for LEAD; however, whether homocystinemia plays an etiologic role in LEAD is unclear. The abnormal metabolism of homocysteine (a thiol-containing amino acid) can be normalized through administration of vitamin B_6, vitamin B_{12}, and/or folic acid. Although some studies show significant improvements in ABI's following therapy to normalize homocysteine levels, more studies are needed before any definitive recommendations can be made (Andras et al, 2013; Liapis et al, 2009; WOCN®, 2008).

Inflammation. Inflammation is known to play a role in the development of atherosclerotic lesions in that endothelial injury triggers an inflammatory response that ultimately results in fibrosis. Some investigators suggest that repeated episodes of tissue ischemia (as evidenced by claudication) may trigger a low-grade inflammatory response that contributes to disease progression. Others have hypothesized that rapid progression of the disease process in a subset of patients may be the result of an underlying inflammatory disorder. The role of inflammation in the progression of the disease seems to be supported by studies demonstrating the presence of inflammatory markers such as C-reactive protein (CRP) within atherosclerotic plaque and by elevated levels of inflammatory markers such as CRP, fibrinogen, and interleukin-6 among patients with advanced PAD. In addition, the potential for therapeutic intervention seems to be supported by data showing an inverse relationship between patients' omega-3 values and inflammatory biomarkers; this suggests that dietary changes or fish oil supplements might possibly reduce the inflammatory process and improve outcomes in patients with LEAD. However, the link between inflammation and the progression of PAD is unclear, and at present there are no recommendations for routine assessment of inflammatory markers such as CRP levels or for intervention (Chaparaia et al, 2009; Grenon et al, 2013; Liapis et al, 2009; van Wijk et al, 2013; WOCN®, 2008).

Infection. Inflammation, specifically both periodontal disease and *Chlamydia pneumoniae* (CPN), has been associated with increased risk and severity of LEAD. Acute CPN infections have been associated with increased lipid abnormalities and endothelial dysfunction. Antibiotic treatment of LEAD resulted in better clinical outcomes in patients who were seropositive for CPN than in seropositive controls who did not receive antibiotic therapy. Although more research is needed, prompt treatment of any infectious process is recommended for all patients (Liapis et al, 2009; WOCN®, 2008).

Kidney Disease. Chronic kidney disease (CKD) is an independent risk factor for development of atherosclerotic disease. In addition, patients with CKD are at greater risk for cardiovascular-associated morbidity and mortality, including limb loss. Revascularization for critical limb ischemia is also less successful in these patients. These facts underscore the importance of aggressive management of all reversible risk factors for patients with CKD, as well as prompt and comprehensive treatment of PAD to minimize the risk of amputation (Garimella et al, 2012; Tamura et al, 2013).

PATHOLOGY OF ARTERIAL ULCERATION

The exact pathologic mechanisms producing ulceration in the ischemic limb have not been clearly defined. Spontaneous ulceration typically involves the toes or distal foot and most likely is the result of progressive occlusion leading to cellular ischemia and tissue necrosis. Arterial ulcers may also be precipitated by minor trauma, which results in nonhealing wounds because the damaged vessels are unable to meet the increased demands for oxygen associated with tissue injury and the healing process (Hirsch et al, 2006; Wennberg, 2013). Patients with LEAD and compromised mobility are at greater risk for pressure ulcer development because they have an existing baseline of diminished blood flow. Therefore heel ulcers may occur rapidly in a bedbound patient with preexisting vascular impairment. It should be emphasized that pressure ulcers in these patients *are* avoidable; they can be prevented with standard interventions such as heel elevation.

ASSESSMENT

A comprehensive assessment provides the data needed for development of an appropriate management plan for any patient with a lower extremity ulcer (Checklist 11-1). In a small percentage of patients, arterial insufficiency is the only etiologic factor; more commonly, arterial insufficiency is a complicating factor for ulcers caused primarily by venous insufficiency or neuropathy or by combined pathologies. The clinician must consider all etiologic and contributing factors when developing and implementing a management plan, and this requires a comprehensive vascular and sensorimotor assessment. For example, the patient with a venous ulcer who has coexisting arterial insufficiency will require modifications in the management plan based on the severity of the coexisting arterial disease. In addition, a comprehensive assessment enables the clinician to identify patients with asymptomatic (early) arterial insufficiency; these patients should be referred for cardiac workup even if the level of LEAD is mild and does not interfere with wound healing (Jude et al, 2010; Wennberg, 2013).

A comprehensive assessment for any patient with a lower extremity ulcer should include the patient's medical/surgical history, ulcer history (to include onset and previous management), pain patterns, vascular and sensorimotor assessment, and ulcer characteristics. Simple noninvasive vascular studies should be conducted on all patients; select patients may require more complex or invasive vascular studies. It should be noted that palpable pulses alone do *not* rule out arterial disease; dependence on such unreliable assessment methods is a major contributing factor to the high incidence of unrecognized and untreated LEAD.

Patient History

The patient interview should include general queries regarding any past illnesses or surgical procedures. Specific questions

CHECKLIST 11-1 Lower Extremity Arterial Disease (LEAD) Assessment

✓ General appearance
- Trophic changes: thin, shiny epidermis
- Hair and nail patterns: loss of hair growth, thickened nails
- Edema: variable based on need to keep leg dependent and coexisting disease
- Skin color: pale or ischemic colors (possibly purpura and petechiae secondary to blood thinners)

✓ Functional sensory status: may be diminished with deformities

✓ Range of motion of ankle joint: stiffness

✓ Pain: ischemic (see Box 11-3)

✓ Perfusion
- Dependent rubor and elevational pallor: present (see Box 10-2)
- Skin temperature: cool
- Capillary refill time: delayed
- Blood flow: abnormal turbulence (bruit)
- Pulses: diminished or absent
- ABI: diminished
- TBI: diminished

✓ Diagnostic tests
- ABI and TBI (see Table 11-3)
- Transcutaneous partial pressure of oxygen
- Skin perfusion pressure
- Pulse volume recording and Doppler waveform study
- Segmental limb pressure measurements
- Magnetic resonance angiography
- Duplex angiography
- Computed tomographic angiography
- Arteriography

ABI, Ankle-brachial index; *TBI,* toe-brachial index.

should be posed regarding history of angina, myocardial infarction, cardiovascular procedures, or "problems with circulation." The patient should be queried regarding the major risk factors for LEAD: history of smoking/tobacco use, including any past attempts to stop smoking and willingness to consider smoking cessation; history of diabetes, including onset, type, management, usual fasting glucose level, and last HbA1c; history of hypertension, including onset, duration, management, and usual BP; and lipid levels (if known), as well as any measures in place to manage dyslipidemia (Hopf et al, 2008). The history must include a review of all medications, including herbal agents, over-the-counter medications, and prescription drugs. The patient should be asked about ulcers, any associated events (e.g., trauma), past treatments, and ulcer response.

Pain History

As described in Chapter 10, a careful pain history must be obtained; pain patterns are critical to differential assessment of ulcer etiology. Specific parameters to be included are the location, duration, and intensity of ulcer-related pain, and factors/activities that make the pain better or worse (see Table 10-2). Pain in the lower extremity is often the first indication of LEAD and becomes progressively worse as the disease process advances; the patient typically reports pain that is worsened by activity or elevation and relieved by rest and dependency. The location of the pain may suggest the level of occlusion; in general, the pain is one joint distal to the stenosis or occlusion (Table 11-2) (Cimminiello, 2002; Wennberg, 2013). As outlined in Box 11-3, the characteristics of the pain reflect the severity of the underlying ischemia.

Unfortunately, the patient with LEAD does not always experience or report "classic" ischemic pain symptoms. Intermittent claudication, for example, is normally described as reproducible pain in the buttock, thigh, or calf muscle that is precipitated by exercise and that rapidly disappears within 10 minutes of rest (Hirsch et al, 2006). However, because the patient with LEAD may unconsciously limit walking or activities to avoid pain, signs of claudication may be absent or reported simply as "leg weakness." It is therefore helpful to query patients regarding usual activities and any pain experienced when they walked from their car to the office (Wennberg, 2013). Patients with sensory neuropathy (e.g., mixed neuropathic and arterial disease) may have absent or blunted awareness of ischemic pain (Hopf et al, 2008).

Advanced LEAD is typically evidenced by rest pain, which is commonly described as a "constant deep aching pain." However, advanced LEAD may be associated with a shift in

TABLE 11-2 Correlation Between Site of Occlusion and Location of Pain

Site of Occlusion	Location of Pain
Iliofemoral arteries	Thighs, buttocks, calves
Superficial femoral artery	Calf
Infrapopliteal artery	Foot

From Cimminiello C: PAD: epidemiology and pathophysiology, *Thromb Res* 106(6):V295–V301, 2002.

BOX 11-3 Categories of Ischemic Pain

Intermittent claudication pain	Occurs with moderate-to-heavy activity; relieved by approximately 10 minutes of rest. Typically occurs when involved vessel is approximately 50% occluded.
Nocturnal pain	Develops as occlusion worsens. Occurs when patient is in bed. Caused by combination of leg elevation (to horizontal position) and reduced cardiac output. Relieved by placing limb in a dependent position.
Rest pain	Occurs in absence of activity and with legs in a dependent position. Rest pain signals advanced occlusive disease (typically >90% occlusion).

pain patterns, from nociceptive pain (described as "aching" or "throbbing") to neuropathic pain (described as "tingling, burning, electric-shock" type pain). Further discussion related to the assessment and management of pain is provided in Chapters 25 and 26.

Lower Extremity Assessment

Comprehensive assessment of the patient with a lower extremity ulcer is described in detail in Chapter 10. Typical assessment findings for the patient with LEAD and an arterial ulcer are as follows:

- Signs of chronic tissue ischemia: thin, shiny skin; recent onset of diminished hair growth; thin, ridged nails. It should be noted that absence of hair is a nonspecific finding and that ischemic changes in the nails are frequently obscured by fungal nail infections.
- Elevational pallor or cyanosis and dependent rubor.
- Prolonged venous filling time (>20 seconds) and prolonged capillary refill (>3 seconds).
- Diminished or absent pulses; absence of both pedal pulses mandates referral to a vascular surgeon. However, the presence or absence of pedal pulses cannot be used as a sole measure of arterial perfusion, because some individuals with normal perfusion lack one or both pedal pulses and many patients with arterial insufficiency retain palpable pulses.
- Abnormal ABI (see section on diagnostic testing). It should be noted that ABI greater than 1.3 is indicative of vessel calcification and mandates referral to a vascular laboratory for further testing. It should also be noted that patients with ABI 0.5 to 0.9 have moderate-to-mild LEAD but retain the potential for healing and would not develop ischemic ulcers, though the LEAD could result in slower healing of ulcers caused by other pathologic processes.
- Functional and sensory deficits, especially if the patient has combined LEAD and lower extremity neuropathic disease (LEND).

Ulcer characteristics that are critical to differential assessment include ulcer location, ulcer contours, type of tissue in wound bed, and volume of exudate. The classic arterial ulcer (see Plate 38) is located distally at the point farthest from the heart (toes and forefoot); arterial ulcers may also present as nonhealing traumatic injuries (because perfusion is insufficient to support healing). Arterial ulcers are frequently described as having a "punched out" appearance with well-defined edges; the wound bed is usually pale or necrotic, and there is minimal exudate. Arterial ulcers are very frequently infected because ischemia compromises bacterial control; however, the infection may be missed because the signs of inflammation are very subtle in ischemic tissue (faint halo of erythema, slight induration). Table 10-3 provides a comparison of arterial, venous, and neuropathic ulcer characteristics.

Checklist 11-1 provides a simple list of assessment findings that are typically observed in the patient with LEAD. However, there are relatively few "pure" arterial ulcers; mixed pathology ulcers are more common (venous/arterial or neuropathic/arterial). Therefore Chapter 10 should be carefully reviewed for a detailed description of lower extremity assessment, regardless of etiology (see Boxes 10-2, 10-3, and 10-4).

NONINVASIVE TESTING FOR LEAD

Ankle-brachial index testing should be completed on all patients with lower extremity wounds in order to determine whether or not arterial insufficiency is a contributing factor and to identify patients who require further vascular assessment. Additional diagnostic tests are indicated when the diagnosis is unclear, the wound fails to improve, or surgical revascularization is being contemplated. The most common diagnostic tests for LEAD are listed in Checklist 11-1. With the exception of the ABI, these tests are performed in vascular laboratories by trained technicians; results are interpreted by vascular radiologists or surgeons.

Ankle-Brachial Index

Ankle-brachial index, also known as *ankle-arm index,* is a simple bedside test in which perfusion pressures in the lower leg are compared with those in the upper arm using a standard BP cuff and a handheld, battery-operated, continuous-wave, Doppler ultrasound device (Figure 11-1). The ultrasound probe should utilize an 8- to 9-MHz frequency for accurate assessment of skin-level vessels (Bonham et al, 2007). A "normal" ABI is considered to range from greater than 0.9 to 1.3. Although an ABI of 0.9 to 0.99 has been considered a normal range, some recent data suggest increased risk of cardiovascular disease and mortality in these patients (Wennberg, 2013). An ABI of 0.90 or less is approximately 95% sensitive for detecting LEAD compared with angiography-proven ischemic disease (Norgren et al, 2007). The ABI is also useful for detecting restenosis after revascularization and for monitoring LEAD progression; a 15% change from the baseline ABI is indicative of disease progression (Hirsch et al, 2006). The Wound, Ostomy and Continence Nurses

FIGURE 11-1 Handheld Doppler probe being used to obtain an ankle-brachial index.

TABLE 11-3   Interpretation of Noninvasive Tests for LEAD

Value	Interpretation/Clinical Significance
ABI	
>1.3	Abnormally high range, typically because of calcification of the vessel wall in patient with diabetes
	Renders ABI test invalid as a measure of peripheral perfusion
	TBI indicated
>0.9–1.3	"Normal" range
≤0.9	LEAD
0.6–0.8	Borderline perfusion
≤0.5	Severe ischemia; wound healing unlikely unless revascularization can be accomplished
TBI	
<0.64	LEAD
TcPO$_2$	
(Obtain if ABI or TP cannot be performed due to calcification or amputations of ankle or toes)	
≥40 mm Hg	Normal
<40 mm Hg	Hypoxia with impaired wound healing
AP	
AP <40 mm Hg	Limb threatened
TP	
<30 mm Hg	Critical limb ischemia (<50 mm Hg in patient with diabetes)
SPP	
>30 mm Hg	Required for healing to occur

ABI, Ankle-brachial index; *AP,* ankle pressure; *LEAD,* lower extremity arterial disease; *SPP,* skin partial pressure; *TBI,* toe-brachial index; *TP,* toe pressure; *TcPO$_2$,* transcutaneous partial pressure of oxygen.

BOX 11-4   Procedure for Obtaining an ABI

1. Place patient in supine position in warm, tranquil environment for at least 10 minutes before the test (prevents vasoconstriction of arteries). Provide blankets if necessary.
2. Obtain brachial pressure in each arm using Doppler probe and 12- to 14-cm cuff placed 3 cm above cubital fossa. Inflate cuff 20 to 30 mm Hg above the last sound; slowly deflate cuff until initial sound is heard. Record highest brachial pressure.
3. Place appropriately sized cuff (10 to 12 cm) around lower leg 3 cm above malleolus.
4. Apply acoustic gel over dorsalis pedis pulse location.
5. Hold Doppler probe over pedal pulse according to manufacturer's guidelines (e.g., pen-style Doppler devices should be held at 45-degree angle). Be careful not to occlude the artery with excessive pressure; hold the probe lightly!
6. Inflate cuff to level 20 to 30 mm Hg above point where pulse is no longer audible.
7. Slowly deflate cuff while monitoring for return of pulse signal. The point at which the arterial signal returns is recorded as the dorsalis pedis pressure.
8. Apply acoustic gel over posterior tibial pulse location and repeat procedure. The higher of the two values is used to determine the ABI.
9. Calculate ABI by dividing the higher of the two ankle pressures by the higher of the two brachial pressures.

ABI, Ankle-brachial index.

Ankle-brachial index provides only an indirect measure of peripheral perfusion and cannot be considered accurate in patients with noncompressible vessels (e.g., patients with diabetes, renal failure, and vessel calcification) (Bonham et al, 2007). Patients who have elevated ABI measurements (>1.3 or 1.4) and patients who have normal ABI measurements but clinical evidence of ischemia should be referred for more definitive testing, such as TBI. For example, the patient who has a normal resting ABI but also has intermittent claudication definitely requires further evaluation, since these findings are consistent with severe arterial stenosis (Bonham et al, 2007). Any patient who has an elevated ABI and any patient who has a clinical picture that is inconsistent with ABI findings should be referred to a vascular laboratory for further testing; this may include TBI, treadmill exercise testing, or segmental pulse volume recordings (PVRs) (Hirsch et al, 2006; Wennberg, 2013).

Toe-Brachial Index

Toe-brachial index, also known as the *toe-arm index,* is indicated when ABI is greater than 1.3 or 1.4, which is suggestive of noncompressible arteries (Wennberg, 2013). In this situation, the TBI is more accurate because the toe vessels are less likely to be calcified. Cold toes and vasospastic disease produce constricted arteries. Therefore continuous-wave Doppler devices are neither reliable nor recommended for measuring toe pressures (Bonham et al, 2007). The TBI is performed by a trained clinician and conducted in the same manner as the ABI test, with a small digit cuff placed around

Society™ (WOCN®, 2008) recommends conducting an ABI test every 3 months in patients suffering from LEAD and a nonhealing wound to identify severe or critical limb ischemia that warrants referral or a change in the plan of care (see Table 11-3).

The procedure for conducting an ABI test is outlined in Box 11-4. Guidelines for interpretation of ABI and toe-brachial index (TBI) are provided in Table 11-3. A research-based protocol should be used to measure ABIs with a handheld Doppler; this approach has been shown to provide results that are valid and reliable compared with results obtained in a vascular laboratory (Bonham et al, 2007). At present there is considerable variability in the approach and skill level of practitioners performing this test at the bedside; thus dissemination of evidence-based protocols and skills training is an urgent need (Sihlangu and Bliss, 2012).

the great toe or the second toe and a photoplethysmography sensor placed on the tip of the toe. The test can be done either in the vascular laboratory or at the bedside with a portable photoplethysmograph (Bonham, 2011; Cao et al, 2011). A TBI less than 0.7 is generally considered indicative of LEAD; however, the clinician should be aware that more research is needed to establish the best cutoff value for normal versus abnormal TBI (Hoyer et al, 2013).

Exercise Stress Testing

Exercise stress testing is an effective diagnostic study for symptomatic patients with normal ABI readings and is sometimes used to assess the functional impact of LEAD. A baseline ABI is performed, and the patient then walks on a treadmill set at a constant speed and grade. A patient who is unable to walk on a treadmill can be asked to stand with knees fully extended and to repeatedly raise the heels off the floor. The stress activity (treadmill walking or repetitive heel raises) is continued until the patient becomes symptomatic or until a set limit is reached (e.g., 5 minutes on the treadmill or 50 heel raises). A repeat ABI is obtained 1 minute after completion of the stress activity. Individuals with normal perfusion exhibit no change or a slight increase in ABI, whereas individuals with LEAD exhibit a clear drop in ABI. Contrast-enhanced ultrasound has also been used to assess perfusion of skeletal muscle at rest and following exercise and was found to accurately reflect severity of vascular impairment (Lindner et al, 2008).

Transcutaneous Oxygen Pressure

Transcutaneous partial pressure of oxygen (TcPO$_2$) measurements provide information about the adequacy of oxygen delivery to the skin and underlying tissues. This test is valuable for determining skin perfusion when a wound fails to improve or when ABI and TBI are not valid or are not possible due to incompressible arteries or amputation of feet or toes. TcPO$_2$ is a simple test that usually is performed in a vascular laboratory, specialty clinic, or hyperbaric oxygen therapy (HBOT) center. To obtain a TcPO$_2$ measurement, an oxygen sensor and a particular electrode are attached to the skin to quantify oxygen diffusion through the skin. Values greater than 40 mm Hg reflect good tissue oxygenation and are predictive of normal healing, whereas values less than 20 mm Hg indicate that healing is unlikely (Wennberg, 2013).

Skin Perfusion Pressure

Laser Doppler skin perfusion pressure (SPP) is another non-invasive measurement used for predicting successful wound healing in critical limb ischemia or for planning the lowest possible level of amputation for maximal preservation of functionality and mobility (Tsuji et al, 2008). Skin perfusion pressure has been identified as an alternative when TBI and ABI measurements cannot be accurately obtained due to incompressible arteries or are impossible due to amputation of feet and toes (Okamoto et al, 2006). Unlike TcPO$_2$, SPP results are not influenced by factors such as local edema and

anemia, and the procedure is less time consuming. An SPP value is obtained by using a laser Doppler probe and placing a cuff around the forefoot (including the 5 metatarsal and 14 phalange bones and surrounding soft tissues); the patient should be lying supine in a thermoregulated room. An SPP greater than 30 mm Hg is requisite for wound healing (Tsuji et al, 2008).

Pulse Volume Recordings and Doppler Waveform Studies

The PVR provides a reflection of actual perfusion volume during the cardiac cycle and is recommended when ABI is greater than 1.3. Pulse volume recordings are obtained with cuffs that incorporate pneumoplethysmograph capability (i.e., the ability to detect changes in blood volume in the underlying arteries). The cuffs are inflated to a preset level, and the machine provides tracings that reflect blood volume within the underlying arteries throughout the cardiac cycle. A similar tracing of flow within a single vessel may be obtained using a Doppler probe; this tracing is commonly referred to as a *Doppler waveform study*. Normal tracings for both PVRs and Doppler waveform studies are triphasic, showing a clearly defined systolic peak, followed by a dicrotic notch that represents reversal of blood flow during early diastole, and finally a diastolic wave (Figure 11-2, A). With mild LEAD, the waveform changes to a biphasic pattern, whereas with advanced LEAD, the waveform becomes monophasic or severely blunted (see Figure 11-2, B and C). Waveforms can also be obtained for the digital vessels by wrapping a cuff around the arch of the foot or the great toe; waveforms that are dampened or flat suggest small vessel disease, and a monophasic waveform for the pedal arteries is predictive of lower extremity amputation in dialysis patients with diabetic foot ulcers (Aronow, 2008; Tsai et al, 2013). However, results can be influenced by factors such as local edema and anemia (Tsuji et al, 2008).

Segmental Limb Pressure

Segmental limb pressure (SLP) measurements are used to determine the location of occlusion when surgical intervention is contemplated for CLI. Cuffs are placed at high and low thigh level, below the knee, and just above the ankle. A Doppler probe is used to localize the most distal pulses (dorsalis pedis and posterior tibialis), and the ankle cuff is inflated until the arterial signal is obliterated. The cuff is then deflated until the arterial signal is again audible. The pressure at which the signal is heard is recorded as the ankle systolic pressure. The procedure is repeated with inflation of the "below-the-knee" cuff and then with the thigh cuff. The pressures are then compared, and a difference of 20 mm Hg or more between two adjacent cuff positions localizes the occlusion to the intervening vessels. A 20 to 30 mm Hg pressure difference between the contralateral positions suggests stenosis or an occlusive lesion in the extremity with the lower pressure (Hirsch et al, 2006).

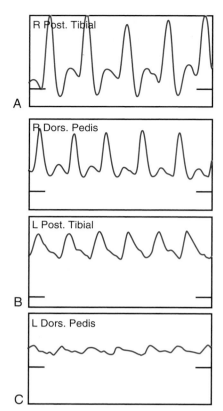

FIGURE 11-2 A, Normal Doppler waveforms from normal vessels (right posterior tibialis and right dorsalis pedis). Signal is triphasic, showing systolic peak, dicrotic notch representing blood flow reversal during early diastole, and a diastolic wave. **B,** Doppler waveform of vessel with moderately severe occlusive disease as evidenced by a monophasic waveform. **C,** Doppler waveform of vessel with advanced occlusive disease. Note that waveform is severely blunted.

Segmental limb pressure and PVR measurements are often obtained in combination. Each one is 85% accurate in detecting and localizing significant occlusive lesions, compared with angiography (see Figure 11-2, A). When SLP and PVR are used together, however, the accuracy is closer to 95%. Additionally, the patient with diabetes and calcified arteries who produces a falsely elevated SLP will be accurately assessed by PVR when the two tests are done in combination (Norgren et al, 2007).

Magnetic Resonance Angiography

Magnetic resonance angiography (MRA), with or without gadolinium enhancement, can be helpful in determining the location and severity of stenosis and is a valid alternative to intraarterial digital subtraction angiography for obtaining the detailed anatomic information required for accurate decision making regarding surgical intervention (Burbelko et al, 2013). Benefits of MRA include its noninvasive nature, its minimal risk, and its ability to provide impressive images of the pedal arteries. Magnetic resonance angiography is not an option for patients with implanted defibrillators, permanent pacemakers, intracranial aneurysm clips, or claustrophobia, and gadolinium enhancement may be contraindicated in patients with chronic renal insufficiency. In addition, MRA does not reliably detect calcification and is not currently able to image endovascular stents constructed of metal alloys (Hirsch et al, 2006; Wennberg, 2013).

Computed Tomographic Angiography

Computed tomographic angiography (CTA) utilizes iodinated contrast agent and x-rays to visualize arterial anatomy and to localize stenosis in patients who are candidates for surgical revascularization or endovascular procedures. The use of CTA is increasing, due in part to improvements in image detail provided by new 64-channel "multidetector" channels. Multidetector CTA can be used to image the arterial system all the way down to the pedal arteries and to evaluate the patency of bypass grafts (Schernthaner et al, 2009). Computed tomographic angiography is faster than MRA and is safer than digital subtraction. Computed tomographic angiography is an alternative for the patient with a pacemaker or implanted defibrillator who cannot undergo MRA. Computed tomographic angiography has reduced accuracy in extensive vessel calcification and cannot be used with the patient who cannot tolerate iodine-based contrast and exposure to ionizing radiation (Hirsch et al, 2006; Wennberg, 2013).

Duplex Angiography (Ultrasound Imaging)

Ultrasonography uses sound waves to reveal characteristics of tissue or organs. By combining ultrasonographic imaging with Doppler assessment of blood flow, duplex angiography provides direct imaging of arteries and the location and severity of stenosis, thrombi, or occlusive lesions (Ajijola and Jaff, 2008; Cao et al, 2011; Hirsch et al, 2006; Wennberg, 2013). Duplex angiography has a sensitivity of 99% and 80% and specificity of 94% and 91% for the femoropopliteal and tibial segments, respectively, compared with arteriography. Results are comparable to contrast-enhanced MRA with lower cost; however, the patient may require more follow-up testing.

INVASIVE TESTING FOR LEAD

Before revascularization, an anatomic roadmap is needed. In many patients, this can be obtained with duplex angiography, MRA, or CTA. However, in selected patients arteriography is still required.

Arteriography

Contrast angiography remains the gold standard when planning surgical intervention, especially for patients in whom MRA and multidetector CTA are contraindicated or would provide insufficient anatomic data. When performed, angiography utilizing digital subtraction technology is the usual choice. A plain film of the involved area is taken before injection of contrast material, and the computer then "subtracts" the plain film image from the postcontrast images. As a result, the final films show only the arteries, allowing for clear identification of the site and severity of stenotic lesions (Norgren et al, 2007; Wennberg, 2013).

MANAGEMENT OF THE PATIENT WITH ARTERIAL ULCERATION

The primary focus in management of the patient with an arterial ulcer is improving perfusion because the ability to heal is directly correlated with the ability to provide sufficient oxygen and nutrients to support the repair process. Secondary concerns include systemic support for wound healing, prevention and management of infection, appropriate topical therapy, and patient education and counseling regarding lifestyle changes and limb preservation. The patient must be monitored carefully for indicators of advancing necrosis, which may mandate amputation.

Measures to Improve Perfusion

Strategies for improving blood flow include surgical revascularization, aggressive management of modifiable risk factors to prevent disease progression, pharmacologic therapy, HBOT, intermittent pneumatic compression devices, and lifestyle modifications. The importance of managing modifiable risk factors cannot be overemphasized, since this is the key to controlling disease progression and to prevention of cardiovascular-related morbidity and mortality. In one study addressing this issue, investigators found insufficient attention to this aspect of care; one month post endovascular intervention for advanced PAD, only 51% of patients had satisfactory control of systolic BP and the percentage of smokers had decreased only 17% (from 41% preop to 24% postop). Fortunately, this same study found that 89% of patients were receiving statins and 98% were receiving antiplatelet drugs or anticoagulants. The authors concluded that secondary prevention is an area where improvement is needed (Alhadad et al, 2013).

Surgical Options

Revascularization is the intervention most likely to provide healing in patients with advanced LEAD and lower extremity ulcers; data indicate that approximately 10% to 20% of individuals with LEAD will require revascularization (Hirsch et al, 2006). Patients who should be referred for surgical evaluation include those with critical limb ischemia and those with ulcers that are not healing with appropriate therapy. According to the American Heart Association/American College of Cardiology (AHA/ACC) guidelines for the management of patients with PAD, patients with incapacitating claudication should be evaluated for revascularization if there is a reasonable likelihood that symptoms will improve and there is an absence of another diagnosis that would limit exercise, such as angina or heart failure (Hennion and Sianok,

2013; Hirsch et al, 2006). Appropriate evaluation is needed to ensure the patency of distal vessels and may involve MRA, multidetector CTA, or contrast angiography using digital subtraction techniques. Options for revascularization include open bypass grafting and endovascular procedures (angioplasty and placement of endovascular stents).

Bypass Grafts. Bypass grafts have been considered the gold standard for revascularization and are most commonly done using the patient's own saphenous vein (autologous saphenous vein bypass) (Figure 11-3). If the saphenous vein is damaged or unavailable, a synthetic graft (e.g., heparin-bonded expanded polytetrafluoroethylene) may be used. Long-term results are generally good, with

FIGURE 11-3 Illustration of bypass grafts using an autologous saphenous vein in a reversed saphenous vein procedure **(A)** and an in situ procedure **(B)**.

5-year patency rates of approximately 70%. Distal bypass procedures involving smaller vessels have slightly lower long-term patency rates. Smoking cessation can improve patency rates and is a key element of a comprehensive management program (Daenens et al, 2009; WOCN®, 2008).

Endovascular Procedures. Endovascular procedures are advantageous because they are less invasive and therefore are associated with lower risk. Although bypass procedures have previously been considered the "optimal" approach, recent advances in endovascular procedures and stent design are increasing their role in the treatment of CLI. Indeed, some authors now state that there is no evidence to support bypass procedures as being superior to endovascular treatment, and others report positive clinical outcomes in endovascular management of patients who would otherwise have required amputation (Albayati and Shearman, 2013; Gazzaruso et al, 2013; Georgakarakos et al, 2013; Kudagi and White, 2013). Meta-analyses of studies addressing outcomes for angioplasty and for bypass revealed similar outcomes. At 36 months post angioplasty, primary patency rates averaged 48.6% and limb salvage averaged 82.4%. The 5-year pooled survival rates of patients post bypass averaged 63.1% primary patency and 77.7% limb salvage (Albers et al, 2006; Romiti, 2008). A systematic review of three randomized controlled trials (RCTs) involving 501 patients found that use of drug-eluting stents significantly improved patency and reduced restenosis; use of these stents was also associated with improved wound healing and longer event-free survival times (Katsanos et al, 2013). Cilostazol may also be of benefit in reducing recurrent stenosis caused by intimal hyperplasia (Dindyal and Kyriakides, 2009).

Management of Modifiable Risk Factors

In addition to managing the primary (causative) contributing risk factors and the emerging risk factors for LEAD (as summarized in Table 11-1), the patient must be counseled regarding simple strategies that improve perfusion, such as maintenance of adequate hydration and avoidance of cold and constriction (Zeymer et al, 2009). Strategies for patients with mild to moderate LEAD and patients who have been effectively revascularized include a supervised graduated walking program (Hopf et al, 2008; WOCN®, 2008).

Supervised Walking Program. Supervised walking programs have been shown to improve walking distance, reduce claudication pain, and reduce cardiovascular morbidity and mortality; mechanisms of action include improved vasoresponsiveness and cellular adaptations that improve oxygen utilization. Patients who are candidates for a walking program should be counseled regarding the benefits and should be strongly encouraged to enroll in a supervised program that provides three to five exercise sessions per week for at least 3 months. Each session should involve 30 to 60 minutes of treadmill or track walking to the point of pain, followed by rest; walking should be resumed once the pain has subsided. There is clear evidence that supervised programs are effective in improving walking distance, but it is frequently difficult for patients to access such programs. Self-directed community-based walking programs may be an alternative to supervised walking programs; however, such programs have generally been shown to be *ineffective* compared with supervised programs, due primarily to their unstructured format. Interestingly, recent studies indicate that such programs can provide comparable outcomes to supervised programs *only when* they incorporate specific recommendations as well as active monitoring and feedback. Supervised walking programs are considered *contraindicated* in patients with CLI, due to the potential for development of new or worsening ulcerations (Diehm et al, 2011; Haas et al, 2012; Hopf et al, 2008; Mays et al, 2013; Sakamoto et al, 2009; WOCN®, 2008).

Pharmacologic Therapy

The mainstays of pharmacologic therapy for LEAD include antiplatelet drugs, cilostazol, statins, and analgesics.

Antiplatelet agents work primarily by reducing platelet aggregation. The most commonly used antiplatelet agent is low- to medium-dose aspirin (75 to 325 mg/day), which may delay the rate at which LEAD progresses and may improve long-term patency of bypass grafts. However, the primary benefit of aspirin is the reduction in morbidity and mortality related to cerebrovascular and cardiovascular disease (stroke and myocardial infarction). Clopidogrel (75 mg/day) is currently recommended as an effective alternative to aspirin (Aronow, 2008; Berger et al, 2009; Hopf et al, 2008; WOCN®, 2008).

Currently recommended *vasodilators* include cilostazol and naftidrofuryl oxalate. Cilostazol has both antiplatelet and vasodilatory effects and is currently the most commonly recommended drug for symptomatic LEAD. Benefits include increased walking distance, reduced intermittent claudication, improved ABI, and possibly a favorable impact on plasma lipoprotein levels (reduced triglyceride levels and increased levels of HDL-C). The recommended dose is 100 mg twice per day, and the drug is generally well tolerated. Approximately one third of patients report mild side effects, which subside in about 6 weeks. New onset of congestive heart failure is generally considered to be a contraindication to vasodilators (Rizzo et al, 2011). Stevens and colleagues (2012) reviewed 26 RCTs addressing the efficacy of cilostazol, naftidrofuryl oxalate, and pentoxifylline; in the studies they reviewed, both cilostazol and naftidrofuryl were effective, but naftidrofuryl was associated with the most significant improvement in pain-free walking distance. Squires and colleagues (2011) conducted a systematic review and concluded that both cilostazol and naftidrofuryl were effective and produced minimal side effects, but noted that more studies are needed to assess long-term effectiveness of these agents.

Statins are lipid-lowering drugs used to treat systemic atherosclerosis. They slow disease progression, improve the ABI, improve walking distance, reduce the risk of adverse cardiovascular events, and may improve patency rates for bypass grafts. In a systematic review and meta-analysis of 46 trials involving 2706 patients, Reriani and colleagues (2011) concluded that statin therapy is associated with significant improvement in endothelial function. Statins are currently considered to be standard therapy for patients with LEAD (Hopf et al, 2008; Liapis et al, 2009; Paraskevas et al, 2013; WOCN®, 2008). Niacin or vitamin B_6 also may be helpful in reducing triglyceride levels and increasing HDL-C levels. The recommended dose of niacin is up to 3 g/day for as long as 60 weeks, as tolerated (WOCN®, 2008).

Analgesics, specifically opioid analgesics, may be required for patients with advanced ischemia to relieve chronic pain and thus improve quality of life. Effective pain management also contributes to improved perfusion by preventing the vasoconstriction caused by sympathetic stimulation (Wipke-Tevis and Sae-Sia, 2004).

Pharmacologic management for the patient with CLI should include antiplatelet agents; anticoagulants are not recommended. There is some evidence that prostanoids may be helpful, especially in patients who are not good candidates for revascularization procedures or who have failed revascularization (Diehm et al, 2011; Lambert and Belch, 2013). *Investigational agents,* such as proangiogenic growth factors, have been used in patients with advanced ischemic disease and ulceration in an attempt to improve perfusion by inducing new vessel growth; however, no clear benefit has been demonstrated (Hamner and Steiner, 2013).

Hyperbaric Oxygen Therapy

Hyperbaric oxygen therapy increases the amount of oxygen dissolved in the plasma, which results in the delivery of "oxygen-enriched" blood to the tissues. Hyperbaric oxygen therapy has been shown to increase tissue oxygen levels in ischemic tissues where positive plasma flow exists; it has also been shown to support angiogenesis and wound healing. Candidates for HBOT include patients with significant ischemic disease who are not candidates for revascularization and patients who have undergone revascularization but who still demonstrate significant tissue hypoxia and impaired healing. Patients should be evaluated carefully to ensure responsiveness to HBOT (i.e., reversal of tissue-level hypoxia). Responsiveness can be evaluated by obtaining $TcPO_2$ measurements while the patient is breathing room air and then repeating $TcPO_2$ measurements while the patient is breathing 100% oxygen. Normally the $TcPO_2$ level will rise to greater than 100 mm Hg when the patient is breathing 100% oxygen, which signifies a good potential for enhanced healing with HBOT. In contrast, a patient who demonstrates minimal response (<10 mm Hg increase) is not likely to benefit from HBOT (Fife et al, 2009).

Hyperbaric oxygen therapy is discussed in greater detail in Chapter 22.

Intermittent Pneumatic Compression

Intermittent pneumatic compression devices (see Figure 12-8) promote venous return without impairing arterial inflow and may actually improve distal perfusion. Further studies are needed to determine the specific mechanisms of action for intermittent pneumatic compression and its potential role in treatment of PAD (Hopf et al, 2008; Sheldon et al, 2013).

Modified Compression for Patients with Mixed Arterial-Venous Disease

Because edema further compromises perfusion, strategies for edema control should be considered when managing the patient with arterial disease complicated by lower limb edema. However, the use of sustained compression devices must be modified based on the severity of the arterial disease. Current evidence supports reduced or modified compression (23 to 30 mm Hg at the ankle) for patients with ABI greater than 0.5 and less than 0.8 (WOCN®, 2008).

Patients with ABI of 0.5 or less should be managed with intermittent pneumatic compression or low-level elevation; they should not receive sustained compression (WOCN®, 2008). Intermittent compression devices are discussed further in Chapter 12.

Systemic Support for Wound Healing

Nutritional support, glucose control, and control of other comorbidities are critical elements of care for the patient with an arterial ulcer (WOCN®, 2008). These issues are discussed in greater depth in Section VI and Chapters 14 and 27.

Prevention and Management of Infection. Ischemia increases the risk for infection, and both ischemia and infection are significant impediments to the repair process. Thus prompt recognition and aggressive treatment of infectious complications are critical to positive outcomes. However, this can be a challenge because signs of infection are frequently muted (and therefore easy to miss) in ischemic conditions. Clinicians must routinely assess for subtle indicators of infection, such as a faint halo of erythema extending circumferentially around the wound edge. In wounds that present with signs of infection, systemic antibiotic therapy should be promptly initiated. When viable tissue is present in the wound bed, a culture should be obtained to ensure appropriate antibiotic selection. Some evidence indicates that "neuroischemic" wounds (wounds caused by a combination of neuropathy and ischemia) may be critically colonized even without obvious indicators; therefore a short course of antibiotic therapy may be appropriate for nonhealing mixed neuroischemic wounds. Effective management of infected ischemic wounds involves revascularization when indicated and possible, aggressive debridement of all necrotic tissue (including any necrotic bone), and appropriate antibiotic therapy. Topical antimicrobial dressings can be used in conjunction with systemic antibiotic therapy and may be helpful in controlling bacterial loads as well as *preventing* infection in clean open wounds. However, antimicrobial dressings should not be used as sole therapy for infected ischemic wounds (WOCN®, 2008).

Topical Therapy. The principles of topical therapy for ischemic ulcers are generally the same as for all other wounds. They involve wound bed preparation (removal of necrotic tissue and control of bacterial burden) followed by moisture-retentive dressings to keep the wound surface clean, moist, and protected. However, specific wound characteristics should be considered when selecting dressings, and distinctly different guidelines for the management of closed necrotic wounds should be followed.

Guidelines for dressing selection. Ischemic ulcers typically have minimal exudate and are at very high risk for infection; therefore hydrating dressings with sustained-release antimicrobial properties and a nonocclusive outer layer are likely to be of particular benefit. In addition, the periwound skin typically is very fragile; thus nonadherent dressings or those with silicone adhesive are frequently indicated, as is protection of the periwound skin with a skin sealant or moisture barrier ointment.

Management of closed necrotic wounds. Although necrotic tissue is clearly a potential medium for bacterial growth, a dry, intact eschar also can serve as a bacterial barrier. A closed wound surface is advantageous when managing a very poorly perfused wound in which any bacterial invasion is likely to result in clinical infection and limb loss. Although research into optimal management of these wounds is clearly needed, there is clinical consensus that a closed wound should be maintained when (1) the involved limb is clearly ischemic with limited or no potential for healing, (2) no indications of infection are present, and (3) the wound surface is dry and necrotic. A sample topical therapy protocol for this type of ulcer is outlined in Box 11-5. Note that this protocol applies only to *uninfected* wounds covered with dry, intact eschar. If the wound develops clinically significant infection, the patient should be promptly referred for surgical evaluation (for debridement and hopefully revascularization) (WOCN®, 2008).

BOX 11-5   Topical Therapy for Dry, Necrotic, Uninfected Ischemic Wound

1. Inspect for subtle indicators of infection. If any signs or symptoms of infection develop, immediate referral for debridement and initiation of antibiotic therapy are critical.
2. Paint with antiseptic solution (e.g., povidone-iodine 10% solution); allow to dry.
3. Apply dry gauze dressing and secure with wrap gauze.

PATIENT EDUCATION

Lifestyle changes may be more difficult for the patient than either a surgical procedure or drug therapy; therefore effective introduction of such changes requires in-depth education and supportive, goal-directed patient counseling. In addition to receiving education regarding the specific plan of care and rationale, the patient should be taught the importance (and specifics) of protective lower limb care (Box 11-6) (Aronow, 2008; WOCN®, 2008).

Amputation

Amputation is reserved as the "treatment of last resort" and is indicated primarily for patients with irreversible ischemia (i.e., tissue necrosis) and invasive infection. $TcPO_2$ measurements may be used to accurately predict the level of amputation at which healing is most likely (Aronow, 2008; Fife et al, 2009; WOCN®, 2008).

BOX 11-6   Limb Preservation Strategies

Routine Skin Care
- Apply emollients after bathing to prevent cracking and fissures.
- Dry carefully between toes to prevent maceration.
- Use lamb's wool or foam toe "sleeves" to prevent interdigital friction and pressure.

Measures to Prevent Mechanical Trauma
- Avoid walking barefoot, even indoors; consistently use protective footwear (e.g., closed-toe shoes) to prevent inadvertent cuts or puncture wounds.
- Inspect shoes before wearing.
- Carefully fit shoes to prevent pressure, friction, and shear injuries.
- If indicated, use protective shin guards when working around house or yard.
- Receive professional foot and nail care (or limit self-care of nails to conservative trimming and filing); no "bathroom surgery."

Measures to Prevent Thermal Trauma
- Wear warm socks during cold weather to prevent vasoconstriction.
- Do not use hot water bottles, heating pads, or other thermal devices.
- Check water temperature with hand or elbow before bathing.

Measures to Prevent Chemical Trauma
- Do not use antiseptic or chemical agents (e.g., corn removers).

General Measures
- Inspect feet and legs daily.
- Promptly report any minor injuries.

CLINICAL CONSULT

A: Consulted for nonhealing leg wound. 66-year old Caucasian female with Type 2 diabetes × 32 years (HbA1c 8.2), atherosclerotic heart disease (stent placement × 3, 18 months ago), hypertension, obesity; 42-year history of cigarette smoking. Patient reports wound started as a tiny "nick" after bumping her leg 2 months ago. She rates rest pain with leg dependent as 3/10 and 9/10 with any significant activity. She sleeps in a recliner. Right lateral shin ulcer 4.5 cm (L) × 2.0 cm (W) × 0.3 cm (D). Ulcer bed 70% gray slough and 30% pale pink; minimal serous exudate; wound edges closed and "punched-out" in appearance; periwound skin mildly erythematous to 3 cm past wound edge circumferentially with slight induration. Lower extremities, absent of hair, with thin shiny skin and thickened fungal nails. Elevational pallor and dependent rubor (R > L), capillary refill of 6 seconds (R) and 5 seconds (L); venous filling time 30 seconds (R) and 26 seconds (L);

diminished DP and PT pulses both feet; ABI 0.32 on right and 0.54 on left.

D: Arterial insufficiency, critical limb ischemia, infected right leg ulcer.

P: Implement interventions to maximize perfusion, eradicate infection and necrosis, promote healing, and prevent further injury.

I: (1) Urgent vascular consult. (2) Smoking cessation program. (3) Collaborate with provider for culture-based treatment of wound infection, effective pain management, and topical therapy that supports debridement and control of bioburden. (4) Collaborate with provider, patient, and dietitian for optimal glucose control. (5) Educate patient regarding preventive foot and lower extremity care.

E: Patient verbalizes understanding and agreement with plan of care. Will follow with care team, review vascular and dietitian consults, and modify topical management, as needed.

SUMMARY

Arterial ulcers are most commonly caused by peripheral arterial occlusive disease and may progress to CLI and limb loss. Risk factors for peripheral arterial occlusive disease and arterial ulcers are the same as those for coronary artery disease and cerebrovascular disease. They include tobacco use, diabetes mellitus, dyslipidemia, and hypertension, as well as family history and age. Arterial ulcers typically present as spontaneous ulceration of the toes and distal foot or as a nonhealing traumatic injury. Ulcers usually are painful, with a pale or necrotic wound bed, well-demarcated edges,

and minimal exudate. Arterial ulcers are commonly infected; however, the signs of infection are muted due to the underlying ischemia. Successful management of an arterial ulcer is dependent on measures to improve perfusion and oxygenation (revascularization, HBOT, and lifestyle measures such as smoking cessation). Positive long-term outcomes are dependent on lifestyle modifications to correct reversible risk factors and a progressive walking program to improve lower limb perfusion, as well as measures to prevent injury.

REFERENCES

Abdulhannan P, Russell D, Homer-Vanniasinkram S: Peripheral arterial disease: a literature review, *Br Med Bull* 104:21–39, 2012.

Ajijola OA, Jaff MR: Noninvasive evaluation of peripheral arterial disease. In Kandarpa K, editor: *Peripheral vascular interventions*, Philadelphia, 2008, Lippincott Williams & Wilkins.

Aksu K, Donmez A, Keser G: Inflammation-induced thrombosis: mechanisms, disease associations, and management, *Curr Pharm Des* 18(11):1478–1493, 2012.

Albayati M, Shearman C: Peripheral arterial disease and bypass surgery in diabetic lower limbs, *Med Clin North Am* 97(5):821–834, 2013.

Albers M, Romiti M, Brochado-Neto F, et al: Meta-analysis of popliteal-to-distal-vein bypass grafts for critical limb ischemia, *J Vasc Surg* 43(3):498–503, 2006.

Alhadad A, Wictorsson C, Alhadad H, et al: Medical risk factor treatment in peripheral artery disease: need for further improvement, *Int Angiol* 32(3):332–338, 2013.

Alzamora M, Fores R, Pera G, et al: Ankle-brachial index and the incidence of cardiovascular events in the Mediterranean low cardiovascular risk population ARTPER cohort, *BMC Cardiovasc Disord* 13:119, 2013.

American Diabetes Association: Standards of medical care in diabetes—2014, *Diabetes Care* 37(Suppl 1):S14–S80, 2014.

Andras A, Stansby G, Hansrani M: Homocysteine-lowering interventions for PAD and bypass grafts, *Cochrane Database Syst Rev* 7:CD003285, 2013.

Apanah S, Rizzolo D: Sickle cell disease: taking a multidisciplinary approach, *JAAPA* 26(8):28–33, 2013.

Aronow H: Peripheral arterial disease in the elderly: recognition and management, *Am J Cardiovasc Drugs* 8(6):353–364, 2008.

Berger J, Krantz MJ, Kittelson JM, et al: Aspirin for the prevention of cardiovascular events in patients with peripheral artery disease: a meta-analysis of randomized trials, *JAMA* 301(18):1909–1919, 2009.

Bevc S, Purg D, Turnsek N, et al: Ankle-brachial index and cardiovascular mortality in nondiabetic hemodialysis patients, *Ther Apher Dial* 17(4):313–317, 2013.

Bonham P: Measuring toe pressures using a portable photoplethysmograph to detect arterial disease in high risk patients: an overview of the literature, *Ostomy Wound Manage* 57(11):36–44, 2011.

Bonham P, Cappuccio M, Hulsey T, et al: Are ankle and toe brachial indices (ABI-TBI) obtained by a pocket Doppler interchangeable with those obtained by standard laboratory equipment? *J Wound Ostomy Continence Nurs* 34(1):35–44, 2007.

Bozkurt A, Cengiz K, Arslan C, et al: A stable prostacyclin analogue (iloprost) in the treatment of Buerger's disease: a prospective analysis of 150 patients, *Ann Thorac Cardiovasc Surg* 19(2):120–125, 2013.

Burbelko M, Augsten M, Kalinowski M, et al: Comparison of contrast-enhanced multistation MR angiography and digital subtraction angiography of lower extremity arterial disease, *J Magn Reson Imaging* 37(6):1427–1435, 2013.

Cao P, Eckstein H, DeRango P, et al: Diagnostic methods, *Eur J Vasc Endovasc Surg* 42(Suppl 2):S13–S32, 2011.

Chaparaia R, et al: Inflammatory profiling of peripheral arterial disease, *Ann Vasc Surg.* 2009 Mar;23(2):172-8. doi: 10.1016/j.avsg.2008.06.005. Epub 2008 Jul 26.

Cimminiello C: PAD: epidemiology and pathophysiology, *Thromb Res* 106(6):V295–V301, 2002.

Daenens K, Schepers S, Fourneau I, et al: Heparin-bonded ePTFE grafts compared with vein grafts in femoropopliteal and femorocrural bypasses: 1 and 2 year results, *J Vasc Surg* 49(5):1210–1216, 2009.

Dargon P, Landry G: Buerger's disease, *Ann Vasc Surg* 26(6):871–880, 2012.

Delaney K, Axelrod K, Buscetta A, et al: Leg ulcers in sickle cell disease: current patterns and practice, *Hemoglobin* 37(4):325–332, 2013.

Dellalibera-Joviliano R, Joviliano E, Silva J, et al: Activation of cytokines corroborate with development of inflammation and autoimmunity in thromboangiitis obliterans patients, *Clin Exp Immunol* 170(1):28–35, 2012.

Diehm N, Schmidli J, Setacci C, et al: Management of cardiovascular risk factors and medical therapy, *Eur J Vasc Endovasc Surg* 42(Suppl 2):S33–S42, 2011.

Dillavou E, Kahn M: Diagnosing and treating the 3 most common peripheral vasculopathies, *Geriatrics* 58(2):37–42, 2003.

Dindyal S, Kyriakides C: A review of cilostazol, a phosphodiesterase inhibitor, and its role in preventing both coronary and peripheral arterial restenosis following endovascular therapy, *Recent Pat Cardiovasc Drug Discov* 4(1):6–14, 2009.

Ergul A: Endothelin-1 and diabetic complications: focus on the vasculature, *Pharmacol Res* 63(6):477–482, 2011.

Fife C, Smart D, Sheffield P, et al: Transcutaneous oximetry in clinical practice: consensus statement from an expert panel based on evidence, *Undersea Hyperb Med* 36(1):43–53, 2009.

Fowkes F, Rudan D, Rudan I, et al: Comparison of global estimates of prevalence and risk factors for peripheral arterial disease in 2000 and 2010: a systematic review and analysis, *Lancet* 382(9901):1329–1340, 2013.

Gaffo A: Thrombosis in vasculitides, *Best Pract Res Clin Rheumatol* 27(1):57–67, 2013.

Gardner A, Afaq A: Management of lower extremity peripheral arterial disease, *J Cardiopulm Rehabil Prev* 28(6):349–357, 2008.

Garimella P, Hart P, O'Hare A, et al: Peripheral artery disease and CKD: a focus on peripheral artery disease as a critical component of CKD care, *Am J Kidney Dis* 60(4):641–654, 2012.

Gazzaruso C, Coppola A, Collaviti S, et al: Percutaneous transluminal angioplasty for critical limb ischemia in very elderly diabetic patients, *Aging Clin Exp Res* 25(2):225–228, 2013.

Georgakarakos E, Papanos N, Papadaki E, et al: Endovascular treatment of critical ischemia in the diabetic foot: new thresholds, new anatomies, *Angiology* 64(8):583–591, 2013.

Gibbons G, Shaw P: Diabetic vascular disease: characteristics of vascular disease unique to the diabetic patient, *Semin Vasc Surg* 25(2):89–92, 2012.

Grenon S, Conte M, Nosova E, et al: Association between N-3 polyunsaturated fatty acid content of red blood cells and inflammatory biomarkers in patients with PAD, *J Vasc Surg* 58(5):1283–1290, 2013.

Haas T, Lloyd P, Yang H, et al: Exercise training and peripheral arterial disease, *Compr Physiol* 2(4):2933–3017, 2012.

Haigh K, Bingley J, Golledge J, et al: Peripheral arterial disease screening in general practice, *Aust Fam Physician* 42(6):391–395, 2013.

Hamner A, Steiner S: Gene therapy for therapeutic angiogenesis in peripheral arterial disease: a systematic review and meta-analysis of randomized controlled trials, *Vasa* 42(5):331–339, 2013.

Hennion D, Siano K: Diagnosis and treatment of peripheral arterial disease, *Am Family Physician* 88(5):306–310, 2013.

Hirsch A, Haskal ZJ, Hertzer NR, et al: ACC/AHA 2005 practice guidelines for the management of patients with peripheral arterial disease (lower extremity, renal, mesenteric, and abdominal aortic), *Circulation* 113(11):1474–1547, 2006.

Hopf H, Ueno C, Aslam R, et al: Guidelines for the prevention of lower extremity arterial ulcers, *Wound Repair Regen* 16(2):175–188, 2008.

Hoyer C, Sandermann J, Paludan J, et al: Diagnostic accuracy of laser Doppler flowmetry versus strain gauge plethysmography for segmental pressure measurement, *J Vasc Surg* 58(6):1563–1570, 2013.

Hus I, Sokolawska B, Waleter-Croneda A, et al: Assessment of plasma prothrombotic factors in patients with Buerger's disease, *Blood Coagul Fibrinolysis* 24(2):133–139, 2013.

Jones W, Patel M, Rockman C, et al: Association of the ankle-brachial index with history of myocardial infarction and stroke, *Am Heart J* 167(4):499–505, 2014.

Jude E, Eleftheriadou I, Tentolouis N: Peripheral arterial disease in diabetes: a review, *Diabetic Med* 27(1):4–14, 2010.

Katsanos K, Spiliopoulos S, Diamantopoulos A, et al: Systematic review of infrapopliteal drug-eluting stents: a meta-analysis of randomized controlled trials, *Cardiovasc Intervent Radiol* 36(3):645–658, 2013.

Katsiki N, Papadopoulou S, Fachantidou A, et al: Smoking and vascular risk: are all forms of smoking harmful to all types of vascular disease? *Public Health* 127(5):435–441, 2013.

Kudagi V, White C: Endovascular stents: a review of their use in peripheral arterial disease, *Am J Cardiovasc Drugs* 13(3):199–212, 2013.

Ladzinski B, Bazakas A, Mistry N, et al: Sickle cell disease and leg ulcers, *Adv Skin Wound Care* 25(9):420–430, 2012.

Lambert M, Belch J: Medical management of critical limb ischemia: where do we stand today? *J Intern Med* 274(4):295–307, 2013.

Liapis C, Avgerinos E, Kadoglou N, et al: What a vascular surgeon should know and do about atherosclerotic risk factors, *J Vasc Surg* 49(5):1348–1354, 2009.

Lindner J, Womack L, Barrett E, et al: Limb stress-rest perfusion imaging with contrast ultrasound in the assessment of peripheral arterial disease severity, *JACC Cardiovasc Imaging* 1(3):343–350, 2008.

Mays R, Rogers K, Hiatt W, et al: Community walking programs for treatment of peripheral arterial disease, *J Vasc Surg* 58(6):1678–1687, 2013.

Mensah G, Bakris G: Treatment and control of high blood pressure in adults, *Cardiol Clin* 28(4):609–622, 2010.

Nassiri N: *Buerger's disease (thromboangiitis obliterans): differential diagnosis and workup,* E-Medicine from Web MD, May 2009. http://emedicine.medscape.com/article/460027-overview. Accessed April 27, 2010.

Norgren L, Hiatt W, Dormandy J, et al: Inter-society consensus for the management of peripheral arterial disease (TASC II), *J Vasc Surg* 45(Suppl S):S5–S67, 2007.

Okamoto K, Oka M, Maesato K, et al: Peripheral arterial occlusive disease is more prevalent in patients with hemodialysis: comparison with the findings from multidetector-row computed tomography, *Am J Kidney Dis* 48(2):269–276, 2006.

Paraskevas K, Giannoukas A, Mikhailidis D: Statins and infrainguinal vascular bypass procedures, *Curr Vasc Pharm* 11(1):51–57, 2013.

Reriani M, Dunlay S, Gupta B, et al: Effects of statins on coronary and peripheral endothelial function in humans: a systematic review and meta-analysis of randomized controlled trials, *Eur J Cardiovasc Prev Rehabil* 18(5):704–716, 2011.

Rizzo M, Corrado E, Patti A, et al: Cilostazol and atherogenic dyslipidemia: a clinically relevant effect? *Expert Opin Pharmacother* 12(4):647–655, 2011.

Rollini F, Franchi F, Muniz-Lozano A, et al: Platelet function profiles in patients with diabetes mellitus, *J Cardiovasc Transl Res* 6(3):329–345, 2013.

Romiti M: Meta-analysis of infrapopliteal angioplasty for chronic critical limb ischemia, *J Vasc Surg* 47(5):975–981, 2008.

Sakamoto S, Yokoyama N, Tamori Y, et al: Patients with peripheral artery disease who complete 12-week supervised exercise training program show reduced cardiovascular mortality and morbidity, *Circ J* 73(1):167–173, 2009.

Schernthaner R, Fleischmann D, Stadler A, et al: Value of MDCT angiography in developing treatment strategies for critical limb ischemia, *AJR Am J Roentgenol* 192(5):1416–1424, 2009.

Sheldon R, Roseguini B, Laughlin M, et al: New insights into the physiologic basis for intermittent pneumatic limb compression as a therapeutic strategy for peripheral artery disease, *J Vasc Surg* 58(6):1688–1696, 2013.

Sigvant B, Wiberg-Hedman K, Bergqvist D, et al: Risk factor profiles and use of cardiovascular drug prevention in women and men with peripheral arterial disease, *Eur J Cardiovasc Prev Rehabil* 16(1):39–46, 2009.

Sihlangu D, Bliss J: Resting Doppler ankle brachial pressure index measurement: a literature review, *Br J Community Nurs* 17(7):318–324, 2012.

Squires H, Simpson E, Meng Y, et al: A systematic review and economic evaluation of cilostazol, naftidrofuryl oxalate, pentoxifylline, and inositol nicotinate for the treatment of intermittent claudication in people with peripheral arterial disease, *Health Technol Assess* 15(40):1–210, 2011.

Stevens J, Simpson E, Harnan S, et al: Systematic review of the efficacy of cilostazol, naftidrofuryl oxalate and pentoxifylline for treatment of intermittent claudication, *Br J Surg* 99(12):1630–1638, 2012.

Tamura K, Tsurumi-Ikeya Y, Wakui H, et al: Therapeutic potential of low-density lipoprotein apheresis in the management of peripheral artery disease in patients with chronic kidney disease, *Ther Apher Dial* 17(2):185–192, 2013.

Tsai C, Chu S, Wen Y, et al: The value of Doppler waveform analysis in predicting major lower extremity amputation among dialysis patients treated for diabetic foot ulcers, *Diabetes Res Clin Pract* 100(2):181–188, 2013.

Tsuji Y, Hiroto T, Kitano I, et al: Importance of skin perfusion pressure in treatment of critical limb ischemia, *Wounds* 20(4):95–100, 2008.

Van Wijk D, Boekholdt M, Wareham N, et al: C-reactive protein, fatal and nonfatal coronary artery disease, stroke, and peripheral artery disease n the prospective EPIC-Norfolk Cohort Study, *Arterioscler Thromb Vasc Biol* 33:2888–2894, 2013.

Wennberg P: Approach to the patient with peripheral arterial disease, *Circulation* 182(20):2241–2250, 2013.

Wipke-Tevis D, Sae-Sia W: Caring for vascular leg ulcers, *Home Healthc Nurse* 22(4):237–247, 2004.

Wound, Ostomy and Continence Nurses Society™ (WOCN®): *Guideline for management of patients with lower extremity arterial disease (WOCN® clinical practice guideline series no. 1)*, Mount Laurel, NJ, 2008, WOCN®.

Xu L, Esparza E, Anadkat M, et al: Cutaneous manifestations of vasculitis, *Semin Arthritis Rheum* 38(5):348–360, 2009.

Zeymer U, Parhofer K, Pittrow D, et al: Risk factor profile, management and prognosis of patients with peripheral arterial disease with or without coronary artery disease: results of the prospective German REACH registry study, *Clin Res Cardiol* 98(4):249–256, 2009.

12

Venous Ulcers

Jane E. Carmel and Ruth A. Bryant

OBJECTIVES

1. Discuss venous ulcers in terms of etiologic factors, risk factors, assessment, diagnostic criteria, pathophysiology, typical presentation, and principles of management.
2. Describe Laplace's law in predicting subbandage pressure and the level of compression applied to the lower leg.
3. Explain the mechanism of action underlying effective compression therapy for the individual with chronic venous insufficiency.
4. Discuss considerations for use of inelastic compression, short-stretch bandages, long-stretch bandages, compression stockings, and intermittent pneumatic compression.
5. Identify adjunctive therapies that may be of benefit to the patient with a venous ulcer.
6. List three key points to teach a patient being treated with a multilayer compression wrap.

Chronic venous disorders include a wide range of morphologic and functional abnormalities of the venous system, ranging from mild conditions (e.g., uncomplicated telangiectasias and varicose veins) to complex conditions (e.g., deep vein thrombosis and venous ulcers). The majority of chronic venous disorders exist in the healthy patient population. The term *chronic venous disease* is used when referring to the subset of chronic venous disorders that are more complicated; those that are associated with signs and symptoms significant enough to require medical care, such as deep vein thrombosis, chronic venous insufficiency, and venous ulcers. Lower extremity venous disease (LEVD) is synonymous with chronic venous disease (CVD). Chronic venous insufficiency (CVI) or CVD refers to leg-related manifestations of venous hypertension and functional abnormalities of the venous system (edema, skin changes, ulceration) (Meissner, 2009). Venous ulcers are the most common lower extremity ulcers, accounting for 80% to 90% of all leg ulcers (Collins and Seraj, 2010; O'Meara et al, 2009). These lesions develop as a result of skin and tissue changes caused by valve dysfunction and the associated ambulatory venous hypertension.

Management of patients with venous ulcers must include measures to optimize wound healing through reduction of edema, prevention of complications, and appropriate topical therapy to promote healing (Moffat et al, 2007; Morton et al, 2013; Robson et al, 2006). Once the ulcer is healed, the emphasis shifts to long-term disease management and prevention of recurrence.

EPIDEMIOLOGY

The exact prevalence of venous ulcers is not known, although prevalence estimates in developed countries range from less than 1% to greater than 3% of the population (Bolton, 2008; Collins and Seraj, 2010; Olyaie et al, 2013; White-Chu and Kerr, 2014). Approximately 2.5 million Americans develop venous ulcers each year, which contributes to 2 million workdays lost annually (Collins and Seraj, 2010; Morton, 2013). Venous disease and venous ulcers occur in individuals as young as 20 years. "Peak" incidence occurs between the ages of 60 and 80 years (Kimmel and Robin, 2013). Although no racial predilection is apparent, most studies report female gender is a risk factor (Collins and Seraj, 2010; Olyale et al, 2013). In addition, an increased incidence of obesity is associated with venous ulcers; 25% of patients with venous ulcers have obesity (Benigni et al, 2006; Collins and Seraj, 2010; Kimmel and Robin, 2013).

Lower extremity venous disease affects approximately 7 million individuals in the United States, and approximately 3 million of these persons will develop ulcerations (WOCN® 2011). The impact of venous disease is tremendous as it relates to the individual and costs to the health care system and society. Individuals with venous disease report pain, itching, anxiety, leakage of exudate and odor, social isolation, and reduced ability to perform usual activities as their areas of greatest concern (Morton et al, 2013; White-Chu and Conner-Kerr, 2014). In contrast, nurses caring for these patients rated pain control as a less important aspect of care than wound healing and limb preservation, which indicates the need for increased awareness and focus on quality-of-life issues on the part of health care providers.

Approximately $2.5 to $3.5 billion is spent annually on the management of venous leg ulcers (VLU) (Morton et al, 2013). In the United Kingdom, the estimated costs of VLU management range from £300 to £600 million per year

(O'Donnell and Balk, 2011). Lifetime costs per individual have been estimated at $40,000 (WOCN®, 2011).

The negative impact of venous ulcers is compounded by recurrence rates. From 6% to 28% recur within 12 months, and as much as 40% recur in 5 years, reflecting the chronicity of venous disease (Kimmel and Robin, 2013; WOCN®, 2011). Frequent recurrence is attributed to a failure to adequately address the primary problems of venous insufficiency and venous hypertension (WOCN®, 2011). Recurrence rates are reduced when ongoing daily compression is provided (Anderson, 2013). Education, support, and access to other compression devices as needed are essential in the management of this patient population.

VENOUS STRUCTURE AND FUNCTION

The veins of the lower extremity venous system include deep veins, superficial veins, and perforator veins. The deep veins include the posterior and anterior tibial and the peroneal veins; these veins are located in the deep tissue adjacent to the calf muscle. The superficial venous system is also known as the *saphenous system* because the two major vessels are the greater saphenous vein and lesser saphenous vein. These two vessels are located just below the superficial fascia and have multiple tributaries located in the superficial tissues (Figure 12-1). The perforator veins "connect" the two systems, transporting blood from the superficial system into the deep system, from which point the blood is propelled back to the heart. The number of perforator veins per leg can vary greatly; the typical patient can have 200 perforator veins below the knee and 20 above the knee (Hussein, 2008).

Veins fill normally via slow capillary inflow, which takes more than approximately 20 seconds. All veins are equipped with one-way valves that support a unidirectional flow of blood toward the heart. Because these valves prevent reflux of blood from the high-pressure deep venous system to the low-pressure superficial venous system, they play an essential role in normal venous function. Further protection is provided by the fact that the perforator veins follow an oblique course through the fascia and muscle layers, which provides additional support for the connecting veins and their valves. The closed valves in the perforator veins prevent transmission of the high resting pressures back into the superficial system, as long as the valves remain competent (Dolibog et al, 2013). Approximately 50% to 60% of patients with venous ulcers have incompetent superficial and perforator vein valves (Agren and Gottrup, 2007).

Returning blood from the feet and legs to the heart is a major physiologic challenge because the blood must flow "uphill" against the forces of gravity. When an individual is standing upright, the gravitational force creates a column of hydrostatic pressure of approximately 90 mm Hg at the ankle. The primary mechanisms by which venous blood is returned to the heart are the smooth muscle tone within the venous walls, the contraction of the calf muscles (gastrocnemius and soleus), and the negative intrathoracic pressure created during inspiration. Of these three mechanisms, contraction of the calf muscle pump is by far the most essential (Meissner, 2009).

The calf muscle pump and one-way valves normally work together to propel venous blood back toward the heart. Calf muscle contraction forces the blood out of the deep veins and into the central circulation. While blood is being pumped from the deep veins, the one-way valves in the perforator system are closed to prevent backflow of the venous blood into the superficial veins. As the calf muscle relaxes, the valves in the perforator veins open to permit the blood in the superficial system to flow into the deep veins. At the onset of calf muscle contraction, the pressures within the deep venous system peak at 120 to 300 mm Hg. These pressures then fall rapidly as the veins empty and the calf muscle relaxes (Figure 12-2). Thus high resting (filling) pressures but low walking (emptying) pressures characterize normal venous function (Figure 12-3).

CHRONIC VENOUS DISEASE

The three elements most essential to normal venous function are competent valves, the physical properties of the venous wall, and the normally functioning calf muscle pump. With the loss of valvular competence, veins no longer fill normally via slow capillary inflow alone. Retrograde flow (reflux or back flow) of venous blood occurs during calf muscle pump relaxation, preventing a reduction in the venous pressure and a rapid (<20 seconds) venous refill time. This sustained high pressure or failure to lower venous pressure in the deep veins via the action of the calf pump muscle can be transmitted into the perforator veins and into the normally low-pressure superficial venous system. Incompetent valves subsequently contribute to venous hypertension and the condition known as CVD. Conditions that cause or contribute to valvular incompetence include those that cause direct damage to the valve leaflets and those that cause venous distention. Distention contributes to valve dysfunction by causing mechanical stretch that results in loss of coaptation of the valve leaflets.

Valve failure changes the normal unidirectional flow of blood into a "bidirectional" flow. As a result, blood refluxes back into the superficial system, causing distention and congestion of the superficial veins and capillaries, which manifest clinically as edema. The deep veins are incompletely emptied, causing increased pressures within the deep system, which create resistance to blood draining from the superficial veins. Resistance to flow creates congestion and distention of the superficial and perforator veins, which cause loss of valve coaptation. The incompetent valves then permit backward transmission of the high pressures in the deep system (Meissner, 2009). The failure to adequately lower venous pressure with the pumping of the calf muscle or by the incompetency of the valves creates ambulatory venous hypertension. Venous ulceration is a direct result of ambulatory

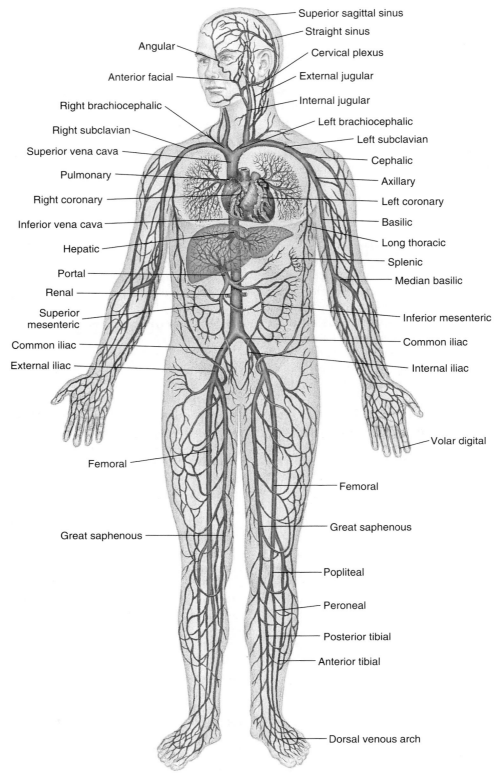

FIGURE 12-1 Systemic circulation: veins. (From Ball JW, Dains JE, Flynn JA, et al: Blood vessels. In *Seidel's guide to physical examination*, ed 8, St. Louis, MO, 2015, Mosby, pp 332–349.)

FIGURE 12-2 Anatomy of the perforating (communicating) veins. During the systolic phase of calf muscle contraction, the one-way valves of the perforating veins are closed, which prevents deep-to-superficial blood flow. During the diastolic phase the valves of the perforating veins are open, allowing superficial-to-deep blood flow to refill the deep veins. (From O'Donnell TF Jr, Shepard AD: Chronic venous insufficiency. In Jarrett F, Hirsch SA, editors: *Vascular surgery of the lower extremities*, St. Louis, MO, 1996, Mosby.)

FIGURE 12-3 Venous valves. **A,** Open valves allow forward blood flow. **B,** Closed valves prevent back flow. **C,** Incompetent valves unable to fully close, causing blood to flow backward and producing venous insufficiency.

venous hypertension from CVD. A clear understanding of the anatomy and physiology of the lower extremity venous system provides the framework for determining the pathology of LEVD, ambulatory venous hypertension, and venous ulceration.

The majority of patients have multisystem valvular incompetence (i.e., incompetent valves in at least two of the three venous systems) (Meissner, 2009). Perforator valve incompetence is particularly common and clinically significant. At least two thirds of patients with venous hypertension and venous ulcers have incompetent perforator valves, which can result in supramalleolar pressures well above 100 mm Hg and a "reflux rate" greater than 60 ml/min. When multiple valves become incompetent, the effect is magnified and clinically evident disease becomes much more likely (Meissner, 2009).

Of the three leg muscle pumps responsible for venous return in lower extremities (foot, calf, and thigh), the calf muscle pump is of greatest importance and generates the highest pressure. Among the venous pumps, the ejection fraction of the calf muscle pump is 65% compared with only 15% from the thigh muscle. In the limb with active ulceration, the ejection fraction can decrease to 35% (Meissner, 2009).

Ultimately, the end result of prolonged ambulatory venous hypertension is damage to the skin and soft tissues that renders these structures vulnerable to minor trauma and susceptible to spontaneous ulceration. Venous ulcers are caused by high venous pressures, venous hypertension, dysfunctional valves, obstruction in veins, or failure of calf muscle pump (Comerota, 2011; Hunter et al, 2013). However, the extent to which the calf muscle pump is impaired corresponds with the severity of the ulceration (White-Chu and Conner-Kerr, 2014). In the past, the cutaneous inflammation observed with venous insufficiency was believed to be the result of blood pooling (thus the term *stasis*) with low oxygen tension in the superficial veins, which precipitated hypoxic damage to the overlying skin. Today, no evidence supports the theories of stasis or hypoxia, and the terms *stasis dermatitis* and *stasis ulcers* are outdated (Hunter et al, 2013).

Classification

Chronic venous disease is classified according to *Clinical* indicators, *Etiologic* factors, *Anatomic* location of the dysfunctional venous structures, and specific *Pathophysiologic* processes (CEAP). This system is presented in Table 12-1 (Agren and Gottrup, 2007; Eklöf, Rutherford, and Bergan, 2004; WOCN®, 2011).

TABLE 12-1 CEAP Classification for Lower Extremity Venous Disease

Clinical Classification*	Etiologic Classification	Anatomic Classification	Pathophysiologic Classification
C_0: No visible or palpable indicators of venous disease	E_c: Congenital	A_s: Superficial veins	P_r: Reflux
C_1: Telangiectases	E_p: Primary	A_d: Deep system	P_o: Obstruction
C_2: Varicosities	E_s: Secondary (postthrombosis)	A_p: Perforator system	P_{ro}: Combination of reflux and obstruction
C_3: Edema	E_n: No venous cause identified	A_n: No venous cause identified	
C_4: Venous skin changes (hemosiderosis, dermatitis, lipodermatosclerosis)			
C_5: Venous skin changes plus healed ulceration			
C_6: Venous skin changes plus active ulceration			

*Clinical Classification is further delineated as to where the patient is symptomatic (i.e., aches, pain tightness, skin irritation) or asymptomatic. For example: $C_{6s}E_pA_{pd}P_r$.

Risk Factors

Risk factors for CVD include a history of major leg trauma, hip or knee surgery, and vein stripping. However, factors that lead to valvular or calf muscle dysfunction are the most common risk factors; they are listed in Table 12-2 along with other key elements of the medical history that must be obtained for the patient with a venous ulcer.

TABLE 12-2 Key Elements of History for Patients with Venous Ulcers

Element	Description
Risk factors for valvular dysfunction	Obesity, pregnancy, thrombophlebitis, leg trauma (e.g., fracture), thrombophilic conditions
Risk factors for muscle dysfunction	Sedentary lifestyle, prolonged standing, advanced age, altered or "shuffling" gait, musculoskeletal conditions and surgeries that compromise calf muscle function (e.g., paralysis, arthritis)
Factors that impede healing	Diabetes, tobacco, malnutrition, unplanned weight loss, medications
Factors that impede treatment	Limited activity and mobility, cardiac disease, heart failure (clinically significant heart failure is contraindication to compression)
Ulcer history	Previous ulcers, onset, duration, precipitating event (duration >6 months is negative predictor for wound healing)
History of prior treatment	Surgical, pharmacologic, compression (venous ulcers that consistently fail to respond to treatment should be evaluated for misdiagnosis, malignant, or mixed disease)
Patient concerns and anticipated barriers	Pain, itching, anxiety, anticipated barriers, transportation, ability to apply compression, job/financial limitations, effect on activities of daily living, treatment goals and priorities

Valvular Dysfunction. Numerous risk factors for valvular dysfunction have been identified and are listed in Box 12-1:
- Obesity, which creates resistance to venous return due to pressure on pelvic veins
- Pregnancy, especially multiple pregnancies or pregnancies that are close together, because of increased pressure against pelvic veins and compromised venous return
- Thrombophlebitis (e.g., deep vein thrombosis, pulmonary embolism), which triggers an inflammatory response that can cause direct damage to the valve leaflets, or chronic partial deep vein obstruction due to incomplete recanalization of the vein, which in turn causes venous distention and valvular compromise
- Leg trauma (e.g., fracture), which suggests undiagnosed damage to the vessel walls and valves
- Thrombophilic conditions (e.g., protein S deficiency, protein C deficiency, factor V [Leiden mutation]), which increase the coagulability of venous blood, thus increasing the risk of deep vein thrombosis and microvascular thrombosis; thrombophilic conditions have been identified in as many as 50% of patients with venous ulcers

Calf Muscle Dysfunction. The dynamics of the calf muscle pump can be adversely affected by changes that accompany major injuries, neurologic disease, and bone or joint pain. The calf muscle becomes weak with disuse; gait changes can exacerbate venous hypertension and calf muscle atrophy

BOX 12-1 Risk Factors for Valve Dysfunction

- Obesity
- Pregnancy
- Thrombophlebitis
- Leg trauma
- Thrombophilic conditions (e.g., protein S deficiency, protein C deficiency, factor V [Leiden mutation])

(Burrows et al, 2007). Risk factors for compromised calf muscle function (Box 12-2) include lifestyle, occupation, musculoskeletal conditions, age, mobility, arthroscopic surgery, extent of calf pump muscle contraction, and injection drug use (Pieper, Templin, Birk, et al, 2008).

Pathology of Venous Ulceration

Whereas CVD is clearly precipitated by ambulatory venous hypertension, the reason for venous ulceration as a consequence of venous hypertension is not well understood. This mystery is compounded by the fact that only a minority of patients with CVD actually progress to ulceration.

Fibrin Cuff Theory. Browse and Burnand (1982) initially postulated that capillary bed distention permitted leakage of large molecules such as fibrinogen into the dermal tissue, and that the fibrinogen then polymerized to form a thick perivascular cuff composed of fibrin, fibronectin, laminin, tenascin, and collagen. These cuffs do not pose any barrier to the diffusion of oxygen and nutrients into the tissues; therefore skin hypoxia cannot be the ultimate factor in the pathogenesis of venous ulcerations (Meissner, 2009). More recent theories on the progression of CVD indicate that chronic inflammation supersedes the "fibrin cuff" theory (Comerota, 2011).

White Blood Cell Activation and Trapping Theory. The trap hypothesis suggests that venous hypertension reduces the velocity of blood flow in the postcapillary bed. When blood flow becomes sluggish, leukocytes begin to adhere to each other (leukocyte aggregation) or to the capillary walls (leukocyte margination). This triggers the release of toxic oxygen metabolites, proteolytic enzymes, and cytokines, causing tissue inflammation and dermal fibrosis (Meissner, 2009). Dermal capillary loops also become plugged with leukocytes so that fibrin and other macromolecules leak out of the permeable capillary beds into the dermis, further aggravating inflammatory and fibrotic changes in the subcutaneous tissues and rendering them very susceptible to ulceration, which can occur spontaneously or as a result of minor trauma. Leukocyte migration and activation and the interaction of leukocytes with the endothelium in the presence of venous hypertension play considerable roles in the pathophysiology of venous ulcerations (Agren and Gottrup, 2007).

ASSESSMENT

Key assessment parameters for patients with a leg ulcer include medical history, ulcer history, previous treatments, clinical examination, inspection of the ulcer, family history, and Doppler assessment of pulses (Winnipeg Regional Health Authority, 2011; WOCN®, 2011). Assessment of Doppler pulses is discussed in Chapters 10 and 11 and illustrated in Figure 11-1.

Patient History

Risk factors for CVI are identified through the patient history. Of particular importance are risk factors that differentiate venous insufficiency from arterial disease and other pathologies that may cause ulceration in the lower extremity (see Table 12-2). Because of the contraindications to sustained compression, pretreatment evaluation must include a cardiac history and any indicators of uncompensated heart failure.

Lower Extremity Assessment

Both legs need to be examined by the clinician to ascertain if the manifestations are bilateral or more severe on one extremity. Findings unique to LEVD include edema, hemosiderosis, dermatitis, lipodermatosclerosis, atrophie blanche, varicose veins, ankle flaring, and scarring from previous ulcers (WOCN®, 2011). Checklist 12-1 gives a list of assessment findings unique to the lower extremity of a patient with CVI.

Arterial Perfusion. Coexisting arterial insufficiency is estimated in 10% to 20% of patients with venous disease (WOCN®, 2011) Therefore an ankle-brachial index (ABI) should be obtained on all patients with venous ulcers to determine whether some degree of arterial insufficiency

---

BOX 12-2 Risk Factors for Calf Pump Muscle Dysfunction

- Sedentary lifestyle
- Occupations that require prolonged standing
- Musculoskeletal conditions that compromise calf muscle function (e.g., paralysis, arthritis)
- Advanced age, which is associated with decreased elasticity of the calf muscle tendon
- Reduced mobility
- Altered or "shuffling" gait
- Arthroscopic surgery
- Injection drug use

CHECKLIST 12-1 Lower Extremity Assessment for Chronic Venous Insufficiency

General appearance
✓ Trophic changes: lipodermatosclerosis
✓ Edema: present from ankle to knee, often pitting
✓ Color: hemosiderin staining, atrophie blanche
✓ Dermatitis or varicosities may be present

Pain
✓ Dull aching (see Table 10-2)
✓ Exacerbates with dependency, improves with compression

Wound characteristics
✓ Gaiter area (see Table 10-3)
✓ Exudative and shallow

Perfusion
✓ Diminished only with coexisting arterial disease
✓ Diagnostic evaluation: duplex ultrasound

is present. An ABI of 0.8 or lower is interpreted to indicate coexisting arterial insufficiency; these ulcers are referred to as *mixed arterial/venous ulcers.* This is an important initial assessment because compression (critical for treatment of venous ulcers) must be modified or, in some cases, omitted. Wounds that begin specifically as a venous ulcer can develop an arterial component, so monitoring for signs of arterial disease at regular intervals is necessary (WOCN®, 2011). It is recommend that the level of compression be closely supervised in patients with an ABI greater than 0.5 to less than 0.8 mm Hg (WOCN®, 2011).

Edema. Edema is a classic indicator of venous disease because of the combination of capillary bed distention and elevated intracapillary pressures. As described in Chapter 10, the severity of edema varies among patients and from time to time throughout the day. The classic pattern is pitting edema (see Figure 10-1) that worsens with dependency and improves with elevation. Box 10-1 describes the assessment of pitting edema. With prolonged disease and gradual fibrosis of the soft tissues, edema may become "brawny," that is, nonpitting. Thus the characteristics of the edema are a clue to the duration of the underlying disease process.

The distribution of edema is also indicative of the underlying process. Venous edema primarily involves the lower leg between the ankle and the knee. In contrast, lymphedema and lipedema involve the entire extremity. Table 10-1 gives a comparison of the edema associated with these three conditions. Measuring the circumference of the calf and gaiter area is another method for assessing edema, especially if it is unilateral. Thus changes in these circumferential measurements provide an indication of the effectiveness of compression therapy (Kimmel and Robin, 2013). Circumferential measurements usually are taken weekly when the compression bandage is changed.

Hemosiderin Staining (Hemosiderosis). Another "classic" indicator of venous insufficiency is hemosiderosis, which is the discoloration of soft tissue located in the gaiter area that results when extravasated red blood cells break down and release the pigment hemosiderin. The result is a gray-brown pigmentation of the skin known also as *hyperpigmentation, skin pigmentation changes,* or *hemosiderin staining* (Kimmel and Robin, 2013; WOCN®, 2011) (see Plates 34, 35, and 39). Hemosiderin plays a significant role in the evolution of skin changes toward lipodermatosclerosis and ulceration (Caggiati et al, 2008; Kimmel and Robin, 2013).

Lipodermatosclerosis. *Lipodermatosclerosis* (see Plate 39), a term used to denote fibrosis, or "hardening," of the soft tissue in the lower leg, is indicative of long-standing venous insufficiency. The fibrotic changes typically are confined to the gaiter, or "sock," area of the leg, which results in an inverted "champagne bottle" or "apple core" appearance of the affected lower leg (WOCN®, 2011). The fibrosis causes abnormal narrowing of the affected area, which contrasts sharply with the normal tissue in the proximal limb, and a "woody," hard texture when the area is palpated. These fibrotic changes are thought to result from a combination of fibrin deposits, compromised fibrinolysis, and deposition of collagen in response to growth factors produced by activated white blood cells (de Araujo et al, 2003). A body mass index greater than 34 has been found to predispose the patient to lipodermatosclerosis (Bruce et al, 2002).

Varicosities. Varicose veins are swollen and twisted veins that appear blue, are close to the skin's surface, may bulge or throb, cause the legs to swell, and precipitate a feeling of heaviness. They are most often seen in the back of the calf or the medial aspect of the leg. Varicosities precede valvular incompetence and appear to develop as a consequence of intrinsic structural and biochemical abnormalities of the vein wall (Meissner, 2009). Patients with varicosities should manage their weight and exercise and avoid crossing their legs and wearing constrictive garments (WOCN®, 2011). *Ankle flaring* has been described in recent guidelines as visible clusters of spider veins around the medial malleolus (WOCN®, 2011).

Atrophie Blanche Lesions. Atrophie blanche lesions (see Plate 35) can be found in as many as one third of patients with LEVD and are more common in women (Sreedharan, 2011). These lesions are smooth, white plaques of thin, "speckled" atrophic tissue with tortuous vessels on the ankle or foot with hemosiderin-pigmented borders. Pathogenesis is unknown, and biopsy is not recommended (Sreedharan, 2011). Sometimes mistaken for scars of healed ulcers, this clinical finding actually represents spontaneously developing lesions. Prompt recognition is important so that a plan can be established to protect these high-risk areas from ulceration due to the thin, atrophic epidermis. Ulcers occurring in this area usually are small, very painful, and hard to heal. Topical steroids should be avoided because they can cause further damage to the very fragile skin.

Venous Dermatitis. Venous dermatitis is a common but distressing inflammation of the epidermis and dermis on the lower extremity of the patient with LEVD (see Plate 39). Often the earliest cutaneous sequelae of CVD, venous dermatitis most commonly affects middle-aged to elderly patients. Manifestations of venous dermatitis include scaling, crusting, weeping, erythema, erosions, and intense itching. Symptoms may be acute or chronic, and this condition may occur on one or both lower legs. The cutaneous inflammation of venous dermatitis is often confused with cellulitis. Factors that distinguish between dermatitis and cellulitis are listed in Table 12-3 (WOCN®, 2011).

Venous dermatitis results from the release of inflammatory mediators from activated leukocytes that are trapped in the perivascular space. Dermal fibrosis, a hallmark of venous dermatitis, develops as a result of fibrin cuff formation, decreased fibrinolysis, and release of transforming growth

TABLE 12-3 Distinguishing Between Dermatitis and Cellulitis

	Dermatitis	Cellulitis
Symptoms	Afebrile Itching Varicose veins/deep vein thrombosis	May have fever Painful No relevant history
Signs	Normal temperature Erythema, inflammation May be tender Vesicles and crusting Lesions on other parts of the body (e.g., other leg, arms) May be unilateral or bilateral	Elevated temperature Erythema, inflammation Tenderness One or a few bullae No crusting No lesions elsewhere Unilateral
Portals of entry	N/A	Usually unknown; breaks in skin, ulcers, trauma, tinea pedis, intertrigo implicated
Laboratory	Normal white blood cell count Negative blood cultures Leukocytosis	Blood cultures usually negative Skin swabs usually negative except for necrotic tissue Skin swabs (*Staphylococcus aureus* common)

DVT, Deep vein thrombosis; *WBC,* white blood cell.
From Wound, Ostomy and Continence Nurses Society™ (WOCN®): *Guideline for management of patients with lower extremity venous disease* (WOCN® clinical practice guideline series no. 1), Glenview, IL, 2005, WOCN®. Data from Quartey-Papafio CM: Lesson of the week: importance of distinguishing between cellulitis and varicose eczema of the leg, *BMJ* 318(7199):1672–1673, 1999.

factor-β_1 (a mediator of dermal fibrosis) by the leukocytes. Potent chemoattractants (intercellular adhesion molecule-1 and vascular cell adhesion molecule-1) keep leukocytes active in the perivascular environment and perpetuate cutaneous inflammation with fibrosis.

Venous dermatitis increases the risk of developing contact sensitivity due to the presence of chronic inflammation of the skin. Exposure to usually benign topical substances (e.g., wound exudate, liquid skin protectants, adhesives, topical antibiotics) easily exacerbates venous dermatitis. Frequent contact allergens include lanolin, balsam of Peru, and fragrances (Romanelli and Romanelli, 2007). Patients also can become sensitized to rubber products contained in some compression wraps and stockings. Allergic contact dermatitis due to topical antibiotics is very common. Neomycin and bacitracin are among the top 10 most common allergens to cause allergic contact dermatitis (Warshaw et al, 2007). Although less common, sensitization of the skin to topical corticosteroids can develop, triggering an allergic contact dermatitis. When the clinical manifestations of the limb affected with venous dermatitis worsen despite appropriate topical therapy, contact dermatitis should be considered.

To prevent venous dermatitis, product ingredients should be carefully scrutinized before topical therapy is selected, and products containing sensitizers should be avoided. Skin moisturizers such as bland, perfume-free topical emollients and white petrolatum can be used to maximize epidermal integrity. An essential component of prevention and treatment of venous dermatitis is graduated compression (discussed later in this chapter), which may require considerable patient education and encouragement due to the discomfort associated with an inflamed, edematous limb. Patients need reassurance that the discomfort should decrease as the edema resolves. Exudate-absorptive dressings (e.g., alginates, hydrofibers, honey) are commonly indicated, often in combination with a secondary foam dressing to adequately absorb and contain exudate.

To reduce inflammation and itching, mild-potency topical corticosteroids (e.g., triamcinolone 0.1% ointment) can be used short term (i.e., 2 weeks) but sparingly because of the risk for skin atrophy. High-potency topical corticosteroids are rarely used because of the risk for skin atrophy and systemic absorption through open denuded skin. Systemic corticosteroids are seldom warranted for treatment of venous dermatitis. Fluocinolone acetonide ointment 0.025% is an example of an intermediate-potency steroid with no preservatives. Cool compresses with Burow's solution (aluminum acetate) 30 to 60 minutes several times a day will soften the dry scaly skin and suppress inflammation (Hess, 2011). Patients with severe or nonresponsive dermatitis should be referred to dermatology for management.

Ulcer Characteristics. The classic venous ulcer is located in the gaiter area and around the medial malleolus, due to the greatest hydrostatic pressure at these sites. Typically, the ulcers are shallow, with moderate to high exudate. The wound bed can be ruddy red with adherent or loose yellow slough and granulation tissue (WOCN®, 2011). Ulcers that are deep and may have exposed tendon are likely not to be of pure venous origin (Nelzen, 2007). Venous ulcers usually have irregular edges and periwound maceration, crusting, scaling, edema, or hyperpigmentation (WOCN®, 2011) (see Plates 34 and 39). See Table 10-3 for a comparison of features that distinguish venous, arterial, and neuropathic ulcers.

Diagnostic Evaluation

In order to effectively diagnose and safely manage the patient with a CVI wound, the patient must first be evaluated for the presence of arterial insufficiency because standard therapy for venous ulcers (compression) may be contraindicated or may require modification of therapy in the presence of arterial disease (AAWC, 2014; Robson et al, 2006). The presence or absence of palpating dorsalis pedis and posterior tibial pulses should not be used in isolation to assess for arterial disease (WOCN®, 2011); an ABI or toe-brachial index (TBI) is warranted. Arterial insufficiency is suspected with an ABI of 0.8 or less or a TBI index of 0.6 or less (AAWC, 2014) (see Table 11-3). Chapter 11 describes diagnostic tests for arterial disease.

Chronic venous insufficiency is the result of either venous reflux or venous obstruction. Noninvasive vascular tests are used to distinguish between these two conditions. Traditionally, tourniquet test, photoplethysmography, and venography were used. However, poor reliability and inability to provide visualization of the venous system compromise the utility of the tests. A hand-held noninvasive photoplethysmography instrument that measures venous filling time is also available, but requires further testing of reliability. The duplex ultrasound imaging has largely replaced these tests (Meissner, 2009).

Duplex Ultrasound. Color duplex ultrasound scanning, including both supine and standing positions to identify anatomic and physiologic data related to venous reflux and/or obstruction, is the preferred method for confirming venous etiology (AAWC, 2014). Duplex ultrasound imaging is noninvasive and has a high degree of sensitivity. Duplex imaging technology uses two-dimensional ultrasound and Doppler shift to produce images of blood flow through the superficial, deep, and perforating veins revealing incompetent perforating veins, pinpointing the anatomic site of reflux, evidence of previous venous thrombosis, obstruction such as deep vein thrombus, and abnormal vein walls, as well as reflux through delicate venous valves (Coleridge-Smith et al, 2006; Kelechi and Bonham, 2008; WOCN®, 2011). This is valuable in providing both anatomic detail and direction of blood flow.

MANAGEMENT

As outlined in the LEVD guideline (WOCN®, 2011), the Association for the Advancement of Wound Care (AAWC) Venous Leg Ulcer guideline (2014), and the Wound Healing Society's guidelines for the treatment of venous ulcers (Robson et al, 2006), key interventions for correcting the underlying cause of venous insufficiency and venous hypertension include lifestyle adaptations and compression therapy. Pharmacologic agents and surgical procedures also play a role in the management of LEVD. A comprehensive treatment plan for the patient with venous disease is multimodal and includes nutritional assessment, exercise, compression therapy, vascular surgery, and advanced wound care modalities (White-Chu and Conner-Kerr, 2014).

Limb Elevation

Limb elevation is a simple but effective strategy for improving venous return by making use of gravitational forces. This is an important component of management for any patient with venous insufficiency, but it is an essential element of therapy for patients who are unable to adhere to a compression therapy regimen. Patients should be taught to lie down and elevate the affected leg above the level of the heart for at least 1 to 2 hours twice daily and during sleep. This position may be difficult for the obese person to manage comfortably. In addition, patients should be taught to strictly avoid prolonged standing or prolonged sitting with the legs dependent. Periods of standing or sitting must be interspersed with walking.

Exercise

Normal function of the calf muscle pump is essential to venous return, and effective contraction of the calf muscle requires a mobile ankle and routine dorsiflexion beyond 90 degrees. The patient with limited mobility is a challenge for clinicians. A patient with reduced ankle mobility or a "shuffling" gait should undergo a physical therapy evaluation to determine whether he or she can benefit from gait retraining and routine exercises to increase ankle strength and range of motion (Burrows et al, 2007). A home-based exercise program that includes isotonic exercise can improve poor calf muscle and calf muscle pump function (WOCN®, 2011). The Wound Healing Society's Prevention of Venous Ulcers Guideline recommends calf muscle pump exercises as helpful in long-term maintenance and venous ulcer prevention (Robson et al, 2006). Patients with venous insufficiency should be encouraged to perform ankle pumps routinely while standing or sitting and to intersperse standing and sitting with walking (Australian Wound Management Association and New Zealand Wound Care Society, 2011). For patients who are ambulatory, a walking program is recommended. Referral to a physical therapist could be beneficial in helping the patient adhere to the exercise program (Whit-Chu and Conner-Kerr, 2014). Primarily used to assess the elderly for fall risk, the Tinetti Balance and Gait Scale (available online) has been found to be reliable and valid in evaluating the walking mobility of patients with venous ulcers using injectable drugs. The wound specialist may find it beneficial to incorporate this scale into the workup of the patient with venous ulcers.

Weight Control

Obesity interferes with venous return, thus increasing the risk for LEVD. Morbid obesity can cause insufficiency in the deep venous system. In addition, significant obesity makes it very difficult for the patient to adhere to compression therapy and to avoid prolonged sitting. With the increase in obesity in younger people, the incidence of venous insufficiency and ulcers is anticipated to continue to rise. Therefore it is important to educate patients regarding the relationship between weight and venous disease and to strongly encourage patients to reduce their weight to a healthy level. Overweight people tend to be less mobile, which can affect calf muscle pump function and venous hypertension (White-Chu and Conner-Kerr, 2014). Patients who are morbidly obese may benefit from a referral to a dietician or a bariatric treatment center for evaluation and management.

Pharmacologic Therapy

Treating venous ulcers with pharmacologic means is based on the hypothesis of venous insufficiency pathogenesis. Inappropriate leukocyte activation, which has been shown to be present in CVD, can lead to the development of a venous ulcer (Coleridge-Smith et al, 2005). Diuretics and topical corticosteroids reduce edema and pain in the short term but offer no long-term treatment. Herbal supplements decrease the inflammatory response to venous hypertension, but are not licensed by the U.S. Food and Drug Administration (FDA) and can vary in efficacy and safety.

The addition of aspirin therapy to compression therapy may be useful in the treatment of VLUs as long as there are no contraindications (Kimmel and Robin, 2013). A daily dose of 300 mg of aspirin was found to shorten the healing time of venous ulcers (del Rio Sola, 2012). Systemic therapies of aspirin and pentoxifylline have been found to improve healing rate, whereas antibiotics do not (Poynter, 2013). Varatharajan et al (2014) reported three clinical studies evaluating aspirin therapy for venous ulcers and found an increased healing rate. Because these studies were small, the beneficial results of aspirin should be interpreted cautiously.

Several pharmacologic agents have demonstrated benefit in the management of venous disease. The three agents with documented efficacy in the management of venous disease are pentoxifylline (Trental), micronized purified flavonoid fraction (MPFF) (Daflon), and horse chestnut seed extract (HCSE).

Pentoxifylline (Trental). In the United States pentoxifylline (Trental) is the drug most commonly prescribed for venous disease and appears to be an effective adjunct to compression therapy. Its mechanism of action appears to be reduced aggregation of platelets and white blood cells, which reduces capillary plugging, and enhanced blood flow in the microcirculation, which reduces tissue ischemia (Jull et al, 2007). Dosages of 400 mg orally three times daily can accelerate healing of venous ulcers and should be considered for slow-healing venous ulcers (Jull et al, 2007; WOCN®, 2011).

Pentoxifylline may also promote healing even in the absence of compression. However, the beneficial effects of pentoxifylline must be balanced against its potential adverse effects (e.g., diarrhea, nausea) and its cost. A Cochran Review identified pentoxifylline to be an effective adjunct to compression bandaging and may even be effective in the absence of compression bandaging (Jull et al, 2012).

Micronized Purified Flavonoid Fraction. Several countries, both in Europe and elsewhere, have approved the phlebotropic drug known as MPFF (Daflon) (which consists of diosmin and flavonoids), for patients with LEVD. The specific mechanisms of action include (1) enhances venous tone, which promotes venous return; (2) reduces capillary permeability, which reduces edema formation; and (3) reduces expression of endothelial adhesion molecules, which reduces margination, activation, and migration of leukocytes (Robson et al, 2006). These mechanisms reduce the release of inflammatory mediators, which is thought to be the primary pathologic event resulting in dermatitis, lipodermatosclerosis, and ulceration. Adhesion of leukocytes at the surface of the endothelium is a starting point of the inflammatory cascade, causing

vein wall remodeling that progresses to valvular incompetence and eventual valve destruction (Perrin and Ramelet, 2011). Micronized purified flavonoid fraction has demonstrated clinical benefits in patients with C4–C6 venous disease (Gohel and Davies, 2010). Adverse effects of flavonoids include gastrointestinal disturbance in 10% of the patients (Australian Wound Management Association and New Zealand Wound Care Society, 2011).

The combination of MPFF with standard therapy (compression plus topical therapy) resulted in a statistically significant improvement in healing rates compared with standard therapy alone or to placebo in a double-blind trial, with a side effect profile comparable to that of placebo (Coleridge-Smith et al, 2005). A meta-analysis of MPFF as adjunct therapy for venous ulcers concluded that venous ulcer healing was accelerated and recommended MPFF use for large and long-standing ulcers (Coleridge-Smith et al, 2005). In addition, compared with conventional therapy, treatment with MPFF has demonstrated a significant reduction in cost of healing and a significant improvement in quality-of-life scores (Coleridge-Smith et al, 2005; Simka and Majewski, 2003).

Horse Chestnut Seed Extract. The herbal agent HCSE, which contains aescin, is commonly used in Europe as a method for managing CVI (Jull, 2007; Leach et al, 2006; Pittler and Ernst, 2012). The mechanism of action appears to be an inhibitory effect on the catalytic breakdown of capillary wall proteoglycans (Suter et al, 2006). Several placebo-controlled trials have demonstrated decrease in leg pain, edema, and pruritus (Pittler and Ernst, 2012). Preliminary evidence suggests comparable outcomes between HCSE and compression therapy. The recommended oral dosage is 300 mg twice daily (Pittler and Ernst, 2012). People with bleeding disorders, kidney disease, or liver disease should avoid HCSE and it is not recommended in combination with Trental, aspirin, or Coumadin (warfarin), unless under medical supervision. Duration of use in clinical trials has been 2 to 16 weeks. A recent Cochran Review reported HCSE an effective and safe short-term treatment for CVI (Pittler and Ernst, 2012).

COMPRESSION THERAPY

Compression therapy is the standard treatment for chronic venous insufficiency (Association for the Advancement of Wound Care, 2014; Australian Wound Management Association and New Zealand Wound Care Society, 2011; Kimmel and Robin, 2013; WOCN®, 2011).

Venous insufficiency is associated with increased hydrostatic pressure in veins in the legs. Compression therapy is used to reduce hydrostatic pressure and aid venous return (Olyaie et al, 2013). Wraps, bandages, garments, or devices are used to provide compression. Compression wraps are products that specifically wrap around the lower extremity. *Bandage* is the more common term used in European literature in place of *wrap* or *compression dressing,* however. *Garment* refers to compression products that are a clothing item, such as compression stockings. The intermittent pneumatic compression device is the only product that is powered.

Venous leg ulcers heal more rapidly with compression wraps compared with no compression wrap (Kimmel and Robin, 2013). Evidence also indicates better healing outcomes with a multicomponent compression system compared with a single compression system (Kimmel and Robin, 2013). Compression products apply pressure externally from the base of the toes to the knee to support the calf muscle pump during ambulation and dorsiflexion. The increased interstitial tissue pressure serves to oppose leakage of fluid into the tissues and to return interstitial fluid to the blood and lymph vessels, thus eliminating edema. Compression of the superficial veins promotes coaptation and normal function of the valves; it also increases the velocity of blood flow,

which reduces the aggregation and extravasation of white blood cells (Weingarten, 2001).

Features

Compression products share many different features, and these features guide the selection of the most appropriate compression option for each individual. Compression therapy can be either sustained (i.e., continuous) pressure or intermittent pressure. Products that remain in place and are removed after several days or only at night provide continuous pressure; the majority of products on the market provide continuous compression (Tables 12-4 and 12-5). Products that provide intermittent compression are applied two to three times per day for 1- to 2-hour intervals; intermittent compression is particularly beneficial to the

TABLE 12-4   Formulary of Compression Therapy Products

Category	Type	Examples*	Elastic	Inelastic	Disposable	Reusable	Therapeutic Pressure	Modified Pressure
Wraps**	Multilayer	Profore/ProGuide (Smith & Nephew) Dyna-Flex (Systagenix Wound Management) Coban 2 Layer (3M) ThreePress (Hartmann-USA Inc.)	X		X		X	X
	Long stretch	SurePress (ConVaTec) Setopress (Mölnlycke Health Care)	X			X	X	X
	Short stretch	Comprilan (BSN Medical) Farrow Wrap (Farrow Medical Innovation)		X		X		X
	Paste	Viscopaste (Smith & Nephew) Unna-Flex (ConVaTec) Gelocast (BSN Medical) Unna Press (Derma Sciences)		X	X			X
**Garments	Reusable inelastic device	CircAid Juxta-Fit (CircAid Medical Products)		X	X	X		X
	Tubular sleeve	Tubigrip (Mölnlycke Health Care) Medigrip (Medline)	X			X		X
	Stockings	Jobst Juzo Sigvaris Medi-Strumpf TheraPress DUO	X			X	X	X
Intermittent pneumatic pumps		Mobility (Derma Science, Inc.)		X		X	X	X

*Not inclusive.
**See also Table 12-5 for important considerations when choosing compressions wraps, stockings, or garments.

TABLE 12-5 Indications for Type of Compression*

Compression Wraps	Compression Stockings	Velcro Wraps
Reducing edema	Minimal shape distortion	Difficulty with dexterity
Reshaping the limb	Intact skin with minimal skin changes	Use as adjunct to stockings
Improving skin changes	Minimal skin folds	When adjustability is needed due to edema
Reducing skin folds	Preventing disease progression	Fragile skin
Improving lymphorrhea	Sequel to compression wraps	Promote self-care
Skin too fragile for hosiery		
Healing ulceration		

*See also Table 12-4 for important considerations in choosing compression wraps, stockings, and garments.
Adapted from Todd M: Venous disease and chronic oedema: treatment and patient concordance, *Br J Nurs* 23(9):466–470, 2014.

patient who cannot tolerate continuous compression or is unable to apply the continuous compression wraps or stockings.

Another feature of compression products is based on the type of material used to deliver the pressure: elastic or inelastic. *Elastic compression* adapts to changes in limb volume. The product exerts external pressure while the leg is at rest and when the calf muscle expands during ambulation, thus continuing to provide external pressure. Elastic compression products are appropriate choices for patients who are relatively sedentary or who have a "shuffling" gait that fails to engage the calf muscle. *Inelastic* (or *nonelastic*) *compression* will not expand during ambulation; they provide very little pressure at rest and high pressure with muscle contraction. As the calf muscle expands while walking, it presses against the "semirigid" bandage/dressing and creates pressure. At rest, when there is no calf pump muscle activity, only limited compression occurs. Therefore inelastic compression products are most appropriate for patients who are actively ambulating.

Compression products can be disposable or reusable. Many compression products are disposable and are used early in treatment when significant edema or an ulcer is present. Reusable compression products can be removed, cleaned, and then reused. The reusable products are nonadhesive wraps or garments. The nonadhesive reusable wraps can be used when edema or an ulcer is present if the patient cannot tolerate a multilayer wrap. The reusable garments are primarily used for "maintenance compression" once the edema has resolved and the ulcer is significantly healed or at least no longer exudative. Short-stretch wraps provide low compression compared with a multilayer compression system.

A key feature of compression wraps/garments is that they can provide a range of pressures. The amount of compression considered "therapeutic" for venous insufficiency (effective in controlling venous hypertension and preventing edema formation) is 30 to 40 mm Hg at the ankle (Marston, 2011; O'Meara

et al, 2009; Vowden and Vowden, 2006). Some clinicians recommend even higher levels of compression (40 to 50 mm Hg) for patients with severe venous insufficiency (Robson et al, 2006). Although the evidence is clear that 30 mm Hg or more is considered high compression and is the preferred level of pressure, many patients experience discomfort with high levels of pressure or are unable to physically apply the garment. In these situations, lower levels of pressure are more appropriate (O'Meara et al, 2009; WOCN®, 2011) (see Table 12-4). A general guide to categories of pressure is as follows: high pressure (30 to 40 mm Hg), medium pressure (20 to 30 mm Hg), and low pressure (14 to 17 mm Hg) (WOCN®, 2014).

Many compression wraps have "indicators" to guide the amount of tension, or stretch, to use when applying the wraps so that the desired amount of pressure can be attained. Similarly, compression stockings are manufactured to provide a specific range of pressure. The use of a pressure-measuring device (e.g., Picopress [Microlab]) that measures applied subbandage pressures is highly recommended for clinicians treating patients with mixed arterial venous ulcers (Marston, 2011).

External compression at high pressures will reduce blood supply to the skin and may lead to pressure damage. Similarly, impaired arterial blood supply to the legs may also result in pressure damage. If the patient expresses complaints about the extremity that is suggestive of device-related pressure damage, the compression may need to be removed so that the extremity can be assessed. Suggestions for correct compression are listed in Box 12-3.

Patients with venous hypertension need to understand that "compression is for life"! It is not a treatment that can be

BOX 12-3 Suggestions for Correct Compression

- Follow manufacturer's instructions for application technique to ensure attaining the appropriate level of compression.
- Measure the extremity accurately when using compression garments.
- Assess patient mobility and activity carefully when selecting elastic versus inelastic compression products. Inelastic compression products will not be effective if the patient is unable to perform very frequent calf muscle pumps, such as with ambulation.
- Compression should be used with caution if the patient has decreased leg sensation, infection in the leg, or allergies to ingredients in the compression materials.
- Screen for arterial disease using a Doppler measurement of the ABI. Use modified or lower levels of compression (23 to 30 mm Hg at the ankle) when coexisting arterial disease is present.
- Compression is contraindicated when the patient with venous insufficiency has an ABI ≤0.5.
- Obtain a toe brachial pressure when the ABI is >1.3 due to diabetes, arthritis or renal failure.
- Monitor the skin around and under the compression wrap or device closely and particularly during dressing changes to prevent pressure ulcers.

discontinued once the ulcer heals or the edema resolves. This ongoing compression is often referred to as "maintenance" compression. When the patient fails to adhere to maintenance compression, a 15% to 70% recurrence rate of venous ulcers has been reported (Kimmel and Robin, 2013). Unfortunately, one of every two patients discontinues compression therapy due to pain and discomfort associated with compression (Briggs and Closs, 2006). Furthermore, a normal ABI can potentially deteriorate over time, thus requiring a modification in the recommended level of compression. It is recommended that ABI be repeated every 3 months (WOCN®, 2011). Diligent monitoring by the wound specialist is essential for continued follow-through with the plan of care (Robson et al, 2006; WOCN®, 2011). The wound specialist is challenged to recommend the most clinically effective and "patient-friendly" system for each patient based on individual assessment, indications, contraindications, advantages and disadvantages, and special considerations of the many available compression products.

Contraindications

Compression is contraindicated in the patient with a coexisting untreated venous thrombosis in the extremity with the ulcer and uncompensated heart failure when the patient's fluid status is not being monitored. Graduated compression of edematous lower legs facilitates mobilization of interstitial fluid back into the circulatory system, potentially increasing preload volume and precipitating pulmonary edema (Collins and Seraj, 2010). During the acute initial treatment of congestive heart failure (CHF), compression may be used in conjunction with diuresis; however, fluid balance, electrolytes, and breath sounds should be monitored closely. In most cases, sustained compression is contraindicated in the presence of severe peripheral vascular disease (i.e., ABI ≤0.6) because sustained tissue pressure could further compromise tissue perfusion and potentially cause ischemic tissue death (Hopf et al, 2006; Marston, 2011). Most experts recommend against high compression in patients with ABI below 0.7 to 0.85. However, recently inelastic compression of up to 40 mm Hg in patients with mixed etiology venous ulcers (ABI > 0.5) was found to not impede arterial perfusion and in fact improved venous pumping function as demonstrated with increased toe pressures and $TcPO_2$ levels (Mosti, Iabichella, and Partsch, 2011). If ABI is below 0.5, revascularization is recommended if possible (Marston, 2011).

COMPRESSION WRAPS

Wraps are one of the most commonly used compression products, especially during the initial phase of treatment when limb volumes are changing rapidly as a result of edema reduction. Compression wraps are referred to by the number of components in the wrap. Single-layer wraps contain a single component, whereas a multilayer wrap may have two, three, or four components that are applied to the extremity. All wraps have a bandage layer; this bandage determines whether the wrap is elastic or inelastic. In addition to the

bandage layer, the two-layer wrap has either an orthopedic wool layer placed against the skin under the bandage wrap or a tubular sleeve over the bandage wrap. The components of a three-layer wrap include the orthopedic wool, a bandage wrap, and a tubular sleeve. The four-layer wrap contains the orthopedic wool, a crepe support bandage, a bandage wrap, and a self-adherent bandage (O'Meara et al, 2012). Multi-component systems containing an elastic bandage appear to be more effective than those mainly composed of inelastic components (O'Meara et al, 2012).

Generally, compression wraps are applied by professionals and left in place for 3 to 7 days. Most wraps are capable of providing modified compression. The most commonly used wraps are inelastic paste wraps, multilayer elastic wraps, and single-layer inelastic (short-stretch) bandages (see Table 12-4). Although individual clinical trials have reported multilayer and single-layer compression systems to be equally effective (Burrows et al, 2007; Castonguay, 2008), a recent systematic review of the literature conducted by the Cochran Collaboration reported that multicomponent systems achieve better healing outcomes than single-component compression (Kimmel and Robin, 2013; O'Meara et al, 2009, 2012). However, the most effective compression is the compression that the patient is able to use consistently.

Application Technique

All compression wraps are designed based on *Laplace's law of physics,* which states that subbandage pressure is directly proportional to the tension and number of bandage layers and inversely proportional to leg circumference and bandage width (Box 12-4). Laplace's law explains why application of a wrap with constant tension will create graduated pressure. Bandage tension is held constant while the circumference of the leg increases steadily from ankle to knee, and subbandage pressure will be highest at the ankle and lowest at the knee (Burrows et al, 2007; Ghosh et al, 2008; Moffat et al, 2007).

Some wraps are designed to be applied with a spiral technique, whereas others require a figure-of-8 application to achieve optimal results. Application techniques must follow the manufacturer's instructions. Some layers require 100% stretch and others 50% stretch; some may incorporate a visual indicator to achieve the correct level of pressure.

BOX 12-4 **Laplace's Law**

$$\text{Subbandage pressure} = \frac{\text{Tension} \times \text{Number of layers}}{\text{Leg circumference} \times \text{width of bandage}}$$

Laplace's law of physics as it applies to compression bandaging. Laplace's law demonstrates how compression therapy is a function of tension, number of layers, leg circumference, and bandage width. Increases in tension and/or layering increase subbandage pressure, whereas increases in leg circumference and/or bandage width decrease subbandage pressure.

The skill of the clinician applying the wrap will affect tension (Moore, 2002; O'Meara et al, 2009). Studies indicate that even when nurses are experienced with application, they frequently wrap with insufficient tension to produce therapeutic pressure levels. Training has been shown to significantly improve accuracy, but further studies are needed to quantify the interval at which this training should be repeated. An accurate and precise subbandage pressure monitor may be an option for assessing the clinician's ability to apply safe, graduated pressure.

The patient with a large calf or uneven contours can experience difficulty in keeping the bandage in place. Slippage of the bandage can lead to a tourniquet effect, which can cause edema above the wrap and injury to the skin. The use of a topical roll-on-adhesive (e.g., It Stays by Jobst) may help with preventing wraps from slipping. Compression wraps must be replaced when slippage occurs. Slippage of wraps is more common when wraps are initially applied due to fluids being shifted out of the tissue. Initially wraps will need to be changed more frequently until edema has stabilized. Another technique for preventing slippage is the use of extra padding to recontour the leg to a normal shape (Moffat et al, 2007). It has been found that bandages applied in a figure-of-8 configuration tend to stay in place better, especially for the person with a large leg. However, the manufacturer's instructions for wrapping must be followed to accommodate differences in product materials and layers, all of which affect the level of compression achieved. The best time of day to apply compression is when the least amount of edema is present: first thing in the morning before getting out of bed and before hanging the legs over the side of the bed. Two clinicians should wrap patients who are unable to lift their leg(s) to ensure an even application (Moffatt et al, 2007).

Multilayer Wraps/Bandages

Multilayer wraps are disposable, are elastic, provide sustained compression, and can be applied to provide either a modified or therapeutic level of pressure. These wraps therefore provide compression when the patient is active and when he or she is at rest (Figure 12-4). Multilayer wraps cannot be reused and should be changed when they begin to loosen, slip, or become saturated (typically in 3 to 7 days). A key feature of multilayer wraps is absorption of exudate. In many settings, these devices have become the product of choice for early intervention because of their ability to absorb exudate, adapt to changes in limb size, and provide sustained compression at rest and with activity.

Paste Wraps. Paste wraps are inelastic wraps that cannot be reused and provide sustained compression at a modified level of pressure. Dr. Paul Unna was the first to introduce use of a zinc paste bandage to create a conformable but inelastic "boot" around the leg; thus a paste-type compression wrap is commonly referred to as an Unna's boot (Weingarten, 2001). Today various inelastic paste wraps exist and are impregnated with any of the following products: zinc, glycerin, gelatin, or calamine (O'Connor and Murphy, 2014). Thus the paste wraps are not identical, and an adverse reaction to one does not predict a reaction to another.

Inelastic paste wraps should be applied without tension, beginning at the base of the toes and extending to the tibial tuberosity below the knee. The patient must be reminded to maintain the foot in a dorsiflexed position while the paste wrap is applied (Box 12-5). Common and appropriate techniques used to ensure a smooth conformable fit include

> **BOX 12-5 Procedure for Paste Bandage Application**
>
> 1. Apply gloves after assembling supplies and washing hands.
> 2. Gently wash and dry extremity. Replace gloves.
> 3. Position patient with affected leg elevated and not in dependent position.
> 4. Foot should be dorsiflexed so foot and leg are at 90-degree angle while applying initial bandage layers around the foot and ankle.
> 5. Open all paste bandage wrappers and cover wrap. Estimate amount of material based on size of leg(s).
> 6. Hold paste bandage roll in nondominant hand. Begin to apply bandage at base of toes.
> 7. If an ulcer is present, apply appropriate topical dressing to ulcer and secondary dressing (if indicated) before applying paste bandage.
> 8. Treat periwound (if indicated) and moisturize rest of leg.
> 9. Wrap twice around base of toes without using tension.
> 10. Continue wrapping bandage around foot, ankle, and heel, using a circular technique, with each strip overlapping previous strip by approximately 50% to 80%. Do not apply tension to the wrap.
> 11. Smooth paste bandage while applying and remove any wrinkles and folds (may pleat, reverse fold, or cut to ensure smooth bandage).
> 12. Wrap up to knee and finish smoothing.
> 13. Remove gloves.
> 14. Apply cover wrap using recommended amount of tension (e.g., 50% stretch) and 50% overlap.
> 15. Remove twice weekly or weekly as indicated by leakage, slippage, hygiene, wound care, complaint of numbness, or anticipated decrease in edema.

FIGURE 12-4 Compression wraps: layered bandage system.

open or closed heel, pleating, reverse folding, and cutting and restarting. When left open to air, the paste layer dries to a "semicast" consistency. Often the paste layer is covered with a self-adherent wrap to protect clothing from the paste. Paste bandages should be changed when they begin to slip, loosen, or become saturated (typically in 3 to 7 days). Problems associated with paste bandages include skin reaction to certain paste ingredients (e.g., calamine), maceration due to lack of an absorptive layer, slippage, poor fit, and inability to bathe (Davis and Gray, 2005; Hess, 2013; O'Connor and Murphy, 2014). As with all inelastic compression devices, paste bandages are most appropriate for actively ambulating patients and are not recommended for people in a wheelchair or bed.

Short-Stretch (Single-Layer) Reusable Wraps. Short-stretch reusable wraps are inelastic, single-layer wraps that provide sustained compression at a modified or therapeutic level. Because they are inelastic, they are most appropriate for the actively ambulating patient. These short-stretch wraps or single-layer wraps must not be confused with *Ace-type bandages,* which provide low levels of compression and are not considered therapeutic for patients with venous hypertension or insufficiency. Ace-type bandages tend to stretch when the calf expands and thus fail to provide calf muscle support during ambulation. In addition, they are very user dependent and are frequently applied incorrectly.

A major advantage of short-stretch reusable wraps is their "wash and reuse" feature. This feature permits more frequent removal of wraps for bathing and dressing changes and contributes to cost-effective care. Many of these wraps incorporate a visual indicator of correct tension, such as printed rectangles that become squares when stretched and applied correctly. This feature is beneficial when teaching caregivers how to apply the wrap correctly to achieve the prescribed level of pressure.

Long-Stretch Reusable Wrap. The long-stretch wrap is also a reusable, single-layer product that provides sustained compression at either a therapeutic or modified level of pressure. However, the distinctive feature of the long-stretch reusable wrap is that it is elastic so it can be used for both the sedentary and the actively ambulating patient. Much like the short-stretch wrap, the long-stretch wrap can be washed and reused and should not be confused with Ace-type bandages.

COMPRESSION GARMENTS

Compression garments are essentially cloth products that can be reused and may be in one of the following forms: stockings, tubular sleeve, and inelastic device.

Stockings

Compression stockings are reusable, elastic garments that are most commonly used for patients with stable venous insufficiency to prevent ulceration (either initial or recurrent).

These garments are appropriate for sedentary and actively ambulating patients. Compression stockings must not be confused with *antiembolism* stockings, which provide 15 to 17 mm Hg of pressure and are therefore not appropriate for therapeutic compression (WOCN®, 2011).

As described in Tables 12-4 and 12-5, stockings are generally not a good choice for compression during the initiation of therapy because of the rapid changes in limb circumference associated with edema reduction. They should be used once the edema has been controlled and limb circumference has stabilized. Another relative contraindication for stocking use is severe lipodermatosclerosis because the "inverted champagne bottle" configuration of the leg typical of this condition makes obtaining a good fit difficult. If necessary, however, customized stockings can be made after a referral to a trained "stocking fitter."

Stockings are available in a variety of colors, styles, and sizes. To obtain a safe size, an accurate measurement of the leg should be obtained after the edema has resolved and with careful review of the manufacturer's instructions. Stockings may be knee high or thigh high; most patients with venous insufficiency are effectively managed with knee-high stockings. Compression stockings are classified according to the pressure produced at the ankle (Kline et al, 2008): class I (light support), class II (medium support), class III (strong support), and class IV (very strong support). The actual amount of pressure (in mm Hg) appointed to each classification varies by country and manufacturer. Compression stockings are produced as either a circular knit or a flat knit garment. The circular knit stocking is a thin, lightweight material without a seam; it is not available in high levels of compression (Moffatt et al, 2007).

Stockings are the "mainstay" of maintenance compression, but are effective only if the patient wears them. Therefore it is critical for the wound specialist to educate the patient and ensure that he or she understands the importance of lifelong compression and is able to correctly don the stocking (Moffatt et al, 2007). If barriers are identified, resources and devices to assist with application or other options for compression must be explored. Tips for applying compression stockings (including assist devices) and other key points for patient education are outlined in Box 12-6. One example of a device that facilitates stocking application is shown in Figure 12-5.

Tubular Sleeve

The knit tubular sleeve is a reusable compression material that, when measured and applied correctly as a double layer, provides sustained compression at a modified level of pressure (18 to 25 mm Hg) (O'Meara et al, 2009). A tubular sleeve may be selected when the patient cannot tolerate other types of compression. It also may be used as a temporary intervention while a more permanent solution is pending. Application and removal are easy and require minimal, if any, education; therefore the tubular sleeve is an excellent option when simplicity is the top priority.

BOX 12-6 Patient Education: Compression Stockings

Tips for Putting On Stockings

- Don stockings immediately upon awakening, before getting out of bed.
- For easier application of stockings, wear rubber gloves; apply talcum powder (light dusting) first to foot and leg.
- Apply heavy stockings over light silk stocking or silky stocking "liner."
- Use commercial device designed to facilitate stocking application:
  - Stocking butler or donning gloves (Jobst)
  - Easy-slide toe sleeves for open-toe stockings (Jobst, Juzo, Sigvaris)
  - Stocking donner (Beiersdorf-Jobst)
  - Doff N Donner (SIGVARIS)
  - Slippie Gator (Juzo)
- Wash new stockings before wearing (follow manufacturer's directions) to reduce stiffness and difficulty in application.
- Use a "layered" approach: either two-piece stockings (TheraPress DUO by Hartmann Conco) or two layers of lower-compression stockings (e.g., two layers of stocking, each of which provides 15 mm Hg compression).
- Turn leg portion of stocking inside-out down to heel. With stocking stretched, slip foot in while pulling stocking by its folded edge over heel. Gently work stocking up leg, gradually turning stocking right-side out.
- Conduct foot exercises with stockings on: move toes in circular motion (make big circles) both clockwise and counterclockwise. Repeat exercise at least 10 times per day.

Care and Management

- Purchase two pairs of stockings to permit laundering.
- Launder with mild detergent and line dry (follow manufacturer's guidelines).
- Replace stockings every 3 to 4 months to maintain therapeutic efficacy.
- If stockings become too tight or too loose, contact wound care nurse, wound program, or physician for refitting.
- For person having problems with stocking sliding down, use roll-on adhesive applicator (It Stays by Jobst).

FIGURE 12-5 Application of a therapeutic support stocking with a "stocking donner."

FIGURE 12-6 An example of an inelastic reusable device. (Courtesy CircAid Medical Products, San Diego, CA.)

Reusable Inelastic Device (Velcro Wraps)

Many of the compression garments and devices used for managing lymphedema can be used to manage the edema associated with venous hypertension. For example, the CircAid (MMAR Sports Medicine), Juxta-Lite (MMAR Sports Medicine), and Juxta-Fitare (MMAR Sports Medicine) inelastic reusable compression devices are secured with overlapping bands. By securing the bands according to the pressure indicators, the device can provide therapeutic or modified levels of pressure (20 to 30, 30 to 40 or 40 to 50 mm Hg) (Figure 12-6). The ability to easily apply and adjust the straps helps prevent slippage as edema fluctuates, permits routine bathing, provides easy access to the wound for dressing changes, and allows the patient to wear shoes of his or her preference—all features that have been reported to improve adherence (Bianchi et al, 2013; Todd, 2014). These products are washable, reusable, and have a 3- to 6-month warranty.

The Cochrane review found multicomponent systems with elastic bandages to be more effective than inelastic systems. Patients heal faster with the four-layer bandage than with the short-stretch bandage. High-compression stocking systems also demonstrated faster healing than short-stretch bandages. More research is needed to study the outcome between high-compression stockings and the four-layer bandage system (O'Meara, 2012).

INTERMITTENT PNEUMATIC COMPRESSION

Intermittent pneumatic compression (IPC) is a reusable compression device that involves the use of an air pump to

FIGURE 12-7 Dynamic compression device: sequential compression therapy.

intermittently inflate a sleeve applied to the lower extremity (Figure 12-7). For over 60 years this therapy has been used for CVI. The basic effects of IPC are to increase venous velocity, reduce edema, increase popliteal artery blood flow, and increase nitric oxide synthase (Comerota, 2009). Initially used to prevent deep vein thrombosis and pulmonary embolism (White-Chu and Conner-Kerr, 2014), this type of therapy is also used for lymphedema and arterial management. Intermittent pneumatic compression may be used for patients with LEVD who are mobile or for those who are immobile and need higher levels of compression than can be provided with stockings or wraps. This is also an alternative for patients unable to tolerate sustained compression or who are too compromised for sustained compression (Robson et al, 2006).

Intermittent compression devices vary in terms of the inflation–deflation cycle, amount of pressure exerted against the leg, and number of compartments in the sleeve. Single-compartment sleeves simply inflate and deflate on a cyclic basis, whereas multicompartment sleeves provide sequential compression. Rapid IPC has been shown to have a greater rate of healing than the slow IPC (Kimmel and Robin, 2013). Typically, patients are instructed to apply the therapy once or twice daily for 1 to 2 hours each time.

Benefits of IPC include mobilization of interstitial (edema) fluid back into the circulation and enhanced venous return without impairing arterial flow (Nelson, Mani, Thomas et al, 2011). In fact, IPC may actually improve distal perfusion, making the therapy safe for patients with coexisting arterial disease (Hopf et al, 2006). Furthermore, IPC therapy may contribute to the healing of long-standing venous ulcers that have "failed" standard compression therapy. Advantages of IPC as a means of compression therapy include (1) ease of use, (2) provision of active and dynamic compression, and (3) the ability to be applied comfortably and consistently at home (Cervantis and Orphey, 2010). Intermittent pneumatic compression is reimbursed in the home setting when the patient has one or more venous ulcers that have failed to heal after a 6-month trial of conservative treatment directed by a physician (Blue Cross/Blue Shield of Kansas, 2013).

Studies report higher levels of patient satisfaction and adherence to IPC therapy, as well as improved wound healing. Nelson (2011) reviewed seven randomized clinical trials to determine whether there was a difference in healing when IPC was used alone or with compression bandages. Intermittent pneumatic compression increased healing when used alone; however, it was not clear if healing was increased when combined with compression wraps. Similarly, Dolibog et al (2013) conducted a pilot study and found that IPC demonstrated a faster reduction in wound surface area than ulcers treated with two-layer short-stretch wrap and standard care only. The updated 2012 Wound Healing Society guidelines recommend the use of IPC, with or without compression, in patients unable to wear an adequate compression system (White-Chu and Conner-Kerr, 2014). More research is needed to determine whether this therapy can increase healing of VLUs, manage edema, and reduce recurrence.

LOCAL WOUND CARE

As with all wounds, topical therapy for the venous wound is selected based on wound characteristics (see Chapter 18). Initially, the venous ulcer may present with copious amounts of exudate. Black necrotic tissue is seldom seen in venous ulcers except when infection, trauma, or significant ischemia is present. Therefore an appropriate rule of thumb is to select dressings that minimize potential allergens while effectively managing the exudate to prevent periwound maceration and control bioburden. O'Meara et al (2013) reported insufficient reliable evidence to support the use of honey or silver-based products; there was some evidence to support cadexomer–iodine use. However, as with all wounds, antimicrobial agents should only be used to treat clinical infection, not bacterial colonization (O'Meara et al, 2013; O'Meara, Al-Kurdi, Ologun et al, 2014).

Topical dressings have also been used to provide topical anesthetics for the control of pain in venous ulcers. In a systematic review of the literature, a lidocaine-prilocaine cream (Eutectic Mixture of Local Anesthetics [EMLA]) was reported to provide effective pain relief during debridement. Patients with ibuprofen slow-release foam dressings achieved greater pain relief when compared with best practice (Briggs et al, 2012).

The periwound skin also requires care in that it must be protected from the maceration that can accompany an exudative wound and from irritants such as adhesives and chemicals. Interventions to prevent and manage venous dermatitis were described earlier in the chapter. As edema decreases, the volume of exudate from the venous ulcer also will diminish, and the types of dressings will need to be modified.

Failure to Progress

When an apparent venous ulcer fails to progress or worsens despite treatment, the entire treatment plan must be reevaluated; if the plan remains appropriate and is consistently implemented, the diagnosis should be reevaluated. The AAWC guidelines recommend a biopsy when the venous ulcer does not improve after 6 weeks of adequate therapy (Morton et al,

2013). Many other causes of lower extremity ulcers can present as venous ulcers, such as mixed venous/arterial, lymphedema, vasculitis, autoimmune disease, and malignancy. If a biopsy and differential diagnosis again confirm a venous etiology, failure to heal may be due to biofilm (discussed in Chapter 16) or the negative cellular environment of a chronic wound. In this case a product or therapy designed to convert the chronic wound environment into an environment that supports repair should be considered. Fogh et al (2012) conducted studies on the use of ibuprofen foam dressing compared with a foam dressing without ibuprofen for painful venous ulcers. The results were that the pain relief was significantly greater with ibuprofen foam dressing.

ADJUNCT THERAPIES

Skin grafts, bioengineered human skin equivalents, negative pressure wound therapy (NPWT), electrical stimulation, and selected growth factors have shown varying degrees of success in the management of refractory venous ulcers once the underlying cause is appropriately addressed (Agency for Healthcare Research and Quality, 2012). The Wound, Ostomy and Continence Nurses Society™ (WOCN®) guideline for management of lower extremity venous ulcers (2011) identifies biologic skin substitutes, electrical stimulation, and ultrasound as a B level of evidence for adjunctive therapies. The AAWC guidelines (2012) algorithm recommends if there are no signs of healing in 30 days, to consider biological dressings, bilayered bioengineered skin, electrical, ultrasound, or radiofrequency stimulation therapies (Figure 12-8). However, Watson et al (2011) concluded the addition of low-dose ultrasound delivered at 1 MHz to the periulcer skin during weekly dressing changes (i.e., low adherent dressings and compression therapy) did not aid healing, improve quality of life, or reduce recurrence.

Among the variety of skin grafts and substitutes available for wound care, sufficient evidence exists to demonstrate significantly more VLUs heal with bilayer artificial skin than with dressings (Jones et al, 2013). A Cochrane review reported that the use of a bilayered living cellular construct (Apligraf [Organogensis, Inc.]) used in conjunction with compression therapy increased the healing of venous ulcers compared with other dressings used with compression (Jones et al, 2013). Biophysical and biologic agents are described in detail in Chapters 19 to 24.

Grafting has also been considered as another form of surgical adjunct therapy. Pinch grafts and split-thickness grafts have been studied, with healing rates of 45% for pinch grafts and 88% to 90% for split-thickness grafts reported (Morton et al, 2013). However, recurrences rates after 4 months have been reported. Grafting along with compression therapy may improve the healing rate.

The effectiveness of NPWT for venous leg ulcers has not been demonstrated. A metaanalysis reported there is no evidence that NPWT improved healing time (Sadat et al, 2008). More recently, in a nonrandomized prospective study with seven patients, Kieser et al (2011) reported NPWT (used in conjunction with compression bandaging) appeared to stimulate rapid wound debridement and granulation tissue formation. However, the early decrease in wound surface area was not sustained. The authors concluded NPWT should be further investigated as a means of preparing venous ulcers for skin grafting.

SURGICAL INTERVENTIONS

Appropriate topical therapy and compression are not sufficient to heal all venous ulcers (Robson et al, 2006). Vascular surgery should be considered when appropriate treatments fail to heal the venous ulcer. Factors associated with failure to heal include increased ulcer size (>5 cm^2), longer duration (>6 months), and failure to show significant progress toward healing during the first 3 to 4 weeks of compression therapy. Coexisting arterial disease, persistence of fibrin throughout the wound bed, reduced mobility, and history of vein ligation or knee or hip replacement have been reported as negative prognostic indicators (Paquette and Falanga, 2002; WOCN®, 2011).

Surgery is indicated to correct superficial venous reflux in patients with chronic venous ulcers that have failed appropriate compression and topical therapy. If conservative treatment fails, AAWC Venous Ulcer Algorithm (2012) recommends corrective vascular surgery be considered to improve vein function, such as minimally invasive subfascial endoscopic perforating vein surgery (SEPS). A number of surgical options are available that can be used to address venous hypertension. Four surgical procedures are available and selection is based on the extent of valvular reflux (Table 12-6): SEPS, laser ablation, radiofrequency ablation (RFA), and sclerotherapy. There is good evidence to support the use of thermal radiofrequency vein ablation and SEPS; however, sclerotherapy is less supported (Morton et al, 2013). With the advancement of minimally invasive techniques there is a decrease in the number and size of incisions, procedure time, and recovery time (Kumar et al, 2009).

Vein stripping was a treatment of choice in the early twentieth century. This procedure was performed to prevent backflow of blood into the lower leg and involved removing the great saphenous vein.

More current options have replaced this procedure that involves destroying the vein while leaving it in place. In the last decade vascular surgery options have increased to correct vein function (White-Chu and Connor-Kerr, 2014). These procedures are venous ablative surgery that is delivered by heat (laser or radiofrequency/sound waves) or sclerotherapy that uses strong burning drugs to destroy the saphenous vein without removal. Patients must have an intact deep venous system to be considered for surgical interventions. Within the past 10 to 15 years these treatments have replaced traditional vein stripping.

Subfascial Endoscopic Perforator Vein Surgery

The SEPS technique was introduced over 15 years ago and involves using an endoscopic video camera and instrumentation placed through small ports remote from the ulcer. Healing rate

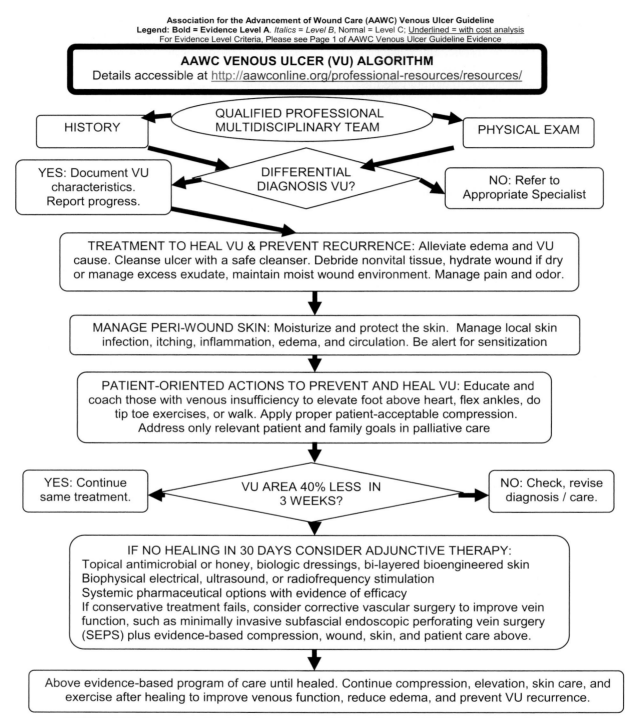

FIGURE 12-8 Association for the Advancement of Wound Care (AAWC) Venous Ulcer Guideline. Malvern, Pennsylvania: Association for the Advancement of Wound Care (AAWC). December 2010. Accessible at http://aawconline.org/professional-resources/resources/

of venous ulcers was reported in 8 weeks with no recurrence in 11.9 months using an ultrasonic scalpel in the SEPS procedure (Kumar et al, 2009). The Wound Healing Society Guidelines recommend the SEPS procedure to address underlining venous etiology of the venous ulcer by preventing backflow from the deep to the superficial venous system. WOCN® Society guidelines

(2011) classified this procedure as level B evidence. The procedure is not effective if the patient has severe deep venous disease with either reflux or obstruction (Robson et al, 2008).

Deep venous insufficiency is due to valvular incompetence. Surgical techniques available for valvular incompetence are artificial venous valve insertion, direct valvuloplasty, and

TABLE 12-6   Surgical Treatments for Chronic Venous Ulcers

Pathology	Surgical Treatment
Superficial vein reflux	RFA
	EVLT
	Vein stripping
Perforator vein reflux	SEPS
	RFA
	Sclerotherapy
Deep vein reflux	Valvuloplasty
	Valve transplantation

autogenous vein valve transplantation. Complications with the SEPS procedure have been reported, including delayed wound healing (0% to 11%), sural paraesthesia (1.9% to 3%), tibial nerve paraesthesia (1%), and a recurrence rate of 8% at 3 years and 18% at 5 years (Di Battista et al, 2012).

Ablation Procedures

Two types of thermal ablation procedures for superficial venous reflux are used: endovenous laser ablation (EVLA) and RFA. Both procedures are performed in an outpatient setting with local anesthetic and usually no sedation. Patients are ambulatory after the procedure, and recovery time is short (Proebstle et al, 2002).

Endovenous laser ablation, also known as *laser surgery,* uses laser to create intense local heat in the incompetent vein. The goal of endovenous laser ablation (ELA) is to deliver sufficient thermal energy to destroy the vascular endothelium layer of the wall of the incompetent vein segment to produce irreversible occlusion of the vein (Proebstle et al, 2002). The amount of thermal energy delivered corresponds with the success of ELA. A catheter is inserted into the vein to be treated, usually just below the knee. Using ultrasound, the surgeon injects a solution of saline and anesthetic agent along the length of the vein to be treated. After this, either laser or RFA is performed. The procedure can take 2 to 3 hours and is performed in an outpatient setting using a local anesthetic. There may be some bruising over the treated site that can last up to 14 days and pain at the site.

Radiofrequency is delivered directly to the vessel wall; the RF energy is delivered both in and around the vessel to be treated. The amount of energy to be delivered is determined to ensure endothelial ablation by thermal sensors. The RF catheter repeats the process along the length of the vein (Subramonia and Lees, 2010). This is a longer procedure to perform, but the results have better outcomes compared with conventional surgery (Subramonia and Lees, 2010). It has been noted that patients have less postoperative pain and can return to their normal routine earlier than patients having the conventional open vein stripping surgery.

Foam sclerotherapy (FS) is another vein ablating procedure. With this technique, a drug mixed with air is administered by a needle into the vein. This drug will burn and scar the inside of the saphenous vein. Ultrasound is used to direct where the drug will go in the vein. The addition of foam to the agent allows for decreased amounts of sclerosing agent injection and improved efficacy (Subramonia and Lees, 2010). This treatment has been used extensively in Europe. Overall effectiveness of this procedure needs further studies.

Surgical intervention of superficial venous reflux with compression therapy has been shown to reduce the recurrence of venous leg ulcers at 4 years (Kimmel and Robin, 2013). *E*ffects of *S*urgery and *C*ompression on *H*ealing *A*nd *R*ecurrence (ESCHAR) studies suggest superficial vein surgery reduces venous ulcer recurrence and should be considered for all patients with chronic venous ulcers (Gohel et al, 2007; Howard et al, 2008; Wright, 2009) Although vein ablative surgery usually has minor complications, there have been some reported complications of nerve damage and deep vein thrombosis (Davies et al, 2008).

FOLLOW-UP AND LIFELONG MAINTENANCE

With recurrence rates of VLUs ranging between 15% and 71%, the emphasis of management must shift to prevention of recurrence once the ulcer is healed (Kimmel and Robin, 2013). Lifelong exercise, weight control, and compression therapy are ongoing challenges. Although compression garments have been demonstrated to increase healing rates (O'Meara et al, 2012) and reduce recurrence rates at 3 years compared with no compression, intolerance of compression is significant (Nelson and Bell-Syer, 2012). Patients fail to utilize compression consistently for a variety of reasons, including the patient's perception of the value of compression, his or her level of comfort/discomfort with the stockings, challenges in application, and modified dress/shoe attire (Defloor, 2010; Shannon et al, 2013). Conditions that can affect the prognosis for invasive and noninvasive procedures are obesity, malnutrition, intravenous drug use, and coexisting medical conditions (Kimmel and Robin, 2013). These findings clearly speak to the importance of patient education regarding lifelong compression, ongoing support and encouragement, and identifying solutions to barriers that jeopardize the patient's adherence (Van Hecke et al, 2013).

Many different strategies can be employed to improve adherence. The patient may be able to tolerate a lower level of compression in terms of pain; he or she may also be able to apply the garment. Although evidence indicates high-level compression stockings are more effective in preventing recurrence, medium-level compression stockings are associated with significantly higher rates of adherence (White-Chu and Conner-Kerr, 2014). The Wound Healing Society's guidelines recommend the use of compression stockings constantly and forever, and attempts must be made to aid the patient's adherence (Robson et al, 2008). The wound clinician needs to recommend a compression device that the person can apply independently. There are more choices available than in the past—the clinician should offer options to meet the individual's needs. The choice may be based on cost issues and the patient's preference (Kimmel and Robin, 2013). Education that includes the families and caregivers, as well as the patient, is critical to achieving optimal outcomes (Burrows et al, 2007; Van Hecke et al, 2013). Chapter 29 provides more strategies for facilitating the patient's ability to adhere to a mutually agreeable plan of care.

In the United Kingdom there are community services, such as the Lindsay Leg Club, that provide quality care and empowerment for patients with leg ulcers, while also supporting and educating nursing staff (Clark, 2010; McKenzie, 2013). This model has been well accepted by patients and has been more economical than traditional visits from the home care nurse. Similarly, The Lively Legs program in the Netherlands is effective in promoting walking and leg exercises, potentially leading to decreased wound healing time (Heinen et al, 2012). Total patient commitment is required for success in managing CVD.

CLINICAL CONSULT

A: Referral for leg ulcer recommendation. 60-year-old Caucasian female with type 2 diabetes, obesity, and history of lower leg edema and venous ulcer of right leg.

Patient has edema of right lower leg, complains of pain with ambulation a short distance and when in bed. Wound assessment revealed a 2 cm x 2.5 cm wound, irregular wound margin, no depth, wound bed has 30% black necrotic tissue with 70% pale pink tissue. Hemosiderin staining present bilateral lower legs in gaitor area. ABI is 1.5.

D: Overall assessment is not consistent with venous ulcer. Risk factors: Diabetes, obesity, patient history. The appearance of the leg ulcer, patient history, and complaint of pain with leg elevation are consistent with mixed arterial venous ulcer. The ABI is a false high reading due to calcification.

P: Referral for vascular testing and vascular surgeon. Manage wound exudate and pain.

I: Plan of care will be as following: (1) Collaborate with vascular and primary provider for developing a treatment plan. (2) Patient and caregivers will be educated on the treatment plan. (3) Use of appropriate topical dressing to manage exudate, facilitate autolysis, and reduce/control pain. Light compression (less than 30 mmHg) or one layer elastic tubular sleeve (Tubigrip). (4) Gradual walking and weight loss program.

E: Will follow to evaluate treatment plan, assess tolerance of compression therapy, and revise interventions as needed.

SUMMARY

Chronic venous disease is a potentially disabling condition accompanied by lower leg edema, venous hypertension, lower leg pain, and ulcerations. To prevent ulceration and to heal existing ulcers, graduated compression is required. Graduated compression therapy via single or multilayer wraps, stockings or intermittent compression provides support to restore near normal vein and calf pump muscle function. Close monitoring with support and encouragement are important to facilitate continued use of these treatment modalities by the patient.

REFERENCES

Agency for Healthcare Research Quality (AHRQ): *Chronic venous ulcers: a comparative effectiveness review of treatment modalities,* 2012. http://effectivehealthcare.ahrq.gov/search-for-guides-reviews-and-reports/?pageaction=displayproduct&productID=995

Agren M, Gottrup F: Causation of venous ulcers. In Morison M, Moffatt CJ, Franks PJ, editors: *Leg ulcers: a problem-based learning approach,* Edinburgh, 2007, Elsevier.

Anderson I: Compression hosiery to reduce leg ulcer recurrence, *Nursing Times* 109(6):18–20, 2013. http://nursingtimes.net. Accessed May 11, 2014.

Association for the Advancement of Wound Care (AAWC): *Venous ulcer guideline,* Malvern, PA, 2010, updated 2014, AAWC. http://aawconline.org/professional-resources/resources. Accessed June 4, 2015.

Australian Wound Management Association and New Zealand Wound Care Society: *Australian and New Zealand clinical practice guideline for prevention and management of venous leg ulcers,* 2011. http://www.awma.com.au/publications/2011_awma_vlug.pdf. Accessed June 10, 2014.

Ball JW, Dains JE, Flynn JA, et al: Blood vessels. In *Seidel's guide to physical examination,* ed 8, St. Louis, MO, 2015, Mosby, pp 332–349.

Benigni JP, Cazoubon M, Mathieu M, et al: Chronic venous disease in the obese male: an epidemiological survey, *Phlebolymphology* 14:47–49, 2006.

Bianchi J, Mahoney K, Nugent L, et al: A fresh way to treat venous leg ulcers with measure compression, *Br J Community Nurs* (Suppl):S34, S36–S40, 2013.

Blue Cross/Blue Shield of Kansas Medical Policy: *Pneumatic compression pumps for treatment of lymphedema and venous ulcers (for home use): current procedural terminology,* American Medical Association, June 7, 2013.

Bolton L: Compression in venous ulcer management, *J Wound Ostomy Continence Nurs* 35(1):40–49, 2008.

Bonham PA, Kelechi T, Mueller M, et al: Are toe pressures measured by a portable photoplethysmograph equivalent to standard laboratory tests? *J Wound Ostomy Continence Nurs* 17(5):475–486, 2010.

Briggs M, Closs SJ: Patients' perceptions of the impact of treatments and products on their experience of leg ulcer pain, *J Wound Care* 15(8):333–337, 2006.

Briggs M, Nelson EA, Martyn-St James M: Topical agents or dressings for pain in venous leg ulcers, *Cochrane Database Syst Rev* 11:CD001177, 2012.

Browse NL, Burnand KG: The cause of venous ulceration, *Lancet* 320(8292):243–245, 1982.

Bruce AJ, Bennett DD, Lohse CM, et al: Lipodermatosclerosis: review of cases evaluated at Mayo Clinic, *J Am Acad Dermatol* 46(2):187–192, 2002.

Burrows C, Miller R, Townsend D, et al: Best practice recommendations for the prevention and treatment of venous ulcers: update 2006, *Adv Skin Wound Care* 20(11):611–621, 2007.

Caggiati A, Rosi C, Franceschini M, et al: The nature of skin pigmentations in chronic venous insufficiency: a preliminary report, *Eur J Vasc Endovasc Surg* 35(1):111–118, 2008.

Castonguay G: Short-stretch or four-layer compression bandages: an overview of the literature, *Ostomy Wound Manage* 54(3):50–55, 2008.

Cervantes C, Orphey S: Pneumatic compression and venous stasis ulcers and implications of lymphedema on delayed wound healing, *Todays Wound Clin* 4(11), 2010.

Clark M: A social model for lower limb care: the Lindsay Leg Club Model, *EMWA J* 10(3):38–40, 2010.

Coleridge-Smith P, Lok C, Ramelet AA: Venous leg ulcer: a meta-analysis of adjunctive therapy with micronized purified flavonoid fraction, *Eur J Vas Endovasc Surg* 30(2):198–208, 2005.

Coleridge-Smith P, Labropoulos N, Partsch H, et al: Duplex ultrasound investigation of the veins in chronic venous disease of the lower limbs: UIP consensus document: part I. Basic principles, *Eur J Vasc Endovasc Surg* 31:83–92, 2006.

Collins L, Seraj S: Diagnosis and treatment of venous ulcers, *Am Fam Physician* 81(8):989–996, 2010.

Comerota A: Intermittent pneumatic compression: physiologic and clinical basis to improve management of venous leg ulcer, *J Vasc Surg* 53(4):1121–1129, 2011.

Comerota A: Treatment of chronic venous disease of the lower extremities: what's new in guidelines? *Phlebolymphology* 16(4):313–320, 2009.

Davies A, Howard A, Howard DPJ, et al: Surgical therapy for chronic venous insufficiency. In Gloviezki P, editor: *Handbook of venous disorders: Guidelines of the American Venous Forum*, ed 3, Boca Raton, FL, 2008, CRC Press, pp 400–409.

Davis J, Gray M: Is Unna's boot bandage as effective as a four-layer wrap for managing venous leg ulcers? *J Wound Ostomy Continence Nurs* 32(3):152–156, 2005.

de Araujo T, Valencia I, Federman DJ, et al: Managing the patient with venous ulcers, *Ann Intern Med* 138(4):326–334, 2003.

Defloor M: Processes underlying adherence to leg ulcer treatment: a qualitative filed study, *Int J Nurs Stud* 48(2):145–155, 2010.

del Rio Sola M, Fajardo A, Vaquero Puerta C: Influence of aspirin therapy in the ulcer associated with chronic venous insufficiency, *Ann Vasc Surg* 26(5):620–629, 2012.

Di Battista L, D'Andrea V, Galani A, et al: Subfascial endoscopic perforator surgery (SEPS) in chronic venous insufficiency. A 14 years experience, *G Chir* 33(3):89–94, 2012.

Dolibog P, Franek A, Taradaj J, et al: A randomized, controlled clinical pilot study comparing three types of compression therapy to treat venous leg ulcers in patients with superficial and/or segmental deep venous reflux, *Ostomy Wound Manage* 59(8):22–30, 2013.

Eklöf B, Rutherford RB, Bergan JJ, et al: Revision of the CEAP classification for chronic venous disorders: consensus statement, *J Vasc Surg* 1248:40–52, 2004.

Fogh K, Andersen MB, Bischoff-Mikkelsen M, et al: Clinically relevant pain relief with an ibuprofen-releasing foam dressing: results from a randomized, controlled, double -blind clinical trial in exuding, painful venous leg ulcers, *Wound Repair Regen* 20(6):815–821, 2012.

Gohel MS, Barwell JR, Taylor M, et al: Long term results of compression therapy alone versus compression and surgery in chronic venous ulceration (ESCHAR): randomised controlled trial, *BMJ* 335(7610):83, 2007.

Gohel MS, Davies AH: Pharmacological treatment in patients with C4, C5 and C6 venous disease, *Phlebology* 25(Suppl 1):35–41, 2010.

Ghosh S, Mukhopadhyay A, Sikka M, et al: Pressure mapping and performance of compression bandage/garment for venous leg ulcer treatment, *J Tissue Viability* 17(3):82–94, 2008.

Heinen M, Borm G, van der Vleuten C, et al: The Lively Legs self-management programme increased physical activity and reduced wound days in leg ulcer patients: results from a randomized controlled trial, *Int J Nurs Stud* 49(2):151–161, 2012.

Hess CT: Venous dermatitis checklist, *Adv Skin Wound* 24(2):96, 2011.

Hopf HW, Ueno C, Aslam R, et al: Guidelines for the treatment of arterial insufficiency ulcers, *Wound Repair Regen* 14(6):693–710, 2006.

Howard DP, Howard A, Kothari A, et al: The role of superficial venous surgery in the management of venous ulcers: a systematic review, *Eur J Vasc Endovasc Surg* 36(4):458–465, 2008.

Hunter S, Langemo D, Thompson P, et al: Observation of periwound skin protection in venous ulcers: a comparison of treatments, *Adv Skin Wound Care* 26(2):62–73, 2013.

Hussein R: Chronic venous ulcer an end of long term suffering, *Internet J Plast Surg* 5(1), 2008.

Jones JE, Nelson EA, Al-Hity A: Skin grafting for venous leg ulcers, *Cochrane Database Syst Rev* 1:CD001737, 2013.

Jull A: An overview of pharmacological treatment options for venous leg ulcers. In Morison MJ, Moffatt CJ, Franks PJ, editors: *Leg ulcers: a problem-based learning approach*, Edinburgh, 2007, Elsevier.

Jull AB, Arroll B, Parag V, et al: Pentoxifylline for treating venous leg ulcers, *Cochrane Database Syst Rev* 12:CD001733, 2012.

Kelechi T, Bonham P: Measuring venous insufficiency objectively in the clinical setting, *J Vasc Nurs* 26(3):67–73, 2008.

Kieser DC, Roake JA, Hammond C, et al: Negative pressure wound therapy as an adjunct to compression for healing chronic venous ulcers, *J Wound Care* 20(1):35–37, 2011.

Kimmel H, Robin A: An evidence-based algorithm for treating venous leg ulcers utilizing the Cochrane Database of Systematic Reviews, *Wounds* 25(9):242–250, 2013.

Kline C, Macias B, Kraus E, et al: Inelastic compression legging produces gradient compression and significantly higher skin surface pressures compared with an elastic compression stocking, *Vascular* 16(1):25–30, 2008.

Kumar A, Agarwal PN, Garg PK: Evaluation of subfascial endoscopic perforator vein surgery (SEPS) using harmonic scalpel in varicose veins: an observational study, *Int J Surg* 7(3):253–256, 2009.

Leach M, Pincombe J, Foster G: Using horse chestnut seed extract in the treatment of venous leg ulcers: a cost-benefit analysis, *Ostomy Wound Manage* 52(4):68–70, 72–74, 76–78, 2006.

Marston W: Mixed arterial and venous ulcers, *Wounds* 23(12): 351–356, 2011.

McKenzie M: The Lindsay Leg Club: supporting the NHS to provide leg ulcer care, *Br J Community Nurs* S2:S16–S20, 2013.

Meissner MH: Pathophysiology of varicose veins and chronic venous insufficiency. In Hallett JW Jr, et al, editors: *Comprehensive vascular and endovascular surgery*, Philadelphia, 2009, Mosby.

Moffatt CJ, Partsch H, Clark M: Compression therapy in leg ulcer management. In Morison M, Moffatt CJ, Franks PJ, et al, editors: *Leg ulcers: a problem-based learning approach*, Edinburgh, 2007, Elsevier.

Moore Z: Compression bandaging: are practitioners achieving the ideal sub-bandage pressures? *J Wound Care* 11(7):265–268, 2002.

Morton LM, Bolton LL, Corbett LQ, et al: An evaluation of the Association for the Advancement of Wound Care venous ulcer guideline and recommendations for future research, *Adv Skin Wound Care* 26(12):553–561, 2013.

Mosti G, Iabichella ML, Partsch H: Compression therapy in mixed ulcers increases venous output and arterial perfusion, *J Vasc Surg* 55:122–128, 2012.

Nelson EA: Venous leg ulcers, *Clin Evid (Online)* 2011:1902, 2011.

Nelson EA, Bell-Syer SE: Compression for preventing recurrence of venous ulcers, *Cochrane Database Syst Rev* 8:CD002303, 2012.

Nelson EA, Mani R, Thomas K, et al: Intermittent pneumatic compression for treatment of venous leg ulcers, *Cochrane Database Syst Rev* 2:CD001899, 2011.

O'Connor S, Murphy S: Chronic venous leg ulcers: is topical zinc the answer? A review of literature, *Adv Skin Wound Care* 27(1):35–44, 2014.

O'Donnell TF Jr, Balk E: The need for an intersociety consensus guideline for venous ulcer, *J Vas Surg* 54:83S–90S, 2011.

Olyaie M, Rad F, Elahifar M, et al: High-frequency and noncontact low-frequency ultrasound therapy for venous leg ulcer treatment: a randomized, controlled study, *Ostomy Wound Manage* 59(8):14–20, 2013.

O'Meara S, Al-Kurdi D, Ologun Y, et al: Antibiotics and antiseptics for venous leg ulcers, *Cochrane Database Syst Rev* 1:CD003557, 2014.

O'Meara S, Cullum NA, Nelson EA: Compression for venous leg ulcers (review), *Cochrane Database Syst Rev* 1:CD000265, 2009.

O'Meara S, Cullum N, Nelson EA, et al: Compression for venous leg ulcers, *Cochrane Database Syst Rev* 11:CD000265, 2012.

Paquette D, Falanga V: Leg ulcers, *Clin Geriatr Med* 18(1):77–88, 2002.

Perrin M, Ramelet A: Pharmacological treatment of primary chronic venous disease: rationale, results and unanswered questions, *Eur J Vasc Endovasc Surg* 41:117–125, 2011.

Pieper B, Templin TN, Birk TJ, et al: Chronic venous disorders and injection drug use, *J Wound Ostomy Continence Nurs* 35(3):301–310, 2008.

Pittler M, Ernst E: Meta-analysis of horse chestnut seed extract studies for chronic venous insufficiency, *Cochrane Database Syst Rev* 11:CD003230, 2012.

Poynter E, Andrews M, Ackerman W: What is the best initial treatment for venous ulcers? *J Fam Pract* 62(8):433–434, 2013.

Proebstle TM, Sandhofer M, Kargl A, et al: Thermal damage of the inner vein wall during endovenous laser treatment: key role of energy absorption by intravascular blood, *Dermatol Surg* 28(7):596–600, 2002.

Robson M, Cooper DM, Aslam R, et al: Guidelines for the treatment of venous ulcers, *Wound Repair Regen* 14:649–662, 2006.

Romanelli M, Romanelli P: Dermatological aspects of leg ulcers. In Morison M, Moffatt CJ, Franks PJ, et al, editors: *Leg ulcers: a problem-based learning approach*, Edinburgh, 2007, Elsevier.

Sadat L, Chang G, Noorani A, et al: Efficacy of TNP on lower-limb wounds: a meta-analysis, *J Wound Care* 17(1):45–48, 2008.

Shannon MM, Hawk J, Navaroli L, et al: Factors affecting patient adherence to recommended measures for prevention of recurrent venous ulcers, *J Wound Ostomy Continence Nurs* 40(3):268–274, 2013.

Simka M, Majewski E: The social and economic burden of venous leg ulcers: focus on the role of micronized purified flavonoid fraction adjuvant therapy, *Am J Clin Dermatol* 4(8):573–581, 2003.

Sreedharan S, Siaha S: Atrophie blanche, *Wound Prac Res* 19(2):74–80, 2011.

Subramonia S, Lees T: Randomized clinical trial of radiofrequency ablation or conventional high ligation and stripping for great saphenous varicose veins, *Br J Surg* 97(3):328–336, 2010.

Suter A, Bommer S, Rechner J: Treatment of patients with venous insufficiency with fresh plant horse chestnut seed extract: a review of 5 clinical studies, *Adv Ther* 23(1):179–190, 2006.

Todd M: Venous disease and chronic oedema: treatment and patient concordance, *Br J Nurs* 23(9):466–470, 2014.

Van Hecke A, Beeckman D, Grypdonck M, et al: Knowledge deficits and information-seeking behavior in leg ulcer patients: an exploratory qualitative study, *J Wound Ostomy Continence Nurs* 40(4):381–387, 2013.

Varatharajan L, Thapar A, Davies A: Adjunctive aspirin for venous ulcer healing, *Phlebology* 29(6):336–337, 2014.

Vowden KR, Vowden P: Preventing venous ulcer recurrence: a review, *Int Wound J* 3:11–21, 2006.

Warshaw EM, Ahmed RL, Belsito DV, et al: Contact dermatitis of the hands: cross-sectional analyses of North American Contact Dermatitis Group data, 1994–2004, *J Am Acad Dermatol* 57(2):301–314, 2007.

Watson JM, Kang'ombe AR, Soares MO, et al: VenUS III: a randomised controlled trial of therapeutic ultrasound in the management of venous ulcers, *Health Technol Assess* 15(13):1–192, 2011.

Weingarten M: State-of-the-art treatment of chronic venous disease, *Clin Infect Dis* 32:949–954, 2001.

White-Chu E, Conner-Kerr T: Overview of guidelines for the prevention and treatment of venous leg ulcers: a U.S. perspective, *J Multidiscip Healthc* 7:111–117, 2014.

Winnipeg Regional Health Authority: *Regional wound care clinical practice guidelines. venous, arterial and mixed lower leg ulcers*, Winnipeg, Manitoba, Canada, 2011, WRHA.

Wound, Ostomy and Continence Nurses Society™ (WOCN®): *Guideline for management of patients with lower-extremity venous disease*, Mt. Laurel, NJ, 2011, WOCN®.

Wright DD: THE ESCHAR trial: should it change practice? *Perspect Vasc Surg Endovasc Ther* 21(2):69–72, 2009.

13

Lymphedema

Catherine R. Ratliff

OBJECTIVES

1. Describe the pathophysiology of lymphedema.
2. Identify and describe two types of lymphedema.
3. Distinguish the difference between lymphedema and lipedema.
4. List two common diagnostic tests used to diagnose lymphedema.
5. Articulate important assessment features for the patient being evaluated for lymphedema.

6. Outline a treatment plan for a patient with lymphedema, including conservative measures and adjunctive therapies such as surgery.
7. Explain prevention and treatment measures for a patient with cellulitis.

Lymphedema is a chronic disease characterized by swelling of the affected body part, usually the limb, because of impaired flow of lymph fluid. Accumulation of lymph fluid results in swelling in the affected limb. The swelling may be mild or it may be severe, such that the individual is unable to use the affected limb. Lymphedema primarily occurs in the subcutaneous fatty tissues of the arms or legs (Lawenda et al, 2009; Sieggreen and Kline, 2004).

The clinical presentation of lymphedema (see Plate 42) results from the subcutaneous accumulation of fluid. With interstitial fluid accumulation comes an inflammatory response; slowed lymphatic flow, which causes lipogenesis; and fat deposition. Patients develop firmer subcutaneous tissue in the limb as fibrosis, as well as hypertrophy of the adipose tissue. These physical changes present clinically as soft and pitting edema, but later progress to induration and fibrosis with nonpitting edema (Warren et al, 2007a).

EPIDEMIOLOGY

As the third component of the vascular system, the lymphatic system receives the least attention. Similarly, lymphedema and related pathologies have received much less attention than the pathologies associated with venous and arterial ulcers. Chronic lymphedema has no cure, and long-term management with patient involvement is critical to control the lymphedema. Lymphedema is frequently undertreated, and an insufficient number of lymphedema centers and specialists are addressing the problem.

Lymphedema prevalence refers to the estimated population who are managing the condition. The prevalence is more than 3 million people in the United States (Cormier et al, 2011). Incidence refers to the number of new cases of lymphedema diagnosed each year. The incidence of secondary lymphedema from malignancies include breast cancer (up to 40%), melanoma (16%), gynecologic (20%), genitourinary (10%), and head/neck cancer (4%) (Cormier et al, 2011). Lymphedema in cancer patients is seen today at more advanced stages of the cancer than in the past because cancer patients are living longer as a result of more effective cancer treatments. With the increased survival of these patients, the numbers of cancer patients with lymphedema are expected to increase. However, these patients may be sicker and less able to care for themselves, including managing their lymphedema (Cheville, 2007).

PATHOPHYSIOLOGY

The lymphatic system is composed of lymphatic vessels and lymphatic tissue, which function as a drainage and transport system. When fluid from the interstitial space enters the lymphatic system, it is considered lymph fluid. Lymph fluid consists of protein, water, fatty acids, salts, white blood cells, microorganisms, and debris. It is absorbed from the interstitial spaces into the lymphatic vessels, where it is transported to the venous system (Holcomb, 2006; Lawenda et al, 2009).

The major function of the lymphatic system is to return fluid and protein from interstitial spaces to the vascular system. Because lymphatic vessels often lack a basement membrane and have thinner vessel walls, they can reabsorb molecules too large for the venous system (Holcomb, 2006; Sieggreen and Kline, 2004). Usually tissue fluid and protein macromolecules filtrated by the arterial capillaries are reabsorbed and returned to the circulation through the lymphatic system. From 50% to 100% of the intravascular proteins are filtered this way in the interstitial space. The lymphatic vessels absorb 2 to 4 L of protein-rich fluid retained in the interstitial space per day. This fluid is picked up by the lymphatic capillaries and returned to the circulation, thus maintaining normal plasma volume and preventing interstitial edema. If the system is overloaded, fluid and protein accumulate in the interstitial space, forming a high-protein edema that triggers an inflammatory response with deposition of collagen (Holcomb, 2006; Macdonald et al, 2003).

Two systems of lymphatic drainage work similarly to the venous system. The superficial system drains the skin and subcutaneous tissues, and the deep system drains the tissues to the fascia and below. The lymphatic vessels in the superficial system are located in the subcutaneous tissues, whereas those of the deep system are aligned with the blood vessels, especially the veins. These two systems of lymphatic drainage are connected by perforating vessels just like the veins (Lawenda et al, 2009; Macdonald et al, 2003).

The lymphatic system is composed of lymphatic capillaries, precollectors, lymph collectors, and lymphatic trunks. Capillaries absorb lymph fluid and transport it to lymph nodes, lymphatic trunks, and lymphatic ducts. The lymphatic capillaries are larger than the blood capillaries, are more permeable with thinner walls, and have no basement membranes allowing them to absorb fluids. The lymphatic capillaries do not have valves, so lymph flows in the direction of the lower pressure. The precollectors connect the lymphatic capillaries with the lymph collectors. The lymph collectors are similar to veins; they have valves and transport lymph fluid to the lymph nodes and lymphatic trunks. The precollectors and collectors are the principal vessels of the lymphatic system and eventually filter through to the lymph nodes (Lawenda et al, 2009; Macdonald et al, 2003).

Lymph drains from the legs into the lumbar lymphatic trunk to the intestinal lymphatic trunk and cisterna chyli to the thoracic duct, which drains into the left subclavian vein (Figure 13-1). The thoracic duct empties approximately 3 L of lymph fluid per day into the venous circulation (Lawenda et al, 2009). From the left side of upper body, the lymphatic vessels of the left arm drain into the left subclavian lymphatic trunk, which then drains into the left subclavian vein. Lymph is drained from the right side of the head, neck, thorax, and right arm into the right subclavian vein by way of the right thoracic duct (Sieggreen and Kline, 2004).

Lymphedema is caused by dysfunction of the lymphatic system, where accumulation or pooling of lymph fluid into the interstitial space occurs. External forces such as surgery, radiation, or infection, which can damage the lymphatic system, most commonly cause the dysfunction. With an impaired lymphatic system, the amount of lymphatic fluid in the interstitial space becomes more than the body's lymph system can handle. Plasma oncotic pressure decreases, oncotic pressure of tissue fluid increases, and lymphatic

blockage or obstruction occurs (Sieggreen and Kline, 2004). With retention of fluid and large protein molecules within this interstitial space, the space swells (Lawenda et al, 2009). With swelling, the large protein molecules leak into the tissues, causing fibrosis. Over time, progressive obstruction to lymphatic flow occurs by distortion or obliteration of the lymphatic channels from the fibrotic changes in the tissues (Macdonald et al, 2003; Sarvis, 2003; Tiwari et al, 2003).

TYPES OF LYMPHEDEMA

Lymphedema may be *acute* or *chronic*. Acute lymphedema is a condition that lasts less than 6 months and is associated with pitting edema with pressure and lack of brawny skin changes. Risk factors for acute lymphedema include surgical drains with extravasation into the surgical site, acute injury to the limb, radiation therapy, infection, and phlebitis (Sieggreen and Kline, 2004). Chronic lymphedema, unlike acute lymphedema, is not reversible and requires lifetime management. Lymphedema may be classified as *primary* (idiopathic) or *secondary* (acquired) (Holcomb, 2006).

Primary (Idiopathic) Lymphedema

Primary lymphedema is caused by congenital absence or abnormalities of lymphatic tissue. It affects between 1 and 2 million individuals in the United States and usually involves the leg (Holcomb, 2006; Rossy, 2015). Primary lymphedema may be classified by time of onset: *congenital lymphedema* is detected at less than 1 year of age, *lymphedema praecox* is detected from ages 1 to 35 years, and *lymphedema tarda* is detected after age 35 (Holcomb, 2006; Kerchner et al, 2008). The congenital type may be sporadic or familial. The familial form is associated with Meige disease, Nonne-Milroy disease, Prader-Willi syndrome, or Turner syndrome for which lymphedema is a clinical manifestation (Tiwari et al, 2012). Congenital lymphedema affects both lower extremities, but can involve the upper extremities as well as the face. The most common type of primary lymphedema is lymphedema praecox (Meige disease). It usually affects adolescent women. Meige disease occurs when some lymphatics that are present at birth become damaged by infection or when the number of lymphatics is inadequate as the individual grows and matures. The condition usually is unilateral, involving the foot and calf. Lymphedema tarda is seen in individuals after age 35 who have congenitally weakened lymphatics so that a precipitating event such as injury can result in lymphedema (Kerchner et al, 2008).

Secondary (Acquired) Lymphedema

Secondary lymphedema affects between 2 and 3 million individuals in the United States (Holcomb, 2006). The most common cause of secondary lymphedema in the United States is related to malignancy and its subsequent treatment (postradiotherapy). The types of cancers associated with secondary lymphedema include breast cancer, gynecologic cancer, lymphoma, melanoma, and urologic cancers. Secondary lymphedema is

FIGURE 13-1 Anatomy of the lymphatic system. (From Monahan FD, Neighbors M: *Medical surgical nursing: foundations for clinical practice,* ed 2, Philadelphia, 1998, Saunders.)

caused by dysfunction or obstruction of the lymphatic system that usually occurs at proximal limb segments (i.e., lymph nodes) due to surgery, radiation, trauma, infection, malignancy, or scar tissue. Surgery may include the removal of one or more lymph nodes. If the remaining lymph nodes and vessels cannot compensate for those that have been removed, then lymphedema can result. The current use of sentinel node biopsy (e.g., with cancer surgery) has helped reduce the risk of patients developing lymphedema because fewer lymph nodes are removed. Radiation can cause scarring and inflammation of the lymph system, which can restrict the flow of lymph fluid, thus increasing the risk for lymphedema. Cancer can block the lymphatic vessels, which also increases the risk for lymphedema. In addition to cancer, chronic diseases such as congestive heart failure, liver disease, and end-stage renal disease can cause chronic edema.

Infection from parasites can infiltrate the lymph vessels and block the flow. The cause of the most common form of infection, called *filariasis,* is the nematode *Wuchereria bancrofti,* which is transmitted to humans by mosquitoes. When the filarial larvae mature into adult worms in the lymphatic channels, they block the lymph channels, causing severe lymphedema in the arms, legs, and genitalia, a condition also known as *elephantiasis*. It infects more than 90 million people globally; occurs mainly in southeast Asia, India, and Africa; and is the most common cause of lymphedema worldwide (Macdonald et al, 2003; Tiwari et al, 2003).

Once damage has occurred to the lymphatic system, transport capacity is permanently decreased, predisposing to lymphedema. The pelvic and inguinal nodes in the lower limbs and the axillary nodes of the upper limbs are the primary sites of obstruction (Sieggreen and Kline, 2004). Lymphedema has been reported 20 to 30 years after the precipitating event (e.g., surgery).

With the rise in obesity rates comes an increase in the number of cases of secondary lymphedema in the morbidly obese. In a review of wound clinic data of approximately 15,000 patients from 17 wound centers in the United States, Fife and Carter (2008) found 74% prevalence of secondary lymphedema in morbidly obese patients. Morbidly obese patients also have been observed to have lymphedema in conjunction with venous ulcer disease. Obesity impedes lymphatic flow, leading to accumulation of lymphatic fluid in the subcutaneous tissue (Kerchner et al, 2008). The risk for lymphedema increases as body mass index (BMI) increases (Dell and Doll, 2006). Sizable weight gain has been shown to increase a woman's risk for lymphedema following breast cancer (Warren et al, 2007a). With the increase of lymphatic fluid in the setting of decreased oxygen tensions, fibrosis with chronic inflammation and increased risk for infection result. In addition to occurring in the extremities, lymphedema can be seen in the overhanging abdominal pannus of the morbidly obese (Kerchner et al, 2008).

Green et al (2012) studied 15 patients with BMIs of greater than 30 with bilateral lower extremity enlargement. Twelve of the 15 were women, and the mean age was 57.9 years; the mean BMI was 51.4 (range, 30.7 to 88.1). None of the patients had a history of primary lymphedema, inguinal lymphadenectomy or radiation, or lower extremity ulcers. The BMI range of the five patients with lymphedema (59.7 to 88.1) was significantly greater than the range of the BMI of the 10 patients without lymphedema; 30.7 to 53.3 ($p < 0.001$). The authors concluded that as BMI increases, there might be a threshold above which lymphatic flow becomes impaired.

STAGES OF LYMPHEDEMA

The International Society of Lymphology recognizes four categories or classifications for staging (Table 13-1). Stage 0 is a subclinical lymphedema in which swelling is not evident despite impaired lymphatic function. Stage 0 (reversible) may exist for months or years before edema occurs. Stage I (reversible) is defined as lymph fluid with a high protein content (in contrast to venous ulcer disease edema) that dissipates after limb elevation. Pitting may occur. Pitting edema is considered present when, 5 seconds after a finger is pressed into the edematous tissue, an indentation remains. In Stage II (irreversible), pitting edema is present but limb elevation

TABLE 13-1	**Stages of Lymphedema**
Stage	**Manifestations**
0	Subclinical lymphedema with edema that is not evident despite impaired lymphatic function
	(Nonvisible, latency stage)
I	Reversible pitting edema that begins distally (at foot)
	Negative or borderline Stemmer sign
	No palpable fibrosis
	(Spontaneously reversible)
II	Minimally pitting or nonpitting (brawny) edema that is not reduced by conservative measures such as elevation
	Positive Stemmer sign
	Pronounced fibrosis
	Hyperkeratosis (thickening of skin)
	Papillomatosis (skin has rough cobblestone appearance and texture)
	(Spontaneously irreversible)
III	Lymphostatic elephantiasis (massive enlargement and distortion of limb caused by breakdown of skin's elastic components)
	Progressive fibrosis, acanthosis, hyperkeratosis, papillomatosis
	Ulceration
	(Spontaneously irreversible)

National Lymphedema Network: *NLN position paper: The diagnosis and treatment of lymphedema.* http://lymphnet.org/resources/nln-position-paper-the-diagnosis-and-treatment-of-lymphedema. Accessed May 31, 2014.

alone does not reduce edema. As Stage II progresses, tissue fibrosis develops, and pitting may or may not be present. Stage III (irreversible) is elephantiasis in which pitting is not present but skin changes in the limb, such as acanthosis (increase in thickness of the epidermis), fatty deposits, and warty growths, may be present. Within each stage, limb volume differences can be categorized as minimal ($<20\%$ increase in size), moderate (20% to 40% increase in size), and severe ($>40\%$ increase in size) (Holcomb, 2006; Macdonald et al, 2003).

LIPEDEMA

Lipedema, often confused with lymphedema, is a syndrome of bilateral adipose deposition that almost always is seen in the lower extremities of overweight/obese women. Excess fatty tissue will affect the lymphatic system by constricting the flow of lymph fluid. It can affect the upper extremities in 30% of cases (Wagner, 2011). In addition, there is a predisposition to orthostatic edema and to hematoma formation after the slightest trauma. Women with lipedema may also complain of increased sensitivity to touch.

Lipedema usually presents around puberty with a familial tendency of enlarged or fatty legs and buttocks (hips and thighs) with sparing of the feet. The leg enlargement is frequently misdiagnosed as lymphedema even when no lymphatic malfunction is present. However, lipedema can eventually result in secondary lymphatic dysfunction leading to lipolymphedema (Fife et al, 2010). Features distinguishing lymphedema from lipedema are listed in Table 13-2 (Fife et al, 2010; Fonder et al, 2007; Warren et al, 2007b). Table 10-1 compares characteristics of venous edema to lipedema and lymphedema.

The diagnosis of lipedema usually is based on history and physical examination. Diagnostic tests, such as those done with lymphedema, may be conducted and usually only show subcutaneous fat hypertrophy. Treatment options for lipedema are mainly dietary and lifestyle modifications. However, despite attempts at losing weight resulting in loss of upper body fat, the size of the legs does not decrease (Fife et al, 2010).

The best treatment options include gentle compression garments to manage the orthostatic component of edema, rigorous weight control, and exercise. There is limited benefit from aggressive compression bandaging and manual lymphatic drainage unless lymphedema has developed. Liposuction can remove fatty deposits, particularly on the upper leg, but some techniques may damage lymphatics (Fife et al, 2010).

Clinical research is also assessing the role of liposuction in treating lipedema patients. Schmeller and Meier-Vollrath (2006) treated 28 female patients with liposuction. Twenty-one patients were reevaluated after an average of 12 months. All patients showed an improvement in body proportions. Eighteen patients suffered from pain before the procedure; 10 patients had improvement in pain levels after liposuction. All patients complained of sensitivity to pressure. After the liposuction, this symptom disappeared in 8 patients and improved in 13 patients. Generally lipedema responds poorly to compression therapy and leg elevation, although low-level compression therapy usually is recommended to prevent the disease from progressing to lipolymphedema, which is a combination of lipedema and lymphedema (Fonder et al, 2007; Kerchner et al, 2008; Schmeller and Meier-Vollrath, 2006).

DIAGNOSTIC TESTS

Diagnosis of lymphedema typically is made through clinical presentation and history. Diagnostic confirmation can be made with isotopic lymphoscintigraphy, in which a radionuclide is injected into the lymphatic tissue between the first and second digits of the affected limb to identify abnormalities of the lymphatic pathways, including enlarged vessels and backflow problems due to obstruction. Lymphoscintigraphy is considered the gold standard for imaging studies for lymphedema (Holcomb, 2006; Kerchner et al, 2008; Lohrmann et al, 2006; Warren et al, 2007a). However, lymphoscintigraphy is expensive and invasive. Because radioactive dye must be injected into an already compromised limb, lymphoscintigraphy generally is indicated only if the patient is a surgical candidate and a definitive diagnosis is needed. Computed tomography scans or magnetic resonance imaging (MRI) can be performed to evaluate for the presence of lymphedema and to show lymph trunk anatomy and causes of obstructive secondary lymphedema. Magnetic resonance imaging can detect a honeycomb pattern of the subcutaneous tissue from fibrosis and lymph fluid, a finding that is not seen with other forms of edema, so it can be helpful for diagnosis (Kerchner et al, 2008; Warren et al, 2007a). Lymph fluid analysis with protein content between 1 and 5.5 g/dl usually indicates lymphedema (Holcomb, 2006). Other laboratory studies, such as serum albumin and urinalysis, should be performed to rule out other causes of edema, such as renal or hepatic impairment. Edema can be classified by its protein content. Low-protein edema is composed of less than 1 g of protein per 100 ml of fluid; high-protein edema is composed of greater than 1 g of protein per 100 ml of fluid (Lawenda et al, 2009). Lymphedema is a high-protein edema. Ultrasound can provide an analysis of soft tissue changes but does not provide any information about the lymphatics. Duplex Doppler studies may be required if venous ulcer disease is also suspected. Genetic testing may be recommended for patients with primary lymphedema.

TABLE 13-2	Comparison of Lymphedema and Lipedema	
	Lymphedema	**Lipedema**
Gender	Male and female	Female
Age	Any age	After or during puberty (10 to 30 years of age)
Edema	Pitting progresses to firm fibrotic	Nonpitting
Epidermal skin changes	Common	Uncommon
Cellulitis	Common	Uncommon
Stemmer sign	Positive	Negative, but positive fat pad sign at ankle (fatty tissue just anterior to lateral malleolus and between Achilles tendon and medial malleolus)
Distribution	Unilateral or bilateral, toes to groin	Always bilateral legs, ends at ankles. Feet usually spared, sometimes arms affected with hands spared
Tenderness	None usually	Tender to palpation. Aching sensation. Bruising common
Magnetic resonance imaging	Honeycomb pattern	Normal

Bioimpedance spectroscopy (BIS) is a procedure in which an electrical current is passed through the limb and impedance flow is measured. This technique, also known as *bioelectrical impedance analysis,* measures the composition of tissues, especially the presence of fluids such as lymph. Reduced impedance values are indicative of lymphedema. In lymphedema management, BIS can be used for early detection and ongoing measurements of fluid buildup in the affected limb to determine the effectiveness of therapy. Warren et al (2007c) studied 15 patients with either upper or lower limb lymphedema who underwent BIS analysis. Participants underwent BIS of both limbs so that they could serve as their own control. The average ratio of impedance to current flow of the affected extremity to the unaffected extremity was 0.9. The authors concluded that BIS can be used as a tool for documenting the presence of lymphedema in patients and may be useful in long-term monitoring of patients (Warren et al, 2007a).

ASSESSMENT

Assessment of the patient with limb enlargement should begin with a history of risk factors for lymphedema, such as surgeries (especially nodal dissections), radiation therapy, trauma, infection, malignancy, obesity, familial history, and travel to areas with endemic filariasis. To determine whether lymphedema is the cause of swelling, knowing the onset of limb enlargement and associated symptoms is important. Symptoms of lymphedema include feelings of heaviness, aching, and fatigue in the affected limb. A history of recurrent infections (e.g., cellulitis) is an important clue to lymphedema. Individuals may report less flexibility in the extremities and difficulty fitting into clothing, hardening of the skin, and paresthesias (Neese, 2000). Brown et al (2013) surveyed long-term cancer survivors and found that 34.5% (37 of 107) reported one or more symptoms of lower leg lymphedema. Symptoms these patients reported included difficulty walking (100%), aching (86%), puffiness (76%), and pain (73%).

Knowing if the patient has a history of comorbid conditions that can cause swelling of the extremities, such as cardiac disease, venous ulcer disease, renal disease, hepatic disease, trauma, and infection, also is important. Patients with rheumatoid arthritis, obesity, lipedema, and venous ulcer disease are at greater risk for lymphedema because these conditions further stress the already impaired lymphatics. Lymph nodes are located around most joints, so patients undergoing surgical procedures such as total knee replacements may be at greater risk for developing lymphedema because these nodes may become damaged during the surgery. Some relatively minor conditions, such as vein stripping, can exacerbate mild lymphedema (Tiwari et al, 2003). Yellow nail syndrome is an uncommon disorder that may be seen with lymphedema. The pathophysiology of the syndrome remains unclear, but lymphatic abnormalities, as well as chronic pulmonary disease and genetic predisposition, may play a role (Maldonada et al, 2009).

Physical Assessment

Physical assessment parameters for lymphedema include skin texture (soft vs. hard), papillomatosis (cobblestone skin appearance), skin color (erythema, unusually dark), lymphangiomas (blisters containing lymph fluid), presence of skin fissures, presence of skin folds, presence of pedal pulses, edema, range of motion of the limb, neurologic deficits, and signs of venous ulcer disease. Mushroomlike papules may be present. In normal persons, leg circumference varies as the leg is measured from ankle to knee. However, in lymphedema patients, the circumference from ankle to knee is almost the same. The Stemmer sign (or Kaposi-Stemmer sign) is another clinical indication of lymphedema. In this test, the examiner is unable to pinch a fold of skin at the base of the second toe on the dorsal aspect of the foot or between the second and third finger. Skin that does not fold up into a pinch is considered a positive sign of lymphedema (Kerchner et al, 2008; Sarvis, 2003).

Physical examination and history usually are sufficient to make a diagnosis of lymphedema. Lymphedema is evaluated by visual inspection and palpation. Initially there will be soft, painless pitting edema, but over time fibrosis, nonpitting edema, and induration may be present in the affected limb. The characteristic lymphatic swelling in the lower extremity is edema from the ankle up toward the knee. Occasionally swelling includes the feet. Depending on the extent of the disease, the edema may extend into the groin. The skin has a roughened leathery appearance resembling an elephant's skin. Because of this appearance, the name *elephantiasis* was coined for the lymphedema caused by the filarial infection. The skin over the lymphedema does not usually have the darkened brown pigment skin changes seen with venous ulcer disease unless the patient has venous ulcer disease. Patients with lymphedema and venous ulcer disease may have a leathery appearance of the skin with dark-brown hemosiderin-pigmented skin changes.

Measuring Limb Size. Two methods for measuring the size of the limb affected by lymphedema are girth and volume. Girth measurements should include 3 cm above the lateral malleolus, 12 cm above the lateral malleolus, and 18 cm above the lateral malleolus. Using a flexible tape to measure circumference around these areas, the clinician should then compare those measurements with the contralateral limb (Fowler and Carson, 2007) and measurements for each assessment recorded. The clinician should measure the limb in the same position each time and try to measure the limb at the same time of day because girth may increase during the day because of swelling. An increase in limb size by 1.5 cm or more is suspicious for lymphedema (Dell and Doll, 2006). Other methods of measurement, such as water displacement of the limb, can be used to determine limb volume. For this method, a container is filled with tepid water and the limb is immersed in the water. The amount of overflow is measured to determine the volume of fluid displaced. Both limbs are assessed and results are compared. A volume difference of

20% or more is considered significant. Even though this method may be more precise than tape measurements and is often considered the gold standard for measuring girth, it is not user friendly for the clinician (Dell and Doll, 2006). To clinically define the presence of lymphedema, Spillane et al (2008) assessed 66 patients who had undergone inguinal or ilioinguinal lymph node dissection for metastatic melanoma. They found that a change in limb volume of 15% or more and an increase of 7% or more in the sum of limb circumferences of the defined points on the limb provided a more standardized definition of lymphedema in those patients (Spillane et al, 2008).

PREVENTION

Prevention of lymphedema in high-risk individuals, especially those undergoing surgery and radiation for cancer, is paramount. The importance of skin integrity in preventing injury and infection cannot be overemphasized (Box 13-1).

Skin Care

Skin care is important in the prevention of infection, dermatitis, and hyperkeratosis. Lanolin or fragrances can

---

BOX 13-1 Teaching Points for the Patient with Lymphedema

- Apply moisturizer to affected limbs daily to prevent dry/cracking skin.
- Protect exposed skin with sunscreen and insect repellent.
- Use care with razors by not shaving on dry skin or areas with skin folds
- Avoid, if possible, blood draws and injections in affected limb.
- Provide good nail care and do not cut cuticles.
- If scratches in the skin occur, wash with soap and water, apply topical antibiotics, and monitor for signs of infection/cellulitis.
- Maintain ideal body weight since obesity is a known risk factor.
- Avoid prolonged (greater than 15 minutes) exposure to heat, such as saunas or hot tubs.
- Avoid exposure to extreme cold, which can cause chaffing and rebound swelling.
- Avoid prolonged standing, sitting, or crossing legs
- Wear gloves when doing activities that may cause skin injury, for example, washing dishes, cleaning, using tools, and gardening.
- Protect lymphedema extremity and foot from all types of trauma.
- Avoid heavy lifting with affected limb (arm); do not carry handbag or other bags on shoulder of affected side.
- Do not restrict fluid or protein intake in attempt to prevent fluid buildup.
- Exercise in moderation wearing compression garment in place.
- Carry lymphedema alert card and wear lymphedema alert bracelet or necklace.

---

cause sensitization in this population and so should be avoided. However, routine use of fragrance-free, lanolin-free emollients to prevent cracking and promote suppleness of the skin is encouraged. Any break in the skin can be an entry site for bacteria, and the protein-rich lymphedema fluid is a great medium for bacterial proliferation. Foot care with daily cleansing and drying of the toe web spaces will help to prevent fungal infections of the edematous feet. A common symptom of lymphedema is pruritus. Scratching from pruritus can cause breaks in the skin, which contribute to infection and cellulitis. Pruritus is thought to be caused by factors in the lymphedematous skin that lower the threshold for degranulation of dermal mast cells. With the degranulation of mast cells comes a subsequent release of histamine, which potentiates the itch. McCord and Fore (2007) evaluated nine patients with mild to severe pruritus associated with lymphedema over a 6-month period who were treated with olivamine-based products. The average pruritus evaluation score before treatment with the products was 2, which corresponds to mild to moderate pruritus; after treatment the average score was 0.11, which corresponds to absent pruritus. Additional research is needed to determine which products work best for the management of pruritus associated with lymphedema (McCord and Fore, 2007).

Protect from Injury

Protecting the limb from injury is important to prevent infection. For example, using an electric razor and wearing gloves when gardening or washing dishes are advisable. Many of the interventions for protection are based on common sense to prevent injury to an already compromised limb. Greene et al (2005) suggests that avoidance of blood pressure measurements and venipuncture in patients at risk for lymphedema does not appear to be evidence based. According to Greene et al, the treatment of lymphedema is compression therapy, including compression pumps, so pumping the cuff for blood pressure readings should not cause injury. They report no cases of cellulitis from venipuncture. In addition, no cases of cellulitis resulting from the use of lymphoscintigraphy (i.e., injection of dye into the compromised limb) in the diagnosis of lymphedema have been reported in the literature (Greene et al, 2005). As we continue to search for evidence that determines best practice, additional common-sense approaches may be challenged.

Promote Lymphatic Flow

Placing limbs in gravity-dependent positions for long periods promotes swelling and should be avoided. The patient should avoid constricting garments, weight gain, heavy lifting, extreme heat (e.g., from heating pad or sauna), and rapid altitude changes seen with flying for 2 hours. Exercises that do not make the patient feel fatigued can increase movement of lymph fluid out of the limb and decrease the risk for lymphedema. Wrapping the limb with bandages can promote lymphatic flow and drainage.

MANAGEMENT

Chronic lymphedema has no known cure. Positive clinical outcomes depend on prompt recognition of lymphedema and initiation of treatment to interrupt the cycle of fluid retention, lymphatic obstruction, and soft tissue fibrosis. Effective management of the patient with lymphedema requires a comprehensive lifelong program of exercise, massage, skin care, and compression garments and is most effectively carried out in a lymphedema center. Patients and care providers need to understand that conservative therapies are aimed at reducing symptoms and will not cure the underlying lymphatic dysfunction.

Ridner et al (2012) conducted a systematic review from 2004 to 2011 on the benefit of specific interventions on lymphedema self-management. The studies on total body exercise, such as aerobics, showed that it may help to stabilize limb volume and may reduce exacerbations in those with lymphedema. Based on expert opinion, complete decongestive physiotherapy (CDT) benefits lymphedema patients. Compression garments and pneumatic compression devices did not have enough evidence to determine whether they would be effective as stand-alone therapy. Aromatherapy was found to be likely ineffective. However, few studies on lymphedema included clinical outcomes, and there were very few randomized controlled trials.

The goals of lymphedema management include (1) moving the "trapped" lymph from the interstitial space, (2) eliminating edema, (3) restoring normal limb contours, (4) maintaining the "restored" limb state, and (5) preventing infection. The components of treatment are highlighted in Table 13-3, with key points discussed by Macdonald et al (2003), Sarvis (2003), and Tiwari et al (2003).

Complete Decongestive Physiotherapy

Complete decongestive physiotherapy is the gold standard for management of moderate to severe lymphedema. Patients should be referred to a lymphedema therapist, who might be an occupational therapist, physical therapist, or nurse practitioner who is specially trained in CDP.

Complete decongestive physiotherapy is a specialized massage technique designed to stimulate the lymph vessels, break up subcutaneous fibrous tissue, and redirect lymph fluid to areas where lymph flow is normal. The therapy involves four steps: manual lymph drainage, compression bandaging, exercises, and skin/nail care. Complete decongestive physiotherapy is administered in two phases. In the initial reductive (restorative) phase, manual lymph drainage involves daily to weekly sessions (3 to 8 weeks). The lymphedema therapist uses specialized massage techniques to (1) activate the lymphatic channels proximal to the affected limb, (2) mobilize lymph in the proximal tissues, and (3) mobilize lymph in the distal

TABLE 13-3 Lymphedema: Treatment Components

Intervention	Desired Effect	Action	Cautions
Complex decongestive physiotherapy Therapeutic massage Compression bandages applied immediately after treatment	Mobilization of retained lymph	Mobilize lymphatic fluid in channels adjacent and proximal to involved site	Performed only by therapist trained in the technique Usually requires treatments daily for 1 to 3 weeks
Sequential compression therapy	Mobilization of retained lymph	Dynamic compression pumps with limb sleeves compress lymphatic fluid and mobilize lymph	Risk of displacing fluid to proximal leg or genitalia Risk of further damage to lymphatics
Limb elevation	Edema reduction	Counter effect of gravity on lymph flow	Effective only in early phase of disease
Compression bandaging	Critical component of maintenance therapy Nonelastic or short-stretch bandages and custom-fitted sleeves or stockings most effective	Apply pressure to tissues to facilitate compression of lymph channels and movement of lymph from interstitial space into circulation	Should provide 40 to 60 mm Hg subbandage pressure Replace regularly to prevent loss of therapeutic effectiveness
Exercise (light movement exercise with compression bandage or garment in place)	Maintenance of lymph reduction	Stimulate intact lymphatics to increase rate of lymph transport	Should not be strenuous or cause fatigue
Skin and nail care (avoid trauma, apply moisturizer, regular nail care)	Infection control during restorative and maintenance phases	Keep skin supple and prevent breaks in skin to reduce risk of infection	Recommend having standing prescription for antibiotic should signs of infection appear Do not cut cuticles

tissues. Manual lymph drainage is accompanied by range-of-motion exercises, short-stretch compression bandages (worn between treatments), and meticulous skin/nail care to prevent skin infections. When the extremity has been reduced in size, a compression garment is ordered and the ongoing maintenance phase begins, which includes self-lymph drainage, exercise, skin care, and compression garments.

Compression wraps and stockings are an important component of therapy for all patients with lymphedema to prevent the reaccumulation of lymph fluid in the limb. Compression garments must be worn between manual lymph drainage treatment sessions during the reductive phase and throughout the day and night thereafter. During the first phase of manual lymph drainage, short-stretch bandages are used in multilayers. These bandages may be difficult to apply for some patients with physical impairments. There are also wraps with nonelastic Velcro straps that can be put on and taken off very easily. These products are especially beneficial for patients who cannot easily bend or have the strength to pull on elastic compression stockings (see Figure 12-6).

Intermittent pneumatic compression pumps (see Figure 12-7) are another method for decreasing the volume of the affected limb. The pump, which can be used in the home, consists of a sleeve with several compartments that are serially inflated to push the fluid out of the extremity from the distal to the proximal portion. After the daily or twice-daily treatments, which last for several hours, the patient should continue with compression through either a garment or bandaging. Reassessment determines frequency and duration of treatments. For example, if the treatments are not effective after 4 weeks of therapy, they should be discontinued.

Pneumatic compression devices are covered in the home setting for the treatment of lymphedema if the patient has undergone a 4-week trial of conservative therapy and the treating practitioner determines that there has been no significant improvement or if significant symptoms remain after the trial. The trial of conservative therapy must include use of an appropriate compression bandage system or compression garment, exercise, and elevation of the limb. The garment may be prefabricated or custom fabricated, but must provide adequate graduated compression (National Government Services, 2011).

Badger et al (2004) examined randomized controlled clinical trials that tested physical therapy modalities with a follow-up of at least 6 months. Only three studies with a total of 150 patients were included. Because none of the studies examined the same intervention, combining the data was not possible. One crossover study of manual lymph drainage followed by self-administered massage versus no treatment concluded that improvements seen in both groups were attributed to compression sleeves and that manual lymph drainage provided no extra benefit. Another trial of hosiery versus no treatment had a high dropout rate, with only 3 of 14 in the treatment group and 1 of 11 in the control group finishing the trial. Clearly more well-controlled clinical trials on the physical therapy modalities used to treat lymphedema are needed.

Lasinski et al (2012) reviewed the research literature from 2004 to 2011 that pertains to the individual components of manual lymph drainage and compression bandaging, as well as CDT. Ninety-nine articles related to lymphedema treatment were reviewed, but only 26 studies met inclusion criteria. Complete decongestive physiotherapy was found to be effective in reducing lymphedema, but the majority of the studies focused on CDT as a bundled intervention that included the two individual components, manual lymph draining and compression bandaging. Additional studies are needed to determine the value and efficacy of the individual components of CDT.

Adjunctive Therapy

Selenium therapy for lymphedema is currently being studied. The hypothesis is that lymphedema is caused by excessive generation of oxygen free radicals and that selenium, an antioxidant, consumes oxygen radicals, which might decrease the damage to the lymph system (Holcomb, 2006). The use of hyperbaric oxygen is also being studied. Hyperbaric oxygen may stimulate growth of new lymphatic channels in breast cancer patients (Holcomb, 2006). The role of thermal therapy and pulsed radiofrequency energy in the treatment of lymphedema remains unclear (Holcomb, 2006).

Kinesio taping is a type of compression therapy that is being tested in trials of lymphedema patients. Kinesio tape is a thin elastic tape invented by Kenzo Kase in 1996. The tape can be stretched up to 140% of its original length, making it very elastic (Fu et al, 2008). The wrapping technique with the Kinesio tape is thought to reduce swelling by improving blood and lymphatic fluid flow and is beginning to be used with lymphedema patients. However, research regarding its effectiveness in lymphedema patients currently is lacking (Fu et al, 2008; Morris et al, 2013).

Barclay et al (2006) described a randomized trial determining the effect of self-massage and skin care using a cream with aromatherapy oils versus a cream without aromatherapy oils on limb volume measurements and symptom relief in 81 people with lymphedema. Results showed that self-massage and skin care significantly improved patient-identified symptom relief and well-being but did not significantly reduce limb volume. Aromatherapy oils did not appear to improve limb volume measurements (Barclay et al, 2006).

Surgery

Surgical treatment of lymphedema has been increasingly utilized. Surgeries, such as excisions, lymphaticovenous anastomosis (LVA), vascularized lymph nodes transfers (VLNT), and lymphatic liposuction, may provide options to treat patients with different lymphedema symptoms and levels of severity. Appropriate surgery can help reduce the size of an affected arm or leg, decrease the need for compression garments, and greatly reduce the occurrences of infections or cellulitis.

Debulking or excisional surgical techniques involve the removal of lymphedematous adipose tissue down to the fascia, followed by skin grafting or skin flaps (Cormier et al, 2012). Resection or debulking procedures remove redundant skin folds and subcutaneous tissue to reduce the size and weight of the limb, resulting in good clinical outcomes with minimal complications (Kerchner et al, 2008; Tiwari et al, 2012). Salgado (2007) reports a 21% volume reduction in the upper extremity at 1 year postoperatively. Complications that have been reported include hematoma formation, skin/flap necrosis, infection, scarring, destruction of remaining lymphatic vessels, loss of limb function, and recurrence of the lymphedema (Cormier et al, 2012).

Microsurgical procedures for lymphatic reconstruction have included anastomosis between lymphatic channels and veins, between lymph nodes and veins, and between distal and proximal lymphatics. Lymphaticovenous anastomoses connect lymphatic channels to subdermal venules of less than 0.8 mm in diameter. It is believed that the subdermal lymphatics are less affected by lymphedema and the small venular pressure is low, decreasing the risk of backflow. The LVA procedures require less time than the debulking procedures since they require minimal dissections and can be performed under local anesthesia, shortening hospitalization times (Cormier et al, 2012; Tiwari et al, 2012). Lympholymphatic anastomosis and lymphatic grafting involve removing normal lymph nodes from an unaffected limb and transplanting them into the lymphedematous area, with end-to-end anastomosis between the transplanted lymph tissue and the lymphedematous lymph node tissue.

Suction-assisted lipectomy, which is the removal of subcutaneous fatty tissue through circumferential liposuction of the affected limb, is less invasive and has been proven effective for volume reduction and increasing blood flow to the limb, decreasing the risk of cellulitis. The most common side effect of the liposuction is transient numbness (Tiwari et al, 2012). Patients undergoing all of these procedures are placed immediately postoperatively in compression garments (Warren et al, 2007a).

Cormier et al (2012) conducted a systematic review of surgical treatment of lymphedema. A total of 20 studies looked at three surgical procedures: excisional procedures (n = 8), lymphatic reconstruction (n = 8), and tissue transfer (n = 4). Most of the studies had small sample sizes with complications rarely reported and so they concluded that any surgical approach should be individualized.

Salgado et al (2007) reviewed 15 patients with lymphedema who had not responded to conventional therapy and were treated by surgical reduction of lymphedema tissue with preservation of perforating skin vessels from posterior tibial and peroneal arteries. This procedure allowed for reduction of lymphedema tissue in a single procedure while preserving blood supply to the skin. In these 15 patients, the average lymphedema reduction was 52%. At follow-up of 13 months, no cases of skin flap necrosis or incisional wound breakdown

were seen. Three patients had cellulitis, and one patient had a seroma and hematoma (Salgado et al, 2007).

Campisi and Boccardo (2004) reviewed 676 patients with lymphedema treated with microsurgical LVAs. They found that of the 447 patients who were available for follow-up, 380 (85%) had been able to discontinue conservative methods for managing the disease, with an average reduction in limb volume of 69%. An 87% reduction in cellulitis after the microsurgery also was noted (Campisi and Boccardo, 2004). Koshima et al (2004) studied the effectiveness of LVAs for lower leg lymphedema in patients under local anesthesia and reported that 17 patients had a greater than 4-cm reduction in leg circumference.

Pharmacology

Medications that are used to treat lymphedema include retinoidlike agents (e.g., acitretin, topical tazarotene), anthelmintic agents (e.g., albendazole), topical skin products (e.g., ammonium lactate lotion, topical urea), and antibiotics (e.g., cefazolin, clindamycin, penicillin) (Rossy, 2013). Diuretics are not beneficial for lymphedema because they may promote volume depletion. Diuretics draw off excess water, but not protein, from the interstitial spaces. As soon as the diuretic is stopped, the concentrated proteins pull more water back into the interstitial space, increasing the edema (Holcomb, 2006). Diuretics act to remove water from the cells. Lymphedema is a high-protein edema, and the high osmotic pressure from the increased protein in the interstitial space causes rapid reaccumulation of edema. In addition, the higher concentration of protein in the edema fluid causes increased fibrosis and induration of the skin. Diuretics are not contraindicated for treatment of other conditions in lymphedema patients, but they should not be used as primary treatment of lymphedema (Neese, 2000).

Benzopyrones (e.g., coumarin) are thought to hydrolyze tissue proteins and facilitate absorption while stimulating lymphatic collectors. Treatment with benzopyrones is thought to decrease fluid formation in the subcutaneous tissues and to reduce pain and discomfort of the affected area. However, in a systematic review published in the *Cochrane Library,* Badger et al (2009) found that there was not enough good-quality evidence to draw conclusions about whether benzopyrones are useful either in reducing lymphedema or the pain and discomfort associated with it.

COMPLICATIONS

Common skin complications seen with lymphedema include lymphangitis and cellulitis. Lymphangitis has a distinctive erythematous linear pattern (red streak) that travels along the lymphatics. Fever, chills, headache, muscle aches, and loss of appetite are common presenting symptoms. Lymphangitis often results from a streptococcal or staphylococcal infection of the skin, which causes the lymph vessels to become swollen and tender. Antibiotics, analgesics, and antiinflammatory drugs may be prescribed and elevation of the extremity recommended.

Cellulitis involves the subcutaneous tissue. It usually has an indistinct border and is characterized by pain, warmth, and edema, with red appearance of the skin. Fever, chills, headache, muscle aches, and fatigue may be presenting symptoms. Cellulitis occurs in approximately 50% of patients with lymphedema and usually occurs when a crack or fissure in the skin serves as the portal entry for bacteria. The most common pathogen is β-hemolytic streptococcus. According to Badger et al (2004), penicillin V is the antibiotic of choice because streptococcus is believed to be the most common infecting organism. Antibiotics should be used at the first sign of cellulitis. Penicillin 250 mg orally four times per day for 7 to 10 days usually is effective. Patients who are prone to cellulitis should have medication on hand at home (Badger et al, 2004; Neese, 2000).

Macdonald et al (2003) reported that compression bandaging is indicated for treatment of cellulitis. However, other sources do not recommend compression bandaging until the patient is afebrile and erythema is resolving (Feldman, 2005). Fungal infections with itching and burning between the toes increase the risk for cellulitis in the lower extremity (Feldman, 2005). Meticulous skin care, including washing with soap and water and applying emollients to dry skin areas, decreases the risk of cellulitis.

CLINICAL CONSULT

A: Referral from primary provider for wound management recommendations. 55-year-old Caucasian male with leg edema, morbid obesity, type 2 diabetes (HbA1c pending), and coronary artery disease. Unemployed; spends most of his day at home computer with legs dependent. Complains of heavy achy legs. Right posterior calf wound 14 cm × 3 cm × 0.25 cm originated from bumping a chair one year ago. Wound base red with large amounts of serosanguineous exudate. No local signs of infection. Legs have leathery appearance with hemosiderin-pigmented skin changes and multiple mushroom papules. Edema non-pitting. Leg circumference measurements almost the same from ankle to knee (see flow sheet). Stemmer sign positive. Primary provider has also consulted a dietician and endocrinologist.

D: History, edema pattern, and positive Stemmer sign indicative of venous insufficiency and lymphedema.
P: Promote lymphatic flow, protect legs from additional injury, weight loss, and local wound care to promote healing and prevent infection.
I: (1) Referral to lymphedema clinic. (2) Educate on skin injury prevention strategies. Discuss the need for life style modifications such as weight loss, exercise, and diabetes management. (3) Calcium alginate followed by foam dressing changes every other day to manage moisture.
E: Wife demonstrates ability to change dressing and able to verbalize signs of infection. Patient states he is motivated to improve his health but is overwhelmed by all of the new information. No plans to return to wound clinic as lymphedema clinic will also help manage local wound care.

SUMMARY

Lymphedema is a chronic disease. Treatment focuses on managing the symptoms, mainly the high-protein edema and its effects on the limb. Lymphedema management crosses all care settings. The numbers of lymphedema patients, especially among the obese and the elderly, are increasing. Management of the disease relies on patients and caregivers assuming lymphedema care practices in the home setting. Most care providers are not familiar with the specialized care required for lymphedema patients, and local resources may be unavailable (Box 13-2). Health care providers need to become more knowledgeable about lymphedema practices because many lymphedema patients have comorbid conditions that necessitate their admission to acute and long-term care.

BOX 13-2 Lymphedema Resources

Circle of Hope Lymphedema Foundation	http://www.lymphedemacircleofhope.org
Lymphology Association of North America	http://www.clt-lana.org
Lymphedema Awareness Foundation	http://www.eLymphNotes.org
Lymphatic Research Foundation	http://www.lymphaticresearch.org
Lymphedema Resources, Inc.	http://www.lymphedemaresources.org/
Lymphedema Treatment Act	http://lymphedematreatmentact.org/
National Lymphedema Network	http://lymphnet.org/resources
Lymphedema Treatment Act	http://lymphedematreatmentact.org/

REFERENCES

Badger C, Preston N, Seers K, et al: Physical therapies for reducing and controlling lymphoedema of the limbs, *Cochrane Database Syst Rev* 1:CD003141, 2009.

Barclay J, Vestey J, Lambert A, et al: Reducing the symptoms of lymphoedema: is there a role for aromatherapy? *Eur J Oncol Nurs* 10(2):140–149, 2006.

Brown JC, Chu CS, Cheville AL, et al: The prevalence of lymphedema symptoms among survivors of long-term cancer with or at risk for lower leg lymphedema, *Am J Phys Med Rehabil* 92:223–231, 2013.

Campisi C, Boccardo F: Microsurgical techniques for lymphedema treatment: lymphatic-venous microsurgery, *World J Surg* 28(6):609–613, 2004.

Cheville AL: Current and future trends in lymphedema management: implications for women's health, *Phys Med Rehabil Clin North Am* 18(3):539–553, 2007.

Cormier JN, Rourke L, Crosby M, et al: The surgical treatment of lymphedema: a systematic review of the contemporary literature (2004-2010), *Ann Surg Oncol* 19(20):624–651, 2012.

Dell DD, Doll C: Caring for a patient with lymphedema, *Nursing* 36(6):49–51, 2006.

Feldman JL: The challenge of infection in lymphedema, *Lymph Link Article* 17(4):1, 2005.

Fife CE, Carter MJ: Lymphedema in the morbidly obese patient: unique challenges in a unique population, *Ostomy Wound Manage* 54(1):44–56, 2008.

Fife CE, Maus EA, Carter MJ: Lipedema: a frequently misdiagnosed and misunderstood fatty deposition syndrome, *Adv Skin Wound Care* 23(2):81–92, 2010.

Fonder MA, Loveless JW, Lazarus GS: Lipedema, a frequently unrecognized problem, *J Am Acad Dermatol* 57(2):51–53, 2007.

Fowler E, Carson S: Management of edema. In Sussman C, Bates-Jensen B, editors: *Wound care: a collaborative practice manual for health professionals*, Baltimore, 2007, Lippincott Williams & Wilkins.

Fu TC, Wong AM, Pei YC, et al: Effect of Kinesio taping on muscle strength in athletes—a pilot study, *J Sci Med Sport* 11(2):198–201, 2008.

Greene AK, Borud L, Slavin SA: Blood pressure monitoring and venipuncture in the lymphedematous extremity, *Plast Reconstr Surg* 116(7):2058–2059, 2005.

Greene AK, Grant FD, Slavin SA: Lower-extremity lymphedema and elevated body-mass index, *N Engl J Med* 366:2136–2137, 2012.

Holcomb SS: Identification and treatment of different types of lymphedema, *Adv Skin Wound Care* 19(2):103–108, 2006.

Kerchner K, Fleischer A, Yosipovitch G: Lower extremity lymphedema update: pathophysiology, diagnosis, and treatment guidelines, *J Am Acad Dermatol* 59(2):324–331, 2008.

Koshima I, Nanba Y, Tsutsui T, et al: Minimal invasive lymphaticovenular anastomosis under local anesthesia for leg lymphedema: is it effective for Stage III or IV? *Ann Plast Surg* 53(3):261–266, 2004.

Lasinski BB, Thrift KM, Squire D, et al: A systematic review of the evidence for complete decongestive therapy in the treatment of lymphedema from 2004 to 2011, *PM R* 4(8):580–601, 2012.

Lawenda BD, Mondry TE, Johnstone PA: Lymphedema: a primer on the identification and management of a chronic condition in oncologic treatment, *CA Cancer J Clin* 59(1):8–24, 2009.

Lohrmann C, Kautz O, Speck O, et al: Chronic lymphedema: detected with high-resolution magnetic resonance lymphangiography, *J Comput Assist Tomogr* 30(4):688, 2006.

Macdonald JM, Sims N, Mayrovitz HN, et al: Lymphedema, lipedema, and the open wound the role of compression therapy, *Surg Clin North Am* 83(3):639–658, 2003.

Maldonada F, Tazelaar HD, Wang CW, et al: Yellow nail syndrome: analysis of 41 consecutive patients, *Chest* 134(2):375–381, 2008.

National Government Services: *LCD for pneumatic compression devices (L27028)*, 2011. http://apps.ngsmedicare.com/applications/Content.aspx?DOCID=37&CatID=3&RegID=51&ContentID=34350. Accessed June 5, 2014.

McCord D, Fore J: Using olivamine-containing products to reduce pruritic symptoms associated with localized lymphedema, *Adv Skin Wound Care* 20(8):441–442, 444, 2007.

Monahan FD, Neighbors M: *Medical surgical nursing: foundations for clinical practice*, ed 2, Philadelphia, 1998, Saunders.

Morris D, Jones D, Ryan H, et al: The clinical effects of Kinesio® Tex taping: a systematic review, *Physiother Theory Pract* 29(4):259–270, 2013.

Neese PY: Management of lymphedema, *Lippincotts Prim Care Pract* 4(4):390–399, 2000.

National Lymphedema Network: *NLN position paper: The diagnosis and treatment of lymphedema*, 2011. http://lymphnet.org/resources/nln-position-paper-the-diagnosis-and-treatment-of-lymphedema. Accessed May 31, 2014.

Ridner SH, Fu MR, Wanchai A, et al: Self-management of lymphedema: a systematic review of the literature from 2004-2011, *Nurs Res* 61(4):291–299, 2012.

Rossy KM: *Lymphedema*, 2015. http://emedicine.medscape.com/article/1087313-overview. Accessed April 10, 2015.

Salgado CJ, Mardini S, Spanio S, et al: Radical reduction of lymphedema with preservation of perforators, *Ann Plast Surg* 59(2):173–179, 2007.

Sarvis C: When lymphedema takes hold, *RN* 66(9):32–36, 2003.

Schmeller W, Meier-Vollrath I: Tumescent liposuction: a new and successful therapy for lipedema, *J Cutan Med Surg* 10(1):7–10, 2006.

Sieggreen MY, Kline RA: Current concepts in lymphedema management, *Adv Skin Wound Care* 17(4):174–178, 2004.

Spillane AJ, Saw RP, Tucker M, et al: Defining lower limb lymphedema after inguinal or ilio-inguinal dissection in patients with melanoma using classification and regression tree analysis, *Ann Surg* 248(2):286–293, 2008.

Tiwari A, Cheng K, Button M, et al: Differential diagnosis, investigation, and current treatment of lower limb lymphedema, *Arch Surg* 138(2):152–161, 2003.

Tiwari P, Corridi M, Lamp S: Lymphedema strategies for investigation and treatment, *Plast Surg Nurs* 32(4):173–177, 2012.

Wagner S: Lymphedema and lipedema—an overview of conservative treatment, *Vasa* 40:271–279, 2011.

Warren AG, Brorson H, Borud LJ, et al: Lymphedema a comprehensive review, *Ann Plast Surg* 59(4):464–472, 2007a.

Warren AG, Janz BA, Borud LJ, et al: Evaluation and management of the fat leg syndrome, *Plast Reconstr Surg* 119(1):9e–15e, 2007b.

Warren AG, Janz BA, Slavin SA, et al: The use of bioimpedance analysis to evaluate lymphedema, *Ann Plast Surg* 58(5):541–543, 2007c.

14

Neuropathic Wounds: The Diabetic Wound

Vickie R. Driver, Jonathan M. LeBretton, Latricia Allen, and Nanjin J. Park

OBJECTIVES

1. Describe three types of neuropathy that may occur in the patient with diabetes.
2. Identify critical factors to be included in the history and physical examination of the patient with lower extremity neuropathic disease.
3. Describe the correlation of protective sensation with risk for diabetic foot ulcer.
4. Distinguish from among the musculoskeletal foot deformities that lead to focal areas of high pressure in the patient with peripheral neuropathy.
5. Identify key components of a patient education program for the patient with lower extremity neuropathic disease.
6. Identify key concepts in effective and appropriate offloading.

Offloading is an essential component needed for effective treatment of diabetic foot ulcers. Clinician treatment choices should be driven by recent best practice guidelines in order to provide the most effective evidence-driven therapy. In 2014 the American Diabetes Association (ADA) recommended a multidisciplinary approach for high-risk patients, as well as long-term preventative visits with a foot specialist. The ADA's Standards of Medical Care in Diabetes are recommendations that are in the form of an evidence-based grading system to guide clinical practice (ADA, 2014).

Lower extremity neuropathic disease (LEND) develops as a result of damage to nerve structures. In the case of diabetic foot ulcers, lower extremity metabolic changes and peripheral arterial disease (PAD) exacerbate neuropathy. Diabetic foot ulcers are sometimes referred to as *neurotrophic, trophic, perforating,* or *mal perforans* ulcers (see Plate 40). The presence of possible coexisting factors, such as impaired perfusion, susceptibility to infection, neuropathy, biochemical abnormalities, repeated or continual trauma, or a combination of these factors, in the patient with LEND who has diabetes creates a particularly challenging situation for ulcer healing (Frykberg, 2003). This chapter presents the assessment, prevention, and management of the diabetic foot ulcer.

EPIDEMIOLOGY

The prevalence of diabetes in the United States is 8.3% of the population, or 25.8 million people (2011 estimate) and is increasing. Of these cases, 7 million are undiagnosed (CDC, 2011). Cases of type 2 diabetes in the United States are steadily increasing. In the 31 years from 1980 to 2011, the prevalence of diagnosed diabetes tripled (CDC, 2012). Data

from 2011 indicate that 79 million adults age 20 years and older qualify as prediabetic, that is, they have fasting glucose levels that are elevated but still below the threshold for a diagnosis of diabetes (CDC, 2011). The increasing prevalence of diabetes is due to a wide variety of causes, with the obesity epidemic and an aging population heading the list. Although population-based prevalence data are lacking, statistics indicate that type 2 diabetes is on the rise among Americans 10 to 19 years old (AAP, 2013). An increase in type 2 diabetes is expected, with an estimated 7% of adolescents in the United States meeting criteria of prediabetes (CDC, 2011). These data lay the foundation for future research into the causative factors and lifetime risk of diabetes.

Using the Behavioral Risk Factor Surveillance System (BRFSS), a national survey database, the Centers for Disease Control (CDC) (2003) estimated a 12.7% prevalence of patients with diabetes who had a history of foot ulcers. In the BRFSS, foot ulcers are defined as "any sores or irritations on the feet that took greater than 4 weeks to heal." Reiber et al (1995) estimated a slightly higher 15% to 20% prevalence of diabetic foot ulcers during the lifetime of a patient with diabetes. Within a given year, the incidence of patients with diabetes who develop foot ulcers ranges from 1.0% to 4.1%, with a potential lifetime risk of 25% (Abbott et al, 2002; Muller et al, 2002; Singh et al, 2005).

Foot ulcers precede lower extremity amputations in 85% of cases (Larsson et al, 1998; Pecoraro et al, 1990). The leading nontraumatic cause of lower extremity amputations in the United States is attributed to diabetes. Of all the nontraumatic amputations in the United States, 50% to 75% are caused by diabetic foot ulcers (Boulton et al, 2005). The national average annual incidence of patients with diabetes

239

having a lower extremity amputation was approximately 3.3 per 1000 (age-adjusted) for the year 2009 (CDC, 2014b).

After decades of steady increase, the percentage of amputations in the diabetic population compared with total amputations appears to be decreasing. Department of Veterans Affairs data show that in 1986, 59% of all amputations were because of diabetes. In 1998, 66% of all amputations were because of diabetes (Mayfield et al, 2000). In 1997 the total number of lower extremity amputations for patients with diabetes in the United States peaked at 84,000 (excluding military health care facilities), and the total figure remained above 80,000 annually until 2007 and then dropped to 68,000 in 2009 (CDC 2014a, 2014b). Presumably, advancements in therapeutic modalities and diagnostics, implementation of multidisciplinary teams, and advanced wound care have supported this downtrend. Although overall lower extremity amputation rates are declining, they continue to rise with patient age (CDC, 2014c). The rate of lower extremity amputation for patients with diabetes is 12 times greater than for individuals without diabetes (Fosse et al, 2009). Furthermore, amputation of the contralateral limb within 2 to 3 years is 50% to 84%, although implementation of a multidisciplinary foot care service has been shown to lower contralateral amputation rates to as low as 7% and to lower the odds ratio for lower extremity amputation in diabetics compared with nondiabetics (Van Gils et al, 1999). Driver et al (2005) reported an 82% reduction in amputations using a multidisciplinary approach, despite a 48% increase in diagnosed diabetics receiving treatment. Three years after a patient with diabetes has a lower extremity amputation, the mortality rate is 20% to 50% (Moulik et al, 2003; Reiber et al, 1995). Five-year survival rates among patients with diabetes who undergo above-knee and below-knee amputations are reported as low as 28% (Aulivola et al, 2004; Corey et al, 2012).

Economic Burden

The economic burden of diabetes in the United States is enormous and is growing. Direct medical and indirect expenditures due to diabetes in 2007 were estimated to be $174 billion (ADA, 2008b). Lower extremity amputations in patients with diabetes and their consequences represent a significant portion of these costs (not to mention the cost in quality of life). Using 1992 to 1995 data from a private health maintenance organization, Ramsey et al (1999) estimated the 2-year medical costs for a middle-aged man with a diabetic foot ulcer to be $27,900. Using Medicare data from 1995 to 1996, Harrington et al (2000) and Stockle et al (2004) found a 20-week healing rate for diabetic foot ulcers to be only 31% and estimated the annual cost for lower extremity ulcer treatment in patients with diabetes to be $15,300, with 74% of the costs from inpatient charges.

The cost of care increases significantly when a diabetic foot ulcer proceeds to amputation. Using 2005 costs, the total event cost ranges from $43,800 for a toe amputation to $66,215 for an above-the-knee amputation (Boulton et al, 2005). An earlier comprehensive study of amputation costs

from Sweden that includes all inpatient, outpatient, and home care costs over a 3-year period estimated a cost of $43,100 for a minor amputation and $63,100 for a major amputation (Apelqvist et al, 2000). Shearer et al (2003) reported that the cost to treat an uninfected foot ulcer was $775 per month, increasing to $2049 per month for an ulcer with cellulitis and $3798 for an ulcer with osteomyelitis. Driver et al (2005) found that hospitalizations involving osteomyelitis were 2.5 times more expensive as diabetic ulcer patients with no infection. Economic data support early identification and intervention of diabetic foot ulcers to prevent not only amputations but also the vast increases in costs associated with recurring infections, comorbid disease progression, and hard-to-close wounds (ADA, 2007).

PATHOGENESIS

The origin and development of a diabetic foot ulcer have several components. An in-depth causal pathway study with two patient cohorts from different parts of the world identified 32 unique causal pathways for developing foot ulcers. The study found three components present in the majority (63%) of the identified pathways: peripheral neuropathy, structural foot problems, and minor trauma (Reiber et al, 1999). In another study, peripheral neuropathy was the major contributing factor leading to the development of 90% of all foot ulcers (Lavery, 2013). The risk of developing a diabetic foot ulcer is seven times more likely in diabetic patients with neuropathy than in their nonneuropathic counterparts (Rathur and Boulton, 2007). Other less prevalent causes were edema, callus, and peripheral ischemia resulting from PAD. Diabetics with PAD have been shown to have more distal disease coupled with poorer mortality and amputation outcomes than nondiabetic patients (Jude et al, 2001; Rathur and Boulton, 2007).

Infection is the most common factor that leads to lower extremity amputation and develops in over half of foot ulcers (Uçkay, 2014).

Neuropathy

Peripheral neuropathy is involved in 78% of diabetic foot ulcers (Reiber et al, 1999). The incidence of neuropathy in patients with diabetes appears to be linked to the duration of diabetes and, to some extent, to glycemic control. Prospective studies comparing patients with standard versus those with tighter control of blood glucose have shown that patients with better glucose control have better nerve conduction velocity and less retinopathy and nephropathy. Lowering hemoglobin A1c values has been shown to decrease the neuropathic and microvascular complications of diabetes (Nathan et al, 2009). The exact etiology of peripheral neuropathy is unknown. In the past, peripheral neuropathy was likely the result of metabolic events, including accrual of glucose, sorbitol, and fructose; reduction in myoinositol (needed for nerve conduction); and nerve ischemia due to reduction in the number and diameter of vessels in the vasa nervosum

(Levin, 2002). Furthermore, recent research done by O'Brien et al (2014) implicates endoplasmic reticulum (ER) stress as a mechanism of diabetic peripheral neuropathy (DPN). Mouse studies show that an increased level of ER stress can cause abnormal metabolic events, which can play a role in cell injury. However, further study into the relationship between ER stress and DPN is required. The predominant structural mechanism affected by the various metabolic components may be the microvascular component. Under normal conditions the arteriole-venule (AV) shunts in the sole of the foot are closed, and blood flows through the nutrient capillaries (capillary dermal papillae loops). With diabetic neuropathy, a decrease in the sympathetic innervation of the highly innervated AV shunts results in a greater dilation in the arterioles, which leads to a shunting away of blood from the capillary dermal papillae loops. This results in lower skin temperature and a decrease in transcutaneous oxygen tension at the skin. Theoretically the metabolic components may be reversible, but structural component changes (shunting) apparently cannot be undone once changed (Tanneberg and Donofrio, 2008). However, recent advances and several randomized clinical trials in various areas of gene therapy and angiogenesis show promise in changing this long-standing convention and expanding our insight into the disease process (Driver and LeBretton, 2008). A more detailed explanation of the many etiologic pathways that lead to diabetic neuropathy is beyond the scope of this chapter.

Neuropathy can be either focal or diffuse. *Focal neuropathies* can be divided into ischemic and entrapment types. *Focal ischemic neuropathies* are caused by an acute event to the nerves. Examples include cranial and femoral neuropathies. These types of neuropathy are characterized by sudden onset and are asymmetric in distribution. Focal entrapment neuropathies occur when a nerve is compressed in a specific area of the body. These neuropathies tend to be more progressive in development and are also often asymmetrically located. Examples include carpal tunnel syndrome and tarsal tunnel syndrome.

Diffuse neuropathies can be divided into *distal symmetric polyneuropathy*, which includes motor and sensory neuropathies and *autonomic neuropathy* (Tanneberg and Donofrio, 2008). Diffuse neuropathies are caused by abnormal structural, vascular, and metabolic conditions. They have a symmetric distribution and are progressive in nature. Diffuse neuropathies are the type encountered frequently in patients with diabetes.

Neuropathy is a frequent risk factor for diabetic foot ulcers and can include (1) sensory nerves (controlling sensation), (2) motor nerves (controlling musculature), and (3) autonomic nerves (controlling functions, e.g., sweating and oil production, vascular flow, and heart rate) (Sumpio, 2000; Tanneberg and Donofrio, 2008). Sensory, motor, and autonomic neuropathies represent the most common complications affecting the lower extremities of patients with diabetes (Mulder et al, 2003; Nathan et al, 2009). Although diabetes is the most common cause of lower extremity

neuropathy, other well-defined causes include uremia, acquired immunodeficiency syndrome (AIDS), nutritional deficiencies, nerve compression, trauma, fractures, prolonged use of crutches, tumors, radiation and cold exposure, certain medicines, systemic lupus erythematosus, and rheumatoid arthritis (NINDS, 2003).

Sensory and Motor Neuropathy. Sensory and motor neuropathies are grouped under the frequently cited category of "peripheral neuropathy" rather than distal symmetric polyneuropathy. The vast peripheral nervous system connects the nerves running from the brain and spinal cord (the central nervous system) and transmits information to the rest of the body (arms, legs, hands, feet). This distal and dying-back progression of neuropathy is often referred to as a "stocking and glove" pattern.

In *sensory neuropathy* the loss of protective sensation leads to a lack of awareness of pain and temperature change, resulting in increased susceptibility to injury. However, the eventual lack of pain awareness is generally preceded by 8 to 10 years of painful neuropathy. Persons with this condition will have worse pain at night, and relief will come from movement rather than rest (Tanneberg and Donofrio, 2008). Once the painful phase ends, minor trauma caused by poorly fitting shoes or an acute injury can precipitate a chronic ulcer. Patients may not realize they have a foot wound for some time because of lack of sensation in their feet. The loss of pain sensation can reach to the knees.

Motor neuropathy affects the muscles required for normal foot movement and can result in muscle atrophy. The distal motor nerves are the most commonly affected and cause atrophy of the small intrinsic muscles of the foot. Often, wasting of the lumbrical and interosseous muscles of the foot will result in collapse of the arch (Alavi et al, 2014; Sumpio, 2000). Cocked-up or claw toes, hammertoes (Figure 14-1), and weight redistribution from the toes to the metatarsal heads lead to increased pressures and subsequent ulceration (Alavi et al, 2014; Levin, 2002). Generally, patients with diabetes develop both kinds of distal symmetric polyneuropathy (Alavi et al, 2014; Sumpio, 2000).

Autonomic Neuropathy. Autonomic neuropathy—a disease of the involuntary nervous system—can affect a wide range of organ systems throughout the body. Diabetic autonomic neuropathy frequently coexists with other peripheral neuropathies and other diabetic complications (Zochodne et al, 2014). Autonomic neuropathy results in decreased sweating and oil production, loss of skin temperature regulation, and abnormal blood flow in the soles of the feet. The resulting xerosis can precipitate fissures, cracks, callus, and finally ulceration (Alavi et al, 2014; Mulder et al, 2003; Tanneberg and Donofrio, 2008).

Musculoskeletal Abnormalities

Foot deformities (Table 14-1) are very common in patients with diabetes and peripheral neuropathy and lead to focal

FIGURE 14-1 A, Hammertoes. **B,** Charcot foot. **C,** Hallux valgus (lateral deviation of hallux) and bunions. (**A, C** From Ball JW, Dains JE, Flynn JA: *Musculoskeletal system.* In *Seidel's guide to physical examination,* ed 8, St. Louis, MO, 2015, Mosby. Courtesy Charles W. Bradley, DPM, MPA, and Caroline Harvey, DPM, California College of Podiatric Medicine. **B** From Bowker JH, Pfeifer MA: *Levin and O'Neal's the diabetic foot,* ed 6, St. Louis, MO, 2001, Mosby.)

TABLE 14-1 Brief Descriptions for Selected Foot Malformations

Malformation	Characteristics
Plantar fasciitis	Heel pain caused by inflammation of long band of connective tissue running from calcaneus to ball of foot
Heel spurs	Bony growths on underside, forepart of calcaneus bone; may lead to plantar fasciitis
Bunions (hallux valgus)	First joint of large metatarsal slants outward, with tip angling toward other toes; may lead to edema, tenderness (see Figure 14-1, *C*)
Hammer (claw) toes	Toes appear bent into clawlike position, often seen in second metatarsal when bunion slants large metatarsal toward and under it (see Figure 14-1, *A*)
Neuromas	Enlarged, benign growths of nerves, most commonly between third and fourth toes; caused by bones or other tissue rubbing against and irritating the nerves
Charcot arthropathy	Disruption or disintegration of some foot and ankle joints; frequently associated with diabetes, resulting in erythema, edema, deformity (see Figure 14-1, *B*)
Pes cavus	High arch or instep
Pes covus	Flat foot

areas of high pressure. These deformities are also associated with thinning of the fat pad under the metatarsal heads. Diabetic foot ulcers generally result from repetitive stress on "hot spots" that develop from bone deformities or callus buildup (Levin, 2002). The areas at the top of the toes, the tips of the toes, under the metatarsal heads, and the heels are vulnerable to ulceration and infection. Atrophied or dislocated fat pads beneath the metatarsal heads increase the pressure under them. This situation can lead to skin loss or callus development and increases the risk of ulceration (Alavi et al, 2014; Sumpio, 2000). A 28% incidence of ulcers among neuropathic patients with elevated plantar pressures has been observed compared with patients with normal plantar pressures. Notably, no ulcers were observed in the normal pressure group (Alavi et al, 2014; Boulton, 2004).

Associated callus can increase foot pressure by as much as 30% (Young et al, 1992). Callus presence has been associated with a 77-fold increase in ulceration in one cross-sectional study. Further follow-up data showed that plantar ulcers in neuropathic patients formed only at callus sites, suggesting an infinite risk for ulcer development (Frykberg et al, 2006; Murray et al, 1996). In the absence of neuropathy, the patient can feel the presence of a fissure, blister, or bony prominence and will take corrective action. However, with neuropathy, the protective response is diminished or even nonexistent. Thus foot ulcers can get progressively worse before any action is taken. Individuals with diabetic neuropathy have been known to walk around for days in shoes containing shoehorns. Abnormalities in foot biomechanics from the previously described deformities and possible ulceration often cause a dysfunctional gait, which leads to further damage to the structure of the foot.

Ankle Joint Equinus. Ankle joint equinus, defined as less than 0 degrees of ankle joint dorsiflexion, occurs in some patients with peripheral neuropathy. With ankle joint equinus the range of motion of the foot joint becomes limited, which increases pressure on the sole of the foot (Caselli et al, 2002). Of all patients with diabetes, 10.3% develop ankle joint equinus; this risk increases with duration of disease (Lavery et al, 2002). High plantar pressures from ankle equinus can increase the incidence of ulceration in patients with diabetes (Caselli et al, 2002).

Foot. Charcot foot or Charcot neuroarthropathy (or arthropathy) is a classic and increasingly common diabetic foot deformity affecting nearly 10% of diabetics with neuropathy and greater than 16% of those with a history of neuropathic ulcer (Reiber et al, 1995). Lavery et al (2003) found the incidence of Charcot arthropathy for non-Hispanic whites with diabetes to be 11.7 per 1000 per year. A long duration of diabetes is an important factor in the development of Charcot neuroarthropathy; greater than 80% of patients with Charcot foot had diabetes for more than 10 years (Cofield et al, 1983; Rajbhandari et al, 2002). The early stage of Charcot is characterized by erythema and edema. This can be similar to the early stage of infection; however, fever and pain can be absent in Charcot foot. Also, laboratory results show normal erythrocyte sedimentation rate (ESR) (Rogers et al, 2011).

The precise neural mechanism causing Charcot foot is unknown, and a number of different theories have been proposed to explain the underlying etiology (Frykberg et al, 2006; Gerald and Hudson, 2002). Despite conventional thinking that many lower extremities of diabetics are ischemic, overwhelming evidence indicates that many patients with diabetic neuropathy have increased blood and pooling in their feet. This condition has been directly correlated with decreased bone density in Charcot foot, possibly as a result of autonomic neuropathy. Charcot foot may well be due to a combination of neurotraumatic and neurovascular mechanisms (Frykberg et al, 2006; Gerald and Hudson, 2002).

Progression of Charcot disease is divided into three radiographically different stages: development, coalescence, and reconstruction. *Development* represents the acute, destructive phase characterized by joint effusions, edema, subluxation, formation of bone and cartilage debris, intraarticular fractures, and bone fragmentation. This period is often initiated by minor trauma and is aggravated by persistent ambulation. The second stage, *coalescence,* is marked by a reduction in edema, absorption of fine debris, and healing of fractures. The final phase of bone healing is *reconstruction,* in which further repair and remodeling of bones take place, along with fusion and rounding of large bone fragments and decreased

joint mobility. Early diagnosis and treatment (i.e., offloading) in the development stage are critical in the treatment of this disease (Sanders et al, 2008).

The Charcot foot is prone to increased pressures because of its deformity and possible bone or joint collapse. The patient with Charcot neuroarthropathy is four times more likely to develop a foot ulcer (Gerald and Hudson, 2002; Jeffcoate and Harding, 2003).

Peripheral Arterial Disease

Peripheral arterial disease is a major risk factor for lower extremity amputation, particularly in patients who have diabetes, because the accompanying inadequate oxygenation and perfusion of tissues significantly impair wound healing (see discussion of PAD in Chapter 11) (Mulder et al, 2003). In a comparison between patients with diabetes and patients without diabetes and PAD, patients with diabetes were five times more likely to have an amputation (Jude et al, 2001).

The incidence of ischemic diabetic foot ulcers is relatively low. However, because more than half of people with PAD are asymptomatic, determining the true prevalence in patients with diabetes is difficult. Peripheral ischemia was present in 35% of ulcerations in a two-center causal pathway study (Reiber et al, 1999). Oyibo et al (2002) found that 11% of diabetic foot ulcers were ischemic (52.3% neuroischemic, 36% neuropathic). In contrast, a study from England found that only 16% of new diabetic foot ulcers were ischemic (24% neuroischemic). Incongruence in ulcer classification rates could indicate greater awareness spawned by the advent of multidisciplinary teams (Rathur and Boulton, 2007), as well as improvements in classification and stratification of ulcer presentation as diagnostic technology, research, and our understanding of causative factors continue to advance. Although ischemic foot ulcers are relatively less common than neuropathic or neuroischemic diabetic foot ulcers, they are more serious and lead to higher rates of amputation in patients with diabetes who do not have peripheral neuropathy (Moulik et al, 2003). Amputations of lower extremities in patients with diabetes are almost always due to multiple causes, including ischemia, infection, and neuropathy. Van Gils et al (1999) found that 55% of amputations required within a high-risk foot clinic were due to the combination of ischemia and infection. Their study supported the findings of Prompers et al (2008), who showed a negative healing impact of infection among patients with PAD and infection compared with patients with infections and no PAD. Additionally, infection was the only predictor of healing in patients with PAD.

Relatively little is known about the biology of PAD in patients with diabetes; however, it is thought to be similar to other manifestations of atherosclerotic disease, such as coronary artery disease and carotid artery disease. Seventy percent of deaths among type 2 diabetics can be attributed to vascular disease (National Diabetes Advisory Board, 1983). Peripheral arterial disease typically results from gradual diameter reduction of the lower extremity arteries and from the progression of atherosclerotic changes in arterial circulation in the lower extremities. Endothelial injury and resulting endothelial dysfunction occur in the earliest stages of the disease. The endothelial surface can be injured by various means, including hyperlipidemia and diabetes (Levy, 2002). The atherosclerotic plaque that develops in the patient with diabetes and PAD is no different from the plaque that develops in the patient without diabetes (Levin, 2002). The pattern of PAD in patients with diabetes is such that medium-size arteries, mainly at the popliteal trifurcation, are affected. However, distal pedal vessels are spared (Steed et al, 2006).

Microvascular tissue perfusion, in contrast to macrocirculation, may present problems for patients with diabetes. Whereas PAD in persons with diabetes normally spares the small pedal arteries, microcirculation abnormalities in the foot as a result of neuropathy are common. Diabetic neuropathy impairs the nerve axon reflex and causes local vasodilation in response to a painful stimulus. The impaired vasodilation in diabetic neuropathic lower extremities can create a functional ischemia.

ASSESSMENT

The components of assessment for any patient with signs or symptoms of LEND include the patient history and risk factors, physical examination, and simple noninvasive tests. Select patients may require more complex studies.

Patient History

The patient history includes general state of health, a record of diabetic complications and treatments, walking difficulties, shoe problems, pain in the extremity, medications (prescribed and over-the-counter), glycosylated hemoglobin level, and risk factors for LEND and diabetic foot ulcers. Because diabetic foot ulcers can occur as a consequence of neuropathy and lower extremity arterial disease (LEAD), specific questions regarding any LEAD risk factors should be posed (see Box 11-1).

Risk Factors.
A number of studies have quantified the relative significance of various risk factors associated with the presence of foot ulceration (Lavery et al, 1998) found that in the patient with diabetes, the relative risk (RR) for foot ulceration increases according to the number and type of risk factor present:
- RR = 1.7 in persons with peripheral neuropathy
- RR = 12.1 in persons with peripheral neuropathy *and* foot deformity
- RR = 36.4 in persons with peripheral neuropathy, foot deformity, *and* a history of previous amputation

In a large multicenter study that lasted 30 months, Pham et al (2000) analyzed the incidence of new foot ulceration in patients with diabetes and various measurable risk factors. Of the patients enrolled in their study, 29% developed one or more foot ulcers over the 30-month period (a very high

incidence). Nearly all (99%) of these patients had a high neuropathy disability score and/or a poor score on the Semmes-Weinstein monofilament examination for sensation. Additional factors that yielded a statistically significant odds ratio for foot ulceration during the study include the following:
- Gender (male)
- Ethnic background (Native American)
- Duration of diabetes (long)
- Palpable pulses
- History of foot ulceration
- High vibration threshold score
- High foot pressures

Foot ulcers often have a multifactorial etiology. Although the earlier studies list the most commonly associated risk factors, the clinician must recognize many other risk factors in order to comprehensively assess a patient. Box 14-1 contains a list of the most commonly recognized risk factors for ulceration (Abbott et al, 2002; Lavery et al, 2012). As with the presence of infection, vascular insufficiency has a much more important role in delaying wound healing and subsequent amputation than as a risk factor contributing to ulceration (Lavery et al, 1998).

Classification of risk. Many specialized foot treatment clinics use a foot risk classification system for patients with diabetes to allocate resources such as therapeutic shoes, education, and frequency of clinic visits (Frykberg et al, 2006; Peters and Lavery, 2001). The International Working Group on the Diabetic Foot (Apelqvist and Larsson, 2000) recommends the "international" system as listed in Box 14-2. Risk classification systems have been shown to be very effective in predicting future diabetic foot ulcers (Lavery et al, 1998; Peters and Lavery, 2001). Additional risk classification systems are provided in Tables 14-2 and 14-3.

BOX 14-1 Diabetic Foot Ulcer Risk Factors

- Absence of protective sensation due to peripheral neuropathy
- Vascular insufficiency
- Structural deformities and callus formation
- Autonomic neuropathy causing decreased sweating and dry feet
- Limited joint mobility
- Long duration of diabetes
- Long history of smoking
- Poor glucose control
- Obesity
- Impaired vision
- Past history of ulcer or amputation
- Male gender
- Increased age
- Ethnic background with high incidence of diabetes (e.g., Native American)
- Poor footwear inadequately protecting skin from high pressures

BOX 14-2 Foot Risk Classification by the International Working Group on the Diabetic Foot

Group 0: Patients have diabetes but no other risk factors
Group 1: Patients have both diabetes and neuropathy
Group 2: Patients have diabetes, neuropathy, vascular disease, and/or foot deformities
Group 3: Patients have a history of foot ulcers or previous amputation and further specified as:
  Group 3A: Patients with history of foot ulcers
  Group 3B: Patients with previous amputation

From Lavery LA, Peters EJ, Williams JR, et al: Reevaluating the way we classify the diabetic foot: restructuring the diabetic foot risk classification system of the International Working Group on the Diabetic Foot, *Diabetes Care* 31(1):154–156, 2008.

Lower Extremity and Foot Physical Examination

Chapter 10 describes how to conduct a comprehensive lower extremity assessment and should be carefully reviewed. The following section discusses the aspects of the lower extremity examination that are unique to the patient with LEND.

Protective Sensation. Screening for neuropathy can be done rapidly and reliably using a Semmes-Weinstein 5.07 (10-g) monofilament test or a vibration tuning fork test with the on-off method (ADA, 2007; Perkins et al, 2001). Biothesiometry expands on the traditional tuning fork, allowing for quantification of the vibration threshold (Figure 14-2, *A*). An electric oscillator is applied to the traditional assessment landmarks (see Figure 14-2, *B*) and "dialed in" until the

patient is able to perceive the vibration (see Figure 14-2, *C*). The value obtained can be used to follow the progression of neuropathy and qualify future assessment findings. As shown in Figure 14-3, the monofilament line used for the Semmes-Weinstein test is normally mounted on a rigid paper holder. The line has been standardized to deliver a 10-g force when pushed against an area of the foot. Regardless of which method is used, the patient should be placed in a room that is quiet and relaxed. Boxes 14-3 and 14-4 provide procedures for conducting these examinations.

Pain. A description of neuropathic pain is an important assessment parameter and may be specific to the disease state. In general, neuropathic pain varies in severity and is described as "burning," "tingling," "shooting," or "pins and needles." Activity can alleviate or exacerbate neuropathic pain. Because of the potential for LEAD, the patient should be assessed for ischemic pain (see Box 11-3). A comparison of pain characteristics of venous, arterial, and neuropathic wounds is given in Table 10-2. Chapters 25 and 26 provide a detailed discussion on the assessment and management of wound-related pain.

Musculoskeletal Abnormalities. Loss of motor nerve function affects the intrinsic foot muscles. When imbalances due to weakening of the intrinsic muscles occur, they can cause changes in foot structure and gait and muscle wasting. Plantar fat pads also become displaced, and the metatarsal heads become prominent. These changes may predispose the patient to ulceration. Each foot has 26 bones, 29 joints, and 42 muscles; thus there are numerous potential locations for

TABLE 14-2 Foot Risk Classification System and Management Considerations

Low-Risk Diabetes	Moderate-Risk Diabetes	High-Risk Diabetes
Classification		
Intact sensation (neurologic)	Intact sensation (neurologic)	Absence of sensation (neurologic)
and/or	and/or	and/or
Intact pulses (vascular)	Intact pulses (vascular)	Absence of pulses (vascular)
Absence of foot deformities	Presence of foot deformities	Presence or absence of foot deformities
Management		
Education emphasizing disease control, proper shoe fit/design, daily self-inspection, early reporting of foot injuries or breaks in skin	Education emphasizing disease control, proper shoe fit/design, daily self-inspection, early reporting of foot injuries or breaks in skin	Education emphasizing disease control, proper shoe fit/design, daily self-inspection, early reporting of foot injuries or breaks in skin
Proper fitting/design footwear with orthotics as needed	Proper fitting/design footwear with orthotics as needed; depth-inlay footwear, molded/modified orthosis may be required	May require modified or custom footwear
Annual follow-up for foot screening	Routine follow-up every 6 months for foot examination	Routine follow-up every 1 to 12 weeks for foot ulcer evaluation and callus/nail care
Follow as needed for skin/callus/nail care or orthosis	Referral to foot and ankle care specialist if deformity is causing pressure point and conservative measures fail	Referral to foot and ankle care specialist

Data from Driver VR, Madsen J, Goodman RA: Reducing amputation rates in patients with diabetes at a military medical center: the limb preservation service model, *Diabetes Care* 28(2):248–253, 2005.

TABLE 14-3 Lower Extremity Amputation Prevention (LEAP) Program and Management Categories for the Foot

Risk Categories	Definition	Management Categories
0	Diabetes, but no loss of protective sensation in feet	Education emphasizing disease control, proper shoe fit/design Follow-up yearly for foot screen Follow as needed for skin, callus, nail care, or orthosis
1	Diabetes, loss of protective sensation in feet	Education emphasizing disease control, fit/design, daily inspection, skin/nail care, early reporting of foot injuries Properly fitting/design footwear with soft inserts/soles Routine follow-up every 3 to 6 months for foot/shoe examination and nail care
2	Diabetes, loss of protective sensation in feet with high pressure (callout/deformity), or poor circulation	Education emphasizing disease control, proper shoe fit/design, daily inspection, skin/nail care, early reporting of foot injuries Depth-inlay footwear, molded/modified orthoses Modify shoes as needed; footwear with soft inserts/soles Routine follow-up every 1 to 3 months for foot/activity/footwear evaluation and callus/nail care
3	Diabetes, history of plantar ulceration or neuropathic fracture	Education emphasizing disease control, properly fitting footwear, daily inspection, skin/nail/callus care, early reporting of foot injuries Depth-inlay footwear, molded/modified orthoses; modified/custom footwear, ankle footwear orthoses as needed Routine follow-up every 1 to 12 weeks for foot/activity/footwear evaluation and callus/nail care

Note: "Loss of protective sensation" is assessed using a 5.07 monofilament at 10 locations on each foot.
From Crawford PE, Fields-Varnado M, WOCN Society: Guideline for the management of wounds in patients with lower-extremity neuropathic disease, *J Wound Ostomy Continence Nurs.* 40(1):34-45, 2012.

FIGURE 14-2 A, Biothesiometer. **B,** Application of biothesiometer oscillator head to patient's foot during peripheral neuropathy assessment. **C,** Oscillator amplitude knob to determine level of sensation. (Courtesy J. LeBretton and V. Driver.)

FIGURE 14-3 A, Monofilament. **B,** Press the monofilament against the skin hard enough so that it bends. (Ball JW, Dains JE, Flynn JA: Examination techniques and equipment. In *Seidel's guide to physical examination*, ed 8, St. Louis, MO, 2015, Mosby.)

BOX 14-3   Procedure for Semmes-Weinstein 5.07 (10-g) Monofilament Examination (SWME)

1. Explain procedure to patient.
2. Position patient in sitting position, resting patient's lower leg on examiner's lap.
3. Demonstrate monofilament on patient's hand so that he or she knows what to expect.
4. Explain to patient that he or she should respond with a "yes" when he or she feels the filament touching the skin.
5. Have the patient close his or her eyes. The five key viability sites should be tested as shown in the illustration (fat pad of 1st and 4th toe, and metatarsal head of 1st, 3rd, and 5th toe).
6. Apply monofilament perpendicular to skin's surface. Apply sufficient force to cause the filament to buckle or bend in C-shape. Use a smooth, not jabbing, motion.
7. Total duration of the approach, skin contact, and departure of filament from each site should be approximately 1 to 2 seconds.
8. Apply filament along margin of callus, ulcer, scar, and/or necrotic tissue; do *not* apply filament over these lesions.
9. Record and, if appropriate, map the results on examination form.

Right foot   Left foot

(From Dehn R, Asprey D: *Essential clinical procedures,* ed 3, St Louis, 2013, Saunders.)

BOX 14-4   Procedure for Biothesiometry Examination (Amplitude of Vibration)

1. Explain procedure to patient.
2. Position patient in sitting position, resting patient's lower leg on examiner's lap.
3. Demonstrate oscillator on patient's hand so that he or she knows what to expect.
4. Explain to patient that he or she should respond with a "yes" when he or she feels the oscillator vibrating.
5. Have the patient close his or her eyes. Sites to be tested should be shown on examination form.
6. Apply oscillator perpendicular to (flat against) skin's surface. Apply just enough force for the oscillator head to make total contact with skin. Use a smooth, not jabbing, motion.
7. The amplitude of the vibration should be slowly increased until the patient perceives the vibration and the value on the meter noted.
8. Apply oscillator along margin of callus, ulcer, scar, and/or necrotic tissue; do *not* apply oscillator over these lesions.
9. Record and, if appropriate, map the results on examination form.

---

problems. A few structural foot deformities are briefly described in Table 14-1. Figure 14-1 provides illustrations of selected structural foot deformities.

Claw, hammer, and mallet toes are signs of distal muscle atrophy and foot neuropathy. When muscles weaken, other muscles can overpower them, leading to contractures. *Hammer toe* is a contracture of the proximal joint, which is further from the front (or top) of the toe. *Mallet toe* refers to the distal joint, closer to the end of the toe, and is almost identical to hammer toe. When both joints are contracted, the condition is called *claw toe.* Prominent metatarsal heads occur if one of the metatarsal bones is longer or lower than its neighboring bones. This may lead to uneven weight distribution between the heads and subsequent pain, callus, and ulceration. Bunions are caused by an enlarged head of the first metatarsal bone just below the first toe joint (ADA, 2004a, 2008a).

When changes in the gait or foot structure are observed, the patient should be referred for more testing. Patients with Charcot foot normally have a rocker-bottom foot that is hot, erythematous, and edematous with bounding pedal pulses and prominent veins (see Figure 14-1). Pain is normally, but not always, minimal in the early stages. The foot may be 10° F to 12° F warmer than the rest of the skin (Frykberg et al, 2006; Gerald and Hudson, 2002). A history including an absence of trauma, a portal of entry for infection, or other signs of infection is suggestive of an acute Charcot foot (Levin, 2002).

Vascular Status. The coexisting calcification of arteries that occurs with diabetes and PAD leaves the blood vessels difficult to compress and therefore difficult to assess (Levin, 2002; Sumpio, 2000). When pulses cannot be palpated, use of a Doppler probe will allow the skilled examiner to determine whether pulses are triphasic, biphasic, or monophasic. The absence of pedal pulses despite the presence of popliteal pulses is a classic finding for patients with diabetes who also have PAD. If pedal pulses are not detectable with a Doppler device, a referral to a vascular specialist is warranted (Hopf et al, 2006).

In the absence of pedal pulses, additional noninvasive vascular tests may be conducted to obtain a better indication of the condition: (1) segmental pressures (i.e., taken at the thigh, calf, and ankle); (2) toe pressures; or (3) transcutaneous oxygen readings (Steed et al, 2006). Transcutaneous oximetry ($TcPO_2$) is an assessment of the microcirculatory system, which can be impaired in persons with diabetes and peripheral neuropathy. Zimny et al (2001a) found that patients with diabetes and neuropathy had significantly higher sitting to supine $TcPO_2$ differences than patients with diabetes only, indicating microcirculatory impairment.

Vasodilation in diabetic, neuropathic lower extremities can create a functional ischemia. Symptoms of impaired microcirculation are discussed in Chapters 10 and 11. Armstrong et al (2003b) showed that skin temperature is a poor indicator of vascular status, neuropathy, or future foot complications in patients with diabetes. The only significant association found in their study was higher skin temperatures in patients with Charcot arthropathy. However, a difference in skin temperature may be an indication of trauma, fracture, and/or infection. Skin temperature should be assessed in both feet using the back of the examiner's hand or an infrared temperature scanner.

Skin and Nail Condition. Skin and nail condition is an important component of the assessment for the patient with LEND. Descriptions of foot lesions and nail disorders are given in Chapter 15. Loss of sweating and oil production may cause cracking of the skin and fissures that can become infected. The presence of eczema, dermatitis, and/or psoriasis should be noted. The web spaces between the toes should be examined for moisture and/or fungal problems. The patient's skin condition should be documented and any corns, calluses, preulcerative lesions (e.g., blisters, hematomas), or open ulcers measured and drawn on the documentation form. If the patient has coexisting vascular disease, additional skin changes may be apparent. Table 10-3 lists characteristics of lower extremities and wounds in patients with LEAD, LEND, and lower extremity venous disease (LEVD).

Callus formation is a natural protective response to repetitive stress. It is characterized by thickened hyperkeratotic skin. The problem with this buildup is that accumulation of callus can increase pressure 25% to 30%, resulting in an ulcer below the callused area that is not visible to the examiner and/or is not palpable. Hemorrhage into a callus is a principal indicator of ulceration (WOCN®, 2012). A callus usually is painless but in some cases can cause pain because nerve endings close to the surface layers are irritated. Callus buildup is a result of a biomechanical problem. Unless the underlying cause is eliminated, callus will continue to occur. Based on the duration and amount of pressure applied, the skin may eventually breakdown and an ulcer will develop.

Thickened nails are common. In addition, any abnormalities under the nail and any sign of nail infections should be noted. Nails bear the brunt of daily activities: running, walking, participating in sports, and just wearing shoes. When feet are abused and/or injured, a portion or all of the nail plate can be damaged. Repeated trauma, improper trimming, and minor injuries can result in nail problems. If the toe box is pressing down on the nails, bleeding may occur under the nail. Some nail disorders are hereditary. Ingrown toenails (onychocryptosis) may have a convex deformity. As pressure is exerted on the tissues, callus builds up. Nails that are red, brown, or black may indicate trauma (acute or chronic). Any discharge from around the nail or under the nail may indicate an infection process. Fungal infections are common. A nail that curves inward in the corners is called a *paronychia*. If present, remove nail polish to better view the nails.

Footwear

Evaluation of the patient's shoes is as important as taking a good history or examining the patient's feet. The majority of injuries to the foot are not recognized by the person with diabetes because of neuropathy. Most skin injuries on the foot of the person with diabetes are located on either the dorsal or the plantar surface. Many ulcers on the dorsum are located at sites of high pressure where the patient's footwear creates a lesion, implying a biomechanical etiology. Due to the lack of clinical outcome studies guiding practice, assessment of footwear should follow a logical progression, observing for pressure points, wear, and areas of friction. Checklist 14-1 outlines the items that should be investigated when evaluating the patient's shoes. Boxes 14-5 and 15-5 provide tips for appropriate footwear selection.

Foot Imprints (Harris Mat). Although a number of commercial devices exist for barefoot or in-shoe plantar pressure measurement, an inexpensive method that can be used to identify areas of increased pressure and unequal weight distribution of the patient's feet is the Harris mat (Tanneberg and Donofrio, 2008). The mat (foot imprint system) has two compartments. One side of the mat is inked. Paper is placed facing the inked surface. Two sheets are required, one

---

CHECKLIST 14-1 Items to Investigate When Evaluating Shoes in a Patient with Diabetes

✓ Bulges on outside of shoes
✓ Wear patterns on soles of shoes
✓ Wearing down on heels
✓ Worn lining inside shoes
✓ Shoe cushioning
✓ Foreign objects in shoes

BOX 14-5   Instructions for Care of Diabetic Feet

Inspection
- Inspect feet and toes daily for blisters, cuts, swelling, redness, and any other discolored areas. If you are unable to see the bottoms of your feet, use a mirror.
- Look for dry areas and cracks in the skin.
- Apply a thin coat of lubricating oil after bathing.
- If your vision is impaired, have a family member inspect your feet daily and trim nails and buff calluses when required.

Bathing
- Wash your feet daily. Dry them carefully, including between the toes. Test the water with hands or elbow to ensure it will not burn your feet.
- Do not soak your feet. Soaking actually dries the skin by removing natural oil and can cause maceration (wrinkled appearance).
- Apply moisturizing cream to feet top to bottom after bathing (not between toes).

Toenail Care
- Cut toenails after bathing, when they are soft and easier to trim.
- Never cut nails too short. Leave one-sixteenth to one-eighth inch of the nail. Nails should be cut straight across the top or shaped to follow the contour of the toe. Sharp edges should be filed smooth with an emery board to avoid cutting adjacent toes.
- Ingrown nails or other problematic nails should be cared for by a foot care provider.
- Avoid using sharp objects to clean under the toenail.

Corns and Calluses
- Do not use chemical corn or callus removers or corn pads. They can damage or burn the skin.
- When feet are dry, file away calluses with a pumice stone.
- Corns and calluses are a response to pressure from poorly fitting shoes. Change footwear to reduce these pressure "hot spots."
- Never use a razor blade yourself to reduce corns or calluses.

Shoes and Socks
- Wear clean socks every day. Avoid nylon socks as much as possible.
- Socks need to fit well, with no tight elastic at the top or seams.
- Do not walk barefoot, even in your home. Wear slippers with a rubber sole. Wear shoes and socks outside at all times.
- In winter, take special precautions to prevent foot damage from the cold.
- Inspect shoes for objects inside before you put them on.
- Buy shoes later in the day when feet are their largest. Do not depend on breaking in shoes.
- Shoes should be sufficiently wide for your feet and should have thick, flexible rubber soles, closed toes, and closed heels, as in running or walking shoes.
- Avoid pointed-toe shoes or boots. Do not wear sandals with a strap between your toes.
- Wear new shoes for short periods each day, from 1 to 2 hours. Watch for signs of poor fit.

Circulation
- Do not smoke. If you do, stop!
- Exercise regularly.
- If your feet are cold, wear socks to keep your feet warm.
- Do not use a heating pad or hot water bottle.

---

for each foot. The inked side is closed, and the mat is reversed. The patient is asked to remove his or her shoes, leaving socks or hose on. The patient is asked to take a normal step down on the side that does not have ink. Stepping on the mat leaves an impression of the foot on the paper that indicates areas of high pressure and uneven weight distribution (Figure 14-4, *A*). Use of the mat identifies high-risk areas and is a good motivator for getting patients to wear their orthotics because they can see where problem areas exist.

Forefoot Test. The forefoot test shows patients how well their shoes fit their feet. First, have the patient remove his or her socks or hose. Instruct the patient to stand on a piece of paper with both feet. Trace the outline of both feet on the paper. Next, take the patient's shoes and just place the edge of the shoe over the traced outline. If any of the lines are visible, the shoes are too tight (see Figure 14-4, *B*). Again, this is a highly visual cue that helps the patient realize the importance of wearing shoes that fit his or her feet.

Diabetic Foot Ulcer Evaluation

The initial description of the foot ulcer is critical for mapping its development during treatment. Detailed wound assessment and evaluation of healing are described in Chapter 6.

FIGURE 14-4 A, Example of Harris ink mat impression. **B,** Patient's shoe laid over traced image of foot. (Courtesy David M. Osterman.)

Characteristics. Common locations and causes of diabetic foot ulcers are listed in Table 14-4. Ulcers with a LEND etiology may resemble a laceration, puncture, or blister with a rounded or oblong shape. The wound base may be necrotic, pink, or pale, with well-defined, smooth edges and small to moderate amounts of serous or clear exudate. The periwound skin often presents with callus.

Diabetic Foot Ulcer with Lower Extremity Arterial Disease. Although ischemic foot ulcers are relatively less common than neuropathic or neuroischemic diabetic foot ulcers, they are more serious and lead to higher rates of amputation in patients with diabetes (Moulik et al, 2003). A comparison of the characteristics of neuropathic, arterial, and venous wounds is given in Table 10-3. Trophic changes for arterial disease alone are not diagnostic of arterial insufficiency and should be interpreted with caution. Characteristics of ischemic foot ulcers include pain, absence of bleeding, presence of an underlying deformity, or history of a trauma (Sumpio, 2000). Ischemic ulcers on the dorsum are uncommon because perfusion usually is better and pressures are reduced at that location (Sumpio, 2000). Additional indicators of ischemia are discussed in detail in Chapter 11.

Diabetic Foot Ulcer Classification. Numerous diabetic foot ulcer classification systems have been reported in the literature

(Ince et al 2008; Lavery et al, 1996; Lipsky et al 2012; Sims et al, 1988; Van Acker et al, 2002; Wagner, 1981). These systems are useful for guiding treatment regimens, facilitating communication among care providers, predicting future outcomes, and conducting clinical trials. The various systems often include location, depth, necrotic characteristics, and presence of infection, ischemia, or neuropathy.

The widely used Wagner foot wound classification system divides foot ulcers into six grades based on the depth of the lesion and the presence of osteomyelitis or gangrene (Wagner, 1981). The Wagner system does not include presence of infection, ischemia, or neuropathy. The Wound, Ostomy and Continence Nurses Society™ (WOCN®) (2012) modified the Wagner system to address ischemia and infection (Table 14-5).

Another popular diabetic foot ulcer classification system, the University of Texas system (Table 14-6), utilizes a matrix structure with four grades of wound depth and four associated stages to specify ischemia, infection, both ischemia and infection, or neither (Lavery et al, 1996). The University of Texas system has been judged superior to the original Wagner system as a predictor of patient outcomes (Oyibo et al, 2001). Another system is the Size (Area and Depth) (SAD) classification system,

---

TABLE 14-4   Common Wound Sites for Neuropathic Wounds

Wound Location	Causative Factor
Toe interphalangeal joints	Limited interphalangeal joint flexibility, rigid toe
Metatarsal head	Increased prominence, limited ankle joint flexibility
Interdigital	Increased moisture, footwear too narrow, toe crowding, deformity
Bunion sites	Footwear too narrow, foot deformity
Dorsal toes	Hammer or claw toe deformity, footwear too shallow in toe box
Distal toes	Poor arterial perfusion, external force, footwear too short, short, toe deformity
Midfoot (dorsal or plantar surface)	Charcot fracture, external trauma, edema blisters
	Heel fissures
	Anhidrosis
Heels	Unrelieved pressure, particularly during bedbound episodes

From Crawford PE, Fields-Varnado M, WOCN Society: Guideline for the management of wounds in patients with lower-extremity neuropathic disease, *J Wound Ostomy Continence Nurs.* 40(1): 34-45, 2012.

TABLE 14-5   Wagner Ulcer Classification System (Modified)*

Grade	Description
0	At-risk foot
	Preulcer
	No open lesions; skin intact
	May have deformities, erythematous areas of pressure, or callus formation
1	Superficial ulcer
	Disruption of skin without extending into subcutaneous fat layer*
	Superficial infection, with or without cellulitis, may be present*
2	Full-thickness ulcer
	Penetrates through fat to tendon or joint capsule, without abscess or osteomyelitis
3	Deep ulcer that may probe to the bone, with abscess, osteomyelitis, or joint sepsis
	Includes deep plantar space infections or abscesses, necrotizing fasciitis, or tendon sheath infections*
4	Gangrene of geographic portion of foot (e.g., toes, forefoot, heel)
	Remainder of foot is salvageable but may be infected*
5	Gangrene of whole foot beyond salvage
	Required limb- or life-sparing amputation*

*Modification was added to the Wagner scale to identify ischemia and infection.

From Crawford PE, Fields-Varnado M, WOCN Society: Guideline for the management of wounds in patients with lower-extremity neuropathic disease, *J Wound Ostomy Continence Nurs.* 40(1): 34-45, 2012.

TABLE 14-6   University of Texas at San Antonio Diabetic Wound Classification System

Stage	0	I	II	III
		GRADE		
A	Preulcerative or postulcerative lesion completely healed	Superficial wound not involving tendon, capsule, or bone	Wound penetrating to tendon or capsule	Wound penetrating to bone or joint
B	Preulcerative or postulcerative lesion completely epithelialized with infection	Superficial wound not involving tendon, capsule, or bone with infection	Wound penetrating to tendon or capsule with infection	Wound penetrating to bone or joint with infection
C	Preulcerative or postulcerative lesion completely epithelialized with ischemia	Superficial wound not involving tendon, capsule, or bone with ischemia	Wound penetrating to tendon or capsule with ischemia	Wound penetrating to bone or joint with ischemia
D	Preulcerative or postulcerative lesion completely epithelialized with infection and ischemia	Superficial wound not involving tendon, capsule, or bone with infection and ischemia	Wound penetrating to tendon or capsule with infection and ischemia	Wound penetrating to bone or joint with infection and ischemia

From Lavery LA, Armstrong DG, Harkless LB: Classification of diabetic foot wounds, *J Foot Ankle Surg* 35:528, 1996.

which grades the wound according to area, depth, sepsis, quality of pulses, and accuracy of sensation (Table 14-7) (Macfarlane and Jeffcoate, 1999).

Infection. Infection rarely causes diabetic foot ulcers. Rather, ulcers provide a portal for the entry of pathogens, which often thrive because of the impaired host response of the person with diabetes (Steed et al, 2006). Infection is a causal component in 59% of diabetic limb amputations (Armstrong et al, 1998; Pecoraro et al, 1990). In a Swedish study, Eneroth et al (1997) found that 42% of patients with diabetes who had deep foot infections required lower extremity amputations and 86% required surgery. However, a recent study done by Frykberg et al (2006) suggested that 20% of patients with foot ulcers will subsequently require an amputation.

The person with diabetes is more prone to infection than is the person without diabetes (Shah and Hux, 2003), most likely due to impaired leukocyte function in patients with chronic hyperglycemia. However, infected diabetic foot wounds often are less symptomatic than nondiabetic wounds, exhibiting only subtle or even a complete absence of signs

(Frykberg, 2003; Lipsky et al, 2012). Recalcitrant hyperglycemia may be one of the clinical findings indicating a severe infection of a diabetic foot ulcer (Frykberg, 2002; Frykberg et al, 2006; Mendes and Neves, 2012). The presence of probable infection needs to be noted during the initial examination, although culturing is best done after surgical debridement.

Wound culture technique is important to ensure surface colonies are not included and therefore confused with infection (see Chapter 16). Wound cultures should be taken by obtaining tissue from the debrided wound base or by aspirating pus. If swabs are the only option, ensure they are taken from the wound base after cleansing. The gold standard for infection assessment is the quantitative biopsy (Frykberg, 2003). Evaluation does not end after initial culturing. Wounds must be continually monitored for bacterial colonization.

Like the classification of diabetic foot ulcers in general, the classification of diabetic foot infections can be useful for determining appropriate treatment. Diabetic foot infections are subdivided into either non–limb-threatening or limb-threatening categories (Table 14-8), with the understanding that the latter classification can become life threatening (ADA,

TABLE 14-7   Size (Area and Depth) (SAD) Classification

Grade	Area	Depth	Sepsis	Arteriopathy	Denervation
0	Skin intact	Skin intact	No infection	Pedal pulses palpable	SWMT (Semmes Weinstein monofilament test) normal (see Box 14-3 for procedure) VPT normal
1	<10 mm²	Skin and subcutaneous tissue	Superficial slough or exudate	Diminution of both pulses or absence of one	Reduced or absent pinprick sensation VPT raised
2	10–30 mm²	Tendon, joint, capsule, periosteum	Cellulitis	Absence of both pedal pulses	Neuropathy dominant, palpable pedal pulses
3	>30 mm²	Bone and/or joint spaces	Osteomyelitis	Gangrene	Charcot foot

VPT, Vibration perception threshold.
From Macfarlane R, Jeffcoate W: Classification of diabetic foot ulcers: the size (area and depth) (SAD) system, *Diabetic Foot* 2(4):123, 1999.

TABLE 14-8 Signs of Limb-Threatening and Non–Limb-Threatening Diabetic Foot Infections

Non–Limb-Threatening	Limb-Threatening
Less than 2 cm of surrounding cellulitis	Greater than 2 cm of surrounding cellulitis
No systemic toxicity signs	Deep abscess or osteomyelitis, gangrene
No deep abscess, osteomyelitis, gangrene	

1999). Research indicates that stratification is warranted to distinguish wounds with vascular insufficiency from those without. Prompers et al (2008) suggest that diabetic foot ulcers with and without PAD be classified as different disease states due to vastly different predictors of healing between diabetic wounds with and those without concomitant PAD.

One of the most important assessments at this stage is wound depth and, more importantly, presence of osteomyelitis, which is surprisingly common. It is found in approximately 60% of moderate to severe diabetic foot ulcers (Berendt et al, 2008; Eneroth et al, 1997). Bone biopsy gives a definitive diagnosis, but less invasive techniques are useful in establishing a diagnosis with a high degree of sensitivity and specificity. Appropriate diagnostic measures include probing the wound, serial x-ray films, magnetic resonance imaging, computed tomography, and radionuclide imaging (Steed et al, 2006). The ulcer normally is examined with a blunt sterile probe. Either direct exposure of bone or a positive "probe to bone" test is used to determine the presence of osteomyelitis (Steed et al, 2006). Probing can also detect sinus tract formations and undermining along the ulcer margins (Frykberg, 2002). X-ray studies are inexpensive, readily available, and useful for *excluding* an inflammatory process such as osteomyelitis. However, evidence of changes on x-ray films generally take about 2 weeks after bone infection, giving x-ray films a sensitivity of approximately 55% (Sinacore and Mueller, 2008a). Magnetic resonance imaging offers high-resolution views not only of bone but also of soft tissue; has a sensitivity and specificity of greater than 90% and 80%, respectively; and, therefore, tends to be the diagnostic procedure of choice.

MANAGEMENT

The level of expertise and knowledge required to manage LEND and diabetic foot ulcers is constantly increasing. Because of the complex nature of diabetic foot ulcers and the numerous comorbidities that can occur in patients with diabetes, a multidisciplinary team approach to management is recommended (ADA, 2007; Driver et al, 2005, 2010; Frykberg, 2002). An ideal foot care team should include the following: (1) podiatric/orthopedic surgeon, (2) vascular surgeon, (3) infectious disease specialist, (4) endocrinologist or family practice or internal medicine provider, (5) orthopedic/podiatric technician, (6) certified wound care nurse,

(7) orthotist, and (8) certified diabetes educator. Numerous references from the U.S. and European literature document improvements in patient outcomes, including reduction of lower extremity amputation rates, as a result of implementing a multidisciplinary approach to diabetic foot care (Driver et al, 2005; Meltzer et al, 2002; Muller et al, 2002; Sanders et al, 2010). Rates of avoidance of lower extremity amputation after implementation of a multidisciplinary team have been shown to be as high as 86.5% after 3 years and 83% after 5 years (Van Gils et al, 1999). However, health care providers frequently work in situations without this level and variety of expertise; thus patients with diabetes who develop a foot problem will often require referral to consultants. In fact, the standards of medical care in diabetes recommend the referral of high-risk patients to foot specialists for surveillance and preventative care (Bowen et al, 2015; Driver et al, 2005).

Diabetic neuropathy is associated with a reduced blood supply to the nerves, a microcirculatory network called the *vasa nervosum*. Currently, no prescription therapy in the United States is approved for treatment of the underlying process of microvascular damage that leads to diabetic peripheral neuropathy, although lowering of HbA1c levels has been shown to decrease the microvascular complications of diabetes (ADA, 2007; Fowler, 2008). Research has demonstrated that capillary vascular perfusion is inversely correlated with the degree of peripheral neuropathy (Nabuurs-Franssen et al, 2002). Nerve ischemia leads to poor nerve function. Based on earlier research in which certain prostacyclins (vasodilators) or their analogs gained approval for treatment of critical limb ischemia in Europe, Remodulin (treprostinil) is being tested in patients with diabetes and neuropathic ulcers. Mohler et al (2000) demonstrated that treatment significantly increased lower limb blood flow in these patients. Furthermore, the study done by Berman et al (2006) showed 62% reduction in mean worst rest pain during use of this medication. The study was open label and it suggested that further controlled studies are needed.

Another new area of investigation for neuropathy treatment of the patient with diabetes involves the enzyme protein kinase C-beta (PKC-β). Current hypotheses concerning the pathogenesis of diabetic neuropathy suggest that PKC-β (which is stimulated by hyperglycemia) may be involved in the process that leads to microvascular dysfunction, impairment of endoneural blood flow, and damage of nerves (Vinik et al, 2005). The PKC-β inhibitor LY333531 (Eli Lilly) is currently being tested and has shown encouraging results in improving DPN (Vinik et al, 2005). Advancements in gene therapy have shown promise as potential treatments of diabetic complications such as neuropathy and neuropathic wounds, and research continues to broaden our understanding of the biochemical and molecular bases of diabetes and associated complications (Driver and LeBretton, 2008; Park et al, 2013).

Early Intervention (Prevention)

Careful and frequent inspection of the diabetic foot is the most effective and least expensive method for preventing diabetic foot ulcers and possibly lower extremity amputations. Abnormalities, whether age related, structural, or pathologic, can be assessed and documented. The ADA (2007) and Boulton et al (2008) recommend patients with a low-risk foot ulcer (no loss of protective sensation, no PAD, no deformity) with well-controlled diabetes undergo a comprehensive annual foot examination.

At least 50% of all amputations due to diabetic neuropathy are preventable with early intervention (Reiber et al, 1995). Given the life-altering and life-threatening risks associated with the development of a diabetic foot ulcer, it is incumbent upon the health care professional to identify patients with lower extremity peripheral neuropathy as early as possible so that preventive interventions can be implemented. Preventive interventions for the patient with LEND must become a routine that the patient incorporates into everyday life. Specific instructions concerning inspection of the foot, bathing, nail care, care of corns and calluses, shoes, socks, and circulation should be enforced in writing and verbally as outlined in Box 14-5. Clearly, one of the most important components of the clinician's role is providing patient education.

Using the patient's foot risk classification, a management plan (i.e., education, diagnostic studies, footwear recommendations, referrals, and follow-up visits) can be developed in order to minimize the odds of developing a foot ulcer (Driver, 2004). Tables 14-2 and 14-3 list programs that correlate specific preventive interventions with each level of risk. Implementing these early interventions and adhering to preventive interventions (e.g., over-the-counter moisturizing cream to moisturize the foot and inspecting the shoe before putting it on) address the first two principles of wound management (i.e., control or eliminate causative factors, and provide systemic support to reduce existing and potential cofactors).

Glycemic Control

In 2010 approximately 7 million people in the United States were undiagnosed with diabetes (CDC, 2011). A similar percentage of people admitted to the hospital for treatment also have undiagnosed diabetes. A study by Umpierrez et al (2002) documented that 31% of persons with diabetes admitted to an urban hospital had no known history of the condition and were diagnosed during their stay.

Inadequate glycemic control is key in the development of neuropathy in the extremities of the person with diabetes (Steed et al, 2006). Hyperglycemia results in leukocyte dysfunction and suppression of lymphocytes, high blood pressure, and impaired endothelial function, among other dangers. Because of their impaired immune response, persons with hyperglycemia will respond poorly to a severe foot infection. Armstrong et al (1996) found that 56% of persons being admitted for diabetic foot infections had normal white blood cell counts. Improved blood glucose levels will increase the immune defenses of patients and thus should be a component of clinical care of infected diabetic foot ulcers. Elevated HbA1c levels in a

patient with diabetes who is infected may be the only sign alerting the provider to the problem (Frykberg, 2003). Thus patients with diabetes must be managed with a high index of suspicion for soft tissue infection, deep space infection, and osteomyelitis.

Offloading

Offloading and redistributing pressure is a basic principle involved in the prevention of foot ulcers and lower extremity amputations, as well as the healing of existing diabetic foot ulcers. Numerous books, references, and websites discuss the various offloading modalities used for patients with diabetic foot ulcers or at risk for developing foot ulcers. Orthotists and pedorthists are frequently consulted for assistance in managing foot problems. Orthotists and pedorthists are trained specifically to make and fit orthopedic footwear (and other appliances) that can accommodate the patient with diabetes. Table 15-5 lists various methods and considerations for offloading the foot. Options for offloading include bed rest, wheelchairs, crutches, surgical shoes, custom sandals, healing shoes, cast shoes, and foam dressings (Steed et al, 2006). The following section discusses total-contact casts, removable cast walkers (RCWs), felted foam dressings (FFDs), orthotics and orthopedic footwear, and surgical offloading procedures.

The total-contact cast (TCC) has been shown to be very effective at relieving pressure and healing diabetic foot ulcers. The cast is designed to equalize pressure loading of the plantar surface by equal "total contact" of the plantar skin with the cast material (Figure 14-5). Repetitive injury to the wound site is reduced while the patient ambulates. Epidemiologic studies have shown that TCC healing rates are between 73% and 100%, with healing times between 30 and 63 days (Bus et al, 2008). A study of the histologic features of patients undergoing ulcerectomy after 20 days in a TCC versus

FIGURE 14-5 Modified total-contact cast applied to offload pressure from neuropathic plantar ulcer that developed after prolonged use of a multipodus boot. A window around the wounds allows dressing changes without cast removal. The cutout portion of the cast is secured with self-adhering wrap. (Courtesy Ted Tomter, RN, CWOCN, St. Joseph's Candler Health System, Savannah, Ga.)

patients undergoing ulcerectomy at presentation showed marked increases in granulation and angiogenesis in the TCC group (Piagessi et al, 2003). Total-contact casts are absolutely contraindicated for patients with acute deep infection, sepsis, or gangrene. Relative contraindications include patients with ulcers with depth greater than width, fragile skin, or excessive edema; noncompliant patients; and those who would be unstable with a cast (Sinacore and Mueller, 2008b).

A test of the effectiveness of TCCs, RCWs, and half-shoes in healing neuropathic diabetic foot ulcers demonstrated that patients with a TCC had significantly better healing rates at 12 weeks than did patients treated with the other two offloading modalities. Interestingly, patients with a TCC were significantly less active than were patients with half-shoes. No activity difference was noted between patients with the TCC and those with the RCW (Armstrong et al, 2001). Armstrong et al (2003a) devised an activity test for patients with diabetic foot ulcers wearing RCWs. Total daily activity was recorded per patient. In addition, unbeknown to patients, the daily activity of the RCW also was recorded. Results showed that patients wore the RCW only 28% of the time.

A study of 50 patients with neuropathic foot ulcerations compared healing rates of wounds offloaded with RCW to wounds offloaded with RCW wrapped with a cohesive bandage. Results showed that the wounds offloaded with the RCW wrapped with a cohesive bandage healed significantly sooner ($p < .05$) than did those with only the RCW, which could be removed more easily (Armstrong et al, 2005a). These studies suggest that protective footwear that is less easily removed may increase the odds of healing

diabetic foot ulcers by increasing patient compliance. Interestingly, a 2008 study showed that only 1.7% of the 895 clinical respondents used a TCC as a treatment modality for diabetic foot ulcer and 45.5% reported no use of a TCC. Patient tolerance and application requirements were the predominant reasons indicated for lack of TCC use (Wu et al, 2008).

Often described as a "poor man's TCC," the felted foam dressing (FFD) has been shown to provide the offloading benefits of a TCC while allowing appropriate management of patients with typical contraindications (Figure 14-6). A 2001 report from German researchers indicates that an FFD reduces plantar loading at the ulcer site while allowing for daily dressing changes (Zimny et al, 2001b). Whether used as an adjunct to a surgical shoe, a healing shoe, or a walking splint, an FFD has been found to be equally as effective as a TCC in time to healing and healing proportion (Birke et al, 2002). An FFD requires less skill to apply and reduces or eliminates some of the inherent challenges and risks of a TCC, such as limited assessment ability (Wu et al, 2008) and edema-related compromise. An FFD helps to foster compliance levels while eliminating the bulk and relative immobility of TCCs. It also allows for direct offloading of a diabetic foot ulcer while permitting the use of orthotics to meet concurrent offloading needs. When felted foam is being applied, all edges must be beveled to prevent improper redistribution of forces (edge effect).

PPT and Plastazote (foam) inserts, custom-molded foot beds, and molded orthotics such as the Charcot restraint orthotic walker (CROW) (Figure 14-7) shoe modifications are the predominant methods of pressure management in the patients with diabetes (Figure 14-8) (Wu et al, 2008). Patients

FIGURE 14-6 A, Felted foam applied to plantar aspect of foot to decrease loading forces directly over an ulcer. **B,** Foam secured in place using cloth mesh tape and rubber cement. A cutout is made in the tape to allow for dressing changes between office visits. **C,** Felted foam dressing with concurrent dressing applied. Gauze roll is used to further secure the dressing in place and then is covered in a sock or stockinette. (Courtesy J. LeBretton and V. Driver.)

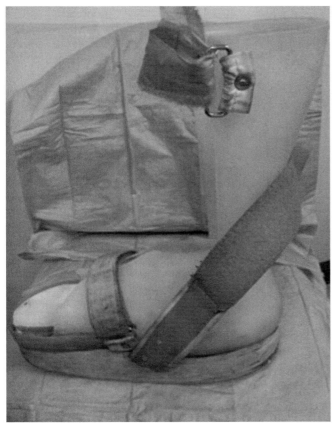

FIGURE 14-7 Customized removable offloading walker (Charcot restraint orthotic walker) boot. (Courtesy J. LeBretton and V. Driver.)

FIGURE 14-8 Custom-molded shoe for a transmetatarsal amputation. (Courtesy J. LeBretton and V. Driver.)

who used a Plastazote arch filler in conjunction with an RCW showed healing of recalcitrant plantar ulcers within 4 months (Ritz et al, 1996). Patients who used various foam inlays applied to their shoes and rocker-bottom outsoles demonstrated a reduction in peak plantar pressures (Praet and Louwerens, 2003).

Offloading can also be achieved with prophylactic and corrective surgical procedures such as Achilles tendon lengthening, sometimes referred to as tendo-Achilles lengthening (TAL); joint arthroplasty; and excision or resection of bony prominences. Patients who may be considered for TAL include those with peripheral neuropathy and equinus contracture. Equinus causes high forefoot pressure that contributes to plantar surface ulceration (LaBorde, 2003). A randomized clinical trial of patients with plantar diabetic foot ulcers compared TCC with and TCC without TAL. The study showed that all ulcers in the TAL plus TCC group healed with a risk of recurrence that was 75% less at 7 months and 52% less at 2 years than in the TCC-only treatment group (Mueller et al, 2003). However, a follow-up to this study found that patients who had undergone the TAL plus TCC procedure had decreased physical functioning compared with the TCC-only patients after 8 months (Mueller et al, 2004). Although joint arthroplasty in combination with TCC showed no difference in healing proportions compared with TCC alone, significantly shorter healing time was observed in the arthroplasty group (Armstrong et al, 2003b; Lin et al, 2003). Metatarsal head resection has also been demonstrated to shorten healing time compared with a control group (Armstrong et al, 2005b). Increases in pressure in other areas of the foot have been observed with metatarsal head resection, necessitating a multidisciplinary approach and accommodative orthotics or other offloading to compensate for changes in pressure and to support prevention of new, recurrent, or recalcitrant ulceration.

Structural Foot Deformities. The traditional treatment for Charcot arthropathy (without ulceration) is cast immobilization. Few patients require surgery for this condition; however, exostectomy has been shown to be an appropriate method of treatment of Charcot prominences (Catanzariti et al, 2000) should nonsurgical interventions fail. Before immobilization, compression bandages are applied at weekly intervals until all edema has subsided. This period can last 2 to 3 weeks. A short non–weight-bearing cast is generally required for 12 to 16 weeks. The cast can be changed one or more times during this period. Gradual weight bearing is started when the surface of the skin has returned to near-normal temperature (Yu and Hudson, 2002). Noninvasive bone stimulation such as electrostimulation can be a valuable adjunctive treatment of Charcot arthropathy (Grady et al, 2000). If edema and inflammation persist, administration of pamidronate is recommended to prevent further deterioration (Guis et al, 1999). Table 14-9 lists the healing phases of Charcot foot.

Wound Management

The principles of wound management and goals of topical therapy are described in Chapter 18. Jeffcoate and Harding (2003) listed the following priorities specifically for treating diabetic foot wounds: (1) aggressively treat infections; (2) establish whether ischemia is present and revascularization is required; (3) relieve pressure to the wound; and

TABLE 14-9 Healing Phases of Charcot Foot

Clinical Presentation	Dissolution Phase	Coalescence Phase	Remodeling Phase
Edema	May be profound	Decreased	Decreased
Erythema	May be severe	Generally absent	Generally absent
Temperature compared with contralateral foot	May be increased 3° C to 7° C	Generally more than compared with 2° C increased	Generally less than compared with 2° C increased
X-ray image	May demonstrate fractures, dislocations, subluxations May not show abnormality during earliest acute phase of injury	May demonstrate early consolidation, formation of bone callus	Demonstrates consolidation stability

From Crawford PE, Fields-Varnado M, WOCN Society: Guideline for the management of wounds in patients with lower-extremity neuropathic disease, *J Wound Ostomy Continence Nurs.* 40(1):34-45, 2012.

(4) improve the wound condition by debridement, dressings, and advanced care treatments where appropriate. Ultimately, the principal goal in the treatment of diabetic foot ulcers is wound closure.

Debridement and Callus Management. Wound and callus debridement is integral in the management of diabetic foot wounds. Key benefits of debridement in the diabetic wound include removal of free-living bacteria and biofilms, stimulation of growth factors, removal of senescent cells, and removal of hyperproliferative nonmigratory tissue (i.e., callus) (Steed et al, 2006). Serial debridement of wounds for the first 4 weeks of treatment has been shown to reduce median wound area by as much as 54% compared with wounds not undergoing serial debridement. Notably, this was the first study to evaluate healing rates and debridement across multiple chronic wound etiologies (Cardinal et al, 2009). Methods of debridement may change over time or may be performed in combination as conditions change. Debridement is repeated as often as needed, depending on the formation of new necrotic tissue (Wilcox et al, 2013). Weekly debridement is common and is generally referred to as *maintenance debridement* (Steed et al, 2006).

Hyperkeratotic callus buildup is frequently seen in the patient with diabetes due to the drying effects of autonomic dysfunction secondary to neuropathy and the natural response to repetitive minor trauma over pressure points. The callus development increases peak plantar pressures, fostering hematoma development and ulceration. A vicious circle is created in which high pressure causes callus buildup, which in turn leads to higher pressures and further callus development. Callus management is integral in the prevention and treatment of diabetic foot ulcer. Callus removal (see Plates 40 and 41) should be performed regularly and combined with effective orthotics or shoe modifications to better distribute pressures and prevent callus buildup. Supportive therapy, such as daily application of moisturizer, will assist in counteracting decreases in skin oil production seen in the patient with diabetes who has neuropathy.

Traditionally, callus has been removed by means of a scalpel or tissue nipper, but difficulty in smoothing the edges of the callus where tissue has been removed can result in areas of micropressure. Rotary files use a small drum covered with sandpaper or various burrs spun at rates of 1000 to 3000 rpm. Due to the high revolution, rotary files allow the skilled clinician to "shape" the callus rather than excise hyperkeratotic tissue, which can create minute pressure points and a potential portal of entry for infection. Removal of dry hyperkeratotic tissue decreases pressure and can reveal ulcerations and undermining of tissue under the callus that otherwise would not be visible.

When selecting a specific method of debridement of diabetic foot ulcers, many factors must be considered: pain, arterial insufficiency, antiembolic medications, patient setting, resources, characteristics of the wound, and the type of debridement. Methods of debridement and factors to consider for selection are discussed in detail in Chapter 17.

Considerations specific to patients with LEND and diabetic foot ulcers are highlighted by the ADA and the WOCN® Society:

- Revascularization and surgical removal of necrotic tissue from an infected wound on an ischemic leg or foot is the treatment of choice for limb salvage.
- All ulcers with extensive cellulitis and/or osteomyelitis should be debrided and referred for pharmacologic (intravenous) intervention.
- Evidence supporting the use of whirlpool or pulsatile jet irrigation in neuropathic ulcers is insufficient.
- Caution must be exercised to prevent immersion burns from whirlpools because of reduced sensitivity in the neuropathic leg.
- Maintain dry, stable eschar on noninfected, ischemic, neuropathic wounds.

Infection. The assessment and treatment of infection is discussed in detail in Chapter 16. The classification of the infection, allergies, medical condition of the patient, and culture results (often not available initially) usually guide antibiotic therapy (Frykberg, 2003). The ADA (1999) and Lipsky et al (2012) cite categories of infection for the patient with diabetes as limb-threatening infections, non–limb-threatening infections, and osteomyelitis.

No antibiotics are recommended for the patient with an ulcer that is not clinically infected. However, remember that the patient with diabetes often does not show common symptoms of infection and thus must be monitored closely. Limb-threatening infections (see Table 14-8) require immediate hospitalization. Additional conditions of limb-threatening infections may include necrotizing fasciitis, ischemia, hyperglycemia, and leukocytosis (ADA, 1999; Berendt et al, 1997; Frykberg, 2003).

Patients with non–limb-threatening infections require immediate antibiotic therapy, generally beginning the same day as the diagnosis is made. For mild and most moderate infections, therapy can be an oral agent, although certain patients may require parenteral therapy. Commonly used oral agents include cephalexin, clindamycin, levofloxacin, and amoxicillin/clavulanate (Lipsky, 2012). Trovafloxacin is appropriate for polymicrobial infections. Patients with mild or moderate infections may be treated on an outpatient basis, but only if certain criteria are met. Those who require surgical procedures, multiple diagnostic tests, or consultations or who are immunocompromised may be better treated and evaluated in a brief hospitalization.

Patients with limb-threatening infections need to be hospitalized and treated parenterally with antibiotics. Empirical therapy for these infections should be broad in spectrum, including aerobic, gram-positive, and gram-negative organisms, as well as resistant organisms. Examples of antibiotic therapies include imipenem/cilastatin or vancomycin plus aztreonam plus metronidazole. Antibiotics should be reassessed when culture results are available.

Healing osteomyelitis with antibiotics alone is difficult but possible. Treatment usually lasts 6 weeks or more, often with 1 to 2 weeks of parenteral therapy. Infected bones that can be easily resected should be removed to speed recovery and reduce the need for antibiotic therapy (Steed et al, 2006). Additional regimens for treating diabetic foot infections can be found in the new international consensus guidelines for diagnosing and treating infected diabetic feet (Lipsky et al, 2012; Richard et al, 2011).

Methicillin-resistant *Staphylococcus aureus* (MRSA) and other resistant bacteria are a major challenge in the treatment of diabetic foot ulcer infections (Frykberg, 2003). Using data from a multihospital study in the United States, Pfaller et al (2001) reported that the percentage of MRSA of all *S. aureus* isolates increased from 22% to 34% from 1997 to 2000. In Korea, the number of MRSA cases was found to be 32% in 2008 and then it rebounded back to 63.7% in 2011 (Huh et al, 2013). Vancomycin or linezolid is frequently prescribed for the control of MRSA. Vancomycin-resistant *S. aureus* (VRSA), the evolution of MRSA in response to current practices in antibiotic therapy, has been reported (Tenover, 2006; Tenover et al, 2004).

Topical Wound Care. Evidence does not support the use of one dressing over the other for the treatment of diabetic foot ulcers (WOCN®, 2012). Topical therapy for diabetic foot ulcers is based on the principles outlined in Chapter 18, and a formulary of multiple dressing options will be necessary to meet the needs of the wound as its characteristics (e.g., size, depth, exudate) change.

The increase in bacterial resistance to antibiotics has changed how some clinicians view the use of topical antimicrobials.

There is a lack of consensus on the use of topical antimicrobial therapy for infected or ischemic neuropathic ulcers (WOCN®, 2012). A short course of a topical antimicrobial may be considered if the ulcer has a high level of bacteria (Steed et al, 2006; WOCN®, 2012). However, wounds treated with topical antimicrobials can develop resistant organisms over time. Topical creams, ointments, and gels containing antimicrobials may also cause sensitivity reactions.

Advanced care has been described as "the use of drugs, devices, or treatment regimens that may be experimental, newly approved, or above and beyond treatment modalities routinely used in the general community for a specific medical problem." Advanced care may sometimes be the only means of rapidly and effectively attaining wound closure (Mulder et al, 2003). Diabetic foot ulcers that are limb threatening (based on ADA criteria) and require hospitalization, antibiotics, and debridement may not progress to this level (or any further) if early advanced care interventions are made. Early, advanced, or "appropriate" care practices may be more cost-effective than standard care practices in decreasing the incidence of lower extremity amputations (Apelqvist et al, 1995; Warriner and Driver, 2006).

When confronted with a wound that fails to progress, the clinician must carefully reevaluate the entire treatment plan to ensure appropriateness and should consider biopsy to rule out malignancy. If the biopsy result is negative and the management plan is appropriate, the most likely reason for failure to heal is the negative cellular environment of a chronic wound. In this case the clinician should consider implementing an interactive wound therapy, that is, a product or therapy designed to convert the chronic wound environment into an environment that supports repair (Driver, 2004). Specific therapies that have shown varying degrees of success in the management of diabetic foot ulcers include contact and noncontact ultrasound technologies, regenerative tissue matrix, electrical stimulation, negative pressure wound therapy, hyperbaric oxygen therapy, angiogenic stimulators, and protease inhibitors (Cullen et al, 2002; Driver and Fabbi, 2009; Driver and LeBretton, 2008; Park et al, 2013; Steed et al, 2006). These therapies are discussed in Chapters 18 through 24.

Pain Control

A variety of interventions can be used for the treatment of neuropathic pain; management of pain is presented in Chapter 26. In some cases, referral of the patient to a pain clinic and to neurologists for pain management may be necessary (WOCN®, 2012).

Education

Basic knowledge assessment of patients with diabetes, regardless of the length of time since their diagnosis, often reveals a lack of understanding about the principles of diabetes self-management. Education must be relevant, simple, complete, and ongoing in order to assist the patient to achieve and maintain the highest possible level of functioning. However, education does not equal knowledge. Achieving understanding often requires presentation of material multiple times in different formats and by different health care team members.

Key components of the patient's education plan require behavioral change on the part of the patient, which can leave the patient feeling overwhelmed. The inability of the patient to follow through with a treatment plan should be carefully scrutinized and explored. The patient's behavior should not be assumed to be intentional, nor should the patient be erroneously labeled as "noncompliant," as many factors can contribute to an individual's ability to succeed or fail in the treatment plan. Key among these factors is expecting the patient to implement a therapy that he or she is physically unable to perform or that conflicts with another activity in his or her life. Probably the best advice to health care professionals was provided by Heisler et al (2002, 2007), who stated that to facilitate patients' self-management, there is a need for a paradigm shift in the relations between provider and patients from directive to a more collaborative interactive style in which problems, treatment goals, and management stratagems are defined together. Strategies for achieving a sustainable plan are discussed further in Chapter 29.

Studies have documented the success of diabetes and foot care education in reducing the incidence of diabetic foot ulcers (Al-Wahbi 2010; Dargis et al, 1999; Ollendorf et al, 1998). However, many of the studies documenting success of educational efforts at reducing diabetic foot problems compared comprehensive programs that may not exist in more operational settings. In real-world situations, both patients and providers face significant challenges in the areas of diabetes and diabetic foot care education. A study in south Texas showed contextual factors such as time constraints, practice economics, and low reimbursement rather than physician knowledge and attitude affected caregivers' performance in delivering diabetes care education. The study also found that patients with a lower income had a decreased awareness of diabetic care principles (Larme and Pugh, 2001).

Appropriate measures should be implemented for patients who have limited mobility, cognitive problems, and visual difficulties. Other family members or friends can assist with visual assessments. Many patients diagnosed with diabetes participate in general diabetes self-management education programs through their primary health care provider (ADA, 2014). Some clinics include a preexamination and a postexamination test on diabetes and foot care knowledge, providing an opportunity to build on the patient's knowledge base. The test is scored at the time of the visit, and the patient is told that the test will be repeated at the end of the visit.

It is imperative that patients understand the importance of daily foot examinations, the implications of losing protective sensation, their risk for ulceration and amputation, and the methods for minimizing or eliminating factors that place them at risk for ulceration and amputation. Box 14-5 provides an example of general foot care instructions that can be given to patients (Steed et al, 2006).

Teaching appropriate footwear selection is essential. All patients need to pay special attention to the fit and style of their shoes. Shoes need to fit the foot, so patients should avoid tight-fitting shoes, pointed-toe or open-toe shoes, flip-flops, and high heels. The shoes should be able to breathe; plastic shoes are inelastic and do not breathe. Finally, shoes should be adjustable with hook and loop closures, laces, or buckles. Shoes with soft insoles that cushion the feet may do well at reducing plantar pressure, but injury to the dorsum may result if the upper part of the shoes does not fit when the insole is inserted (Cavanagh and Ulbrecht, 2008).

CLINICAL CONSULT

A: Referral received for wound care consult for a 50-year-old male with diabetes presenting with a large demarcated ulceration on the posterior aspect of the plantar surface of the right calcaneous. Patient's type 1 diabetes first diagnosed at age 15 and appears to have overall good level of knowledge of DM and self-care needs. Lower leg without edema, hair present, warm to touch, all pedal pulses palpable. Small amount of callous present lateral to ulceration and over plantar surface of first metatarsal head. Loss of protective sensation present (0/10 with monofilament testing both feet). Reports walking barefoot in his home and in yard; often does not wear socks. Has never seen a podiatrist or foot specialist. Three days ago a rock fell out of his shoe as it was being removed and he discovered a large, red, open wound on the bottom of his foot. Ulcer measures 4 × 3 cm × 1 cm. Wound base is 90% red, viable tissue with 10% yellow slough. No surrounding erythema or callous; minimal exudate present. Dry gauze in place over wound and adherent to wound bed.

D: Neuropathic diabetic foot ulcer in patient with high risk diabetes; ulceration due to undetected object in shoe.

P: Promote moist wound healing, stimulate cellular activity, avoid repetitive stress and trauma to ulcer site, review essentials of foot care in insensate feet; refer to foot specialists to assess for appropriate foot wear and provide ongoing routine monitoring.

I: (1) Review teaching materials for "Care of the Diabetic Foot" to include foot inspection before applying and after removing shoes, daily washing and drying well between toes, routine and appropriate nail care, no "bare-feet," and wear cotton socks. (2) Foot specialist to recommend appropriate foot wear after ulcer heals. (3) TBI while in clinic and if >0.5 will notify mid-level provider to proceed with sharp debridement. (4) Initiate platelet derived growth factor (becaplermin) 7 inches (length × width × 0.6) to cover wound bed, cover with normal saline moistened gauze, then telfa and secure with roll gauze. Apply becaplermin at 7 PM. Remove at 7 AM, rinse wound and apply hydrogel impregnated gauze covered with telfa, secure with island dressing. (5) Return to Bry-Nix Wound Clinic weekly to monitor for changes and debride as needed. (6) No weight bearing on right heel to protect ulcer from stress/friction. (7) Consult with PT to address ambulation needs. May use crutches.

E: Monitor wound dimensions weekly; anticipate at least 30% reduced size by week 10 and healed by week 20. Will reevaluate need for contact cast if unable to adequately offload wound site or healing slower than anticipated.

SUMMARY

Peripheral neuropathy, structural foot problems, and minor trauma are the primary causative factors for a diabetic foot ulcer in the patient with LEND, and 25% of patients with a diabetic foot ulcer require lower extremity amputation. The ultimate goals of care of the patient with LEND and a diabetic foot ulcer are to reduce the incidence of lower extremity amputations and to increase the frequency of minor or partial foot amputations as a percentage of all lower extremity amputations. A team approach is required for comprehensive management of the patient with LEND to adequately address the complex needs of this patient population: prevention of injury or trauma, frequent inspection, diligent daily foot care, education and support, and appropriate offloading (i.e., use of shoes and orthotics).

REFERENCES

Abbott CA, Carrington AL, Ashe H, et al: The North-West Diabetes Foot Care Study: incidence of, and risk factors for, new diabetic-foot ulceration in a community-based patient cohort, *Diabetes Med* 19(5):377–384, 2002.

Alavi A, Sibbald RG, Mayer D, et al: Diabetic foot ulcers: Part 1: pathophysiology and prevention, *J Am Acad Dermatol* 70(1): e1–e18, 2014.

Al-Wahbi AM: Impact of a diabetic foot care education program on lower limb amputation rate, *Vasc Health Risk Manage* 6: 923–934, 2010.

American Academy of Pediatrics: *Management of newly diagnosed type 2 diabetes mellitus (T2DM) in children and adolescents,* 2013. http://www.pediatrics.org/content/131/2/364.full. Accessed January 28, 2013.

American Diabetes Association (ADA): Consensus Development Conference on Diabetic Foot Wound Care, 7-8 April 1999, Boston, Mass, *Diabetes Care* 22(8):1354–1360, 1999.

American Diabetes Association (ADA): Standards of medical care in diabetes—2007, *Diabetes Care* 30(Suppl 1):S4–S41, 2007.

American Diabetes Association (ADA): Comprehensive foot examination and risk assessment, *Diabetes Care* 31(8):1679–1685, 2008a.

American Diabetes Association (ADA): Economic costs of diabetes in the U.S. in 2007, *Diabetes Care* 31(3):596–615, 2008b.

American Diabetes Association (ADA): Standards of medical care in diabetes, *Diabetes Care* 37(Suppl 1):S14–S80, 2014.

Apelqvist J, Larsson J: What is the most effective way to reduce incidence of amputation in diabetic foot? *Diabetes Metab Res Rev* 16(Suppl 1):S75–S83, 2000.

Apelqvist J, Ragnarson-Tennvall G, Larsson J, et al: Long-term costs for foot ulcers in diabetic patients in a multidisciplinary setting, *Foot Ankle Int* 16:388–394, 1995.

Armstrong DG, Lavery LA, Harkless LB: Validation of a diabetic wound classification system: the contribution of depth, infection, and ischemia to risk of amputation, *Diabetes Care* 21(5):855–859, 1998.

Armstrong DG, Lavery LA, Kimbriel HR, et al: Activity patterns with diabetic foot ulceration: patients with active ulceration may not adhere to a standard pressure off-loading regimen, *Diabetes Care* 26(9):2595–2597, 2003a.

Armstrong DG, Lavery LA, Vazquez JR, et al: Clinical efficacy of the first metatarsophalangeal joint arthroplasty as a curative procedure for hallux interphalangeal joint wounds in patients with diabetes, *Diabetes Care* 26(12):3284–3287, 2003b.

Armstrong DG, Lavery LA, Wu S, et al: Evaluation of removable and irremovable cast walkers in the healing of diabetic foot wounds: a randomized controlled trial, *Diabetes Care* 28(3):551–554, 2005a.

Armstrong DG, Lavery LA, Wunderlich RP, et al: Skin temperatures as a one-time screening tool do not predict future diabetic foot complications, *J Am Podiatr Med Assoc* 93(6):443–447, 2003b.

Armstrong DG, Nguyen HC, Lavery LA, et al: Off-loading the diabetic foot wound: a randomized clinical trial, *Diabetes Care* 24(6):1019–1022, 2001.

Armstrong DG, Perales TA, Murff RT, et al: Value of white blood cell count with differential in the acute diabetic foot infection, *J Am Podiatr Med Assoc* 86(5):224–227, 1996.

Armstrong DG, Rosales MA, Gashi A: Efficacy of fifth metatarsal head resection for treatment of chronic diabetic foot ulceration, *J Am Podiatr Med Assoc* 95(4):353–356, 2005b.

Aulivola B, Hile CN, Hamdan AD, et al: Major lower extremity amputation: outcome of a modern series, *Arch Surg* 139(4): 395–399, 2004.

Ball JW, Dains, JE, Flynn JA: Musculoskeletal system. In *Seidel's guide to physical examination,* ed 8, St. Louis, MO, 2015, Mosby.

Berendt AR, Peters EJ, Bakker K, et al: Diabetic foot osteomyelitis: a progress report on diagnosis and a systematic review of treatment, *Diabetes Metab Res Rev* 24(Suppl 1):S145–S161, 2008.

Berman S, Quick R, Yoder P, et al: Treprostinil sodium (Remodulin), a prostacyclin analog, in the treatment of critical limb ischemia: open-label study, *Vascular* 14(3):142–148, 2006.

Birke JA, Pavich MA, Patout CA Jr, et al: Comparison of forefoot ulcer healing using alternative off-loading methods in patients with diabetes mellitus, *Adv Skin Wound Care* 15(5):210–215, 2002.

Boulton AJM: Pressure and the diabetic foot: clinical science and offloading techniques, *Am J Surg* 187(5A):17S–24S, 2004.

Boulton AJM, Armstrong DG, Albert SF, et al: Comprehensive foot examination and risk assessment: a report of the Task Force of the Foot Care Interest Group of the American Diabetes Association, with endorsement by the American Association of Clinical Endocrinologists, *Diabetes Care* 31(8):1679–1685, 2008.

Boulton AJM, Vilekyte L, Ragnarson-Tennvall G, et al: The global burden of diabetic foot disease, *Lancet* 366:1719–1724, 2005.

Bowen GC: *screening and treatment of early complications in the diabetic foot, management of diabetic foot complications,* In Shearman C.P (ED) Management of Diabetic Foot Complications Springr-Verlag London 2015, pp 9–22.

Bowker JH, Pfeifer MA: *Levin and O'Neal's the diabetic foot,* ed 6, St. Louis, MO, 2001, Mosby.

Bus SA, Valk GD, van Deursen RW, et al: The effectiveness of footwear and offloading interventions to prevent and heal foot ulcers and reduce plantar pressure in diabetes: a systematic review, *Diabetes Metab Res Rev* 24(Suppl 1):S162–S180, 2008.

Cardinal M, Eisenbud DE, Armstrong DG, et al: Serial surgical debridement: a retrospective study on clinical outcomes in chronic lower extremity wounds, *Wound Repair Regen* 17(3):306–311, 2009.

Caselli A, Pham H, Giurini JM, et al: The forefoot-to-rearfoot plantar pressure ratio is increased in severe diabetic neuropathy and can predict foot ulceration, *Diabetes Care* 25(6):1066–1071, 2002.

Catanzariti AR, Mendicino R, Haverstock B: Ostectomy for diabetic neuroarthropathy involving the midfoot, *J Foot Ankle Surg* 39(5):291–300, 2000.

Cavanagh PR, Ulbrecht JS: The biomechanics of the foot in diabetes mellitus. In Bowker JH, Pfeiffer MA, editors: *Levin and O'Neal's the diabetic foot*, ed 7, St. Louis, MO, 2008, Mosby.

Centers for Disease Control and Prevention (CDC): History of foot ulcer among persons with diabetes—United States, 2000–2002, *MMWR Morb Mortal Wkly Rep* 52(45):1098–1102, 2003.

Centers for Disease Control and Prevention: *Diabetes Report Card 2012.* Atlanta, GA: Centers for Disease Control and Prevention, U.S. Department of Health and Human Services, 2012. http://www.cdc.gov/diabetes/pubs/pdf/diabetesreportcard.pdf. Accessed April 27, 2015.

Centers for Disease Control and Prevention (CDC): *Age-adjusted hospital discharge rates per 1,000 diabetic population, by level of amputation, United States, 1993–2009*, 2014a. http://www.cdc.gov/diabetes/statistics/lealevel/fig8.htm. Accessed April 27, 2015.

Centers for Disease Control and Prevention (CDC): *Crude and age-adjusted hospital discharge rates for nontraumatic lower extremity amputation per 1,000 diabetic population, United States, 1988-2009*, 2014b. http://www.cdc.gov/diabetes/statistics/lea/fig3.htm. Accessed April 27, 2015.

Centers for Disease Control and Prevention (CDC): *Hospital discharge rates for nontraumatic lower extremity amputation per 1,000 diabetic population, by age, United States 1988-2009*, 2014c. http://www.cdc.gov/diabetes/statistics/lea/fig4.htm. Accessed April 27, 2015.

Centers for Disease Control and Prevention (CDC): *National diabetes fact sheet*, 2011. http://www.cdc.gov/diabetes/pubs/pdf/ndfs_2011.pdf. Accessed January 6, 2014.

Cofield RH, Morrison MJ, Beabout JW: Diabetic neuroarthropathy in the foot: patient characteristics and patterns of radiographic change, *Foot Ankle* 4(1):15–22, 1983.

Corey MR, St Julien J, Miller C, et al: Patient education level affects functionality and long term mortality after major lower extremity amputation, *Am J Surg* 204(5):626–630, 2012.

Cullen B, Smith R, McCulloch E, et al: Mechanism of action of PROMOGRAN, a protease modulating matrix, for the treatment of diabetic foot ulcers, *Wound Repair Regen* 10(1):16–25, 2002.

Dargis V, Pantelejeva O, Jonushaite A, et al: Benefits of a multidisciplinary approach in the management of recurrent diabetic foot ulceration in Lithuania: a prospective study, *Diabetes Care* 22(9):1428–1431, 1999.

Driver VR: Treating the macro and micro wound environment of the diabetic patient: managing the whole patient, not the hole in the patient, *Foot Ankle Q* 16(2):47–56, 2004.

Driver VR, Fabbi M: Recent advances in the use of ultrasound in wound care. In Sed CK, editor: *Advances in wound care,* vol 1, 2010, pp 550–555. Mary Ann Liebert, Inc. publishers New Rochelle, NY

Driver VR, Fabbi M, Lavery LA, et al: The costs of diabetic foot: the economic case for the limb salvage team, *J Vasc Surg* 52(3): 17S–22S, 2010.

Driver VR, LeBretton JM: "Gene therapy"-therapeutic angiogenesis—does it have an impact for wound healing and limb preservation? *Podiatry Today* 2008(August):74–78.

Driver VR, Madsen J, Goodman RA: Reducing amputation rates in patients with diabetes at a military medical center: the limb preservation service model, *Diabetes Care* 28(2):248–253, 2005.

Eneroth M, Apelqvist J, Stenström A: Clinical characteristics and outcome in 223 diabetic patients with deep foot infections, *Foot Ankle Int* 18(11):716–722, 1997.

Fosse S, Hartemann-Heurtier A, Jacqueminet S, et al: Incidence and characteristics of lower limb amputations in people with diabetes, *Diabet Med* 26:391–396, 2009.

Fowler MJ: Microvascular and macrovascular complications of diabetes, *Clin Diabetes* 26(2):77–82, 2008.

Frykberg RG: Diabetic foot ulcers: pathogenesis and management, *Am Fam Physician* 66:1655–1662, 2002.

Frykberg RG: An evidence-based approach to diabetic foot infections, *Am J Surg* 186(5A):44S–54S, 2003.

Frykberg RG, Zgonis T, Armstrong DG, et al: Diabetic foot disorders—a clinical practice guideline, *J Foot Ankle Surg* 45(Suppl 5):S1–S66, 2006.

Gerald YV, Hudson JR: Evaluation and treatment of stage 0 Charcot's neuroarthropathy of the foot and ankle, *J Am Podiatr Med Assoc* 92(4):210–220, 2002.

Grady JF, O'Connor KJ, Axe TM, et al: Use of electrostimulation in the treatment of diabetic neuropathy, *J Am Podiatr Med Assoc* 90(6):287–294, 2000.

Guis S, Pellissier JF, Arniaud D, et al: Healing of Charcot's joint by pamidronate infusion, *J Rheumatol* 26(8):1843–1845, 1999.

Harrington C, Zagari MJ, Corea J, et al: A cost analysis of diabetic lower-extremity ulcers, *Diabetes Care* 23(9):1333–1338, 2000.

Heisler M, Bouknight RR, Hayward RA, et al: The relative importance of physician communication, participatory decision making, and patient understanding in diabetes self-management, *J Gen Intern Med* 17(4):243–252, 2002.

Heisler M, Cole I, Weir D, et al: Does physician communication influence older patients' diabetes self-management and glycemic control? *J Gerontol A Biol Sci Med Sci* 62 (12):1435–1442, 2007.

Hopf HW, Ueno C, Aslam R, et al: Guidelines for the treatment of arterial insufficiency ulcers, *Wound Repair Regen* 14(6):693–710, 2006.

Huh KM, Kim J, Cho SY, et al: Continuous increase of the antimicrobial resistance among gram-negative pathogens causing bacteremia: a nationwide surveillance study by the Korean Network for Study on Infectious Disease (KONSID), *Diagn Microbiol Infect Dis* 76:477–482, 2013.

Ince P, Abbas ZG, Lutale JK, et al: Use of the SINBAD classification system and score in comparing outcome of foot ulcer management on three continents, *Diabetes Care* 31(5): 964–967, 2008.

Jeffcoate WJ, Harding KG: Diabetic foot ulcers, *Lancet* 361(9368):1545–1551, 2003.

Joseph WS, Lipsky BA: Medical therapy of diabetic foot infection, *J Vasc Surg* 52(Suppl 3):S67–S71, 2010.

Jude EB, Oyibo SO, Chalmers N, et al: Peripheral arterial disease in diabetic and nondiabetic patients: a comparison of severity and outcome, *Diabetes Care* 24(8):1433–1437, 2001.

Laborde JM: Treatment of forefoot ulcers with tendon lengthenings, *J South Orthop Assoc* 12(2):60–65, 2003.

Larme AC, Pugh JA: Evidence-based guidelines meet the real world, *Diabetes Care* 24(10):1728–1733, 2001.

Larsson J, Agardh CD, Apelqvist J, et al: Long-term prognosis after healed amputations in patients with diabetes, *Clin Orthop Relat Res* 350:149–158, 1998.

Lavery LA: Preventing the first or recurrent ulcers, *Med Clin North Am* 97(5):807–820, 2013.

Lavery LA, Armstrong DG, Boulton AJ, et al: Ankle equinus deformity and its relationship to high plantar pressure in a large population with diabetes mellitus, *J Am Podiatr Med Assoc* 92(9):479–482, 2002.

Lavery LA, Armstrong DG, Harkless LB: Classification of diabetic foot wounds, *J Foot Ankle Surg* 35(6):528–531, 1996.

Lavery LA, Armstrong DG, Vela SA, et al: Practical criteria for screening patients at high risk for diabetic foot ulceration. *Arch Intern Med* 158:157–162, 1998.

Lavery LA, Armstrong DG, Wunderlich RP, et al: Diabetic foot syndrome: evaluating the prevalence and incidence of foot pathology in Mexican Americans and non-Hispanic whites from a diabetes disease management cohort, *Diabetes Care* 26(5):1435–1438, 2003.

Levin ME: Management of the diabetic foot: preventing amputation, *South Med J* 95(1):10–20, 2002.

Levy PJ: Epidemiology and pathophysiology of peripheral arterial disease, *Clin Cornerstone* 4(5):1–15, 2002.

Lin SS, Bono CM, Lee TH: Total contact casting and Keller arthroplasty for diabetic great toe ulceration under the interphalangeal joint, *Foot Ankle Int* 21:588–591, 2000.

Lipsky BA: A report from the international consensus on diagnosing and treating the infected diabetic foot, *Diabetes Metab Res Rev* 20(Suppl 1):S68–S77, 2004.

Lipsky BA, Berendt AR, Cornia PB, et al: 2012 Infectious Diseases Society of America clinical practice guideline for the diagnosis and treatment of diabetic foot infections, *Clin Infect Dis* 54(12):e132–e173, 2012.

Macfarlane R, Jeffcoate W: Classification of diabetic foot ulcers: the size (area and depth) (SAD) system, *Diabetic Foot* 2(4):123, 1999.

Maser RE, Steenkiste AR, Dorman JS, et al: Epidemiological correlates of diabetic neuropathy. Report from Pittsburg Epidemiology of Diabetes Complications Study, *Diabetes* 38(11):1456–1461, 1989.

Mayfield JA, Reiber GE, Maynard C, et al: Trends in lower limb amputation in the Veterans Health Administration, 1989–1998, *J Rehabil Res Dev* 37(1):23–30, 2000.

Meltzer DD, et al: Decreasing amputation rates in patients with diabetes mellitus. An outcome study, *J Am Podiatr Med Assoc* 92(8):425–428, 2002.

Mendes JJ, Neves J: Diabetic foot infections: current diagnosis and treatment, *J Diabet Foot Complications* 4(2):26–45, 2012.

Mohler ER 3rd, Klugherz B, Goldman R, et al: Trial of a novel prostacyclin analog, UT-15, in patients with severe intermittent claudication, *Vasc Med* 5(4):231–237, 2000.

Moulik PK, Mtonga R, Gill GV: Amputation and mortality in new-onset foot ulcers stratified by etiology, *Diabetes Care* 26(2):491–494, 2003.

Mueller MJ, Sinacore DR, Hastings MK, et al: Effect of Achilles tendon lengthening on neuropathic plantar ulcers. A randomized clinical trial, *J Bone Joint Surg Am* 85(8):1436–1445, 2003.

Mueller MJ, Sinacore DR, Hastings MK, et al: Impact of Achilles tendon lengthening on functional limitations and perceived disability in people with a neuropathic plantar ulcer, *Diabetes Care* 27(7):1559–1564, 2004.

Mulder G, Armstrong D, Seaman S: Standard, appropriate, and advanced care and medical-legal considerations. Part one—diabetic foot ulcerations, *Wounds* 15(4):92, 2003.

Muller IS, de Grauw WJ, van Gerwen WH, et al: Foot ulceration and lower limb amputation in type 2 diabetic patients in Dutch primary health care, *Diabetes Care* 25(3):570–574, 2002.

Murray HJ, Young MH, Hollis S, et al: The relationship between callus formation, high pressures and neuropathy in diabetic foot ulceration, *Diabet Med* 13:979–982, 1996.

Nabuurs-Franssen MH, Houben AJ, Tooke JE, et al: The effect of polyneuropathy on foot microcirculation in type II diabetes, *Diabetologia* 45(8):1164–1171, 2002.

Nathan DM, Buse JB, Davidson MB, et al: Medical management of hyperglycemia in type 2 diabetes: a consensus algorithm for the initiation and adjustment of therapy. A consensus statement of America Diabetes Association and the European Association for the Study of Diabetes, *Diabetes Care* 32(1):193–203, 2009.

National Diabetes Advisory Board: *The prevention and treatment of five complications of diabetes: a guide for primary care practitioners* (HHS publication no. 83-8392), Atlanta, GA, 1983, Centers for Disease Control.

National Institute of Neurological Disorders and Stroke (NINDS), National Institutes of Health: *NINDS peripheral neuropathy information page*, 2003, http://www.ninds.nih.gov/disorders/peripheralneuropathy/peripheralneuropathy.htm. Accessed 7-26-2015

O'Brien PD, Hinder LM, Sakowski SA, et al: ER stress in diabetic peripheral neuropathy: a new therapeutic agent, *Antioxid Redox Signal* 21(4):621–633, 2014.

Ollendorf DA, Kotsanos JG, Wishner WJ, et al: Potential economic benefits of lower-extremity amputation prevention strategies in diabetes, *Diabetes Care* 21(8):1240–1245, 1998.

Oyibo SO, Jude EB, Tarawneh I, et al: A comparison of two diabetic foot ulcer classification systems: the Wagner and the University of Texas wound classification systems, *Diabetes Care* 24(1):84–88, 2001.

Oyibo SO, Jude EB, Voyatzoglou D, et al: Clinical characteristics of patients with diabetic foot problems: changing patterns of foot ulcer presentation, *Pract Diabetes Int* 19:10–12, 2002.

Park N, Allen L, Driver VL: Updating on understanding and managing chronic wound, *Dermatol Ther* 26(3):236–256, 2013.

Pecoraro RE, Reiber GE, Burgess EM: Pathways to diabetic limb amputation. Basis for prevention, *Diabetes Care* 13(5):513–521, 1990.

Perkins BA, Olaleye D, Zinman B, et al: Simple screening tests for peripheral neuropathy in the diabetes clinic, *Diabetes Care* 24(2):250–256, 2001.

Peters EJG, Lavery LA, International Working Group on the Diabetic Foot: Effectiveness of the diabetic foot risk classification system of the, *Diabetes Care* 24(8):1442–1447, 2001.

Peters EJG, Lipsky BA: Diagnosis and management of infection in the diabetic foot, *Med Clin North Am* 97(5):911–946, 2013.

Pfaller MA, Diekema DJ, Jones RN, Messer SA, Hollis RJ, SENTRY Participants Group. 2002. Trends in antifungal susceptibility of Candida spp. isolated from pediatric and adult patients with bloodstream infections: SENTRY Antimicrobial Surveillance Program, 1997 to 2000. *J. Clin. Microbiol* 40: 852–856, 2002.

Pham H, Armstrong DG, Harvey C, et al: Screening techniques to identify people at high risk for diabetic foot ulceration: a prospective multicenter trial, *Diabetes Care* 23(5):606–611, 2000.

Piagessi A, Viacava P, Rizzo L, et al: Semiquantitative analysis of the histopathological features of the neuropathic foot ulcer: effects of pressure relief, *Diabetes Care* 26(11):3123–3128, 2003.

Praet SF, Louwerens JW: The influence of shoe design on plantar pressures in neuropathic feet, *Diabetes Care* 26(2):441–445, 2003.

Prompers L, Schaper N, Apelqvist J, et al: Prediction of outcome in individuals with diabetic foot ulcers: focus on the differences between individuals with and without peripheral arterial disease. The EURODIALE Study, *Diabetologia* 51(5):747–755, 2008.

Rajbhandari SM, Jenkins RC, Davies C, et al: Charcot Neuroarthropathy in diabetes mellitus, *Diabetologia* 45(8):1085–1096, 2002.

Ramsey SD, Newton K, Blough D, et al: Incidence, outcomes, and cost of foot ulcers in patients with diabetes, *Diabetes Care* 22(3):382–387, 1999.

Rathur HM, Boulton AJM: The diabetic foot, *Clin Dermatol* 25:109–120, 2007.

Reiber GE, et al: Lower extremity foot ulcers and amputations in diabetes, In *Diabetes in America*, ed 2, Bethesda, MD, 1995, National Institutes of Health.

Reiber GE, Vileikyte L, Boyko EJ, et al: Causal pathways for incident lower-extremity ulcers in patients with diabetes from two settings, *Diabetes Care* 22(1):157–162, 1999.

Richard JL, Sotto A, Lavigne JP: New insights in diabetic foot infection, *World J Diabetes* 2(2):24–32, 2011.

Ritz G, Rowland WD, Rowland JW: Use of the Cam Walker in treating diabetic ulcers, a case report, *J Am Podiatr Med Assoc* 86(6):253–256, 1996.

Rogers LC, Frykberg RG, Armstrong DG, et al. The Charcot foot in diabetes. *Diabetes Care* 34(9):2123–2129, 2011.

Sanders LJ, et al: The Charcot's foot (pied de Charcot), in Bowker JH, Pfeiffer MA, editors: *Levin and O'Neal's the diabetic foot*, ed 7, St. Louis, MO, 2008, Mosby.

Sanders LJ, Robbins JM, Edmonds ME: History of the team approach to amputation prevention: Pioneers and milestones, *J Vasc Surg* 52(Suppl 3):S3– S16, 2010.

Shah BR, Hux JE: Quantifying the risk of infectious diseases for people with diabetes, *Diabetes Care* 26(2):510–513, 2003.

Shearer A, Scuffham P, Gordois A, et al: Predicted costs and outcomes from reduced vibration detection in people with diabetes in the U.S., *Diabetes Care* 26(8):2305–2310, 2003.

Sims DS, Cavanagh PR, Ulbrecht JS: Risk factors in the diabetic foot: recognition and management, *Phys Ther* 68(12):1887–1902, 1988.

Sinacore DR, Mueller MJ: Infectious problems of the foot in diabetic patients, In Bowker JH, Pfeiffer MA, editors: *Levin and O'Neal's the diabetic foot*, ed 7, St. Louis, MO, 2008a, Mosby.

Sinacore DR, Mueller MJ: Off loading for diabetic foot disease. In Bowker JH, Pfeiffer MA, editors: *Levin and O'Neal's the diabetic foot*, ed 7, St. Louis, MO, 2008b, Mosby.

Singh N, Armstrong DG, Lipsky BA: Preventing foot ulcers in patient with diabetes, *JAMA* 293(2):217–228, 2005.

Steed DL, Attinger C, Colaizzi T, et al: Guidelines for the treatment of diabetic ulcers, *Wound Repair Regen* 14(6):680–692, 2006.

Stockl K, Vanderplas A, Tafesse E, et al: Cost of lower-extremity ulcers among patients with diabetes, *Diabetes Care* 27(9): 2129–2130, 2004.

Sumpio B: Primary care: foot ulcers, *N Engl J Med* 343(1):787–793, 2000.

Tanneberg RJ, Donofrio PD: Neuropathic problems of the lower limbs in diabetic patients. In Bowker JH, Pfeiffer MA, editors: *Levin and O'Neal's the diabetic foot*, ed 7, St. Louis, MO, 2008, Mosby.

Tenover FC: Mechanisms of antimicrobial resistance in bacteria, *Am J Med* 119(6):S3–S10, 2006.

Tenover FC, Weigel LM, Appelbaum PC, et al: Vancomycin-resistant Staphylococcus aureus isolate from a patient in Pennsylvania, *Antimicrob Agents Chemother* 48(1):275–280, 2004.

Uçkay L, Gariani K, Pataky Z, et al: Diabetic foot infection: state of the art, *Diabetes Obes Metab* 16(4):305–316, 2014.

Umpierrez GE, Isaacs SD, Bazargan N, et al: Hyperglycemia: an independent marker of in-hospital mortality in patients with undiagnosed diabetes, *J Clin Endocrinol Metab* 87(3):978–982, 2002.

Van Acker K, De Block C, Abrams P, et al: The choice of diabetic foot ulcer classification in relation to the final outcome, *Wounds* 14(1):16, 2002.

Van Gils CC, Wheeler LA, Mellstrom M, et al: Amputation prevention by vascular surgery and podiatry collaboration in high-risk diabetic and nondiabetic patients, *Diabetes Care* 22(5):678–683, 1999.

Vinik AI, Bril V, Kempler P, et al: Treatment of symptomatic diabetic peripheral neuropathy with the protein kinase C β-inhibitor ruboxistaurin mesylate during a 1-year, randomized, placebo-controlled, double-blind clinical trial, *Clin Ther* 27(8):1164–1180, 2005.

Wagner FW: The dysvascular foot: a system for diagnosis and treatment, *Foot Ankle* 2(2):64–122, 1981.

Warriner RA, Driver VR: The true cost of growth factor therapy in diabetic foot ulcer care, *Wounds* (Suppl):1–11, July 2006.

Wilcox JR, Carter MJ, Covington S. Frequency of Debridements and Time to Heal: A Retrospective Cohort Study of 312 744 Wounds. *JAMA Dermatol* 2013;149(9):1050–1058. doi:10.1001/jamadermatol.2013.4960.

Wound, Ostomy and Continence Nurses Society™ (WOCN®): *Guideline for management of wounds in patients with lower-extremity neuropathic disease (WOCN® clinical practice guideline series no. 3)*, Glenview, IL, 2012, WOCN®.

Wu SC, Jensen JL, Weber AK, et al: Use of pressure offloading devices in diabetic foot ulcers, *Diabetes Care* 31(11):2118–2119, 2008.

Young MJ, Cavanagh PR, Thomas G, et al: The effect of callus removal on dynamic plantar foot pressures in diabetic patients, *Diabetic Med* 9(1):55–57, 1992.

Yu GV, Hudson JR: Evaluation and treatment of stage 0 Charcot's neuropathy of the foot and ankle, *J Am Podiatr Med Assoc* 92(4):210–220, 2002.

Zimny S, Dessel F, Ehren M, et al: Early detection of microcirculatory impairment in diabetic patients with foot at risk, *Diabetes Care* 24(10):1810–1814, 2001a.

Zimny S, Reinsch B, Schatz H, et al: Effects of felted foam on plantar pressures in the treatment of neuropathic diabetic foot ulcers, *Diabetes Care* 24(12):2153–2154, 2001b.

Zochodne DW, Malik RA: Diabetic autonomic neuropathy, *Handb Clin Neurol* 126:63-67, 2014.

15

Foot and Nail Care

Sheila Howes-Trammel and Ruth A. Bryant

OBJECTIVES

1. Correlate medical conditions with potential foot problems.
2. Describe the structure and function of the foot and nails.
3. Compare and contrast foot malformations addressing key features, prevention, and management.
4. Describe common foot lesions, including their etiology, manifestations, treatment, and prevention.
5. Distinguish between two toenail disorders and their treatments.
6. Develop an appropriate plan for routine care of the foot.

Foot problems occur in at least 75% of Americans (Menz and Lord, 2001). The five most common problems in the elderly population are *toenail disorders* (75%); *toe deformities* (60%); *corns and calluses* (58%); *bunions* (37%); and *dry skin, fungal infections,* or *maceration between the toes* (36%). Most of these foot problems can be prevented by proper foot care performed on a regular basis (Badlissi et al, 2005).

Age-related changes (e.g., impaired vision, inability to reach feet, thinning of epidermis and dermis), vascular-related skin changes (e.g., trophic, edema), and deformed hardened toenails affect foot hygiene. An age-related change of the foot and lower extremity is loss of hair, which leads to increased dry skin. Trophic changes in the skin are related to loss of vasculature (e.g., pigmentation changes; shiny, red skin; hair loss).

Chronic foot problems (i.e., those lasting more than 2 weeks) are associated with diabetes, peripheral vascular disease, neuropathy, atherosclerosis, arthritis, and obesity. In fact, the signs and symptoms of many of these systemic disorders manifest initially in the feet. Improper shoe wear, overuse, or systemic disease can trigger chronic foot pain. These issues magnify the importance of a good foot assessment (Popoola and Jenkins, 2004).

QUALITY OF LIFE

Foot diseases and their treatments have a tremendous impact on quality of life (Katsambas et al, 2005). In fact, patients with diabetes who have foot ulcers report a poorer quality of life than patients with diabetes who have amputations (Price and Harding, 2000). In a large-scale, quality-of-life survey of 45,593 patients with various foot diseases representing 17 countries (the Achilles Project), the researchers found that 40.3% of the respondents experienced discomfort in walking,

30.7% had pain, 27.3% had embarrassment, and 19.6% experienced limitations in their activities of daily living (Katsambas et al, 2005).

Overall, foot disease has a significantly greater effect on the quality of life of women than of men with regard to their experience of pain, discomfort in walking, and embarrassment (Katsambas et al, 2005; Leveille et al, 1998). One explanation is that the many types of shoes typically worn by women are tighter fitting, which increases their risk of developing toenail onychomycosis, which is associated with pain and discomfort in walking.

STRUCTURE AND FUNCTION

Feet are excellent at collecting information. Thousands of neurologic receptors in the feet send valuable feedback to the brain to tell your body where it is in space and what the terrain is like. Actively stimulating these receptors improves balance, increases circulation, and enhances overall foot health. There are three main elements of the body that send information to the central nervous system: the joints, skin, and muscles/tendons. Collectively they are otherwise called mechanoreceptors. When all three are firing properly and able to send accurate and precise information about pressure, joint orientation, rate of movement, and range of movement about the joint, the body works with greater synergy.

The foot has two key functions: weight bearing and propulsion. To perform properly, the foot requires a high degree of stability and must be flexible to adapt to uneven surfaces. The numerous bones and joints in the foot provide flexibility; these bones also form the arch to support weight (Quinn, 2014). Each foot contains 26 bones; 33 joints; and a network of more than 100 tendons, muscles, ligaments, blood vessels, nerves, and nails. Together, the feet comprise a quarter of the 206 bones in the body. An average day of walking brings a force equal to several hundred tons to bear on the feet. As such, feet are more subject to injury than any other part of the body (Cavanagh and Ulbrecht, 2008; Mix, 1999).

Skeletal Components

The three functional units of the foot are the hindfoot (2 bones), midfoot (5 bones), and forefoot (19 bones). All units must work together to provide both flexibility and stability (Figure 15-1).

Within the forefoot are the phalanges (toes) and the five metatarsal bones. Each toe (phalanx) is made up of several bones. The great toe (also called the hallux) consists of two phalanx bones: proximal and distal; these phalanges are larger than all the other phalanges. Phalanges two through five have three phalanx bones each: proximal, distal, and intermediate (an additional middle bone). Each phalanx is connected to a metatarsal at the metatarsophalangeal (MTP) joint; together the MTP joints form the ball of the foot. The proximal portion of a metatarsal is called the *base*, the middle is the *shaft*, and the distal is the *head* (Figure 15-2). Each of the five metatarsals is unique in size. The first metatarsal is the shortest in length, the largest in diameter, bears the most weight, and plays the most important role in propulsion (Quinn, 2014). At the head of the first metatarsal bone on the plantar surface of the foot are two sesamoid bones that serve to attach small muscles and aid in stabilizing the first MTP joint. (A sesamoid bone is a bone imbedded within a tendon and functions to protect the tendon where it passes over a bony prominence.) The second, third, and fourth metatarsal bones are the most stable metatarsal bones. At the fifth metatarsal base is an eminence on the lateral aspect called the *tuberosity of fifth metatarsal* or *styloid process*. This area is easily palpated on the lateral aspect of the foot.

In the midfoot, five of the seven tarsal bones are located (see Figure 15-2). These irregularly shaped tarsals (the navicular, cuboid, and three cuneiform) form the arch and contain multiple joints. The three cuneiform bones articulate with the navicular bone in the proximal midfoot. The midfoot connects with the forefoot at the five tarsometatarsal (TMT) joints and connects to the hindfoot by muscles and ligaments.

The hindfoot links the midfoot to the ankle and consists of two of the seven tarsal bones: the talus and the calcaneus. The talus sits on top of the calcaneus and articulates with the tibia and fibula at the calcaneus and navicular bones, allowing the foot to move up and down. The calcaneus forms the heel and is the largest tarsal and the largest bone in the foot. It allows the foot to become rigid or loose to accommodate the process of walking. It is also the cause of numerous heel-related pains (Jolly et al, 2005).

Ligaments hold the bones together at the joints. The Achilles tendon stretches from the calf muscle to heel and is the largest, strongest tendon in the foot. The planter fascia is the longest ligament and forms an arch on the sole of the foot from the heel to the toes. These long fibrous strands are vulnerable to injury (e.g., a strain or sprain in the foot or ankle) because the ligaments can overstretch, break, and curl back on themselves. Over time the strain heals with scar tissue; however, the scar is never as strong as the original fibers of the ligament.

Muscular Components

The foot is constructed of 20 muscles. These muscles hold the bones in place, providing the foot with its shape and contracting and relaxing to allow for movement. Key muscles are the anterior tibial (moves foot upward), posterior tibial (supports arch), peroneal tibial (controls lateral ankle movements), extensors (help ankle raise toes to begin walking), and flexors (stabilizes to the ground).

Neurovascular

The feet are innervated by the sciatic nerve, which branches off the spinal cord at the sacral level. As it descends, the sciatic

FIGURE 15-1 Anatomic structures of the foot. (Courtesy Fort Worth Orthopaedics.)

Distal
Middle ⎱ Phalanges
Proximal ⎰

Sesamoids

Head
Shaft ⎱ Metatarsals
Base ⎰

Lateral
Intermediate ⎱ Cuneiforms
Medial ⎰

Tuberosity of fifth metatarsal

Groove for fibularis longus

Tuberosity of cuboid

Calcaneus

Tuberosity of navicular

Head of talus

Sustentaculum tali

Groove for flexor hallucis longus

Calcaneal tuberosity

FIGURE 15-2 Dorsal view of anatomic structures of foot. (From Jenkins DB: *Hollinshead's functional anatomy of the limbs and back*, ed 9, St. Louis, MO, 2009, Elsevier, p 333.)

nerve divides into the tibial and common peroneal nerves and further subdivides into numerous branches.

Branching off the popliteal artery in the lower leg are the anterior tibial artery and the posterior tibial artery. The anterior tibial artery becomes the dorsalis pedis (dorsum of the foot). The posterior tibial artery passes posterior to the medial malleolus, divides into the peroneal and plantar arteries, and then feeds into the lateral plantar and medial plantar arteries. The two most dominant arteries in the foot are the dorsalis pedis and the posterior tibial artery. Two sets of veins drain the leg and foot: the deep veins and superficial veins.

As shown in Figure 10-2, the dorsalis pedis pulse is palpated or auscultated over the navicular and middle cuneiform bones. The posterior tibial pulse is palpated over the medial malleolus of the tibia.

Cutaneous and Subcutaneous Components

The skin on the plantar surface of the foot is thick and hairless and contains numerous sweat glands. *Eccrine* sweat glands are densely populated on the soles of the feet, palms, and axillae. Their primary function is thermoregulation through evaporation of sweat. The sebaceous and apocrine sweat glands empty into the upper portions of the hair follicles. Sebaceous glands produce lipid-rich sebum that prevents the skin and hair from drying out. Because the foot has little hair growth and therefore very few *sebaceous* glands, the foot is extremely vulnerable to dryness and xerosis.

Three anatomic areas on the plantar surface of the foot have increased fat in the form of fat pads: the calcaneus, the metatarsals, and the lateral longitudinal arch. Contained by the subcutaneous tissue, the fat pad absorbs impact and tolerates weight bearing as a means of protecting the underlying bones. With age, these fat pads thin and provide less shock absorbency. More pressure is then exerted over the calcaneus and metatarsal. Thinning of the fat pad is accelerated by obesity, diabetes, and constant high impact. The thinning process begins as early

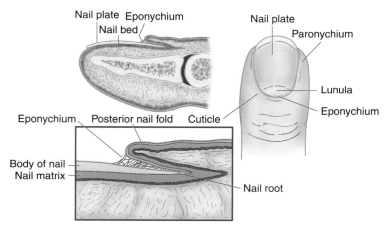

FIGURE 15-3 Anatomic structures of the nail. (From Thompson JM, et al: *Mosby's clinical nursing*, ed 5, St. Louis, MO, 2002, Mosby.)

as 30 years of age. An orthotic or insole cushioning can be used to provide additional shock absorption (Ozdemir et al, 2004).

Nail Structure

Nails are made of epidermal cells converted to hard plates of keratin. The function of the toenail is to provide protection to the soft tissue of the toe. The nail measures one sixteenth of an inch in thickness and is composed of three layers: a dorsal thin covering, a thicker middle layer, and a deep inner layer derived from the nail bed. The nail bed, or the matrix, is made up of epithelium, a rough surface of longitudinal waves that interface with grooves on the underside of the nail plate, facilitating adherence of the plate to the bed. The distal aspect of the matrix is the lunula, or the moons, which is the crescent-shaped white area. Normal nail color is translucent with a pink tinge reflecting the highly vascular matrix. As the nail grows, extending beyond the nail root or matrix, the translucent color is lost and becomes white. The stratum corneum layer of the skin covering the nail root is the eponychium (cuticle), which forms a seal between the nail and the digit to prevent foreign matter from entering. The hyponychium smoothly seals the border between the distal end of the nail and the bed. The perionychium creates a seal on the lateral folds. These three parts of the nail prevent infection from occurring under the nail bed. The normal nail is composed of six parts: nail root (under the skin), nail bed (under the nail plate), nail plate, eponychium (cuticle), perionychium (nail fold), and hyponychium (skin under the front edge of the nail) as illustrated in Figure 15-3 and described in Box 15-1.

Nails grow all the time, but their rate of growth slows with age and poor circulation. Fingernails grow faster than toenails. They grow at a rate of 3 mm per month and take 6 months to grow from root to free edge. Toenails grow approximately 1 mm per month and require 12 to 18 months to be completely replaced. Actual growth rate is dependent on age, gender, season, exercise level, diet, and hereditary factors (Sinni-McKeehen, 2007).

BOX 15-1 Nail Anatomy

Nail Root (Matrix): Root of fingernail is also known as the matrix. The matrix begins 7 to 8 mm under proximal nail fold to lunula (white crescent at distal nail). Fingernail root produces most of volume of nail plate and nail bed.

Nail Bed: Part of nail matrix, under the nail plate. Extends from lunula (white crescent at distal nail) to hyponychium. Nail bed contains blood vessels, nerves, and melanocytes or melanin-producing cells. As nail is produced by root, it streams down along the nail bed, which adds material to the undersurface of the nail, making it thicker.

Nail Plate: The actual fingernail, made of translucent keratin. Pink appearance of nail comes from blood vessels underneath nail. Underneath surface of nail plate has grooves along length of nail that help anchor it to the nail bed.

Eponychium (Cuticle): Fold at proximal end of nail plate. Nail plate has very firm adhesion to the cuticle. Both epidermal structures are directly continuous with one another, overlapping the lunula. Fusing of these structures provides a waterproof barrier.

Perionychium: Skin that overlies nail plate on its sides. Also known as the paronychial edge. Site of hangnails, ingrown nails, and infection of skin called *paronychia.*

Hyponychium: Area between free edge of nail plate and epidermis of toe. Continuous fusing of these areas to epidermal structures provides waterproof barrier.

Periungual: Tissue around nail plate.

Subungual: Tissue under nail plate.

Ungual: Pertaining to the nail.

From Mix G: *The salon professional's guide to foot care,* Albany, NY, 1998, Milady Salon Ovations.

PHYSICAL ASSESSMENT

Components of an initial evaluation of the patient with an actual or potential foot disorder are listed in Checklist 15-1. Because so many patients with foot disorders have concomitant lower extremity disease, perfusion and sensation must be assessed (see Chapters 10, 11, 12, and 14), and a baseline

CHECKLIST 15-1 Components of Initial Evaluation of Patient with Foot Disorder

History

✓ Presenting complaint, including detailed description of pain
✓ General: vision, strength, dexterity, mobility
✓ Blood glucose readings for past month, HbA1c
✓ Personal or family history: skin, hair, or nail disease (especially rashes); lichen planus; psoriasis; diabetes; heart or vascular disease; obesity
✓ Specific history of foot problems: foot malformations, lesions, skin alterations, nail disorders, changes in sensation, foot/ankle strength
✓ Current and prior treatments and medications (including over the counter) used to treat nail and foot problems
✓ Health habits: smoking, exercise, hygiene, nutrition, weight management

Physical Assessment

✓ Overall skin condition
✓ Lesions on foot
✓ Foot malformations
✓ Condition of nails
✓ Perfusion and sensation, pulses, blanching, capillary refill, microvascular function (laser Doppler flowmetry), ankle-brachial index or toe-brachial index, temperature, hair growth
✓ Musculoskeletal function: gait, mobility, balance, hand strength and dexterity, visual cognition

Risk Assessment

✓ Ulceration risk (see Table 14-1)
✓ Amputation risk

Equipment

✓ Footwear (including socks)
✓ Mobility aids (canes, walkers)

health history is essential. The following discussion presents the unique assessment parameters for the foot and nail.

Specific information should be elicited about routine care of the foot, any history of foot and nail problems, and how these problems were treated either personally or by a health care provider. Effects of prior treatments, including prescription and over-the-counter medications, should be assessed (Piraccini et al, 2004; Sprecher, 2005). Quality-of-life-information should be solicited (Garrow et al, 2004; Vileikyte et al, 2003).

Musculoskeletal Function

Musculoskeletal function of the foot involves assessment of range of motion, deformities, and strength. Passive range of motion of the first MTP joint and the subtalar joint should be assessed. Maximal range of motion is determined from maximal inversion to maximal eversion of the subtalar joint of the foot (Figure 15-4). If available, a goniometer can be used to quantify the arc or range of motion (Badlissi et al, 2005) (Figure 15-5). Range of motion can also be tested by supporting the heel with the hand and grasping the foot with the other hand, then moving the foot in dorsiflexion, plantar flexion, eversion, and inversion. The dorsiflexion position tests for shortening of the Achilles tendon. Inversion will be limited by a spasm of the peronei. Eversion will be limited with a rigid flat foot. Restrictions in range of motion of the ankle might limit the ability to correct a loss of balance (Duthie, 2007).

The strength of the anterior leg muscles can be tested by having the patient stand on the heels. Muscle strength can also be assessed by comparing both feet as the patient walks a few steps on the toes and then the heels. If the patient has difficulty with balance, cannot walk, or both, strength can be assessed with the patient sitting. With the clinician's hand under the patient's foot, the patient is asked to flex and extend the foot against resistance by "pressing down on the

FIGURE 15-4 Range of motion of the foot and ankle. **A,** Dorsiflexion and planter flexion. **B,** Inversion and eversion. **C,** Abduction and adduction. (From Ball JW, Dains JE, Flynn JA: *Seidel's guide to physical examination*, ed 8, St. Louis, MO, 2015, Mosby.)

FIGURE 15-5 Goniometer. (From Ball JW, Dains JE, Flynn JA: *Seidel's guide to physical examination*, ed 8, St. Louis, MO, 2015, Mosby.)

should be stopped. The heel should be able to drop below the level of the stair without causing strain in the calf. Some strain can be improved with flexibility exercises (Frey, 2005).

To examine the medial longitudinal arch, have the patient stand with feet parallel, separated by 4 inches. Note if the arch flattens with weight bearing and if it resumes to normal shape without weight bearing.

Muscle strength reflexes (deep tendon reflexes) usually show no changes in the elderly patient, although nearly half have a diminished Achilles tendon reflex. This is likely due to slow nerve conduction and decreased tendon elasticity. Hyperactive deep tendon reflexes suggest upper motor neuron disease; hypoactive reflexes suggest lower motor neuron dysfunction. Tone is assessed through passive motion. Increased tone is suggestive of upper motor neuron dysfunction; decreased tone is suggestive of lower motor neuron dysfunction.

Functional Ability

The patient's functional ability is a significant factor influencing his or her ability for self-care and safety. Assessments of functional ability should address cognition, vision, strength–hand dexterity, coordination, balance, proprioception, and gait. Because key interventions in the prevention and management of foot and nail disorders are patient education and self-care, the patient will need adequate cognition to conduct self-care or communicate pain. Vision and strength–hand dexterity are essential so that patients will be able to inspect their feet and remove footwear (Duthie, 2007). Many of these

gas pedal." Next, with the clinician's hand positioned on the top of the patient's foot and the clinician's thumbs underneath, the patient is instructed to pull the "toes toward the nose" while the clinician applies gentle pressure downward. Any differences in strength currently or in the past 6 months should also be recorded (Frey, 2005).

To assess toe flexibility, the patient can be instructed to pick up a marble or a small dishtowel with the toes (Table 15-1). To test ankle flexibility, the patient is instructed to stand on a stair step, hang his or her heel off a step, and let the heel drop below the level of the stair. If this motion causes pain, the exercise

TABLE 15-1	Foot Flexibility Exercises		
	Exercise	**Instructions**	**Recommendations**
	Toe raise, toe point, toe curls	Hold each position for 5 seconds and repeat 10 times.	Individuals with hammer-toes or toe cramps
	Golf ball roll	Roll a golf ball under the ball of your foot for 2 minutes—great massage for bottom of foot.	Individuals with plantar fasciitis (heel pain), arch strain, or foot cramps
	Towel curls	Place small towel on floor and curl it toward you, using only your toes. You can increase resistance by putting a weight on end of towel. Relax and repeat exercise five times.	Individuals with hammer-toes, toe cramps, and pain in the ball of the foot
	Marble pick up	Place 20 marbles on floor. Pick up one marble at a time with your toes and put it in a small bowl. Do this exercise until you have picked up all 20 marbles.	Individuals with pain in the ball of the foot, hammer-toes, and toe cramps
	Sand walking	Any chance you get, take off your shoes and walk in the sand at the beach. This not only massages your feet, but also strengthens your toes.	Good for general foot conditioning Watch out for glass!

Modified from American Orthopaedic Foot and Ankle Society: *Keep your foot flexible*, http://www.aofas.org/Scripts/4Disapi.dll/4DCGI/cms/review.html?Action=CMS_Document&DocID=71. Accessed September 2, 2010.

functional abilities can be assessed through observation and demonstration return.

Coordination can be determined with a rapid alternating movement that includes heel to shin testing. Another test in which the patient taps the feet rhythmically against the floor will assess the accuracy and reproducibility of endpoints, as well as the ability to maintain motor movements over time. The coordination testing is documented qualitatively because no quantification guidelines are available (Duthie, 2007).

Proprioception is the awareness of the body's position in context with the surrounding environment. Disturbed proprioception (loss of position sense) in the feet is disabling; the patient may be clumsy, bump into things, or have an abnormal gait. In practice, the patient often comes down hard on the heels and then slaps the sole of the foot (high stepping and stamping) in an attempt to increase sensory feedback and restore proprioception. Proprioception disturbances are always worse in the dark when vision cannot be used to compensate for loss of position sense.

The Romberg test (Box 15-2) is positive in the patient with proprioception disturbances (Jarvis, 2004). In addition, the patient's gait may be slightly wide, whereas the stride length is normal or a little reduced (Willacy, 2008). Gait should be assessed without an assistive device if possible so as not to mask deviations. Proprioception and vibration sense are carried by the same nerve pathways. Therefore testing vibration may reveal proprioception disturbances. To test vibration sense, a 128-Hz tuning fork is applied over a bony prominence such as the medial malleolus and the patient is asked to report when the vibration stops (Jarvis, 2004).

Condition of Legs, Feet, Toes, and Nails

Lower extremity assessment should include all of the components discussed in Chapter 10. In addition to examining skin integrity, color changes, sensation, pain, and vascular conditions, the foot must be inspected for skin that is too dry or too moist, evidence of fungal or bacterial infection, lesions, foot malformations, and nail conditions (Boulton and Armstrong, 2008). All surfaces (dorsal, plantar, medial, lateral, posterior surfaces) of the heel, areas between the toes (interdigitally), and each nail should be examined. Note the character of skin changes from the proximal leg to the distal foot. Compare the skin on the lower extremity and feet to the skin on the arms and hands.

Ulceration and Amputation Risk

The data collected during the examination will assist in identifying risk for ulceration and amputation. Risk assessment

tools with management strategies are given in Tables 14-2 and 14-3. Risk factors include history of plantar ulcer, presence of foot deformity, presence of protective sensations, and presence of diseases that lead to decreased sensation. Risk categories range from 0 (no risk) to 3 (greatest risk). The level of risk determines the patient's management strategy. International guidelines recommend foot examinations every 3-6 months once loss of sensation develops, every 1-3 months once a callous also develops, and every 1-12 weeks when history of ulcer is present (see Table 14-3).

PREVENTION AND ROUTINE MANAGEMENT

Maintaining healthy nails and feet requires daily attention to the skin of the foot and ankle, nails, and footwear. Routine over-the-counter remedies can be used to correct common problems and hopefully prevent deterioration into a serious condition.

Routine Foot Hygiene

Routine foot care includes daily inspection and moisturizing. Daily cleansing or bathing should be based on the individual needs of the patient and should consist of mild skin cleansers and lukewarm water to minimize drying effects. After bathing, the feet must be dried completely, especially between the toes. The patient should use a mirror to view the bottom of the foot for inspection of any alterations in the skin. No moisturizers should be used between the toes. Patients should wear socks to provide extra padding to bony prominences and to wick away moisture from the skin. Socks may need to be changed more than once per day if feet sweat excessively. The use of an occlusive moisturizer can be applied to the feet at night and covered with socks for additional moisturizing.

Maceration between the toes (interdigital) and under the toes (subdigital) is a very common foot problem. Such over-hydration of the skin, characterized by a white, "waterlogged" appearance, weakens collagen, promotes overgrowth of bacterial and fungal species of skin flora, and decreases the skin's ability to resist trauma (Kelechi, 2005; Stroud and Kelechi, 2006). Pseudomonas and gram-negative organisms are common etiologic agents (Schwartz, 2013). Overhydration of the skin can occur with excessive perspiration (hyperhidrosis) related to endocrine, neurologic, or sweat gland disorders.

Maceration is prevented by keeping the skin dry and protected. After bathing, the patient should pay special attention to drying the interdigit spaces; using a hair dryer on a cool setting may be helpful. The treatment interventions can include separating the toes with the use of lamb's wool, the use of an absorbent foot powder (e.g., Zeasorb) twice per day, the use of skin sealants to protect the skin from moisture, or use of an antiperspirant (e.g., Drysol). If maceration persists after 1 week of care, consider the presence of interdigital tinea (Table 15-2) or superimposed bacterial infection. Treatment includes drying the interdigital web spaces, topical econazole, and local application of Castellani paint (a drying agent containing 1.5% phenol in a water and alcohol base) daily to three times a day (Schwartz, 2013).

BOX 15-2	Romberg (Equilibrium) Test

- Have patient stand with arms at side and feet together.
- Have patient maintain position for 20 seconds with only minimal swaying.
- Have patient perform initially with eyes open and then with eyes closed.
- Stand close to patient to prevent falls.

TABLE 15-2 **Assessment, Prevention, and Management of Common Foot Lesions and Infections**

Name	Description	Common Locations	Prevention	Treatment
Soft corn (heloma molle)	Enlarged interphalangeal joint causing friction to the opposing surface Aggravated by tight shoes and ambulation	Between fourth and fifth toes	Properly fitting shoes, offload with interdigit foam or gel pads, or lamb's wool	Pumice, file Wider shoes Surgically reshape phalange
Hard corn (heloma durum)	Toes curl inside of shoes, creating pressure between toes against the sole Aggravated by narrow-toed shoes	Sides and tops of toes	Offload pressure with pads (aperture or crest pads)	Use wider shoes or sandals Reduce corn with file, pumice, rotary tool Assess for underlying ulceration Offload and pad as needed Surgically straighten toes
Callus (keratoma or tyloma) generalized pressure (see Plate 41A)	Thickened areas of skin without distinct borders caused by repeated pressure Aggravated by narrow-toed shoes and high heels	Planter surface, heel, under metatarsal head	Padding, properly fitting shoes	Reduce with file, pumice, rotary tool, or paring Assess for underlying ulceration Moisturize and exfoliate (best applied to damp skin after bathing) Offload and pad as needed Use shoes with soft soles, lower heels, arch support, extra width
Planter wart (*Verruca plantaris*)	Caused by a contagious viral infection (human papillomavirus) Overproliferation of skin and mucosa growing downward (iceberg effect) Single lesion or clustered Yellow, brown, gray, or black Vesicular inclusion from dried capillary ends leads to black/red appearance	Pressure points on sole, heel, ball of foot	Change socks and shoes daily Do not share shoes Keep feet clean and dry Avoid direct contact with warts on other people Use water-resistant footwear in showers, locker rooms, pools	Reduce with file or pumice Salicylic acid podophyllin, or cryotherapy/electrocautery Surgical curettage or laser removal Human papillomavirus dies within 1 to 2 years and wart disappears
Tinea pedis (interdigital)	Dermatophyte infection White, macerated, denuded, vesicles, scales, or fissures	Between fourth and fifth toes		Topical antifungal twice daily for minimum of 1 week (gel product to reduce the moisture) Urea cream for scaling, itching
Tinea pedis (plantar)	Dermatophyte infection Itchy, hyperkeratotic scaling, cracking, peeling, dry patches Chronic, diffuse, noninflammatory	Sole, heel, side of foot (moccasin)		Topical antifungal twice daily for minimum of 1 week Urea cream for scaling, itching
Tinea pedis (vesiculobullous)	Dermatophyte infection Acute, highly inflammatory eruptions	Arch, side of foot		Topical or systemic antifungals and corticosteroids (depending on severity)

Foot odor (bromhidrosis) is caused by excessive perspiration from the more than 250,000 sweat glands in the foot. Bacteria living in shoes and socks metabolize the sweat to form isovaleric acid, which is responsible for foot odor. In addition to washing the feet and changing shoes and socks even more frequently than daily, the patient can dust the feet with a nonmedicated spray, foot powder, or antiperspirants. Soaking feet in vinegar and water can help lessen odor (American Podiatric Medical Association, 2010). The shoes should be treated by freezing, washing in hot water, or discarding. Severe cases of foot odor may be caused by hyperhidrosis (excessive perspiration formation related to endocrine, neurologic, or sweat gland disorders). The prescription-strength antiperspirant Drysol can be used if over-the-counter antiperspirants or sprays fail (Hill, 2008). In severe cases, the nerve controlling the sweat glands in the feet may be surgically severed, but compensatory sweating in other areas of the body may occur after surgery.

Anhidrosis (inability to produce sweat) is associated with autonomic dysfunction caused by endocrine or neurologic disorders, environmental conditions, and aging. Xerosis is a consequence of the skin's loss of natural moisturizing factors and loss of moisture from the stratum corneum and intercellular matrix (Hill, 2008). Clinically, xerosis appears as excessively dry, rough, uneven, and cracked skin. Raised or uplifted skin edges (scaling), desquamation (flaking), chapping, and pruritus may be present. This condition occurs particularly on the heels and bottoms of the feet. A person who has a decrease or loss of function of the sweat glands on the plantar surface of the foot will experience xerosis or anhidrosis of the feet (Kelechi, 2005). *Xerosis* can lead to fissures (linear cracks in the skin), which may serve as a portal of entry for bacteria. Consequently, fissures are associated with increased risk of cellulitis and foot ulceration (Hill, 2008). *Fissures* are treated with humectants and exfoliant moisturizers or liquid adhesive bandage, such as Dermabond, Nexcare, or Liquiband. Prevention includes ongoing use of moisturizers and exfoliants and wearing shoes that do not flop at the heel. Hyperkeratotic tissue is common around fissures and often necessitates debridement and exfoliation. Table 15-3 provides a formulary of products for the prevention and treatment of dry skin.

Cuticles and Nails

About half of the foot care professional's activity is nail care and specifically nail debridement. Nail trimming can be done by a nurse or caregiver when the nail is normal in thickness and appearance. The nail should be trimmed straight across, no lower than one sixteenth to one eighth of an inch from the end of the toe, to prevent ingrown toenails. This should be followed by the smoothing of the nail with a rasp or nail file. The cuticle should not be trimmed or manipulated.

Nail debridement should only be provided by a nurse who is qualified based on the individual state's nurse practice. Nail debridement begins with nipping small areas of the nail, starting at one edge and completing to the other side of the nail, following the contour of the top of the toe. The shape and length will depend on the individual patient history and assessment. A hyperkeratotic nail or areas of hyperkeratosis (corns or calluses) on the toes or bottom of the foot should be debrided and a treatment plan developed. Nail debridement and trimming can be accomplished with manual nippers (Box 15-3) or with a mechanical rotary tool (Box 15-4). The use of proper and professional-quality instruments is key to providing proper foot and nail care. Five basic instruments are recommended for providing foot and nail care: toenail nippers, curette, rasp, ingrown nail shaver, and cuticle nippers.

Toenail Nippers. Podiatry toenail cutters or pedicure nail nippers are best suited for trimming thicker toenails and lateral curves of the nail. This instrument should be used like scissors. The nail should be removed incrementally to avoid injuring the hyponychium and thus breaking the seal on the nail plate, which would open a portal of entry for fungal or bacterial infections (Godfrey, 2006). There is much debate regarding the best methods for debriding or trimming

TABLE 15-3	Formulary of Moisturizing Products: Descriptions, Examples, and Indications		
Moisturizer	**Indications and Actions**	**Ingredient Examples***	**Product Examples***
Emollients	Prevent dry skin Fill in cracks between clusters of desquamating corneocytes Not occlusive unless applied heavily	Lipids Oils Dimethicone	Keri Original (Bristol Myers Squibb) Cavilon Emollient Cream (3M) Cetaphil Lotion (Galderma Laboratories)
Occlusives	Treat dry skin Reduce transepidermal water loss by creating hydrophobic barrier over skin Has most pronounced effect when applied to slightly damp skin	Petrolatum Lanolin Mineral oil Dimethicone	Cetaphil Cream (Galderma Laboratories) Remedy Skin Repair Cream (Medline) Sween 24 Cream (Coloplast)
Humectants and exfoliants	Treat dry skin, xerosis, fissures, ichthyoses Contains urea, lactic acid, or both, which are naturally present in healthy skin and markedly reduced in dry skin Enhance water absorption by drawing and absorbing water from environment and retaining moisture within skin cells Keratolytic effects soften scales to be easily released from skin surface Urea has antipruritic effects	Urea Lactic acid	Eucerin 10% Urea Lotion (Beiersdorf) Lac-Hydrin Lotion (Bristol Myers Squibb) Atrac-Tain Lotion (Coloplast)

*Concentrations and total formulation determine actions and effectiveness. List is not all inclusive.
Data from Pham HT, Exelbert L, Segal-Owens AC, et al: A prospective, randomized, controlled double-blind study of a moisturizer for xerosis of the feet in patients with diabetes, *Ostomy Wound Manage* 48(5):30–36, 2002; Milne CT: *Wound Source.* 17th ed. Hinesburg: Kerstel Health Information, 2014; Lodén M: Role of topical emollients and moisturizers in the treatment of dry skin barrier disorders, *Am J Clin Dermatol* 4:771–788, 2003.

BOX 15-3 **Basic Cuticle and Nail Trimming Using Toenail Nippers**

1. Begin cuticle and nail care after bathing when nails are softer.
2. Examine nails.
   a. Observe for presence of hyponychium that has hypertrophied, hypergranulation tissue, ingrowing corners of nail borders, hyperkeratosis, or other abnormal findings. Patients with very thick or ingrown nails require referral to foot care professional.
   b. Define the free nail border by assessing the tissue underneath the nail, using beveled edge of orangewood stick.
   c. Unhealthy nails should be trimmed last to prevent the transmission of infection.
3. Remove any loose debris from under the nail.
4. Gently trim excessively thick or loose cuticles with cuticle nippers.
   a. Avoid excess manipulation of the cuticle, which may lead to infection.
5. Decide between slightly rounded cut and straight across cut:
   a. *Straight across* (not too short) for puffy or thick skin folds prone to ingrown toenails
   b. *Slightly rounded* for problems with nail corners curving and causing pain and thickening of skin at distal aspect of nail groove
6. Remove free edge of nail.
   a. Do not trim nail off in one clip; make small cuts.
   b. Begin at one edge of nail, nip smoothly working across entire nail border no lower than one sixteenth to one eighth of an inch from end of toe (lateral plate should extend beyond nail fold).
   c. Do not cut deeply into lateral corners of nail bed.
   d. Avoid cutting skin; openings in skin are avenues of entry for bacteria and other infectious agents. If small cuts occur, cleanse thoroughly and apply an antibiotic ointment while educating the patient on follow-up care.
7. Use fine point of nipper to trim out sharp edge of lateral aspect of nail that curves deeply in nail margin.
8. For hyperkeratotic nails, the use of either nippers or a Dremel is effective in debriding the thickened nail plate. Smooth the top and edges of nail with nail rasp or nail file.

BOX 15-4 **Nail Debridement Using Mechanical Rotary Tool**

1. Before using a Dremel drill, patients should be informed that they will feel a vibration while the nail is being debrided.
2. Don appropriate personal protective equipment.
3. Remove most of fungal nail with quality nippers before using drill to minimize dust.
4. Support toe between index finger and thumb of nondominant hand to prevent toe from moving during debridement. The other toes should be held away from the bur during the procedure.
5. Set grinder speed to 10,000 to 15,000 rpm.
6. Debride nail by slowly and gently applying pressure as grinder is moved from proximal to distal portion of plate.
7. Keep nail plate visible at all times. Frequently stop grinding to wipe away dust with a cloth (do not blow).
8. Stop grinding when nail is thin or when dust becomes very fine and is not visibly produced during debridement.
9. *Do not grind through nail plate!* Soft underlying layers of plate can be abraded, possibly resulting in subungual wound to nail bed.
10. Avoid surrounding tissue, which can become abraded.

Equipment Options
- Drill with attached vacuum
- Room air circulators with high-efficiency particulate air (HEPA) filters
- Tungsten carbide burs and bits are preferable because they run cold, do not abrade skin, and produce big particles rather than dust
- Ruby carvers and diamond bits are preferable to steel

Equipment Sterilization
- Proper cleansing of equipment between patients is single most important task in reducing or eliminating spread of infection
- Sterilize in autoclave or use antifungal cold soaking solution (glutaraldehyde, phenol, sodium hypochlorite, sodium bromide, iodophors)
- Alcohol does not kill fungus and should not be used for cleansing nail equipment

Personal Protective Equipment and Back Safety
- Gloves, mask, goggles, gown, hair covering
- Height-adjustable chair or examination table for patient
- Height-adjustable chair for clinician
- Change positions frequently; stretch back muscles

---

toenails: straight across versus rounding, or following the shape or contouring of the top of the toe. If the patient has a problem with nail corners curving and causing pain and thickening of the skin at the distal aspect of the nail groove, it is recommended that the corners be slightly rounded. Patients who have puffy or a thick skin fold might require nails that are cut straight across so that the corners grow up out of the grooves to prevent ingrown toenails (Katoh, 2008). Box 15-3 gives a procedure for basic cuticle and nail trimming using a nipper.

Curette. The dull-edged curette is a small spoon-shaped instrument that allows for removal of debris under the nail margins. A scooping motion is used along the nail plate to remove debris from the nail groove. This process may need to be repeated until all the debris is removed.

Nail Rasp or Nail File. The medical field calls the nail file a *nail rasp*. It is used to smooth the distal edges of the nail in the nail groove. The file is placed gently in the nail groove against the free (distal) edges of the nail plate. The rasp is then pulled along the edges of the rough nail plate. Each nail should be smoothed with the nail rasp, beginning with healthy nails to prevent transmission of infection.

Ingrown Nail Shaver and Cuticle Nippers. These tools are used when a little more nail needs to be removed from the lateral nail margins. The nail shaver is shaped like a small paddle and has a slot in the middle of the paddle; the end of the slot is filed to a sharp cutting edge. The paddle portion of the nail shaver is placed in the nail groove so that the end of the nail edge is in the slot to trim the spicule of nail present (Mix, 1999).

Mechanical Rotary Tool. The mechanical rotary tool (Dremel drill, cordless or plug-in) is a standard tool used for nail debridement. Use of a rotary tool disperses nail dust into the air, which can be inhaled by the patient and the clinician and can settle on surfaces throughout the room. Aerosol nail dust, particularly from onychomycotic toenails, can lead to conjunctivitis, rhinitis, asthma, coughing, hypersensitivity, and impaired lung function (Ward, 2005). Personal protection equipment reduces the risk of exposure to the resulting small particles. The hazards associated with these aerosolized small particles have resulted in a great deal of controversy related to the appropriate selection and use of mechanical nail avulsion and debridement tools (Rees, 2008). For example, a drill with an attached vacuum is available that will automatically contain large particles. Box 15-4 lists equipment options and sterilization tips that enhance safety and effectiveness.

Footwear

The main purpose of the shoe is to protect and cushion the foot. Incorrectly fitting footwear is common in older people and is strongly associated with forefoot pathology (hallux valgus, lesser toe deformities, corns, calluses), foot pain, skin breakdown, abnormal foot pressures, ischemia, and inflammation from repetitive stress (Menz and Morris, 2005; Ward, 2005). Although foot size increases with age, surprisingly, many people continue to wear the same size shoe throughout their lifespan. As a result, the foot will take on the shape of the shoe, regardless of the fit. A proper shoe fit requires appropriate length and width measurements, as well as an assessment of the person's style of arch. Box 15-5 provides several considerations for selecting and maintaining appropriate footwear.

Any patient with foot or ankle problems should have his or her shoes evaluated. Assessment parameters include wear pattern; a tracing of the weight-bearing foot; footprints; and use of heels, arch supports, and heel cushions. Normal wear patterns occur on the outsole and slightly medial at the great toe and lateral calcaneus. Different wear patterns may be indicative of underlying foot problems or problems with

---

BOX 15-5 Selecting and Maintaining Appropriate Footwear

Shoe Size
- Do not select shoes by size marked inside shoe; sizes vary among shoe brands and styles.

Measurement
- Measure *both* feet regularly; size of feet change with age.

Fitting
- Fit to larger foot.
- Fit at end of the day when feet are at their largest.
- Stand during fitting process.
- Hold new shoe over foot tracing to be certain entire tracing is covered by shoe.
- There should be ⅜ inch to ½ inch between longest toe and end of each shoe.
- Stand next to shoes to determine whether shoes are shaped like feet or if there are areas of constriction.
- Shoe should conform as much as possible to shape of foot.
- Heel should fit comfortably in shoe with minimum amount of slippage.
- Ball of foot should fit comfortably into widest part (ball pocket) of shoe.
- Do not purchase shoes that feel too tight, expecting them to "stretch" to fit.
- Examine inside of shoe by hand to check for seams, tacks, rough places.
- Walk in shoe to make sure it fits and feels right.

Shoe Type
- A healthy shoe is one that is shaped like the foot. Shoe has deep, roomy, and rounded or square toe box (area of shoe over toes).
- Shoe should be made of very soft material similar to glove leather.

- Flat shoes (with heel height of 1 inch or less) are the healthiest shoes for feet. If high-heeled shoes are needed, keep to heel height of 2 inches or less; limit wearing of shoes to 3 hours at a time; and take shoes off coming to and from work, dinner, or church.
- Soles should be shock absorbing and skid resistant (rubber rather than smooth leather).
- Avoid shoes that have seams over areas of pain (e.g., bunion).
- Avoid shoes with heavy rubber soles that curl over top of toe area (e.g., some running shoes) because they can catch on carpets and cause accidental falls.
- Lace-up rather than slip-on shoes provide more secure fit and can accommodate insoles and orthotic devices.
- Select and wear shoe appropriate to activity (e.g., steel-toed boots for farm work, running shoes for running).

Additional Tips
- Wear new shoes initially for short intervals (e.g., 20 minutes twice per day) and check feet and toes upon removal.
- Indentations, skin discoloration, warmth may be signs of mechanical trauma (pressure points, friction, repetitive stress).
- Do not wear same pair of shoes every day.
- Before putting on shoes, shake them and feel inside them to remove any foreign objects
- Note lumpy insoles or torn linings. Replace worn-out shoes as soon as possible.
- White or light-colored socks are preferred so that any drainage (suggestive of ulceration) is readily apparent.
- Avoid walking barefoot, even at home, because feet are more susceptible to injury and infection.
- Apply sun block to feet when wearing sandals or at the beach.
- Discard socks with holes, socks that have been darned.
- Tops of socks should not restrict circulation.

Data from Orthopaedic Foot and Ankle Society, the National Shoe Retailers Association, and the Pedorthic Footwear Association (Am Orthop Foot Ankle Soc, 2003).

FIGURE 15-6 How to "read" your shoes. **1,** Wear on the ball of the foot. **2,** Wear on the inner sole. **3,** Toe-shaped ridges on the upper toe box. **4,** Outer sole wear. **5,** Bulge and wear to the side of the big toe. **6,** Wear on the surface distal to metatarsal head and toes. (Modified from American Orthopaedic Foot & Ankle Society: *How to "read" your shoes,* 2014. http://www.aofas.org/footcaremd/how-to/footwear/Pages/How-to-Read-Your-Shoes.aspx. Accessed April 17, 2015.)

alignment and gait, as illustrated in Figure 15-6. For example, wear on the ball of the foot may indicate that the heel tendon is tight, in which case heel-raising exercises can be recommended to release this tendon. Toe-shaped ridges on the upper toe box may indicate that the shoes are too small or that hammertoes are developing. A bulge and wear to the side of the great toe may indicate that the shoe is too narrow or that a bunion is present. Finally, unridged wear on the upper toe box generally indicates that the front of the shoe is too low (Ward, 2005).

A tracing of the weight-bearing foot is useful in assessing the fit of the shoe in terms of length and width. The foot tracing is compared with the current shoe to objectively reveal the flaw in the fitting, whether the foot is wider or longer than the shoe (see Figure 14-4). For example, toe box width plays an enormous role in the development of bunions, toe deformities, and corns. This type of foot tracing will also reveal the source of any foot pain. This tracing can be used to reinforce teaching to the patient about proper shoe fitting. Because the proper fitting of shoes is not an exact science, the patient should be encouraged to take the tracing to the shoe store when purchasing new shoes.

To evaluate the arch, a footprint can be made by placing the foot into a bucket of water and making a footprint on a piece of brown paper (Figure 15-7). A footprint that is very wide in the middle is indicative of flat feet (pes planus). With flat feet, the foot rolls excessively to the inside (i.e., overpronation), which leads to arch strain and pain on the inside of the knee. Adaptations to overcome flat feet and overpronation include molded leather arch supports (available over the counter) and athletic shoe styles. These types of shoes are designed with "control" features that aid in preventing the rolling-in motion of the ankle. If arch supports or sports shoes are ineffective, a foot specialist can fabricate a custom-molded orthotic shoe insert.

If the footprint shows little or no connectedness between the heel and the forefoot, the person has a high arch (pes cavus) (underpronation). In this case the foot rolls too much laterally, with a lot of weight landing on the outside edge of the foot. With this type of situation, the ankle becomes more susceptible to sprains and stress fractures. Again, athletic shoes are most appropriate because (1) "stability" athletic shoes are built with extra cushioning and (2) high-top athletic shoes cover the foot and ankle snugly to reduce the risk

Normal foot

Flat foot

High arch

FIGURE 15-7 How to "read" your footprint. (From American Orthopaedic Foot & Ankle Society: *How to "read" your footprint.* http://www.aofas.org/footcaremd/how-to/foot-health/Pages/How-to-Read-Your-Footprint.aspx. Accessed April 17, 2015.)

of ankle sprains and minimize damage to the ankle from twists (American Orthopaedic Foot & Ankle Society, 2015).

High heels increase torque on the knee and increase pressure on the forefoot. In addition, women naturally pronate more than men and naturally rely heavily on heel cushioning and arch support to reduce pronation. Unfortunately, high heels and arch supports restrict the natural movement of the ankle. Furthermore, by reducing pronation, the natural function in ankle motion also increases torque on the knee (Godfrey, 2006).

Offloading and Padding

Offloading and padding are used to protect bony structures of the foot, such as prominent metatarsal heads, or toe deformities from mechanical trauma caused by seams in the socks or shoes. Offloading techniques such as those summarized in Table 15-4

TABLE 15-4 Offloading Repetitive Stress for Foot and Nail

Anatomic Location	Offloading Method	Advantages/Disadvantages
All sites	Bed rest	Total non–weight-bearing Patient adherence is difficult Presents quality-of-life issues Promotes hyperglycemia Promotes patient debilitation Increases risk of posterior heel pressures (therefore must float heels)
All sites	Total contact cast (see Figure 14-5)	Forces adherence Allows for limited ambulation Requires specialized skill to make Not advisable for infected or highly exudative wounds
All sites	Walking splints/removable casts (see Figure 14-7)	Allows for daily wound surveillance and care Requires strict patient adherence
Forefoot ulcers	Football dressing	Forces compliance Ease of use with dressings Simple to make Inexpensive Can create balance issues
Forefoot sites	Wedge-soled shoe (aka custom molded shoe) (see Figure 14-8)	Commercially available Can be customized May cause balance problems
Plantar/posterior heel ulcers	Heel sole shoe with removable offloading pegs	Commercially available Can be customized May cause balance problems
All wound sites	Healing shoe with large toe box and customized inserts	Provides offloading to specific wound locations Requires specialized equipment Requires specialized skill to make
Metatarsal head sites	Adhesive felt pad	Simple to make Inexpensive Easy to use with dressings Requires at least weekly dressing changes
Metatarsal head sites	Felted foam or gel pads	Simple to make Inexpensive Easy to use with dressings Requires replacement every 3 to 4 days
Toes	Crest pads	Simple to make Adjunct for hammertoes or claw toes Commercially available Inexpensive May be used for wound prevention Requires frequent replacement
Toes	Silicone or foam Interdigital pads Lamb's wool	Commercially available Especially useful for crowded toes and crossed toes and interdigital wounds May be used for wound prevention Ineffective if shoes are too narrow Monitor for toe constriction Inexpensive
Bony deformities all sites on foot	Padded socks	Commercially available May be cause of foot pressure and/or toe constriction if shoe fit does not allow for increased padding
All bony deformities	Ball and ring shoe stretcher	Simple to use Pressure relief on leather shoes at specific sites of deformity

Modified from Wound, Ostomy and Continence Nurses Society™ (WOCN®): *Guideline for management of wounds in patients with lower-extremity neuropathic disease* (WOCN® clinical practice guideline series no. 3), Glenview, IL, 2012, WOCN®.

and illustrated in Figures 14-5, 14-6, 14-7, and 14-8 include total-contact casts; removable splints and casts; and customized shoes, pads, and inserts.

Over-the-counter and custom-molded padding and inserts can be used to redistribute pressure, reduce hyperkeratotic lesions, and eliminate repetitive stress and friction (Freeman, 2002; WOCN®, 2012). Pads can be used to protect diminished fat pads on the plantar surface of the foot. However, pads with aggressive adhesives should be avoided on fragile elderly skin. Nonadherent silicone pads should be used and can be held in place with socks over prominent metatarsal heads. Tubular pads can be fit on the tips of toes to protect at-risk areas or used between toes where interdigital calluses may form. Lamb's wool can be woven between all toes or placed between at-risk toes. The wool provides inherent moisturizing from the lanolin while also absorbing perspiration and excess moisture (Kelechi and Lukacs, 1996; Ozdemir et al, 2004).

MANAGEMENT OF SPECIFIC CONDITIONS

Many conditions and circumstances can greatly affect the integrity and function of the foot, such as obesity, anemia, renal insufficiency, impaired circulation, gout, warfarin therapy, Raynaud disease, immunosuppression, and recurrent cellulitis. The 33 joints in each foot must accommodate an extraordinary weight load, making the feet particularly susceptible to arthritic inflammation and swelling of the cartilage and lining of the joints. Individuals older than 50 years are at greatest risk for arthritis. Osteoarthritis is the most common form of arthritis and is associated with aging, injury, or overuse. The foot is one of the first places for osteoporosis to appear; a stress fracture of the foot is often its first sign. A variety of normal age-associated changes occur in the foot: the foot becomes wider, longer, and flatter; the fat pad on the bottom of the calcaneus thins; and the foot and ankle lose some degree of range of motion and become stiff, which contributes to some loss of balance with ambulation (Ozdemir et al, 2004; Willacy, 2008). Impaired circulation due to lower extremity arterial disease or lower extremity venous disease, as well as decreased foot sensation due to lower extremity neuropathic disease, syphilis, leprosy, myelomeningocele, syringomyelia, hereditary neuropathies, or traumatic nerve injury, contribute to problems with the foot (Adler et al, 1999; Younes et al, 2004). Superficial as well as deep lesions and skin alterations can potentially lead to significant infection.

Skin Conditions

A variety of skin conditions (e.g., vesicles, bullae, or ulcers) can develop on the feet due to repetitive friction and prolonged pressure from ill-fitting shoes. Infection can develop in the foot triggered by a moist environment and require treatment with appropriate medications (antifungal, antibacterial, or antiviral). Hyperkeratotic lesions (corns and calluses) are among the most common foot problems in older people (Figure 15-8). Ulcers can develop under these hyperkeratotic lesions with long-term, low-level insult and become

FIGURE 15-8 Selected lesions and skin alterations. **A,** Corn. **B,** Callus. (From Ball JW, Dains JE, Flynn JA: *Seidel's guide to physical examination*, ed 8, St. Louis, MO, 2015, Mosby.)

particularly problematic in the person with loss of protective sensation (Spink et al, 2009).

Warts *(Verruca papilloma)* are common dermatologic infections. Plantar warts, specifically, are caused by the human papillomavirus, affect persons of all ages, are contagious, and will spread to other people, especially where the epidermal barrier is disrupted (Watkins, 2006). Plantar warts can also spread to other histologically similar sites (Lichon and Khachemoune, 2007).

Fungal infections may develop and include candida (rarely seen on the feet) and dermatophytes. More commonly called tinea, dermatophyte lesions are discussed in detail in Chapter 5. Dermatophyte symptoms may be less pronounced in elderly individuals and in individuals with altered sensation (Hill, 2008). The moccasin type of tinea pedis is often mistaken for dry skin on the plantar surface of the foot, but does not respond to emollient application (Crawford, 2004). Tinea pedis may coexist with a secondary bacterial infection (Erbagci, 2004).

Table 15-2 summarizes the assessment, prevention, and management of common foot lesions. The variety of interventions includes properly fitting shoes; offloading; positioning; and topical agents such as emollients, antifungals, and, in some cases, corticosteroids. Offloading and padding, as described previously, is needed to interrupt the presence of the stressors causing vesicles, ulcers, and corns. In general, a vesicle or bulla should be left intact. Topical care of open lesions should be selected based on the needs of the wound, as described in Chapter 18.

As with all interventions, reevaluation of the effectiveness is needed. If the problem deteriorates or fails to respond to treatment within a reasonable period of time (i.e., 7 days), reassessment and modification of the treatment should be conducted. For example, topical antibiotics and corticosteroids may need to be delivered systemically rather than topically. However, use of these medications should be recommended only by a practitioner who is well informed of their potential complications and side effects, which can include conditions such as skin reactions, liver enzyme abnormalities, diarrhea, and visual and taste disturbances.

Foot Conditions (Malformations)

Foot malformations can affect all three sections of the foot: forefoot, midfoot, and hindfoot. Charcot arthropathy (see Figure 14-1, *B)* is a fairly rare but serious condition caused by the disruption or disintegration of some of the foot and ankle joints. Redness, swelling, and deformity may develop and may be misinterpreted as cellulitis. Charcot arthropathy is frequently associated with diabetes (discussed in greater detail in Chapter 14).

Forefoot. The forefoot area has the highest prevalence of foot malformations. The most common problems that arise in the forefoot are hallux valgus (bunions), bunionettes, hallux rigidus, claw toes, hammertoes and mallet toes, metatarsalgia, and interdigit neuromas (Morton neuroma). Forefoot problems are painful and are generally accompanied by ingrown toenail, calluses, and corns (Hsi et al, 2005). Forefoot problems occur nine times more often in women than in men and are most commonly associated with wearing shoes with high heels and a narrow toe box. Once forefoot problems develop, finding footwear can be difficult. Brief descriptions of forefoot malformations are provided in Table 15-5 and illustrated in Figure 14-1 (Ferrari et al, 2004; Larson et al, 2005; Thomson

TABLE 15-5	Types of Forefoot Malformations	
Name	**Description**	**Common Location(s)**
Hallux valgus (bunion) (see Figure 14-1, *C)*	Lateral deviation of great toe (hallux) Produces abnormal hypertrophic bursa over medial eminence of first metatarsal Diagnostic testing includes examination and radiograph to determine degree of deviation Symptoms include pain, redness, and swelling at or near the joint; as toe devastation progresses, bunion becomes more painful	First MTP joint
Bunionette (tailor's bunion)	Less common than bunion; see previous description	Fifth MTP joint
Hallux rigidus	Degenerative arthritis of MTP joint Presents with pain in great toe with activity, especially in toe-off phase of gait Stiffness of great toe and loss of extension at MTP joint Toe in normal alignment Radiographs show narrowing of MTP joint of great toe	First MTP joint
Interdigit neuroma (Morton neuroma)	Not a true neuroma Perineural fibrosis of common digital nerve as it passes through metatarsal head; fibrosis results from repeated irritation of nerve that may be caused by bones or other tissue rubbing against and irritating the nerves Plantar pain in forefoot is most common presenting symptom Pain usually is alleviated by rubbing ball of the foot after removing shoes	Metatarsal head
Claw toe	Usually associated with neurologic disorder or inflammatory arthritis	Lesser toes
Hammertoe (see Figure 14-1, *A)*	Fixation of proximal dorsiflexion, middle joint is fixed in plantar flexion, distal joint is moveable Usually bilateral Often accompanied by hallux valgus	Lesser toes
Mallet toe	Distal interphalangeal joint is plantarflexed on intermediate phalanx with rest of joint in normal position	Lesser toes
Charcot arthropathy (see Figure 14-1, *B)*	Fairly rare but serious; associated with diabetes Caused by disruption or disintegration of some of the foot and ankle joints Redness, swelling, and deformity may develop and may be misinterpreted as cellulitis (Discussed in greater detail in Chapter 14)	Foot

MTP, Metatarsophalangeal.

et al, 2004). Forefoot pain, specifically metatarsalgia, results from an abnormal metatarsal length with alteration of the weight-bearing forces. Symptoms of metatarsalgia include callus formation and localized pain in the plantar aspect of the forefoot over the metatarsal heads. Treatment of forefoot pain involves the application of a metatarsal pad and paring down of calluses (Hsi et al, 2005).

Midfoot. The primary midfoot problem is pain. Midfoot pain is commonly caused by arthritis in the midfoot joints, including the TMT joint, subtalar joint, and talonavicular joint. The exact area of pain is easily pinpointed with palpation. The palpation of a bony prominence that is an osteophyte or dorsal bossing corresponds with the joint with the arthritis. Although less common, soft tissue pain can be present on the plantar aspect of the midfoot, which occurs with plantar fasciitis; this is discussed in more detail in the "Hindfoot" section (Frey, 2005).

Hindfoot. Heel pain, a typical hindfoot problem, is caused by stress on the calcaneus and results from poorly made footwear and walking or jumping on hard surfaces. Common causes include plantar fasciitis, heel spur, tarsal tunnel syndrome, and Achilles tendonitis (Labib et al, 2002). Additional causative factors include arthritis, gout, ankylosing spondylitis, Reiter syndrome, radiculopathy, inferior calcaneal bursitis, calcaneal fracture, foreign bodies, circulatory problems, and obesity. Calcaneus pain can be palpated directly over the plantar medial calcaneal tuberosity. A heel spur, an osteophyte bony growth on the underside, foremost part of the calcaneus bone, is commonly associated with plantar fasciitis, as illustrated in Figure 15-9 (Frey, 2005).

Plantar fasciitis is the most common condition causing heel pain. This pain occurs with weight bearing or faulty biomechanics that place too much stress on the calcaneus bone, ligaments, or nerves in the area (Jolly et al, 2005; La Porta and La Fata, 2005). Plantar fasciitis is essentially an inflammation of the long band of connective tissue running from the calcaneus to the ball of the foot that forms the arch of the foot (Lemont et al, 2003). Symptoms include pain on the plantar surface of the heel and pain that is worse upon arising or after sitting a long time and increases over a few months. Plantar fasciitis is most likely to develop in people with either overly flat feet or high arched feet.

Posterior heel pain causes symptoms behind the foot rather than underneath, is likely related to irritation from shoes, and presents with a prominence over the superior process of the calcaneus. A common cause of posterior heel pain is Achilles tendonitis, considered a jumping injury. The Achilles tendon connects the calf muscle to the heel bone and facilitates walking by helping raise the heel off the ground. Symptoms of Achilles tendon pathology include pain along the tendon (aching, stiff, soreness) and pain that begins upon arising and after periods of rest, improves slightly with movement, then worsens with increased activity. Athletes are at high risk for developing Achilles tendon pathology. Tarsal tunnel syndrome causes heel pain similar to carpal tunnel syndrome in the hand and is a repetitive motion injury (Badlissi et al, 2005).

The cause of heel pain must be determined before a plan of treatment is initiated. General treatments include rest or avoiding the precipitating activity (e.g., jogging), icing the heel, exercises and stretches, and nonsteroidal antiinflammatory medications. An orthotic device, such as a silicone heel pad insert with shock-absorbing soles, is often key to successful treatment of calcaneus pain. Exercises such as "alphabet exercise," where the patient moves the ankle in multiple planes of motion by drawing both lowercase and uppercase

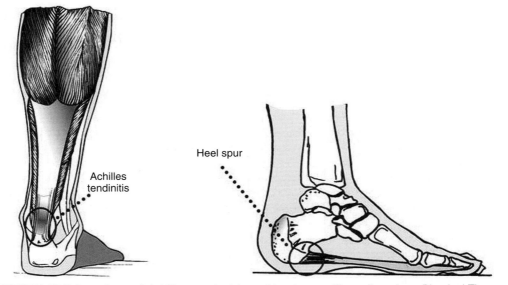

Achilles
tendinitis

Heel spur

FIGURE 15-9 Locations of Achilles tendonitis and heel spur. (From American Physical Therapy Association, 1996.)

letters of the alphabet with the foot, is particularly beneficial for heel spurs. Cortisone injections and over-the-counter heel cups or custom-made orthotics also may be warranted.

Nail Conditions (Onychopathy)

Onycho means "nail." Onychopathy is any disease or deformity of the nail. Abnormal nails are clues to multisystem diseases. The growth rate, discoloration, thickness, and structural changes can be equated to specific disease processes. Nails should be inspected for general appearance; nail plate for length, color, thickness, presence of subungual debris, odor, hyponychium or eponychium for separation from the nail plate; and paronychial edge for infection, ingrown nails, hangnails, and pain. The toenails should be assessed for changes in color, continuity of the nail plate, missing nails or nail malformations, and infection. Selected nail disorders, descriptions, symptoms, and causes are listed in Table 15-6. This section describes management strategies.

Onychocryptosis (Ingrown Nail). Management of onychocryptosis includes education on proper nail trimming and proper fitting of shoes. The lateral plate should be allowed to grow well beyond the nail fold before trimming horizontally. The mild to moderate ingrown nail with minimal pain and erythema and no discharge can be treated with the application of a cotton wedge or dental floss underneath the lateral nail plate. This separates the nail plate from the lateral nail fold, which relieves the pressure. The moderate to severe ingrown toenail with substantial erythema and pustular discharge (Figure 15-10, *B*) will require a digital block and removal of the involved nail wedge with a hemostat. Cleansing the area with 1:1 peroxide and water two to three times per day followed by the application of a topical antibiotic is recommended (Rounding and Bloomfield, 2005).

Onychomycosis (Fungal Infection of Nail). Fungal infections account for only 50% of the dystrophic nails. Nail conditions such as psoriasis, lichen planus, dermatitis, dyshidrosis, and other infections may mimic onychomycosis (Baran and Kaoukhov, 2005). Therefore culturing the nail has become a standard of practice before treatment with an antifungal. The antifungal chosen is usually driven by insurance reimbursement of the medication. The highest cure rates are associated with oral terbinafine and itraconazole. Topical nail lacquer containing ciclopirox is used for mild to moderate onychomycosis that does not involve the lunula (see Figure 15-3). The lacquer is applied once daily to the affected nail, 5 mm of surrounding skin, the nail bed (hyponychium), and the undersurface of the nail plate. Once per week, the nail lacquer is wiped off with alcohol. Studies have showed increased efficacy with the combination treatment (Sidou and Soto, 2004).

TABLE 15-6	Selected Nail Disorders		
Name	**Description**	**Symptoms**	**Cause**
Paronychia (see Figure 15-10, *A*)	Painful infection of tissue around base of nail (perionychium)	Swelling and tenderness posterior or lateral to nail folds May progress to superficial abscess	Bacteria enter break in skin caused by damage, trauma (e.g., nail biting, chemical irritants)
Onychocryptosis (ingrown nail) (see Figure 15-10, *B*)	Penetration of segment of nail plate into nail sulcus and subcutaneous tissue	Acute inflammation, edema, exudate, pain Can evolve into infection (paronychia, cellulitis), ulceration, necrosis Most commonly affects large toes	Improper nail trimming Shoe pressure Injury or fungal infection Poor foot structure Onychogryposis Higher risk: male, increasing age, immunosuppression, diabetes, PVD
Onychomycosis (fungal infection)	Tinea unguium or dermatophyte infection Occurs in three distinct forms: distal subungual, proximal subungual, white superficial	Painless, dystrophic changes (thick, brittle discoloration) of one or many toenails Psoriasis, lichen planus, dermatitis, dyshidrosis may mimic onychomycosis	Infectious agent present on susceptible host Chronic exposure to moisture Hyperhidrosis Tinea pedis Poor hygiene
Onychogryposis (ram's horn nail)	Large, deformed, hypertrophic nail	Thick hard nails that curl like horn of ram	Nail was permitted to grow without trimming or debridement
Onychophosis	Localized or diffuse hyperkeratosis on lateral or proximal nail folds, in space between nail folds and nail plate	First and fifth toes are commonly affected	Poor-fitting shoes
Onychatrophia	Atrophy of nails	Softer, thinner, smaller nails Nail detachment	Skin diseases, underlying diseases

PVD, Peripheral vascular disease.

FIGURE 15-10 Selected nail disorders: **A,** Paronychia **B,** Onychocryptosis (ingrown nail). (**A,** From Ball JW, Dains JE, Flynn JA: *Seidel's guide to physical examination,* ed 8, St. Louis, MO, 2015, Mosby. **B,** From White GM: *Color atlas of regional dermatology,* St. Louis, MO, 1994, Mosby.)

Paronychia. Paronychia is inflammation of the cells that grow the nail (matrix) (see Figure 15-10, *A*), resulting in edema and erythema from many of the disorders described in Table 15-6. For chronic paronychia, treatment consists of warm soaks and topical antifungal agents. Treatment of acute paronychia includes warm compresses for 20 minutes three times per day and topical antibiotics (triple antibiotic) applied after the warm soaks. For more severe infections, oral antibiotics with gram-positive coverage may be necessary (Billingsley, 2014).

Referral

Numerous specialists (e.g., primary care provider, podiatry, orthopedics, dermatology, endocrinology, vascular surgery, general surgery, physical therapy, occupational therapy, pedorthist/orthotist, home health, pain management, diabetes education, smoking cessation, case/care manager, social worker, wound specialist) may be required to provide comprehensive foot and nail care. Results of the foot screening must be communicated to the appropriate health care provider, along with the patient's foot ulceration risk and a record of the educational materials given to the patient and family (Boulton and Armstrong, 2008; Patout et al, 2001).

Patient and Caregiver Education

Involving patients in their own care decreases foot complications; therefore it is important to provide education on foot and nail care to the patient and caregiver (Howell and Thirlaway, 2004). Box 15-6 lists the components of patient and family education related to foot care. Patients should be taught that they can protect the health of their feet by maintaining a normal weight to lessen changes due to osteoporosis (Neno, 2007; Woodrow et al, 2005). Additional foot care instructions can be found in Box 14-5. The patient should be taught to call the health care professional when problems listed in Box 15-6 arise (American Orthopaedic Foot & Ankle Society, 2015; Gemmell et al, 2005; van Os et al, 2005).

Home Remedies

Many over-the-counter and home remedies are used for treatment of foot and nail problems. Four products are most commonly used: Vicks VapoRub, vinegar, vegetable oil, and Vaseline. Vaseline and vegetable oil (Crisco) are inexpensive options and can be used to moisturize the skin. Vegetable oil has a risk of bacterial growth while in the container and the risk of allergic dermatitis. Vaseline (petroleum) comes in different grades, which vary depending on composition, purity (depending on stock), production, and packaging. Petrolatum-based products have been identified as clinically effective and cost-effective. However, allergic dermatitis can occur from petroleum products (Kelechi, 2004).

Vinegar, tea tree oil, and mentholated topical petrolatum-based gel (such as Vicks VapoRub) are used to treat fungal and bacterial infections. In various dilutions, vinegar is effective in reducing or eliminating growth of bacteria. Evidence for the use of vinegar in treating fungal infection is limited. The literature has reported vinegar (one part vinegar and two parts water for 15 minutes per day) used as treatment of toenail fungus, athlete's foot, and foot odor and as an exfoliant. Long-term use of vinegar (regardless of concentration) is contraindicated, however, due to the drying effect and potential for skin irritation. Tea tree oil is an antiseptic/tinneacide. Anecdotally, Vicks VapoRub applied topically to the nail daily has been used for treatment of toenail fungus (Kelechi, 2004).

Unsupervised home remedies for foot ailments should be avoided. Self-treatment has the potential for turning a minor problem into a major one. Persons with diabetes, poor circulation, or heart problems should not treat their own feet because they are more prone to infection. It is vital that older individuals see a foot care specialist at least once per year for a checkup (Neno, 2007; Woodrow et al, 2005).

CLINICAL CONSULT

A: Patient referred by nursing home nurse to evaluate a 63-year-old Caucasian male for scratching LE and open area on right great toe. Current medical history includes insulin-dependent diabetes, hypothyroid, hepatitis C, hypertension, major depression, and skin picking disorder. Upon exam patient states that he is not having any scratching, admits to picking/cutting his toenails. Ambulates independently. Wears orthotic shoes. Excoriation on bilateral lower extremities with no redness or drainage. Right great toe lateral nail fold has small purulent discharge, erythema, and edema present; painful to touch. Blood sugar 246, afebrile.

D: Paronychia, heel fissure, interdigit toe maceration.

P: Apply antibacterial ointment three times daily; cover with nonadherent dressing and secure with roll gauze. Start doxycycline 100 mg twice a day ×10 days.

I: (1) Use healing shoe until infection resolved to prevent further trauma. (2) Wear padded socks. (3) Schedule foot and nail care nurse visits for callus removal and nail debriding. (4) Remove nail-clipping tools from patient's room. (5) Education on diabetic foot care. (6) Apply Lac-Hydrin to lower extremities daily. Redirect if patient is seen scratching. (7) Lamb's wool between toes and changed daily. (8) Pedorthist to reevaluate orthotic shoes for proper fitting. (9) Joint collaboration with mental health care provider for potential antianxiety medications and behavior therapy to diminish picking behavior.

E: Recheck visit in 3 days.

SUMMARY

Foot and nail disorders are predominantly a reflection of the patient's overall health status. By conducting a regular and routine foot and nail assessment in conjunction with a routine skin assessment, preventive interventions can be identified that will prevent the discomfort and secondary complications that arise from foot and nail disorders. Routine foot care should be integrated into everyday practice, thus keeping the skin healthy and intact and minimizing the risk of trauma or malformation (Howell and Thirlaway, 2004).

REFERENCES

Adler AL, Boyko EJ, Smith DG: Lower-extremity amputation in diabetes. The independent effect of peripheral vascular disease, sensory neuropathy and foot ulcers, *Diabetes Care* 22(7):1029–1035, 1999.

American Orthopaedic Foot and Ankle Society: *How to "read" your footprint*, 2015. http://www.aofas.org/footcaremd/how-to/foot-health/Pages/How-to-Read-Your-Footprint.aspx. Accessed April 17, 2015.

American Podiatric Medical Association: *Your podiatric physician talks about foot health*, 2010. http://www.apma.org/files/ProductPDFs/Foot_Health.pdf. Accessed April 17, 2015.

Badlissi F, Dunn JE, Link CL, et al: Foot musculoskeletal disorders, pain, and foot-related functional limitation in older persons, *J Am Geriatr Soc* 53:1029–1033, 2005.

Ball JW, Dains JE, Flynn JA: *Seidel's guide to physical examination*, ed 8, St. Louis, MO, 2015, Mosby.

Baran R, Kaoukhov A: Topical antifungal drugs for the treatment of onychomycosis: an overview of current strategies for monotherapy and combination therapy, *J Eur Acad Dermatol Venereol* 19:21–29, 2005.

Billingsley E, Vidimos A: *Paronychia treatment and management*, updated November 17, 2014. http://emedicine.medscape.com/article/1106062-treatment. Accessed July 27, 2015.

Boulton A, Armstrong D: Comprehensive foot examination and risk assessment, *Diabetes Care* 31:1679–1685, 2008.

Cavanagh PR, Ulbrecht JS: The biomechanics of the foot in diabetes mellitus. In Bowker JH, Pfeiffer MA, editors: *Levin and O'Neal's the diabetic foot*, ed 7, St. Louis, 2008, Mosby.

Crawford F: Athlete's foot and fungally infected toenails, *Clin Evid* 11:2128–2132, 2004.

Duthie EH: History and physical exam. In Duthie EH, et al, editors: *Practice of geriatrics*, ed 4, Philadelphia, 2007, Saunders.

Erbagci Z: Topical therapy for dermatophytoses: should corticosteroids be included? *Am J Clin Dermatol* 5:375–384, 2004.

Ferrari J, Higgins JP, Prior TD: Interventions for treating hallux valgus (abductovalgus) and bunions, *Cochrane Database Syst Rev* 1:CD000964, 2004.

Freeman DB: Corns and calluses resulting from mechanical hyperkeratosis, *Am Fam Physician* 65:2277–2280, 2002.

Frey C: Plantar fasciitis. In Griffin LY, editor: *Essentials of musculoskeletal care*, ed 3, Rosemont, IL, 2005, American Academy of Orthopaedic Surgeons.

Garrow AP, Silman AJ, Macfarlane GJ: The Cheshire foot pain and disability survey: a population survey assessing prevalence and associations, *Pain* 110:378–384, 2004.

Gemmell H, Hayes B, Conway M: A theoretical model for treatment of soft tissue injuries: treatment of an ankle sprain in a college tennis player, *J Manipulat Physiol Therapeut* 28:285–288, 2005.

Godfrey JR: Toward the optimal health. D. Casey Kerrigan, M.D., discusses the impact of footwear on the progression of osteoarthritis in women, *J Womens Health (Larchmt)* 15:894–897, 2006.

Hill MJ: Fungal infections, *Dermatol Nurs* 20:137–138, 2008.

Howell M, Thirlaway S: Integrating foot care into the everyday clinical practice of nurses, *Br J Nurs* 13:470–473, 2004.

Hsi WL, et al: Optimum position of metatarsal pad in metatarsalgia for pressure relief, *Am J Phys Med Rehabil* 84:514, 2005.

Jarvis C: Neurologic system. In Jarvis C, editor: *Physical examination and health assessment*, St. Louis, MO, 2004, Saunders.

Jolly GP, Zgonis T, Hendrix CL: Neurogenic heel pain, *Clin Podiatr Med Surg* 22:101–113, 2005.

Katoh T: Outpatient foot care by dermatologist and specially trained nurse, *Jpn J Mycol* 49:173–174, 2008.

Katsambas A, Abeck D, Haneke E, et al: The effects of foot disease on quality of life: results of the Achilles project, *J Eur Acad Dermatol Venereol* 19:191–195, 2005.

Kelechi T, Lukacs K: Intrapreneurial nursing: the comprehensive lower extremity assessment form, *Clin Nurse Spec CNS* 10: 266–274, 1996.

Kelechi T, Stroud S: The four V's of footcare, *Adv Nurse Pract* 12:67–70, 2004.

La Porta GA, La Fata PC: Pathologic conditions of the plantar fascia, *Clin Podiatr Med Surg* 22:1–9, 2005.

Labib SA, Gould JS, Rodriguez-del-Rio FA, et al: Heel pain triad (HPT): the combination of plantar fasciitis, posterior tibial tendon dysfunction and tarsal tunnel syndrome, *Foot Ankle Int* 23:212–220, 2002.

Larson EE, Barrett SL, Battison B, et al: Accurate nomenclature for forefoot nerve entrapment: a historical perspective, *J Am Podiatr Med Assoc* 95:298–306, 2005.

Lemont H, Ammirati KM, Usen N: Plantar fasciitis: a degenerative process (fasciosis) without inflammation, *J Am Podiatr Med Assoc* 93:234–237, 2003.

Leveille SG, Gurainik JM, Ferrucci L, et al: Foot pain and disability in older women, *Am J Epidemiol* 148:657–665, 1998.

Lichon V, Khachemoune A: Plantar warts: a focus on treatment modalities, *Dermatol Nurs* 19(4):372–375, 2007.

Menz HB, Lord SR: The contribution of foot problems to mobility impairment and falls in community-dwelling older people, *J Am Geriatr Soc* 49:1651–1656, 2001.

Menz HB, Morris ME: Footwear characteristics and foot problems in older people, *Gerontology* 51:346–351, 2005.

Mix G: *Salon professional's guide to foot care*, Albany, NY, 1999, Milady Salon Ovations.

Neno R: Feet for purpose? *Nurs Older People* 19(8):5–6, 2007.

Ozdemir H, Söyüncü Y, Ozgörgen M, et al: Effects of changes in heel fat pad thickness and elasticity on heel pain, *J Am Podiatr Med Assoc* 94:47–52, 2004.

Patout CA Jr, Birke JA, Wilbright WA, et al: A decision pathway for the staged management of foot problems in diabetes mellitus, *Arch Phys Med Rehabil* 82:1724–1728, 2001.

Piraccini BM, Iorizzo M, Antonoucci A, et al: Drug-induced nail abnormalities, *Expert Opin Drug Saf* 3:57–65, 2004.

Popoola MM, Jenkins L: Caring for the foot mobile, *Holistic Nurs Pract* 19:222–227, 2004.

Price P, Harding K: The impact of foot complications on health-related quality of life in patients with diabetes, *J Cutan Med Surg* 4:45–50, 2000.

Quinn E: *Foot anatomy and physiology*. Sports Medicine About, 2014. http://sportsmedicine.about.com/cs/foot_facts/a/foot1.htm. Accessed April 17, 2015.

Rees HG: World at work: evidence-based risk management of nail dust in chiropodists and podiatrists, *Occupat Environ Med* 65:216–217, 2008.

Rounding C, Bloomfield S: Surgical treatments for ingrowing toenails, *Cochrane Database Syst Rev*, 2:CD001541, 2005.

Schwartz R: *Gram-negative toe web infection*, 2013. http://emedicine.medscape.com/article/1055306-diagnosis. Accessed April 17, 2015.

Sidou F, Soto P: A randomized comparison of nail surface remanence three nail lacquers, containing amorolfine 5%, ciclopirox 8% or tioconazole 28%, in healthy volunteers, *Int J Tissue Reactions* 26(1–2):17–24, 2004.

Sinni-McKeehen B: Nursing assessment. Integumentary system. In Lewis SL, et al, editors: *Medical-surgical nursing. Assessment and management of clinical problems*, St. Louis, MO, 2007, Elsevier.

Spink MJ, Menz HB, Lord SR: Distribution and correlates of plantar hyperkeratotic lesions in older people, *J Foot Ankle Res* 30:8, 2009.

Sprecher E: Genetic hair and nail disorders, *Clin Dermatol* 23: 47–55, 2005.

Stroud S, Kelechi T: Itching and sores between the toes. Maceration and fungal infection, *Adv Nurse Pract* 16(7):26, 2006.

Thomson CE, Gibson JN, Martin D: Interventions for the treatment of Morton's neuroma, *Cochrane Database Syst Rev* 3:CD003118, 2004.

van Os AG, Bierma-Zeinstra SM, Verhagen AP, et al: Comparison of conventional treatment and supervised rehabilitation for treatment of acute lateral ankle sprains: a systematic review of the literature, *J Orthop Sports Phys Ther* 35:95–105, 2005.

Vileikyte L, Peyrot M, Bundy C: The development and validation of a neuropathy- and foot ulcer-specific quality of life instrument, *Diabetes Care* 26:2549–2555, 2003.

Ward SA: Diabetes, exercise, and foot care, *Physician Sports Med* 33:33–38, 2005.

Watkins P: Identifying and treating plantar warts, *Nurs Stand* 20(42):50–54, 2006.

Willacy H: *Abnormal gait*, version 20, updated April 24, 2008. http://www.patient.co.uk/doctor/Abnormal-Gait.htm. Accessed December 8, 2009.

Woodrow P, Dickson N, Wright P: Foot care for non-diabetic older people, *Nurs Older People* 17(8):31–32, 2005.

Wound, Ostomy and Continence Nurses Society™ (WOCN®): *Guideline for management of wounds in patients with lower-extremity neuropathic disease (WOCN® clinical practice guideline series no. 3)*, Glenview IL, 2012, WOCN®.

Younes NA, Albsoul AM, Awad H: Diabetic heel ulcers: a major risk factor for lower extremity amputation, *Ostomy Wound Manage* 50:50–60, 2004.

16

Wound Infection: Diagnosis and Management

Nancy A. Stotts

OBJECTIVES

1. Compare and contrast the signs and symptoms and treatment of the continuum of bacterial bioburden, including contamination, colonization, critical colonization, biofilm, and wound infection.
2. Identify risk factors for chronic wound infection.
3. Describe the processes used in obtaining a wound culture by biopsy, aspiration, and swab and the strengths and limitations of each.

4. Interpret laboratory data indicative of a wound infection.
5. Propose interventions to prevent biofilm redevelopment.
6. Propose interventions to treat wound infection.

Intact skin is the body's greatest defense against infection. It is a mechanical barrier to microorganisms, and its normal flora and acidic pH control invasion of the skin by other microorganisms. When skin integrity is breached, tissue quickly becomes contaminated by body fluids and normal skin flora (Fonder et al, 2008). The effects of microorganisms' burden, called *bioburden,* on the wound are numerous and complex.

There is much we do not understand about the role of microorganisms in wound healing. Until recently, all organisms in wounds were thought to be free-floating bacteria, called *planktonic phenotype.* Costerton's group was the first to identify biofilm and, over time, the scientific community came to appreciate that biofilms composed of organisms aggregated and embedded a matrix of sugars, protein, and lipids were present on chronic wounds (Costerton et al, 1999). This became known as *biofilm phenotype.* The biofilms develop multiple layers of organisms, and the organisms are able to communicate with each other (quantum sensing) and send messages that alter the organisms' phenotype and genotype. The gene modulation allows the organisms deep in the biofilm to reduce their metabolism (even become dormant) so they can live in the nutrient- and oxygen-deficient environment found at the base of the wound. Importantly, organisms in the biofilm become tolerant to antibiotics (Gottrup et al, 2013).

The biofilm matrix also is important in this process. It provides the environment in which the organisms live, mutate, and die. Much information about what takes place in biofilm has been provided by studies that include two common organisms: *Staphylococcus aureus* and *Pseudomonas aeruginosa.* *S. aureus* is often present in wounds with delayed healing, but it is not always linked to infection. *P. aeruginosa* is associated with ulcers that are larger than wounds without the organism (Zhao et al, 2010) and in large pressure ulcers (Madsen et al, 1996). *P. aeruginosa* produces rhamnolipids that impair neutrophil function and, combined with the influx of dead neutrophils and degraded enzymes (reactive oxygen species) and metaloproteinases (Fazli et al, 2011), contribute to delayed healing. Analyses of these data have led to speculation that the organisms present in biofilm may be more important than the number of them (Gottrup et al, 2013). The virulence of hemolytic staphylococcus type A and G is well known. It is possible that *P. aeruginosa* should be added to the list.

Our understanding of infection has been of planktonic phenotype organisms that compete for the limited nutrients and oxygen present in the wound. In addition, they produce endotoxins and exotoxins that destroy or alter normal cellular activities, such as collagen deposition and cross-linking. *Endotoxins* are lipids and polysaccharides that are located in the cell wall of gram-negative organisms. When released, they activate the regulatory systems of the body (e.g., clotting, inflammation). *Exotoxins* are proteins released from bacteria that enzymatically inactivate or modify cells, causing them to die or disrupt their normal cellular functioning (Edwards and Harding, 2004). Under normal regulatory conditions, the body is able to compensate and wound healing takes place, with the anticipated time and healing sequence for acute wounds.

In contrast, regulation of the healing processes sometimes gets out of control and results in chronic wounds. These chronic wounds contain some degree of bacterial bioburden and exhibit significantly elevated proinflammatory cytokines (interleukin-1, tumor necrosis factor-α, γ-interferon), matrix metalloproteinases (MMP-2, MMP-8, MMP-9), and neutrophils (Wolcott et al, 2009). In response to the proinflammatory proteins, neutrophils continue to arrive at the wound and release cytotoxic enzymes, free oxygen radicals, and inflammatory mediators, triggering additional degradation of extracellular matrix and growth factors. Eventually, protein lysis exceeds the synthesis of proteins essential to wound repair so that the wound remains in the inflammatory phase and is unable to advance into the proliferative phase (Bjarnsholt et al, 2008; Woo and Sibbald, 2009), thus delayed healing results (Expert Working Group, 2008). Chronic wounds are costly in finances and human suffering, and they have the potential to deteriorate into infection, sepsis, multisystem organ failure, and death.

CONTINUUM OF MICROORGANISM BIOBURDEN

All wounds have some level of bacterial burden; few wounds are infected. The presence of organisms in the wound is an expectation. The continuum of bacterial bioburden has been subdivided into progressive microbial states: contamination, colonization, critical colonization, biofilm, and infection (Box 16-1).

Contamination

Contamination is the presence of nonreplicating microorganisms on the wound surface (Sibbald et al, 2006). Because all open wounds are contaminated by normal skin flora, the body is continually challenged to defend itself against invasion (Basu et al, 2009). Contaminating microorganisms may be endogenous (e.g., normal skin and gastrointestinal flora) or exogenous, present in the external environment (e.g., bed linen, devices, hospital personnel) (Woo and Sibbald, 2009).

Early contaminants usually are gram-positive organisms (*S. aureus, Corynebacterium, Streptococcus*). They are followed by gram-negative organisms (*Escherichia coli, Klebsiella, Proteus*) from the urogenital area. Days to weeks later, anaerobic organisms, such as *Prevotella, Bacteroides,* and *Peptostreptococcus,* and fungi arrive. The third wave of organisms is difficult to isolate with routine culture techniques because they typically lodge deep in the wound (Landis, 2008; Daeschlein, 2013). Local or systemic antibiotics are not utilized for contaminated wounds.

Colonization

With colonization, the microorganisms adhere to the surface of the wound and replicate. Colonization does not impair healing (Edwards and Harding, 2004). There are no signs or symptoms of colonization. Inappropriate use of antibiotics during this phase has contributed to the prevalence of antibiotic-resistant organisms (Landis, 2008).

BOX 16-1   Glossary of Terms

Antibiotic: Agent that can destroy or inhibit organisms.

Antimicrobial: General term for a substance that destroys or inhibits growth and replication of microorganisms in wound or on intact skin.

Antiseptic/Antibacterial: Topical substance that inhibits growth and reproduction of organisms. Can be used on open wounds and intact skin. Strong biocidal agents and multiple pharmaceutical targets; little resistance developed to them; examples are iodine and silver. Duration of use limited to 2 weeks.

Bioburden: Presence of microorganisms on or in a wound. Continuum of bioburden ranges from contamination, colonization, critical colonization, biofilm, and infection. Bioburden includes the quantity of microorganisms present, as well as their diversity, virulence, and interaction of the organisms with each other and with the body (synergism).

Biofilm: Complex community of aggregated bacteria embedded in a self-secreted extracellular polysaccharide matrix. Bacteria within biofilm respond to signals from other bacteria in the community to change their phenotype. Highly resistant to and poorly penetrated by antimicrobials. Can be removed with debridement. Reformation is prevented with antimicrobials and maintenance debridement (including autolysis).

Colonization: Replicating microorganisms adherent to the wound surface without a host reaction. Antimicrobials are not indicated.

Contamination: Nonreplicating microorganisms on the wound surface without a host reaction. All open wounds are contaminated by normal skin flora. Antimicrobials are not indicated.

Critical Colonization: Replicating microorganisms present on the wound and attached to the cells and structures in the wound. Level of bacteria inhibits wound healing. No systemic signs of infection are present. Topical antimicrobials are indicated.

Disinfectant: Chemical that destroys, neutralizes, or inhibits growth of microorganisms. Usually used on inanimate objects and intact skin; harmful to open tissue. Examples include alcohol and hydrogen peroxide.

Infection: Microorganisms invade tissue and yield a systemic response. Cultures are obtained to direct antibiotic selection.

Osteomyelitis: Bone infection characterized by a mixture of inflammatory cells, fibrosis, bone necrosis, and new bone formation.

Planktonic Bacteria: Free-floating (not anchored) bacteria, such as occurs with contamination and colonization.

Critical Colonization

The classification of critical colonization was developed to explain wounds with delayed healing that responded to topical antimicrobial treatment (Sotto et al, 2012; White and Cutting, 2006). This level of bioburden describes a level of bacterial presence that affects skin cell proliferation and tissue repair; however, there is no systemic response (i.e., fever or leukocytosis) (Landis, 2008). Several authors (Percival et al, 2012; Phillips et al, 2011) suggest that this phase is more appropriately described as colonization with polymicrobial biofilm communities.

Clinical Manifestations. In an effort to help clinicians identify wounds that are critically colonized, Sibbald et al, (2006) offered the acronym NERDS: nonhealing (N), increased exudate (E), red and bleeding wound (R), debris (D), and smell (S) (Box 16-2). The presence of three or more of the NERDS signs is considered diagnostic of critical colonization. When critical colonization is identified, topical antimicrobials and antiinflammatory dressings are recommended (Sibbald et al, 2011; Gottrup et al, 2013). Some authors also recommend topical antibiotics (Daeschlein, 2013). However, if a topical antibiotic is used, it should target a specific organism and its effect on that organism monitored to document effectiveness (Gottrup et al, 2013).

Biofilm

Biofilm has been described conceptually as a complex community of microorganisms embedded in an extracellular matrix of protein, lipids, and polysaccharides that is adherent to a wound or surface (Costerton, 1999; Percival et al, 2012). Planktonic organisms present on the surface of the wound attach to the wound surface, and initially there is no invasion of the tissues by the organisms (Leaper et al, 2012). The bacteria and/or fungi undergo phenotypical changes with attachment and begin to develop a biofilm (Percival et al, 2014).

Early on, the communities are increasingly biologically active and their attachment is reversible (phase 1). Biologic activity is important because for antibiotics and antiseptics to be effective, the organisms must be biologically active. When the biofilm is not disrupted in the first 24 hours, the biofilm becomes more permanently attached (phase 2) to the biologic or nonbiologic surface (Daeschlein, 2013; Percival et al, 2012). The longer the duration of the biofilm, the more resistant it is to removal and the greater the risk of infection (Daeschlein, 2013; Percival et al, 2012).

Importantly, biofilms are pervasive in chronic wounds. Data show that about 60% of chronic wounds have a biofilm present, whereas only 6% of acute wounds have documented biofilm (James et al, 2008). This raises the question of how the biofilm contributes to a chronic wound developing and persisting. Although seemingly important, biofilm is not the only factor that contributes to the development and persistence of chronic wounds.

Biofilm has a number of defenses that protect it. The extracellular matrix is a mechanical and chemical barrier to antibiotics. Also, the biofilm organisms present as an altered phenotype and communicate via quantum sensing, signaling molecules to alter their DNA pattern and change the biofilm organisms' metabolism. This change in the phenotype and genotype due to signaling increases the difficulty of identifying an antibiotic that is effective in eradicating the organisms in the biofilm. Biofilm communities are resilient and able to replace a wound's biofilm within hours of it being debrided (Wolcott and Rhodes, 2008) or slow their metabolism so they can live on the nutrients available in the extracellular matrix. These defenses also protect the biofilm organisms from invasion by other organisms, the phagocytic activity of polymorphonuclear neutrophils, oral or topical antibiotics, and the majority of topical antiseptics.

Clinical Manifestations. Some authors suggest that experienced clinicians can identify biofilm as translucent, shiny patches or layers of an opaque yellow-green substance on the surface of the wound (Metcalf et al, 2014). Others describe biofilm as slough and shiny with signs/characteristics that include necrotic tissue, malodor, and being unresponsive/recalcitrant to antimicrobial intervention (Percival et al, 2012).

Currently biofilm is identified primarily by scanning electron microscopy, confocal microscopy, and molecular modalities (Leaper et al, 2012; Percival et al, 2012). However, availability and cost currently are roadblocks to their widespread use (Attinger and Wolcott, 2012; Jones and Kennedy, 2012). Point of care diagnostic and therapeutic sensors are being developed and tested that may aid the clinician in the near future (Dargaville et al, 2013).

BOX 16-2   Criteria for Colonization and Infection

Critical Colonization (NERDS)
N = Nonhealing wound
E = Exudative wound
R = Red and bleeding wound
D = Debris
S = Smell from the wound

Deep Tissue Infection (STONEES)
S = Size is bigger
T = Temperature increased
O = Os (probes to or exposed bone)
N = New area of breakdown
E = Erythema/Edema
E = Exudate
S = Smell

Data from Sibbald RG, Goodman L, Woo KY, et al: Special considerations in wound bed preparation 2011: an update, *Adv Skin Wound Care* 24(9):415–436; quiz 437–438, 2011; Sibbald RG, Woo K, Ayello EA: Increased bacterial burden and infection: the story of NERDS and STONES, *Adv Skin Wound Care* 19(8):447–461, 2006; Woo KY, Sibbald RG: A cross sectional validation study of using NERDS and STONEES to assess bacterial burden, *Ostomy Wound Manage* 55(8):40–48, 2009.

Infection

Wound infection occurs when microorganisms on the wound surface penetrate into the wound tissues. A local or systemic response is indicative of an infection (Table 16-1), which may include increased exudate, erythema, odor, local warmth, edema, induration, pain, tenderness, fever, chills, and leukocytosis (Cutting and Harding, 1994; Gardner et al, 2001; Sibbald et al, 2006). Infection develops when the wound bioburden is significant enough to overwhelm the body's defenses. A quantitative bacterial count of $>10^5$ in the wound is the gold standard for diagnosing a wound infection (Leaper et al, 2012; Robson and Heggers, 1969).

The concept of wound bioburden, however, encompasses more than the number of bacteria present. Bioburden includes diversity, virulence, and interaction of the organisms with each other and with the body (synergism). Because more than one species of microorganisms exists in the wound, infection can develop with fewer than 10^5 microorganisms due to the interaction among them. More than 90% of chronic wounds have polymicrobial flora containing up to four species (Woo and Sibbald, 2009).

Appreciation of the role of biofilm in chronic wounds raises the question of whether the classic definition of infection ($>10^5$ CFU [colony-forming units]) will require revision in the near future. Additional issues have been identified on the accuracy of the results showing $>10^5$ CFU. Specific concerns are that laboratory protocols differ, the number of organisms within a wound varies depending on where in the wound the culture is obtained, whether the culture is taken by biopsy or swab, the depth of the biopsy, and methods to identify the organisms in biofilm are

not readily available in clinical practice (Gottrup et al, 2013)

Infection depends on the adherence of the organism to the host's body. Attachment requires that the organism bond with a receptor using a ligand. Some receptors are site specific (e.g., mucous membranes), some are cell specific (e.g., T lymphocytes), and others are nonspecific (e.g., moist surface). Colonization and ultimately invasion of the tissue by microorganisms cannot occur without attachment. Microorganisms have invasive factors that allow penetration of the host tissue, including enzymes (e.g., proteases) that lyse cells.

The local wound environment is important in the genesis of a wound infection. Organisms proliferate in an environment rich in necrotic tissue, foreign bodies (e.g., sutures, dirt), and hematomas. These serve as a nidus for infection, providing a medium for the growth of invading microorganisms. Inflammatory mediators and cytokines are stimulated, and enzymes released lyse proteins, such as fibrin, that are essential for fibroblast migration and maintenance of macrophage activity. The inflammatory response is augmented and prolonged. Exotoxins are released from the organisms and inhibit migration of keratinocytes and fibroblasts. The organisms use oxygen and contribute to the relative hypoxia as seen in infected wounds (Falanga, 2004). In addition, if the environment is warm, moist, and slightly hypoxic, anaerobic organisms proliferate (Edwards and Harding, 2004; Falanga, 2004).

Clinical Manifestations. Diagnosis of a wound infection is based primarily on clinical assessment (see Table 16-1). The classic signs of infection are erythema, increased temperature,

TABLE 16-1	Data-Based Paradigms of Infection in Chronic Wounds		
	Classic Work in Identifying Wound Infection*#	**Clinical Signs and Symptoms Checklist****	**NERDS and STONEES*****
Pain	X	X	
Erythema	X	X	X
Edema		X	X
Increased temperature	X	X	X
Exudate	X	X	X
Delayed healing	X	X	X
Discoloration of tissue	X	X	
Friable granulation tissue	X	X	X
Pocketing in the wound	X	X	
Odor	X	X	X
Wound breakdown		X	X
Increased wound size			X
Bone involved			X

* Cutting KF, Harding KGH: Criteria for identifying wound infection, *J Wound Care* 3:198, 1994.
** Gardner SE, Frantz RA, Doebbeling BN: The validity of the clinical signs and symptoms used to identify localized chronic wound infection, *Wound Repair Regen* 9(3):178–186, 2001.
*** Sibbald RG, Woo K, Ayello EA: Increased bacterial burden and infection: the story of NERDS and STONES, *Adv Skin Wound Care* 19(8):447–461, 2006.
\# Additional items: abscess, cellulitis, bridging of the epithelium or soft tissue.

increased exudate, delayed healing, friable granulation tissue, and odor. Others are present (e.g., pain, edema) but not as consistently identified in the research literature. The classic signs of infection may be muted or absent when the inflammatory response is impaired, as in cases of malnutrition, steroid therapy, immunosuppression, and wound chronicity (Gardner and Frantz, 2008; Leaper et al, 2012). Infection must be diagnosed in the context of the patient's history and risk factors (Box 16-3).

Researchers have explored the reliability and validity of signs and symptoms of infection and critical colonization of the chronic wound. The Clinical Signs and Symptoms Checklist, derived from the early work by Cutting and Harding (1994), was tested and extended by Gardner et al (2001, 2007). Later, the acronym NERDS for identifying critical colonization (Nonhealing wound, Exudative wound, Red and bleeding wound, Debris, Smell from the wound) and the acronym STONEES (Size is bigger, Temperature increased, Os [probes to bone or exposed bone]), New area of breakdown, Erythema/ Edema, Exudate, Smell) (see Box 16-2) were validated (Woo and Sibbald, 2009).

Infection in each type of chronic wound may be defined by its own set of signs and symptoms (Cutting and White, 2005; Gardner et al, 2009). For example, the criteria used to define infection in diabetic foot ulcers (anything below the malleolus) are purulence plus two cardinal signs of inflammation (Lipsky et al, 2008). Data from a Delphi study have delineated criteria for infection in major types of wounds: acute, venous, arterial,

BOX 16-3 Risk Factors for Wound Infection Elicited Through History

- History of prior wounds
- Family history of chronic wounds/poor healing
- Systemic conditions:
  - Human immunodeficiency virus/acquired immunodeficiency syndrome
  - Rheumatoid disease
  - Malnutrition: weight loss, obesity
  - Diabetes
  - Immune deficiency
  - Hypoxic conditions: chronic obstructive pulmonary disease, anemia
  - Ischemic disease: peripheral artery disease, congestive heart failure, shock, dehydration
  - Organ failure: heart, kidney, liver
  - Remote infection
- Health habits
  - Drug use/abuse
  - Smoking
- Drugs that impair healing
  - Corticosteroids
  - Antiinflammatory drugs
  - Chemotherapeutic agents

*Data from Fonder MA, Lazarus GS, Cowan DA, et al: Treating chronic wounds: a practical approach to the care of nonhealing wounds and wound care dressings, *J Am Acad Dermatol* 58(2):185–206, 2008; Stojadinovic A, Carlson JW, Schultz GS, et al: Topical advances in wound care, *Gynecol Oncol* 111(2 Suppl):S70–S80, 2008.

pressure ulcer, diabetic ulcer, and acute wound (Expert Working Group, 2008). Further research is needed to develop construct validity before these criteria are considered diagnostic of wound infection in various types of wounds.

Laboratory Tests and Cultures. Laboratory tests may reveal an increase in the number of white blood cells when infection is present. The differential may show an increase in bands or immature neutrophils. This "shift to the left" denotes increased immature leukocytes are released from the bone marrow into the bloodstream to fight invading organisms. Ongoing evaluation of inflammation can be monitored with erythrocyte sedimentation rate and C-reactive protein levels, which are elevated with inflammation.

Cultures are indicated when clinical signs of infection are present (see Table 16-1) or when a clean wound does not show any progress in healing with 2 weeks of topical treatment (Robson et al, 2006; Steed et al, 2006; Whitney et al, 2006). However, it is acknowledged that culture results underrepresent the number and type of organisms present (Leaper et al, 2012; Percival et al, 2013). A wound culture is performed primarily to identify the specific aerobic and anaerobic organisms present and their susceptibility to antibiotics, recognizing that only planktonic phenotype organisms can be identified. Wound culture also is used to obtain a specimen for Gram staining, a rapid diagnostic technique for identifying infection (Duke et al, 1972; Levine et al, 1976). For a Gram stain, the tissue fluid is placed on a slide, treated with various stains, and viewed under a microscope. Gram stain identifies whether more than 10^5 organisms are present and whether they are gram positive or gram negative. Results from a Gram stain can be expected in 20 minutes, a preliminary culture report in 24 hours, and a final culture and sensitivity within 48 hours. A Gram stain provides information about the type of organism present in the wound and allows the provider to prescribe a preliminary antibiotic.

A wound culture must be taken from clean, healthy-appearing tissue. Because infection involves the tissue, it is important to culture the tissue rather than pus, slough, eschar, or necrotic material (Gardner et al, 2006). Although a laboratory report will be produced if pus, eschar, or necrotic tissue is cultured, the results will reflect the microflora of that site but will not provide an accurate profile of the microflora in the tissue. In fact, the results will be a false report—the only question is the type of error. It could be false positive (organisms present in the area that is cultured but not present in the tissue), false negative (organisms not present in the area that is cultured but present in the tissue), or a chance agreement (area that is cultured and tissue have the same result). A false negative is problematic in that the patient has an infection and needs to receive treatment. In this case the patient's condition may deteriorate if the patient is not treated. A false positive is problematic if the patient is treated when there is not a need, increasing the risk of side effects and organisms developing antibiotic resistance. The culture underestimates the number and type of organisms in the wound because it only assesses the planktonic phenotype organisms (Daeschlein et al, 2013; Leaper et al, 2012). Data indicate that even within the same wound tissue, the number and types of organisms vary (Leaper et al, 2012; Levine et al, 1976; Percival et al, 2012). In general, a wound infection is present when the culture results show greater than 10^5 organisms or the presence of *any* β-hemolytic streptococcus (Robson et al, 2006; Steed et al, 2006; Whitney et al, 2006).

Three techniques are used in the clinical arena to obtain a wound culture: biopsy, needle aspiration culture, and swab culture.

Tissue biopsy for culture is removal of a piece of tissue with a scalpel or punch biopsy. Caution should be exercised in the use of local anesthetic because some data show that local anesthetics have antibiotic properties and may result in false-negative results (Johnson et al, 2008). The open wound is cleansed with a nonantiseptic sterile solution. A biopsy specimen is taken from clean tissue with a scalpel or punch biopsy, and bleeding is controlled. Once in the laboratory, the specimen is processed and plated (Gardner et al, 2006; Robson and Heggers, 1969).

The tissue biopsy is considered the gold standard for wound culture (Gardner et al, 2006; Robson and Heggers, 1969; Leaper et al, 2012; WOCN®, 2008, 2010). A physician or wound care specialist with appropriate training performs the biopsy. One of the limitations of the technique is that many facilities do not process tissue for culture, so the method cannot be used. In addition, obtaining a tissue culture requires disruption of the wound, which may cause the patient pain because living tissue is severed when obtaining the sample or may introduce contamination into the wound. Patients who are therapeutically anticoagulated are at risk of bleeding.

The second technique, *needle aspiration,* involves insertion of a needle in the tissue adjacent to the wound to aspirate tissue fluid. It is performed by a physician or appropriately prepared provider. Organisms present in the tissue are detected in the aspirated tissue fluid (Lee et al, 1985). Intact skin next to the wound is disinfected and allowed to dry. Fanning the area to speed drying is not recommended because organisms in the environment are stirred up and may settle on the biopsy site. Using a 10-ml disposable syringe and a 22-gauge needle, about 0.5 ml of air is drawn into the syringe, and the needle is inserted through intact skin adjacent to the wound. Suction is applied by withdrawing the plunger to the 10-ml mark. The needle is moved backward and forward at different angles for two to four explorations. After the needle is withdrawn from the tissue, excess air is removed from the syringe and the syringe is capped. The aspirated fluid is plated in the laboratory. If tissue is extracted using this technique, it is processed as described for tissue biopsy.

With the aspiration technique, the operator needs to understand the structures being penetrated by the needle. The major risk of this technique is inadvertent damage caused by the needle. Compared with tissue biopsy, needle aspiration tends to underestimate the number of organisms (Rudensky et al, 1992).

The *swab technique* is the third type of culture and is the most commonly performed. Two approaches have been used: the Levine technique and a Z technique, in which the base of the wound is cultured by moving the swab back and forth over the surface of the wound in as criss-cross pattern. Comparison of these two swab techniques to tissue biopsy showed the Levine technique had a 91% sensitivity and 57% specificity compared with the Z technique (63% sensitivity and 53% specificity) (Levine et al, 1976). The procedure for a swab culture using the Levine technique is outlined in Box 16-4. The swab technique probably is the most frequently used because it requires the fewest clinical skills and most laboratories are accustomed to performing the analysis. Recent reviews recommend the Levine technique over the Z technique (Leaper et al, 2012; Rondas, 2013). National guidelines on management of various types of chronic wounds (venous, diabetic, pressure) recommend determining the level of suspected infection by either tissue biopsy or validated quantitative swab technique (Robson et al, 2006; Steed et al, 2006; Whitney et al, 2006; WOCN®, 2010). The decision of which technique to use is made by the provider, considering the available equipment, the speed with which the specimen can be transported to the laboratory, and the ability of the laboratory to perform the requested culture.

MANAGEMENT OF BIOBURDEN

As described in Chapter 18, the three principles of wound management are to eliminate or reduce causative factors, minimize cofactors, and provide an optimal physiologic wound environment. In this section, only treatment of bacterial burden is discussed, with the understanding that appropriate interventions will be implemented to satisfy the first two principles of wound management.

BOX 16-4   Procedure for Swab Wound Culture Using Levine Technique

1. Collect specimen before starting antibiotics.
2. Collect specimen using sterile technique. If a Gram stain will be performed, obtain a second swab from the same clean tissue site.
3. Identify 1 cm² of *clean wound tissue* (infection resides in viable tissue; culturing epidermis, periwound skin, or necrotic tissue will lead to false-positive results).
4. Clean wound with nonantiseptic sterile solution.
5. Moisten swab or applicator with normal saline without a preservative (moist swab provides more precise data than dry swab).
6. Apply pressure and rotate applicator within 1 to 2 cm² of clean wound tissue to elicit tissue fluid.
7. Insert tip of saturated swab into appropriate sterile container (do not contaminate specimen when placing it in sterile container).
8. Complete the laboratory slip to provide clinical data to the microbiologist, including wound site, time collected, and prior antibiotics.
9. Transport culture specimen quickly (within 1 hour) to laboratory to keep the specimen stable.

Appropriate topical therapy focuses on removing pathogenic organisms from the wound. In conjunction with cleansing, debridement, and moist wound healing (see Chapters 17 and 18), topical antimicrobials are used to kill or inhibit microorganisms and to prevent reformation of biofilm (Gottrup et al, 2013; Vowden et al, 2011). It should be noted that topical antimicrobials are not sufficiently absorbed when applied topically to effectively treat systemic infections (Landis, 2008).

Critical Colonization and Biofilm

Management of critical colonization is recommended for 14 to 21 days and then the need for continued treatment is evaluated (Vowden et al, 2011). Topical antimicrobials were out of favor for a period of time, but as the number of antibiotic-resistant organisms have increased and the role of bioburden in chronic wounds has been appreciated, practitioners have realized that early control of bioburden with topical antimicrobials has the potential to reduce the need for antibiotics, while preventing the development of resistant bacteria strains, and biofilm (Sibbald et al, 2011; Leaper et al, 2012). With that said, it is anticipated that resistance to topical agents can and will occur as their use increases (Table 16-2) (Gottrup et al, 2013).

Wounds not responding to topical antiseptics may be covered with mature biofilm that cannot be penetrated by most antiseptics. The goals in the management of biofilm are (1) removal of the biofilm and (2) prevention of its recurrence without causing tissue injury or development of drug resistance (Gottrup et al, 2013; Leaper et al, 2012; Sibbald et al, 2011).

Surgical (or aggressive sharp) debridement is the cornerstone of physical biofilm control, as it quickly and efficiently removes the biofilm and disrupts its integrity (Daeschlein, 2013; Leaper et al, 2012). Conservative sharp debridement is not adequate (Attinger and Wolcott, 2012). Although there is no standard approach to surgical (aggressive sharp) debridement, the protocol used by Wolcott and Rhodes (2008) offers a good model of the extent of sharp debridement. They describe opening all the surfaces of the wound (e.g., tunnels, undermining) and resecting them so no surfaces touch. Devitalized tissue and slough are removed until normal tissue with a good blood supply is visible. This includes bone, which is debrided down to bleeding bone; bone involvement indicates the presence of osteomyelitis.

Recent data show that the effectiveness of debridement is time dependent (Wolcott et al, 2010). Data show that biofilm is most susceptible to antimicrobial treatment in the first 24 hours after debridement, less susceptible in the 24- to 48-hour period, and resistant by 72 hours. Serial surgical/sharp debridement opens a potential window for breaking the biofilm growth cycle.

These data support repeated surgical or aggressive sharp debridement, called by some *continued maintenance debridement,* to keep wound biofilm in a weakened and susceptible state (Leaper, 2012; Wolcott et al, 2009). Findings also suggest that early treatment is most effective (Jones and Kennedy, 2012; Wolcott et al, 2010).

Ultrasound is used to debride biofilm or as an adjunct to sharp debridement. This form of mechanical debridement employs electrical current, which piezoelectric crystals convert to mechanical vibrations, and results in acoustic energy that is transferred to the wound bed. Saline is used as the transfer media, and the air bubbles in the fluid expand and collapse, causing shockwave formation, cavitation, and erosion and fragmentation of the dead tissues (Wendelken et al, 2010). Ultrasound is especially useful for biofilm removal, given that the biofilm spreads below the surface via perivascular channels that need to be disrupted to remove the biofilm (Attinger and Wolcott, 2012). A systematic review showed that low frequency, low-intensity noncontact or low-frequency, high-intensity contact ultrasound improved healing in patients with chronic wounds (venous ulcers and diabetic ulcers), although the authors note that the quality of the data may be threatened by researcher biases (Voigt et al, 2011).

Topical Antiseptics. These may be biocides or biostatic; they may be bactericidal, fungicidal, virucidal, or sporicidal when they kill organisms and bacteriostatic, fungistatic, sporistatic, or virustatic when they inhibit the organisms' growth. However, the use of various antiseptics has had mixed support in the literature (Gottrup et al, 2013). The selection of an antimicrobial is based on provider preference, availability, cost, the agent's mechanism of action, and its overall effectiveness (Gottrup et al, 2013; Leaper and Durani, 2008). Antiseptics frequently used to manage bioburden are silver, iodine, and polyhexamethylene biguanide (PHMB) (Phillips et al, 2010; Sibbald et al, 2011; Vowden et al, 2011).

Iodine. Although a number of antiseptics have been found to reduce biofilm colony forming units (CFU) logs, sustained release cadexomer iodine is the only antiseptic known to kill biofilm. Iodine has long been used in wound care and, although elemental iodine is toxic, the iodophors (povidone iodine and cadexomer iodine) are not (Leaper et al, 2012). Metaanalysis showed that greater healing occurred in patients with venous ulcer when cadexomer iodine was used compared with standard care. Complete healing was not different when cadexomer iodine was compared with hydrocolloid dressing, paraffin gauze dressing, dextranomer, and silver-impregnated dressings (O'Meara et al, 2014). The same review also showed no between-group differences in complete healing or in growth factors when povidone-iodine was compared with hydrocolloid, moist, or foam dressings.

Much of the literature on cadexomer iodine is older and therefore does not specifically address biofilm. Recent work, however, indicates that cadexomer iodine is effective against *P. aeruginosa* biofilm in laboratory studies (Phillips et al, 2010) and is more effective than silver or PHMB in pig skin explants (Phillips et al, 2014). Because cadexomer iodine dries the wound, it is especially useful in moderately and highly exudative wounds. Its onset of action is rapid (within 24 hours) and sustained up to 72 hours (Phillips et al, 2014).

TABLE 16-2 Topical Antimicrobials*

Topical Agent	Action	Comments
Acetic acid 0.25% to 0.5%	Bactericidal	Effective against *P. aeruginosa*, gram-positive and gram-negative organisms Used as irrigant or soak Protect periwound skin Changes pH
Cadexomer iodine	Denatures protein Bacteriostatic and bactericidal	Effective against methicillin-resistant *Staphylococcus aureus* (MRSA) and organisms (*S. aureus*) Concentrations are nontoxic to fibroblasts Microspheres absorb bacteria and exudate while slowly releasing iodine to remove inhibitory cytokines Not effective in dry wounds Confirm patient is not allergic to iodine before use
Chlorhexidine 0.02%	Inhibits enzymes associated with cell membranes so contents leak out	Effective against *S. aureus* and *E. coli* Consider use in patients allergic to iodine Use as irrigant solution
Ethylenediamine tetraacetic acid (EDTA)	Bactericidal Chelates ions essential (Ca^{++}, Fe^{+++}) to bacterial function	Effective against gram-negative organisms and to a lesser degree to gram-positive organisms
Honey (medical grade)	Acidic pH Hyperosmolarity Produces H_2O_2 Contains antioxidants	Broad antibacterial action Effective against fungi, protozoa, and viruses Releases antiinflammatory products Reduces odor through bacterial metabolism that yields lactic acid instead of ammonia or sulfur Confirm patient is not allergic to honey, bee products, or bee stings before use
Hydrofera blue	Bacteriostatic Combination of methylene blue and gentian violet	Effective against methicillin-resistant *Staphylococcus epidermidis* (MRSE), vancomycin-resistant enterococcus (VRE), *S. aureus*, *S. epidermidis*, *Serratia*, and *E. coli* Important to keep dressing moist and remoisten before removal if dry
Hydrogen peroxide	Forms free radicals when necrotic tissue/debris present in wound	Effective against biofilms (*S. epidermidis*, *Streptococcus mutans*) Useful in removing debris because of its effervescent effects Use with care in closed cavities because of gas release
Mupirocin 2% ointment	Blocks activity of enzyme in bacteria responsible for making proteins	Antibiotic effective against MRSA, β-hemolytic streptococcus, *Streptococcus pyogenes* Contraindicated for large burns Contains polyethylene glycol, which may damage kidneys if absorbed through skin
Polyhexamethylene biguanides (PHMB)	Biocide Binds to cell wall to increase cell wall permeability	Broad spectrum against gram-positive and gram-negative organisms.
Povidone-iodine 1% to 10%	Broad spectrum	Effective in gram-positive and gram-negative bacteria, fungi, viruses, protozoa, bacterial spores No reported resistance Do not use scrub in open wounds Confirm patient is not allergic to iodine before use
Silver	Broad-spectrum cell membrane Denatures protein Alters nucleic acids Disrupts key enzyme systems in microorganisms	Broad-spectrum action Effectiveness depends on rate of release of ionic silver Effective against MRSA, VRE Incorporated into cream, mesh, transparency, hydrogel, hydrocolloid, foam, alginate dressings, with selection based on wound characteristic and patient's needs (see Chapter 18) Minimal allergic response Potential for tissue staining (see Plate 44)

TABLE 16-2	Topical Antimicrobials—cont'd	
Topical Agent	**Action**	**Comments**
Sodium hypo-chlorite (Dakin's solution)	Chlorine action kills organisms	0.005% to 0.025% exerts antimicriobial effects without cytotoxicity to fibroblasts (Heggars et al, 1985) 0.125 % = 1/4 strength concentration 0.5% = full strength (may be use in palliative wound to control odor Various dilutions may be used to manage drainage, diminish bacterial burden, promote debridement and reduce odor (Cornwall et al, 2010)

*Note: Bacitracin zinc-neomycin, gentamycin sulfate, polymyxin B, and garamycin for topical wound care are not frequently prescribed due to frequent development of sensitization.
EPS, Extracellularpolymeric substance.
Data in part from Percival SL, Cooper RA, Lipsky BA: Antimicrobial interventions for wounds. In Percival S, Cutting K, editors: *Microbiology of wounds,* Boca Raton, FL, 2010, CRC Press; Cornwell P, Arnold-Long M, Barss SB, Varnado MF: The use of Dakin's solution in chronic wounds: A clinical perspective case series. *JWOCN:* January/February 2010, 37(1), 94–104.

However, the efficacy of iodine in vivo remains to be established (Ammons, 2010)

Silver. Silver acts to bind with protein and causes structural changes in cell walls and intracellular and nuclear membranes (Leaper et al, 2012). Its composition varies (e.g., nanocrystalline, silver sulfadiazine), as do the rate and quantity of silver released in the wound bed, making evaluation of its efficacy challenging (Ammons, 2010; Leaper et al, 2012). Moisture is needed so inert silver becomes ionized and acts to kill microorganisms. When wound exudate is sparse, water should be used to activate the silver; use of sodium chloride should not be used.

Silver has been shown to improve wound healing, reduce odor, decrease excess exudate, and have a long wear time (Lo et al, 2009). Silver dressings reduce a few biofilm CFU logs in vitro (Percival et al, 2008) and a wide range of pathogens (Ammons, 2010). In a systematic review of treatments for patients with venous leg ulcers, there were no between-group differences in complete healing when 1% silver sulfadiazine ointment was compared with standard care/placebo and tripeptide copper complex or with various brands of silver-impregnated dressings, or when silver-impregnated dressings were compared with nonantimicrobial dressings (O'Meara et al, 2014). Oil-based products (e.g., zinc oxide, petrolatum) interfere with the ionization of the silver (Sibbald et al, 2011) and should be kept away from the wound. Some concern exists about the potential damage silver might cause to host cells when high–silver-containing wound dressings are used (Poon and Burd, 2004). Silver is advantageous in that many dressings may be left in place for a longer period of time, topical application is not painful, skin staining is temporary, and side effects rarely have been reported (Sibbald et al, 2011).

Polyhexamethylene biguanide exerts its antimicrobial effects by binding with microorganisms' cell membranes (a mechanism similar to naturally occurring antimicrobial peptides) and breaking down cell walls to kill organisms (PHMB, 2010). It has been used for 60 years as a disinfectant, more recently on contact lenses and in swimming pools. Its role as an antiseptic has received increased attention, as there

was appreciation of antibiotic resistance and little to no anticipation of new antibiotics in the future, as well as its low toxicity and low cost. In fact, it is the firstline antiseptic in Europe (PHMB, 2010).

Polyhexamethylene biguanide (PHMB) is available as a solution, gel, and dressing. A consensus statement from the United Kingdom reviewed many studies that show its effectiveness as a disinfectant and topical antiseptic. It reduces slough and is painless (PHMB, 2010). It is more effective than silver in reducing bioburden (Eberlein et al, 2012). It is used with negative pressure wound therapy to reduce bioburden (Daeschlein, 2013). Importantly, it also has been shown to reduce bioburden in vitro (Harbs and Siebert, 2007). When used as a dressing, it should be kept moist. If it does become dry, it should be moisturized with saline.

Among the biologic agents, honey has been used to treat chronic wounds. It makes the wound pH more acidic, acts as an osmotic agent, and generates hydrogen peroxide to kill organisms. A Cochrane review concluded that topical honey may improve healing of partial-thickness burns (O'Meara et al, 2014). However, compared with usual care in patients with venous ulcers, honey-based preparations showed no between-group differences in time to healing or complete healing (O'Meara et al, 2014). Manuka-type honey has been shown to penetrate biofilm and kill various strains of *S. aureus* and reduce biofilm CFU logs (Lu et al, 2014). It is important to use medical-grade honey (Lu et al, 2014) and apply it only to the wound, not to the skin surface. Honey is used in patients with thick eschar; scoring of the eschar allows the honey to penetrate the area, and absorptive dressing is required to contain the digested tissue (Sibbald et al, 2011).

Lactoferrin and xylitol are other biologic treatments for biofilm. Lactoferrin is an iron-chelating protein that destabilizes the cell wall of biofilm phenotype organisms (Ammons and Copié, 2013). Xylitol is an alcohol that has been studied primarily in oral biofilm (e.g., mouthwash) (Ammons, 2010). A combination of lactoferrin and xylitol on *P. aeruginosa* biofilms inhibits the *P. aeruginosa* biofilms and its ability to respond to ambient iron restriction (Ammons et al, 2011).

Many agents are being tested for their effects on biofilm (e.g., octenidine, dihydrochloride) (Daeschlein, 2013). In addition, various strategies to inhibit/kill biofilm phenotype organisms are being explored—for example, bacteriophages (viruses that infect bacteria), quantum sensing inhibitors (approaches to keep organisms within the biofilm from communicating with each other) (Ammons, 2010), and altering pH (Percival et al, 2014). Research offers new vistas for treating biofilm and reducing the effect of biofilm on chronic wounds.

Infection

Systemic antibiotics are the primary treatment of wound infection (Lavery et al, 2009). Culture and Gram stain are obtained before initiating antibiotic therapy to avoid false-negative culture results. Topical antimicrobials (as described in Table 16-2) may also be used in conjunction with systemic antibiotics to reach ischemic tissue or granulation tissue, which systemic antibiotics cannot reach (Leaper et al, 2012; WOCN®, 2010). In difficult situations, consultation with an infection disease specialist and pharmacologist may be warranted.

Osteomyelitis

Osteomyelitis, infection of the bone, develops as a complication of a wound infection and is not easily diagnosed. It is characterized by a mixture of inflammatory cells, fibrosis, bone necrosis, and new bone formation (Lavery et al, 2009; Rennert et al, 2009). The bone marrow, cortex, periosteum, and surrounding soft tissue all can be affected. Osteomyelitis can be categorized as acute (first episode resolves in less than 6 weeks) or chronic (recurs after initial infection or lasts longer than 6 weeks).

When a wound has visible signs of infection in combination with exposed bone, osteomyelitis should be suspected (Rennert et al, 2009). In diabetics, other factors that should raise suspicion that osteomyelitis is present include positive probe-to-bone test, ulcer present for more than a month, recurrent foot ulcer, traumatic foot wound, peripheral vascular disease, prior lower extremity amputation, neuropathy, renal insufficiency, and history of walking barefoot (Lipsky et al, 2012).

Bone biopsy that yields microorganisms with histologic findings of inflammatory cells and osteonecrosis is the gold standard for diagnosing osteomyelitis (Lipsky et al, 2008, 2012). However, this requires a surgical procedure, and one of the risks is seeding the wound with organisms.

A metaanalysis of diagnostic tests for osteomyelitis in diabetic foot ulcers summarized sensitivity and specificity (Table 16-3). The authors concluded that exposed bone or a positive probe-to-bone test result is moderately predictive of osteomyelitis, and magnetic resonance imaging (MRI) is the most accurate imaging test for diagnosis of osteomyelitis (Dinh et al, 2008). More recent data from the Infectious Diseases Society of America (IDSA) clinical practice guidelines for diabetic ulcers recommend a probe-to-bone test for any open diabetic foot wound to help diagnose or exclude osteomyelitis. They go on to recommend plain radiographs of the foot for confirming or excluding osteomyelitis, even though they have low sensitivity and specificity, and suggest considering

TABLE 16-3 Sensitivity and Specificity of Tests for Osteomyelitis

Test	Sensitivity	Specificity
Plain radiography	0.54	0.68
Exposed bone or probe-to-bone	0.60	0.91
Bone scan	0.81	0.28
Leukocyte scan	0.74	0.28
MRI	0.90	0.79

MRI, Magnetic resonance imaging.
Data from Dinh MT, Abad CL, Safdar N: Diagnostic accuracy of the physical examination and imaging tests for osteomyelitis underlying diabetic foot ulcers: meta-analysis, *Clin Infect Dis* 47(4): 519–527, 2008.

using serial plain radiographs to diagnose or monitor suspected osteomyelitis. The IDSA recommends using MRI to diagnose osteomyelitis and, if MRI is not available or contraindicated, they suggest a leukocyte or antigranulocyte scan, ideally combined with a bone scan. No other nuclear medicine investigations are recommended (Lipsky et al, 2012).

EVALUATION

As with all wounds, ongoing surveillance at regular intervals is essential; signs of critical colonization should abate within a 2-week period (Robson et al, 2006; Steed et al, 2006; Whitney et al, 2006). When the wound is infected, a response (decreased erythema) should be observed within 24 to 48 hours. The wound size should decrease, quality of the granulation tissue improve, volume of exudate decrease, odor resolve, and pain intensity decrease.

The absence of a response to treatment, further deterioration, or recurrence of signs and symptoms warrants reassessment of the wound and of the interventions. When the patient has an intact immune system and the subtle signs of critical colonization are still present but no local or systemic signs of infection are seen, interventions should be modified to (1) assess adequate relief from the underlying etiology, (2) ensure adequate resolution of cofactors (e.g., low tissue oxygenation, poor nutrition, high serum glucose), and (3) alter the physiologic wound environment by using a different antiseptic dressing and increasing the frequency of dressing changes. If a quantitative tissue biopsy can be obtained, sites different from the ones that were sampled in the original biopsy should be used. Reculturing will determine whether the pathogens have changed, thereby indicating a need for a different antibiotic. Given that much of the treatment of wound infection is provided on an outpatient basis, it is critical that patients/families be given detailed instructions about what they should observe and for how long, as well as how to contact the provider for continued follow-up. With a wound that is unresponsive, biopsy may be indicated to differentiate infection from atypical lesions such as cancer, calciphylaxis, or vasculitis.

CLINICAL CONSULT

A: Wound clinic referral for nonhealing leg wound. 60-year-old female with Parkinson disease and right posterior leg pressure ulcer just below the knee. Patient states she noted it a month ago when she had her cast removed after a leg fracture from a fall. Provider ordered hydrocolloid dressing changes every 4 days. She returned 10 days later with no progress and started silver hydrocolloids. After 2 weeks and no progress, patient was referred to wound clinic. Posterior right leg wound 4 × 2 cm thick yellow adherent base, moderate exudate, wound edges attached, periwound skin intact. Patient denies pain now that the cast is off and she can wear shoes. BMI within normal limits,

denies any problems eating or recent weight loss. No known allergies and no history of kidney or thyroid disease.
D: Medical device related unstageable pressure ulcer non-healing despite complete pressure relief, optimal wound care and trial of broad spectrum antimicrobial therapy. Suspect biofilm.
P: Penetrate, eradicate, and prevent reformation of biofilm.
I: (1) Sharp debridement. (2) Codexemier iodine dressing changed every other day, sooner if exudate strikes through cover dressing.
E: Small amounts of nonviable tissue removed and remaining scored. Wound remains unstageable. Return to clinic in 1 week for evaluation of local wound care and debridment.

SUMMARY

Creating an optimal wound environment requires diligent management of the wound bioburden. Failure to recognize and treat the manifestations of the continuum of bioburden conditions will lead to inflammation, delay of healing, and infection. The wound care provider must be vigilant for early signs of critical colonization and wound infection. Treatment focuses on antibiotics, antiseptics, and strategies to disrupt bioburden.

REFERENCES

Ammons MC: Anti-biofilm strategies and the need for innovations in wound care, *Recent Pat Antiinfect Drug Discov* 5(1):10–17, 2010.

Ammons MC, Copié V: Mini-review: Lactoferrin: a bioinspired, anti-biofilm therapeutic, *Biofouling* 29(4):443–455, 2013.

Ammons MC, Ward LS, Dowd S, et al: Combined treatment of Pseudomonas aeruginosa biofilm with lactoferrin and xylitol inhibits the ability of bacteria to respond to damage resulting from lactoferrin iron chelation, *Int J Antimicrob Agents* 37(4):316–323, 2011.

Attinger C, Wolcott R: Clinically addressing biofilm in chronic wounds, *Adv Wound Care* 1(3):127–132, 2012.

Basu S, Ramchuran Panray T, Bali Singh T, et al: A prospective descriptive study to identify the microbiological profile of chronic wounds in outpatients, *Ostomy Wound Manage* 55(1):14–20, 2009.

Bjarnsholt T, Kirketerp-Møller K, Jensen PØ, et al: Why chronic wounds will not heal: a novel hypothesis, *Wound Repair Regen* 16(1):2–10, 2008.

Costerton JW, Stewart PS, Greenberg EP: Bacterial biofilms: a common cause of persistent infections, *Science* 284(5418): 1318–1322, 1999.

Cutting KF, Harding KGH: Criteria for identifying wound infection, *J Wound Care* 3:198, 1994.

Cutting KF, White RJ: Criteria for identifying wound infection—revisited, *Ostomy Wound Manage* 51(1):28–34, 2005.

Daeschlein G: Antimicrobial and antiseptic strategies in wound management, *Int Wound J* 10(Suppl 1):9–14, 2013.

Dargaville TR, Farrugia BL, Broadbent JA, et al: Sensors and imaging for wound healing: a review, *Biosens Bioelecton* 41:30–42, 2013.

Dinh MT, Abad CL, Safdar N: Diagnostic accuracy of the physical examination and imaging tests for osteomyelitis underlying diabetic foot ulcers: meta-analysis, *Clin Infect Dis* 47(4):519–527, 2008.

Duke WF, Robson MC, Krizek TJ: Civilian wounds, their bacterial flora and rate of infection, *Surg Forum* 23:518–520, 1972.

Eberlein T, Haemmerle G, Signer M, et al: Comparison of PHMB-containing dressing and silver dressings in patients with critically colonised or locally infected wounds, *J Wound Care* 21(1):12, 14–16, 18–20, 2012.

Edwards R, Harding KG: Bacteria and wound healing, *Curr Opin Infect Dis* 17(2):91–96, 2004.

Expert Working Group: Wound infection, *Int Wound J* 5(3):1–11, 2008.

Falanga V: The chronic wound: impaired healing and solutions in the context of wound bed preparation, *Blood Cells Mol Dis* 31:88–94, 2004.

Fazli M, Bjarnsholt T, Kirketerp-Møller K, et al: Quantitative analysis of the cellular inflammatory response against biofilm bacteria in chronic wounds, *Wound Repair Regen* 19:387–391, 2011.

Fonder MA, Lazarus GS, Cowan DA, et al: Treating chronic wounds: a practical approach to the care of nonhealing wounds and wound care dressings, *J Am Acad Dermatol* 58(2):185–206, 2008.

Gardner SE, Frantz RA: Wound bioburden and infection-related complications in diabetic foot ulcers, *Biol Res Nurs* 10(1):44–53, 2008.

Gardner SE, Frantz RA, Doebbeling BN: The validity of the clinical signs and symptoms used to identify localized chronic wound infection, *Wound Repair Regen* 9(3):178–186, 2001.

Gardner SE, Frantz RA, Park H, et al: The inter-rater reliability of the clinical signs and symptoms checklist in diabetic foot ulcers, *Ostomy Wound Manage* 53(1):46–51, 2007.

Gardner SE, Frantz RA, Saltzman CL, et al: Diagnostic validity of three swab techniques for identifying chronic wound infection, *Wound Repair Regen* 14(5):548–557, 2006.

Gardner SE, Hillis SL, Frantz RA: Clinical signs of infection in diabetic foot ulcers with high microbial load, *Biol Res Nurs* 11(2):119–128, 2009.

Gottrup F, Apelqvist J, Bjarnsholt T, et al: EWMA document: Antimicrobials and non-healing wounds—evidence, controversies and suggestions, *J Wound Care* 22(Suppl 5):S1–S92, 2013.

Harbs N, Siebert J: In vitro efficacy of octenidine and polihexanide against biofilms composed of Pseudomonas aeruginosa, *GMS Krankenhaushyg Interdiszip* 2(2): Doc 45, 2007.

James GA, Swogger E, Wolcott R, et al: Biofilms in chronic wounds, *Wound Repair Regen* 16(1):37–44, 2008.

Johnson SM, Swogger E, Wolcott R: Local anesthetics as antimicrobial agents: a review, *Surg Infect (Larchmt)* 9(2):205–213, 2008.

Jones CE, Kennedy JP: Treatment options to manage wound biofilm, *Adv Wound Care (New Rochelle)* 1(3):120–126, 2012.

Landis SJ: Chronic wound infection and antimicrobial use, *Adv Skin Wound Care* 21(11):531–540, quiz 541–542, 2008.

Lavery LA, Peters EJ, Armstrong DG, et al: Risk factors for developing osteomyelitis in patients with diabetic foot wounds, *Diabetes Res Clin Pract* 83(3):347–352, 2009.

Leaper DJ, Durani P: Topical antimicrobial therapy of chronic wounds healing by secondary intention using iodine products, *Int Wound J* 5:361–368, 2008.

Leaper DJ, Schultz G, Carville K, et al: Extending the TIME concept: what have we learned in the past 10 years? *Int Wound J* (Suppl 2):1–19, 2012.

Lee P, Turnidge J, McDonald PJ: Fine-needle aspiration biopsy in diagnosis of soft tissue infections, *J Clin Microbiol* 22(1):80–83, 1985.

Levine NS, Lindberg RB, Mason AD Jr, et al: The quantitative swab culture and smear: a quick, simple method for determining the number of viable aerobic bacteria on open wounds, *J Trauma* 16(2):89–94, 1976.

Lipsky BA, Berendt AR, Cornia PB, et al: 2012 Infectious Diseases Society of America clinical practice guideline for the diagnosis and treatment of diabetic foot infections, *Clin Infect Dis* 54(12):e132–e173, 2012.

Lipsky BA, Holroyd KJ, Zasloff M: Topical versus systemic antimicrobial therapy for treating mildly infected diabetic foot ulcers: a randomized, controlled, double-blinded, multicenter trial of pexiganan cream, *Clin Infect Dis* 47(12):1537–1545, 2008.

Lo SF, Chang CJ, Hu WY, et al: The effectiveness of silver-releasing dressings in the management of non-healing chronic wounds: a meta-analysis, *J Clin Nurs* 18(5):716–728, 2009.

Lu J, Turnbull L, Burke CM, et al: Manuka-type honeys can eradicate biofilms produced by Staphylococcus aureus strains with different biofilm-forming abilities, *Peer J* 2:e326, 2014.

Madsen SM, Westh H, Danielsen L, et al: Bacterial colonization and healing of venous leg ulcers, *APMIS* 104:895–899, 1996.

Metcalf DG, Bowler PG, Hurlow J: A clinical algorithm for wound biofilm identification, *J Wound Care* 23(3):137–138, 140–142, 2014.

O'Meara S, Al-Kurdi D, Ologun Y, et al: Antibiotics and antiseptics for venous leg ulcers, *Cochrane Database Syst Rev* 1:CD003557, 2014.

Percival SL, Bowler P, et al: Assessing the effect of an antimicrobial wound dressing on biofilms, *Wound Repair Regen* 16(1):52–57, 2008.

Percival SL, Cooper RA, Lipsky BA: Antimicrobial interventions for wounds. In Percival S, Cutting K, editors: *Microbiology of wounds*, Boca Raton, FL, 2010, CRC Press.

Percival SL, Hill KE, Williams DW, et al: A review of the scientific evidence for biofilms in wounds, *Wound Repair Regen* 20(5):647–657, 2012.

Percival SL, McCarty S, Hunt JA, et al: The effects of pH on wound healing, biofilms, and antimicrobial efficacy, *Wound Repair Regen* 22(2):174–186, 2014.

Phillips PL, Wolcott Fletcher J, et al: Biofilms made easy, *Wounds Int* 1(3):1–6, 2010. http://www.woundsinternational.com. Accessed April 2014.

Phillips P, Yang Q, Gibson D, et al: Assessing the bioburden in poorly healing wounds, *Wounds International* 2(2):1–4, 2011. http://www.woundsinternational.com/practice-development/assessing-the-bioburden-in-poorly-healing-wounds. Accessed April 2014.

PHMB and its potential contribution to wound management. Aberdeen, 2010, Wounds UK.

Poon VK, Burd A: In vitro cytotoxology of silver: implications for clinical wound care, *Burns* 30(2):140–147, 2004.

Rennert R, Golinko M, Yan A, et al: Developing and evaluating outcomes of an evidence-based protocol for the treatment of

osteomyelitis in stage IV pressure ulcers: a literature and wound electronic medical record database review, *Ostomy Wound Manage* 55(3):42–53, 2009.

Robson MC, Cooper DM, Aslam R, et al: Guidelines for the treatment of venous ulcers, *Wound Repair Regen* 14(6):649–662, 2006.

Robson MC, Heggers JP: Bacterial quantification of open wounds, *Mil Med* 134(1):19, 1969.

Rondas AA: Swab versus biopsy for the diagnosis of chronic infected wounds, *Adv Skin Wound Care* 26(5):211–219, 2013.

Rudensky R, Lipschits M, Isaacsohn M, et al: Infected pressure sores: comparison of methods for bacterial identification, *South Med J* 85(9):901–903, 1992.

Sibbald RG, Goodman L, Woo KY, et al: Special considerations in wound bed preparation 2011: an update, *Adv Skin Wound Care* 24(9):415–436; quiz 437–438, 2011.

Sibbald RG, Woo K, Ayello EA: Increased bacterial burden and infection: the story of NERDS and STONES, *Adv Skin Wound Care* 19(8):447–461, 2006.

Sotto A, Richard JL, Messad N, et al: Distinguishing colonization from infection with Staphylococcus aureus in diabetic foot ulcers with miniaturized oligonucleotide arrays: a French multicenter study, *Diabetes Care* 35:617–623, 2012.

Steed DL, Attinger C, Brem H, et al: Guidelines for the treatment of diabetic ulcers, *Wound Repair Regen* 14(6):680–692, 2006.

Stojadinovic A, Carlson JW, Schultz GS, et al: Topical advances in wound care, *Gynecol Oncol* 111(Suppl 2):S70–S80, 2008.

Voigt J, Wendelken M, Driver V, et al: Low-frequency ultrasound (20-40 kHz) as an adjunctive therapy for chronic wound healing: a systematic review of the literature and meta-analysis of eight randomized controlled trials, *Int J Low Extrem Wounds* 10(4):190–199, 2011.

Vowden P, Vowden K, Carville K: Antimicrobial dressings made easy, *Wounds Int* 2(1):1–6, 2011.

Wendelken ME, Markowitz L, Alvarez OM: A closer look at ultrasound debridement, *Podiatry Today* 23(8):2, 2010.

White RJ, Cutting KF: Critical colonization—the concept under scrutiny, *Ostomy Wound Manage* 52(11): 50–56, 2006.

Whitney J, Phillips L, Aslam R, et al: Guidelines for the treatment of pressure ulcers, *Wound Repair Regen* 14(6):663–679, 2006.

Wolcott RD, Rhodes DO: A study of biofilm-based wound management in subjects with critical limb ischemia, *J Wound Care* 17(4):145–155, 2008.

Wolcott RD, Rhoads DD: A study of biofilm-based wound management in subjects with critical limb ischaemia, *J Wound Care* 17(4):145–148, 150–152, 154–155, 2008.

Wolcott RD, Rumbaugh KP, James G, et al: Regular debridement is the main tool for maintaining a healthy wound bed in most chronic wounds, *J Wound Care* 18(2):54–56, 2009.

Wolcott RD, Rumbaugh KP, James G, et al: Biofilm maturity studies indicate sharp debridement opens a time-dependent therapeutic window, *J Wound Care* 19(8):320–328, 2010.

Woo KY, Sibbald RG: A cross sectional validation study of using NERDS and STONEES to assess bacterial burden, *Ostomy Wound Manage* 55(8):40–48, 2009.

Wound, Ostomy and Continence Nurses Society™ (WOCN®): *Guideline for management of patients with lower-extremity arterial disease*, Mt. Laurel, NJ, 2008, WOCN®.

Wound, Ostomy and Continence Nurses Society™ (WOCN®): *Guideline for prevention and management of pressure ulcers*, Mt. Laurel, NJ, 2010, WOCN®.

Zhao G, Hochwalt PC, Usui ML, et al: Delayed wound healing in diabetic (db/db) mice with Pseudomonas aeruginosa biofilm challenge: a model for the study of chronic wounds, *Wound Repair Regen* 18(5):467–477, 2010.

17

Wound Debridement

Janet M. Ramundo

OBJECTIVES

1. Describe the role of debridement in the wound-healing process.
2. List contraindications to debridement.
3. Distinguish between selective and nonselective debridement.
4. Compare and contrast four methods of debridement: autolysis, chemical, mechanical, and sharp.
5. Describe the appropriate use of debridement using wet-to-dry dressings, conservative sharp debridement, and high-pressure wound irrigations.

6. List debridement options for the infected wound.
7. Describe at least five factors to consider when selecting a debridement approach.
8. For each method of debridement, list two advantages, disadvantages, and relevant special considerations.

Debridement is the removal of nonviable tissue and foreign matter from a wound and is a naturally occurring event in the wound repair process. During the inflammatory phase, neutrophils and macrophages digest and remove "used" platelets, cellular debris, and avascular injured tissue from the wound area. However, with the accumulation of significant amounts of damaged tissue, this natural process becomes overwhelmed and insufficient. Buildup of necrotic tissue then places considerable phagocytic demand on the wound, coupled with the continued presence of proinflammatory cells, both of which ultimately retard wound healing (Robson, 1997; Stotts and Hunt 1997). Consequently, debridement of necrotic tissue is an essential objective of topical therapy and a critical component of optimal wound management. Debridement not only is an integral component of wound bed preparation, it also facilitates bacterial balance and moisture balance (Hopf et al, 2006; Robson et al, 2006; Steed et al, 2006; Whitney et al, 2006).

Debridement is believed to achieve several objectives:

1. Reduce the bioburden of the wound. Because devitalized tissue supports the growth of bacteria, the presence of necrotic tissue places the patient at risk for wound infection and sepsis. Using external measures to remove the necrotic tissue and foreign matter reduces the volume of pathogenic microbes present in the wound.
2. Control and potentially prevent wound infections, particularly in the deteriorating wound.

3. Facilitate visualization of the wound wall and base. In the presence of necrotic tissue, accurate and thorough assessment of the viable tissue is hampered.
4. At the molecular level, debridement interrupts the cycle of the chronic wound so that protease and cytokine levels more closely approximate those of the acute wound (Schultz et al, 2003).

Necrotic tissue can appear in various forms. Eschar has the firm, dry, leathery appearance of desiccated and compressed tissue layers (see Plates 24 and 32c). When the tissue is kept moist, the devitalized tissue, called slough, remains soft and may be brown, yellow, or gray in appearance (see Plates 14, 25, 26A, and 32). Slough may be adherent to the wound bed and edges or loosely adherent and stringy (see Plate 25). Components of slough include fibrin, microorganisms, intact leukocytes, cell debris, and serous exudate (Thomas, 1990). Once the eschar is removed, slough is often visible covering the wound bed. Maintaining a moist wound environment is essential because continued exposure to air dehydrates slough, causing it to return to a hard, leathery state.

Debridement is indicated for any wound, acute or chronic, when necrotic tissue (which may be slough or eschar) or foreign bodies are present. It is also indicated when the wound is infected. In the absence of biofilm, once the wound bed is clean with viable tissue present, debridement is no longer indicated. Stable eschar (attached, noninfected, dry) on a poorly perfused limb or on a pressure ulcer on the heel should not be debrided (Hopf et al, 2006; Robson et al, 2006; Steed et al, 2006; Whitney et al, 2006; WOCN® 2010, 2014).

METHODS OF DEBRIDEMENT

Several methods of debridement are available for removal of devitalized tissue from necrotic wounds. Debridement methods are classified as either selective (only necrotic tissue is removed) or nonselective (viable tissue is removed along with the nonviable tissue) (Box 17-1). More specifically, debridement is classified by the actual mechanism of action: autolysis, chemical, mechanical, biologic, or sharp (conservative or surgical). Although one method of debridement may be the primary approach selected to rid the wound of necrotic tissue, debridement typically involves a combination of methods.

Autolysis

Autolysis as a natural, highly selective, painless method of debridement. Specifically, autolysis is the lysis of necrotic tissue by the body's white blood cells and natural enzymes, which enter the wound site during the normal inflammatory process. The body's proteolytic, fibrinolytic, and collagenolytic enzymes are released to digest the devitalized tissue present in the wound while leaving the healthy tissue intact (Rodeheaver et al, 1994). As a naturally occurring physiologic process, autolysis is stimulated by a moist, vascular environment with adequate leukocyte function count. Therefore autolysis is contraindicated in patients with compromised immunity. Autolysis as a sole method of debridement is not recommended for actively infected wounds or wounds with extensive necrotic tissue or significant tunneling and undermining (NPUAP, EPUAP, PPPIA, 2014).

A moist environment is facilitated by the application of a moisture-retentive dressing left undisturbed for a reasonable length of time, typically 24 to 72 hours. Maintaining a moist wound environment allows the cellular structures that are essential for phagocytosis (neutrophils and macrophages) to remain intact and avoid premature destruction through desiccation. An important role of macrophages is production of growth factors, so the presence of healthy macrophages in the wound fluid supports continued production of growth factors. Once autolysis is initiated, eschar will loosen from the edges, become soft, change to a brown or gray color, and eventually transform into stringy yellow slough. It is critical to monitor the wound closely during the autolysis process because as the wound is debrided, the full wound bed and walls are exposed and the true extent of the wound is revealed; consequently, the wound will increase in length, width, and depth, necessitating a change in topical therapy. Plate 26 shows the appearance of a wound before and after autolysis.

Clinicians, patients, and family members unfamiliar with the process of autolysis can misinterpret the collection of wound exudate and the accompanying odor as indicative of an infection. It is important to emphasize that the wound exudate contains enzymes and growth factors that are essential to wound repair. In fact, wounds treated with moisture-retentive dressings are less likely to become infected than are wounds treated with conventional dressings because moisture-retentive dressings are impermeable to exogenous bacteria. In addition, viable neutrophils and other natural substances in wound fluid inhibit bacterial growth (Hutchinson, 1989; Lawrence, 1994).

The use of moisture-retentive dressings to create and maintain a moist wound environment launched the use of autolysis as an alternative to surgical debridement. Moisture-retentive dressings trap enzyme-rich wound exudate at the wound site (Chen, 1992), which is very effective at detaching nonviable tissue from the surrounding skin and wound base. Selection of dressings that promote autolysis is based on the condition of the wound base, depth of the wound, presence of tunnels or undermining, volume of wound exudate, and the patient's condition. When the wound base is dry, a dressing that will add moisture, such as a hydrogel, should be used. If absorption is needed, a dressing should be selected that will absorb excess exudate without dehydrating the wound surface, such as an alginate dressing for a highly exudative wound or a hydrocolloid for the minimally exudative wound. Chapter 18 provides an in-depth discussion on dressing selection to promote autolysis while matching the needs of the wound.

Comparison studies for methods of debridement are difficult due to the focus on healing as an endpoint rather than the effectiveness of debridement (Jull et al, 2013). König and colleagues (2005) report that autolysis compares favorably with other methods of debridement in terms of effectiveness. However, the process is slower than alternative methods such as mechanical and sharp. A multicenter randomized trial conducted by Burgos et al (2000) showed no significant difference in healing of Stage III pressure ulcers with the use of a hydrocolloid for autolysis compared with a commercially prepared topical enzyme product. Another randomized study comparing the same products found the enzyme to be faster when used to treat Stage IV pressure ulcers on the heel after surgical debridement (Müller et al, 2001). Milne (2010) reported similar slower results when autolysis with hydrogel was compared with enzymes in a study of 27 patients with pressure ulcers.

BOX 17-1 Selective versus Nonselective Debridement Methods

Selective	Nonselective
Autolysis	Surgical
Enzyme	Hydrotherapy
Conservative sharp	Wet-to-dry gauze
debridement	Surgical sharp
Biosurgical (maggot)	
Ultrasonic mist	

More recently introduced to the market, both medical-grade honey (Al-Waili et al, 2011; Bilgari et al, 2013; Gethen and Cowman, 2009; Jull et al, 2013) and polyacrylate dressings containing Ringer's solution may be effectively used to enhance autolysis, particularly in the home care setting since less frequent dressing changes are required (Paustian and Stegman, 2003). The timeframe for the occurrence of autolysis varies depending on the size of the wound and the amount and type of necrotic tissue. Generally, the softening and separating of necrotic tissue are observed within days. If significant debridement is not apparent in 1 to 2 weeks, another method of debridement should be used (Hopf et al, 2006; Robson et al, 2006; Steed et al, 2006; Whitney et al, 2006).

Autolysis can be used in combination with other debridement techniques. In fact, promotion of autolysis is an important adjuvant to all debridement modalities for ongoing maintenance debridement and prevention of tissue dehydration and cellular desiccation. For example, after surgical sharp debridement of a pressure ulcer, the application of a hydrogel-impregnated gauze maintains a moist wound environment, thus preventing tissue desiccation and promoting continued softening and loosening of residual necrotic tissue. It often becomes necessary to combine dressings to achieve debridement while meeting all the needs of the patient and the wound. For example, a transparent dressing is inappropriate for debridement of a wound that has depth or is heavily exudative. Instead, a dressing such as an alginate is warranted because it will fill the wound depth and absorb the exudate (see Chapter 18).

Chemical

Necrotic wound tissue can be removed through a chemical process using enzymes. Silver nitrate is another method of chemical debridement (also referred to as *chemical cauterization*); however, it is more commonly used on closed wound edges (described in Chapter 4 and shown in Figure 4-6 and Plate 4) and hypergranulation tissue (described in Chapter 6 and shown on Plate 27).

Enzymes. Topical application of exogenous enzymes is a selective method of debridement. Over the years, various sources have been used to manufacture enzymes (e.g., krill, crab, papaya, bovine extract, bacteria). Today the only enzyme available in the United States is collagenase, which is derived from Clostridium bacteria. Collagenase digests collagen in necrotic tissue by dissolving the collagen "anchors" that secure the avascular tissue to the underlying wound bed (NPUAP, EPUAP, PPPIA, 2014).

Similar to autolysis, enzymatic debridement is considered slower than mechanical or sharp debridement, but is frequently used for initial debridement when anticoagulant therapy renders surgical debridement unfeasible (König et al, 2005; Ramundo and Gray, 2009). Despite the cost of the enzyme, which is a prescription item, it has shown to be cost-effective (Milne, 2013; Woo et al, 2013). The length of time required to achieve debridement may range from several days to weeks. Unlike autolysis, enzymes may also be used to debride a wound with significant bacterial bioburden or infection (Ramundo and Gray, 2009). Although some topical antibiotics such as polymyxin B/bacitracin, mupirocin, or neomycin may be safely used in conjunction with collagenase, other antibiotics may inhibit the enzymatic activity (Jovanovic et al, 2012). Specific ions, including several commonly used antimicrobial dressings and antiseptic solutions, inhibit or inactivate collagenase. Silver dressings and cadexomer iodine have been reported to reduce collagenase activity by more than 50% and 90%, respectively. Antiseptic cleansers that have a pH level below 6.0 or above 8.0 also reduce the activity of collagenase. Most sodium hypochlorite–based cleansers may be safely used with collagenase (Jovanovic et al, 2012).

A secondary dressing is required when an enzyme is used and should be selected based on the needs of the wound. With the previously mentioned exceptions, manufacturers state that most dressings can be used safely with enzymes, including gauze, hydrogels, and transparent film dressings; however, silver-impregnated dressings should be avoided. Iodine dressings or those containing zinc should not be used with collagenase (Shi et al, 2010). Frequency of enzyme application is at least daily and may be twice daily; therefore the secondary dressing also should be appropriate for daily or twice-daily changes (Shi et al, 2010). Enzymatic debridement can be augmented by using a moisture-retentive dressing that will hold moisture at the wound bed, such as a transparent film or hydrogel. Enzymes require a prescription, so their use has cost and reimbursement implications. In addition, daily or twice-daily dressing changes dictate considerable commitment on the part of the caregiver (patient, family, or staff) that may not always be reasonable or acceptable.

When collagenase is used on a wound with intact eschar, the eschar must be cross-hatched to allow penetration of the enzyme, and the wound surface must be kept moist. Cross-hatching the eschar is achieved by using a no. 10 blade to make several shallow slits in the eschar without damaging the viable wound base. Once the eschar begins to separate or demarcate from the surrounding skin, the enzyme can be applied to the wound edges along the line of demarcation to hasten separation. At this point, conservative sharp debridement can be used to remove softened necrotic tissue. Enzyme treatment can then be continued, or another debridement technique such as autolysis can be instituted. Because these enzymes are selective, damage to viable tissue in the wound bed should not occur if the dressing is continued once debridement is completed and viable tissue is exposed. However, enzyme application typically is discontinued when the wound bed is free of necrotic tissue. More appropriate dressings are available at a fraction of the cost and should be implemented once the wound is debrided. A transient stinging or burning sensation, particularly when the enzyme comes into contact with intact skin, has been reported (Ramundo and Gray, 2008). Barrier ointments can be used to protect the periwound skin.

Biosurgical (Maggots)

Originating from the battlefield, maggots have been used to achieve a biologic method of debridement. Providers noted anecdotal reports from medics who observed the rapid removal of necrotic tissue when maggots were present on the wound bed. Today, therapeutic maggot therapy involves sterilizing the eggs of *Lucilia sericata* (greenbottle fly). Once the eggs hatch (again, under sterile conditions), the sterile larvae are introduced into the wound bed.

It is theorized that larvae secrete proteolytic enzymes, including collagenase, allantoin, and other agents, which rapidly break down necrotic tissue (NPUAP, EPUAP, PPPIA, 2014). It is also believed that the larvae ingest microorganisms, which are then destroyed. Some researchers are investigating the effects of maggots on fibroblasts and extracellular matrix interaction and enhancement of healing beyond the debridement effects (Chambers et al, 2003; Horobin et al, 2003). Because of this reported action and the emergence of resistant organisms, there is renewed interest in maggot therapy in some centers, and more research supporting this therapy is available (Sherman, 2002, 2003; Wallina et al, 2002; Wolff and Hansson, 2003). In a study of 119 patients with slough-filled wounds, debridement was achieved faster with maggot therapy than wounds treated with sharp debridement and autolysis combined during the first week of treatment. However no statistical significance was noted after 2 weeks of therapy (Opletalová et al, 2012).

Despite the renewed interest in clinical centers and reports in the literature, maggot therapy is still generally considered a last-resort option when the patient is not a surgical candidate and the wound has not responded to conventional methods of debridement. Recent reviews and metaanalysis have concluded that maggot therapy, although a promising therapy, offers no more overall effectiveness than other methods of debridement (Gray, 2008; Hoppe, 2012; Tian et al, 2013; Zarchi and Jemec, 2012).

Biosurgical therapy should not be used with wounds that are poorly perfused; require frequent inspection; or have exposed blood vessels, necrotic bone, or limb-threatening infections (Cowan, 2013; Mexican Association for Wound Care and Healing, 2010). Care should be taken to prevent the larvae from coming in contact with healthy skin because the proteolytic enzymes can cause damage. Pain and bleeding have been reported, so the patient should be monitored for both, particularly with the widespread use of antiplatelet therapy (Steenvoorde and van Doorn, 2008; Steenvoorde et al, 2005). The main disadvantage to maggot therapy is the sensation of crawling that some patients experience, but confinement of the larvae to the wound bed decreases this sensation. Various dressings have been described; most involve periwound protection with mesh or nylon net to contain the larvae and an absorbent pad to absorb exudate; some dressings incorporate the maggots into a layered dressing, which allows ease of application and removal, and eliminates concerns about containment (Opletalová et al, 2012).

Mechanical

Mechanical modes of debridement include wet-to-dry gauze dressings, irrigation, and hydrotherapy. These techniques represent selective and nonselective modes of debridement. Historically, whirlpool has been used as a mechanical method of debridement. However, most recent guidelines do not mention whirlpool as a recommended option for debridement (Hopf et al, 2006; NPUAP, EPUAP, PPPIA, 2014; Robson et al, 2006; Steed et al, 2006; WOCN® 2010, 2011, 2012a). Information about the use of hydrotherapy in burn care can be found in Chapter 32.

Wet-to-Dry Gauze. Experts agree that wet-to-dry dressings for debridement may induce mechanical separation of eschar. However, the method can be painful, as well as nonselective, resulting in damage to newly formed viable tissue (Hopf et al, 2006; Robson et al, 2006; Steed et al, 2006; Whitney et al, 2006; WOCN®, 2010). If wet-to-dry debridement must be used, it is most appropriate with heavily necrotic and infected wounds without visible granulation tissue. Wet-to-dry dressings have not been shown to be effective with removal of biofilm in a chronic wound (Phillips et al, 2013). Correct technique consists of lightly packing moistened (not dripping wet) open-weave cotton gauze in the wound bed and allowing it to dry on the wound to trap debris and necrotic tissue. Once dry, usually 4 to 6 hours after application, the dressing is pulled off the wound along with the trapped debris and necrotic tissue; moistening the gauze before removal will not facilitate mechanical debridement. Finally, the wound is cleansed, and the process is repeated. If the procedure is performed correctly, wet-to-dry gauze debridement requires dressing changes for several days to weeks, three to six times per day. The perception that wet-to-dry debridement is cost-effective may not be accurate once caregiver time is factored into the equation, as well as the potential for delayed healing if the nonselective nature of the procedure leads to damage of healthy tissue. Woo and associates (2013) compared the cost of various methods of debridement and noted mechanical wet-to-dry debridement as one of the most costly methods.

Wound Irrigation and Pulsatile Lavage. Wound irrigation and pulsatile lavage involve debridement of necrotic tissue using fluid and between 4 and 15 pounds per square inch (psi) of pressure, which is adequate to remove debris from the wound bed without damaging healthy tissue or inoculating the underlying tissue with bacteria (Hopf et al, 2006; Robson et al, 2006; Steed et al, 2006; Whitney et al, 2006).

Delivering fluid under pressure to the wound bed can cause dissemination of wound bacteria over a wide area, exposing the patient and care provider to potential contamination. Consequently, the care provider should wear personal protective equipment (mask, gloves, gown, goggles) during this procedure when "splash" is expected (NPUAP, EPUAP, PPPIA, 2014).

Wound irrigation is accomplished using a 19-gauge angiocatheter and a 35-ml syringe (a bulb syringe does not provide enough pressure). Prepackaged canisters of pressurized saline and products that attach to saline bags for continuous acceptable pressures are available for irrigation.

A pulsatile lavage machine combines intermittent high-pressure lavage with suction to loosen necrotic tissue and facilitate its removal by other methods of debridement (Morgan and Hoelscher, 2000). Pulsatile lavage is effective for removing larger amounts of debris and should be discontinued once the wound is clean. Pulsatile lavage should be used with caution to avoid blood vessels; graft sites; and exposed muscle, tendon, and bone. Patients on anticoagulant therapy should be observed carefully for any bleeding and treatment discontinued immediately if bleeding occurs. Disadvantages of debridement with pulsatile lavage include cost and time. The hose and tip are designed for one-time use, and large necrotic wounds may require twice-daily treatments. Pulsatile lavage treatment should be delivered in an enclosed area separate from any other patients to prevent contamination with mist (Maragakis et al, 2004).

Ultrasonic Mist. Ultrasound uses acoustic energy to remove necrotic tissue from the wound bed and promote healing. Ultrasound mist therapy uses saline coupled with the acoustic wave to produce mechanical and thermal effects. When the probe delivering the mist is in contact with the wound, destruction of fibrin may occur (Stanisic et al, 2005). This debridement effect is not seen when contact with the wound is avoided, as in low-frequency, low-intensity, noncontact ultrasound. A review of the literature on the use of ultrasound noted insufficient evidence to determine the effectiveness of debridement (Ramundo and Gray, 2008). Ultrasound use for wound care is discussed in greater detail in Chapters 16 and 24.

Sharp Debridement

Sharp debridement is a rapid process that uses sterile instruments. Sharp debridement can be done sequentially in a conservative fashion (conservative sharp wound debridement), or it can be done surgically (surgical sharp debridement). Any method of sharp debridement must be performed by a specially trained, competent, qualified, and licensed health care professional consistent with local legal and regulatory statutes (NPUAP, EPUAP, PPPIA, 2014; WOCN®, 2005). Sharp debridement is considered cost-effective and rapid in time to debride compared with enzymatic, autolytic, mechanical, and biologic methods of debridement (Woo

et al, 2013). The role of sharp debridement in the management of biofilm is discussed briefly later in this chapter and in detail in Chapter 16.

Conservative Sharp Wound Debridement. Conservative sharp wound debridement, also known as *conservative instrumental debridement,* is a selective debridement method for the removal of loosely adherent, nonviable tissue using sterile instruments (e.g., forceps or "pick-ups," scissors, and scalpel with no. 10 or no. 15 blade). When done correctly, the procedure is not aggressive enough to harm viable tissue and is not likely to result in blood loss.

Conservative sharp debridement has several advantages. It removes the necrotic tissue more quickly than the previously discussed methods, and it can be accomplished in a serial manner. This method of debridement can be combined with other debridement techniques (autolysis or enzymatic) to shorten this phase of wound care. Theoretically, a more rapid approach to debridement decreases the body's expenditure of energy during a time of high resource use.

Because of the low risk involved, conservative sharp debridement in many states is a delegated medical function that can be performed in a variety of settings by a clinician who is competent and credentialed in the technique. Therefore conservative sharp debridement is a viable option for patients residing in nonacute care settings without the need for transfer to a hospital. A variety of requirements may need to be satisfied, depending on the nurse practice act specific to the state and the employer's requirements. Checklist 17-1 contains factors to consider before performing conservative

---

CHECKLIST 17-1   Factors to Consider Before Performing Conservative Sharp Debridement

✓ Is conservative sharp debridement covered under the clinician's state practice act?

✓ Are specialty education, training, and credentials in conservative sharp debridement required by the state or the employer?

✓ What formal knowledge and skill updates are required and how often?

✓ Has the individual's professional organization or employer delineated specific guidelines related to conservative sharp debridement?

✓ Are policies, procedures, and protocols in place for conservative sharp debridement?

✓ Is conservative sharp debridement considered part of the clinician's clinical privileges, or is a provider's order required for each incident of conservative sharp debridement?

✓ What level of provider supervision, if any, is required for conservative sharp debridement?

✓ Does the employer provide malpractice insurance coverage for conservative sharp debridement?

✓ Does the clinician carry malpractice insurance to cover conservative sharp debridement?

sharp debridement. Box 17-2 provides a sample policy and procedure for conservative sharp debridement.

A disadvantage of conservative sharp debridement is that, depending on the size of the ulcer and the amount of necrotic tissue involved, it could conceivably take weeks to remove all of the nonviable tissue. The procedure may be uncomfortable for the patient, so the need for analgesia should be considered. Blood loss is not expected during conservative sharp debridement but remains a possibility. As a result, the patient should be assessed for factors that place him or her at risk for clotting problems if a vessel is accidentally severed. Factors to consider include medications (e.g., anticoagulants, high-dose nonsteroidal antiinflammatory drugs) and pathologic conditions (e.g., thrombocytopenia, impaired hepatic function, vitamin K deficiency, malnutrition). When any of these factors are present, the wound specialist should confer with the provider before proceeding with conservative sharp debridement.

Infected wounds present unique considerations for conservative sharp debridement. In general, there is the potential for transient bacteremia after debridement of a wound (Bryan et al, 1983), particularly when the wound is infected. Transient bacteremia in a patient who is nutritionally compromised, leukopenic, or otherwise immunocompromised can be devastating.

Surgical sharp debridement is the preferred method for debriding most infected wounds. (NPUAP, EPUAP, PPPIA, 2014). However, if surgical sharp debridement is not an option because of the patient's condition or the care setting, serial conservative sharp debridement can be conducted by the non–physician wound care provider, but only in conjunction with appropriate antibiotic coverage. Although systemic antibiotics may not penetrate the necrotic tissue to reduce the bacterial load in the wound, they should reduce the potential for systemic dissemination of the pathogens. Topical antiseptic solutions may also be instrumental in reducing the bioburden of the wound. The wound specialist should be in compliance with the policies of the facility or agency on the management of infected wounds.

Surgical Sharp Wound Debridement. Surgical debridement is the fastest method for removing large amounts of

---

BOX 17-2   Policy and Procedure: Conservative Sharp Wound Debridement

I. Purpose

The purpose of this policy and procedure is to outline the process by which an RN with certification in wound care may remove devitalized tissue by conservative sharp wound debridement.

II. Policy

1. Any RN performing conservative sharp wound debridement will have additional didactic education in the skill.
2. Any RN performing conservative sharp wound debridement will have additional laboratory education to develop the skill.
3. Any RN performing conservative sharp wound debridement will participate in a clinical practicum involving patients with wounds.
4. Documentation of the first three items will be filed with the individual's other credentialing information. (This is determined by practice setting.)

III. Authority and Responsibility

1. The individual performing conservative sharp wound debridement will provide documentation of education and competency.
2. An order from the provider will be obtained before the procedure, or provider practice protocols permitting the procedure will be in effect.
3. Consent will be obtained from the patient or appropriate representative. (This is determined by practice setting.)

IV. Definitions

Conservative sharp wound debridement is the removal of loose, avascular tissue using surgical instruments (e.g., scissors, scalpel, forceps) without inflicting pain or precipitating bleeding.

V. Procedure

1. Explain procedure to patient.
2. Obtain consent. (This is determined by practice setting.)
3. Assemble equipment:
   - Sterile forceps with teeth
   - Sterile scalpel handle with no. 15 blade
   - Silver nitrate sticks
   - Curved iris scissors
   - Surgical gel foam or silver nitrate stick
   - Gauze sponges
   - Normal saline
   - Clean gloves
4. Wash hands.
5. Prepare work surface.
6. Position patient for procedure.
7. Ensure adequate lighting.
8. Apply clean gloves.
9. Remove old dressing and discard.
10. Wash hands and apply clean gloves.
11. Clean wound with normal saline or appropriate surgical scrub/solution.
12. Grasp loosely adherent tissue with forceps; pull taut, exposing a clear line of dissection.
13. Cut or snip loose tissue, avoiding all vascular tissues and tissues that are not clearly identified.
14. Irrigate wound with normal saline.
15. For minor bleeding, apply silver nitrate, gel foam, or pressure.
16. Apply appropriate dressing.
17. Document procedure and patient's response to procedure and type of dressing applied.

Data from Wound, Ostomy and Continence Society™ (WOCN®): *Conservative sharp wound debridement: best practice for clinicians,* Mt. Laurel, NJ, 2005, WOCN®.

RN, Registered nurse.

necrotic tissue, but is outside of the scope of practice of most providers. This method not only removes necrotic tissue and its attached bacterial burden, but it also can result in removal of senescent cells and bleeding, thus converting a chronic wound to a pseudoacute wound (Steed et al, 1996). In many cases, surgical debridement is performed at the bedside. However, international guidelines for the care of pressure ulcers recommend performing debridement in the operating room in the following cases (NPUAP, EPUAP, PPPIA, 2014):

- Presence of advancing cellulitis
- Wound-related sepsis
- Extensive necrotic tissue
- Inability to establish degree of undermining and tunneling
- Infected bone or hardware that may need to be removed

Disadvantages of surgical debridement include the potential for negative effects from anesthesia, excess bleeding, and transient bacteremia that may progress to systemic infection and patient death. The condition of the patient, aggressive nature of this procedure, and higher level of care required after debridement may require the patient to spend more time in the hospital.

Laser and Water Debridement. *Laser debridement,* a form of surgical debridement, uses focused beams of light to cauterize, vaporize, or slice through tissue. Several light sources for lasers are available (Habif, 1996); each type of laser emits light at a specific wavelength, and different body tissues absorb different wavelengths. The part of the tissue that absorbs the light is called the *chromophore.* When the chromophore absorbs the light, it is quickly heated and vaporized. When the beam of light is tightly focused, it is capable of cutting through human tissue like a knife (Raz, 1995).

Advantages of laser debridement are that the wound bed is sterilized and most severed vessels are cauterized (Flemming et al, 1986). Animal studies using a laser to debride partial-thickness burns have demonstrated results similar to those of surgical debridement with a scalpel, but with hemostasis and no disturbance of periwound skin (Graham et al, 2002; Lam et al, 2002). Disadvantages of laser debridement include risk of injury to adjacent healthy tissue and therefore delayed healing. Work with pulsed laser beams rather than continuous laser beams has decreased these negative effects (Glatter et al, 1998; Smith et al, 1997). Unfortunately, this method is not available in all settings.

The *hydrosurgical water knife* is a method of surgical debridement that dispenses normal saline at a high power, which enables debridement and cleansing of the wound base. This water jet device is regulated so that the clinician is able to precisely control the depth of debridement. The high-velocity stream runs parallel to the wound surface and creates a vacuum, which then cleanses and removes debris into a collection container. This device is designed for use only in the operating room. Limited studies have shown some promise compared with traditional surgical debridement in the treatment of burns and lower extremity ulcers due to the shorter time to debridement with similar outcomes (Caputo et al, 2008; NPUAP,

EPUAP, PPPIA, 2014); additionally, it may be cost-effective compared with traditional surgery (Gravante et al, 2007).

SELECTION OF DEBRIDEMENT METHOD

Three general parameters guide the selection of the most appropriate debridement process: (1) overall condition and goals for the patient, (2) status of the wound and urgency of the need for debridement, and (3) skill level of the care provider. Algorithms are available to guide the clinician in selecting the appropriate debridement method. Although they are based on expert opinion and have not been validated, these algorithms can serve as a useful starting point for decision making (Figure 17-1).

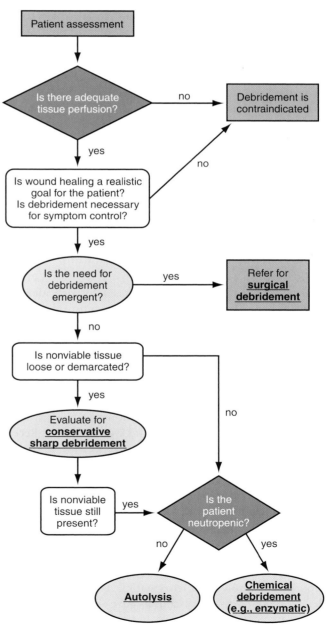

FIGURE 17-1 Debridement algorithm.

Overall Condition and Goals for the Patient

Occasionally, it may be necessary to forgo debridement if it is not consistent with the patient's wishes and overall goals for care (NPUAP, EPUAP, PPPIA, 2014). Such a decision must include input from the patient, the patient's significant others, and the primary care provider. Even if the goal is not to heal the wound, debridement of necrotic tissue will control infection and unpleasant wound odors, making the environment more comfortable for the patient, family, and caregivers.

The patient's history and coexisting morbidities affect the selection of debridement method. For example, awareness of any clotting disorders or anticoagulant medications used is critical when considering sharp debridement. When a patient has severe neutropenia (absolute count less than 500) and therefore at risk for severe sepsis, autolysis is not realistic or safe because of the insufficient number of neutrophils available to respond to the wound demands (Bodey et al, 1966). Generally, the wound will appear stagnant during this time. Debridement by autolysis should be postponed until the neutrophil count climbs over 1000 mm³. Chemical debridement using enzymes is an effective option in the presence of severe neutropenia.

The risk for transient bacteremia in conjunction with any debridement technique should be considered. The release of microorganisms from the necrotic tissue of even a noninfected wound may be sufficient to overwhelm the patient's immune system, and the procedure may need to be postponed for the patient who is critically ill or neutropenic.

Wound Status (Infection, Perfusion, Pain, and Biofilm)

When there is no urgent clinical need for debridement, then mechanical, autolytic, enzymatic, or biosurgical methods of debridement can be used. Ulcer-related cellulitis, crepitus, or sepsis dictates rapid surgical debridement (NPUAP, EPUAP, PPPIA, 2014). Surgical (or aggressive sharp) debridement is the cornerstone of biofilm management (Daeschlein, 2013; Leaper et al, 2012). Ultrasound can be a useful adjunct given that biofilm spreads below the surface via perivascular channels that need to be disrupted to remove the biofilm (Attinger and Wolcott, 2012). Recent data suggest that in order to be effective, the timing of interventions for biofilm management is critical (Wolcott et al, 2010). Chapter 16 is a must read to understand the complexities and most recent management strategies for biofilm, including maintenance or serial debridement to break the biofilm growth cycle.

Wound pain is another critical determinant of debridement method selection. Patients who are experiencing wound pain may benefit from the less painful debridement modalities (autolysis or enzymatic). The other types of debridement (wet-to-dry, conservative sharp, and surgical sharp) may trigger or exacerbate pain. The patient's pain status during dressing changes and while resting should be assessed. Prophylactic analgesia should be administered topically or systemically.

Dry, stable (i.e., noninfected or nonfluctuant) ischemic wounds or those with dry gangrene should not be debrided until perfusion to the extremity has improved (Hopf et al, 2006; NPUAP, 2009; Robson et al, 2006; Steed et al, 2006; Whitney et al, 2006; WOCN®, 2014). As described in Chapter 11, measurement of vascular status, including an ankle-brachial index, is an important component of the assessment process when considering debridement in a patient with lower leg ulceration. Debridement is also contraindicated for stable eschar-covered heels. Treatment goals should be consistent with the goals and lifestyle of the individual (AWMA, 2012; Hopf et al, 2006; NPUAP, 2009; Robson et al, 2006; Steed et al, 2006; Whitney et al, 2006).

Clinician Experience and Competence

Although debridement methods such as autolysis, wound irrigation, wet-to-dry dressings, and enzymes ideally are initiated under the direction of the provider or wound care specialist, they are procedures that can be performed by nurses, physical therapists, the patient, and caregivers. However, the more aggressive methods of debridement, specifically sharp debridement, require a greater level of skill and competence. Conservative sharp debridement should be performed only by a wound specialist or provider with demonstrated and documented competence. The wound care specialist must be in compliance with his or her scope of practice, state nurse practice act, and institutional policies. Surgical sharp debridement and laser debridement are performed only by providers.

Clinicians performing sharp debridement in the outpatient setting are encouraged to work closely with experienced coders and billing personnel. Accurate coding and billing will ensure the provider is adequately reimbursed and that errors are avoided. Guidelines are provided and should be followed carefully for the advanced practice provider, as well as certified wound care nurses who are billing "incident to" the licensed provider (WOCN®, 2012b). Coding errors for debridement are common. A review by the Office of Inspector General (OIG) noted an error rate of 66% in Medicare claims from 2004 when the codes specific to debridement were examined (OIG, 2007).

Progression and Maintenance of Debridement

The methods of wound debridement typically used by the wound specialist do not immediately yield a completely clean wound; therefore the wound must be closely monitored for indicators of progression of the debridement process. Maintenance debridement for diabetic foot ulcers and biofilm management are discussed in Chapters 14 and 16, respectively.

Deterioration of the wound requires reevaluation of the treatment selected. Assessment parameters include wound dimensions, volume of exudate, odor, type of tissue present, and condition of the periwound skin. Wound dimensions typically increase as the necrotic tissue is removed from the wound. Early in the debridement process, the wound is commonly exudative; this should decrease as the necrotic tissue is removed. As the underlying tissue is exposed, healthy viable tissue in the wound base should be present. When using autolysis, enzymes, or wet-to-dry dressings, a gradual transition in the type of necrotic tissue present in the wound base should be observed and documented. Hydrated eschar becomes gray and soft; firmly adherent slough becomes loose and stringy. When the wound is infected, a decrease in periwound erythema and induration should be observed after debridement. If the patient was febrile or had leukocytosis before initiating debridement, a decrease should be observed as the necrotic tissue is removed and the bacterial load is reduced. However, these clinical changes may also be attributed to antibiotic therapy.

Traditionally, the clinician discontinues sharp or enzymatic debridement when the wound base is clean and free of necrotic tissue. At that point, moisture-retentive dressings are critical to the wound to maintain a clean vascular wound bed. Without this moist vascular wound environment, the wound bed will become dry, cellular desiccation will occur, and necrotic tissue will begin to re-form. Maintaining a moist wound environment with moisture-retentive dressings will prevent these negative consequences. Inevitably cellular by-products will accumulate on the wound surface. By utilizing moisture-retentive dressings, autolysis will naturally occur and therefore essentially achieve maintenance debridement by keeping the wound bed moist.

Some clinical experts propose continuing sharp debridement even when the wound bed is visibly free of necrotic tissue, particularly in recalcitrant wound beds (Falanga et al, 2008). This theory of maintenance debridement is based on findings from clinical trials that noted improved healing rates when more frequent debridement was performed (Steed et al, 1996). This concept requires further study to determine efficacy and to guide the clinician in the decision to continue debridement, select the appropriate method of debridement, and differentiate between selection of advanced wound therapy and maintenance debridement.

CLINICAL CONSULT

A: Referred to wound care team for evaluation of an unstagable pressure ulcer present on admission. 84-year-old Caucasian female admitted from home with pneumonia and urinary tract infection. Cared for by elderly husband. History of congestive heart failure, hypertension, and type 2 diabetes mellitus. Weight 168 lbs, 5 feet 4 inches, husband reports recent 15 lb weight loss. Currently febrile (oral temp 101° F). Altered mental status; restless in bed, does not respond to commands. Left trochanter pressure ulcer 5 cm × 4 cm; no measurable depth, wound base is 75% eschar beginning to lift from the wound; 25% adherent yellow slough. Mild periwound erythema and induration, small amount of yellow exudate.

D: Unstagable pressure ulcer with possible infection.

P: Remove nonviable tissue, confirm and treat infection, prevent further skin breakdown.

I: (1) Surgical consult for sharp wound debridement. (2) Collagenase ointment to wound to promote removal of slough and lifting of the eschar, cover with hydrogel saturated dressing and change twice daily. (3) Redistribute pressure and friction with low air loss support and every two hours, repositioning schedules off trochanters. (4) Float heels. (5) Nutrition consult. (6) Consult social work to assist with discharge planning.

E: Nurse and husband verbalize understanding of plan. Will meet with husband tomorrow for more teaching, review surgical consult and adjust local wound care as needed to control bioburden and promote autolysis and moist wound healing.

SUMMARY

Debridement is a critical component of topical therapy for necrotic wounds. The wound specialist should be knowledgeable about the various methods available for debridement and should discuss the options with the patient and with the patient's provider so that the most appropriate wound management choice can be made. Debridement methods are not used in isolation; rather, they are used in combination and are modified as the wound conditions change. For example, an eschar-covered, noninfected wound may be cross-hatched and covered with a hydrogel sheet. As the eschar softens, it may become possible to use conservative sharp debridement to facilitate removal of the bulk of the residual eschar and then continue use of the hydrogel or select another moisture-retentive dressing, depending on the wound needs. Close supervision of the patient and accurate wound assessments during the debridement phase are essential to ensure an outcome consistent with the stated wound goals.

REFERENCES

Al-Waili N, Salom K, Al-Ghamdi AA: Honey for wound healing, ulcers, and burns; data supporting its use in clinical practice, *Sci World J* 11:766–787, 2011.

Attinger C, Wolcott R: Clinically addressing biofilm in chronic wounds, *Adv Wound Care* 1(3):127–132, 2012.

Australian Wound Management Association: *Pan Pacific clinical practice guideline for the prevention and management of pressure injury*, Osborne Park, Western Australia, 2012, Cambridge Media.

Bilgari B, Moghaddam A, Santos K, et al: Multicentre prospective observational study on professional wound care using honey, *Int Wound J* 10(3):252–259, 2013.

Bodey GP, Buckley M, Sathe YS, et al: Quantitative relationship between circulating leukocytes and infection in patients with acute leukemia, *Ann Intern Med* 64(2):328–340, 1966.

Bryan CS, Dew CE, Reynolds KL: Bacteremia associated with decubitus ulcers, *Arch Intern Med* 143(11):2093–2095, 1983.

Burgos A, Giménez J, Moreno E, et al: Cost, efficacy, efficiency and tolerability of collagenase ointment versus hydrocolloid occlusive dressing in the treatment of pressure ulcers: a comparative, randomised, multicenter study, *Clin Drug Invest* 19(5):357–365, 2000.

Caputo WJ, Beggs DJ, DeFede JL, et al: A prospective randomised controlled clinical trial comparing hydrosurgery debridement with conventional surgical debridement in lower extremity ulcers, *Int Wound J* 5(2):288–294, 2008.

Chambers L, Woodrow S, Brown AP, et al: Degradation of extracellular matrix components by defined proteinases from the greenbottle larva Lucilia sericata used for the clinical debridement of non-healing wounds, *Br J Dermatol* 148:14–23, 2003.

Chen WY, Rogers AA, Lydon MJ: Characterization of biologic properties of wound fluid collected during early stages of wound healing, *J Invest Dermatol* 99(5):559–564, 1992.

Cowan L, Stechmiller J, Phillips P, et al: Chronic wounds, biofilms and the use of medicinal larvae, *Ulcers* 2013(2013):487024. http://dx.doi.org/10.1155/2013/487024. Accessed April 18, 2015.

Daeschlein G: Antimicrobial and antiseptic strategies in wound management, *Int Wound J* 10(Suppl 1):9–14, 2013.

Falanga V, Brem H, Ennis WJ, et al: Maintenance debridement in the treatment of difficult to heal wounds, recommendations of an expert panel, *Ostomy Wound Manage* (Suppl):2–13, 2008.

Flemming A, Frame J, Dhillon R: Skin edge necrosis in irradiated tissue after carbon dioxide laser excision of tumor, *Lasers Med Sci* 1:263–265, 1986.

Gethen G, Cowman C: Manuka honey vs. hydrogel-a prospective, open label, multicentre, randomized controlled trial to compare desloughing efficacy and healing outcomes in venous ulcers, *J Clin Nurs* 18(3):466–474, 2009.

Glatter RD, Goldberg JS, Schomacker KT, et al: Carbon dioxide laser ablation with immediate auto-grafting in a full-thickness porcine burn model, *Ann Surg* 228(2):257–265, 1998.

Graham JS, Schomacker KT, Glatter RD, et al: Efficacy of laser debridement with autologous split-thickness skin grafting in promoting improved healing of deep cutaneous sulfur mustard burns, *Burns* 28:719–730, 2002.

Gravante G, Delogu D, Esposito G, et al: Versajet hydrosurgery versus classic escharectomy for burn débridement: a prospective randomized trial, *J Burn Care Res* 28(5):720–724, 2007.

Gray M: Is larval (maggot) debridement effective for removal of necrotic tissue from chronic wounds? *J Wound Ostomy Continence Nurs* 35(4):378–384, 2008.

Habif TP, editor: *Clinical dermatology: a color guide to diagnosis and therapy,* ed 3, St. Louis, MO, 1996, Mosby.

Hopf HW et al: Guidelines for the treatment of arterial insufficiency ulcers, *Wound Repair Regen* 14(6):693–710, 2006.

Hoppe I, Granick M: Debridement of chronic wounds: A qualitative systematic review of randomized controlled trials, *Clin Plast Surg* 39:221–228, 2012.

Horobin AJ et al: Maggots and wound healing: an investigation of the effects of secretions from Lucilia sericata larvae upon interactions between human dermal fibroblasts and extracellular matrix components, *Br J Dermatol* 148:923–933, 2003.

Hutchinson JJ: Prevalence of wound infection under occlusive dressings: a collected survey of reported research, *Wounds* 1(2):123–133, 1989.

Jovanovic A, Ermis R, Mewaldt R, et al: The influence of metal salts, surfactants, and wound care products on enzymatic activity of collagenase, the wound debriding enzyme, *Wounds* 24(9):242–253, 2012.

Jull AB, Walker N, Deshpande S: Honey as a topical treatment for wounds, *Cochrane Database Syst Rev* 2:CD005083, 2013.

König M, Vanscheidt W, Augustin M, et al: Enzymatic versus autolytic debridement of chronic leg ulcers: a prospective randomized trial, *J Wound Care* 14(7):320–323, 2005.

Lam DG, Rice P, Brown RF: The treatment of Lewisite burns with laser debridement— "lasablation," *Burns* 28(1):19–25, 2002.

Lawrence JC: Dressings and wound infection, *Am J Surg* 167(1A):S21–S24, 1994.

Leaper DJ, Schultz G, Carville K, et al: Extending the TIME concept: what have we learned in the past 10 years? *Int Wound J* Suppl 2:1–19, 2012.

Mexican Association for Wound Care and Healing: *Clinical practice guideline for the treatment of acute and chronic wounds with maggot debridement therapy*, Mexico City, 2010, AMCICHAC.

Milne CT: A comparison of collagenase to hydrogel dressings in wound debridement, *Wounds* 22(11):270–274, 2010.

Milne CT: Clinical and economic benefit of enzymatic debridement of pressure ulcers compared to autolytic debridement with a hydrogel dressing, *J Med Econ* 16(7): 976–986, 2013.

Morgan D, Hoelscher J: Pulsed lavage: promoting comfort and healing in home care, *Ostomy Wound Manage* 46(4):44–49, 2000.

Müller E, van Leen MW, Bergemann R: Economic evaluation of collagenase-containing ointment and hydrocolloid dressing in the treatment of pressure ulcers, *Pharmacoeconomics* 19(12):1209–1216, 2001.

National Pressure Ulcer Advisory Panel (NPUAP), European ressure Ulcer Advisory Panel (EPUAP) and Pan Pacific Pressure Injury Alliance (PPPIA): *Prevention and Treatment of Pressure Ulcers: Clinical Practice Guideline*, Emily Haesler, editor: Perth, Australia, 2014, Cambridge Media.

Office of Inspector General (OIG): *Medicare payments for surgical debridement services in 2004*, OEI-02-05-00390, May 2007. available at https://oig.hhs.gov/oei/reports/oei-04-99-00460.pdf. Accessed 8.1.2015

Opletalová K, Blaizot X, Mourgeon B, et al: Maggot therapy for wound debridement: a randomized multicenter trial, *Arch Dermatol* 48:432–438, 2012.

Paustian C, Stegman MR: Preparing the wound for healing: the effect of activated polyacrylate dressing on debridement, *Ostomy Wound Manage* 49(9):34–42, 2003.

Phillips P, Yang Q, Davis S, et al: Antimicrobial dressing efficacy against mature pseudomonas aeruginosa biofilm on porcine skin explants, *Int Wound J*, Sep 13, 2013, Accessed April 26, 2014. doi: 10.111/iwij.1214.

Ramundo J, Gray M: Is ultrasonic mist therapy effective for debriding chronic wounds? *J Wound Ostomy Continence Nurs* 35(6):579–583, 2008.

Ramundo J, Gray M: Collagenase for enzymatic debridement, a systematic review, *J Wound Ostomy Continence Nurs* 36 (Suppl 6):S4–S11, 2009.

Raz K: Laser physics, *Clin Dermatol* 13:11, 1995.

Robson M: Wound infection: a failure of wound healing caused by an imbalance of bacteria, *Surg Clin North Am* 77(3):637–650, 1997.

Robson MC, Cooper DM, Aslam R, et al: Guidelines for the treatment of venous ulcers, *Wound Repair Regen* 14(6):649–662, 2006.

Rodeheaver GT, Baharestani MM, Brabec ME, et al: Wound healing and wound management: focus on debridement, *Adv Wound Care* 7(1):22–24, 26–29, 32–36, 1994.

Schultz G, Sibbald RG, Falanga V, et al: Wound bed preparation, a systemic approach to wound bed management, *Wound Rep Regen* 11(Suppl 1):S1–S28, 2003.

Sherman R: Maggot vs conservative debridement therapy for the treatment of pressure ulcers, *Wound Repair Regen* 10(4): 208–214, 2002.

Sherman R: Maggot therapy for treating diabetic foot ulcers unresponsive to conventional therapy, *Diabetes Care* 26(2):446–451, 2003.

Shi L, Ermis R, Kiedaisch B, et al: The effect of various wound dressings on the activity of debriding enzymes, *Adv Skin Wound Care* 23(10):456–462, 2010.

Smith K, Skelton HG, Graham JS, et al: Depth of morphologic skin damage and viability after one, two, and three passes of a high-energy, short pulse CO2 laser (Tru-Pulse) in pig skin, *J Am Acad Dermatol* 37(2):204–210, 1997.

Stanisic MC, Provo BJ, Larson DL, et al: Wound debridement with 25 kHz ultrasound, *Adv Skin Wound Care* 18(9):484–490, 2005.

Steed DL, Attinger C, Colaizzi T, et al: Guidelines for the treatment of diabetic ulcers, *Wound Repair Regen* 14(6):680–692, 2006.

Steed DL, Donohoe D, Webster MW, et al: Effect of extensive debridement and treatment on the healing of diabetic foot ulcer, *J Am Coll Surg* 183:61–64, 1996.

Steenvoorde P, Budding T, Oskam J: Determining pain levels in patients treated with maggot debridement therapy, *J Wound Care* 14(10):485–488, 2005.

Steenvoorde P, van Doorn LP: Maggot debridement therapy: serious bleeding can occur: report of a case, *J Wound Ostomy Continence Nurs* 35(4):412–414, 2008.

Stotts N, Hunt T: Managing bacterial colonization and infection, *Clin Geriatr Med* 13(3):565–573, 1997.

Thomas S: *Wound management and dressings*, London, 1990, Pharmaceutical Press.

Tian X, Liang XM, Song GM, et al: Maggot debridement therapy for the treatment of diabetic foot ulcers: a meta-analysis, *J Wound Care* 22(9):462–469, 2013.

Wallina U, Liebold K, Schmidt WD, et al: Biosurgery supports granulation and debridement in chronic wounds—clinical data and remittance spectroscopy measurement, *Int J Dermatol* 41(10):635–639, 2002.

Whitney J, Phillips L, Aslam R, et al: Guidelines for the treatment of pressure ulcers, *Wound Repair Regen* 14(6):663–679, 2006.

Wolcott RD, Rumbaugh KP, James G, et al: Biofilm maturity studies indicate sharp debridement opens a time-dependent therapeutic window, *J Wound Care* 19(8):320–328, 2010.

Wolff H, Hansson C: Larval therapy—an effective method of ulcer debridement, *Clin Exp Dermatol* 28(2):134–137, 2003.

Woo K, Keast D, Parsons N, et al: The cost of debridement: a Canadian perspective, *Int Wound J*, 12:402–407 Jul 9, 2013. doi: 10.1111/iwj.12122.

Wound, Ostomy and Continence Nurses Society™ (WOCN®): *Conservative sharp wound debridement: best practice for clinicians*, Mt. Laurel, NJ, 2005, WOCN®.

Wound, Ostomy and Continence Nursing Society™ (WOCN®): *Guideline for prevention and management of pressure ulcers*, Mt. Laurel, NJ, 2010, WOCN®.

Wound, Ostomy, and Continence Nurses Society™ (WOCN®): *Guideline for management of wounds in patients with lower-extremity venous disease*, Mt. Laurel, NJ, 2011, WOCN®.

Wound, Ostomy and Continence Nurses Society™ (WOCN®): *Guideline for management of patients with lower extremity neuropathic disease* (WOCN® clinical practice guideline series no. 1), Mt. Laurel, NJ, 2012a, WOCN®.

Wound, Ostomy and Continence Nurses Society™ (WOCN®): Introduction to Reimbursement of Advanced Practice Registered Nurse Services and Understanding Medicare Part B Incident to Billing, *J Wound Ostomy and Continence Nurs* 39(Suppl 2): S7–S16, 2012b.

Wound, Ostomy and Continence Nurses Society™ (WOCN®): *Guideline for management of patients with lower extremity arterial disease* (WOCN® clinical practice guideline series no. 1), Mt. Laurel, NJ, 2014, WOCN®.

Zarchi K, Jemec, G: The efficacy of maggot debridement therapy—a review of comparative clinical trials, *Int Wound J* 9(5): 469–477, 2012.

18

Principles of Wound Healing and Topical Management

Ruth A. Bryant and Denise P. Nix

OBJECTIVES

1. Identify three principles of wound management.
2. Describe the characteristics of a physiologic wound environment.
3. Identify at least five objectives in creating a physiologic wound environment.
4. Define the terms occlusive, semiocclusive, moisture retentive, primary dressing, and secondary dressing.
5. List two indications and one contraindication for each dressing category.
6. Describe the factors to consider when selecting a wound dressing.

The wound dressings for topical management discussed in this chapter have been used extensively, with positive outcomes when used appropriately (Brölmann et al, 2012; Carter et al, 2010; Dumville et al, 2013; Jull et al, 2008; Lo et al, 2008, 2009; Vermeulen et al, 2005). However, several published randomized control trials (RCTs), Cochrane reviews, and metaanalyses conclude that there is insufficient evidence to show that these dressings improve healing rates (Dumville et al, 2012; Jull et al, 2013; Michaels et al, 2009; O'Meara et al, 2013; Storm-Versloot et al, 2010; Vermeulen et al, 2007;). This disparity is often due to the use of complete healing as an endpoint. Wound care experts realize that most dressings are not intended to provide complete healing, from wound onset to healing; rather, the type of dressing must change as the needs of the patient and characteristics of the wound evolve toward healing (Gottrup and Apelqvist, 2010; Leaper and Drake, 2011; Rolstad, Bryant and Nix, 2012; White et al, 2010). More appropriate endpoints to measure are the characteristics of a physiologic wound environment listed in Table 18-1 and described in this chapter.

PRINCIPLES OF WOUND MANAGEMENT

Numerous factors affect the process of wound healing, all of which must be addressed to achieve wound closure. Topical wound management is determined based on many of these factors. Topical wound management is the manipulation of the wound to positively influence the physiologic local wound environment. Three principles of wound management provide comprehensive and holistic guidance to optimize the patient's ability to heal.

Wounds do not occur as an isolated event within a patient. Consequently, the principles of effective wound management must incorporate a holistic approach that identifies and intervenes to minimize or abate the underlying etiology and any coexisting contributing factors. Box 18-1 lists the three principles of wound management and examples of how these principles can be addressed. To control or eliminate causative factors and potential cofactors, diagnostic or laboratory tests are often required. Failure to address causative factors will result in delayed healing or a nonhealing wound despite appropriate systemic and topical therapies. No dressing can compensate for an uncorrected pathologic condition. The various possible etiologies of acute or chronic wounds and the cofactors that impair wound healing are discussed throughout this textbook. This chapter focuses solely on the third principle of wound management: create a physiologic wound environment.

Characteristics of a Physiologic Wound Environment

Topical wound management is the manipulation of the wound to restore a physiologic wound environment; an environment that is "characteristic of an organism's healthy or normal functioning." Key features of a physiologic wound environment are adequate moisture level, temperature control, pH regulation, and control of bacterial burden. These various conditions create a milieu that is conducive to a successful and expedient journey from compromised skin to skin repair and restoration of function. Wound care dressings are used to mimic the skin so that a physiologic local wound environment can be created. Objectives and interventions

TABLE 18-1   Objectives of a Physiologic Wound Environment

Objectives	Interventions
(1) Prevent and manage infection	Cover wound with dressings impermeable to bacteria to protect from outside contaminants, with the most appropriate dressing or combination of dressings based on wound assessment and overall goals for the patient Infection control precautions, no-touch dressing application Appropriate wound cleansing and debridement Antimicrobials when indicated Appropriate wound culture technique (see Chapter 16)
(2) Cleanse wound	Normal saline with 4 to 15 psi of pressure/force to remove debris without harming healthy tissue
(3) Remove nonviable tissue	Most appropriate debridement method or combination of debridement methods based on patient's condition and wound assessment (see Chapter 17) Method of debridement consistent with patient's overall goals
(4) Maintain appropriate level of moisture	Dressing with high moisture vapor transmission rate will allow moisture to escape and evaporate to manage minimally exudative wounds Moderate to heavily exudative wounds require absorptive dressings Select topical dressings that maintain moist wound environment to prevent tissue desiccation
(5) Eliminate dead space	Hydrating or absorbent-impregnated gauze for large, deep wounds Fluff packing material and loosely place into wound using cotton-tipped applicator Ensure packing material is in contact with wound edges and can be easily retrieved
(6) Control odor	Appropriate dressing change frequency Cleansing with each dressing change Debridement and antimicrobials as indicated Charcoal dressings
(7) Eliminate or minimize pain	Semiocclusive dressings Nonadherent dressings Dressings that require fewer changes Pain control interventions as described in Chapters 25 and 26
(8) Protect wound and periwound skin	Skin barriers (liquid, ointments, wafers) to protect the periwound skin from moisture and adhesives as described in Table 5-4 Appropriate interval for dressing changes so that exudate does not pool on surrounding skin or undermine adhesive of wound dressing

BOX 18-1   Wound Management Principles and Examples

1. Control or eliminate causative factors
   - Offload pressure
   - Reduce friction and shear
   - Protect from moisture
   - Compression to improve venous return
   - Prevent trauma to insensate foot
2. Provide systemic support to reduce existing and potential cofactors
   - Optimize nutrition
   - Provide adequate hydration
   - Reduce edema
   - Control blood glucose levels
   - Promote blood flow (avoid cold, control pain, eliminate nicotine and caffeine)
3. Maintain physiologic local wound environment (see Table 18-1)
   - Prevent and manage infection; remove biofilm
   - Cleanse wound
   - Remove nonviable tissue (debridement)
   - Maintain appropriate level of moisture
   - Eliminate dead space
   - Control odor
   - Eliminate or minimize pain
   - Protect periwound skin

for creating a physiologic wound environment are given in Table 18-1.

Moisture Level. The human body is more than 65% water; the primary means of maintaining this level of moisture is located within the epidermis (Spruitt, 1972). The stratum corneum layer of the epidermis prevents loss of excessive amounts of water in the form of water vapor to the external environment. Therefore moisture levels of healthy skin are maintained by an intact stratum corneum. When the stratum corneum has been removed or compromised, tissues and cells are subject to increased loss of moisture and may desiccate and eventually die. Wound healing is slowed significantly in such a dry environment because epithelial cells must burrow below the dry surface to reach a moist surface over which they can migrate (Hinman and Maibach, 1963; Winter, 1962,

2006). A moist environment physiologically favors cellular migration and extracellular matrix formation, which facilitates healing of wounds, reduces pain and tenderness, reduces fibrosis, decreases wound infection, and produces a better cosmetic outcome (Hopf et al, 2006; Robson et al, 2006; Steed et al, 2006; Whitney et al, 2006). However, the moisture level of the wound surface can range from dry (particularly nonviable tissue) to an excessively moist surface. Topical dressings are used to establish and maintain a moist—not wet—wound environment. They maintain adequate moisture in the wound by one of three mechanisms: containing wound fluids, absorbing excess moisture, or donating moisture. Semiocclusive dressings can keep a wound moist, even when no additional moisture is supplied, by "catching" and retaining moisture vapor that is being lost by the wound on a continual basis. Their ability to maintain tissue hydration can be characterized by a measurement known as the moisture vapor transmission rate (MVTR). Dressings transmit less moisture vapor than the average wound loses, thus facilitating moisture retention in the tissue as opposed to desiccation. In general, if the dressing material transmits less moisture vapor than the wound loses, the wound will remain moist. If the dressing material transmits more moisture vapor than the wound loses, the wound may dry out. For this reason, transparent dressings designed for intravenous sites have a higher MVTR than the transparent dressings intended for wound management.

In a wound that has excess moisture, the topical dressing must have moisture-absorptive capacity to prevent the wound from becoming overly saturated and the periwound skin macerated. The process of absorption physically moves drainage away from the wound's surface and edges and into the dressing material. At the other end of the hydration spectrum, wound tissue that is dry may need to be actively rehydrated using dressing materials that donate water to the tissue (i.e., hydrogel).

Normal Body Temperature. One of the functions of the skin is to provide thermoregulation. All cellular functions are affected by temperature, including chemical reactions (e.g., metabolism, enzymatic catalysis, production of growth factors interleukin-1α and interleukin-2, protein synthesis, and oxidation) and processes. The consequences of local hypothermia on phagocytes include decreased phagocyte activity, decreased production of reactive oxygen products, impaired ability to migrate, and an increased risk of infection by causing vasoconstriction and increasing hemoglobin's affinity for oxygen, both of which result in a decreased availability of oxygen to phagocytes (MacFie et al, 2005).

In order for wound healing to occur without delay, a normal core body temperature and a body surface temperature above 33° C and below 42° C is needed. Studies show that each time a dressing is changed, the wound temperature drops and takes 30 minutes to restore after an appropriate dressing is reapplied. Therefore wound cleansing solutions must not be too cold and the dressings selected need to restore the insulating effect formerly provided by the skin

by reducing moisture loss, remaining intact, and requiring fewer dressing changes to prevent frequent local cooling (McGuinness et al, 2004).

Bacterial Balance. The importance of bacterial balance for a physiologic wound environment and interventions to control bioburden (including biofilm) are discussed in Chapters 16 and 17. Strategies include (1) debridement, (2) appropriate wound cleansing, (3) appropriate infection control precautions, (4) use of antimicrobials, and (5) use of moisture-retentive dressings.

Semiocclusive dressings reduce wound infections by more than 50% compared with traditional gauze dressings. This finding supports the theory that semiocclusive dressings optimize the phagocytic efficiency of endogenous leukocytes by maintaining a moist wound environment and reduce airborne dispersal of bacteria during dressing changes. Semiocclusive dressings provide a mechanical barrier to the entry of exogenous bacteria. In contrast, bacteria have been reported to penetrate up to 64 layers of gauze (Lawrence, 1994; Ovington, 2001).

pH. A neutral pH similar to the pH of blood (7.4) is required to provide a physiologic wound environment. In fact, successful skin grafting requires a wound bed with pH values above 7.3 (Schneider et al, 2007). The consequence of an altered pH is an increased risk of bacterial invasion and impaired function of matrix metalloproteinases (MMPs) (Ovington, 2002). The pH of a wound is a dynamic factor that fluctuates with therapeutic interventions; most notably, the kind of dressing applied to the wound affects the pH of the wound bed. Wound exudate under nonocclusive dressings is more alkaline than exudate under occlusive dressings. The more acidic environment under the occlusive dressing is thought to inhibit bacterial growth while promoting fibroblast growth. Any method of wound debridement is also known to raise the pH of the wound bed (Schneider et al, 2007).

TYPES OF DRESSINGS

Wound dressings include both primary dressings and secondary dressings. The *primary dressing* is a therapeutic or protective covering applied directly to the wound bed to meet the needs of the wound. The *secondary dressing* serves a therapeutic or protective function and is used to increase the ability to adequately meet the wound needs and/or secure the primary dressing. For example, a hydrocolloid dressing is the primary dressing when it is used over a shallow, minimally exudative wound, but it functions as a secondary dressing when it is used over a wound filler.

Most wound dressings today are semiocclusive rather than occlusive. Semiocclusive dressings (also known as *moisture-retentive dressings*) emerged in the 1970s and currently are staples in the wound care portfolio. North America dominates the wound care market. Globally, the wound care market is expected to reach $18.3 billion by

2019 (from $15.6 billion in 2014). The largest area of growth is anticipated to be in anti-infective wound dressings (Market and Market, 2015). The wound care market is constantly changing with an extensive variety of dressings that vary by shape, size, and ingredients. They are selected based on the needs of the wound, the patient, and the care setting.

Common ingredients in wound dressings include glycerin, polymers, carboxymethylcellulose, collagen, alginate, cellulose, cotton or rayon, and polyurethane. Wound care dressings may be *single-component* dressings containing, for example, only alginate, hydrogel, or hydrocolloid, or *multicomponent* dressings in which components are mixed together, such as an alginate and a hydrocolloid, to increase absorptive capacity. Multicomponent dressings are categorized and reimbursed according to the clinically predominant component (e.g., alginate, collagen, foam, gauze, hydrocolloid, hydrogel). Most of the dressing categories are available in an antimicrobial form such as silver (as discussed in Chapter 16); however, reimbursement is still based upon their clinically prominent component. The effects of these products and components have been reported by a number of studies (Hopf et al, 2006; NPUAP, EPUAP, PPPIA, 2014; Robson et al, 2006; Steed et al, 2006; Whitney et al, 2006).

Wound care needs may change frequently throughout the various phases of wound healing. Therefore a variety of products must be accessible. In general, dressing selection and utilization are guided by the Medicare Part B Surgical Dressing Policy (CMS, 2011). Table 18-2 is a formulary of wound care products and provides examples in addition to the Medicare Part B utilization parameters and codes. Before using specific products, providers should refer to the manufacturer's product insert for the most current information on contraindications, interactions, and utilization. The policy also contains a category for pouching wounds. These products are described in Chapter 38.

Alginate and Fiber Gelling/Hydrofiber

These highly absorptive products are gelling dressings made of spun fibers of brown seaweed (alginate dressings) or carboxymethylcellulose (fiber gelling/hydrofiber dressings). They act via an ion exchange mechanism to absorb serous fluid or exudate, forming a nonadhesive, nonocclusive hydrophilic gel that conforms to the shape of the wound (Sweeney et al, 2012). Alginates have hemostatic properties as well. Alginates interact with the wound by donating calcium ions to the bed in exchange for sodium ions present in wound exudate, facilitating blood coagulation, thus assisting hemostasis (Timmons, 2009). Because these dressings absorb and hold exudate, they create a moist environment, thus promoting autolysis, granulation, and epithelization. Chaby and colleagues (2007) conducted a systemic review of dressings and concluded that alginates debride necrotic wounds better than other autolytic debriding dressings. The authors also reported that hydrofibers and foam dressings reduced time to

heal for acute wounds when compared with other traditional and silver dressings.

These versatile dressings are available in the form of sheets or ropes that can be cut to the size of the wound or loosely packed into wound dead space (see Plates 45 and 46). Alginate and fiber gelling/hydrofiber dressing covers are indicated for moderately to highly exudative full-thickness wounds (e.g., Stage III or IV ulcers). Filler versions are indicated for moderately to highly exudative full-thickness wound cavities. Alginates may be considered for infected pressure ulcers as long as appropriate concurrent treatment for infection is implemented (NPUAP, EPUAP, PPPIA, 2014). They are not medically indicated for dry wounds or wounds covered with eschar. Usual dressing change is up to once per day. One wound cover sheet of the approximate size of the wound or up to 2 units of wound filler (1 unit = 6 inches of alginate or other fiber gelling dressing rope) is usually used at each dressing change. It is usually inappropriate to use this category of dressing in combination with hydrogels (CMS, 2011).

Alginates and fiber gelling/hydrofiber dressings are primary dressings changed as often as daily, or they are left on for several days depending on the volume of exudate and the secondary dressing used. For example, transparent films used as secondary dressings will not add to the absorptive capacity of an alginate or fiber gelling/hydrofiber product, whereas foams used as secondary dressings with alginates will increase overall absorptive capacity and facilitate a longer wear time. Some alginates become almost amorphous gels in the wound and will require irrigation for removal, whereas others retain their structural integrity as they "gel" and can be lifted out of the wound. Removal of the dressing need not be aggressive, as the residual fibers are biocompatible. If an alginate is used inappropriately (e.g., used with minimally exudative wounds), the wound bed may become desiccated with alginate fibers embedded in the wound. The alginate dressing should not be moistened before application. If the dressing is dry at the scheduled dressing change, the dressing change frequency should be decreased or an alternative product selected (Belmin et al, 2002; NPUAP, EPUAP, PPPIA, 2014).

Collagen Matrix

Collagen, the most prevalent body protein, is essential in wound healing. However, collagen is also degraded in chronic wounds by MMPs common in the healing wound. Collagen dressings chemically bind to members of the MMP family, thus reducing the levels of proteases in chronic wounds (Cullen, 2002; Nisi et al, 2005; Ovington, 2002) and allowing the healthy intrinsic collagen to remain intact. Collagen is typically formulated with type I bovine (cowhides or tendon) or avian collagen or with type III porcine collagen. Collagen products are nonadhesive, nonocclusive primary dressings available in a variety of formulations: particles encapsulated in nonadherent pouches or vials, gels loaded in a syringe, pads, and freeze-dried sheets. A collagen dressing

TABLE 18-2 Wound Dressing Formulary

Product and Examples	Description	Indications for Use	Instructions for Use	Coverage Guidelines/HCPCS
Antimicrobial: antiseptics, cadexomer iodine, honey, hydrofera blue, mupirocin ointment, silver cream, silver dressings (see Plate 43)	See Chapter 16 for complete descriptions	Partial- or full-thickness wound Critical colonization, infection or high risk of infection Odorous wound Usually not recommended for long-term use	Cleanse wound *Avoid* saline in nanocrystalline silver products Apply to wound Apply appropriate secondary dressing as needed and secure in place	No reimbursement for antiseptics Silver dressings coded by function (i.e., silver hydrogel A6242-A6248, honey alginate A6196-A6199)
Calcium alginate: Restore CalciCare (Hollister), Sea-Sorb (Coloplast), Algisite (Smith & Nephew) (see Plates 45 and 46)	Polysaccharide derived from brown seaweed Highly absorbent Converts to viscous, hydrophilic gel Provides moist environment Hemostatic properties	Full-thickness wound with or without depth Moderate to heavily exudative wounds Contraindicated in third-degree burns Not medically indicated for dry wounds, wounds covered with eschar, or in combination with hydrogels	Cleanse wound base Place or lightly pack into wound Apply appropriate secondary dressing and secure in place Change as needed, usually every 24 to 48 hours	One dressing per day Fillers up to 2 per day Cover when used on full-thickness wound with moderate-to-heavy exudate Coded as alginate or other fiber gelling/hydrofiber dressing A6196–A6199
Charcoal: CarboFlex odor control (ConvaTec), Lyofoam C (Molnlycke, ConvaTec)	Activated carbon (charcoal) Absorbs toxins and wound degradation products Absorbs volatile amines and fatty acids responsible for odor	Malodorous wound (e.g., infected, fungating) Fecal fistula Pressure ulcer	Apply as a "filter" for odor control If absorbing exudate, may need to be changed daily Weekly if no exudate Can be reused if filter only	Coded by predominant ingredient (i.e., CarboFlex is coded as an alginate and Lyofoam C is coded as a foam)
Collagen: Puracol collagen (Medline), Biostep (Smith & Nephew), Cellerate gel (Hymed Group), CollaSorb (Hartmann)	May enhance deposition of organized collagen fibers Chemoattractant to granulocytes and fibroblasts Bioresorbable Hemostatic properties Most processed from bovine or porcine sources	Full-thickness wound, with or without depth Noninfected wound Light-to-moderate drainage Contraindicated in bovine sensitivities and third-degree burns	Packaged as gels, alginates, sheets, powders Cleanse wound as appropriate Apply to wound base Apply appropriate secondary dressing Secure as necessary	Collagen fillers (once a day) A6010 to A6011 Collagen dressings A6021 to A6024 Dressing change frequency depends on product used and amount of exudate; check manufacturer's recommendations
Promogran (Systagenix Wound Management)	Some collagens also inactivate matrix metalloproteinases	Chronic wound free of necrotic tissue	Read manufacturer's instructions carefully; some may need to be moistened with saline if wound bed dry	

Composite: Tegaderm absorbent clear acrylic dressing (3M), Alldress (Molnlycke), Covaderm Plus (DeRoyal)	Combine physically distinct components into single dressing Functions as bacterial barrier Absorptive layer distinct from alginate, foam, hydrocolloid, hydrogel Semiadherent or nonadherent	Partial- or full-thickness wound without depth Dry-to-heavy exudate (depends on dressing components) Product selection varies based on wound characteristics	Cleanse wound as appropriate Dressing application dependent on product selected Can function as either primary or secondary dressing May be used with topical medications	Up to 3 per week A6203 to A6205
Contact layer: Restore TRIACT technology (Hollister), Mepitel (Molnlycke)	Protects wound bed from direct contact with other agents and dressings Conforms to wound shape Porous to allow exudate to pass or medication to absorb into wound	Partial- or full-thickness wounds, with or without depth Infected wounds Donor sites Split-thickness skin grafts	Cleanse wound as appropriate Line wound bed Apply topical agent over contact layer *or* apply secondary dressing for absorption Not intended to be changed with each dressing change	One contact layer per week A6206 to A6208
Fiber Gelling/Hydrofiber: Aquacel Hydrofiber (ConvaTec)	Carboxymethylcellulose Absorbs heavy exudate Converts to a gel Keeps wound base moist	Partial- or full-thickness wound, with or without depth Moderate to heavily exudative wound	Cleanse wound base Place or lightly pack into wound Apply appropriate secondary dressing and secure in place Change every 24 to 48 hours	One dressing per day Coded as alginate or other fiber gelling/hydrofiber dressing A6196 to A6199
Foam: Biatain (Coloplast), Hydrocell (Derma Sciences), PolyMem (Ferris Mfg Corp) (see Plates 47 and 48)	Absorptive and nonadherent Consists of hydrophilic polyurethane or film-coated layer	Partial- or full-thickness wound without depth (sheets) or with depth (fillers) Moderate to heavily exudative wound Contraindicated in ischemic wound with dry eschar and third-degree burns Frequently a secondary dressing	Cleanse wound base and dry well Apply topical agent or primary dressing to wound base Place foam dressing in wound Apply appropriate secondary dressing and secure in place Change every 24 hours or as needed	Three dressings per week Covered when used on full-thickness wound with moderate-to-heavy exudate Foam filler: one per day Sheets covered as primary or secondary dressing A6209 to A6215
Gauze: Hypertonic saline Curasalt (Tyco Healthcare/Kendal), Mesalt (Molnlycke Health Care)	Gauze impregnated with dry sodium chloride by the manufacturer	Full-thickness, heavily exudating wound and nonviable wound base, with or without infection	Cleanse wound Apply to the wound dry Cover with secondary dressing	Coded as gauze impregnated with products *other than* water, normal saline, and hydrogel A6222 to A6224

Continued

TABLE 18-2 Wound Dressing Formulary—cont'd

Product and Examples	Description	Indications for Use	Instructions for Use	Coverage Guidelines/ HCPCS
Hydrocolloid: DuoDERM (ConvaTec), Exuderm (Medline), Replicare (Smith & Nephew) (see Plates 49 to 51)	Contains gel-forming agents (gelatin, pectin, carboxymeth-ylcellulose) Forms gelatinous mass Impermeable to contaminants, reducing risk of infection Promotes autolysis Reduces pain and protects Promotes moist wound Molds to body contours Adhesive	Partial- or full-thickness wound without depth Light to moderately exudative wound Avoid acutely infected wound Avoid dry eschar Use with caution in persons with diabetes Contraindicated in third-degree burns	Cleanse wound and dry periwound area well Select dressing 1 to 2 inches larger than wound Apply light pressure to allow body heat to promote adhesion Change every 3 to 5 days as needed Use periwound skin preparation product	Three dressings per week per wound A6234 to A6241
Hydrogel: Skintegrity (Medline), Elasto-Gel (Southwest Technolo-gies), Vigilon (Bard) (see Plates 52 to 54)	Maintains clean, moist wound Nonadherent Little or no absorption Various formulations: amor-phous gel, sheet, impreg-nated gauze Cool and soothing Decreases pain Aggressive debridement by autolysis	Full-thickness wounds without depth (sheet or gel) or with depth (impregnated gauze) Dry to lightly exudative wound Sterile gel for every 3-day dressing changes Nonsterile gel can be used for daily dressing changes Contraindicated in third-degree burns	Cleanse wound Wounds without depth: apply to cover wound base Wounds with depth: use hydrogel-impregnated gauze (do not use hydrogel alone as a wound filler) Use appropriate secondary dressing Cover/secure as necessary Change daily	Hydrogel wound covers without adhesive border or hydrogel wound fillers up to once per day (3 oz/30 days/wound) Hydrogel sheets or wound covers with adhesive border up to three times per week. A6231 to A6233, A6242 to A6248
Transparent film: Tega-derm (3M) Suresite (Medline), Opsite (Smith & Nephew) (see Plates 56 to 58)	Permeable to oxygen and water vapor Protects from environmental contaminants—good shield Maintains moist wound Creates "second skin" Reduces friction Nonabsorbent Promotes autolysis	Shallow partial-thickness or closed wound Dry to minimally exudative wound Not recommended for acutely infected wound Contraindicated in third-degree burns	Cleanse wound and dry peri-wound area Allow for 1- to 2-inch border around wound Apply without stretching or tension Change every 4 to 7 days or as needed Use skin sealant around wound edges	Three dressings per week per wound A6257 to A6259
Wound fillers: Flexigel strands (Smith & Nephew), Multidex maltodextrin (DeRoyal)	Pastes, granules, powders, beads, gels	Full-thickness wound with depth Minimal-to-moderate exudate Infected or noninfected	Cleanse wound as appropriate Apply directly to wound Use appropriate secondary dressing to optimize moist wound environment Change every 1 to 2 days	A6261 (gel/paste) A6262 (dry form) Usual dressing change is up to once per day

HCPCS, Healthcare Common Procedure Coding System.
Examples of product brand names within this formulary are not inclusive or intended as a product endorsement.

requires the use of a secondary cover dressing and can be safely used for a partial-thickness or full-thickness wound with granular or nonviable tissue. International pressure ulcer guidelines recommend considering the use of collagen dressings for nonhealing Stage III and IV pressure ulcers (NPUAP, EPUAP, PPPIA, 2014). However, they also describe a randomized controlled trial comparing collagen and hydrocolloid dressings that found no significant difference in the healing rate of Stage II and III pressure ulcers after adjusting for baseline depth (Graumlich et al, 2003). The guidelines also point out that collagen dressings are more expensive and time consuming to apply than hydrocolloid dressings.

Composite

Composite dressings are used as primary or secondary dressings. They combine physically distinct components into a single dressing that provides multiple functions. The component in the center of the composite dressing is placed over or in contact with the wound base, and the attached adhesive border secures the dressing. Composite dressings should not be cut because the structure of the dressing design will be compromised. Composites should be sized to have at least 2.5 cm (1 inch) of dressing that extends onto intact surrounding skin.

Up to three composite dressing changes per week are considered medically necessary, one wound cover per dressing change, unless it is documented that more frequent changes are medically necessary. Because composite dressings, foam and hydrocolloid wound covers, and transparent film, when used as secondary dressings, are meant to be changed at frequencies less than daily, appropriate clinical judgment should be used to avoid their use with primary dressings, which would require more frequent dressing changes. For these dressings, changes greater than once every other day are not considered medically necessary (CMS, 2011). Although a highly exudative wound might require such a combination initially, with continued proper management, the wound should progress to a point where the appropriate selection of these products should result in the less frequent dressing changes that they are designed to allow.

Contact Layers

Contact layers are nonadherent sheets that are woven or perforated. They are intended for placement over the wound bed to protect the tissue from direct contact with other dressings. Contact layers are porous to allow wound fluid to pass through for absorption by an overlying separate or attached dressing. A single contact layer is generally applied as a liner over a granular or epithelial wound surface overlapping onto surrounding skin. The contact layer stays in place during dressing changes, protecting the wound bed from trauma while allowing for passage of exudate through its mesh or perforations. Contact layers usually are changed once per week. They are not recommended for dry wounds, those with thick viscous exudate, and wounds with tunneling and extensive undermining.

Soft Silicone Contact Layers. Soft silicone contact layers are polymer dressings that are insoluble to wound exudate, not intrinsically absorbent, and do not interact chemically with the wound. Soft silicone dressings are manufactured as single contact layers, or they are added to the wound-facing layer of an absorbent dressing (e.g., foam) for management of an exuding wound (Dykes and Heggie, 2003). An international advisory group of scar management experts recommends the use of silicone gel sheeting for the prevention and treatment of hypertrophic scars and keloids in select situations (Mustoe et al, 2002). Silicone dressings are easily removed and therefore do not traumatize the wound or the surrounding skin (Maume et al, 2003; NPUAP, EPUAP, PPPIA, 2014).

Foam

Polyurethane foam dressings are sheets of foamed polymers that contain variably sized, small, open cells capable of holding wound exudate away from the wound bed. A moist environment is created by maintaining the exudate in the wound space. Foam dressings are adhesive or nonadhesive, primary or secondary dressings, and available in widely variable formulations (see Plates 47 and 48). Nonadhesive foam dressings can be secured in position with a secondary dressing, such as a transparent film dressing, or a nonadhesive wrap, such as roll gauze. The foam may be of traditional thickness (4 to 7 mm) or thin (<1 mm). Generally, the thin foam dressing has an adhesive wound surface and an outer layer of a transparent film dressing that provides a waterproof barrier but less MVT. The traditional-thickness nonadhesive foam dressings may or may not have an adhesive border or an outer transparent layer that helps prevent strikethrough exudate. Foams are available as wafers, rolls, and cavity dressings, as well as shapes to fit the heel, elbow, or sacrum. *Polymeric membrane* foams combine glycerin (to soften devitalized tissue), starch (to wick away exudate), and a surfactant (to loosen necrotic tissue) (Yastrub, 2004).

The appropriately sized foam dressing extends onto the periwound skin at least 2.5 cm (1 inch). Foam other than cavity dressings can be cut or contoured to fit anatomic areas. The manufacturer's instructions should be consulted to determine which side of the dressing is applied to the wound surface. The usual dressing change for an open-cell foam dressing is up to three times per week. Foam cavity dressings used as wound fillers may be changed as often as once per day.

Because traditional-thickness open-cell foam is one of the most absorbent materials available, foam dressings are appropriate for moderate to heavy exudative wounds, with or without a clean granular wound bed (Diehm and Lawall, 2005). International pressure ulcer guidelines recommend considering foam dressings for use on exudative Stage II and shallow Stage III pressure ulcers (NPUAP, EPUAP, PPPIA, 2014). The traditional-thickness nonadhesive foam dressing is particularly useful for management of exudate under compression in venous ulcers and in any wound with friable or fragile periwound skin. Foam dressings can be used as secondary dressings to absorptive primary dressings (e.g., alginate, collagen, or fiber gelling/hydrofiber) to enhance absorption of wound exudate. Only very thin foam can be used to manage the superficial wound with minimal exudate and protect intact vulnerable skin. When applied to a dry or minimally exudative wound, the traditional-thickness foam dressing may adhere to the wound surface and require irrigation to minimize trauma and pain during removal. Not surprisingly, if foams are used appropriately, studies show that patients report less pain with use of foams than with traditional gauze dressings (Vermeulen et al, 2005).

When a cavity foam dressing is used to fill depth, the size of the product should be determined carefully, leaving sufficient room in the wound for the cavity dressing to expand as it absorbs wound exudate. Single small pieces of foam dressings should not be placed in cavities (NPUAP, EPUAP, PPPIA, 2014). Foam must be packaged to cut into one continuous strip to fill tunnel. As previously described, Chaby and colleagues (2007) found faster healing times in acute wounds with use of foam or hydrofiber dressings compared with traditional and silver dressings. Similar to many recent Cochrane reviews of topical dressings, O'Meara and colleagues (2013) reported that there was no evidence to suggest that polyurethane foam dressings were significantly better or worse than other types of dressings with respect to healing rates. The authors were unable to draw conclusions related to adverse events, quality of life, costs, or pain, due to low or unclear methodological quality of the studies reviewed. Foam dressings do not redistribute pressure, but have been shown to be effective in reducing shear (NPUAP, EPUAP, PPPIA, 2014; Ohura et al, 2005).

Hydrocolloid

Hydrocolloid dressings are a formulation of elastomeric, adhesive, and gelling agents. The most common absorbent ingredient in the hydrocolloid is carboxymethylcellulose, which was adapted from ostomy skin barriers. Early versions of hydrocolloid dressings were described as being fully occlusive. Today hydrocolloids are backed with a semiocclusive film layer that renders them impermeable to fluids and bacteria and semipermeable to gas and water vapor. The wound side of this dressing is adhesive and adheres to moist surfaces as well as dry skin, but does not adhere to moist wound beds. Hydrocolloid dressings are waterproof and provide a great degree of conformability and flexibility. Some hydrocolloid dressings are formulated to contain an alginate, which increases the dressing's absorptive capacity. As wound fluid is absorbed, the hydrocolloid forms a viscous, colloidal gel in the wound bed, which enhances the moist wound environment and reduces local pH. Upon removal of a hydrocolloid, the gel mixed with wound fluid may create a slight odor and deceptively resemble pus that an inexperienced caregiver might mistake for infection. However, the gel is easily irrigated

out of the wound, so an appropriate wound assessment of actual wound tissue (rather than the byproducts of the dressing) can be made (Sweeney et al, 2012).

As a primary dressing, the hydrocolloid is available as a wafer in several shapes and sizes. Contoured dressings also are available that enhance adherence to anatomically challenging sites, such as the sacrum, heel, knee, and elbow (see Plates 49 to 51). Many hydrocolloid dressings have an adhesive border that extends beyond the actual hydrocolloid surface. This design prevents shear and friction from loosening the edges of the hydrocolloid and circumvents the need for additional tape along the borders of the dressing.

The correct size of hydrocolloid dressing should extend onto intact periwound skin at least 2.5 cm (1 inch). If the hydrocolloid is cut from a larger piece, the edges should be taped to avoid rolling or adhering to clothing or sheets. Because hydrocolloids are most effective at body temperature, the dressing should be held in place with the hand for a short period of time (30 to 60 seconds) after application. Dressings should be changed when the wound gel appears to have migrated beyond the margins of the wound, the seal is leaking so that periwound skin is in contact with exudates, or the wound is contaminated with feces or urine.

Traditional-thickness hydrocolloid dressings are indicated as primary dressings for minimally to moderately exudate partial- and full-thickness wounds without depth. Hydrocolloids can be used as a secondary dressing over filler materials such as hydrocolloid powders, pastes, and alginates. International pressure ulcer guidelines advocate the use of hydrocolloids for clean Stage II and noninfected shallow Stage III pressure ulcers in anatomic locations where the product does not roll or melt (NPUAP, EPUAP, PPPIA, 2014). Due to its prescribed wear time and reimbursement, wounds that require assessment more often than twice per week should not be treated with a hydrocolloid. As with thin foams, thin hydrocolloids absorb minimal exudate but have a lower profile and are more flexible. Therefore thin hydrocolloid dressings are indicated for the partial-thickness wound with minimal exudate or for intact skin that needs protection against friction or skin stripping.

Multiple metaanalyses confirm what is widely accepted in clinical practice—that hydrocolloids result in better (statistically significant) wound-healing outcomes compared with gauze (Bouza et al, 2005; Chaby et al, 2007; Singh et al, 2004). Studies have also shown that hydrocolloids result in healing rates similar to other moist wound-healing dressings such as alginates, foams, and collagens (Belmin et al, 2002; Dumville et al, 2012; Graumlich et al, 2003).

Hydrogel

Hydrogel dressings contain hydrated (glycerin- or water-based) hydrophilic polymers that are primarily and uniquely designed to hydrate or donate moisture to the wound, thus facilitating moist wound healing and autolysis. Therefore hydrogel dressings are indicated for dry to minimally exudative wounds, with or without depth, and are a good choice for painful wounds because hydrogel dressings do not adhere to the base of the wound. International pressure ulcer guidelines recommend considering the use of hydrogels for dry to minimally exudative pressure ulcers that are noninfected and granulating (NPUAP, EPUAP, PPPIA, 2014). Hydrogel dressings are formulated as sheets or amorphous gel (see Plates 52, 53, and 54).

Amorphous hydrogels are similar in formulation to the hydrogel sheet, except that the polymer has not been cross-linked to form a sheet. However, because of the absence of cross-linking, the amorphous hydrogel does not provide the same cooling effect as the sheet hydrogel. These dressings vary widely in viscosity and are available in a foil package, tube, spray bottle, impregnated gauze (see Plate 53), or ribbon gauze strips. The ability to hydrate the wound surface and resist drying out has been among the most salient selling points of hydrogel dressings, making them excellent replacements for saline-moistened gauze (Eisenbud et al, 2003). Unlike saline-moistened gauze, however, amorphous hydrogel usually needs only to be changed daily. Amorphous hydrogels can be applied to shallow wounds or may be impregnated into gauze to pack wounds with depth, undermining, or tunneling (impregnated into gauze and strips). Amorphous gels are clinically preferred over sheets for ulcers in moving and/or dependent anatomic locations because they are less likely to migrate or slip like a sheet would (NPUAP, EPUAP, PPPIA, 2014). Because of the high water content of amorphous gels, care must be taken to protect the periwound skin from maceration, which can be achieved with careful placement of the product solely over the wound or by applying a skin barrier to the periwound tissue.

Hydrogel sheets are three-dimensional networks of cross-linked, hydrophilic polymers intended for use on dry or minimally exudative shallow wounds. They are clinically preferred over amorphous gels for ulcers in nonmoving and nondependent anatomic locations that are not at risk for dressing migration (NPUAP, EPUAP, PPPIA, 2014). The cross-linked polymer (polyethylene oxide, polyacrylamide, or polyvinylpyrrolidone) physically traps water to form a solid sheet. Although the hydrogel sheet may contain up to 96% moisture and feel moist, water is not released when the sheet is squeezed. Hydrogel sheets have a cooling effect that can be further enhanced with refrigeration, a particularly effective intervention when a sustained "cooling sensation" is the priority (e.g., with a sunburn). Sheets may be packaged with a polymer film on one or both sides; one side is removed before the sheet is placed on the wound bed. Hydrogel sheets that are composed primarily of water should be cut to the size of the wound to avoid overlapping and maceration of intact periwound skin (see Plate 54). A skin barrier ointment or skin sealant (see Plate 55) can be applied to the immediate periwound skin to further prevent maceration. The hydrogel sheet that is predominantly glycerin can be applied to the wound and overlap onto the periwound skin with minimal risk of periwound maceration. Hydrogel sheets can be sterile or nonsterile and are formulated with or without an adhesive border. Sheets without borders require secondary dressings.

Hydrogel sheets are generally changed daily to three times per week. More than one type of hydrogel dressing (filler, cover, or impregnated gauze) on the same wound at the same time is not medically necessary (CMS, 2011)

The findings from a review (Jones and Vaughan, 2005) support the use of hydrogels in promoting natural debridement, hydrating necrotic tissue, and loosening and absorbing slough and exudate in a variety of wounds. Some evidence was found in a Cochrane review (Dumville et al, 2013) to suggest that hydrogel dressings are more effective in healing (lower-grade) diabetic foot ulcers than basic wound contact dressings. None of the studies that met the research criteria showed that hydrogel was more effective than larval therapy or platelet-derived growth factors in healing diabetic foot ulcers, nor that one brand of hydrogel is more effective than another in ulcer healing. No RCTs comparing hydrogel dressings with other advanced dressing types were found.

Medical-Grade Honey

In 2007, the U.S. Food and Drug Administration approved a honey-based wound dressing that uses active Manuka honey (*Leptospermum scoparium*), derived from tea plants, and *Leptospermum polygalifolium,* known as the jelly bush (Pieper, 2009). The strong osmotic action of honey has demonstrated the ability to promote autolysis by pulling lymph fluid from surrounding tissues, thus adding moisture to the wound. Honey's production of hydrogen peroxide may also provide broad-spectrum antibacterial effect and facilitate autolysis by activating MMPs (Lusby et al, 2002; Pieper, 2009; WOCN®, 2010). Odor is reduced because it releases lactic acid rather than ammonia and sulfur during metabolism (NPUAP, EPUAP, PPPIA, 2014). Honey for wound care can be formulated into gels that are spread onto a dressing before application or purchased (and reimbursed) as impregnated pads, gels, or alginates (CMS, 2011). Contraindications for using a honey dressing reported by Pieper (2009) include (1) using a honey product that is not indicated for wound care; (2) sensitivity to bee venom/stings or honey; (3) dressings that cannot be changed within a specific time; (4) wounds requiring surgical debridement; and (5) following an incision and drain of an abscess. Sweeney and colleagues (2012) state that honey cannot be applied to large wounds of patients with diabetes, as their blood glucose may rise to dangerous levels.

A review of 19 RCTs with a total of 2554 participants suggested that honey improved healing times in mild to moderate superficial and partial-thickness burns compared with conventional dressings (Jull et al, 2008). This was supported by a metaanalysis of systematic reviews that found that honey reduces healing times in burns (Brölmann et al, 2012). In contrast, a Cochrane review (Jull et al, 2013) of 25 RCTs (with a total of 2987 participants) looking at healing rates only reported that honey might be superior to some conventional dressing materials, but there is considerable uncertainty about the replicability and applicability of this evidence, and health services may wish to consider avoiding routine (meaning firstline) use of honey dressings.

Specialty Absorptive

Specialty absorptive dressings are multilayer dressings, with or without an adhesive border, that provide either (1) a semiadherent quality or nonadherent layer or (2) highly absorptive layers of fibers, such as absorbent cellulose, cotton, or rayon. Specialty absorptive dressings are indicated for wounds with moderate to heavy exudate and are usually changed up to once per day for a dressing without an adhesive border and up to every other day for a dressing with a border (CMS, 2011). Examples of specialty absorptive dressings are Abdominal Pads, Multipads, and Xtrasorb.

Transparent Film

Transparent film dressings are polyurethane sheets coated on one side with an acrylic, hypoallergenic adhesive. The adhesive is inactivated by moisture and will not adhere to a moist surface. Film dressings are available in a variety of sizes and features (see Plates 56, 57, and 58).

Film dressings have no absorbent capacity and are impermeable to fluids and bacteria. However, they are semipermeable to gas, such as oxygen and water vapor. The extent of semipermeability, measured as MVTR, is variable. Traditional film dressings have a low MVTR that ranges from 400 to 800 $g/m^2/day$. A "high-permeability" film dressing has an MVTR of 3000 $g/m^2/day$ and higher and is specifically designed to be used over an intravenous site. High-permeability film dressings will allow an excessive amount of moisture to escape if they are used over a wound and precipitate desiccation. A collection of purulent-appearing fluid is typical when using a transparent film dressing (particularly in the presence of nonviable tissue) and should not be misinterpreted as indicative of an infection (see Plate 58).

Film dressings are commonly used as secondary dressings to other products, such as alginates and foam. Film dressings are indicated as a primary dressing for (1) prophylaxis on high-risk intact skin; (2) superficial wounds with minimal or no exudate; and (3) eschar-covered wounds when autolysis is indicated, appropriate, and safe (NPUAP, EPUAP, PPPIA, 2014). For example, if the patient is immunocompromised or blood flow to the wound is impaired, autolysis will not be possible and the moist environment created in that situation would not be safe for the patient. When a transparent dressing is being used to facilitate autolysis in an eschar-covered wound, it should be used alone as a primary dressing. It is not recommended for use over enzymes, gels, or ointments (NPUAP, EPUAP, PPPIA, 2014), and it must be monitored closely in case it needs to be changed more frequently to avoid periwound maceration. During the autolysis process, the eschar will liquefy, and the fluid that accumulates potentially can undermine the film's adhesive. As the eschar softens, liquefies, and is removed, the depth of the wound becomes apparent, and alternative dressings will be indicated to fill dead space and absorb exudate.

A film dressing should be selected that allows a 2.5-cm (1-inch) perimeter of intact surrounding skin. A liquid skin barrier can be applied to the periwound skin before dressing application to prevent skin stripping, particularly in the presence of fragile skin. When removing the transparent film dressing, stretch the film in a direction parallel to the wound rather than pulling upward. The stretching action gently breaks the seal. Film dressings should be changed when the exudate extends beyond the edges of the wound onto periwound skin (see Plate 58). The typical dressing change frequency for the transparent dressing is every 3 days.

Transparent dressings should be avoided in the management of arterial ulcers and infected wounds that require frequent monitoring. Because transparent films do not fill dead space, they should not be used as a primary dressing on wounds with depth, undermining, or tunneling.

Gauze

Gauze is available woven or nonwoven, as cotton or synthetic blends, sterile or nonsterile, in many forms (pads, ribbon, strips, and rolls), and plain or impregnated. Nonwoven cotton-filled gauze is particularly useful for scrubbing, prepping, wiping, absorption, and protection. To increase versatility and applicability, gauze may be impregnated by the manufacturer with substances such as iodinated agents, petrolatum, zinc paste, crystalline sodium chloride, chlorhexidine gluconate, bismuth tribromophenate, water, aqueous saline, hydrogel, or other agents. Impregnated gauze provides additional functions, such as hydrating the wound (e.g., hydrogel or aqueous saline impregnated), absorbing exudate (e.g., crystalline sodium chloride formulations), or delivering antimicrobial agents and nutrients.

Because of their low unit cost, gauze dressings are often viewed as the least expensive and most cost-effective dressing. However, when analyzing cost-efficacy, it is important to take into consideration health care provider time, frequency of dressing changes, ease of use, patient discomfort, and healing rate, as well as the unit cost of the dressing (Hopf et al, 2006; NPUAP, EPUAP, PPPIA, 2014; Robson et al, 2006; Steed et al, 2006; Whitney et al, 2006). Gauze does not maintain a moist wound environment unless the wound is heavily exudative, which often necessitates more frequent dressing changes. When numerous dressing changes are required each day to manage moisture, alternative dressing options are indicated to decrease pain, caregiver time, and the potential for dispersal of bacteria during dressing changes (Hopf et al, 2006; Ovington, 2001).

The many disadvantages of gauze use are summarized in Table 18-3. Unlike semiocclusive dressings, gauze lacks a mechanical barrier to the entry of exogenous bacteria. Compared with semiocclusive dressings, gauze has been associated with a 50% greater infection rate (Ovington, 2001). The Wound Healing Society states that wet-to-dry dressings are not an appropriate wound dressing selection because they are not continuously moist (Whitney et al, 2006). Indications for use of dry gauze in wound management is also constrained by the fact that dry gauze does not maintain a moist wound environment unless the wound is heavily exudative.

TABLE 18-3 Disadvantages of Gauze Dressings

Disadvantage	Potential Consequences
Moisture evaporates quickly and dressing dries out	Painful removal Impaired cell migration Desiccation of viable tissue Impaired autolysis Removal of healthy tissue upon removal
Requires frequent dressing changes	Dispersal of bacteria with each dressing change Increased patient discomfort and need for pain medications Increased caregiver time and costs
Associated with increased infection rates compared with semiocclusive dressings	Increased cost for antimicrobials Slower healing rates Increased pain Decrease in patient satisfaction Increased caregiver time

International pressure ulcer guidelines recommend avoiding gauze dressings with open pressure ulcers that have been cleaned and debrided because they are labor intensive, cause pain upon removal if dry, and lead to desiccation of viable tissue if they dry. However, when other forms of moisture-retentive dressings are not available, continuously moist gauze is preferable to dry gauze (NPUAP, EPUAP, PPPIA, 2014).

Continuously Moist Saline Gauze. Continuously moist saline gauze dressings can be effective in terms of healing rate, but may have other drawbacks, such as maceration of the periwound skin, practicality of use, and cost-effectiveness (Robson et al, 2006). The ability of saline-moistened gauze dressings to keep a wound from drying out depends on the amount of exudate from the wound and the frequency with which the gauze is changed or moistened. It is possible to extend the ability of saline-moistened gauze to prevent loss of moisture by incorporating petrolatum-impregnated gauze into the dressing as an upper layer. The hydrophobic nature of petrolatum will block transmission of moisture through

BOX 18-2 Guide to Appropriate Use of Gauze Dressing

- Avoid gauze dressings for clean pressure ulcers because these dressings are labor intensive and dry out easily, leading to painful removal and tissue desiccation.
- When other forms of moisture-retentive dressings are not available, use continuously moist gauze.
  - Loosely fill dead space to avoid pressure on the wound.
  - Fill dead space with single gauze piece or roll (small pieces may be left behind, creating a potential infection source).
- Use loosely woven gauze for highly exudative wounds.
- Use tightly woven gauze for minimally exudative wounds.

the upper dressing. Box 18-2 contains a guide to appropriate use of gauze dressings (NPUAP, EPUAP, PPPIA, 2014).

Hypertonic Saline–Impregnated Gauze. Hypertonic saline gauze is impregnated with dry sodium chloride. The product is applied to the wound dry, requires a secondary dressing, and is dependent on heavy wound exudate for a moist environment. Once moistened with wound exudate, the dressing becomes isotonic and uses a wicking action to draw fluid and debris out of the wound, thereby decreasing interstitial edema, an ideal dressing for infected, exudative cavity wounds. Because they are dependent on wound exudate for moisture, hypertonic saline dressings should not be used for dry or minimally exudative wounds. Conversely, they may not be cost-effective if too many dressing changes are required. Hypertonic saline gauze should be discontinued when new growth of granulation tissue in sufficient amount is present. Hypertonic saline gauze should not be confused with normal saline– or sterile water–impregnated gauze. If normal saline– or sterile water–impregnated gauze dressings are billed, they will be denied as unreasonable and unnecessary (CMS, 2011).

Wound Filler

Wound fillers are dressing materials that are placed into open wounds to eliminate dead space, absorb exudate, or maintain a moist wound surface. Wound fillers come in hydrated forms (e.g., pastes, gels), dry forms (e.g., powder, granules, beads), and other forms (e.g., ropes, spirals, pillows). Up to one dressing change per day is considered medically necessary, unless it is documented that more frequent changes are needed.

COMPONENTS OF A DRESSING CHANGE

In general, the components of a dressing change are the same: infection control, atraumatic removal, cleansing, light filling or packing, periwound skin protection, dressing application, and securement.

Infection Control

Although the wound surface is contaminated, infection control measures are needed to prevent bacteria from inoculating or escalating to an infection. This is particularly important in light of studies identifying health care workers (nurses, providers, technicians) as the source of methicillin-resistant *Staphylococcus aureus* (MRSA). Results from studies of health care workers colonized with MRSA ranged from 15% to 50% (Bisaga et al, 2008; Johnston et al, 2007).

Standard universal precautions (gloves, eye protection when splashes are possible, etc.) and handwashing should be routinely followed during dressing changes (Stotts et al, 1997). Although handwashing is the most effective infection control practice, it is the most frequently overlooked precaution. Caregivers should wash their hands (1) before and after patient contact, (2) after contact with a source of microorganisms (e.g., body fluid and substances, mucous membranes, broken skin, soiled dressings), and (3) after removing gloves. An easily overlooked opportunity for handwashing is between care of a dirty body site and a clean body site; an analogy is the removal of a dirty wound dressing and application of a new dressing. Although the practice has not been researched specifically, two sets of gloves should be used: one set for dressing removal and wound cleansing and another set for dressing application.

Bioburden can be affected by the techniques used to apply and remove dressings and topical agents. There is no evidence that sterile techniques as opposed to clean techniques for changing dressings on chronic wounds is warranted or improves outcomes (Ferreira and de Andrade, 2008). There is also a lack of agreement as to what actually constitutes sterile as opposed to nonsterile technique. *No-touch* technique is a method of changing surface dressings without directly touching the wound or any surface that might come in contact with the wound (WOCN® and APIC, 2011). Sterile devices are used to hold and administer sterile irrigant solution. Sterile cotton-tipped applicators are used to probe the wound and insert wound fillers, gauze, or packing. Clean (rather than sterile) gloves are used to apply sterile dressings; however, the surface of the dressing that will contact the wound bed is not touched.

Atraumatic Dressing Removal

During dressing removal, the periwound skin and the wound base must be protected from trauma. Adhesives are removed in the direction of hair growth. An edge of the dressing is gently rolled or lifted to obtain a starting edge. The tissue adjacent to the dressing is supported as the dressing is gently released from the skin. Moistened gauze can be used to support the skin during dressing removal to minimize the potential for stripping. If the dressing material is attached to the wound base, saline or a wound cleanser can be used to moisten the dressing and allow gentle release of the dressing material from the tissue. Difficult or painful removal must also facilitate an alternative wound care plan (i.e., skin sealant or nonadhesive product) to decrease pain and trauma to the wound with future dressing changes (McNichol et al, 2013). Dressing changes are performed on a scheduled basis depending on the type of dressing in use; dressings that are oversaturated or leaking should be changed promptly. Dressing materials and contaminated gloves are disposed of in accordance with agency policies and procedures.

Cleansing and Irrigation

Every open wound, regardless of size or depth, requires cleansing with each dressing change. Wound cleansing is necessary to physically remove surface bacteria and debris from the wound bed without damaging healthy tissue or inoculating the underlying tissue with bacteria by using a force between 4 and 15 pounds per square inch (psi) (Hopf et al, 2006; Robson et al, 2006; Steed et al, 2006; Whitney et al, 2006). This is accomplished with the use of normal saline, a 19-gauge angiocatheter, and a 35-ml syringe (bulb syringes

do not provide enough pressure). For most wounds, tap water (safe for drinking) or normal saline is appropriate (Fernandez and Griffiths, 2012; NPUAP, EPUAP, PPPIA, 2014). Aseptic technique using sterile products should be considered with immunocompromised patients, when the wound enters a sterile body cavity, or when the wound-healing environment is compromised (NPUAP, EPUAP, PPPIA, 2014).

Commercially prepackaged canisters of pressurized saline and wound cleansers with surfactants that deliver a safe range of pressure to the wound are available. The shelf life of solutions once they are opened is based on manufacturers' recommendations and the policy of the health care institution providing the care. Although normal saline is generally the wound cleanser of choice in hospitals, it does not contain a preservative to prevent bacteria from growing in the container. Therefore, once opened, saline bottles must be discarded in a short period (i.e., 24 hours) (WOCN®, 2011).

When the wound is suspected of having critical colonization or infection, an irrigant with a surfactant, antiseptic, or antimicrobial agent is indicated. Antiseptic solutions are generally diluted and discontinued when the condition of the wound improves. Cleansers cytotoxic to fibroblast should be avoided or only used for a short period of time. Cleansers designed for intact skin such as incontinent care cleansers or bath products are not indicated for wound cleansing. (NPUAP, EPUAP, PPPIA, 2014). To date, there is no wound-cleansing product that can remove suspected biofilm. Chapter 16 provides a detailed discussion related to wound infection, diagnosis and management, including descriptions and indications for antimicrobials and antiseptic solutions.

Periwound Skin Cleansing and Protection

After dressing removal and wound cleansing, the surrounding skin is gently cleansed and dried. Wound exudate and dressing adhesives place the periwound skin at risk for maceration, skin stripping, and infection. Periwound maceration and continuous contact with wound exudate can enlarge the wound and impede healing (Robson et al, 2006; Steed et al, 2006; Whitney et al, 2006). In addition, the pathophysiologic impact of an underlying etiology such as arterial insufficiency may leave the periwound skin dry, cracked, or friable. Measures to maintain the integrity of the periwound skin include use of moisturizers when the skin is dry, use of skin sealants to protect the skin from moisture and adhesives (see Table 5-4 and Plate 55), and use of nonadhesive dressings (see Tables 18-2 and 18-4). Dressings should be changed or modified when the wound exudate is no longer contained by the dressing and is encroaching on the intact skin. Chapter 5 provides a detailed discussion of additional steps to prevent and manage skin stripping and candidiasis.

Dressing Application

The selected dressing is applied according to manufacturer's instructions without stretching the skin. In the gluteal fold, wafer dressings are folded in half before application to ensure

TABLE 18-4	**Dressing Options Based on Wound Needs**					
Dry to Minimal Exudate, Shallow	**Moderate to Heavy Exudate, Shallow**	**Dry to Minimal Exudate with Depth**	**Moderate to Heavy Exudate with Depth**	**Nonadherent**	**Conformable**	**Recalcitrant**
Foam (thin)	Specialty absorptive	Hydrogel-impregnated gauze	Alginate/hydrofiber	Foam (nonadhesive brand)	Alginate	Antimicrobials (see Chapter 16)
Hydrocolloid	Foam (standard)	Continuously moist gauze	Foam cavity	Contact layer	Transparent	Collagen
Transparent	Hydrocolloid (moderate exudate)		Loosely woven gauze	Hydrogel	Hydrocolloid	
Hydrogel	Alginate/hydrofiber		Hypertonic saline gauze		Thin foam	

that the adhesive seals into the anatomic contours. Applications of dressings at the heel or elbow may require cutting and shaping the dressing to customize the fit. Position the heel or elbow in the bent position during application so that the dressing does not pull the skin when the limb is extended.

Packing or Filling. The purpose of filling or packing the wound is to fill dead space and avoid the potential of abscess formation by premature closure of the wound. Packing materials should be conformable to the base and sides of the wound. In the presence of undermining, impregnated gauze, alginate rope, or fiber gelling/hydrofiber dressings may be used to gently pack the space. When tunneling is apparent in the wound, strip gauze packing may be used to fill narrow areas so that the complete dressing can be easily removed during dressing changes. Absorbent packing dressings (e.g., alginate, hydrofera blue, fiber gelling/hydrofiber, dry gauze) are appropriate for wounds that are exudative. Conversely, for wounds that are dry, the packing material must be hydrating so that it provides moisture to the wounds (e.g., hydrogel-impregnated gauze, collagen dressings, continuously moist gauze). For large deep wounds, hydrating or absorbent-impregnated gauze is effective and usually requires fewer dressing changes than dry gauze. The packing material is fluffed and loosely placed into the wound with a cotton-tipped applicator so that the packing material is in contact with the wound edges and base. Gauze dressings may be necessary to act as an additional absorbent layer. "Overpacking" the wound should be avoided. A secondary cover dressing is then applied and secured.

Securing the Dressing

A method of securing nonadhesive dressings is necessary to keep such dressings in place. Self-adhesive wraps, tape, Montgomery straps, gauze wraps, or tubular mesh dressings may be used. If the wound is located on the leg, a gauze wrap can be taped upon itself to avoid applying tape to the skin. Again, see Chapter 5 for appropriate selection and use of medical adhesive if an adhesive product is needed to secure the dressing (McNichol et al, 2013).

DRESSING SELECTION

Topical dressing selection is based on the wound characteristics and dressing functions. The process of dressing selection is guided by a series of questions and assessments (Checklist 18-1). Two key wound assessment parameters that most influence dressing selection are the amount of wound exudate and the depth of the wound. Not all dressings are intended or appropriate to be used continuously until closure. Therefore dressings should be reevaluated for appropriateness based on the wound characteristics and patient response. As always, it is important to follow manufacturers' instructions for use of their products.

Does the Wound Have Exudate?

The volume and type of wound exudate are such sufficiently significant factors in selecting a wound dressing that the presence of exudate is the first question posed. Dry wounds require a dressing that will hydrate the tissue. Conversely, exudative wounds require absorbent dressing materials. Several dressings are available that are designed to manage the full range of exudate volume, from minimal to heavy amounts (see Tables 18-2 and 18-4). Adequate containment of exudate is critical to managing bioburden, maintaining a seal, protecting the periwound skin, controlling odor, and avoiding overuse of wound care products. In addition, the prolonged presence of excessive amounts of moisture in the wound may

---

CHECKLIST 18-1 Questions for Appropriate Dressing Selection

✓ Is the wound dry or does it have exudate?
✓ Does the wound have depth, tunneling, or undermining?
✓ What type of tissue is present in the base of the wound?
✓ What is the condition of the periwound skin?
✓ Are there any compatibility issues to consider?
✓ What is the location of the wound?
✓ Are topical antimicrobials indicated?
✓ Is senescence suspected?
✓ Are there any special patient or caregiver considerations?

increase the patient's risk for developing hyperplasia or hypergranulation tissue in the base of the wound (see Plate 27). Methods of exudate management include moisture vapor transmission, as with transparent dressings, and wicking, as with alginate or foam dressings.

Does the Wound Have Depth, Tunneling, or Undermining?

Tissue that is not exposed to treatment agents cannot be expected to respond to the regimen and proceed to healing (Whitney et al, 2006). Once depth, tunneling, or undermining is identified, the dressing selected must be able to reach the extent of the wound base, as well as fill the dead space to prevent abscess and premature closure of the wound. For example, a hydrocolloid paste can fill a very small amount of depth, whereas a deeper wound may require layers or strips of packing agents such as impregnated gauze to adequately fill dead space.

What Type of Tissue Is Present in the Base of the Wound?

When granulation is the primary tissue in the wound, a dressing that maintains a moist wound surface usually is ideal. The presence of slough or eschar in the wound will dictate the need for some form of debridement to decrease the bioburden in the wound and remove physical obstacles to wound closure. Moisture-retentive dressings promote autolysis by maintaining a moist wound–dressing interface. The type of dressing used to achieve or assist with debridement varies depending on the form of debridement selected. All of the dressing categories in the formulary, except for dry gauze, are moisture retentive. The dressing selected is also based on the volume of exudate and the architecture of the wound. For example, when the wound is minimally exudative and eschar covered, one option for autolysis is to apply an amorphous hydrogel over the wound and cover with a transparent dressing. Within 24 hours the eschar typically is rehydrated and loosening from the wound edges. At that time, sharp debridement may be indicated and the hydrogel may continue to be appropriate, or another dressing may be indicated if the wound depth is revealed.

What Is the Condition of the Periwound Skin?

The periwound skin can be intact, dry, cracked, macerated, erythematous, or infected (e.g., candidiasis). Dry and cracked skin may require a moisturizer before dressing application. Skin that is vulnerable to adhesives may require a nonadhesive dressing or can be protected from adhesives with the use of skin protectants, sealants, and barriers. Skin integrity is also affected by the technique used to apply and remove adhesives. When appropriate, less frequent dressing changes are preferred to prevent unnecessary exposure of the skin to adhesive removal. As previously described, less aggressive adhesives such as silicones may be indicated. Caregivers should be taught techniques for gentle removal of dressings to prevent skin stripping.

The presence of maceration indicates that wound exudate is not adequately contained or managed. Prolonged contact of wound fluid with the periwound skin predisposes the patient to development of fungal infection (most commonly candidiasis) or erythema at the periwound site. To correct this situation, either the type of dressing used should be modified to a more absorbent type (see Tables 18-2 and 18-4) or the frequency of dressing changes should be increased. A liquid skin barrier will protect the periwound skin from damp or saturated wound dressings. Occasionally the patient will require an antifungal powder or lotion to treat a fungal infection, although milder cases may resolve spontaneously when the excessive wound exudate is managed effectively. Absorbent dressings and pouching techniques are used to manage wound exudate, thus preventing or reducing periwound maceration, erythema, and candidiasis.

Are There Compatibility Issues to Consider?

Safety features of wound care dressings indicate that products be free from toxic chemicals and fibers and that product biocompatibility has been tested and reported by the manufacturers. Safety should also demonstrate that the product does not increase the patient's risk of morbidity or mortality. The wound specialist's role in safety includes correct use of the product as recommended by the manufacturer (including FDA-approved clinical indications) and proper education of the caregiver. Systemic cofactors and sensitivities must be taken into consideration and may prohibit use of some dressing ingredients. For example, honey on large wounds of patients with diabetes or iodine products for individuals with renal failure should not be used (NPUAP, EPUAP, PPPIA, 2014).

The wound specialist should be cautious about mixing different topical agents for use in a wound because ingredients in one agent may interact with ingredients in another. For example, the enzymatic activity of collagenase is adversely affected by certain detergents and heavy metal ions (e.g., mercury, silver), which are used in some antiseptics, and is inactivated by povidone-iodine. If the collagenase enzyme is used in combination with a secondary cover dressing that releases silver ions, the silver ions would inactivate the enzyme, resulting in no enzymatic debridement and little or no antibacterial effect of the silver. Similarly, certain foams are degraded by hydrogen peroxide, and the two should not be used sequentially. It is vitally important to thoroughly read product package inserts and instructions for use when dressings, ointments, and solutions are being used together or sequentially in the same wound.

Finally, compatibility with concurrently used therapies and procedures is an important consideration in selecting the optimal dressing. For example, some products are not compatible with electrical stimulation, hyperbaric oxygen therapy, or radiation therapy. Because various compression therapy methods have change frequencies ranging from daily to weekly, the patient with a venous insufficiency wound requires a dressing with a compatible wear time. The patient with an ostomy close to a midline incision wound will require a dressing that does not interfere with the patient's ability to empty and change the ostomy pouch.

What Is the Location of the Wound?

The dressing selected should stay in place, minimize shear and friction, and not cause additional tissue damage (Robson et al, 2006; Steed et al, 2006; Whitney et al, 2006). Wound location combined with patient activity can significantly affect the dressing's ability to stay intact. Digit dressings are useful for the toes and fingers. In some situations, flexible dressing options shaped to fit heels, elbows, and sacrum may provide better coverage and wear time than a standard square or rectangular dressing. Wounds in locations exposed to friction and shear from sheets, clothing, or braces may require thin adhesive dressings with smooth backings and tapered edges to keep from rolling. In the presence of incontinence, wounds close to the perineal region will benefit from waterproof dressings.

Are Topical Antimicrobials Indicated?

Bacterial bioburden influences decisions on topical wound management. Therefore with each dressing change, the wound should be assessed for signs and symptoms of infection. When the wound is overcolonized or infected, a complete systemic assessment and appropriate treatment must be instituted. Chapter 16 provides a detailed discussion related to wound infection, diagnosis, and management, including descriptions and indications for antimicrobial dressings and antiseptic solutions. Generally, nonocclusive dressings are indicated as the most conservative topical wound care approach; semiocclusive dressings are not recommended for infected wounds. Semiocclusive dressings should be monitored closely and changed more frequently than generally anticipated.

Odor is also commonly associated with infected or highly colonized wounds, such as fungating lesions or pressure ulcers with necrotic debris. Improvement is generally noted as odor-causing bacteria are eliminated through the use of debridement, antimicrobials, and antiseptics. However, a slight odor noted during a dressing change may not be indicative of an infection. Odor is associated with the use of certain types of dressings (e.g., hydrocolloids), strikethrough exudate and leakage, poor hygiene, and inappropriate use of dressings (e.g., extending dressing wear time beyond that which is recommended). In these situations, patient and caregiver education is indicated. Chapter 37 presents interventions (including topical dressing options) that are available when odor is an ongoing problem, such as with a fungating wound.

Is Senescence Suspected?

If a wound is not progressing despite optimal care, cellular senescence (a decrease in proliferation potential of dermal fibroblasts and inability of cells to respond to growth factors) may be a factor. In the case of senescence, biophysical and biologic agents (e.g., growth factors, electrical stimulation, negative pressure wound therapy) may be considered to manipulate the repair process for successful "recruitment" of nonsenescent cells to the wound bed. These therapies are discussed in greater detail in Chapters 19 through 24.

Are There Special Patient or Caregiver Considerations?

During the initial patient interview, it is valuable to obtain a history of the patient's wound, including what dressings thus far have been used for the wound and the effect of those interventions. This information can be used to identify dressings to avoid, dressings that may require extra encouragement for the patient to use again, or dressings that will require additional periwound skin protection, such as a skin barrier ointment, cream, or sealant. Realistic goals for the wound and for the patient must be identified (WOCN®, 2010). For example, the patient with a wound on a limb with an ankle-brachial index (ABI) of 0.6 that cannot be revascularized may not have enough blood flow to promote autolysis; thus keeping the wound dry with Betadine treatments is a more appropriate plan than promoting moist wound healing.

A holistic assessment of the patient requires identifying who is (or will be) providing care and in what care setting. Box 18-1 shows the numerous variables that affect product selection and potential outcomes of care. Clearly, the caregiver has a significant impact on the ability to achieve positive wound-related outcomes. As the plan of care is being developed and dressing choices are being made, the availability, level of skill, and care-related concerns of the caregiver will be important to ascertain and explore. A primary concern of the caregiver is ease of use.

Reimbursement for supplies (and therefore access to products) is dependent on the type of health care setting and how the setting is paid for services. When the patient needs to pay out-of-pocket expenses for wound care supplies, the risk of nonadherence with the plan of care is increased. Therefore treatment decisions should be made considering what is financially reasonable for the patient so that the patient is able to implement the plan of care. Wound care items that are not reimbursed are listed in Box 18-3. For more discussion of facilitating cooperation and establishing a sustainable plan of care, see Chapter 29.

Pain at the wound site must be adequately described and objectively quantified before the wound specialist can understand the origin of the pain and identify appropriate pain control measures. Chronic pain, as occurs with ischemia, requires maintenance pain control measures. Pain at the wound site may be relieved or minimized by the use of nonadhesive, moisture-retentive dressings. Analgesics given before the dressing change also may be indicated. However, pain that occurs during dressing changes should prompt a reevaluation of dressing change technique and wound care product choices. Liquid skin sealants will protect skin from mechanical forces during dressing removal. Nonetheless, caregiver technique in the removal of tape (i.e., proper use of adhesives and supporting the tissue during dressing removal) has a dramatic effect on the patient's pain experience. Wound pain and control measures are discussed in greater detail in Chapters 25 and 26.

DOCUMENTATION AND REIMBURSEMENT

On a per-patient basis, local wound management interventions should be planned with consideration of product

BOX 18-3 Wound Care Items that Are Not Reimbursed

- Dressings for drainage from a cutaneous fistula that has not been caused by or treated by a surgical procedure
- Dressings for Stage I pressure ulcers
- Dressings for first-degree burns
- Dressings for wounds caused by trauma that do not require surgical closure or debridement (skin tears, venipuncture, arterial puncture site)
- Skin sealants or barriers, wound cleansers or irrigating solutions, solutions used to moisten gauze (e.g., saline), topical antiseptics, and topical antibiotics
- Gauze or other dressings used to debride a wound, but not left on the wound
- Dressing kits (all dressings must be individualized for each patient)
- More than one type of wound filler or wound cover in a single wound
- Use of some combinations of a hydrating dressing and an absorptive dressing (e.g., hydrogel, alginate) on the same wound at the same time
- More than a 1-month supply at a time

Data from Aetna: Surgical dressings (wound care supplies), *Clinical Policy Bulletin* no. 0526. http://www.aetna.com/cpb/medical/data/500_599/0526.html. Accessed April 22, 2015.

CHECKLIST 18-2 Documentation Requirements for Coverage and/or Medical Necessity

Wound Care Orders
✓ Written wound care orders every 3 months, when a new dressing is added, or if quantity increases
✓ Order must be signed and dated by health care provider
✓ Order must specify the following:
   a. Type of dressing
   b. Size of the dressing
   c. Number/amount to be used at one time
   d. Frequency of dressing changes
   e. Expected duration of need

Documentation
✓ Monthly documentation by nurse, provider, or other health care professional
✓ More frequent documentation (e.g., weekly) for patients in nursing facility or patients with heavily draining or infected wounds
✓ Documentation must include the following:
   a. Number of wounds being treated with a dressing
   b. Type of wound (e.g., surgical wound, debrided wound)
   c. Whether dressing is being used as primary or secondary dressing
   d. Location, size (length × width, in centimeters), depth of wound; amount of exudate
   e. Additional relevant information

Data from Aetna: Surgical dressings (wound care supplies), Clinical Policy Bulletin no. 0526. http://www.aetna.com/cpb/medical/data/500_599/0526.html. Accessed April 25, 2015.

reimbursement for the patient. Documentation, product selection, and the care setting affect how reimbursement occurs. Some wound care items, such as skin and wound cleansers, moisturizers, and skin barriers, are not reimbursed by Medicare. If the patient is paying out of pocket for these supplies, wound care may be jeopardized. Guidelines for utilization as established by Medicare Part B require documentation of medical necessity as defined in Checklist 18-2. Guidelines for utilization and Healthcare Common Procedure Coding System (HCPCS) codes are given in Table 18-2

and Box 18-3 (CMS, 2011). Dressing size must be based on, and appropriate to, the size of the wound. For wound covers, the pad size usually is about 2 inches greater than the dimensions of the wound. No more than a 1-month supply of dressings may be provided at one time.

CLINICAL CONSULT

A: Home care referral received to provide wound consult for a 78-year-old male who lives in a trailer with his son and his nursing assistant daughter-in-law. Patient was recently discharged following a lengthy hospital stay for pneumonia during which he required prolonged periods of head of bed elevation and supplemental oxygen. Respiratory status is much improved. He is afebrile and on oral antibiotics. Developed hospital acquired pressure ulcer left buttock near gluteal cleft. Pressure ulcer encompasses a 5 × 6 cm area of nonblanchable erythema with a centrally located 2 × 1.5 × 0.5 cm full-thickness wound of red, viable tissue. Currently using a hydrocolloid dressing with instructions to change dressing twice weekly. Patient has noticed drainage from dressing onto underwear and tries to reduce this seepage by covering dressing with paper towels. Wound edges are open; periwound skin macerated; no periwound erythema. Patient spends much of his day on the couch reading or watching TV while his adult children are at work.

D: Stage III pressure ulcer with moderate exudate inadequately contained.

P: Implement absorptive wound filler and consult with PT regarding activity and seating surface support device.

I: (1) Calcium alginate rope into wound bed. (2) Cover with foam dressing with border adhesive. (3) Change every Monday and Thursday or if loosens. (4) Physical therapy to assess for pressure redistribution chair cushion, weight shifts, and safe use of his walker to stand and walk about the trailer each hour. (5) Dietary consult to assess nutritional needs and counsel patient/family.

E: Home care to continue to follow twice weekly. Wound care to return in 2 weeks to reassess wound progress and modify topical therapy as needed.

SUMMARY

Wounded skin is a complex pathophysiologic condition that necessitates a specific and intricate knowledge base, which includes assessments and interventions to achieve appropriate outcomes for the wound. Unfortunately, nonphysiologic approaches and inappropriate product use remain commonplace and are likely to delay wound closure, thus increasing the overall cost of wound care.

A frequently stated axiom in wound care is "All wounds are not the same." Consequently, many aspects of local wound management differ, and numerous factors affect local wound treatment decisions. One treatment protocol is not appropriate for all wounds, and seldom does a wound progress to healing with only one type of dressing used. Most

wounds require numerous modific
teristics change.

This chapter reviewed the pr
management with an emphasis on maintain
wound environment. Even when a physiologic wou
ronment is maintained, realistic and appropriate goals for the patient with a wound can be obtained only when causative factors are controlled or eliminated and systemic support of the patient is provided. Furthermore, understanding the principles of wound management prepares the wound specialist to partner with interdisciplinary teams, to articulate underlying rationale, and to use a research-based approach to provide cost-effective care to the patient with a wound.

REFERENCES

Belmin J, Meaume S, Rabus MT, et al: Sequential treatment with calcium alginate dressings and hydrocolloid dressings accelerates pressure ulcer healing in older subjects: a multicenter randomized trial of sequential versus nonsequential treatment with hydrocolloid dressings alone, *J Am Geriatr Soc* 50(2):269–274, 2002.

Bisaga A, Paquette K, Sabatini L, et al: Prevalence study of methicillin-resistant Staphylococcus aureus colonization in emergency department health care workers, *Ann Emerg Med* 52(5):525–528, 2008.

Bouza C, Saz Z, Muñoz A, et al: Efficacy of advanced dressings in the treatment of pressure ulcers: a systematic review, *J Wound Care* 14(5):193–199, 2005.

Brölmann FE, Ubbink DT, Nelson EA, et al: Evidence-based decisions for local and systemic wound care, *Br J Surg* 99(9):1172–1183, 2012.

Carter MJ, Tingley-Kelley K, Warriner RA: Silver treatments and silver-impregnated dressings for the healing of leg wounds and ulcers: a systematic review and meta-analysis, *J Am Acad Dermatol* 63:668–679, 2010.

Centers for Medicare and Medicaid Services (CMS): *Local coverage determination (LCD): surgical dressings (L11449)*, 2011. http://www.medicarenhic.com/viewdoc.aspx?id=2304. Accessed April 27, 2015.

Chaby G, Senet P, Vaneau M, et al: Dressings for acute and chronic wounds. A systemic review, *Arch Dermatol* 143:1297–1304, 2007.

Cullen B: The role of oxidized regenerated cellulose/collagen in chronic wound repair. Part 2, *Ostomy Wound Manage* 48 (Suppl 6):8–13, 2002.

Diehm C, Lawall H: Evaluation of Tielle hydropolymer dressings in the management of chronic exuding wounds in primary care, *Int Wound J* 2(1):26–35, 2005.

Dumville JC, Deshpande S, O'Meara S, et al: Hydrocolloid dressings for healing diabetic foot ulcers, *Cochrane Database Syst Rev* 2:CD009099, 2012.

Dumville JC, O'Meara S, Deshpande S, et al: Hydrogel dressings for healing diabetic foot ulcers, *Cochrane Database Syst Rev* 7:CD009101, 2013.

Dykes PJ, Heggie R: The link between the peel force of adhesive dressings and subjective discomfort in volunteer subjects, *J Wound Care* 12(7):260–262, 2003.

Eisenbud D, Hunter H, Kessler L, et al: Hydrogel wound dressings: where do we stand in 2003? *Ostomy Wound Manage* 49(10):52–57, 2003.

Fernandez R, Griffiths R: Water for wound cleansing, *Cochrane Database Syst Rev* 2:CD003861, 2012.

Ferreira AM, de Andrade D: Integrative review of the clean and sterile technique, agreement and disagreement in the execution of dressing, *Acta Paul Enferm* 21:117–121, 2008.

Gottrup F, Apelqvist J: The challenge of using randomized trials in wound healing, *Br J Surg* 97:303–304, 2010.

Graumlich JF, Blough LS, McLaughlin RG, et al: Healing pressure ulcers with collagen or hydrocolloid: a randomized controlled trial, *J Am Geriatr Soc* 51(2):147–154, 2003.

Hinman CD, Maibach H: Effect of air exposure and occlusion on experimental human skin wounds, *Nature* 200:377–378, 1963.

Hopf HW, Ueno C, Aslam R, et al: Guidelines for the treatment of arterial insufficiency ulcers, *Wound Repair Regen* 14(6):693–710, 2006.

Johnston CP, Stokes AK, Ross T, et al: Staphylococcus aureus colonization among healthcare workers at a tertiary care hospital, *Infect Control Hosp Epidemiol* 28:1404–1407, 2007.

Jones A, Vaughan D: Hydrogel dressings in the management of a variety of wound types: a review, *J Orthopaedic Nurs* 9:S1–S11, 2005.

Jull AB, Rodgers A, Walker N, et al: Honey as a topical treatment for wounds, *Cochrane Database Syst Rev* 4:CD00508, 2008.

Jull AB, Walker N, Deshpande S: Honey as a topical treatment for wounds, *Cochrane Database Syst Rev* 2:CD005083, 2013.

Lawrence CL: Dressings and wound infection, *Am J Surg* 167(1A):S21–S24, 1994.

Leaper D, Drake R: Should one size fit all? An overview and critique of the VULCAN study on silver dressings, *Int Wound J* 8(1):1–4, 2011.

Lo S-F, Chang CJ, Hu WY, et al: The effectiveness of silver-releasing dressings in the management of non-healing chronic wounds: a meta-analysis, *J Clin Nurs* 18:716–728, 2009.

Hayter M, Chang CJ, et al: A systematic review of silver-releasing dressings in the management of infected chronic wounds, *J Clin Nurs* 17:1973–1985, 2008.

Lusby PE, Coombes A, Wilkinson JM: Honey: a potent agent for wound healing? *J Wound Ostomy Continence Nurs* 29:295–300, 2002.

MacFie CC, Melling AC, Leaper DJ: Effects of warming on healing, *J Wound Care* 14(3):133–136, 2005.

Markets and Markets: *Wound care market by type (traditional (wound closure, anti infective), basic (films, cleansing), advanced (hydrogels, hydrocolloids, alginate, collagen), active (artificial skin & skin substitutes), pressure relief devices, NPWT) - Global Forecast to 2019*, Report Code: MD 2611, August 2015. http://www.marketsandmarkets.com/Market-Reports/wound-care-market-371.html?gclid=CNLv37GAmMUCFQmRaQodnTAAGQ. Accessed July 26, 2015.

Maume S, Van De Looverbosch D, Heyman H, et al: A study to compare a new self-adherent soft silicone dressing with a self-adherent polymer dressing in Stage II pressure ulcers, *Ostomy Wound Manage* 49(9):44–51, 2003.

McGuinness W, Vella E, Harrison D: Influence of dressing changes on wound temperature, *J Wound Care* 13(9):383–385, 2004.

McNichol L, Lund C, Rosen T, et al: Medical adhesives and patient safety: state of the science: consensus statements for the assessment, prevention, and treatment of adhesive-related skin injuries, *J Wound Ostomy Continence Nurs* 40(4):365–380, 2013.

Michaels JA, Campbell B, King B, et al: Randomized controlled trial and cost-effectiveness analysis of silver-donating antimicrobial dressings for venous leg ulcers, *Br J Surg* 96(10):1147–1156, 2009.

Mustoe TA, Cooter RD, Gold MH, et al: International clinical recommendations on scar management, *Plast Reconstr Surg* 110(2):560–571, 2002.

National Pressure Ulcer Advisory Panel (NPUAP), European Pressure Ulcer Advisory Panel (EPUAP), Pan Pacific Pressure Injury Alliance (PPPIA): *Prevention and treatment of pressure ulcers: clinical practice guideline*. In Haesler E, editor: Perth, Australia, 2014, Cambridge Media.

Nisi G, Brandi C, Grimaldi L, et al: Use of a protease-modulating matrix in the treatment of pressure sores, *Chir Ital* 57(4):465–468, 2005.

Ohura N, Ichioka S, Nakatsuka T, et al: Evaluating dressing materials for the prevention of shear force in the treatment of pressure ulcers, *J Wound Care* 14(9):401–404, 2005.

O'Meara S, Martyn-St James M: Foam dressings for venous leg ulcers, *Cochrane Database of Syst Rev* 5:CD009907, 2013.

Ovington LG: Hanging wet-to-dry dressings out to dry, *Home Healthc Nurse* 19:477–484, 2001.

Ovington LG: Overview of matrix metalloproteinase modulation and growth factor protection in wound healing. Part 1, *Ostomy Wound Manage* 48(Suppl 6):3–7, 2002.

Pieper B: Honey-based dressings and wound care, *J Wound Ostomy Continence Nurs* 36(1):60–66. 2009.

Robson MC, Cooper DM, Aslam R, et al: Guidelines for the treatment of venous ulcers, *Wound Repair Regen* 14(6):649–662, 2006.

Rolstad BS, Bryant RA, Nix DP: Topical management. In RA Bryant and DP Nix (eds): *Acute & Chronic Wounds. Current Management*, 4th ed. Elsevier, St. Louis, 2012, pp 289–306.

Schneider AK, Korber A, Grabbe S, et al: Influence of pH on wound-healing: a new perspective for wound-therapy? *Arch Dermatol Res* 298:413–420, 2007.

Singh A, Halder S, Menon GR, et al: Meta-analysis of randomized controlled trials on hydrocolloid occlusive dressing versus conventional gauze dressing in the healing of chronic wounds, *Asian J Surg* 27(4):326–332, 2004.

Spruitt D: The water barrier and its repair. In Maebashi H, Rovee D, editors: *Epidermal wound healing*, Chicago, 1972, Yearbook Medical.

Steed DL, Attinger C, Colaizzi T, et al: Guidelines for the treatment of diabetic ulcers, *Wound Repair Regen* 14(6):680–692, 2006.

Storm-Versloot MN, Vos CG, et al: Topical silver for preventing wound infection, *Cochrane Database Syst Rev* 17(3):CD006478, 2010.

Stotts NA, Barbour S, Griggs K, et al: Sterile versus clean technique in postoperative wound care of patients with open surgical wounds: a pilot study, *J Wound Ostomy Continence Nurs* 24:10–18, 1997.

Sweeney IR, Miraftab M, Collyer G: A critical review of modern and emerging absorbent dressings used to treat exuding wounds, *Int Wound J* 9(6):601–612, 2012.

Timmons J: Alginates as haemostatic agents: worth revisiting? *Wounds UK* 5:122–125, 2009.

Vermeulen HH, Ubbink DT, Goossens A, et al: Systematic review of dressings and topical agents for surgical wounds healing by secondary intention, *Br J Surg* 6:665–672, 2005.

Vermeulen H, van Hattern JM, Storm-Versloot MN, et al: Topical silver for treating infected wounds, *Cochrane Database Syst Rev* 24(1):CD005486, 2007.

White R, Cutting K, Ousey K, et al: Randomized controlled trial and cost-effectiveness analysis of silver-donating antimicrobial dressings for venous leg ulcers (VULCAN trial) (Br J Surg 2009; 96: 1147-1156), *Br J Surg* 97(3):459–460, 2010.

Whitney J, Phillips L, Aslam R, et al: Guidelines for the treatment of pressure ulcers, *Wound Repair Regen* 14(6):663–679, 2006.

Winter GD: Formation of the scab and the rate of epithelization of superficial wounds in the skin of the young domestic pig, *Nature* 193(4812):293–294, 1962.

Winter GD: Some factors affecting skin and wound healing, *J Tissue Viability* 16(2):20–23, 2006.

Wound, Ostomy and Continence Nurses Society™ (WOCN®): *Guideline for management of pressure ulcers (WOCN® clinical practice guideline series no. 2)*, Glenview, IL, 2010, WOCN®.

Wound, Ostomy Continence Nurses Society™ (WOCN®), Association for Professionals in Infection Control and Epidemiology (APIC): *Clean vs. sterile dressing techniques for management of chronic wounds: a fact sheet*, 2011. http://journals.lww.com/jwocnonline/pages/articleviewer.aspx?year=2012&issue=03001&article=00007&type=Fulltext. Accessed April 17, 2015.

Yastrub D: Relationship between type of treatment and degree of wound healing among institutionalized geriatric patients with Stage II pressure ulcers, *Care Manage J* 5(4):213–218, 2004.

Cellular- and/or Tissue-Based Products for Wounds

Sharon Saim, Ann B. Heintzelman, and Ruth A. Bryant*

OBJECTIVES

1. Describe the indications and role of cellular- and tissue-based products (CTPs) for wounds.
2. Identify the significance of a CTP being cellular or acellular.
3. Differentiate the function and composition of epidermal, dermal, extracellular matrix (ECM) scaffolds, and bilayer CTPs.

4. Outline the guiding principles for the process of patient and wound bed preparation, CTP application, method of securement, and frequency of follow-up and reapplication.
5. Discuss the issues related to regulatory and reimbursement policies by CMS and insurance carriers that must be addressed/explored when planning CTP utilization.

Optimum care utilizing moist wound-healing dressings and comprehensive systemic support (i.e., offloading, glucose management, nutritional support) will not be adequate to heal all chronic wounds. Furthermore, this approach may be inadequate or too slow for wounds with extensive tissue loss. In these situations tissue-engineered products are often indicated. Tissue engineering is defined as "the use of methods that promote biological repair or regeneration of tissues or organs by providing signaling, structural or cellular elements with or without systems that contain living tissue or cells" (Hashimoto, 2000). Historically a variety of names have been used to describe these products: bioengineered skin equivalents, tissue-engineered skin, biologic skin substitutes, and living skin replacements. For clarity, accuracy, and consistency, the term *culture- and tissue-based products (CTPs) for wounds* is recommended because no product is currently available that is a permanent replacement for lost or damaged skin.

INDICATIONS FOR USE

Culture- and tissue-based products act as protective dressings that limit bacteria colonization and fluid loss and/or stimulate

healing depending on the layer of skin they are designed to replace (Greaves et al, 2013). These products are designed to mimic native tissues to promote healing. Numerous CTPs are available, and appropriate utilization requires an understanding of their composition and function. For example, the majority of CTPs are a scaffold (or matrix) product created from a collagen source and used as a temporary extracellular matrix (ECM) implant. This ECM provides a structure into which native blood vessels, cytokines, and growth factors can migrate. Some of these ECMs are also seeded with growth factors and deliver supplemental growth factors to the wound bed. Still other ECMs will also be seeded with fibroblast cells simulating the composition of the dermis. A much smaller number of CTPs deliver keratinocytes to the wound bed and are described as epidermal CTPs. Bilayer CTPs are products that contain live keratinocytes on a dermal matrix seeded with fibroblasts; these may be bioengineered or cadaveric.

All CTPs must be safe for the patient (nontoxic, nonimmunogenic, cause low level of inflammation if at all, and no or low level of transmissible disease risk), clinically effective, and convenient in handling and application (Shevchenko et al, 2009). Ideally CTPs should also be biodegradable, support reconstruction of normal tissue that functions similar to the skin it replaces, provide pain relief, and be readily available with a long shelf life. Just as topical dressings are selected based on wound manifestations and needs that change over the healing time period, CTPs are selected to achieve specific

*The authors and editors acknowledge Susie Seaman for her work on developing content of this chapter in the 4th edition of *Acute and Chronic Wounds: Current Management Concepts.*

objectives: (1) protection by providing a mechanical barrier to microorganisms and vapor loss; (2) protection by providing a temporary wound covering while awaiting permanent wound closure via skin grafting or cultured autologous keratinocytes; (3) delivery of dermal matrix components, cytokines, and growth factors to stimulate and enhance wound-healing activity of host cells; and (4) delivery of structures (i.e., dermal collagen or cultured cells) that are integrated into the wound (Catalano, Cochis, and Varoni, 2013; Shevchenko et al, 2009). The components of the CTP (e.g., collagen) are derived from human (autologous or allogeneic), animal (e.g., bovine, porcine, marine), and synthetic sources.

Culture- and tissue-based products are used as adjuncts to excellent wound and patient care, with the goal of improving patient outcomes by facilitating closure of chronic wounds or large areas of skin loss. Ultimately, the success in using these products depends on appropriate product selection for the wound condition; meticulous wound bed preparation; diligent patient preparation and correction of systemic cofactors that impair healing; aggressive correction of the underlying wound etiology; proper CTP application; appropriate cover dressings; and consistent, regular monitoring of both the cover dressings and the wound bed. It is critical that the wound bed be debrided of nonviable tissue, sinus tracts, or tunnels and that there are no clinical signs of infection. Many CTPs require reapplication, and this should be anticipated when planning CTP use. Checklist 19-1 lists essential steps in the appropriate use of CTPs.

CHECKLIST 19-1 Essential Steps to Using CTPs

1. Address underlying pathology.
   ✓ Revascularize patients with peripheral arterial disease.
   ✓ Correct peripheral edema.
   ✓ Offload plantar ulcers.
   ✓ Redistribute pressure in patients with pressure ulcers.
2. Correct systemic factors interfering with wound healing.
   ✓ Ensure adequate nutrition.
   ✓ Normalize blood glucose.
   ✓ Encourage smoking cessation.
   ✓ Collaborate with other clinicians on systemic medication changes to promote wound healing (e.g., decreasing steroid dose, if possible).
3. Identify and treat clinical infection.
4. Debride all necrotic tissue, fibrinous slough, and surrounding callus.
   ✓ Many wounds may require surgical debridement in the operating room.
5. Ensure complete contact of product with wound bed.
   ✓ Eliminate any bubbles or wrinkles.
   ✓ Use pressure dressings/bolsters to maintain contact.
6. Fenestrate product (if not already packaged that way) to allow wound fluid to escape and prevent accumulation of fluid under product.
7. Keep products without synthetic backings moist.
8. Follow package insert for directions specific to individual products.

Food and Drug Administration (FDA)-approved indications for CTPs in chronic wound management vary by the specific CTP, as shown in the tables of this chapter. The range of indications includes burns, diabetic foot ulcers, venous ulcers, and epidermolysis bullosa. Contraindications to the use of CTPs include known allergy to bovine collagen or hypersensitivity to components in the CTP product shipping or packaging ingredients. In preparation for utilization, patients should be adequately informed of the source and composition of bioengineered skin out of respect for personal, cultural, ethnic, or religious preferences.

Another decision point when considering a CTP is the cost of the product and reimbursement. The Centers for Medicare & Medicaid Services (CMS) 2014 Hospital Outpatient Prospective Payment System (HOPPS) rule bundled the widely diverse CTPs used in a surgical procedure into a high-cost group and low-cost group (Schuam, 2014). It is important to be familiar with this ruling and the impact on product selection and reimbursement for CTP utilization in hospital outpatient departments and ambulatory surgery centers. The wound care clinician should also be aware of the insurance carrier's policy for CTP utilization (including frequency of reapplication), reimbursement, and medical necessity. In addition, although there are many CTPs on the market, not all are approved for use by Medicare and insurance companies. Culture- and tissue-based products that are ruled as experimental or investigational by that insurance carrier or Medicare will not be reimbursed. Some insurance carriers may also require prior approval. The local coverage determination (LCD) outlines appropriate utilization to optimize reimbursement and should be closely reviewed and followed for all Medicare patients. These LCDs are updated frequently and require close monitoring. In general, physicians with special training, surgeons, and advanced practice nurses are approved providers for the application of CTPs, although this should be verified with the insurance provider. Documentation should clearly address medical necessity, outline the treatment plan, and ideally include serial photographs to span the time period before application until the wound has healed. If a CTP application is denied for reimbursement, the provider may need to consider billing the patient for the service, which involves asking the patient to sign an advanced beneficiary notice (ABN). Preauthorization is recommended so that the financial aspect of providing optimal wound care is not a burden to the patient or health care provider.

CLASSIFICATION OF PRODUCTS

Several classification schemes are used to describe CTPs: cellular composition, anatomic structure, duration of product, source of CTP components, and processing (Box 19-1).

Culture- and tissue-based products are either *cellular* (i.e., containing living cells) or *acellular*. Cellular CTPs contain cultured keratinocytes and/or fibroblasts situated on a "delivery system," usually a bioabsorbable matrix, and derived from either autologous or allogeneic sources. The

BOX 19-1	Classification Schemes for CTPs
Cellular composition	**Source of CTP components**
Cellular	Biologic (autologous,
Acellular	allogeneic, xenogeneic)
Anatomic structure	Synthetic
Epidermal	**Processing**
Dermal	In vitro
Bilayer (composite, der-	In vivo
moepidermal)	
Scaffold	
Duration of product	
Temporary	
Permanent	

majority of cellular products used in chronic wound care are produced with allogeneic cells. The primary purpose of allogeneic CTPs is to deliver healthy living cells to the wound, where they secrete multiple growth factors and other ECM proteins that stimulate the host cells to proceed with wound repair.

Anatomically, *cellular* CTPs are designed to stimulate or function as specific skin layers: epidermal, dermal, or bilayered (or composite). Epidermal CTPs consist of keratinocytes; dermal CTPs contain fibroblasts that are embedded in a matrix; and bilayered skin substitutes have some type of both keratinocytes and the matrix-embedded fibroblasts to form epidermal and dermal layers. Cellular skin substitutes do not contain skin structures such as blood vessels, hair follicles, sweat glands, or many skin cells such as melanocytes, Langerhans cells, macrophages, and lymphocytes. Human neonatal foreskin is the common source for allogeneic cellular products. Both the donating neonate and its mother are thoroughly screened for infectious diseases before use in the manufacture of these products.

Acellular CTPs are an *ECM scaffold*. In addition to providing a moist wound environment, these products can actively interact with the wound environment to reduce high levels of matrix metalloproteinases (MMPs) (Límová, 2010). These products all contain collagen that is commonly derived from nonhuman sources (e.g., porcine, bovine, equine, avian), biosynthetic sources (a combination of biologic and manufactured materials), or synthetic (manufactured materials) (Ågren and Werthén, 2007; Shores et al, 2007). Acellular CTPs are available as sheets (which may have to be rehydrated), gels, or granules. Some acellular CTPs retain native growth factors and other polypeptides, such as fibronectin, which may retain some activity in the wound bed.

Autologous cellular CTPs (i.e., skin grafts) are expected to "take," or survive. In contrast, allogeneic cell-based CTPs are temporary and biodegrade (Griffiths et al, 2004; Metcalfe and Ferguson, 2007). Allogeneic fibroblasts have been reported to survive in the host for 3 to 8 weeks, whereas the host will reject and slough allogeneic keratinocytes within a few weeks

(i.e., 2 to 3) (Shevchenko et al, 2009). However, CTPs that are engineered to resist degradation will more likely evoke an inflammatory response and, while enhancing wound closure, will result in scar tissue formation. In contrast, products that provide controlled degradation while allowing infiltration of and replacement by native tissue have the potential to reduce scar formation (Badylak, 2007; Greaves et al, 2013; Shores et al, 2007; van Winterswijk and Nout, 2007). The tables in this chapter provide examples, descriptions, and indications for known cellular and acellular products, including those that are not available in the United States. In the following sections, products that are available in the U.S. market are presented.

Epidermal Culture- and Tissue-Based Products

Epidermal CTPs (Table 19-1) are cultured keratinocytes taken as a biopsy either from the patient's healthy skin (autologous) or from another human (allogeneic) and then expanded and enlarged in a laboratory setting. They are manufactured as sheets, gels, sprays, and suspensions. However, only cultured epidermal autograft sheets are currently available in the United States (Kulkarni et al, 2014; Shevchenko et al, 2009).

One of the first skin substitutes on the market was *Epicel*, a cultured epidermal autograft with FDA approval for deep partial-thickness and full-thickness burns affecting 30% or greater total body surface area. Currently it is processed into sheets that are attached to petrolatum gauze backing using surgical stainless-steel clips. Epicel is not used in chronic wound care. The main advantage of Epicel in burn care is the ability to cover large wounds with permanent skin that will not be rejected because the graft is autologous (Kamolz, 2008). Disadvantages to Epicel include the 2- to 3-week wait for product availability and its fragility. It is only two to eight cells thick, so it can be difficult to handle and apply. It also lacks long-term strength, which can lead to spontaneous blistering months after grafting (Woodley et al, 1998). Table 19-1 lists other epidermal skin substitutes that are not yet available in the United States.

Dermal and Bilayered Culture- and Tissue-Based Products: Living Cellular

Epidermal CTPs (Table 19-2) are insufficient for optimal wound healing when the dermis is absent because the dermis provides elasticity and mechanical resistance. In the absence of the dermis, the epidermis is fragile and vulnerable to blistering, scar formation, and contractures (Greaves et al, 2013). Dermal CTPs contain fibroblasts seeded and cultured on a three-dimensional bioabsorbable matrix, along with the ECM proteins and growth factors that they produce. The presence of viable cells seeded onto the matrix ensures that important growth factors are secreted into the wound bed and incorporated into the wound-healing process (Greaves et al, 2013; Jang et al, 2013). They may be delivered fresh or cryopreserved, although only the latter is available in the United States.

TABLE 19-1 Epidermal CPTs

Product	Description
CellSpray XP* (Avita Medical, Cambridge, United Kingdom)	Autologous preconfluent keratinocytes in suspension, sprayed on wound. Requires larger biopsy. Suspension ready in 2 days.
CellSpray* (Avita Medical, Cambridge, United Kingdom)	Autologous preconfluent keratinocytes in suspension, sprayed on wound. Requires small biopsy. Suspension ready in 5 days.
Epicel (Genzyme, Cambridge, MA, USA)	Cultured from autologous keratinocytes obtained from skin biopsy of patient. Delivered as 30-cm^2 sheets, attached to a petrolatum gauze backing. Autologous cells; therefore no risk of rejection; high incidence of uptake. Fragile. One-day shelf life. Inferior cosmesis in many patients. FDA approved for deep partial-thickness and full-thickness burns.
Keragraf* (Smith & Nephew Inc., Florida, USA; Advanced Tissue Sciences Inc., La Jolla, California, USA)	Cultured from autologous adult stem and precursor cells derived from hair plucked from the patient.
Laserskin* (Fidia Advanced Polymers, Abano Terme, Italy)	Sheet of biodegradable matrix composed of a benzyl esterified hyaluronic acid derivative with laser-created perforations seeded with autologous keratinocytes that are cultured directly on the matrix. The graft can be removed from culture without disturbing the arrangement of basement membrane proteins. Duration of contact permanent.

Products listed are not inclusive, and other products may be available.
*Currently not available in the United States.
FDA, Food and Drug Administration.

TABLE 19-2 Dermal and Bilayered CTPs

Trade Name	Description	U.S. FDA-approved indications
Apligraf (Organogenesis Inc., Canton, Massachusetts USA)	Allogeneic Bilayered fibroblasts mixed with bovine collagen gel and cultured keratinocytes seeded and cultured on gel 44 cm^2 Delivered fresh Apply dermal side toward wound Five-day shelf life	Venous ulcers over 1-month duration Full-thickness diabetic neuropathic foot ulcers > 3 weeks' duration but without tendon, muscle, capsule, or bone exposure. Venous/diabetic ulcers
CDS (Cultured Dermal Substitute) (Kitasato University, Japan)	Allogeneic dermal fibroblasts seeded onto two-layered sponge of lyophilized hyaluronic acid and bovine collagen, then cryopreserved.	None
Dermagraft (Organogenesis, Canton, MA, USA)	Allogeneic dermal fibroblasts obtained from neonatal foreskin seeded and cultured on bioabsorbable polyglactin mesh for several weeks then cryopreserved; delivered on dry ice 5 × 7.5 cm Apply either side to wound Duration of contact permanent Mimics function of dermis	Nonhealing full-thickness diabetic foot ulcers > 6 weeks' duration, extending through dermis, but without tendon, muscle, joint, or bone exposure Ulcers secondary to epidermolysis bullosa
GammaGraft (Promethean LifeSciences, Pittsburgh, PA, USA)	Gamma-irradiated human cadaver skin Stored at room temperature up to 2 years May stay in place until wound heals if it remains adherent to wound bed Left in place while new host skin grows in under dressing Gradually dries out and edges peel away	Chronic wounds and burns
OrCel (Ortec International Inc., New York, New York, USA)	Allogeneic Bilayered fibroblasts seeded on porous side of bovine collagen sponge; keratinocytes seeded on nonporous side Has been used fresh or cryopreserved Duration of contact permanent Mimics cytokine expression of healing skin Nine-month shelf life Cryopreserved; requires cryopreserved storage	Hand reconstruction surgery in patients suffering from recessive dystrophic epidermolysis bullosa and for healing of autograft donor sites in burn patients

Products listed are not inclusive, and other products may be available.

Dermagraft is a cryopreserved, allogeneic dermal substitute with fibroblasts seeded on a bioabsorbable polyglactin mesh (Roberts and Mansbridge, 2002). Once thawed at the bedside in an easy step-by-step process, a 5×7.5-cm living dermal substitute can be applied onto clean, debrided wounds that are free of infection.

Dermagraft is approved by the FDA for the treatment of full-thickness diabetic foot ulcers of greater than 6 weeks' duration that extend through the dermis and are without tendon, muscle, joint capsule, or bone exposure. In a randomized controlled trial of 314 patients with diabetic foot ulcers of over 6 weeks' duration, 30% of Dermagraft-treated patients were healed at 12 weeks versus 18.3% in the control group ($p = .023$) (Marston et al, 2003). Dermagraft is also recommended for use in the treatment of nonhealing diabetic foot ulcers by the Wound Healing Society (Steed et al, 2006).

Dermagraft must be used only as an adjunct to standard care, which includes offloading the ulcer, debridement, treatment of infection, glucose control, and assurance of adequate blood flow for healing. Optimal healing rates are associated with aggressive offloading, not only with footwear, but also with crutches or wheelchairs. Dermagraft is applied with either side toward the wound bed and is covered with a nonadherent contact layer. To ensure good contact of Dermagraft with the wound bed, the wound should be lightly filled with saline-moistened gauze or a soft foam dressing. Although Dermagraft was applied weekly for up to 8 weeks in clinical trials, this frequent application should not be necessary with most patients.

Acellular Extracellular Matrix Scaffolds

Acellular scaffolds (also referred to as acellular dermal replacements) do not contain living cells and thus minimize the risk of an immunologic response (Greaves et al, 2013). Components of these products originate from allogeneic, xenographic, biosynthetic, or synthetic materials. Although most acellular products are commonly referred to as *ECM scaffolds,* those with a synthetic epidermal layer are considered to be bilayer or composites (Table 19-3). The goal in using ECM scaffolds in chronic wound care is to promote rapid healing while minimizing scar tissue formation (Kahn, Beers, & Lentz, 2011). The ideal ECM scaffold provides for host cell attachment and migration of keratinocytes, fibroblasts, endothelial cells, and other cells involved in wound healing. Depending on the signaling that occurs in response to the type of ECM scaffold used, marrow-derived stem cells may be recruited to the area, differentiating into various cell types that manufacture original host tissue instead of scar (Clark et al, 2007). Angiogenesis and neovascularization occur, and as the implanted scaffold is infiltrated by new host tissue, the scaffold undergoes controlled degradation. Products such as collagen-based dressings, which degrade almost immediately, do not last long enough to function as a scaffold for cell ingrowth. Products that have been altered to withstand degradation to the point that they persist for many months may elicit a chronic inflammatory response, which results in scar tissue formation (Badylak, 2007). Although the goal in the use of ECM scaffolds is the regeneration of normal tissue, most products available today result in varying degrees of regenerated and repaired (scarred) tissue.

The products presented here are used primarily for wound management. However, multiple acellular products, both allogeneic and xenographic, are used for surgical indications such as hernia repair, breast reconstruction, and other reconstructive surgeries.

Allogeneic ECM Scaffolds

AlloDerm is an acellular dermal matrix derived from cadaveric human skin. It has a distinct basement membrane side and a dermal side. It is used to serve as a scaffold for normal tissue remodeling. The collagen framework provides strength to the skin and contains no cells that can cause rejection or irritation. AlloDerm is available in multiple sizes and thicknesses. The orientation of AlloDerm into a defect and the thickness used depend on what is being treated (e.g., hernia vs. soft tissue defect); therefore the package insert should be checked for application instructions. AlloDerm has been studied for treatment of multiple surgical defects and wound repair procedures. No randomized controlled trials have examined the use of AlloDerm in chronic wound care.

Cymetra is an injectable, micronized particulate form of AlloDerm. Only case reports and case series on the use of Cymetra in chronic wounds unresponsive to conventional therapy have been published. Although these cases are interesting and appear to indicate that Cymetra stimulates healing in chronic ulcers, no randomized controlled trials have compared this product to standard care in the treatment of chronic wounds. Therefore no strong conclusions regarding its efficacy can be made.

GraftJacket regenerative tissue matrix is essentially the same product as AlloDerm. Unlike AlloDerm, GraftJacket is meshed and is available in only two sizes and one thickness for chronic wound care. GraftJacket is applied to clean, debrided ulcers with the dermal reticular side against the wound bed. It should cover the entire wound and be sutured or stapled in place. GraftJacket must be kept moist with mineral oil–soaked gauze packing, which is used to ensure that the product does not dry out and maintains good contact with the wound base. The dressing is left in place for 5 days without being disturbed and then changed every 3 to 5 days after that. Two small pilot studies have demonstrated enhanced healing of diabetic foot ulcers compared with control (Brigido, 2006; Brigido et al, 2004). A study of 86 patients with diabetic foot ulcers demonstrated complete healing at 12 weeks in 67% of patients treated with GraftJacket versus 46% in the control group, a statistically significant difference ($p = .03$) (Reyzelman et al, 2009).

GraftJacket Xpress is essentially the same product as Cymetra. It is processed by LifeCell for Wright Medical and is marketed for the treatment of wounds with depth. The

TABLE 19-3 Acellular ECM Scaffolds

Trade Name	Description	U.S. FDA-Approved Indications
AlloDerm (LifeCell Inc., Woodlands, TX, USA)	Allogeneic Derived from cadaveric human skin from tissue banks Epidermis and all cellular components removed, leaving dermal matrix Freeze-dried; rehydrate to use Contains intact collagen fibers to support ingrowth of new tissue, elastin filaments to provide strength, and hyaluronan and proteoglycans for cell attachment and migration Duration of contact permanent Two-year shelf life Lacks cellular components	Burns, traumatic, or oncologic wounds with deep structure exposure, hernia repair, breast, and other tissue reconstruction
Cymetra (LifeCell)	Allogeneic injectable micronized particulate form of AlloDerm Dry form, packaged in syringe, rehydrated before use with either normal saline or lidocaine for injection	Cosmetic soft tissue augmentation and treatment of vocal cord paralysis by injection laryngoplasty
GraftJacket Regenerative Tissue Matrix (Wright Medical Technology, Inc., Arlington, TN, USA) (licensed to KCI USA, Inc.)	Allogeneic Same as AlloDerm, but meshed 1:1 to allow wound exudate to pass through; available in two sizes (4 × 4 cm and 4 × 8 cm) and one thickness (0.4 to 0.8 mm) for chronic wound care Available nonmeshed and thicker for tendon and ligament repair	Diabetic foot ulcers and other chronic wounds, ligament and tendon repair
EZ Derm (Molnlycke Health Care, US, LLC, Norcross, GA)	Porcine-derived xenograft (nonhuman skin graft) of collagen that has been chemically cross-linked with aldehyde to provide strength and durability Relatively long shelf life Potential immune response and/or disease transmission	Partial-thickness burns, venous ulcers, diabetic ulcers, pressure ulcers
GraftJacket Xpress (Wright Medical Technology Inc., Arlington, TN, USA) (licensed to KCI USA, Inc.)	Allogeneic Same as Cymetra Available in a prefilled 5-cc syringe Once rehydrated, is injected to fill the entire dead space of a sinus tract or deep wound	Deep wounds, tunnels, or sinus tracts
DermaMatrix (Synthes CMF, West Chester, PA, USA)	Allogeneic Cadaver human skin from tissue banks Donor skin is processed to remove all cellular components, including epidermis, and then is freeze dried Rehydrate to use	Similar to indications for AlloDerm: soft tissue repair, breast reconstruction, abdominal hernia repair, head and neck reconstruction
Biovance (Alliqua Biomedical, Langhorn, PA)	Allogeneic Derived from the placenta of a healthy, full-term human pregnancy Supplied as a single dehydrated sterile sheet to be applied and secured to a clean wound followed by a secondary, nonadherent dressing Five-year shelf life Store at room temperature Contains no antigens	Acute and chronic wounds
Oasis Matrix (Smith & Nephew Inc., Florida, USA; Advanced Tissue Sciences Inc., La Jolla, CA, USA)	Xenographic and acellular Porcine small intestinal submucosa (SIS) with complex matrix of collagen, glycosaminoglycans, proteoglycans, cell adhesive glycoproteins, and growth factors; freeze dried Available in multiple sizes, fenestrated, or meshed Acts as a wound covering One-and-a-half-year shelf life Potential immune response	Partial- and full-thickness wounds, chronic ulcers, traumatic wounds, superficial and second-degree burns, surgical wounds

TABLE 19-3	Acellular ECM Scaffolds—cont'd	
Trade Name	**Description**	**U.S. FDA-Approved Indications**
MatriStem (ACell Inc., Columbia, MD, USA)	Xenographic porcine urinary bladder matrix (UBM) with intact basement membrane; composed of collagen matrix, glycosaminoglycans, glycoproteins, and proteoglycans Available as fenestrated sheets of variable sizes or as powder Must be rehydrated before use and cut to size of wound	Partial- and full-thickness wounds, traumatic wounds, surgical wounds, chronic wounds
PriMatrix (TEI Biosciences, Boston, MA, USA)	Xenographic fetal bovine dermis that has been decellularized, freeze dried, and sterilized Must be rehydrated Available nonfenestrated in various sizes and thicknesses Must fenestrate for high-exudative wounds	Skin ulcers, second-degree burns, surgical wounds
Xelma (Mölnlycke, Göteborg, Sweden)	Xenographic Consists of amelogenin proteins derived from the enamel matrix of developing porcine teeth, mixed with propylene glycol alginate and water Administered as a gel Promotes cell migration via ECM and cell adhesion properties	None
MatriDerm (Dr. Suwelack Skin & Health Care, Billerbeck, Germany)	Xenographic Engineered three-dimensional matrix consisting of native structured collagen from bovine dermis and elastin from bovine nuchal ligament Available in three sizes with 1- or 2-mm thickness, based on grafting needs of wound	None
Biobrane (UDL Laboratories, Sugar Land, TX, USA)	Biosynthetic very thin sheet of semipermeable silicone bonded to a knitted trifilament nylon or monofilament nylon (Biobrane-L) coated with type 1 porcine collagen, which creates hydrophilic coating that facilitates adherence to wound Silicone membrane has water vapor loss rate similar to that of intact skin; once Biobrane has adhered to a wound, it provides moist, protected environment that minimizes water loss	Partial-thickness burns, skin graft donor sites, superficial wounds after surgery, laser resurfacing, dermabrasion Lesions secondary to toxic epidermal necrolysis and pemphigus, as coverage for chronic wounds
Integra (Integra LifeSciences Corp., Plainsboro, NJ, USA)	Bilayered (two layers) membrane system made of a porous matrix of fibers that cross-link bovine tendon collagen and glycosaminoglycan The epidermal substitute layer is made of a thin polysilicone layer to control moisture Duration of contact permanent Moderate shelf life Operative removal of silicone layer required	Deep partial- or full-thickness burns, contracture release procedures, reconstructive surgery of complex wounds and surgical defects
Hyalomatrix PA (Fidia Anika Therapeutics Inc., Bedford, MA, USA)	Synthetic Bilayered with thin moisture vapor–permeable silicone sheet adhered to nonwoven pad composed of the benzyl ester of hyaluronic acid (Hyaff-11) Provides matrix for cell migration, and silicone maintains protected moist environment	Most chronic wounds, partial- and full-thickness burns, surgical wounds, traumatic wounds Widely used in Europe
Suprathel (BioMed Sciences, Allentown, PA, USA)	Synthetic epidermal substitute composed of copolymer of polylactide, trimethylene carbonate, and ε-caprolactone Completely dissolves within 4 weeks	Used in Germany since 2004 for deep partial-thickness burns, superficial full-thickness burns, skin graft donor sites, abrasions, scar revision

Products listed are not inclusive and other products may be available.
ECM, Extracellular matrix.

cover dressing should maintain a moist environment and apply gentle pressure to keep the matrix in place. It should be left in place for 3 to 5 days and then changed as needed to manage exudate. No randomized controlled trials have examined the use of GraftJacket Xpress in the treatment of chronic wounds.

Xenographic Extracellular Matrix Scaffolds

Oasis Wound Matrix is derived from porcine small intestinal submucosa (SIS). It has been examined in numerous preclinical studies; in the clinical treatment of soft tissue defects, wounds, and hernias; and in urologic, gynecologic, and orthopedic reconstructive surgeries (Badylak, 2007; Cook Biotech, 2010; Hodde et al, 2005). In a prospective randomized controlled trial, 55% of 120 patients with venous ulcers healed at 12 weeks compared with 34% in the control group ($p < .02$) (Mostow et al, 2005). In clinical practice, Oasis acts as a wound covering. It should be applied to clean, debrided wounds that are free of infection; cut slightly larger than the wound; secured with Steri-strips, glue, staples, or sutures; and then moistened with normal saline. A nonadherent contact layer is then applied, and the cover dressing is based on the amount of exudate. Foam dressings work well to absorb exudate and provide local compression to maintain good contact of Oasis to the wound bed. Secondary dressings may be changed as needed, but any remnants of Oasis, which may appear as an amber gelatinous material in the wound, should be left undisturbed. Additional Oasis can be reapplied weekly as needed.

MatriStem is derived from porcine urinary bladder. There are no published studies of the use of MatriStem in chronic wound care. Although animal studies indicate potential for this product to stimulate tissue regeneration (Gilbert et al, 2008; Nieponice et al, 2006), and it has been used with burns (Ryssel, Gazyakan, Germann, et al, 2008) and necrotizing fasciitis defects (Ryssel, Germann, Czermak, et al, 2010), clinical trials in chronic wounds are needed to establish efficacy. It may be used in the clinical setting in the same fashion as Oasis.

Unite Biomatrix is derived from decellularized equine pericardium. It is rehydrated and cut 2 to 4 mm larger than the wound size so that it will slightly overlap the edges and then is secured with the clinician's method of choice. Stapling the product in place is ideal. A nonadherent contact layer should then be applied and covered with a gauze bolster or foam dressing to ensure good contact of the product with the wound bed. Mineral oil should not be used to moisten this product. Silver dressings can be used to decrease bacterial counts. The initial cover dressing should be left undisturbed for 5 days, and then subsequent dressings can be changed every 3 to 7 days as needed. If exudate is low, the outer aspect of Unite Biomatrix may dry out, but the product will maintain a moist interface at the wound surface. Unite Biomatrix should not be removed from the wound; the edges can be trimmed as they lift. There are case reports and case series on the use of this product in multiple types of chronic wounds

(Mulder and Lee, 2009a–c), but no randomized controlled trials have been published.

PriMatrix is derived from fetal bovine dermis and is processed to preserve the natural structure and biologic properties of its native collagen. It should be applied with either side down to clean, debrided wounds, with a 1-mm overlap onto surrounding skin, and then secured with the clinician's choice of fixation. It can be fenestrated for heavily draining wounds. After application, PriMatrix should be covered with a nonadherent contact layer and then moist dressings, based on the amount of exudate. There are no published reports or studies testing the efficacy of PriMatrix in the care of patients with chronic wounds.

Mediskin and *E-Z Derm* are porcine xenografts that have been used for years for temporary coverage of burns, surgical wounds, and partial- and full-thickness wounds of variable etiologies (Davis and Arpey, 2000). They are applied to freshly debrided wounds and left in place for 1 to 2 weeks. During that period, the underlying tissue granulates and, frequently upon removal of the xenograft, a split-thickness skin graft is immediately applied. No large randomized controlled trials have demonstrated the efficacy of xenografts in the treatment of chronic wounds.

Biosynthetic Extracellular Matrix Scaffolds

Biobrane consists of a very thin sheet of semipermeable silicone bonded to nylon fabric. It has been used for over 25 years in the treatment of superficial burns and has good data supporting its use for this indication (Whitaker et al, 2008). Because of its ease of use, Biobrane may be particularly useful in pediatric burn care (Mandal, 2007).

Biobrane should be applied to freshly debrided, noninfected wounds with the dull fabric side down and then secured with staples, sutures, or tape. It should be covered firmly with a gauze bolster to prevent movement of the dressing for 24 to 36 hours. The gauze dressing should be removed at 24 to 36 hours for assessment and again at 48 to 72 hours. Adherence of Biobrane is the goal. After 72 hours, if the Biobrane is loose or fluid or purulence is present under the dressing, the Biobrane may need to be removed, the tissue debrided, and a new piece of Biobrane applied if no infection is present. Once there is good adherence after 3 days, then the secondary dressings can be removed and the patient can resume normal activity and bathing as desired. Biobrane should be removed once the underlying tissue is healed, usually 7 to 14 days later. Removal should be delayed if excessive pain or bleeding occurs when attempting to take the Biobrane off an apparently healed area. Further studies are needed before wide use of Biobrane can be recommended in chronic wound care.

Integra Dermal Regeneration Template (IDRT) (Integra Life Sciences) is a bilayered product composed of an outer semipermeable silicone sheet and an inner ECM scaffold. The outer layer provides protection from bacterial invasion and significant fluid loss. The inner layer facilitates cell migration and tissue ingrowth, which leads to dermal regeneration, usually within 2 to 3 weeks of application. As the neodermis is formed, the ECM matrix of IDRT degrades. Once the new dermis is present, the silicone layer is removed and a very thin autograft can be applied, if required. There are no randomized controlled trials of IDRT in the treatment of chronic wounds.

Integra Bilayer Matrix Wound Dressing (BMWD) is the exact same product as Integra Dermal Regeneration Template, but is renamed for use and marketing in chronic wound care; therefore available data are the same for both products. Bilayer Matrix Wound Dressing is available meshed or unmeshed in various sizes. Wounds should be thoroughly debrided and meticulous hemostasis achieved before application of BMWD. The BMWD is rinsed in normal saline for 1 to 2 minutes before application and applied to the wound bed with the ECM matrix side down. All air bubbles and wrinkles should be eliminated from the dressing to achieve intimate contact of the product with the wound. It then should be secured with either staples or sutures. An antimicrobial dressing should be applied next, consisting of a silver product, silver nitrate 0.5% soaks, or mafenide acetate 5% soaks, followed by a bulky pressure dressing and a compression bandage. Alternatively, negative pressure wound therapy can be used over meshed BMWD to hold it in place. Dressings over the product should be changed every 2 to 3 days or more often if needed to manage exudate or to remoisten antimicrobial dressings. Any blood or fluid accumulation under the dressing should be gently aspirated or wicked away with a gauze pad (if a meshed product is not being used, the silicone layer should be incised). Generally, the matrix will be completely vascularized in about 3 weeks, as evidenced by blanching of the underlying tissue when gentle pressure is applied to the BMWD. At this point, the silicone can be removed and a thin autograft can be applied. Conversely, the underlying wound may completely heal within 3 to 4 weeks. As healing progresses, the silicone portion of the product will loosen and can be removed.

Integra Matrix Wound Dressing is the ECM matrix without the silicone covering and is used alone or with BMWD for deeper wounds. When used alone, the Integra Matrix Wound Dressing should be applied in a similar fashion as noted for the BMWD and covered with a nonadherent contact layer, followed by an antimicrobial dressing and a pressure dressing. Postapplication care is the same for both products.

Integra Flowable Wound Matrix has the same ingredients (minus the silicone layer) as the other Integra products; however, the ECM matrix is provided in a syringe as dry granules that are hydrated with saline before use. It has the same indications as BMWD, but its use focuses on application to wounds with deep tunnels or undermining. It is available for one-time use in a 3-cc syringe. It is injected directly into wounds with depth or undermining until the wound is filled and then is covered with a dressing of choice to hold the matrix in place and absorb exudate. Dressing change frequency is based on the amount of exudate. There are no published studies on Integra Flowable Wound Matrix in chronic wound care.

Synthetic Extracellular Matrix Scaffolds

Hyalomatrix PA is a bilayered product consisting of a thin moisture vapor–permeable silicone sheet adhered to a nonwoven pad composed entirely of the benzyl ester of hyaluronic acid (Hyaff-11). It does not contain any animal-derived products. When the Hyaff-11 contacts the wound bed, it provides a scaffold for cell attachment and migration, and the silicone backing maintains a moist wound bed and protects against bacterial contamination (Price et al, 2006). The Hyaff-11 degrades over time as host tissue infiltrates the matrix. Case series have been published on the use of Hyalomatrix PA in deep partial-thickness burns and diabetic foot ulcers (Caravaggi et al, 2009; Gravante et al, 2007). It is intended for one-time use and is indicated for the treatment of most chronic wounds, partial- and full-thickness burns, surgical wounds, and traumatic wounds. Hyalomatrix PA is widely used in Europe. It received 510K clearance by the FDA in 2007 and is now available in the United States.

BILAYERED CTPs

Living Cellular

Apligraf, a living, allogeneic, bilayered CTP, consists of keratinocytes and fibroblasts. Fibroblasts are cultured in a type 1 bovine collagen gel. Keratinocytes are then seeded on this gel, cultured, and air exposed to stimulate differentiation into the layers of the epidermis, including the stratum corneum. This process results in a 44-cm^2, 0.75-mm-thick skin substitute delivered fresh on a Petri dish containing nutrient medium and sealed in an airtight bag.

Apligraf, when used in conjunction with compression therapy, has been demonstrated to achieve closure of hard-to-heal venous ulcers at a significantly higher rate than seen with compression alone (Falanga and Sabolinski, 1999; Falanga et al, 1998). Apligraf is FDA approved for the treatment of venous ulcers of greater than 1 month's duration that have not adequately responded to standard care, including debridement, infection control, assurance of adequate arterial flow, and compression therapy. National guidelines support the use of bilayered skin substitutes in conjunction with compression bandaging to improve healing rates of venous ulcers (Robson et al, 2006).

Apligraf has also demonstrated efficacy in the treatment of diabetic foot ulcers. In a trial of 208 patients with diabetic neuropathic foot ulcers, Veves et al (2001) found that 56% of patients treated with Apligraf were healed at 12 weeks versus 38% in the control group, a statistically significant difference ($p = .0042$). Apligraf is FDA approved for the treatment of diabetic neuropathic foot ulcers of at least 3 weeks' duration that extend through the dermis without tendon, muscle, joint capsule, or bone exposure and that have not adequately responded to standard care, including debridement, infection control, glucose control, offloading, and assurance of adequate arterial flow.

Like Dermagraft, Apligraf is an adjunct to standard wound care. Apligraf is applied to the wound with the dermal side contacting the wound bed. Many clinicians fenestrate Apligraf with a scalpel before application to allow exudate to pass through it onto bandages because pooled exudate under the product may decrease its efficacy. Once applied, it may be anchored with Steri-strips, staples, or skin adhesive. Negative pressure wound therapy (NPWT) can also be used to not only stabilize the graft to the wound bed but also enhance the direct contact and adherence of these fragile grafts to the wound bed. Apligraf should be covered with a nonadherent contact layer and a secondary bandage of choice. Foam dressings work well over venous ulcers because they absorb exudate and apply local pressure under the compression wrap to keep the Apligraf in good contact with the wound bed. Secondary dressings are changed as needed based on the amount of exudate; the contact layer over the Apligraf can be replaced in 7 to 10 days, being careful to cleanse the surface without disrupting any attached retained Apligraf. Best practice algorithms guiding the use of Apligraft in the treatment of diabetic foot ulcers and venous leg ulcers have been published (Cavorsi, Vicari, Wirthlin, et al, 2006).

OrCel is a bilayered allogeneic product first developed by an Australian physician in the 1980s to treat his son, who suffered from epidermolysis bullosa. This bilayered cellular matrix is made of human dermal cells (containing neonatal foreskin–derived cultured keratinocytes and fibroblasts) cultured in bovine collagen sponge. Fresh and cryopreserved OrCel is FDA approved under a humanitarian device exemption (HDE) for the treatment of surgical wounds and donor sites in patients with epidermolysis bullosa undergoing reconstructive hand surgery. In a study of split-thickness autograft donor site treatment in burn patients, donor sites treated with OrCel healed an average of 7 days faster versus treatment with Biobrane-L ($p < .0006$) and were ready for recropping for more autografts an average of 5 days faster (Still et al, 2003). This has also been used in combination with split thickness autografts (Eisenberg and Llewelyn, 1998) (see Table 19-2).

Dermal and Bilayered Cellular- and Tissue-Based Products: Nonliving Cellular

Cadaveric human skin has been used for years as temporary wound coverage in burn care (Britton-Byrd et al, 2008; Kagan et al, 2005). This nonliving product facilitates the short-term coverage of large tissue defects when autografts are not yet available, leading to reduced loss of fluid, electrolytes, and protein; decreased risk of infection; decreased wound desiccation and pain; and improved success of later autografting. One disadvantage of using cadaveric skin is the possibility of disease transmission, despite donor screening regulations by the FDA and quality control

standards developed by the American Association of Tissue Banks (AATB) (Humphries and Mansavage, 2006). Another disadvantage is the fact that the host rejects cadaveric skin within 2 to 4 weeks. Cadaveric human skin is available fresh (used within 14 days of harvesting), cryopreserved (stored in a freezer for 3 to 6 months or in liquid nitrogen for up to 10 years), or irradiated (stored at room temperature).

GammaGraft is gamma-irradiated human cadaver skin that provides wound coverage for chronic wounds or burns. It can remain in place until the wound is healed, depending on wound size and depth of tissue damage. GammaGraft is placed on a clean, debrided wound that is free of infection and is covered with a nonadherent dressing for 1 to 2 days. At that time, the graft should be adherent to the wound base. If the graft is not adherent, the wound may be infected and the graft should be removed. If GammaGraft is adherent, it should be left uncovered; it will dry out and appear much like a scab. It is left in place while new host skin covers the wound underneath. As the wound heals, the edges of the GammaGraft will peel away and can be cut off. Treatment of the underlying problem, such as compression for edema or offloading for pressure redistribution, must be continued throughout the treatment period. GammaGraft may be used on any chronic wound. However, although there are case reports of GammaGraft use in chronic wounds (Rosales et al, 2004), no randomized controlled trials have demonstrated the efficacy of this product in wound healing compared with standard care.

FUTURE DIRECTIONS

Additional products for providing cell therapy in the treatment of chronic wounds are in development (Ehrenreich and Ruszczak, 2006; Hrabchak et al, 2006). Next-generation products may extend beyond the relative simplicity of providing keratinocytes and/or fibroblasts with their secreted growth factors and ECM proteins to a chronic wound. Melanocytes for repigmentation, endothelial cells for neovascularization, and stem cells for regeneration of tissue all may be included in future products. Genetically engineered cells may be used that express specific growth factors to stimulate a particular aspect of wound healing (e.g., neovascularization) identified to be deficient in an individual patient. "Smart" CTPs may be developed in which genetically engineered cells respond to the wound environment by secreting or restricting secretion of certain cytokines, depending on what the wound requires to progress through repair or, better yet, regeneration (Metcalfe and Ferguson, 2007). Cells can be engineered to secrete increased levels of natural bactericidal chemicals to decrease risk of infection (Schurr et al, 2009). As these products become available, clinicians must critically analyze data to ensure that the use of these products enhances healing while reducing complications compared with standard care.

CLINICAL CONSULT

A: Referral received for a 50-year-old female with diabetes who has an ulcer on the dorsal surface of her right foot. No foot deformities present. Ulcer has failed to close with serial debridements and robust topical management. Insensate foot; able to detect 2/9 points with monofilament testing. Toe-brachial index 0.8. Wound bed is clean, red, with healthy granulation tissue. Pressure points noted surrounding ulceration due to a poorly fitted shoe and last appointment with orthotic specialist was 8 months ago. HbA1c is 4.6 indicating good glycemic control. No pedal or lower leg edema.

D: Nonhealing foot ulcer due to repetitive stress in patient with diabetes. Level 1 LEAP risk category and high risk diabetes due to absence of sensation in foot. Circulation in foot adequate for healing.

P: Debride lightly and apply allogeneic dermal graft; secure and stabilize with a border adhesive foam nonadherent wound dressing. No shoe on foot for 12 weeks following graft.

I: (1) Procedure will be explained and consent obtained. (2) Will schedule for procedure in 3 days after PT has consulted to provide recommendations for appropriate off-loading Velcro closure boot and dietician has seen patient for assessment of protein and vitamin needs. (3) Will continue with current topical therapy until patient returns for graft.

E: Return to NixBry Wound clinic in 1 week for graft. Will follow weekly for dressing changes and to assess graft.

SUMMARY

The days of simply covering a wound with a moisture-retentive dressing and treating the underlying pathology are over for recalcitrant, nonresponsive wounds. When a wound does not improve with optimal care within 2 to 4 weeks of treatment, the use of adjunctive modalities such as CTPs should be considered for select wounds. The clinicians will need to be knowledgeable about the types of products available, how the product functions, the objective for the wound, the CTP application process, how the dressing is stabilized, and frequency of reapplication. In addition, the wound care clinician needs to understand the cellular components of the CTP and moral, ethical, and religious implications for the patient. Many of these products need more research to substantiate their effectiveness and efficacy. When used in conjunction with good care, these products may increase the probability of ultimate wound closure for recalcitrant chronic wounds, as well as acute wounds affecting large surface areas.

REFERENCES

Ågren MS, Werthén M: The extracellular matrix in wound healing: a closer look at therapeutics for chronic wounds, *Int J Low Extrem Wounds* 6:82–97, 2007.

Badylak SF: The extracellular matrix as a biologic scaffold material, *Biomaterials* 28:3587–3593, 2007.

Brigido SA: The use of an acellular dermal regenerative tissue matrix in the treatment of lower extremity wounds: a prospective 16-week pilot study, *Int Wound J* 3:181–187, 2006.

Brigido SA, Boc SF, Lopez RC: Effective management of major lower extremity wounds using an acellular regenerative tissue matrix: a pilot study, *Orthopedics* 27:s145–s149, 2004.

Britton-Byrd BW, Lynch JP, Williamson S, et al: Early use of allograft skin: are 3-day microbiologic cultures safe? *J Trauma* 64:816–818, 2008.

Caravaggi C, De Giglio R, Pritelli C, et al: Hyaff 11-based autologous dermal and epidermal grafts in the treatment of noninfected diabetic plantar and dorsal foot ulcers: a prospective, multicenter, controlled, randomized clinical trial, *Diabetes Care* 26:2853–2859, 2003.

Caravaggi C, Sganzaroli AB, Pogliaghi I, et al: Safety and efficacy of a dermal substitute in the coverage of cancellous bone after surgical debridement for severe diabetic foot ulceration, *EWMA J* 9:19–22, 2009.

Catalano E, Cochis A, Varoni E, et al: Tissue-engineered skin substitutes: an overview, *J Artif Organs* 16:397–403, 2013.

Cavorsi J, Vicari F, Wirthlin DJ, et al: Best-practice algorithms for the use of a bilayered living cell therapy (Apligraf) in the treatment of lower-extremity ulcers, *Wound Repair Regen* 14:102–109, 2006.

Clark RA, Ghosh K, Tonnesen MG, et al: Tissue engineering for cutaneous wounds, *J Invest Dermatol* 127:1018–1029, 2007.

Cook Biotech: *Cook Biotech reference page,* 2014 http://www.cook-biotech.com/technology.php. Accessed May 9, 2010.

Davis DA, Arpey CJ: Porcine heterografts in dermatologic surgery and reconstruction, *Dermatol Surg* 26:76–80, 2000.

Ehrenreich M, Ruszczak Z: Update on tissue-engineered biological dressings, *Tissue Eng* 12:2407–2424, 2006.

Eisenberg M, Llewelyn D: Surgical management of hands in children with recessive dystrophic epidermolysis bullosa: use of allogeneic composite cultured skin grafts, *Br J Plast Surg* 51:608–613, 1998.

Falanga V, Margolis D, Alvarez O, et al: Rapid healing of venous ulcers and lack of clinical rejection with an allogeneic cultured human skin equivalent, *Arch Dermatol* 134:293–300, 1998.

Falanga V, Sabolinski M: A bilayered living skin construct (Apligraf) accelerates complete closure of hard-to-heal venous ulcers, *Wound Repair Regen* 7:201–207, 1999.

Gilbert TW, Nieponice A, Spievack AR, et al: Repair of the thoracic wall with an extracellular matrix scaffold in a canine model, *J Surg Res* 147:61–67, 2008.

Gravante G, Delogu D, Giordan N, et al: The use of Hyalomatrix PA in the treatment of deep partial-thickness burns, *J Burn Care Res* 28:269–274, 2007.

Greaves N, Iqbal SA, Baguneid M, et al: The role of skin substitutes in the management of chronic cutaneous wounds, *Wound Repair Regen* 21:194–210, 2013.

Griffiths M, Ojeh N, Livingstone R, et al: Survival of Apligraf in acute human wounds, *Tissue Eng* 10:1180–1195, 2004.

Hashimoto K: Regulation of keratinocyte function by growth factors, *J Dermatol Sci* 24:S46–S50, 2000.

Hodde JP, Ernst DM, Hiles MC: An investigation of the long-term bioactivity of endogenous growth factor in OASIS Wound Matrix, *J Wound Care* 14:23–25, 2005.

Hrabchak C, Flynn L, Woodhouse KA: Biological skin substitutes for wound cover and closure, *Expert Rev Med Devices* 3:373–385, 2006.

Humphries LK, Mansavage VL: Quality control in tissue banking-ensuring the safety of allograft tissues, *AORN J* 84:385–398, 2006.

Jang JC, Choi RJ, Han SK, et al: Effect of fibroblast-seeded artificial dermis on wound healing, *Ann Plast Surg*, 74(4):501–507, 2015.

Kagan RJ, Robb EC, Plessinger RT: Human skin banking, *Clin Lab Med* 25:587–605, 2005.

Kahn S, Beers RJ, Lentz CW: Use of acellular dermal replacement in reconstruction of nonhealing lower extremity wounds, *J Burn Care Res* 32(1):124–128, 2011.

Kamolz LP, Lumenta DB, Kitzinger HB, et al: Tissue engineering for cutaneous wounds: an overview of current standards and possibilities, *Eur Surg* 40:19–26, 2008.

Kulkarni M, O'Loughlin A, Vazquez R, et al: Use of a fibrin-based system for enhancing angiogenesis and modulating inflammation in the treatment of hyperglycemic wounds, *Biomaterials* 35:2001–2010, 2014.

Límová M: Active wound coverings: bioengineered skin and dermal substitutes, *Surg Clin North Am* 90:1237–1255, 2010.

Mandal A: Paediatric partial-thickness scald burns—is Biobrane the best treatment available? *Int Wound J* 4:15–19, 2007.

Marston WA, Hanft J, Norwood P, et al: The efficacy and safety of Dermagraft in improving the healing of chronic diabetic foot ulcers: results of a prospective randomized trial, *Diabetes Care* 26:1701–1705, 2003.

Metcalfe AD, Ferguson MWJ: Tissue engineering of replacement skin: the crossroads of biomaterials, wound healing, embryonic development, stem cells and regeneration, *J R Soc Interface* 4:413–437, 2007.

Mostow EN, Haraway GD, Dalsing M, et al: Effectiveness of an extracellular matrix graft (OASIS Wound Matrix) in the treatment of chronic leg ulcers: a randomized clinical trial, *J Vasc Surg* 41:837–843, 2005.

Mulder G, Lee D: Case presentation: xenograft resistance to protease degradation in a vasculitic ulcer, *Int J Low Extrem Wounds* 8:157–161, 2009a.

Mulder G, Lee D: A retrospective clinical review of extracellular matrices for tissue reconstruction: equine pericardium as a biological covering to assist with wound closure, *Wounds* 21:254–261, 2009b.

Mulder G, Lee D: Use of equine derived pericardium as a biological cover to promote closure of a complicated wound with associated scleroderma and Raynaud's disease, *Wounds* 21:297–301, 2009c.

Nieponice A, Gilbert TW, Badylak SF: Reinforcement of esophageal anastomoses with an extracellular matrix scaffold in a canine model, *Ann Thorac Surg* 82:2050–2058, 2006.

Price RD, Das-Gupta V, Leigh IM, et al: A comparison of tissue-engineered hyaluronic acid dermal matrices in a human wound model, *Tissue Eng* 12:2985–2995, 2006.

Reyzelman A, Crews RT, Moore JC, et al: Clinical effectiveness of a acellular dermal regenerative tissue matrix compared to standard wound management in healing diabetic foot ulcers: a prospective, randomized multicentre study, *Int Wound J* 6:196–208, 2009.

Roberts C, Mansbridge J: The scientific basis and differentiating features of Dermagraft, *Can J Plast Surg* 10(Suppl A):6A–13A, 2002.

Robson MC, Cooper DM, Aslam R, et al: Guidelines for the treatment of venous ulcers, *Wound Repair Regen* 14:649–662, 2006.

Rosales MA, Bruntz M, Armstrong DG: Gamma-irradiated human skin allograft: a potential treatment modality for lower extremity ulcers, *Int Wound J* 1:201–206, 2004.

Ryssel H, Gazyakan E, Germann G, et al: The use of MatriDerm in early excision and simultaneous autologous skin grafting in burns—a pilot study, *Burns* 34:93–97, 2008.

Ryssel H, Germann G, Czermak C, et al: Matriderm® in depth-adjusted reconstruction of necrotising fasciitis defects, *Burns* 36(7):1107–1111, 2010.

Schaum KD: More 2014 code changes and medicare payment changes for wound care providers, *Adv Skin Wound Care* 27(3):108–110, 2014.

Schurr MJ, Foster KN, Centanni JM, et al: Phase I/II clinical evaluation of StrataGraft: a consistent pathogen-free human skin substitute, *J Trauma* 66:866–874, 2009.

Shevchenko R, James SL, James SE: A review of tissue-engineered skin bioconstructs available for skin reconstruction, *J R Soc Interface* 7:229–258, 2009.

Shores JT, Gabriel A, Gupta S: Skin substitutes and alternatives: a review, *Adv Skin Wound Care* 20:493–508, 2007.

Steed DL, Attinger C, Colaizzi T, et al: Guidelines for the treatment of diabetic ulcers, *Wound Repair Regen* 14:680–692, 2006.

Still J, Glat P, Silverstein P, et al: The use of a collagen sponge/living cell composite material to treat donor sites in burn patients, *Burns* 29:837–841, 2003.

van Winterswijk PJ, Nout E: Tissue engineering and wound healing: an overview of the past, present, and future, *Wounds* 19:277–284, 2007.

Veves A, Falanga V, Armstrong DG, et al: Graftskin, a human skin equivalent, is effective in the management of noninfected neuropathic diabetic foot ulcers: a prospective randomized multicenter clinical trial, *Diabetes Care* 24:290–295, 2001.

Whitaker IS, Prowse S, Potokar TS: A critical evaluation of the use of Biobrane as a biologic skin substitute: a versatile tool for the plastic and reconstructive surgeon, *Ann Plast Surg* 60:333–337, 2008.

Woodley DT, Peterson HD, Herzog SR, et al: Burn wounds resurfaced by cultured epidermal autografts show abnormal reconstitution of anchoring fibrils, *JAMA* 259:2566–2571, 1998.

20

Molecular and Cellular Regulators

Gregory Schultz, Priscilla L. Phillips, and Daniel J. Gibson

OBJECTIVES

1. Describe the importance of adhesion and migration of leukocytes in inflammation.
2. Distinguish between growth factors and cytokines.
3. Identify important processes in wound healing that are regulated by growth factors, cytokines, proteases, or hormones.
4. Describe the molecular environment that growth factors need to promote wound healing.
5. For each growth factor family, list one member, a key target cell, one main action, and one therapeutic use.
6. Describe the molecular differences between acute, healing wounds and chronic, nonhealing wounds.
7. Review two key updated points for wound bed preparation, biofilms, and point-of-care diagnostics and their application for the removal of barriers to wound healing.

At the cellular level, the complex process of the healing of skin wounds involves platelets, leukocytes, epidermal cells, fibroblasts, and vascular endothelial cells. At the molecular level, many growth factors, cytokines, proteases, and hormones regulate most of the key actions of cells during wound healing, such as the directed movement of cells into a wound (chemotactic migration), replacement of damaged epidermal and dermal cells (mitosis), growth of new blood vessels (neovascularization), formation of scar tissue (synthesis of extracellular matrix proteins), and remodeling of scar tissue (proteolytic turnover of extracellular matrix proteins) (Bennett and Schultz, 1993a, 1993b). Any condition that disrupts the normal actions of these molecular regulators in wounds will directly disrupt healing and promote the establishment and maintenance of chronic wounds (Mast and Schultz, 1996; Tarnuzzer and Schultz, 1996). By identifying abnormalities in the actions of molecular regulators in chronic wounds, therapies can be designed that will reestablish an environment that permits molecular regulators to function normally and achieve healing.

BIOLOGIC ROLES OF CYTOKINES AND GROWTH FACTORS

Growth factors are polypeptide proteins produced by the body to regulate proliferation, migration, and differentiation of target cells (e.g., expression of specialized genes) by binding to receptors on the cell surface. Specifically, proliferation and differentiation of non–immune system cells are regulated primarily by growth factors. In contrast, cytokines are protein molecules that primarily regulate the interactions between cells that participate in the immune response (Frenette and Wagner, 1996a, 1996b; Springer, 1990).

Cytokines are a unique family of growth factors that are small signaling proteins that mediate and regulate immunity, inflammation, and hematopoiesis. Produced in response to an immune stimulus, cytokines are secreted primarily from leukocytes, although other wound cells can also secrete cytokines. Cytokines function at very low concentration and act over short distances. After the cytokines bind to specific membrane receptors, secondary messengers are triggered that signal the cell to alter its behavior by increasing or decreasing membrane proteins, proliferation, and secretion of molecules. The same cytokine may be secreted by different types of cells, and the same cytokine may act on several different cell types.

General Phases of Wound Healing

The four phases of acute wound healing are hemostasis, inflammation, repair, and remodeling. There is considerable temporal overlap of these phases of healing, and the entire process lasts for several months. Immediately after injury, the process of blood clotting is initiated by activation of a proteolytic cascade, which ultimately converts fibrinogen into fibrin. As the fibrin molecules self-associate into a weblike net, red blood cells (RBCs) and platelets become entrapped. The aggregate of fibrin, RBCs, and platelets quickly grows large enough to form a stable clot that acts as a tamponade to physically block an injured capillary and stop the flow of blood.

The process of blood clotting also induces platelet degranulation, which releases a burst of preformed growth factors stored in platelet granules. These include platelet-derived growth factor (PDGF), transforming growth factor-β (TGF-β), epidermal growth factor (EGF), and insulinlike growth factor-1 (IGF-1). These growth factors initiate two major processes: inflammation and tissue repair. The growth factors released from platelets quickly diffuse from the wound into the surrounding tissues and attract leukocytes into the injured area (Bennett and Schultz, 1993a, 1993b).

Adhesion Molecules and Adhesion Receptors in Inflammation

The chemotactic attraction of leukocytes to a wound and the movement of leukocytes from the blood into wounded tissue (extravasation) involve expression and activation of adhesion molecules and adhesion receptors on leukocytes, platelets, and vascular endothelial cells. Cytokines and growth factors play key roles in these processes (Arai et al, 1990; Frenette and Wagner, 1996a, 1996b; Springer, 1990). Among the many types of adhesion molecules and receptors on the cell surface, four major families of transmembrane proteins stand out in the process of inflammation: integrins, selectins, cell adhesion molecules, and cadherins (Figure 20-1).

Integrins are glycoproteins composed of two different types of subunits, designated α and β. In simple terms, integrins are cellular receptors for extracellular matrix proteins, as shown with $\alpha_5\beta_1$, which is a receptor for fibronectin. A short amino acid sequence, such as arginine-glycine-aspartate (RGD), is often the site of recognition by the integrin receptor. Integrins are important because they are capable of generating signals inside cells when the integrin receptor binds to a specific extracellular matrix protein, in much the same way the insulin receptor generates intracellular signals, which regulate glucose transport into a cell when insulin binds to its cellular receptor. Expression of β_2 integrins is limited to leukocytes, whereas β_1 integrins are expressed on most cell types. β_1 integrins primarily bind to extracellular matrix components such as fibronectin, laminin, and collagens. (These substances are discussed in more detail in Chapter 4.)

Selectins are proteins that have a unique structure called a *lectin domain* at the distal end, which can bind specific carbohydrate groups of glycoproteins or mucins on adjacent cells. Thus, unlike other adhesion proteins, which recognize specific protein structures, selectins recognize and bind to carbohydrate ligands on leukocytes and vascular endothelial cells. E-selectin appears on endothelial cells after they have been activated by inflammatory cytokines, and P-selectin is stored in the α-granules of platelets and

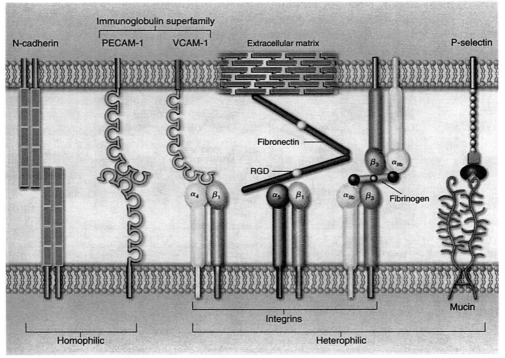

FIGURE 20-1 Four major classes of adhesion proteins and adhesion receptors embedded in a theoretic plasma membrane: integrins, selectins, cell adhesion molecules (platelet-endothelial cell adhesion molecule [PECAM-1] and vascular cell adhesion molecule VCAM-1]), and cadherins. (From Frenette PS, Wagner DD: Adhesion molecules. Part I, *N Engl J Med* 334:1526, 1996.)

the storage granules of endothelial cells (Weibel-Palade bodies).

Cell adhesion molecules (CAMs) are members of the immunoglobulin superfamily of proteins. Cell adhesion molecules can bind to other CAMs or to integrins on cells. Cell adhesion molecules that are important in inflammation include the platelet-endothelial cell adhesion molecule (PECAM), vascular cell adhesion molecule (VCAM), and intercellular adhesion molecule-1 (ICAM-1).

Cadherins are important in establishing molecular links between adjacent cells, especially during embryonic development. They form zipper-like structures of dimers at specialized regions of contact between neighboring cells called *adherens junctions.* Cadherins are linked to the cytoskeleton through molecules called *catenins,* which associate with actin microfilaments.

During the process of extravasation of inflammatory cells into a wound, important interactions occur between blood vessels and blood cells (Arai et al, 1990; Frenette and Wagner, 1996a, 1996b; Springer, 1990). Initially, circulating leukocytes begin rolling on endothelial cells through the binding of glycoproteins expressed on their cell surface to selectins, transiently expressed by activated endothelial cells of venules (Figure 20-2). The binding affinity of selectins is relatively low, but is enough to serve as a biologic brake, making leukocytes quickly decelerate by rolling on endothelial cells. While rolling, leukocytes can become activated by chemoattractants (cytokines, growth factors, or bacterial products). After activation, leukocytes firmly adhere to endothelial cells as a result of the binding between their β_2 class of integrins and ligands, such as VCAM and ICAM expressed on activated endothelial cells. Chemotactic signals present outside the venule induce leukocytes to squeeze between endothelial cells of the venule and migrate into the inflammatory center by using their β_1 class of integrins to recognize and bind to extracellular matrix components.

Adhesion and degranulation of platelets at sites of vascular injury also use a system of adhesion molecules and adhesion receptor proteins. Vascular injury immediately induces endothelial cells to release the contents of their storage granules (Weibel-Palade bodies), including the proteins P-selectin and von Willebrand factor. P-selectin promptly moves to the plasma membrane of endothelial cells, where it induces rolling of platelets on endothelial cells, and von Willebrand factor is quickly deposited on the exposed extracellular matrix, where it plays a crucial role in the adhesion of platelets to the damaged site.

Inflammatory Cell Proteases

When the inflammatory cascade is activated, neutrophils enter the wound initially, followed by macrophages. Neutrophils and macrophages become activated and engulf and destroy bacteria through their production of reactive oxygen species (super oxide anion, oxygen free radicals, or hydrogen peroxide). Activated neutrophils and macrophages also release several proteases, including neutrophil elastase (a serine type of protease), neutrophil collagenase (a matrix metalloproteinase [MMP] type of protease designated MMP-8), and

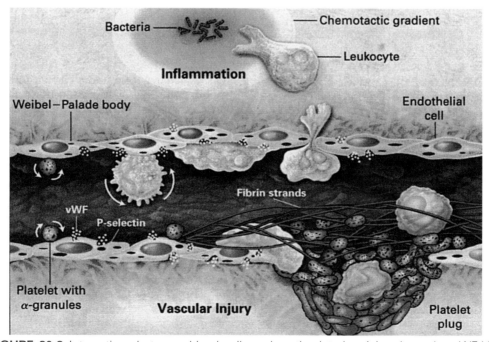

FIGURE 20-2 Interactions between blood cells and a stimulated or injured venule. *vWF,* Von Willebrand factor. (From Frenette PS, Wagner DD: Adhesion molecules. Part II: Blood vessels and blood cells, *N Engl J Med* 335:43, 1996.)

macrophage metalloelastase (MMP-12). These proteases play important, beneficial roles in initiating normal wound healing by removing proteolytically degrading, damaged extracellular matrix components, which must be replaced by new, intact extracellular matrix molecules for wound healing to proceed. These proteases also are important for enabling inflammatory cells to move through the basement membrane that surrounds capillaries.

Inflammatory Cell Cytokines and Growth Factors in Proliferation and Repair

The growth factors released by platelets diffuse away from a wound within a few hours, but they are replaced by growth factors and cytokines that are produced by neutrophils, macrophages, activated fibroblasts, vascular endothelial cells, and epidermal cells that are drawn into the wound area. For example, activated macrophages secrete several important cytokines, including tumor necrosis factor-α (TNF-α) and interleukin-1β (IL-1β), which have a variety of actions on different cells. TNF-α and IL-1β are potent inflammatory cytokines, which further stimulate inflammation. Tumor necrosis factor-α also induces macrophages to produce IL-1β, which is mitogenic for fibroblasts and upregulates expression of MMPs. Both TNF-α and IL-1β directly influence deposition of collagen in the wound by inducing synthesis of collagen by fibroblasts and by upregulating expression of MMPs. In addition, these cytokines down-regulate expression of the tissue inhibitors of metalloproteinases (TIMPs), which are the natural inhibitors of MMPs. Interferon-γ (IFN-γ), produced by lymphocytes attracted into the wound, inhibits fibroblast migration and down-regulates collagen synthesis (Table 20-1).

Inflammatory cells secrete other growth factors, including TGF-β, TGF-α, heparin-binding epidermal growth factor (HB-EGF), and basic fibroblast growth factor (bFGF). The growth factors secreted by macrophages continue to stimulate migration of fibroblasts, epithelial cells, and vascular endothelial cells into the wound. As the fibroblasts, epithelial cells, and vascular endothelial cells migrate into the site of injury, they begin to proliferate, and the cellularity of the wound increases. This begins the proliferative and repair phase, which often lasts several weeks. If the wound is not

TABLE 20-1 Growth Factor Families

Growth Factor Family	Cell Source	Actions	Relevant Research
Transforming growth factor-β (TGF-β₁, TGF-β₂, TGF-β₃)	Platelets Fibroblasts Macrophages	Fibroblast chemotaxis and activation ECM deposition Collagen synthesis TIMP synthesis MMP synthesis Reduces scarring Collagen synthesis Fibronectin synthesis	Chronic skin ulcers (Robson et al, 1995)
Platelet-derived growth factor (PDGF-AA, PDGF-BB, vascular endothelial growth factor)	Platelets Macrophages Keratinocytes Fibroblasts	Activation of immune cells and fibroblasts ECM deposition Collagen synthesis TIMP synthesis MMP synthesis Angiogenesis	Pressure ulcers (Robson et al, 1992b) Diabetic ulcers (Steed, Diabetic Ulcer Study Group, 1995)
Fibroblast growth factor (acidic FGF, basic FGF, keratinocyte growth factor)	Macrophages Endothelial cells Fibroblasts	Angiogenesis Endothelial cell activation Keratinocyte proliferation and migration ECM deposition	Pressure ulcers (Robson et al, 1992a) Second-degree burns (Fu et al, 1998)
Insulinlike growth factor (IGF-1, IGF-2, insulin)	Liver Skeletal muscle Fibroblasts Macrophages Neutrophils	Keratinocyte proliferation Fibroblast proliferation Endothelial cell activation Angiogenesis Collagen synthesis ECM deposition Cell metabolism	No published reports evaluating IGF-1 for treatment of wounds
Epidermal growth factor (EGF, heparin-binding epidermal growth factor, transforming growth factor-α, amphiregulin, betacellulin)	Keratinocytes Macrophages	Keratinocyte proliferation and migration ECM deposition	Burns, donor sites (Brown et al, 1986, 1989) Venous ulcers (Falanga et al, 1992)
Connective tissue growth factor (CTGF)	Fibroblasts Endothelial cells Epithelial cells	Mediates action of TGF-βs on collagen synthesis	No published reports evaluating CTGF for treatment of wounds

ECM, Extracellular matrix; *MMP*, matrix metalloproteinase; *TIMP*, tissue inhibitor of metalloproteinase.

infected, the number of inflammatory cells in a wound begins to decrease after a few days. Other types of cells, such as fibroblasts, endothelial cells, and keratinocytes, are drawn into the wound and begin to synthesize growth factors. Fibroblasts secrete IGF-1, bFGF, TGF-β, PDGF, and keratinocyte growth factor (KGF). Endothelial cells produce vascular endothelial growth factor (VEGF), bFGF, and PDGF. Keratinocytes synthesize TGF-α, TGF-β, and IL-1β. These growth factors continue to stimulate cell proliferation and synthesis of extracellular matrix proteins and to promote formation of new capillaries.

Remodeling Phase

After the initial scar forms, proliferation and neovascularization cease and the wound enters the remodeling phase, which can last for many months. During this last phase, a new balance is reached between the synthesis of extracellular matrix components in the scar and their degradation by metalloproteinases such as collagenase, gelatinase, and stromelysin. Fibroblasts synthesize a majority of the collagen, elastin, and proteoglycans that compose the dermal scar matrix. Fibroblasts also are a major source of the MMPs that degrade the scar matrix, as well as their inhibitors, the TIMPs. They also secrete lysyl oxidase, an enzyme that covalently cross-links components of the extracellular matrix, such as collagen and elastin molecules, producing a stable extracellular matrix. Keratinocytes secrete much of the type IV collagen that re-forms the basement membrane, which separates the epidermal and dermal layers and forms the surface on which keratinocytes prefer to migrate. Angiogenesis ceases and the density of capillaries decreases in the wound site as a result of programmed cell death (apoptosis) of the vascular endothelial cells. Eventually, remodeling of the scar tissue reaches equilibrium, although the mature scar is never as strong as uninjured skin.

CYTOKINES

Cytokines are produced extensively by activated T cells and macrophages, although non–immune system cells such as keratinocytes and vascular endothelial cells also produce some cytokines. Studies have revealed that cytokines generally induce multiple biologic activities (pleiotropic) and that a single cytokine can act as both a positive signal and a negative signal, depending on the type of the target cell. Cytokines such as IL-1, IL-2, IL-3, IL-4, IL-5, IL-6, and IL-10; granulocyte-macrophage colony-stimulating factor (GM-CSF); granulocyte colony-stimulating factor (G-CSF); IFN-γ; and TNF-α are key mediators of immune and inflammatory responses. A cytokine is also referred to as a *lymphokine* (cytokine made by lymphocytes), *monokine* (cytokine made by monocytes), *chemokine* (cytokine with chemotactic action), and *interleukin* (cytokines made by one leukocyte and acting on other leukocytes). Two cytokines in particular, TNF-α and IL-1β, have activities that substantially influence skin wound healing through their ability to increase production of MMPs and suppress production of TIMPs. Table 20-2 lists the cytokines involved in wound healing, along with cell source, biologic activity, and their subclassification as proinflammatory or antiinflammatory.

Cytokines have not been investigated extensively in human wound-healing studies. Interleukin-1β was evaluated in a prospective, randomized, double-blind, placebo-controlled trial performed on 26 patients with Stage III and IV pressure ulcers (Robson et al, 1994). No statistically

TABLE 20-2 Cytokines Involved in Wound Healing

Cytokine	Cell Source	Biologic Activity
Proinflammatory Cytokines		
TNF-α	Macrophages	PMN margination and cytotoxicity; collagen synthesis; provides metabolic substrate
IL-1	Macrophages Keratinocytes	Fibroblast and keratinocyte chemotaxis; collagen synthesis
IL-2	T lymphocytes	Increases fibroblast infiltration and metabolism
IL-6	Macrophages PMNs Fibroblasts	Fibroblast proliferation; hepatic acute-phase protein synthesis
IL-8	Macrophages Fibroblasts	Macrophage and PMN chemotaxis; keratinocyte maturation
IFN-γ	T lymphocytes Macrophages	Macrophage and PMN activation; retards collagen synthesis and cross-linking; stimulates collagenase activity
Antiinflammatory Cytokines		
IL-4	T lymphocytes Basophils Mast cells	Inhibition of TNF, IL-1, IL-6 production; fibroblast proliferation; collagen synthesis
IL-10	T lymphocytes Macrophages Keratinocytes	Inhibition of TNF, IL-1, IL-6 production; inhibits macrophage and PMN activation

IFN, Interferon; *IL,* interleukin; *PMN,* polymorphonuclear leukocyte; *TNF,* tumor necrosis factor.

significant differences were seen in the percentage decrease of wound volumes between the treatment groups.

GROWTH FACTORS

Discovery, Purification, and Cloning of Growth Factors

Protein growth factors were discovered as a consequence of their ability to stimulate multiple cycles of cell growth (mitosis) when added to cultures of normal, quiescent cells. This process distinguishes growth factors from essential nutrients such as vitamins, cofactors, and trace minerals (e.g., selenium), which are required for metabolic processes but are not sufficient to initiate cell division by themselves. Both nutrients and growth factors are necessary for mitosis, but only growth factors can initiate mitosis of quiescent cells.

Based on the ability of growth factors to stimulate continuous mitosis of cells in culture, it is not surprising that many growth factors initially were isolated from medium conditioned by tumor cells. Other sources of growth factors included platelets, macrophages, and normal tissues that can proliferate rapidly, such as ovarian follicles and placenta. Although growth factors were present in minute quantities from these natural sources, tiny amounts eventually were purified using traditional biochemical methods. The amino acid sequences of the proteins were determined, which permitted cloning and sequencing of the growth factor genes. With the development of recombinant DNA technology, large amounts of synthetic human growth factors were produced from cultures of bacteria, yeast, or human cells that carried the gene for the growth factor. The availability of large amounts of the synthetic growth factors enabled research that led to a better understanding of the biologic roles of growth factors in wound healing and other physiologic processes, such as fetal development, aging, and cancer. Ultimately, this led to experiments that evaluated the effects of synthetic growth factors in animal wound-healing models and eventually to clinical trials in patients.

Autocrine and Paracrine Action of Growth Factors

Growth factors are synthesized and secreted by many types of cells involved in wound healing, including platelets, inflammatory cells, fibroblasts, epithelial cells, and vascular endothelial cells. Moreover, growth factors usually act either on the producer cell (autocrine stimulation) or on adjacent cells (paracrine stimulation). In contrast to classic endocrine hormones, growth factors generally do not enter the bloodstream and act on cells at a great distance (Figure 20-3) (Barrientos et al, 2008).

Receptors

All peptide growth factors initiate their effects on target cells by binding to specific, high-affinity receptor proteins located in the plasma membrane of target cells (Fantl et al, 1993). Only cells that express the specific receptor protein can

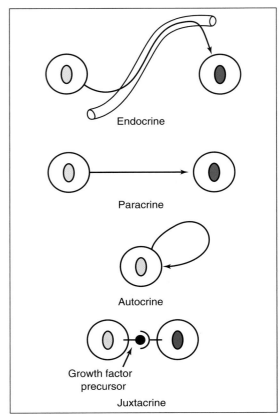

FIGURE 20-3 Growth factor action. Secreted growth factors act predominately by an autocrine (self-stimulation) or a paracrine (adjacent cells) pathway and usually not by classic endocrine pathways. Membrane-bound growth factors may also interact with adjacent cells by juxtacrine stimulation. (From Bennett NT, Schultz GS: Growth factors and wound healing: biochemical properties of growth factors and their receptors, *Am J Surg* 165:728, 1993.)

respond to the growth factor. Binding of the growth factor to its receptor activates a region of the receptor protein called a *kinase domain*, which is located inside the cell (Figure 20-4). Kinase domains have the enzymatic ability to covalently transfer a phosphate group from the high-energy adenosine triphosphate (ATP) molecule to an amino acid, such as tyrosine, serine, or threonine, in a protein. The activated receptor protein is the "first messenger" in the response system of a cell to a growth factor.

The activated receptor kinase domain then phosphorylates amino acids on a small number of specific cytoplasmic proteins. These cytoplasmic proteins become activated when phosphorylated and are the first in a series of "second messenger" proteins that eventually generate a response in the cell to the growth factor. Second messenger proteins also typically contain kinase domains that are activated when the proteins are phosphorylated. The activated cytoplasmic kinase proteins in turn phosphorylate other cytoplasmic proteins in a sequential cascade of phosphorylations and activations that eventually leads to activation of special proteins

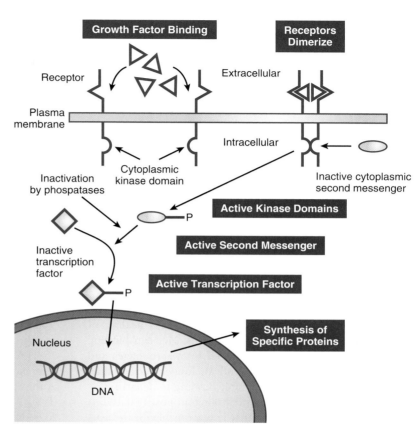

FIGURE 20-4 Growth factor receptor signal generation. Growth factors typically affect cells by binding to specific, high-affinity receptor proteins located in the plasma membrane of target cells, which then dimerize and activate tyrosine or serine/threonine kinase domains located in the cytoplasmic region of the receptor. The activated receptor then phosphorylates second messenger proteins, which frequently also are kinases that participate in a cascade of phosphorylation/activation steps that ultimately activate an RNA transcription factor, which selectively initiates synthesis of proteins that alter the behavior of the target cell. The second messenger system is turned off by enzymes called phosphatases that remove phosphate groups from proteins.

called *RNA transcription factors*. Activated RNA transcription factors bind with selected regions of the DNA to help initiate transcription of genes into messenger RNAs (mRNAs), which are translated into proteins that ultimately alter the functions of the target cell.

Another system of cytoplasmic proteins acts to turn off the transcription of genes that are turned on by growth factors. These proteins are called *phosphatases*. They remove the phosphate groups that were added to the amino acids of the second messenger kinase proteins and to the RNA transcription factors. Removal of the phosphate groups inactivates the second messenger proteins and the transcription factors. Thus the effects of growth factors on target cells require an integrated balance among receptor proteins, second messenger kinase proteins, RNA transcription factors, and phosphatases.

MAJOR FAMILIES OF GROWTH FACTORS

The first attempt to use growth factors to promote healing of human wounds was based on the concept that platelets contained numerous growth factors that were released at the time of injury. Furthermore, substantial amounts of activated platelet supernatant could be obtained from individual patients with chronic skin ulcers or from apheresis donors. This would permit patients to be treated with their own activated platelet supernatant or from carefully screened platelet

donors. To test this concept, a U.S. Food and Drug Administration (FDA)–approved, randomized, controlled, multicenter, dose-response trial of topically applied activated platelet supernatant in 97 patients with a chronic, nonhealing diabetic wound was conducted (David et al, 1992; Holloway et al, 1993).

The use of placebo treatment, combined with good basic wound care, reduced wound area 77% and reduced wound volume 83% from baseline to final visit, although only 29% of the placebo group healed completely compared with 63% of the patients treated with platelet releasate. All healing parameters were significantly improved in the patients who were treated with all doses of platelet releasate. These results demonstrated the benefit of treatment of chronic diabetic wounds with a mixture of growth factors and proteins released from platelets. Table 20-1 presents an overview of the major families of growth factors, including those growth factors that have been shown to play roles in wound healing in animals or humans (not all known growth factors are included).

Epidermal Growth Factor Family

Epidermal growth factor was the first growth factor to be purified and biochemically characterized (Carpenter and Cohen, 1990). Other members of the EGF family that influence wound healing are TGF-α (Massague, 1990) and HB-EGF (Higashiyama et al, 1992). Members of the EGF family are small single-chain proteins that bind to a common receptor protein (EGF receptor) that has tyrosine kinase activity and is expressed on almost all types of cells. Members of the EGF family have similar, but not identical, biologic effects on target cells. They are chemoattractants and mitogens for epidermal cells, fibroblasts, and vascular endothelial cells, but are most effective for epidermal cells.

Epidermal growth factor and TGF-α are synthesized as membrane-bound precursors that are released by proteolysis in a wide range of cells, including cells of the lacrimal and salivary glands. Epidermal growth factor and TGF-α are present in saliva and tears, and data from many different types of experiments strongly suggest that EGF and TGF-α play important roles in both the normal turnover of epithelial cells of the gut and cornea and in the healing of wounds in these tissues. Specifically, in the skin, epidermal cells synthesize large amounts of TGF-α. Mice that lack TGF-α or EGF receptors have abnormal hair and skin architecture. Levels of EGF receptor are elevated in the leading edge of epidermal cells in burn wounds (Nanney and King, 1996). Specific inhibition of the EGF receptor delays healing of partial-thickness skin injuries in animals. Heparin-binding epidermal growth factor is produced by macrophages and presumably is retained in a wound for longer periods than EGF or TGF-α because of reversible binding to heparin.

Current models of skin wound healing propose that TGF-α is the growth factor that is primarily responsible for the normal maintenance and turnover of epidermal cells of the skin. When a skin injury occurs, epidermal cell proliferation and migration are stimulated by TGF-α produced by epidermal cells; EGF produced by epithelial cells lining the hair follicles, sweat glands, and sebaceous glands; and HB-EGF produced by macrophages that enter the wound. In addition, fibroblasts surrounding the wound secrete KGF, a member of the fibroblast growth factor system, which exclusively promotes migration and mitosis of keratinocytes.

Injections of recombinant human EGF into the dermal tissue at the edge of chronic diabetic foot ulcers promoted healing and reduced amputations compared with standard care of wet-to-dry gauze dressings (Acosta et al, 2006).

Platelet-Derived Growth Factor Family

The PDGF family comprises two major proteins, PDGF and VEGF, which influence wound healing (Heldin and Westermark, 1996). Platelet-derived growth factor and VEGF share about 25% of the amino acid sequence homology, and both are composed of two subunits that are covalently linked by disulfide bonds. Platelet-derived growth factor has two different subunits (designated types A and B). Human platelets contain high levels of PDGF, and many types of human cells important in skin wound healing can secrete PDGF, including fibroblasts, vascular smooth muscle cells, and vascular endothelial cells.

Platelet-derived growth factor and VEGF bind to different receptor proteins (both are tyrosine kinases) and stimulate different biologic actions. Two distinct PDGF receptors have been characterized. The PDGF-α receptor recognizes both α and β subunits of PDGF, whereas the PDGF-β receptor only recognizes the β subunit of PDGF.

Platelet-derived growth factor is a chemoattractant and mitogen primarily for fibroblasts, whereas VEGF is a chemoattractant and mitogen primarily for vascular endothelial cells. Vascular endothelial growth factor is one of the most effective angiogenic factors yet discovered, and synthesis of VEGF by vascular endothelial cells is increased by hypoxia.

Transforming Growth Factor-β Family

The TGF-β family of proteins is the newest family to be discovered (Roberts and Sporn, 1996). Three distinct TGF-βs have been identified in humans: TGF-β₁, TGF-β₂, and TGF-β₃. All three are synthesized as inactive proteins that must be activated by proteolytic removal of a segment of the proteins. The TGF-βs are synthesized by a variety of cell types, including platelets, macrophages, lymphocytes, fibroblasts, bone cells, and keratinocytes, and nearly all nucleated cells have TGF-β receptors. Thus TGF-βs probably are the most broadly acting of all the families of growth factors.

Three different TGF-β receptor proteins have been identified and are designated type I, type II, and type III receptors. Although all three TGF-β isoforms bind to all three types of TGF-β receptors, they do not appear to have the same biologic effects on target cells. Two of the most important actions of TGF-βs in the context of skin wound healing are their ability to stimulate chemotaxis of inflammatory cells and to stimulate synthesis of extracellular matrix. Elevated, chronic production of TGF-β has been strongly implicated in nearly all fibrotic diseases, including hepatic cirrhosis, pulmonary fibrosis, kidney glomerulonephritis, and pelvic adhesions (Border and Noble, 1994). This has stimulated research into methods for inhibiting the action of TGF-β in vivo. For example, neutralizing antibodies to TGF-βs has been reported to reduce scar formation in rat skin incisions (Shah et al, 1992, 1994; Stromberg et al, 1992).

Connective Tissue Growth Factor

Transforming growth factor-β has been shown to induce synthesis of another important protein, connective tissue growth factor (CTGF) (Bradham et al, 1991; Frazier et al, 1996). Connective tissue growth factor is a potent inducer of extracellular matrix synthesis, and much of the increase in extracellular matrix that occurs in the skin after treatment with TGF-β probably is due to the action of CTGF. Many human fibrotic diseases have been reported to contain elevated levels of CTGF protein (Ito et al, 1998; Kucich et al, 2001). Macrophages, fibroblasts, and epithelial cells all secrete CTGF. The receptor for CTGF has not been conclusively identified. No clinical studies of CTGF have been performed, but adding exogenous CTGF to stimulate healing of chronic wounds is logical. Conversely, inhibiting CTGF action by adding neutralizing antibodies or antisense oligonucleotides (ASO) to wounds should reduce fibrosis.

Recent animal studies reported injections of ASO targeting CTGF mRNA dramatically reduced hypertrophic scarring of full-thickness skin excisions that extended to the cartilage layer in rabbit ears (Sisco et al, 2008). More importantly, phase II clinical studies assessing the effect of injections of ASO CTGF into the edges of surgically excised hypertrophic scars reported significant reduction of the visible appearance of the new incisional scars compared with no treatment or treatment with negative-control ASO with scrambled nucleotide sequence (personal communication, R. Galiano).

Fibroblast Growth Factor Family

Three proteins of the FGF family are thought to be important regulators of wound healing: acidic fibroblast growth factor (aFGF or FGF-1), bFGF (or FGF-2), and KGF (FGF-7) (Abraham and Klagsbrun, 1996). More than 30 synonyms have been reported in the literature describing proteins that eventually were shown to be either aFGF or bFGF. As their names imply, aFGF and bFGF are potent mitogens for fibroblasts that share many similar biochemical and biologic properties. The mechanism of release for aFGF and bFGF from cells is not clear.

Fibroblast growth factors have the ability to bind the glycosaminoglycan heparin and the proteoglycan heparan sulfate. When FGF is associated in the extracellular matrix and in basement membranes with heparan sulfate, it is protected from proteolytic degradation. The binding of FGF to heparin or to heparan sulfate proteoglycans in the membranes of cells results in a substantial increase in cell division. The activity of FGF appears to be regulated by the binding FGFs by heparin-containing components of the extracellular matrix.

Fibroblast growth factors appear to play major roles in wound healing. They stimulate proliferation of the major cell types involved in wound healing, including fibroblasts, keratinocytes, and endothelial cells. Fibroblast growth factors and VEGF probably are the major angiogenic factors in wound healing. Many of the cells that respond to FGF also synthesize the peptide, including fibroblasts, endothelial cells, and smooth muscle cells.

Keratinocyte growth factor shares the ability to bind to heparin. In contrast to aFGF and bFGF, synthesis of KGF is restricted to fibroblasts, and KGF expression is rapidly upregulated in fibroblasts after an injury (Werner et al, 1992). More importantly, KGF only stimulates mitosis of keratinocytes and not fibroblasts, as the receptor for KGF is not expressed by fibroblasts. This has led to the concept that KGF is a paracrine effector of epithelial cell growth. Palifermin, a recombinant derivative of human KGF, is the first active agent approved by the FDA for the prevention of severe oral mucositis in patients undergoing hematopoietic stem cell transplantation (Vadhan-Raj et al, 2013).

Four FGF receptors have been identified: FGFR-1, FGFR-2, FGFR-3, and FGFR-4. However, the receptors differ in their ability to bind bFGF and KGF. Expression of different FGF receptor variants by cells may provide another method for regulating the response of cells to FGFs.

Insulinlike Growth Factor Family

Insulinlike growth factor-1 and IGF-2 have substantial amino acid sequence homology to proinsulin, and both are synthesized as precursor molecules that are proteolytically cleaved to generate active monomeric proteins of approximately 7000 molecular weight. Insulinlike growth factor-2 is synthesized more prominently during fetal development, whereas IGF-1 synthesis persists at high levels in many adult tissues, especially in the liver in response to stimulation by pituitary-derived growth hormone. Many of the biologic actions originally attributed to growth hormone, such as cartilage and bone growth, are mediated in part by IGF-1. However, combinations of growth hormone and IGF-1 are more effective than either hormone alone.

Unlike other growth factors, IGF-1 is present in substantial levels in plasma, which primarily reflects hepatic synthesis. High-affinity IGF-binding proteins reversibly bind almost all the IGF-1 in plasma. Because the IGFs are inactive while bound to their binding proteins, the dynamic balance between free and bound IGFs has a substantial influence on the effects of IGF-1 in wound healing. Insulinlike growth factor-1 is also found in high levels in platelets and is released during platelet degranulation. It is a potent chemotactic agent for vascular endothelial cells, and IGF-1 released from platelets or produced by fibroblasts may promote migration of vascular endothelial cells into the wound area, resulting in increased neovascularization. Insulinlike growth factor-1 stimulates mitosis of fibroblasts and may act synergistically with PDGF to enhance epidermal and dermal regeneration.

Insulinlike growth factor-1 and IGF-2 each has distinct receptor proteins. The IGF-1 receptor is similar in structure to the insulin receptor. It consists of two α subunits that contain the IGF-1 binding site linked by disulfide bonds to the two β subunits that contain the transmembrane and cytoplasmic regions with the tyrosine kinase domain. The IGF-1 receptor binds IGF-1 with high affinity, binds IGF-2 with lower affinity, and binds insulin weakly. The IGF-2 receptor is a monomeric protein that has no kinase activity but binds proteins that contain the sugar mannose-6-phosphate. The IGF-2 receptor binds IGF-2 with high affinity, binds IGF-1 with low affinity, and does not bind insulin.

There are no published reports of clinical studies evaluating IGF-1 treatment of wounds. However, IGF-1 and growth hormone may act synergistically to promote wound healing. Two small double-blind, placebo-controlled studies showed improved healing with topical application of growth hormone to leg ulcers and systemic administration of growth hormone to severely burned pediatric patients (Gilpin et al, 1994; Rasmussen et al, 1991).

INTEGRATING GROWTH FACTORS INTO CLINICAL PRACTICE

Recombinant human PDGF-BB protein (becaplermin or Regranex) has been approved by the FDA for treatment of chronic diabetic foot ulcers, but concerns about an increased rate of mortality secondary to malignancy that was observed in patients treated with three or more tubes of Regranex gel in a postmarketing retrospective cohort study led to a black box warning on the product label. However, a more extensive postmarketing retrospective cohort study did not find this association.

Although no growth factor has received approval for pressure ulcer treatment, national and international guidelines suggest considering PDGF use for pressure ulcers that are not responsive to comprehensive therapy or before surgical repair (EPUAP, NPUAP, 2009; Whitney et al, 2006). Efficacy data are insufficient for national and international guidelines to recommend the application of topical growth factors with other wound types. However, isolated reports (listed in Table 20-1) suggest potential usefulness (Hopf et al, 2006; Robson et al, 2006; Steed et al, 2006).

From a practical clinical perspective, whether manipulating the wound topically with growth factors or with semiocclusive dressings (as discussed in Chapter 18), the three principles of wound management remain the same and must be followed:

1. The underlying condition that caused the wound must be controlled or alleviated.
2. Cofactors that impair healing must be corrected. Similar to the concept of "barren soil," the cells in or adjacent to the wound must be properly prepared so that they can respond to stimulation by growth factors. For example, the cells must have adequate levels of oxygen, nutrients, and intact extracellular matrix components to be able to support cell mitosis, migration, and attachment.
3. A physiologic wound environment (both cellular and molecular) must be created for topical growth factors to be effective, also referred to as *wound bed preparation* (Schultz et al, 2003).

To create a physiologic wound environment, molecular imbalances that are common to chronic wounds (Box 20-1) and detrimental to healing must be corrected. The level of protease activities has emerged as one of the most important

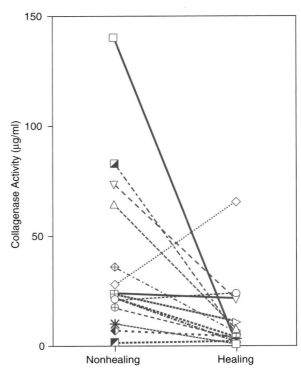

FIGURE 20-5 Protease levels in fluids from chronic venous ulcers before and after initiating healing. Protease activity was measured in fluids collected from nonhealing venous leg ulcers of 15 patients at the start of hospitalization and 2 weeks later, after the ulcers had clinical evidence of healing. Lines connecting the protease levels measured in the two samples from each patient (nonhealing and healing) indicate that protease activity tends to decrease as ulcers begin to heal. (From Schultz GS, Mast BA: Molecular analysis of the environment of healing and chronic wounds: cytokines, proteases and growth factors, *Primary Intention* (7)1:7-14, 1999)

factors preventing chronic wounds from healing because the protease will degrade proteins that are essential for healing, such as growth factors, their receptors, and extracellular matrix proteins. Growth factors added to chronic wound fluids are quickly degraded by the proteases (MMPs and serine proteases such as neutrophil elastase) present in the fluid. Fortunately, levels of protease activity decrease in chronic wounds as they begin to heal (Figures 20-5 and 20-6).

Numerous interventions are available to facilitate wound bed preparation and the creation of a physiologic wound environment. The acronym "TIME," as described in Table 20-3, identifies clinical interventions that should be used. For example, sharp debridement to remove nonviable tissue may be necessary to convert the detrimental chronic wound environment into a pseudoacute wound environment in which growth factors can function more effectively. Topical dressings that contain collagen (e.g., Promogran or Endoform) are designed as "sacrificial substrates" for wound proteases (MMPs and elastase) and thereby "spare" proteolytic destruction of the proteins in the wound bed that are essential for healing, such as growth factors, receptors, and extracellular matrix proteins.

BOX 20-1   Molecular Imbalances in Chronic Wounds

- Chronic wound fluid does not consistently stimulate growth (mitosis) of skin fibroblasts (Alper et al, 1985; Bucalo et al, 1993; Katz et al, 1991).
- Ratios of proinflammatory cytokines (tumor necrosis factor-α and interleukin-1β) and natural receptors are significantly increased (Harris et al, 1995; Mast and Schultz, 1996).
- Protease activity is significantly elevated (Bullen et al, 1995; Harris et al, 1995; Mast and Schultz, 1996; Nwomeh et al, 1998; Rogers et al, 1995; Tarnuzzer and Schultz, 1996; Yager et al, 1996, 1997).
- Cells may be unable to respond or may be senescent (Hopf et al, 2006; Robson et al, 2006; Steed et al, 2006; Whitney et al, 2006).

MOLECULAR ENVIRONMENT OF WOUNDS

FIGURE 20-6 Imbalanced molecular environments of healing and chronic wounds. *MRSA,* Methicillin-resistant Staphyloccocus aureus; *RNS,* reactive nitrogen species; *ROS,* reactive oxygen species.

TABLE 20-3   TIME: Principles of Wound Bed Preparation

Clinical Observations	Proposed Pathophysiology	WBP Clinical Actions	Effect of WBP Actions	Clinical Outcomes
*T*issue nonviable or deficient	Defective matrix and cell debris impair healing	Debridement (episodic or continuous) • Autolytic, sharp, surgical, enzymatic, mechanical, or biologic agents	Restoration of wound base and functional extracellular matrix proteins	Viable wound base
*I*nfection or inflammation	High bacterial counts or prolonged inflammation ↑ Inflammatory cytokines ↑ Protease activity ↓ Growth factor activity	Remove infected foci Implement topical/systemic • Antimicrobials • Antiinflammatories • Protease inhibition	Low bacterial counts or controlled inflammation: ↓ Inflammatory cytokines ↓ Protease activity ↑ Growth factor activity	Bacterial balance and reduced inflammation
*M*oisture balance	Desiccation slows epithelial cell migration Excessive fluid causes maceration of wound margin	Apply moisture-balancing dressings Compression, negative pressure, or other methods for removing fluid	Restoration of epithelial cell migration, desiccation avoided Edema, excessive fluid controlled, maceration avoided	Moisture balance
*E*dge of wound (nonadvancing or undermined)	Nonmigrating keratinocytes Nonresponsive wound cells and abnormalities in extracellular matrix or abnormal protease activity	Reassess cause or consider corrective therapies: • Debridement • Skin grafts • Biologic agents • Adjunctive therapies	Migrating keratinocytes and responsive wound cells Restoration of appropriate protease profile	Advancing edge of wound

TIME, Tissue, Infection, Moisture, Edge; *WBP,* wound bed preparation.

An added benefit to sharp debridement is that it will help to remove bacterial biofilms, which have been reported to be present in over 60% of chronic wounds (James et al, 2008). Biofilm is discussed in Chapter 16. Specific aspects of wound bed preparation were updated in 2012 to include new information that was generated in the 10 years since the original publication on wound bed preparation (Leaper et al, 2012). Biophysical and biologic agents can be used to alter the wound environment and correct senescent cells. These agents are described in detail in Chapters 19 through 24.

CLINICAL CONSULT

A: A 50-year-old female with a lower right extremity leg ulcer referred to wound clinic by friend. Patient wants growth factors because they worked so well on her friend's diabetic foot wound. Pitting edema and hemosiderin staining present on right lower leg gaiter area. Ulcer is irregular-shaped $2 \times 1 \times 0.4$ cm with clean, red, viable wound base. No history of diabetes. ABI and foot sensation within normal limits, no signs of neuropathy. Ulcer has been present for 9 months and patient indicates she is "tired of it being there". Uses several layers of gauze over ulcer and has to change twice daily to prevent soaking through to socks.
D: Venous ulceration.

P: Graduated compression, absorptive topical dressings, collagen wound dressing to reduce breakdown of desirable wound proteins and growth factors.
I: (1) Provide education related to venous insufficiency and need for compression. (2) Recommend collagen wound dressing to attract MMPs and preserve growth factors. (3) Alginate followed by foam cover dressing over collagen to absorb exudate. (4) Wrap with 2 layer compression. (5) Change dressing and apply compression dressing twice weekly in clinic.
E: Patient verbalizes understanding and rationale for plan of care. Return to clinic in 4 days to evaluate effectiveness of compression and local wound care.

SUMMARY

Increased knowledge of the molecular regulation of normal wound healing has led to a better understanding of the molecular imbalances that occur frequently in chronic wounds and that impair healing. One of these is the presence of bacterial biofilms in a high percentage of chronic wounds that stimulate chronic inflammation, which leads to elevated levels of proteases that destroy proteins essential for healing. New dressings that contain collagen help to reduce elevated levels of destructive proteases and improve effectiveness of endogenous growth factors and exogenously applied recombinant growth factors (PDGF, EGF), as well as other advanced therapies, including biologically active, engineered, artificial skin substitutes. These advanced therapies only function optimally when they are applied to wound beds that are properly prepared and contain cells that are able to respond to them. A high percentage of chronic wounds contain bacterial biofilms that stimulate chronic inflammation, which leads to elevated levels of destructive proteases. This understanding has filled in some of the key gaps in the knowledge base of the molecular pathology that impairs healing. For high-priced technologies to find broad application, they must ultimately be shown to have a significant positive effect (e.g., decreased duration of confinement, reduced cost of supplemental therapies, reduced amputation rate). Thus the wound specialist must stay abreast of new discoveries in these areas of wound research to be able to effectively integrate these new advances into clinical practice.

REFERENCES

Abraham J, Klagsbrun M: Modulation of wound repair by members of the fibroblast growth factor family. In Clark RAF, editor: *The molecular and cellular biology of wound repair*, New York, 1996, Plenum Press.

Acosta J, Savigne W, Valdez C, et al: Epidermal growth factor intralesional infiltrations can prevent amputation in patients with advanced diabetic foot wounds, *Int Wound J* 3:232, 2006.

Alper JC, Tibbetts LL, Sarazen AA Jr: The in vitro response of fibroblasts to the fluid that accumulates under a vapor-permeable membrane, *J Invest Dermatol* 84:513, 1985.

Arai K, Lee F, Miyajima A, et al: Cytokines: coordinators of immune and inflammatory responses, *Annu Rev Biochem* 59:783, 1990.

Barrientos S, Brem H, Stojadinovic O, et al: Growth factors and cytokines in wound healing, *Wound Repair Regen* 16:585, 2008.

Bennett NT, Schultz GS: Growth factors and wound healing: biochemical properties of growth factors and their receptors, *Am J Surg* 165:728, 1993a.

Bennett NT, Schultz GS: Growth factors and wound healing. II. Role in normal and chronic wound healing, *Am J Surg* 166:74, 1993b.

Border WA, Noble NA: Transforming growth factor-β in tissue fibrosis, *N Engl J Med* 10:1286, 1994.

Bradham DM, Igarashi A, Potter RL, et al: Connective tissue growth factor: a cysteine-rich mitogen secreted by human vascular endothelial cells is related to the SRC-induced immediate early gene product CEF-10, *J Cell Biol* 114(6):1285, 1991.

Brown GB, Curtsinger L 3rd, Brightwell JR, et al: Enhancement of epidermal regeneration by biosynthetic epidermal growth factor, *J Exp Med* 163:1319, 1986.

Brown GL, Nanney LB, Griffen J, et al: Enhancement of wound healing by topical treatment with epidermal growth factor, *N Engl J Med* 321:76, 1989.

Bucalo B, Eaglstein WH, Falanga V: Inhibition of cell proliferation by chronic wound fluid, *Wound Repair Regen* 1:181, 1993.

Bullen EC, Longaker MT, Updike DL, et al: Tissue inhibitor of metalloproteinases-1 is decreased and activated gelatinases are increased in chronic wounds, *J Invest Dermatol* 104:236, 1995.

Carpenter G, Cohen S: Epidermal growth factor, *J Biol Chem* 265:7709, 1990.

David LS, Goslen JB, Holloway GA, et al: Randomized prospective double-blind trial in healing chronic diabetic foot ulcers, *Diabetes Care* 11:1598, 1992.

European Pressure Ulcer Advisory Panel (EPUAP), National Pressure ulcer Advisory Panel (NPUAP): *Prevention and treatment of pressure ulcers*, Washington DC, 2009, NPUAP.

Falanga V, Eaglstein WH, Bucalo B, et al: Topical use of human recombinant epidermal growth factor (h-EGF) in venous ulcers, *Phlebology* 18:604, 1992.

Fantl WJ, Johnson DE, Williams LT: Signaling by receptor tyrosine kinases, *Annu Rev Biochem* 62:453, 1993.

Frazier K, Williams S, Kothapalli D, et al: Stimulation of fibroblast cell growth, matrix production, and granulation tissue formation by connective tissue growth factor, *J Invest Dermatol* 107:404, 1996.

Frenette PS, Wagner DD: Adhesion molecules, blood vessels and blood cells, *N Engl J Med* 335:43, 1996a.

Frenette PS, Wagner DD: Molecular medicine, adhesion molecules, *N Engl J Med* 334:1526, 1996b.

Fu X, Shen Z, Chen Y, et al: Randomised placebo-controlled trial of use of topical recombinant bovine basic fibroblast growth factor for second-degree burns, *Lancet* 352:1661, 1998.

Gilpin DA, Barrow RE, Rutan RL, et al: Recombinant human growth hormone accelerates wound healing in children with large cutaneous burns, *Ann Surg* 220:19, 1994.

Harris IR, Yee KC, Walters CE, et al: Cytokine and protease levels in healing and non-healing chronic venous leg ulcers, *Exp Dermatol* 4:342, 1995.

Heldin C, Westermark B: Role of platelet derived growth factor in vivo. In Clark RAF, editor: *The molecular and cellular biology of wound repair*, New York, 1996, Plenum Press.

Higashiyama S, et al: Structure of heparin-binding EGF-like growth factor, *J Biol Chem* 267:6205, 1992.

Holloway GA, Steed D, DeMarco M, et al: A randomized, controlled, multicenter, dose response trial of activated platelet supernatant, topical CT-102 in chronic, nonhealing, diabetic wounds, *Wounds* 5:198, 1993.

Hopf HW, Ueno C, Aslam R, et al: Guidelines for the treatment of arterial insufficiency ulcers, *Wound Repair Regen* 14(6):693, 2006.

Ito Y, Aten J, Bende RJ, et al: Expression of connective tissue growth factor in human renal fibrosis, *Kidney Int* 53:853, 1998.

James G, Swogger E, Wolcott R, et al: Biofilms in chronic wounds, *Wound Repair Regen* 16:37, 2008.

Katz MH, Alvarez AF, Kirsner RS, et al: Human wound fluid from acute wounds stimulates fibroblast and endothelial cell growth, *J Am Acad Dermatol* 25:1054, 1991.

Kucich U, Rosenbloom JC, Herrick DJ, et al: Signaling events required for transforming growth factor–beta stimulation of connective tissue growth factor expression by cultured human lung fibroblasts, *Arch Biochem Biophys* 395:103, 2001.

Leaper D, Schultz G, Carville K, et al: Extending the TIME concept: what have we learned in the past 10 years? *Int Wound J* 9 (Suppl 2):S1, 2012.

Massague J: Transforming growth factor alpha. A model for membrane anchored growth factors, *J Biol Chem* 265(35):21393, 1990.

Mast BA, Schultz GS: Interactions of cytokines, growth factors, and proteases in acute and chronic wounds, *Wound Repair Regen* 4:411, 1996.

Nanney LB, King LE: Epidermal growth factor and transforming growth factor-α. In Clark RAF, editor: *The molecular and cellular biology of wound repair*, New York, 1996, Plenum Press.

Nwomeh BC, Liang HX, Diegelmann, RF, et al: Dynamics of the matrix metalloproteinases MMP-1 and MMP-8 in acute open human dermal wounds, *Wound Repair Regen* 6:127, 1998.

Rasmussen LH, Karlsmark T, Avnstorp C, et al: Topical human growth hormone treatment of chronic leg ulcers, *Phlebology* 6:23, 1991.

Roberts AB, Sporn MB: Transforming growth factor-beta. In Clark RAF, editor: *The molecular and cellular biology of wound repair*, New York, 1996, Plenum Press.

Robson MC, Abdullah A, Burns BF, et al: Safety and effect of topical recombinant human interleukin-1β in the management of pressure sores, *Wound Repair Regen* 2:177, 1994.

Robson MC, Cooper DM, Aslam R, et al: Guidelines for the treatment of venous ulcers, *Wound Repair Regen* 14(6):649, 2006.

Robson MC, Phillips LG, Lawrence WT, et al: The safety and effect of topically applied recombinant basic fibroblast growth factor on the healing of chronic pressure sores, *Ann Surg* 216:401, 1992b.

Robson MC, Phillips LG, Thomason A, et al: Recombinant human platelet-derived growth factor-BB for the treatment of chronic pressure ulcers, *Ann Plast Surg* 29:193, 1992a.

Rogers AA, Burnett S, Moore JC, et al: Involvement of proteolytic enzymes—plasminogen activators and matrix metalloproteinases—in the pathophysiology of pressure ulcers, *Wound Repair Regen* 3:273, 1995.

Schultz G, Sibbald R, Falanga V, et al: Wound bed preparation, a systemic approach to wound bed management, *Wound Repair Regen* 11(Suppl 1):S1, 2003.

Shah M, Foreman DM, Ferguson MW: Control of scarring in adult wounds by neutralising antibody to transforming growth factor beta, *Lancet* 339:213, 1992.

Shah M, Foreman DM, Ferguson MW: Neutralising antibody to TGF-beta1,2 reduces cutaneous scarring in adult rodents, *J Cell Sci* 107:1137, 1994.

Sisco M, Kryger Z, O'Shaughnessy K, et al: Antisense inhibition of connective tissue growth factor (CTGF/CCN2) mRNA limits hypertrophic scarring without affecting wound healing in vivo, *Wound Repair Regen* 16:661, 2008.

Springer TA: Adhesion receptors of the immune system, *Nature* 346:425, 1990.

Steed DL: Diabetic Ulcer Study Group: Clinical evaluation of recombinant human platelet-derived growth factor for the treatment of lower extremity diabetic ulcers, *J Vasc Surg* 21:71, 1995.

Steed DL, Attinger C, Colaizzi T, et al: Guidelines for the treatment of diabetic ulcers, *Wound Repair Regen* 14(6):680, 2006.

Stromberg S, Collins, TJ, Gordon AQ, et al: Transforming growth factor-alpha acts as an autocrine growth factor in ovarian carcinoma cell lines, *Cancer Res* 52:341, 1992.

Tarnuzzer RW, Schultz GS: Biochemical analysis of acute and chronic wound environments, *Wound Repair Regen* 4:321, 1996.

Vadhan-Raj S, Goldberg J, Perales M, et al: Clinical applications of palifermin: amelioration of oral mucositis and other potential indications, *J Cell Mol Med* 17:1371, 2013.

Werner S, Peters KG, Longaker MT, et al: Large induction of keratinocyte growth factor expression in the dermis during wound healing, *Proc Natl Acad Sci USA* 89:6896, 1992.

Whitney J, Phillips L, Aslam R, et al: Guidelines for the treatment of pressure ulcers, *Wound Repair Regen* 14(6):663, 2006.

Yager DR, Zhang LY, Liang HX, et al: Wound fluids from human pressure ulcers contain elevated matrix metalloproteinase levels and activity compared to surgical wound fluid, *J Invest Dermatol* 107:743, 1996.

21

Negative Pressure Wound Therapy

Debra S. Netsch, Denise P. Nix, and Vicki Haugen

OBJECTIVES

1. Compare and contrast two different types of negative pressure wound therapy (NPWT).
2. Discuss three mechanisms for the effects of NPWT on wound healing.
3. Describe three indications, contraindications, and precautions for NPWT.
4. Describe the application of NPWT, including undermined or sinus areas.

Negative pressure wound therapy (NPWT) is the application of subatmospheric (negative) pressure to a wound through suction to facilitate healing and collect wound fluid (Campbell et al, 2008; Vikatmaa et al, 2008). The use of NPWT as an open wound therapy was developed during the 1940s in Germany (Vikatmaa et al, 2008). During the 1970s and 1980s, the concept was applied to the management of draining wounds, such as an open wound with a co-existing enteric fistula, by placing a suction catheter or fenestrated drain tube on a moist, gauze-covered wound bed, connecting the catheter to wall suction, and covering the wound (and exit site of the catheter) with a transparent adhesive dressing (Chariker et al, 1989; Irrgang and Bryant, 1984; Orringer et al, 1987). This technique was referred to as *closed suction wound drainage,* with the primary objective of containing drainage.

During the 1990s, NPWT was refined by Morykwas et al (1997) to include a porous polyurethane foam as the filler dressing. Today NPWT has become a common modality for the temporary management of a wide variety of acute and chronic wounds. Numerous NPWT systems are commercially available, each consisting of the following components: a wound filler dressing, a negative pressure device (disposable or reusable), a cover dressing or drape, a source for negative pressure (e.g., pump), and a fluid containment mechanism (i.e., a container or highly absorbent dressing). As shown in Table 21-1, components vary by manufacturer and product. For example, wound fillers range from open cell foam, silicone tubing wrapped with gauze (either plain or antimicrobial), honeycomb configured nonadherent matrix, nonwoven superabsorbent polymer, hydrocolloid, to gauze. Table 21-1 lists NPWT features and options. Available combinations of features and options are contingent on the manufacturer and device. Due to considerable fluctuation, specific brand names are not listed.

MECHANISM OF ACTION

Negative pressure wound therapy is hypothesized to facilitate wound healing through the use of controlled subatmospheric pressure to trigger and enhance the body's wound-healing response at a cellular level (Ubbink et al, 2008). Through animal and in vivo models, the mechanisms of action have been identified as yielding primary and secondary effects (Saxena et al, 2004). Primary effects include (1) edema reduction and fluid removal, (2) macrodeformation and wound contraction, and (3) microdeformation and mechanical stretch perfusion. Secondary effects include increased angiogenesis, granulation tissue formation, and reduction in bacterial bioburden (Orgill et al, 2009).

Edema Reduction and Removal of Wound Fluid

Removal of exudate containing toxic cytokines, bacteria, and matrix metalloproteinases and reduction of interstitial edema is a primary benefit of NPWT (Ubbink et al, 2008). By reducing tissue edema, the compressive effects of edema upon the periwound vasculature are decreased, thereby improving tissue perfusion, delivery of nutrients, and uptake of oxygen, culminating in the wound's ability to resist bacterial proliferation and microbial penetration (Orgill et al, 2009). A decrease in wound bacterial load was first described in the porcine model by Morykwas et al (1997) and is attributed to the following mechanisms: (1) removal of stagnant wound fluid, (2) direct removal of bacteria from the wound bed, (3) removal of third-space fluid, and (4) increased blood flow and thus increased immunity and oxygenation (Orgill et al, 2009). A significant decrease in nonfermentative, gram-negative bacilli has been reported with the use of NPWT compared with moist saline dressings (Moues et al, 2004). However, it is important to note that an increase in *Staphylococcus aureus* compared with the wounds managed

TABLE 21-1	NPWT Features and Options*
Wound Filler	Green foam
	Nonadherent gauze
	Oil immulsing nonadherent gauze
	Polyurethane black foam
	Polyvinyl alcohol white foam
	Proprietary hydrocolloid dressing over antimicrobial gauze or foam interface dressing
	Silver-impregnated polyurethane foam
Canister Volume (ml)	45
	60 ml cartridge
	No canister; absorb up to 140 ml
	250
	500
	1200
Setting Variability	Continuous
	Continuous and dynamic/variable
	Continuous and intermittent
	Continuous, dynamic/variable, and instill irrigant
	Continuous, intermittent, and instills irrigant
Pump Weight (lb)	< 0.5
	1.9
	2.4
	3.2
	4.5
	5.5 lb
	7.4 lb
	12.3 lb
	14.5 lb
Settings (mm Hg)	10 to 200
	40 to 125
	50 to 100
	60 to 200
	70, 120 or 150
	75, 100 or 125
Battery Life (hr)	4
	6
	9
	12
	14
	24
	8 days
	3 weeks alkaline batteries
	No battery proprietary spring mechanism

*Examples only, list not inclusive. Available combinations of features and options are contingent on the manufacturer and device. *NPWT,* Negative pressure wound therapy.

with moist saline dressings was also reported, suggesting close monitoring is warranted. Removal and collection of wound exudate via a closed containment system may also facilitate bioburden reduction by decreasing the frequency of dressing changes and exposure to potential external contaminants (Hinck et al, 2010; Pham et al, 2006).

Macrodeformation and Wound Contraction

Intact skin and soft tissue have a natural tension that, when disrupted, causes skin and soft tissues to typically pull apart (separate). Distractive tissue forces may act to keep a wound open, with vectors that oppose contraction, thereby delaying healing. Negative pressure wound therapy provides a mechanism to oppose these distractive soft tissue vectors (Franz et al, 2008). The application of negative pressure facilitates contraction, or pulling together, of the wound edges, simulating the application of an abdominal binder. The pulling together of the wound edges (contraction) promotes earlier wound healing by delayed primary or secondary intention. This contraction process occurs three dimensionally through mechanical forces, thus allowing decreased wound volume symmetrically and facilitating faster wound closure (Orgill et al, 2009; Ubbink et al, 2008).

Microdeformation and Mechanical Stretch

Histologic wound sections have demonstrated microdeformations of the wound surface present with NPWT that is not present underneath occlusive dressings alone (Saxena et al, 2004). Mechanically, deformation results in fluid flow within the matrix and strain where the matrix cells are anchored. Thus cells are subjected to both mechanical stretch mediated by their attachments to the matrix and shear stresses due to fluid flow. Fluid shear stresses are known to regulate cellular proliferation (Ubbink et al, 2008).

Wound surface microdeformations appear to stimulate increased vascular growth. The stretching of the wound surface is hypothesized to stimulate cell division, proliferation, and angiogenesis (Orgill et al, 2004). In vivo models have demonstrated that cells respond to tension with directional growth and specific gene release (vascular endothelial growth factor) when mechanical tension has been applied (Orgill et al, 2004; Saxena et al, 2004). Researchers also hypothesize that application of mechanical force initiates a cellular response, inducing a cascade of cellular proliferation, angiogenesis, and promotion of wound healing. The term *mechanotransduction* has been adopted to denote this cellular and physiologic response to mechanical strain (Orgill et al, 2009). An in vivo porcine study has found the degree of microdeformation and macrodeformation to be similar between gauze- and foam-based NPWT (Borgquist et al, 2010). In terms of the effect of NPWT on surrounding skin perfusion, it is hypothesized that increased perfusion occurs with the treatment, although the testing mechanism (laser Doppler) was criticized as being an indirect measure of blood flow (Morykwas et al, 2006; Orgill et al, 2009).

Morykwas et al (1997) reported an increase of more than 60% in granulation tissue formation using NPWT in comparison to moist gauze in porcine wounds. Numerous human studies have found increased and/or faster closure rates of wounds when treated with NPWT versus standard practice (Vuerstaek et al, 2006). Comparison of NPWT to standard compression therapy in primarily venous lower leg ulcerations revealed faster wound bed preparation (7 vs. 17 days) and faster healing rates (29 vs. 45 days) (Vuerstaek et al, 2006). Faster granulation tissue coverage over diabetic foot wounds resulted in accelerated wound closure when NPWT was used (Blume et al, 2008).

INDICATIONS AND USES

Negative pressure wound therapy is approved by the Food and Drug Administration (FDA) for use with chronic, acute, traumatic, subacute, and dehisced wounds; partial-thickness burns; ulcers (e.g., diabetic or pressure); flaps and grafts once nonviable tissue is removed; and select high-risk postoperative surgical incisions (e.g., orthopedic, sternal). The modality is used clinically with wounds of all sizes and depths, but most favorably in complicated deep wounds. Negative pressure wound therapy can be used in wounds with tunnels, undermining, or sinus tracts as long as the wound filler can fill the dead space and is easily retrieved (Andros et al, 2006).

Acute Wounds

The use of NPWT has been reported in acute wounds, including the intact postoperative surgical incision, open surgical wounds, contaminated surgical wounds, and burns. The prophylactic application of incisional NPWT (INPWT) in the operating room over a sterile incision is used on "at-risk" incisions to bolster the incision by keeping the cutaneous, dermal, and subcutaneous wound edges approximated and reducing horizontal and vertical shear forces. Physiologically, INPWT reduces lateral stresses on the wound up to 50%. The macrodeformation created by INPWT mimics intact skin elasticity forces. Although findings are inconsistent, the reported benefits of INPWT in high-risk surgical patients include reduced incidence of surgical site infection and reduced seroma and hematoma formation and dehiscence (Ingargiola et al, 2013; Kubec et al, 2013). However, numerous study design limitations with the existing research on INPWT have been noted in a recent Cochrane review (2013), which indicates these findings cannot be conclusively attributed to the INPWT and that further research employing a methodological design to reduce the potential for bias is warranted (Webster et al, 2013).

Negative pressure wound therapy can be used with clean or contaminated surgical wounds and over orthopedic hardware, tendons, bone, and Gor-Tex sheets. It can also be used in the presence of wound infection or osteomyelitis *after* appropriate debridement and antibiotics have been initiated (Andros et al, 2006). Complicated open abdominal wounds with exposed fascia can be managed with NPWT. Safety and efficacy have been reported in the septic patient with an acute, contaminated wound in whom NPWT was placed after the first surgical debridement (Shweiki and Gallagher, 2012).

Negative pressure wound therapy in the open abdominal wound is often used as a "bridge" until the patient is stabilized and the wound is amenable to closure. In addition to providing stabilization of the wound edges, containment of

exudate, and a moist wound environment and promoting granulation tissue formation, NPWT has been reported to improve wound closure rates in the repair of hernias with infected mesh (Baharestani and Gabriel, 2011; DeFranzo et al, 2001). Evidence also suggests that NPWT increases the chance of successful delayed primary fascial closure and reduced negative clinical outcomes (e.g., ventral hernias, prolonged hospitalization), compared with select alternative temporary abdominal closure (TAC) methods (Mouës et al, 2011; Roberts et al, 2012; Stevens, 2009). National Institute for Health and Care Excellence (NICE) guidelines (2013) recommend NPWT as a viable option for the management of the open abdominal wound.

The use of NPWT in burn management has been minimally investigated. One NPWT has received FDA approval for partial-thickness burns, although a Cochrane review found only one randomized controlled trial (RCT) addressing this indication (Dumville and Munson, 2012). The physiologic advantages to using NPWT are similar as in other wounds; however, the reduced edema mediated capillary stasis and improved blood flow, particularly within the first 12 to 24 hours postburn, and has been noted to reduce the progression to full-thickness burns. In addition, with the removal of wound fluid containing proteolytic enzymes, acute-phase protein, and metalloproteinases, a reduced systemic inflammatory response has been observed (Bovill et al, 2008). The use of NPWT for full-thickness burns is unclear and should be explored within the scope of the specialist burn center following a rigorous study protocol.

Chronic Ulcers

Multiple studies have found efficacious and safe use of NPWT with treatment of chronic wounds. Among national evidence-based guidelines for chronic wounds, NPWT is recommended for the treatment of nonhealing venous ulcers and diabetic wounds when conventional therapies have failed (Dowsett, 2012; Mouës et al, 2011; Steed et al, 2006; Whitney et al, 2006). Negative pressure wound therapy may have an adjunct role in the management of arterial ulcers when there is adequate perfusion for healing (Hopf et al, 2006; Mouës et al, 2011). International pressure ulcer guidelines recommend NPWT as an early adjuvant for the treatment of deep Stage III and IV pressure ulcers (NPUAP, EPUAP, PPPIA, 2014). Adequate wound debridement remains an important precursor to the implementation of NPWT with chronic wounds.

The use of NPWT for the management of diabetic foot ulcers after debridement is increasingly prevalent. Armstrong et al (2002) reported that in patients with refractory diabetic foot ulcers, 90.3% (n = 28) of wounds healed after debridement and NPWT within a mean of 8.1 weeks (+/− 5.5 weeks). The remaining three patients required a transmetatarsal amputation or below-the-knee amputation. Enhanced wound healing, reduced time to healing, and fewer amputations have been reported (Armstrong et al, 2007; Blume et al, 2008). Negative pressure wound therapy is recognized in national guidelines as a recommended treatment of diabetic foot ulcers with and without partial foot amputations (Crawford et al, 2013; Steed et al, 2006; WOCN®, 2013).

Flaps and Grafts

Negative pressure wound therapy has also been used to prepare a granular wound bed to receive a graft and to manage the donor, graft, and flap site postoperatively (Gray and Peirce, 2004; Murphy and Evans, 2012; Robson et al, 2006). Stimulation of angiogenesis, granulation formation, and reduction of edema all prepare the wound and improve the success for surgical repair. Additionally, NPWT provides the opportunity of scheduling the elective surgical procedure at a time that is optimal for the patient and does not jeopardize outcomes (Dowsett, 2012; Murphy and Evans, 2012; Robson et al, 2006; Venturi et al, 2006).

Enteric Fistulas

Negative pressure wound therapy has become an increasingly common technique used with acute enterocutaneous fistulas and enteroatmospheric fistulas after they have been explored and evaluated (as described in Chapter 38 and shown in Plate 77). Typically when managing an enterocutaneous fistula, the actual fistula orifice is separated from the wound and the fistula effluent is contained by a pouching system. The remainder of the wound is then managed with NPWT to promote granulation tissue formation and wound contraction.

Although containment of fistula effluent is neither a recommended nor intended use of the vacuum-assisted closure (VAC) sponge method, it is an appropriate indication for most NPWT systems using gauze wound-filler dressings. To minimize trauma to the fascia in the bed of an open abdominal wound and potential fistula formation, NPWT should be used cautiously by applying a lower amount of pressure (i.e., 75 to 90 mm Hg), utilizing a nonadherent wound liner between the wound bed and filler dressing, and/or positioning the catheter so that it does not contact the wound bed (Mouës et al, 2011; Stevens, 2009). Chapter 38 provides more detail about fistula management.

SAFETY, CONTRAINDICATIONS, AND PRECAUTIONS

Negative pressure wound therapy is generally considered to be a safe advanced-practice wound dressing, with rare serious adverse events (Peinemann et al, 2011; Sullivan et al, 2009; Ubbink et al, 2008; Vikatmaa et al, 2008). Between the years 2007 and 2011, however, the FDA received reports of 12 deaths and 174 injuries related to NPWT. Most adverse events and deaths occurred either at home or in a long-term care facility. Bleeding was the most serious complication, with reports of bleeding associated with nine of the overall deaths. According to these reports, extensive bleeding has occurred in patients
- with blood vessel grafts in the leg
- with breastbone or groin wounds
- receiving medication for blood clots
- during removal of dressings attached to the tissues

Patients with bleeding required emergency room visits and/or hospitalization and were treated with surgery and blood transfusions. Wound infection occurred in many of the additional cases, the majority of which were related to the retention of foam dressing pieces in the wounds. Most of these patients required surgery, additional hospitalization, and antibiotics (FDA, 2011).

Contraindications and precautions for NPWT listed by the FDA can be found in Checklist 21-1. Negative pressure wound therapy is contraindicated in the presence of untreated osteomyelitis, necrotic tissue, exposed blood vessels, exposed organs, nonenteric or unexplored fistulas, and malignancy in the wound (select manufacturers). Precautions and close monitoring are indicated with the use of NPWT in the presence of treated infection, treated osteomyelitis, potential for hemorrhage, anticoagulation therapy, postsurgical malignancy excision, and patients who have poor adherence to follow up for monitoring of wound progress by the care provider (Andros et al, 2006; FDA, 2011).

CHECKLIST 21-1 Negative Pressure Wound Therapy: Contraindications and Precautions

Contraindications to NPWT
- ✓ Necrotic tissue with eschar present
- ✓ Untreated osteomyelitis
- ✓ Nonenteric and unexplored fistulas
- ✓ Malignancy in the wound
- ✓ Exposed vasculature
- ✓ Exposed nerves
- ✓ Exposed anastomotic site
- ✓ Exposed organs

Patient Risk Factors/Characteristics to Consider Before NPWT Use
- ✓ Patients at high risk for bleeding and hemorrhage
- ✓ Patients on anticoagulants or platelet aggregation inhibitors
- ✓ Patients with:
  - Friable vessels and infected blood vessels
  - Vascular anastomosis
  - Treated infected wounds
  - Treated osteomyelitis
  - Exposed organs, vessels, nerves, tendons, and ligaments
  - Sharp edges in the wound (i.e., bone fragments)
  - Spinal cord injury (stimulation of sympathetic nervous system)
  - Enteric fistulas
- ✓ Patients requiring:
  - Magnetic resonance imaging
  - Hyperbaric chamber
  - Defibrillation
- ✓ Patient size and weight
- ✓ Use near vagus nerve (bradycardia)
- ✓ Circumferential dressing application
- ✓ Mode of therapy (intermittent vs. continuous negative pressure)

Debridement and appropriate antibiotics should be implemented before using NPWT in an infected wound or when osteomyelitis is present. It is essential that all infected and nonviable tissue or bone be debrided in conjunction with appropriate antibiotic coverage before NPWT placement. To help minimize the risk of retained dressing pieces, keep track of the number of dressing pieces placed in the wound, and do not cut the dressing directly over the wound in order to avoid dressing fragments or debris falling into the wound area while cutting (FDA, 2011).

As shown in Table 21-2, when the potential for hemorrhage exists, NPWT can be used, but cautiously. If the patient's coagulation tests cannot be maintained within a therapeutic range, ecchymosis develops in the wound or periwound area or wound drainage becomes bloody, the pressure setting of the NPWT should be reduced. A nonadherent contact layer or a less adherent, higher-density, moist NPWT foam may be indicated (Andros et al, 2006).

Manufacturers' instructions state that NPWT dressing must be removed if defibrillation is required in the area of dressing placement because it may inhibit transmission of electrical energy and/or patient resuscitation. Some NPWT electrical units are not designed or compatible with hyperbaric oxygen therapy (HBO) or magnetic resonance imaging (MRI) environments. Typically dressings can remain in place, but the electrical NPWT unit should not be taken into the area.

After surgical excision of the malignancy, all NPWT systems can be implemented in the acute surgical wound to aid in closure. Negative pressure wound therapy has been used for palliative care purposes (e.g., reduced frequency of painful dressing changes, containment of exudate and odor); however, it is important to again check the manufacturer's guidelines for that device (Ford-Dunn, 2006). In addition, the insurance provider may not approve use of NPWT for palliative outcomes (as opposed to healing outcomes), and the wound care specialist may need to advocate strongly on the behalf of the patient and family for this type of intervention.

CLINICAL APPLICATION

Clinical application considerations for NPWT include the patient's need for and access to assistance and supplies, pain management, product selection, and amount of negative pressure.

Pain Management

Pain during dressing change removal and application of vacuum has been frequently noted and is cited as a common cause for NPWT discontinuation (Malmsjö et al, 2012; Sullivan et al, 2009). Pain has been associated with the type of wound filler used and may be more pronounced in the acute wound such as the fasciotomy and explant pacer sites. Multiple studies, including one systemic review, confirmed that there is less pain with gauze-based NPWT (Hurd, 2010; Malmsjö et al, 2012; Upton and Andrews 2015). Malmsjö and colleagues (2011) reported significantly higher levels of neuropeptides (calcitonin gene-related peptide [CGRP] and substance P) with the use of foam-based NPWT; both are known to cause inflammation and signal pain when tissue trauma occurs. Instillation of 2% lidocaine solution diluted 50/50 with normal saline into the NPWT tubing with dressing changes or directly into the foam can be used to reduce the pain during the dressing change procedure (Franczynk et al, 2009). The solution should be allowed to dwell in the wound bed for at least 15 minutes to attain the desired effect. Often simply instilling normal saline into the foam will facilitate easier lifting of the wound filler from the wound bed. Conscious sedation may be warranted for the pediatric patient to minimize emotional and physical trauma of the dressing

TABLE 21-2	**Examples of Wound Characteristics Matched with Wound Filler**					
Wound Characteristic	NPWT Open-Cell Foam	NPWT Higher-Density, Moist, Open-Cell Foam	Gauze-Based Filler	Contact Layer (Under Filler)	Antibacterial Layer Under Filler or Silver-Coated Cell Foam	Irrigation with Open-Cell Foam
Deep but visible wound cavity	x		x			
Wound cavity with tunnels or deep undermining		x	x			
Infected wound					x	x
Wound with exposed structures		x		x		
Skin graft bolster	x			x		
Fragile wounds (bleeding potential, friable tissue)		x		x		

Birke-Sorensen et al, 2011; Dowsett, 2012; Glass et al, 2012; Vig et al, 2011.
NPWT, Negative pressure wound therapy.

BOX 21-1 Reducing Pain upon Dressing Removal

- Instill normal saline to moisten wound-filler dressing and allow it to loosen the wound-filler dressing from granulation tissue (either with or without adherent cover dressing in place).
- Decrease pressure setting.
- Change from intermittent to continuous cycling.
- Use nonadherent contact layers (e.g., silicone mesh dressing, impregnated wide-mesh dressings).
- Instill topical diluted lidocaine without epinephrine into wound-filler dressing and/or use systemic analgesics per prescriber's directions.
- Change wound-filler dressing to one less likely to allow granulation growth into dressing.
- Change type of NPWT system.

NPWT, Negative pressure wound therapy.

---

change. Premedication before the dressing change should also be considered. Box 21-1 offers additional interventions for reducing pain upon dressing removal (Franczynk et al, 2009; Gupta et al, 2004; NPUAP-EPUAP, 2009; Pham et al, 2006; Sullivan et al, 2009).

Product Selection

Each system uses the same basic principles of negative pressure despite wound-filler dressing differences. Although each company denotes the nuances of their product, more research is needed to compare effectiveness between different products and wound-filler dressings. One in vivo study found that the pressure delivered with gauze and foam was similar and concluded that the overall NPWT impact should be the same (Malmsjo et al, 2009). Wall suction–based gauze NPWT compared with standard foam NPWT were found to have no statistical significance in healing (Hu et al, 2009). Therefore until research suggests otherwise, NPWT product selection should be based on features, availability, reimbursement, and cost (Campbell et al, 2008; Glass and Nanchahal, 2012; Long and Blevins, 2009). Systematic reviews of NPWT correlating with different wound types have been performed (Birke-Sorenson et al, 2011; Glass and Nanchahal, 2012; Krug et al, 2011; Sullivan et al, 2009; Vig et al, 2011). The recommendations for NPWT selection based upon wound characteristics are summarized in Table 21-2. This table is based upon the summarization of multiple systematic reviews and not from anecdotal experience or case studies (Birke-Sorensen et al, 2011; Dowsett, 2012; Glass et al, 2012; Vig et al, 2011).

Adjunctive Interventions for NPWT. Adjunct wound dressings (e.g., antimicrobial dressings, enzymatic debridement agents, impregnated wide-mesh gauze, silicone mesh dressings, collagen wound dressings, skin substitutes, skin grafts), may be used in conjunction with NPWT, although research regarding their combined use is limited. Instillation of fluids,

including topical or antibiotic solutions, can be used with the NPWT tubing clamped for short periods of time to hold the fluids at the wound site. Initial experiences with instillation of topical solutions in conjunction with NPWT indicate low bioburden maintenance in wounds (Lessing et al, 2013). Instillation of fluid (saline) with NPWT compared with intermittent, dynamic or variable, and continuous modes of NPWT suggests in early in vivo preclinical trials a faster rate of granulation proliferation in NPWT saline instillation than NPWT in continuous and noncontinuous modes (Lessing et al, 2013).

In addition, the use of topical or antimicrobial solutions or silver, including silver-coated polyurethane foam, also may provide improved bioburden reduction than NPWT alone (Glass et al, 2012; Orgill et al, 2009). As such, the combined use of NPWT with antimicrobial products (e.g., solutions, silver, and impregnated gauze) may provide a mechanism for reducing the bioburden of the wound (Orgill et al, 2009). The adjunct use of nonsilver bacterial binding dressings is also becoming commonplace.

Intermittent vs. Continuous Pressure

Negative pressure can be delivered intermittently or continuously, most often continuously. Review of evidence by national guidelines have concluded that there is improved microvascular blood flow and granulation tissue formation with intermittent therapy compared with continuous therapy delivered at 125 mm Hg (WOCN®, 2010). However, the potential loss of seal and subsequent backflow of wound fluid onto the wound, as well as the increased caregiver supervision required to monitor the intermittent therapy, increase the "work" of providing intermittent therapy and consequently outweigh its benefits. Studies have shown that after pressures fall, reexpansion of sponge fillers can lead to tissue disruption and increased pain (Ahearn, 2009). Variable/dynamic pressure is instrumental to intermittent pressure. Variable/dynamic pressure cycles between a higher pressure and a lower pressure, but does not allow the pressure to drop to zero. The premise is that this allows for the aforementioned benefits without the problems of intermittent pressure. In vivo studies of variable/dynamic pressure compared with intermittent and continuous pressures found similar results in efficacy between the variable/dynamic pressure and intermittent pressure for both gauze- and foam-based NPWT (Glass et al, 2012; Malmjso et al, 2012). Continuous therapy delivered at 125 mm Hg is most routinely used; however, variable/dynamic pressure is currently becoming more popular (Glass et al, 2012). In addition to the interventions listed in Box 21-1, lower levels of pressure (75 to 80 mm Hg) can be used to reduce pain without compromising effectiveness (Isago et al, 2003; NPUAP-EPUAP, 2009).

Procedure Components

Once it has been determined that NPWT is appropriate, principles and procedures for application of most brands are similar.

BOX 21-2   NPWT Application and Use

Preparation
1. Assessment of wound and periwound is the initial step to NPWT application.
2. Debridement of eschar or slough, if present, should be performed for removal of devitalized tissue as a step in wound bed preparation.
3. Measurement of wound is necessary as a key assessment of wound-healing progression in addition for justification of continuation of NPWT with third-party payers.

Dressing Application
1. Cover exposed structures (e.g., bone, surgical mesh, tendon) with a nonadherent contact dressing (e.g., silicone or impregnated mesh).
2. Fill wound with wound-filler dressing.
3. Cover with adherent dressing.
4. Mark on adherent dressing the number of wound-filler pieces used.
5. Typically change entire dressing, including wound filler, every 48 hours or three times per week.

Negative Pressure Activation
1. Apply negative pressure device per manufacturer's recommendations.
2. Secure all tubing connections.
3. Ensure that all clamps are open.
4. Activate negative pressure with settings ordered according to patient tolerance, type of wound, and underlying structures.
5. Verify negative pressure settings and maintenance of seal.
6. Change canister weekly unless wound drainage collection necessitates earlier changes.
7. Ensure therapy for at least 20 hours of every 24 hours with disruption no more than 2 hours at a time.
8. Disconnect suction from the NPWT before defibrillation, magnetic resonance imaging, or hyperbaric oxygen therapy.

Documentation
1. Removal process: Ease of removal, wound-filler dressing type, and number of wound-filler dressing pieces removed
2. Assessment process: Assessment of periwound skin, wound, exudate
3. Application process: Nonadherent dressing type and number of pieces, if used; wound-filler dressing type and number of wound-filler dressing pieces used; negative pressure settings; patient's tolerance of procedure

NPWT, Negative pressure wound therapy.

However, it is important to follow the specific manufacturer's instructions. Box 21-2 contains general considerations for application and use of NPWT devices (Gupta et al, 2004).

Prepare the Skin. The cover dressing requires an airtight seal to allow NPWT to function properly (Figure 21-1). Most air leaks can be prevented by (1) drying the periwound skin; (2) framing the periwound area with skin sealant, skin barrier, hydrocolloid, or transparent film dressing; and (3) filling

uneven skin surfaces (e.g., creases, scars, and folds) with a skin barrier product (paste, strip, etc.) or hydrocolloid. Contact dermatitis may result if negative pressure is applied directly to the skin (see Plate 60). This can be prevented by protecting skin near or under suction with a hydrocolloid or transparent film dressing framed over the vulnerable area (Gupta et al, 2004).

Fill Wound Depth, Undermining, Tunneling, or Sinus Tracts. Nonviable tissue should be removed and exposed structures (e.g., bone, surgical mesh, tendon) protected with a contact layer before applying the wound-filler dressing. The brand of NPWT or specific wound-filler dressing may need to be adjusted based on undermining, tunneling, or sinus tracts present. Infections from retained pieces of foam filler that subsequently required surgery and antibiotics have been reported by MedWatch (FDA, 2011). Therefore it is imperative that products are selected, prepared, and used to ensure retrieval of the wound-filler dressing. Undermining, tunneling, or sinus tracts should *not* be packed tightly. Rather, the wound-filler dressing should be gently placed all the way into the undermined, tunneled, or sinus area. Then 1 to 2 cm of the wound filler dressing should be withdrawn from the opening of the undermined, tunneled, or sinus area. The higher pressures will collapse the undermined portion together and promote granulation of the undermined area from the innermost aspect of the wound toward the exterior surface. Progressively smaller amounts of wound filler dressing should be used to allow for contraction and decrease in wound volume over time.

Bridge Multiple Wounds/Areas. If more than one wound/area requires NPWT, these areas can be Y-connected together to the same NPWT device. If a Y-connector is not feasible or available, these multiple areas can be "bridged together" (see Figure 21-1).

Prevent Pressure from Device/Tubes. Pressure ulcers associated with the device, and with the drainage tubing in particular, have been reported, particularly over a bony prominence. Prevention can be achieved by creating a path for the tubing and suction device that leads to an area without pressure points and away from the wound. Apply a thin dressing to the skin (such as a hydrocolloid or transparent dressing) starting at the wound edge and leading toward the site where the negative pressure device can be safely applied. Over this lay a strip of the wound filler (Figure 21-2). The transparent cover dressing then is applied over the wound itself and the wound-filler dressing path. This transparent cover dressing or drape can also be applied in two sections, one to the wound and one to the path separately. Bridging dressings may also be available with the commercial NPWT company.

Maintain a Seal. Although many NPWT systems compensate for small air leaks, it is important that significant air leaks are found and sealed. Air leaks can be identified with the use of a

FIGURE 21-1 Bridging three wounds with one device instead of three. **A,** Wound filler dressing placed in each wound. Transparent dressing applied to protect intact skin under the intended bridge from negative pressure. **B,** Wound filler strips applied to connect/bridge the wounds. **C,** Transparent drape is applied over the entire configuration. An opening is made to accommodate the suction. Note foam is bubbled up above skin level because suction has not yet been applied. **D,** Dressing attached to suction; airtight seal achieved. (Courtesy Debra S. Netsch.)

stethoscope and repaired with the transparent cover dressing or drape. Although one or two additional layers of the transparent cover dressing will repair large air leaks, multiple layers will potentially reduce moisture vapor transmission and cause maceration of the wound and periwound area.

Patient Discharge or Transfer of Care

Most hospitals and long-term care facilities rent specific NPWT systems based on contracts and formularies. Vendor selection and specific system type may not transfer from one facility to another or to the home care venue. Having access to vendor-supported education for both staff and physicians with annual competencies may be necessary for safe NPWT practice.

Transfer of care must be initiated with clear communication related to vendor, system, procedure, supplies, and follow-up. Who (e.g., patient, family member, home care) and when dressing changes need to be done should be discussed and pre-arranged. Staff, patient, and/or caregivers must be educated about how to operate the device, respond to alarms, and how and why to turn off or disconnect therapy (Ousey and Milne, 2014).

When discharging to the community, there must be an assessment of the family's or patient's ability to safely navigate the device in the new environment. The wound specialist will need to obtain information about the physical environment (e.g., stairways, electrical outlets) and the patient's ability to see the device controls and hear the alarms. Cognitive ability to respond appropriately to the alarms and identify when and who to call for complications and emergencies must be assessed. Patients with high-output wounds will need to change or have immediate access to having their canister changed before filling so the dressing seal is not compromised. In the absence of constant supervision by trained staff or caregivers, NPWT may not be an appropriate option for the patient who is unable to cooperate with keeping the system intact (e.g., dementia, agitation).

FIGURE 21-2 Patient laying on left side with pressure ulcer evident over right ischial tuberosity. Bridge created from ischial ulcer to position tubing and negative pressure device on right lateral buttock to avoid vulnerable pressure points near ulcer. (Courtesy Julie Freyberg.)

Checklist 21-2 provides a list of questions and factors to consider during discharge planning for the patient with NPWT (Ousey and Milne, 2014). Checklist 21-3 provides questions for patients and/or their caregivers to ask health care providers before transitioning from receiving NPWT in a health care facility to using it at home (FDA, 2011).

CHECKLIST 21-2 NPWT Factors to Consider before Discharge

✓ Patient mobility—does the patient use a walking aid?
✓ Is the patient able to carry the device and manage the weight and tubing?
✓ Is the patient at risk of falling because of the device?
✓ Is the patient/carer cognitively able to manage the therapy?
✓ Does the patient have sufficient hearing/vision to manage the system and to hear alarms and read the controls?
✓ Is the patient in a psychological and social situation appropriate for NPWT?
✓ Is the patient's home electricity supply safe?
✓ Are there stairs or other obstacles that the patient will need to negotiate with the device?
✓ Does the patient know who to contact in an emergency and what would constitute an emergency?
✓ Is there a risk of potential loss of equipment?
✓ Does community staff have access to the equipment with or without funding?

NPWT, Negative pressure wound therapy.
Adapted from Ousey KJ, Milne J: Exploring portable negative pressure wound therapy devices in the community, *Br J Community Nurs* 19(Suppl 1):S14–S20, 2014.

CHECKLIST 21-3 NPWT: Transitioning from inpatient to Home

✓ Am I using the NPWT device correctly?
✓ How long should I expect to use the NPWT device?
✓ What serious complications might occur in my situation?
✓ What should I do if any of those complications occur?
  • Whom do I contact?
  • How do I recognize bleeding?
  • How do I recognize serious infection?
  • How do I recognize if my wound condition is worsening?
✓ Do I need to stop taking aspirin or any other medicines that affect my bleeding system or platelet function? What's the risk associated with stopping or avoiding such medicines?
✓ Can you provide me with patient instructions or tell me where I can find them?

NPWT, Negative pressure wound therapy.
Source: FDA, 2011.

CLINICAL CONSULT

A: Wound care referral received for a 43-year-old male with diabetic neuropathic ulceration of the left dorsal foot. Patient reports that the ulcer developed due to swelling in his foot and rubbing on his shoe. The wound was surgically debrided 24 hours ago following arterial blood flow testing. Ulcer is 3 cm x 2 cm x 2 cm; 90% red vascular tissue, 10% slough; no tunneling, undermining, periwound erythema, induration, or crepitus.
D: Diabetic neuropathic ulceration, left dorsal foot.
P: Optimize nutrition and management of blood glucose, offload pressure and repetitive stress, initiate NPWT for rapid wound contraction and containment.

I: (1) Dietician referral. (2) Continue with the postoperative offloading shoe. (3) Elevate left foot when sitting. (4) Noninvasive peripheral arterial testing. (5) Home care referral for 3× weekly dressing changes.
E: Patient verbalizes understanding and agreed to the plan once he learned we could use a smaller device than the one he saw in the hospital. Return to clinic in 2 weeks to reevaluate.

SUMMARY

Negative pressure wound therapy has introduced another modality to the toolbox for managing acute and chronic wounds. As with other topical therapies, the efficacy of NPWT is contingent upon correcting host cofactors (e.g., nutritional status, oxygenation, perfusion, pressure redistribution). Negative pressure wound therapy has become an interim adjunctive intervention to prepare the acute wound for definitive closure, such as the fasciotomy, dehisced sternal or abdominal surgical wounds, and donor sites. Negative pressure wound therapy as a wound-healing modality is a significant component of the current wound-healing arsenal and should be considered an option for topical wound management of select wounds for a certain period of time. Additional well-designed comparative studies with standardized protocols are needed to further explore clinical outcomes, the patient's experience, and effectiveness of alternative NPWT systems.

REFERENCES

Ahearn C: Intermittent negative pressure wound therapy and lower negative pressures—exploring the disparity between science and current practice: a review of the literature, *Ostomy Wound Manage* 55(6):22–28, 2009.

Andros G, Armstrong DG, Attinger CE, et al: Consensus statement on negative pressure wound therapy (VAC therapy) for the management of diabetic foot wounds, *Ostomy Wound Manage* 52(Suppl):S1–S32, 2006.

Armstrong DG, Lavery LA, Abu-Rumman P, et al: Outcomes of subatmospheric pressure dressing therapy on wounds of the diabetic foot, *Ostomy Wound Manage* 48(4):64–68, 2002.

Armstrong DG, Lavery LA, Boulton AJ: Negative pressure wound therapy via vacuum-assisted closure following partial foot amputation: what is the role of wound chronicity? *Int Wound J* 4:79–86, 2007.

Baharestani MM, Gabriel A: Use of negative pressure wound therapy in the management of infected abdominal wounds containing mesh: an analysis of outcomes, *Int Wound J* 8:118–125, 2011.

Birke-Sorensen, et al: Evidence-based recommendations for negative pressure wound therapy: treatment variables (pressure levels, wound filler and contact layer)—Steps towards an international consensus, *J Plast Reconstr Aesthet Surg* 64(Suppl 1):S1–S16, 2011.

Blume PA, Walters J, Payne W, et al: Comparison of negative pressure wound therapy using vacuum-assisted closure with advanced moist wound therapy in the treatment of diabetic foot ulcers: a multicenter randomized controlled trial, *Diabetes Care* 31(4):631–636, 2008.

Borgquist O, Gustafsson L, Ingemansson R, et al: Micro- and macro-mechanical effects on the wound bed of negative pressure wound therapy using gauze and foam, *Ann Plast Surg* 64(6):789–793, 2010.

Bovill E, Banwell PE, Teot L, et al: Topical negative pressure wound therapy: a review of its role and guidelines for its use in the management of acute wounds, *Int Wound J* 5(4):511–529, 2008.

Campbell P, Smith G, Smith J: Retrospective clinical evaluation of gauze-based negative pressure wound therapy, *Int Wound J* 5(2):280–286, 2008.

Chariker ME, Jeter KF, Tintle TE, et al: Effective management of incisional and cutaneous fistulae with closed suction wound drainage, *Contemp Surg* 34:59–63, 1989.

Crawford PE, Fields-Varnado M: Guideline for the management of wounds in patients with lower-extremity neuropathic disease, *J Wound Ostomy Continence Nurs* 40(1):34–45, 2013.

DeFranzo AJ, Argenta LC, Marks MW, et al: The use of vacuum-assisted closure therapy for the treatment of lower-extremity wounds with exposed bone, *Plast Reconstr Surg* 108(5):1184–1191, 2001.

Dowsett C: Clinical research/audit: recommendations for the use of negative pressure wound therapy, *Wounds UK* 8(2):48–59, 2012.

Dumville JC, Munson C: Negative pressure wound therapy for partial-thickness burns, *Cochrane Database Syst Rev* 12:CD006215, 2012.

Food and Drug Administration (FDA): *Negative pressure wound therapy (NPWT): preliminary public health notification*, February 24, 2011. http://www.fda.gov/Safety/MedWatch/SafetyInformation/SafetyAlertsforHumanMedicalProducts/ucm190704.htm. Accessed July 1, 2014.

Ford-Dunn S: Use of vacuum assisted closure therapy in the palliation of a malignant wound, *Palliat Med* 20(4):477–478, 2006.

Franczyk M, Lohman RF, Agarwal JP, et al: The impact of topical lidocaine on pain level assessment during and after vacuum-assisted closure dressing changes: a double-blind, prospective, randomized study, *Plast Reconstr Surg* 124(3):854–861, 2009.

Franz MG, Robson MC, Steed DL, et al: Guidelines to aid healing of acute wounds by decreasing impediments of healing, *Wound Repair Regen* 16(6):723–748, 2008.

Glass G, Nanchahal J: The methodology of negative pressure wound therapy: separating fact from fiction, *J Plast Reconstr Aesthet Surg* 65:989–1001, 2012.

Gray M, Peirce B: Is negative pressure wound therapy effective for the management of chronic wounds? *J Wound Ostomy Continence Nurs* 31(3):101–105, 2004.

Gupta S, Baharestani M, Baranoski S, et al: Guidelines for managing pressure ulcers with negative pressure wound therapy, *Adv Skin Wound Care* 17(Suppl 2):1–16, 2004.

Hinck D, Franke A, Gatzka F: Use of vacuum-assisted closure negative pressure wound therapy in combat-related injuries—literature review, *Mil Med* 175(3):173–181, 2010.

Hopf H, Ueno C, Aslam R, et al: Guidelines for the treatment of arterial insufficiency ulcers, *Wound Repair Regen* 14(6):693–710, 2006.

Hu KX, Zhang HW, Zhou F, et al: A comparative study of the clinical effects between two kinds of negative-pressure wound therapy, *Zhonghua Shao Shang Za Zhi* 25(4):253–257, 2009. [Article in Chinese].

Hurd T, Chadwick P, Cote J, et al: Impact of gauze-based NPWT on the patient and nursing experience in the treatment of challenging wounds, *Int Wound J* 7(6):448–455, 2010.

Ingargiola MJ, Daniali LN, Lee ES: Does the application of incisional negative pressure therapy to high-risk wounds prevent surgical site complications? A systematic review, *Eplasty* 13:e49, 2013.

Irrgang S, Bryant R: Management of the enterocutaneous fistula, *J Enterostomal Ther* 11(6):211–228, 1984.

Isago T, Nozaki M, Kikuchi Y, et al: Effects of different negative pressures on reduction of wounds in negative pressure dressings, *J Dermatol* 30(8):596–601, 2003.

Krug E et al: Evidence-based recommendations for the use of negative pressure wound therapy in traumatic wounds and reconstructive surgery: steps towards an international consensus, *Injury* 42(Suppl 1):S1–S12, 2011.

Kubec E, Badeau A, Materazzi S, et al: Negative-pressure wound therapy and the emerging role of incisional negative pressure wound therapy as prophylaxis against surgical site infections. In Méndez-Vilas A, editor: *Microbial pathogens and strategies for combating them: science, technology and education*, Badajoz, Spain, 2013, Formatex.

Lessing CM, James RB, Ingram SC: Comparison of the effects of different negative pressure wound therapy modes—continuous, noncontinuous, and with instillation—on porcine excisional wounds, *Eplasty* 13(October 1):443–454, 2013.

Long MA, Blevins A: Challenges in practice: options in negative pressure wound therapy. Five case studies, *J Wound Ostomy Continence Nurs* 36(2):202–211, 2009.

Malmsjö M, Gustafsson L, Lindstedt S, et al: The effects of variable, intermittent, and continuous negative pressure wound therapy, using foam or gauze, on wound contraction, granulation tissue formation, and ingrowth into the wound filler, *Eplasty* 12:e5, 2012.

Malmsjö M, Ingemansson R, Martin R, et al: The physical properties of gauze and polyurethane open cell foam in negative pressure wound therapy, *Wound Repair Regen* 17(2):200–205, 2009.

Morykwas M, Argenta LC, Shelton-Brown EI, et al: Vacuum-assisted closure: a new method for wound control and treatment: animal studies and basic foundation, *Ann Plast Surg* 38(6):553–562, 1997.

Morykwas M, Simpson J, Punger K, et al: Vacuum-assisted closure: state of basic research and physiologic foundation, *Plast Reconstr Surg* 117(Suppl 7):S121– S126, 2006.

Mouës CM, Heule F, Hovius SE: A review of topical negative pressure therapy in wound healing: sufficient evidence? *Am J Surg* 201(4):544–556, 2011.

Mouës CM, Vos MC, van den Bemd GJ, et al: Bacterial load in relation to vacuum-assisted closure wound therapy: a prospective randomized trial, *Wound Repair Regen* 12(1):11–17, 2004.

Murphy, Patrick S., and Gregory R. D. Evans. "Advances in Wound Healing: A Review of Current Wound Healing Products." *Plastic Surgery International 2012* (2012): available at http://www.ncbi.nlm.nih.gov/pmc/articles/PMC3335515/ accessed 14 Aug. 2015.

National Institute for Health and Care Excellence (NICE): *Negative pressure wound therapy for the open abdomen (NICE interventional procedure guidance no. 467)*, November 2013. website https://www.nice.org.uk/guidance/ipg467 accessed Aug. 14, 2015.

National Pressure Ulcer Advisory Panel (NPUAP), European Pressure Ulcer Advisory Panel (EPUAP) and Pan Pacific Pressure Injury Alliance (PPPIA): *Prevention and treatment of pressure ulcers: Clinical Practice Guideline*. In Emily Haesler, editor: Perth, Australia, 2014, Cambridge Media.

Orgill DP, Austen WG, Butler CE, et al: Guidelines for treatment of complex chest wounds with negative pressure wound therapy, *Wounds* 16(Suppl B):1–23, 2004.

Orgill DP, Manders EK, Sumpio BE, et al: The mechanisms of action of vacuum assisted closure: more to learn, *Surgery* 146(1):40–51, 2009.

Orringer JS, Mendeloff EN, Eckhauser FE: Management of wounds in patients with complex enterocutaneous fistulas, *Surg Gynecol Obstet* 165(1):79–80, 1987.

Ousey K, Milne J: Exploring portable negative pressure wound therapy devices in the community, *Br J Community Nurs* 19(Suppl 1):S14–S20, 2014.

Peinemann F, Sauerland S: Negative-pressure wound therapy: systematic review of randomized controlled trials, *Dtsch Arztebl Int* 108(22):381–389, 2011.

Pham C, Middleton P, Maddern G: The safety and efficacy of topical negative pressure in non-healing wounds: a systematic review, *J Wound Care* 15(6):240–250, 2006.

Roberts DJ, Zygun DA, Grendar J, et al: Negative-pressure wound therapy for critically ill adults with open abdominal wounds: a systematic review, *J Trauma Acute Care Surg* 73:629–639, 2012.

Robson M, Cooper DM, Aslam R, et al: Guidelines for the treatment of venous ulcers, *Wound Repair Regen* 14(6):649–662, 2006.

Saxena V, Hwang CW, Huang S, et al: Vacuum-assisted closure: microdeformations of wounds and cell proliferation, *Plast Reconstr Surg* 114(5):1086–1096, 2004.

Shweiki E, Gallagher KE: Negative pressure wound therapy in acute, contaminated wounds: documenting its safety and efficacy to support current global practice, *Int Wound J* 10:13–43, 2013.

Steed D, Attinger C, Colaizzi T, et al: Guidelines for the treatment of diabetic ulcers, *Wound Repair Regen* 14(6):680–692, 2006.

Stevens P: Vacuum-assisted closure of laparostomy wounds: a critical review of the literature, *Int Wound J* 6(4):259–266, 2009.

Sullivan N, Snyder DL, Tipton K, et al: *Negative pressure wound therapy devices technology assessment report (Project ID: WNDT1108)*, Rockville, MD, 2009, Agency for Healthcare and Research Quality.

Ubbink DT, Westerbos SJ, Evans D, et al: Topical negative pressure for treating chronic wounds, *Cochrane Database Syst Rev* 3:CD001898, 2008.

Upton D, Andrews A: Pain and trauma in negative pressure wound therapy: a review, *Int Wound J* 12(1):100–105, 2015.

Vikatmaa P, Juutilainen V, Kuukasjärvi P, et al: Negative pressure wound therapy: a systematic review on effectiveness and safety, *Eur J Vasc Endovasc Surg* 36(4):438–448, 2008.

Vig S, Dowsett C, Berg L, et al, Evidence-based recommendations for the use of negative pressure wound therapy in chronic wounds: steps towards an international consensus, *J Tissue Viability* 20(Suppl 1):S1–S18, 2011.

Vuerstaek J, Vainas T, Wuite J, et al: State of the art treatment of chronic leg ulcers: a randomized controlled trial comparing vacuum-assisted closure (V.A.C.) with modern wound dressings, *J Vasc Surg* 44(5):1029–1038, 2006.

Webster J, Scuffham P, Sherriff KL, et al: Negative pressure wound therapy for skin grafts and surgical wounds healing by primary intention, *Cochrane Database Syst Rev* 4:CD009261, 2012.

Whitney J, Phillips L, Aslam R, et al: Guidelines for the treatment of pressure ulcers, *Wound Repair Regen* 14(6):663–679, 2006.

Wound, Ostomy and Continence Nurses Society™ (WOCN®): *A quick reference guide for lower-extremity wounds, Venous, Arterial, and Neuropathic*, Mt. Laurel, NJ, 2013, WOCN®.

Wound, Ostomy and Continence Nurses Society™ (WOCN®): *Guideline for prevention and management of pressure ulcers (WOCN® clinical practice guideline series no. 2)*, Glenview, IL, 2010, WOCN®.

22

Hyperbaric Oxygenation

Craig L. Broussard

OBJECTIVES

1. List at least two indications for hyperbaric oxygen therapy.
2. List at least two contraindications for hyperbaric oxygen therapy.
3. Explain the physiologic effects of electrical hyperbaric oxygen therapy.

Hyperbaric oxygenation (HBO) is the systemic, intermittent administration of oxygen delivered under pressure. A hyperbaric environment exists when atmospheric pressure is greater than 1 atmosphere absolute (ATA) (Hammarlund, 1995). A medically significant hyperbaric exposure occurs when atmospheric pressure is increased to greater than 1.4 ATA or 10.2 pounds per square inch gauge pressure (psig) (UHMS, 1996). The typical HBO treatment takes place at a pressure of 2.0 to 2.5 ATA, or 14.7 to 22.0 psig. For HBO to occur, the patient must breathe 100% oxygen while physically exposed to the hyperbaric environment.

Just as wound care is not a subspecialty of HBO, neither is HBO a subspecialty of wound care. In addition to wound management, HBO is indicated for many other conditions, such as carbon monoxide poisoning, osteomyelitis, soft tissue radiation injury, and decompression sickness. Oxygen under pressure functions as a pharmacologic agent in that it has a therapeutic dose, a toxic dose, side effects, contraindications, interactions with other drugs, and incompatibilities with other drugs (Heimbach, 1998).

HISTORY

Much of what is known about the effects of hyperbaric treatment comes from observations and studies of caisson workers and divers. The first description of a pressurization vessel dates to 1662, when Henshaw used bellows to increase and decrease pressures to treat respiratory problems. The nineteenth century saw the advent of caisson workers for bridge construction and the subsequent description of caisson's disease (or decompression sickness), bubble theory, and oxygen toxicity by Paul Bert in 1878 (Elliott, 1995). Eleven years later, Moir used recompression to treat decompression sickness in caisson workers building the Hudson River tunnel. The twentieth century also brought about extensive research and application of hyperbaric therapy for decompression sickness

by the military. As we enter the twenty-first century, research is being conducted on a variety of disorders, including stroke, myocardial infarction, and autism.

Modern use of HBO to potentiate the effects of radiation in cancer patients began in 1955 (Kindwall, 1995). The National Academy of Science–National Research Council appointed a committee to review the physiologic basis for HBO in 1962. In 1966 this group published *Fundamentals of Hyperbaric Medicine,* which describes the physical and physiologic effects of HBO. However, it did not address clinical conditions treated with hyperbaric treatment (UHMS, 1996). The Undersea Medical Society (UMS) was founded in 1967 and was primarily devoted to diving and undersea medicine. The UMS became the Undersea and Hyperbaric Medical Society (UHMS) in 1986. The UHMS is the primary, worldwide source of information on hyperbaric and diving medicine. The mission of the UHMS is to "develop and promote educational activities, symposia and workshops that improve the scientific knowledge of matters related to undersea exposures and hyperbaric oxygen therapy" and "to raise the quality of care across the spectrum of hyperbaric medicine by promoting high standards of patient care and operational safety through clinical hyperbaric facility accreditation" (UHMS, 2015).

PHYSIOLOGIC EFFECTS

The mechanical effect of HBO follows the physical law described by Boyle, which states that as pressure increases, volume decreases. Therefore, in the case of decompression sickness or air/gas embolism, hyperbaric treatment is used to decrease the size of the air bubble or embolism. Physiologic effects of HBO use the physical law described by Henry's law, which states that the amount of gas dissolved in a liquid is directly proportional to the partial pressure of the dissolved gas. As a result, oxygen tensions can be raised

10 to 13 times higher than oxygen breathed at ambient pressure (Hammarlund, 1995). With these increases in oxygen tension, oxygen acts as a drug and has several effects on wound healing (Table 22-1).

Hyperbaric oxygenation increases the capacity of blood to carry and deliver oxygen to tissues. This hyperoxygenation occurs because oxygen is administered under pressure to the patient. Consequently, hyperbaric treatment significantly enhances oxygen delivery to compromised tissues, increases oxygenation to the tissues, and may restore perfusion to compromised areas. The increased capacity of blood to carry oxygen assists in the restoration of cellular function. The volumetric levels of diffusion achieved with HBO are two to three times those obtained under normobaric conditions.

Oxygen is a powerful vasoconstrictor and can be helpful in managing edema related to traumatic wounding or crush injuries. Although HBO may seem injurious in that it decreases blood supply to an injured area, the increase in diffusion of oxygen more than compensates for the decrease in circulation associated with vasoconstriction. In addition, leukocytes have an impaired ability to generate reactive oxygen species in a hypoxic environment, so the delivery of increased tissue oxygenation also enhances leukocyte function and the penetration of concomitant antibiotic therapy (Dauwe et al, 2014). The effect of HBO in blood is instantaneous, with a subsequent plateau in soft tissues approximately 1 hour after exposure. The effect of HBO declines steadily over 2 to 4 hours after exposure (Hammarlund, 1995).

INDICATIONS

The UHMS continuously reviews scientific data regarding the therapeutic benefit of HBO. It currently has designated the conditions or disease processes listed in Box 22-1 as indications for hyperbaric therapy (Gesell, 2008). Hyperbaric oxygenation is the primary therapy for arterial gas embolism, carbon monoxide poisoning, and decompression sickness. When used for any other indication, hyperbaric therapy must be incorporated as part of the plan of care that includes appropriate clinical and surgical treatments (Cianci and Sato, 1994; Gesell, 2008; Hopf et al, 2006; Marx, 1995). The effects of HBO on wound healing and the mechanisms for those effects are listed in Table 22-1. Patient selection should focus on the origin and hypoxic nature of the wound. For example, a pressure ulcer is best treated with pressure reduction; a hypoxic wound is best treated by maximization of oxygen to the wound. Indications specific to wound management recommended by national organizations and guidelines are listed in Table 22-2.

Hyperbaric oxygenation may be considered for the treatment of patients with limb-threatening diabetic and vascular insufficiency wounds of the lower extremity (Hopf et al, 2006; Norgren, et al 2007; Steed et al, 2006; UHMS, 2010; WOCN®, 2008). Löndahl (2012) also recommended HBO as an adjunctive therapy in patients with diabetic foot ulcers not responding to optimal treatment. A Cochrane review reported there was some evidence that in patients with diabetic foot ulcers, the use of HBO in conjunction with appropriate wound care resulted in significant healing by 6 weeks (Kranke et al, 2012). Unfortunately, this effect does not appear to be sustained at 1 year or greater follow-up and further research is needed. To meet Centers for Medicare and Medicaid Services (CMS) criteria, the

TABLE 22-1 Effects and Mechanisms of Hyperbaric Oxygen Therapy on Wound Healing	
Effect	**Mechanism**
Hyperoxygenation	Improved oxygen-carrying capacity Increased distance of diffusion Improved local tissue oxygenation Vasoconstriction and decreased local tissue edema Improved cellular energy metabolism
Improved growth factor expression	Upregulation of platelet-derived growth factor receptor Increased angiogenesis Increased extracellular matrix formation and granulation tissue (may see clinical signs of granulation tissue within 2 weeks of treatment) Enhanced epithelial cell proliferation and migration
Fibroblast proliferation	Increased collagen deposition Improved collagen cross-linking Increased production of fibronectin
Increased nitric oxide production	Enhanced neutrophil activity Enhanced macrophage activity Increased leukocyte-killing ability Enhanced effectiveness of antibiotics

BOX 22-1 Indications for Hyperbaric Oxygen Therapy

- Air/gas embolism*
- Carbon monoxide/cyanide poisoning*
- Central retinal artery occlusion
- Crush injury, compartment syndrome, acute traumatic ischemia
- Clostridial myonecrosis (gas gangrene)
- Compromised skin grafts and/or flaps
- Decompression sickness*
- Exceptional blood loss (severe anemia)
- Intracranial abscess
- Necrotizing soft tissue infections
- Delayed radiation injury (soft tissue and bony necrosis)
- Acute thermal burn injury
- Osteomyelitis (refractory)
- Enhancement of healing in selected problem wounds
- Idiopathic sudden sensorineural hearing loss

*Primary therapy.
Adapted from Undersea and Hyperbaric Medical Society (UHMS): *Indications for hyperbaric oxygen therapy*, http://www.uhms.org/Default.aspx?tabid=270. Accessed July 25, 2014.

TABLE 22-2   Wound-Related Indications for Hyperbaric Oxygen Therapy

Indication	Source
Thermal burns	UHMS (2010)
Acute traumatic ischemia	UHMS (2010)
Necrotizing infections	UHMS (2010)
Osteomyelitis (refractory)	UHMS (2010)
Delayed radiation injury (soft tissue and bony necrosis)	UHMS (2010)
Compromised skin grafts and/or flaps	UHMS (2010)
Selected problem wounds that fail to respond to established medical and surgical management	UHMS (2010)
Diabetic Wagner grade 3 or higher lower extremity wounds not responsive to established medical and surgical management	CMS (2002)
Diabetic limb-threatening lower extremity wound	WOCN® Society (2004) WHS (Steed et al, 2006)
Arterial limb-threatening lower extremity wound	WOCN® Society (2008) WHS (Hopf et al, 2006) Society for Vascular Surgery (Norgren et al, 2007)

UHMS, Undersea and Hyperbaric Medical Society; *WHS,* Wound Healing Society; *WOCN®,* Wound, Ostomy and Continence Nurses™.

lower extremity diabetic wound must be Wagner grade 3 or higher and not responsive to standard wound care, including assessment and correction of vascular insufficiency, maximization of nutritional status, optimization of glycemic control, debridement of nonvital tissue, and maintenance of moist wound healing with the use of topical dressings. Whereas other classification systems are recommended for use with diabetic foot ulcers, for reimbursement purposes, the National Coverage Determination (NCD) continues to insist that the Wagner Classification System be used (CMS, 2006). Infection should be resolving, and the wound must be appropriately offloaded, as described in Chapter 14. Transcutaneous oximetric values greater than 400 mm Hg during HBO exposure indicates a likely successful outcome in the diabetic lower extremity wound. Transcutaneous oximetric values less than 15 mm Hg when breathing room air and less than 100 mm Hg during HBO exposure are predictive of wound healing failure (Broussard, 2003; Fife et al, 2002). Although it is understood that not all wounds heal, consideration for hyperbaric treatment should be given to those patients with lower extremity wounds when it is known that these wounds may not heal. Hyperbaric treatment could mean the difference between limb salvage and a transmetatarsal, below-the-knee or above-the-knee amputation if appropriate circulatory assessment, intervention, and pre-amputation preparation are part of the comprehensive workup.

Crush injury, compartment syndrome, and acute traumatic ischemia benefit from HBO because of the improved oxygen tension in tissue that is inadequately perfused because of a disruption of blood supply and edema associated with injury. Hyperbaric oxygenation helps to decrease edema through its vasoconstrictive action. In addition, it helps to decrease reperfusion injury. The use of HBO in these cases is emergent, and patients should be treated as early as possible (within 4 to 6 hours after injury or surgery) for the best outcome (Latham, 2013). It is recommended that treatment (2 to 2.5 ATA for 60 to 90 minutes) be repeated three times daily for 2 to 3 days, then twice daily for 2 to 3 days, and then daily for 2 to 3 days. However, a recent Cochrane review reported there was insufficient evidence to support or refute the effectiveness of HBO for acute wounds, and further quality randomized controlled trials are needed (Eskes et al, 2010).

Clostridial myonecrosis and necrotizing fasciitis are emergent conditions treated with surgical excision and HBO. Clostridial myonecrosis is an anaerobic bacterial infection where clostridial toxins cause tissue death in advance of the bacteria. Hyperbaric oxygenation helps to neutralize the effects of the toxins and halts the progression of tissue destruction. Necrotizing fasciitis is an acute bacterial infectious process that may include anaerobic and aerobic bacteria that act synergistically to cause rapid tissue destruction. Using HBO as an adjunct to surgical intervention improves oxygenation and may have a direct effect on anaerobic bacteria, as well as improving neutrophil activity.

Chronic osteomyelitis occurs when repeated attempts of standard interventions have failed. It is thought that HBO improves available oxygen at the bone site to improve leukocyte killing ability through oxidative mechanisms. In addition, antibiotic activity may be enhanced. It is also thought that osteoclastic activity and osteogenesis are improved with the use of HBO.

Delayed radiation injury results from endarteritis and subsequent tissue hypoxia. There typically is a latent period of at least 6 months before the effects of delayed injury are seen. Injury may not be seen for many years and often is precipitated by injury or surgical procedures. Hyperbaric oxygenation is used prophylactically before oromaxillary surgical procedures to prevent osteoradionecrosis. Soft tissue radiation injuries, including proctitis and cystitis, can be treated with HBO. The rationale for the use of HBO is induction of neovascularization in the irradiated area.

Compromised grafts and flaps benefit from HBO by facilitating increased distance of oxygen diffusion, thereby supporting the ischemic graft or flap. In addition, it now is believed that graft and flap failure may have a component of reperfusion injury that is overcome with the administration of HBO. Hyperbarics is not indicated in uncomplicated grafts or flaps, nor is it indicated in bioengineered tissues.

Hyperbaric oxygenation has been and is being used for many other disease processes and conditions, as outlined in Box 22-2. However, these are currently not recognized by the UHMS as indicated for hyperbaric treatment. In a systematic

---

BOX 22-2 Situations for Hyperbaric Oxygen Therapy Under Investigation

- Acute myocardial infarction
- Acute cerebrovascular accident
- Closed head injury
- Spinal cord injury
- Sickle cell crisis
- Rheumatic diseases
- Migraine/cluster headache
- Multiple sclerosis
- Radiation cystitis/proctitis
- Human immunodeficiency virus/acquired immunodeficiency syndrome
- Cerebral palsy
- Autism
- Bell palsy
- Fibromyalgia
- Traumatic brain injury
- Posttraumatic stress disorder
- Insulin resistance
- Near-drowning/anoxic brain injury
- Crohn's disease
- Ulcerative colitis
- Preconditioning before vascular surgery (diabetics)

---

review of the literature, the WOCN® Society (2010) concluded there is insufficient evidence to support the use of HBO in the treatment of pressure ulcers.

CONTRAINDICATIONS

Rigorous assessment of the patient must be completed to rule out contraindications to hyperbaric therapy (Box 22-3). Any air-filled cavity must be assessed. The gas law described by Boyle states that as pressure increases, volume decreases, and

---

BOX 22-3 Contraindications to Hyperbaric Oxygen Therapy

Absolute Contraindications
- Untreated pneumothorax
- History of bleomycin
- Adriamycin
- Disulfiram
- Cis-platinum
- Sulfamylon (mafenide acetate)

Relative Contraindications
- Pregnancy
- Upper respiratory infection
- Emphysema with CO_2 retention
- Hyperthermia
- Seizure disorder
- Spherocytosis
- History of spontaneous pneumothorax
- History of optic neuritis
- History of surgery for otosclerosis

---

vice versa. This guides the practitioner to assess air-filled body cavities, such as ears and sinus cavities, and the patient's ability to equalize pressure to prevent barotrauma. A chest x-ray examination will rule out trapping of air in the lungs. Patients with a history of seizure activity should be assessed for seizure control. Hyperbaric treatment is absolutely contraindicated for patients who have a history of receiving bleomycin because of its lifelong increased risk for oxygen toxicity. Hyperbaric treatment also is contraindicated for patients receiving cis-platinum, mafenide acetate (Sulfamylon), or disulfiram. Chemotherapeutic medications that generate oxygen-free radicals, such as cyclophosphamide and the anthracyclines daunorubicin and doxorubicin, are contraindicated with hyperbaric oxygen therapy (Dougherty, 2013). Another absolute contraindication is an untreated pneumothorax. Relative contraindications to hyperbaric treatment include pregnancy, known malignancy, emphysema, pneumonia, bronchitis, and hyperthermia (Foster, 1992; Heimbach, 1998).

PROTOCOLS AND CLINICAL APPLICATION

Hyperbaric treatment protocols depend on the specific disease process. The UHMS has outlined acceptable protocols for hyperbaric exposure. However, this does not preclude physician preference and individualization to meet the patient's needs. Typically, a patient will receive a daily hyperbaric exposure five to seven times per week. The treatment will last for 90 minutes at 2.0 to 2.5 ATA. The patient generally receives 40 to 60 treatments. Continuous assessment of the patient's progress assists the physician in determining when the maximum benefit from HBO therapy has been reached (Gesell, 2008).

Staff Education and Certification

The UHMS and the American College of Hyperbaric Medicine (ACHM) offer certification and a method for physicians to set themselves apart as hyperbaric specialists (ACHM, 2009). The American Board of Medical Specialties offers an examination for hyperbaric medicine that requires completion of a fellowship in hyperbaric medicine (after a grandfather period expired in 2004). The Baromedical Nurses Association (BNA) provides guidance for providing nursing care in the hyperbaric environment. Nurses may obtain national certification in hyperbaric nursing through the Baromedical Nurses Association Certification Board (BNACB), an association that promotes the status and standards of baromedical nursing practice. Three levels of certification are available, depending on practice participation and educational background (BNA, 2009).

Methods and Chambers

To achieve a hyperbaric state, the patient is placed into either a monoplace chamber or a multiplace chamber. The monoplace chamber (Figure 22-1) has rapidly become the predominant chamber seen in outpatient settings. A monoplace chamber typically is compressed with oxygen. These chambers are rated for a maximum clinical pressurization of 44 psi, or 3 ATA. The

FIGURE 22-1 HBO Sechrist 3200 monoplace chamber. (Courtesy Sechrist Industries, Anaheim, Calif., USA.)

FIGURE 22-3 HBO Gulf Coast Multiplace Chamber, inside view. (Courtesy Gulf Coast Hyperbarics, Inc., Panama City, Fla., USA.)

major advantage of using monoplace chambers is that they are relatively inexpensive. The chamber can be placed anywhere an adequate gas supply is available and can be housed in most areas without significant construction costs. Another advantage is that the monoplace chamber can be staffed by either a nurse or technician and a physician. Current reimbursement guidelines dictate that a physician must be available for the duration of a hyperbaric treatment.

Disadvantages of the monoplace chamber include the lack of direct patient contact and the difficulty involved in monitoring the patient other than visually. Methods are available to monitor electrocardiogram, arterial blood pressure, pulmonary artery pressure, wedge pressure, central venous pressure, cuff blood pressure, temperature, and transcutaneous partial pressure of oxygen ($TcPO_2$) monitoring. It also is possible to ventilate a patient in the monoplace chamber; however, most hyperbaric chambers that are integrated within an outpatient wound care clinic do not have the ability to provide support to the critically ill patient.

The multiplace chamber (Figures 22-2 and 22-3) allows a caregiver to enter the chamber with the patient. The caregiver, or *tender*, may be a technician, nurse, or physician. The multiplace chamber can accommodate multiple patients in a single treatment, or *dive*. The number of patients who can be treated simultaneously depends on the size of the chamber and whether the patients are ambulatory or chair-bound or bed-bound. The multiplace chamber can easily be equipped to handle the critically ill. The critically ill patient can be monitored the same as in the monoplace chamber. To breathe oxygen, the patient wears either a mask or a hood. The major disadvantages of the multiplace chamber are the cost and the housing of the chamber. The American Society of Mechanical Engineers (ASME) provides standards for pressure vessels for human occupancy (PVHO-2). The National Fire Protection Association (NFPA, 2002) sets forth construction requirements for the physical structure containing the chamber. A disadvantage of the multiplace chamber is the need to abort a multioccupant dive if a patient is unable to equalize pressure during pressurization. A final consideration of the multiplace chamber is staffing. The multiplace chamber requires a greater expenditure for staff than does the monoplace chamber. The multiplace chamber is staffed with a chamber operator, tender, nurse, and physician.

Patient Preparation and Safety

Two factors dictate the need to follow rigorous procedures for patient preparation and patient safety. The first factor is the nature of hyperbarics (i.e., atmospheric pressure changes). Patient instruction should include air equalization techniques to prevent aural or sinus barotrauma. The patient should be instructed not to hold his or her breath during ascent to prevent pneumothorax. The caregiver responsible for assessing the patient before treatment should assess breath sounds to prevent exposing the patient with compromised pulmonary status to the hyperbaric environment. A random blood sugar measurement before treatment should be obtained for all patients with diabetes because HBO can significantly lower blood sugar levels. Vital signs are obtained to assess for hypertension and hyperthermia. Hyperbaric oxygenation is a potent vasoconstrictor and can predispose the patient to a hypertensive crisis; an oral temperature greater than 102° F (38.9° C) predisposes the patient to an oxygen toxicity seizure.

The second factor affecting patient preparation and safety is the pressurized high-oxygen environment. This is significant in any hyperbaric environment and is of extreme importance when the patient is pressurized in a 100% oxygen environment. This situation poses a significant fire safety issue. In May 2009,

FIGURE 22-2 HBO Gulf Coast Multiplace Chamber, outside view. (Courtesy Gulf Coast Hyperbarics, Inc., Panama City, Fla., USA.)

a chamber fire occurred at the Ocean Hyperbaric Oxygen Neurologic Center, a free-standing hyperbaric facility in Lauderdale-by-the Sea, Florida. The hyperbaric facility specialized in neurologic applications of hyperbaric oxygen for the treatment of conditions including stroke, brain injury, cerebral palsy, and multiple sclerosis. The fire resulted in the deaths of a 62-year-old woman and her 4-year-old grandson who was receiving treatment for cerebral palsy. Neither the grandmother or the grandchild died in the fire, but died later as a result of burn injuries received due to a spark from static electricity; the patient and the grandmother who was accompanying the grandson in the chamber were not wearing a grounding bracelet to dissipate static electricity (Ortega, 2009; Roustan, 2012). Patients should be instructed not to use products that have a petroleum or alcohol base before they go into the chamber. Checklist 22-1 provides a list of materials banned in the hyperbaric chamber. Cosmetic products such as hair spray, hair creams, lotions, petroleum jelly, deodorants, and perfumes must be removed before treatment. All skin care products pose a risk and should be removed before treatment. Only cotton linens and clothing are allowed into the chamber to decrease spark potential. Prosthetics, including hearing aids, should be removed. Although glasses, contact lenses, and dentures are not absolutely contraindicated in the hyperbaric environment, they should be removed if the patient is at risk for seizure activity or has an altered mental condition (Hart, 1995; Larson-Lohr and Norvell, 2002; Weaver and Straas, 1991).

Side Effects

The most common side effect or complication of HBO is claustrophobia. Patients who experience claustrophobia should be reassured, and a tender should be present and in contact with the patient at all times. In the multiplace chamber, the tender can offer direct physical comfort. In the monoplace chamber, the tender should maintain both visual

and verbal contact with the patient. Benzodiazepines offer relief of claustrophobia in most cases. Occasionally, a treatment is aborted and subsequent hyperbaric therapy is discontinued as a result of claustrophobia.

Aural barotrauma, referred to as an *ear squeeze,* will manifest as ear pain and may result in a hematoma to the tympanic membrane, hemorrhage in the middle ear, or tympanic rupture. If a patient experiences an ear squeeze, a myringotomy, or placement of pressure equalization tubes, may be necessary. Sinus barotrauma, or sinus squeeze, results in extreme sinus pain and may lead to hemorrhage of the sinus. The patient who comes for a hyperbaric treatment and has a congested nasal passage may benefit from nasal decongestant sprays before the treatment. Oral decongestants may be indicated for a more long-term approach (Capes and Tomaszewski, 1996; Kidder, 1995; Vrabec et al, 1998).

Visual acuity changes during hyperbaric therapy are not rare. Myopia may worsen after 20 or more hyperbaric exposures. Frequently, a patient who uses glasses to correct presbyopia will find that he or she is able to read without corrective lenses. The exact mechanism behind these visual changes is not known. The patient who experiences a visual change should be instructed not to change prescription eyewear for 2 to 3 months after hyperbaric treatment because the visual change usually is temporary (Maki, 1996).

A physiologic anomaly, breath holding, or cessation of respiration can cause air to be trapped in the lungs. This trapped air can lead to a tension pneumothorax. Should this occur in a multiplace chamber, the patient can be recompressed and the pneumothorax corrected within the chamber before decompression of the chamber. In a monoplace environment, the patient should be recompressed to treatment depth until supplies, equipment, and personnel are available. Once the team and supplies are assembled, the patient should be decompressed and treated immediately upon removal from the chamber.

Seizure activity from oxygen toxicity, although ominous in appearance, is self-limiting and benign. The patient in the monoplace environment should be maintained at pressure until seizure activity has stopped. If the patient is breathing oxygen by mask or hood, the oxygen should be stopped and the patient placed on air. Once the seizure has stopped, the patient can be removed from the chamber. Generally, no further precautions or anticonvulsant medications are necessary for subsequent treatments. Patients with a known history of seizure or who are predisposed to seizure activity would benefit from periodic, scheduled discontinuation of oxygen breathing (air breaks) during the treatment (Clark, 1995).

TOPICAL OXYGEN IS NOT HBO

Various methods for providing topical oxygen have been created, including plastic chambers over a limb; continuous oxygen flow through a battery-operated system or a reservoir within a bandage; and gas dissolved or saturated within saline, gel, or foam (Hopf et al, 2006). Topical oxygen at the wound surface has been shown to enhance cytokine production and

---

CHECKLIST 22-1 Materials Banned from the Hyperbaric Chamber

- ✓ Cosmetic products, including the following:
  - • Hair spray
  - • Hair cream
  - • Skin care products, including lotions and barrier ointments
  - • Deodorant
  - • Perfume
  - • Lipstick
  - • Fingernail polish
- ✓ Petrolatum and products containing petrolatum and paraffin
- ✓ Mineral oil and products containing mineral oil
- ✓ Dressing products containing synthetic fibers (e.g., nylon)
- ✓ Elastic products (e.g., compression wraps)
- ✓ Any device with a battery (e.g., hearing aid)
- ✓ Dentures if patient at risk for seizure activity
- ✓ All jewelry
- ✓ Magnesium eyeglass frames

wound healing in normal animal studies (Fries et al, 2005). A limited number of case studies and clinical series suggest a benefit of topical oxygen in the treatment of a variety of ulcers (Edsberg et al, 2002; Gordillo and Sen, 2003; Heng et al, 2000a, 2000b; Kalliainen et al, 2003). However, until further rigorous studies are performed, there is insufficient evidence to recommend topical oxygen for the treatment of wounds (EPUAP, NPUAP, PPPIA, 2014; Hopf et al, 2006; Robson et al, 2006; WOCN®, 2010).

Published information related to topical oxygen can be confusing when the modality is inaccurately labeled topical hyperbaric oxygen (THBO). Topical therapy literature further confuses the consumer by using HBO to demonstrate its value. In fact, topical oxygen therapy is not HBO; the route of delivery and the mode of action are different. It is important to distinguish between the two modalities in order to clarify the discussion of efficacy (Hopf et al, 2006) and reimbursement; topical oxygen is not reimbursed for wound management (CMS, 2002).

Topical oxygen may produce transient, slight elevations in ambient pressure applied to the wound (as high as 1.03 ATA). The degree of pressure that can be applied is significantly limited by the possibility of occluding arterial inflow or venous outflow with high pressure. In contrast, HBO (systemic) is defined medically as the application of pressures greater than atmospheric to a patient who is entirely enclosed within the pressurized chamber, at pressures of 1.5 to 6 ATA (generally 2 to 3 ATA for wound-healing indications) (Hopf et al, 2006).

CLINICAL CONSULT

A: 55-year-old male referred to wound clinic by provider for small right hip wound after falling 15 feet off a ladder at home. No significant medical history except an inguinal hernia repair 2 years ago. Patient admits to being intoxicated when he fell. Right hip wound 1x1 cm, 0.5 cm depth, 6 cm tunnel at 6 o'clock, 6 cm of periwound erythema with a grey hue, mild edema and 1x1 cm bulla. Oral temperature is 102° F. Patient states it was only just a little when he saw his provider 2 days ago. Pain was 4/10 yesterday now 9/10 today.

D: Right hip wound infection suspicious of necrotizing fasciitis.
P: Urgent referral to ED to rule out necrotizing fasciitis. Pain management.
I: (1) Applied gauze dressing moistened with Dakin's solution, covered with ABD. (2) Transferred to ED; called ahead to alert staff of need for urgent pain control, surgical consult, and probable admission to hospital.
E: Patient verbalizes understanding of plan and called his wife to meet him in the ED. Will follow up with ED. If admitted, will arrange a low air loss pressure redistribution mattress.

SUMMARY

Oxygen is a powerful and versatile agent used in many aspects of medicine. The therapeutic use of oxygen under pressure has been used for many years for multiple medical conditions, including wound healing. Hyperoxygenation of tissue, vasoconstriction, downregulation of inflammatory cytokines, upregulation of growth factors, and antibacterial effects of HBO can benefit patients with specific wound types. As with other biophysical modalities used in wound care today, more research is needed before expanding the list of indications.

REFERENCES

American College of Hyperbaric Medicine (ACHM): *Certification*, February 2, 2009. http://www.hyperbaricmedicine.org. Accessed April 2, 2009.

Asamoto S, Sugiyama H, Doi H, et al: Hyperbaric oxygen (HBO) therapy for acute traumatic cervical spinal cord injury, *Spinal Cord* 38(9):538–540, 2000.

Baromedical Nurses Association (BNA): *The certification process for registered nurses in the hyperbaric field*, March 4, 2009. http://www.hyperbaricnurses.org/certification.html. Accessed March 4, 2009.

Broussard CL: Hyperbaric oxygenation and wound healing, *J Wound Ostomy Continence Nurs* 30(4):210–216, 2003.

Capes JP, Tomaszewski C: Prophylaxis against middle ear barotrauma in U.S. hyperbaric oxygen therapy centers, *Am J Emerg Med* 14(7):645–648, 1996.

Centers for Medicare and Medicaid Services (CMS): *Coverage of hyperbaric oxygen (HBO) therapy for the treatment of diabetic wounds of the lower extremities (Program memorandum intermediaries/carriers, Transmittal AB-02-183)*, Washington, DC, December 27, 2002, Department of Health and Human Services. http://www.cms.gov/transmittals/downloads/AB02183.pdf.

Centers for Medicare and Medicaid Services (CMS): *National coverage determination (NCD) for hyperbaric oxygen therapy (20.29) (Publication no. 100-3), Manual section no. 20.29*, Vol. 3, 2006. http://www.cms.gov/medicare-coverage-database.

Cianci P, Sato R: Adjunctive hyperbaric oxygen therapy in the treatment of thermal burns: a review, *Burns* 20(1):5–14, 1994.

Clark JM: Oxygen toxicity. In Kindwall EP, editor: *Hyperbaric medicine practice*, Flagstaff, AZ, 1995, Best.

Dauwe PB, Pulikkottil BJ, Lavery L, et al: Does hyperbaric oxygen therapy work in facilitating acute wound healing: a systematic review, *Plast Reconstr Surg* 133(2):208e–215e, 2014.

Dougherty JE: The role of hyperbaric oxygen therapy in crush injuries. *Critical Care Nursing Quarterly* 36(3):299–309, 2013.

Edsberg LE, Brogan MS, Jaynes CD, et al: Topical hyperbaric oxygen and electrical stimulation: exploring potential synergy, *Ostomy Wound Manage* 48(11):42–50, 2002.

Elliott DH: Decompression sickness. In Kindwall EP, editor: *Hyperbaric medicine practice*, Flagstaff, AZ, 1995, Best.

Eskes A, Ubbink D, Lubbers M, et al: Hyperbaric oxygen therapy for treating acute surgical and traumatic wounds, *Cochrane Database Syst Rev* 10:CD008059.

Fife CE, Buyukcakir C, Otto GH, et al: The predictive value of transcutaneous oxygen tension measurement in diabetic lower extremity ulcers treated with hyperbaric oxygen therapy: a retrospective analysis of 1144 patients, *Wound Repair Regen* 10:198–207, 2002.

Foster JH: Hyperbaric oxygen treatment contraindications and complications, *J Maxillofac Surg* 50(10):1081–1086, 1992.

Fries RB, Wallace WA, Roy S, et al: Dermal excisional wound healing in pigs following treatment with topically applied pure oxygen, *Mutat Res* 579(1-2):172–181, 2005.

Gesell LB: *Hyperbaric oxygen therapy indications*, ed 12, Durham, NC, 2008, Undersea and Hyperbaric Medical Society.

Gordillo GM, Sen CK: Revisiting the essential role of oxygen in wound healing, *Am J Surg* 186(3):259–263, 2003.

Hammarlund C: The physiologic effects of hyperbaric oxygen. In Kindwall EP, editor: *Hyperbaric medicine practice*, Flagstaff, AZ, 1995, Best.

Hart GB: The monoplace chamber. In Kindwall EP, editor: *Hyperbaric medicine practice*, Flagstaff, AZ, 1995, Best.

Heimbach RD: Physiology and pharmacology of HBO2. In Jefferson C, editor: *Davis Wound Care and Hyperbaric Medicine Center [Course]*, San Antonio, TX, March 4, 1998, Hyperbaric Medicine Team Training, Southwest Texas Methodist Hospital and Nix Medical Center.

Heng MCY, Harker J, Bardakjian VB, et al: Enhanced healing and cost effectiveness of low pressure oxygen therapy in healing necrotic wounds: a feasibility study of technology transfer, *Ostomy Wound Manage* 46(3):52–62, 2000a.

Heng MCY, Harker J, Csathy G, et al: Angiogenesis in necrotic ulcers treated with hyperbaric oxygen, *Ostomy Wound Manage* 46(9):18–32, 2000b.

Hopf HW, Ueno C, Aslam R, et al: Guidelines for the treatment of arterial insufficiency ulcers, *Wound Repair Regen* 14(6):693–710, 2006.

Kalliainen LK, Gordillo GM, Schlanger R, et al: Topical oxygen as an adjunct to wound healing: a clinical case series, *Pathophysiology* 9(2):81–87, 2003.

Kidder TM: Myringotomy. In Kindwall EP, editor: *Hyperbaric medicine practice*, Flagstaff, AZ, 1995, Best.

Kindwall EP: A history of hyperbaric medicine. In Kindwall EP, editor: *Hyperbaric medicine practice*, Flagstaff, AZ, 1995, Best.

Kranke P, Bennett MH, Martyn-St. James M, et al: Hyperbaric oxygen for chronic wounds, *Cochrane Database of Syst Rev* 4:CD004123, 2012.

Larson-Lohr V, Norvell H, editors: *Hyperbaric nursing*, Flagstaff, AZ, 2002, Best.

Latham E: Hyperbaric oxygen therapy, *Medscape*, 2013. Updated: Dec 19, 2014 available at http://emedicine.medscape.com/article/1464149-overview#a2. Accessed Aug. 14, 2015.

Löndahl M: Hyperbaric oxygen therapy as treatment of diabetic foot ulcers, *Diabetes Metab Res Rev* 28(Suppl 1):78–84, 2012.

Maki RD: Ophthalmic side effects of hyperbaric oxygen therapy, *Insight* 21(4):114–117, 1996.

Marx RE: Radiation injury to tissue. In Kindwall EP, editor: *Hyperbaric medicine practice*, Flagstaff, AZ, 1995, Best.

National Fire Protection Association: *NFPA 99: standard for health care facilities*, Quincy, MA, 2002, NFPA.

National Pressure Ulcer Advisory Panel (NPUAP), European Pressure Ulcer Advisory Panel (EPUAP) and Pan Pacific Pressure Injury Alliance (PPPIA): *Prevention and Treatment of Pressure Ulcers: Clinical Practice Guideline*. In Emily, editor: Perth, Australia, 2014, Cambridge Media.

Norgren L, Hiatt WR, Dormandy JA, et al: Inter-Society Consensus for the Management of Peripheral Arterial Disease (TASC II), *J Vasc Surg* 45(Suppl S):S5–S67, 2007.

Ortega J: Child in blast dies from injuries, *Sun Sentinel* June 12, 2009. http://articles.sun-sentinel.com/2009-06-12/news/0906110581_1_hyperbaric-italian-boy-boy-s-family. Accessed January 3, 2014.

Robson MC, Cooper DM, Aslam R, et al: Guidelines for the treatment of venous ulcers, *Wound Repair Regen* 14(6):649–662, 2006.

Roustan WK: Two charged in deadly 2009 hyperbaric chamber fire, *Sun Sentinel* April 25, 2012. http://articles.sun-sentinel.com/2012-04-25/news/fl-hyperbaric-chamber-deaths-0426-20120425_1_francesco-martinisi-hyperbaric-clinic-pure-oxygen. Accessed 8-14-2015.

Steed DL, Attinger C, Colaizzi T, et al: Guidelines for the treatment of diabetic ulcers, *Wound Repair Regen* 14(6):680–692, 2006.

Undersea and Hyperbaric Medical Society (UHMS): *Hyperbaric oxygen therapy: a committee report*, Kensington, MD, 1996, UHMS.

Undersea and Hyperbaric Medical Society (UHMS): *About the UHMS*. https://www.uhms.org/about/about-the-uhms.html. Accessed May 11, 2015.

Undersea and Hyperbaric Medical Society (UHMS): *Indications for hyperbaric oxygen therapy*, 2015. https://www.uhms.org/resources/hbo-indications.html. Accessed May 11, 2015.

Vrabec JT, Clements KS, Mader JT: Short-term tympanostomy in conjunction with hyperbaric oxygen therapy, *Laryngoscope* 108(8):1124–1128, 1998.

Weaver LK, Straas MB, editors: *Monoplace hyperbaric chamber safety guidelines: report to the Hyperbaric Chamber Safety Committee of the Undersea and Hyperbaric Medical Society*, Kensington, MD, 1991, UHMS.

Wound, Ostomy and Continence Nurses Society™ (WOCN®): *Guideline for management of patients with lower extremity neuropathic disease (WOCN® clinical practice guideline series no. 1)*, Glenview, IL, 2004, WOCN®.

Wound, Ostomy and Continence Nurses Society™ (WOCN®): *Guideline for management of patients with lower extremity arterial disease (WOCN® clinical practice guideline series no. 1)*, Glenview, IL, 2008, WOCN®.

Wound, Ostomy and Continence Nurses Society™ (WOCN®): *Guideline for the prevention and management of pressure ulcers (WOCN® clinical practice guideline series no. 2)*, Glenview, IL, 2010, WOCN®.

23

Electrical Stimulation

Rita A. Frantz

OBJECTIVES

1. Explain the physiologic effects of electrical stimulation.
2. List at least two indications for electrical stimulation.

3. List at least two contraindications for electrical stimulation.

Electrical stimulation is a physical wound care modality that uses the transfer of electrical current to tissues to support wound healing. Devices used for wound-healing applications consist of a source of electrical current, a minimum of two wires or leads, and their corresponding electrodes (Figure 23-1). One lead is connected to the negative jack of the device and is the source of negatively charged electrons in an electrical circuit; this is referred to as the *cathode*. The other is connected to a positive jack on the device that serves as an electron depository for the flow of electrons in the electrical circuit; this is called the *anode*. Electrodes are attached to the patient end of the wires and placed on either the patient's wound bed or the adjacent skin. When the device is operating, a unidirectional current flows through this circuit, causing positively charged ions (Na^+, K^+, H^+) in the tissues and positively charged cells (activated neutrophils and fibroblasts) to migrate toward the cathode; negatively charged ions (Cl^-, HCO_3^- P^- and negatively charged cells (epidermal, neutrophils, and macrophages) migrate toward the anode. To understand the basis of electrical stimulation as an adjunctive therapy for wounds, it is important to understand several terms. Table 23-1 provides definitions of relevant terms.

EFFECTS OF ELECTRICAL STIMULATION

In an effort to examine the entire body of evidence on electrical stimulation and chronic wound healing, Gardner et al (1999) conducted a metaanalysis of 15 studies that assessed the efficacy of electrical stimulation. Studies included in the metaanalysis were limited to randomized controlled trials (n = 9) and nonrandom controlled trials (n = 6). Metaanalysis procedures were applied to a total of 24 electrical stimulation samples (n = 591 wounds) and 15 control wound samples (n = 212). The calculated average rate of healing for the electrical stimulation samples was 22% per week compared with 9% for the control samples. The net effect of electrical stimulation therapy was 13% per week, a 144% increase over the control rate. These data provide substantive evidence that electrical stimulation can produce substantial improvement in the healing of chronic wounds. The physiologic effects of electrical stimulation that contribute to its wound-healing efficacy include galvanotaxic, stimulatory, antibacterial, blood flow, and tissue oxygenation.

The underlying physiologic effects of electrical stimulation are mediated by the endogenous bioelectric system in the human body and its response to positive and negative polarity. Several investigators have demonstrated the existence of transepithelial potentials on the skin surface (Barker et al, 1982; Illingsworth and Barker, 1980). These transepithelial potentials arise from Na channels on the mucosal surface of the skin that allow Na to diffuse from the area surrounding epidermal cells to the inside of the cells. As a result of the movement of Na from the skin surface to the interior of epidermal cells, the exterior of the skin maintains a variable level of negative electrical charge (Foulds and Barker, 1983). Jaffe and Vanable (1984) demonstrated that when the epidermis is injured, current flows as ions are transmitted through the tissue fluid between the damaged regions of the epidermis. This "current of injury" has a positive polarity, whereas the adjacent intact skin retains its negative polarity, producing a unidirectional force sufficient to attract reparative cells to the wound bed during the inflammatory and proliferative phases of healing (Vanable, 1989). Once reepithelialization has closed the wound, the current of injury disappears, suggesting that it does not play a role in the remodeling phase of healing. It is important to note that the flow of current out of the wound is blocked if the wound bed is allowed to desiccate and form a scab (Alvarez et al, 1983).

Galvanotaxic Effects

Positively and negatively charged cells are attracted toward an electric field of opposite polarity, a process termed *galvanotaxis*. Multiple in vitro studies have established that cells essential to tissue repair will migrate toward the anode or cathode created by an electric field within a tissue culture (Bourguignon and Bourguignon, 1987; Eberhardt et al, 1986; Orida and Feldman, 1982; Stromberg, 1988). Preliminary

FIGURE 23-1 Example of a high-voltage pulsed current electrical stimulation device. (Courtesy Rich-Mar Corporation, Inola, Okla., USA.)

evidence from in vivo studies has demonstrated that electrical stimulation creates a similar galvanotaxic response. Eberhardt et al (1986) showed that treating wounds with electrical stimulation for 30 minutes increased the relative number of neutrophils in the wound exudate compared with control wounds. Using the pig model, Mertz et al (1993) treated experimentally induced wounds with two 30-minute sessions of monophasic pulsed current (PC) using varying polarity. They found that wounds initially treated with negative polarity (day 0) followed by positive polarity on days 1 to 7 showed 20% greater epithelialization compared with wounds that received only one type of polarity. In the wounds treated by alternating polarity daily (negative one day, positive the next), epithelialization was limited by 45%. Although the influence of polarity on cell migration in human wounds remains to be elucidated more completely, these findings suggest that bioelectric signals play a role in facilitating the phases of healing.

Stimulatory Effects on Cells

Basic science studies have shown that electrical current has a stimulatory effect on fibroblasts. Using the pig model, Cruz et al (1989) demonstrated the presence of significantly more fibroblasts in burn wounds treated with electrical stimulation than in controls. Alvarez et al (1983), also using the pig model, documented more fibroblasts and increased collagen synthesis in partial-thickness wounds, thus substantiating previous findings. Castillo et al (1995) found significant increases in collagen density with burn wounds in the rat model. The stimulatory effect of electrical current on fibroblasts, reported by Bourguignon and Bourguignon (1987), was observed when fibroblasts in culture increased DNA and protein (including collagen) synthesis in response to electrical stimulation. This effect was most noticeable near the negative electrode.

TABLE 23-1	**Terms and Definitions for Electrical Stimulation**
Terms	**Definitions**
Alternating current	Uninterrupted, bidirectional current flow
Amperage	Measure of rate of flow of current; expressed as amperes (A), milliamperes (mA), or microamperes (μA)
Amplitude	Maximum (peak) excursion of voltage or current pulse
Charge	Property of matter determined by proportion of electrons (negatively charged particles) contained by the matter; substance may be neutral, positively charged, or negatively charged; measured in units of coulombs (C) or microcoulombs (μC)
Current	Rate of flow of charged particles (ions or electrons); measured in units of amperes (A) or milliamperes (mA)
Direct current	Uninterrupted, unidirectional current flow
Frequency	Number of pulses delivered per unit of time; also termed *pulse rate;* frequency is the reciprocal of cycle time; usually measured as pulses per second (pps) or hertz (Hz); 0.1 Hz is on for 10 seconds, and a pulse of 1000 Hz is on for 1 ms
Interpulse interval	Time between pulses when no voltage is applied and no current is flowing
Polarity	Property of possessing two oppositely charged electrodes in an electrical circuit (positive and negative); negative electrode (cathode) provides electrons in a circuit; positive electrode (anode) serves as depository to which electrons flow
Pulse duration	Time during which current is flowing
Voltage	Measure of force of flow of electrons through a conductor (wound tissue) between two or more electrodes; created by difference of charges between two electrodes (one with excess in relation to the other); electrodes are polarized in comparison to each other (negative electrode and positive electrode)
Waveform	Graphic representation of current flow; may be monophasic (current that deviates from isoelectric zero line in one direction and then returns to baseline) or biphasic (current that deviates above and below isoelectric zero line); may be symmetric or asymmetric

Blood Flow and Tissue Oxygen Effects

Accumulating evidence indicates that electrical stimulation exerts a positive influence on blood flow and localized tissue oxygen. Hecker et al (1985) showed that negative polarity increased blood flow in the upper extremity as measured by plethysmography. In a sample of patients diagnosed with Raynaud disease and diabetic polyneuropathy, Kaada (1982) demonstrated that application of distant, low-frequency, transcutaneous electrical stimulation (TENS) produced pronounced and prolonged cutaneous vasodilation. Using skin temperature as a measurement of peripheral vasodilation, Kaada found a rise in the temperature of ischemic extremities from 71.6° F to 75.2° F (22° C to 24° C) to 87.8° F to 93.2° F (31° C to 34° C). The latency from stimulus onset to the abrupt rise in temperature averaged 15 to 30 minutes with a duration of response ranging from 4 to 6 hours. Kaada (1983) subsequently reported successful treatment of 10 patients with 19 leg ulcers, previously resistant to treatment, by applying a TENS device to the web space between the first and second metacarpals of the ipsilateral wrist. Using the burst mode, Kaada delivered 15 to 30 mA of pulsed direct current by the cathode for 30 to 34 minutes three times per day. He proposed that the remote application of electrical stimulation enhanced microcirculation in the tissues of the ipsilateral lower extremity, as demonstrated by the increase in toe temperature and ulcer healing. Based on findings from subsequent basic research, Kaada suggested that the improvement in tissue microcirculation was the result of activation of a central serotonergic link that inhibits sympathetic vasoconstriction (Kaada and Helle, 1984; Kaada et al, 1984).

Additional evidence of increased blood flow in wounds treated with electrical stimulation is provided by reports of increasing capillary density after implementation of this therapy. Fifteen venous leg ulcers, previously resistant to healing, were treated for 30 minutes daily for an average of 38 days (Jünger et al, 1997). Using light microscopy to measure capillary density, they found densities increased from a prestimulation baseline of 8.05 capillaries/mm^2 to 11.55 capillaries/mm^2 after stimulation ($p < .039$). Transcutaneous oxygen in the periwound skin was noted to increase from 13.5 to 24.7 mm Hg.

Although research on the effects of electrical stimulation on wound oxygenation has been minimal, preliminary studies demonstrate that cutaneous oxygen can be improved with electrical stimulation. In separate studies, investigators showed that application of electrical stimulation improved cutaneous oxygen in the lower extremity of elderly patients, subjects with diabetes, and patients with spinal cord injuries (Gagnier et al, 1988; Peters et al, 1998). These works provide indirect evidence of the potential for electrical stimulation to increase wound oxygenation.

Antibacterial Effects

Evidence indicates that electrical stimulation has bacteriostatic and bactericidal effects on microorganisms that are known to infect chronic wounds (Daeschlein, 2007). In a study of 20 patients with burn wounds that had been unresponsive to conventional therapy for 3 months to 2 years, Fakhri and Amin (1987) showed a quantitatively lower level of organisms after treatment for 10-minute intervals twice weekly. This decrease in bacterial count was accompanied by epithelialization of the wound margins within 3 days of beginning electrical stimulation. Although the mechanism underlying the bactericidal or bacteriostatic effects remains unclear, the galvanotaxic effect on macrophages and neutrophils has been implicated (Eberhardt et al, 1986; Orida and Feldman, 1982). These studies suggest that the anodal attraction of neutrophils to tissue with high bacterial levels may be a primary mode of action, rather than destruction of pathogens by electrolysis or elevation of tissue pH. However, these studies used direct current, which is not as commonly used in wound management as the PC type (see section on types of electrical stimulation). It appears that the voltage required to produce an antibacterial effect with PC would create profound muscle contractions and therefore would not be applicable in clinical practice (Guffey and Asmussen, 1989; Kincaid and Lavoie, 1989; Szuminsky et al, 1994).

INDICATIONS AND CONTRAINDICATIONS

The U.S. Food and Drug Administration (FDA) has not yet approved any type of electrical stimulation device for wound healing. Consequently, devices cannot be marketed for this indication, although they can be marketed for other already approved indications, such as edema and pain, and subsequently used as an off-label treatment of wound healing.

Among national guidelines disseminated by professional societies dedicated to wound care, recommendations related to electrical stimulation as therapy for chronic wounds vary considerably. The Wound, Ostomy and Continence Nurses Society™ (2010) reports electrical stimulation as being effective in enhancing the healing of recalcitrant Stage II pressure ulcers and the healing of Stage III and IV pressure ulcers. In separate guidelines on treatment of pressure ulcers, diabetic foot ulcers, venous ulcers, and arterial ulcers, the Wound Healing Society states that electrical stimulation may be useful as adjuvant therapy to promote healing, but the society stops short of making specific recommendations for its use (Hopf et al, 2006; Robson et al, 2006; Steed, 2006; Whitney, 2006). International guidelines on pressure ulcer treatment report sufficient evidence exists to support the use of electromagnetic agents, including electrical stimulation, in the management of recalcitrant Stage II, as well as Stage III and IV pressure ulcers (NPUAP-EPUAP, PPPIA, 2014).

As is the case with most therapies, certain contraindications apply to the use of electrical stimulation (Checklist 23-1). It should not be used when basal or squamous cell carcinoma is suspected in the wound or surrounding tissue or when osteomyelitis is present. Patients with electronic implants, such as pacemakers, should not be treated with electrical stimulation.

Electrical stimulation is also contraindicated for use over the heart or when iodine or silver ion residues are present in the wound.

TYPES OF ELECTRICAL STIMULATION

Although several electrotherapy modalities are cited in the literature, the two basic types of electrical current are direct current and alternating current. In general, alternating current is not used for wound treatment and is not described in this chapter. Direct current (DC) is characterized as continuous and monophasic (unidirectional) in which the voltage does not vary with time. The parameters used to stimulate wound healing typically are 200 to 300 μA at a low voltage ($<100\,V$). The polarity that is selected determines the direction of current flow delivered to the wound tissue, with positively charged ions migrating toward the negative electrode (cathode) and negatively charged ions migrating toward the positive electrode (anode). Small, older clinical trials have demonstrated benefits from the use of DC with chronic wounds (Carley and Wainapel, 1985; Gault and Gatens, 1976). However, charged ions of Na^+ and Cl^- in the wound tissue move toward the cathode and anode, respectively, producing a chemical reaction with caustic end-products at the interface of the electrode and tissue. In the case of the cathode, Na^+ reacts with H_2O to form $NaOH$ and H_2, whereas the anode reacts with Cl^- and H_2O to form HCl and O_2. Even when DC is delivered at therapeutic doses, these products form at the electrode tissue interface, creating acid–base changes. If the dosage of DC is delivered at high amplitude over an extended period, the acid–base changes lead to tissue irritation that varies in intensity from erythema to blistering due to electrochemical burning. This side effect can be diminished to some extent by using current amplitudes in the microamperage (μA) range.

Pulsed Current Electrical Stimulation

Devices used to deliver the DC are also capable of delivering PC, a pattern or flow that has become the predominant type of electrical stimulation used for wound healing. Electrodes placed on the tissues deliver the PC as a series of pulses, with each pulse separated by a period in which no current is flowing. Pulsed current can be visually constructed as a waveform that plots amplitude and time.

Waveform Patterns (Monophasic and Biphasic). Two waveform patterns are available as PC (Figure 23-2). Monophasic (unidirectional) PC is the movement of current in one direction away from the isoelectric zero line. Monophasic (bidirectional) PC has been applied to clinical treatment of wounds using a rectangular waveform (Feedar et al, 1991; Gentzkow et al, 1991, 1993; Jünger et al, 1997) and twin-peak waveform of high voltage (Fitzgerald and Newsome, 1993; Griffin et al, 1991; Kloth and Feedar, 1988). Biphasic PC is the movement of current in two directions on either side of the isoelectric zero line. Biphasic PC is configured as charged particles moving above and below the isoelectric zero line in brief succession. The biphasic waveform may be symmetric or asymmetric with respect to the isoelectric zero line. The biphasic symmetric waveform is characterized by amplitude, duration, and rate of rise and decays of current that are identical in relation to the isoelectric zero line. This creates a balanced electrical charge. In contrast, with the biphasic asymmetric waveform, one or more of these elements of the current are unequal in relation to the isoelectric zero line. This produces waveforms that may be electrically balanced or unbalanced. Both biphasic symmetric (Baker et al, 1996, 1997; Debreceni et al, 1995) and asymmetric (Baker et al, 1996, 1997) waveforms have been studied as a modality for promoting wound healing.

Application and Administration Methods. Regardless of the waveform of PC selected for treatment, the electrodes are applied using one of two methods (Baker et al, 1996; Kloth and Feedar, 1988). The first method involves placing one electrode in direct contact with a clean, electrically conductive material (commonly a saline-moistened gauze dressing) that is positioned in the wound; then the second electrode is placed on intact skin approximately 15 to 30 cm from the wound edge. With the second method, the electrodes are positioned on the skin at the wound edges on opposite sides of the wound. The treatment protocol is similar whether the device is a low-voltage or a high-voltage stimulator. The pulse frequency is set to 100 pulses per second, with a current or voltage sufficient to produce a comfortable tingling sensation or, in insensate skin, at a level just below the motor threshold (Feedar et al, 1991; Gentzkow et al, 1991, 1993; Griffin et al, 1991; Kloth and Feedar, 1988). The polarity is determined by the status of the wound and the specific cells that are to be targeted for migration into the wound (Bourguignon and Bourguignon, 1987). Treatments are administered for 1 hour, 5 to 7 days per week, and are continued as long as the wound is progressing toward closure.

Research identifies a range of electrical charge that has supported positive wound-healing outcomes. This dosage of current, defined in microcoulombs (μC), is between 250 and 500 $\mu C/s$ (Feedar et al, 1991; Gentzkow et al, 1991, 1993; Griffin et al, 1991; Jünger et al, 1997; Kloth and Feedar, 1988). The evolution of electrical stimulation devices led to the evaluation of two different types of PC for treatment of chronic wounds: low-voltage amplitude and high-voltage

FIGURE 23-2 Waveforms used in electrical stimulation. **A,** Direct current. **B,** Monophasic pulsed current. **C,** Monophasic high-voltage pulsed current. **D,** Symmetric biphasic pulsed current (balanced). **E,** Asymmetric biphasic pulsed current (balanced). **F,** Asymmetric biphasic pulsed current (unbalanced). (Modified from Dyson M: Adjuvant therapies: ultrasound, laser therapy, electrical stimulation, hyperbaric oxygen and negative pressure therapy. In Morison MJ, Ovington LG, editors: *Chronic wound care: a problem-based learning approach,* Edinburgh, Scotland, 2004, Mosby.)

amplitude. Low-voltage amplitude devices deliver PC with either a monophasic or a biphasic waveform. Their pulse durations are relatively long, so low driving voltages (<150 V) are adequate. High-voltage amplitude devices provide only monophasic PC. Their pulses are of short duration (10 to 20 μs), so these devices must have a high driving voltage (>150 V). Each voltage type of electrical stimulation devices has been examined in clinical studies of wound healing (Table 23-2).

PAYMENT COVERAGE

Policies related to payment coverage for treatment of chronic wounds with electrical stimulation differ dramatically among third-party payers. In 2002 the Centers for Medicare and Medicaid Services (CMS) approved payment for electrical stimulation when used for treatment of chronic Stage III or Stage IV pressure ulcers and for wounds of the lower extremity caused by arterial and venous insufficiency and diabetes, if no measurable improvement is evidenced after at least 30 days of standard wound therapy. National coverage determination (NCD) became effective in July 2004 (CMS, 2004). Generally, electrical stimulation is only reimbursed when the treatment is performed by a physical therapist, although local coverage determinations (LCDs) vary in defining practice parameters that will be reimbursed. In contrast to CMS policies, a health technology assessment of electrical stimulation as an adjuvant treatment of chronic wounds conducted by Blue Cross Blue Shield Association (Lefevre and Samson, 2005) in April 2005 concluded that the available evidence does not demonstrate convincingly that electrical stimulation results in clinically significant improvement in the most relevant outcome—the percentage of patients whose wounds heal completely.

TABLE 23-2 **Studies Using Pulsed Current Electrical Stimulation of Chronic Wounds**

Type of Pulsed Current	Study	Results
Low-voltage monophasic Example: Dermapulse	Feedar et al, 1991	RCT 50 chronic wounds Weekly healing rate 14% vs. 8.25% in control group
	Gentzkow et al, 1991	4-week RCT 40 pressure ulcers Healing rate 12.5% vs. 5.8% in control group $p = .042$
	Gentzkow et al, 1993	7.3-week, prospective, baseline controlled study 61 pressure ulcers 55 (82%) of 61 showed improvement in two or more wound characteristics
	Wood et al, 1993	8-week, multisite, double-blind clinical trial 74 Stage II and III pressure ulcers 25 healed vs. 31 in placebo group
	Jünger et al, 1997	38-day trial of 15 venous leg wounds Wound history: 79 months of standard compression therapy Mean area decreased by 63% $(p < .01)$
	Jünger et al, 2008	Prospective, placebo-controlled, double-blind study 39 venous leg wounds Wound history: 3 months of standard compression therapy Rapid, lasting reduction in pain, no significant difference in wound size
Low-voltage, biphasic	Baker et al, 1996	185 pressure ulcers in patients with spinal cord injury Significantly faster healing rates with asymmetric waveform (compared with symmetric waveform and microcurrent stimulation)
	Baker et al, 1997	80 subjects with diabetic foot ulcers Significantly faster healing rates with asymmetric waveform (compared with symmetric waveform and microcurrent stimulation)
High-voltage asymmetric Example: Figure 23-1	Kloth and Feedar, 1988	16 subjects with Stage IV pressure ulcers Sham group: increase in ulcer size (29% over 7.4 weeks) Treatment group: 100% healing in mean period of 8 weeks (mean healing rate 44.8%)
	Griffin et al, 1991	20-day trial 17 subjects with spinal cord injury Stage II, III, and IV pressure ulcers Significant decrease in wound surface area by days 5, 15, 20 $(p < .05)$ vs. placebo
	Alon et al, 1986	12 of 15 subjects with diabetic foot ulcers achieved closure in mean period of 2.6 months

RCT, Randomized controlled trial.

CLINICAL CONSULT

A: Consulted for unresponsive left trochanter pressure ulcer. 70-year-old Caucasian female bedridden with Parkinson's disease. History and physical reveals hypertension managed with diuretics, negative for cardiac, renal or metabolic disorder. Wound has been unresponsive to standard therapy for over a month including low airloss, repositioning to avoid left trochanter, optimal nutrition per dietitian and tube feedings, and bioburden management with debridement and antimicrobial dressings. Medical history includes Parkinson's disease. Wound dimensions remains 4.8 × 8.2 × 1 cm Stage III, wound bed clean and smooth, absent of granulation. Wound edges attached, periwound skin intact, scant serous exudate, and no local signs of infection. Current local wound care includes daily hydrogel impregnated gauze and covered with nonadherent border cover dressing.

D: Stage III pressure ulcer resistant to healing despite conventional therapy.

P: Initiate daily high-voltage pulsed current electrical stimulation.

I: (1) Continue all current interventions including daily hydrogel dressings to maintain a continuously moist environment. (2) Set voltage between 75 and 200 volts to create a tingling paresthesia at a frequency of 100 pps.

E: Benefits and risks explained to family and they want to proceed. Family understands that therapy can be administered by qualified wound clinic staff only while nurses will continue to manage dressings as indicated. If healing progress ceases, the polarity will be switched daily.

SUMMARY

The transfer of electrical stimulation to mainstream wound care practice continues to be variable and inconsistent. In addition to the lack of consensus regarding the strength of evidence supporting the efficacy and payment for electrical stimulation, several system-level factors are barriers to implementation in practice. Many clinicians and wound specialists are unfamiliar with the therapy. Furthermore, many clinical settings do not have personnel with the necessary expertise to administer the treatment. Finally, the FDA has not approved any electrical stimulation device for wound healing (it is an off-label use).

REFERENCES

Alon G, Azaria M, Stein H: Diabetic ulcer healing using high voltage TENS (Abstract), *Phys Ther* 66:775, 1986.

Alvarez OM, Mertz PM, Smerback RV, et al: The healing of superficial skin wounds is stimulated by external electrical current, *J Invest Dermatol* 81(2):144, 1983.

Baker L, Chambers R, DeMuth SK, et al: Effects of electrical stimulation on wound healing in patients with diabetic ulcers, *Diabetes Care* 20(3):405, 1997.

Baker L, Rubayi S, Villar F, et al: Effect of electrical stimulation waveform on healing of ulcers in human beings with spinal cord injury, *Wound Repair Regen* 4(1):21, 1996.

Barker A, Jaffe LF, Vanable JW Jr: The glabrous epidermis of cavies contains a powerful battery, *Am J Physiol* 11:R358, 1982.

Bourguignon G, Bourguignon L: Electric stimulation of protein and DNA synthesis in human fibroblasts, *FASEB J* 1(5):398, 1987.

Carley PJ, Wainapel SF: Electrotherapy for acceleration of wound healing: low intensity direct current, *Arch Phys Med Rehabil* 66(7):443, 1985.

Castillo E, Sumano H, Fortoul TI, et al: The influence of pulsed electrical stimulation on the wound healing of burned rat skin, *Arch Med Res* 26(2):185, 1995.

Center for Medicare and Medicaid Services (CMS): *National Coverage Determination (NCD) for Electrical Stimulation (ES) and Electromagnetic Therapy for the Treatment of Wounds (270.1) Publication Number 100-3, Manual Section Number 270.1*, July 1, 2004. http://www.cms.gov/medicare-coverage-database/details/ncd-details.aspx?NCDId=131&ncdver=3&bc=BAABAAAAAAAA. Accessed May 24, 2015.

Cruz N, Bayron F, Suarez A: Accelerated healing of full-thickness burns by the use of high-voltage pulsed galvanic stimulation in the pig, *Ann Plast Surg* 23(1):49, 1989.

Daeschlein G: Antibacterial activity of positive and negative polarity low-voltage pulsed current (LVPC) on six typical gram-positive and gram-negative bacterial pathogens of chronic wounds, *Wound Repair Regen* 15(3):399, 2007.

Debreceni L, Gyulai M, Debreceni A, et al: Results of transcutaneous electrical stimulation (TNS) in cure of lower extremity arterial disease, *Angiology* 46(7):613, 1995.

Dyson M: Adjuvant therapies: ultrasound, laser therapy, electrical stimulation, hyperbaric oxygen and negative pressure therapy. In Morison MJ, Ovington LG, editors: *Chronic wound care: a problem-based learning approach*, Edinburgh, Scotland, 2004, Mosby.

Eberhardt A, Szczypiorski P, Korytowski G: Effect of transcutaneous electrostimulation on the cell composition of skin exudate, *Acta Physiol Pol* 37(1):41, 1986.

Fakhri O, Amin M: The effect of low-voltage electric therapy on the healing of resistant skin burns, *J Burn Care Res* 8(1):15, 1987.

Feedar J, Kloth LC, Gentzkow GD: Chronic dermal ulcer healing enhanced with monophasic pulsed electrical stimulation, *Phys Ther* 71(9):639, 1991.

Fitzgerald GK, Newsome D: Treatment of a large infected thoracic spine wound using high voltage pulsed monophasic current, *Phys Ther* 73(6):355, 1993.

Foulds I, Barker A: Human skin battery potentials and their possible role in wound healing, *Br J Dermatol* 109:515, 1983.

Gagnier KA, Manix N, Baker L, et al: The effects of electrical stimulation on cutaneous oxygen supply in paraplegics (Abstract), *Phys Ther* 68(5):835, 1988.

Gardner S, Frantz RA, Schmidt FL: The effect of electrical stimulation on chronic wound healing: a meta-analysis, *Wound Repair Regen* 7(6):495, 1999.

Gault W, Gatens P: Use of low intensity direct current in management of ischemic skin ulcers, *Phys Ther* 56(3):265, 1976.

Gentzkow GD, Alon G, Taler GA, et al: Healing of refractory Stage III and IV pressure ulcers by a new electrical stimulation device, *Wounds* 5(3):160, 1993.

Gentzkow GD, Pollack SV, Kloth LC, et al: Improved healing of pressure ulcers using Dermapulse®, a new electrical stimulation device, *Wounds* 3(5):158, 1991.

Griffin JW, Tooms RE, Mendius RA, et al: Efficacy of high voltage pulsed current for healing of pressure ulcers in patients with spinal cord injury, *Phys Ther* 71(6):433, 1991.

Guffey JS, Asmussen MD: In vitro bactericidal effects of high voltage pulsed current versus direct current against Staphylococcus aureus, *J Clin Electrophysiol* 1(1):5, 1989.

Hecker B, Carron H, Schwartz DP: Pulsed galvanic stimulation: effects of current frequency and polarity on blood flow in healthy subjects, *Arch Phys Med Rehabil* 66(6):369, 1985.

Hopf HW, Ueno C, Aslam R, et al: Guidelines for the treatment of arterial insufficiency ulcers, *Wound Repair Regen* 14(6):693, 2006.

Illingsworth CM, Barker AT: Measurement of electrical currents emerging during the regeneration of amputated finger tips in children, *Clin Phys Physiol Meas* 1:87, 1980.

Jaffe L, Vanable J: Electric fields and wound healing, *Clin Dermatol* 2(3):34, 1984.

Jünger M, Arnold A, Zuder D, et al: Local therapy and treatment costs of chronic, venous leg ulcers with electrical stimulation (Dermapulse®): a prospective, placebo controlled, double blind trial, *Wound Repair Regen* 16(4):480, 2008.

Jünger M, Zuder D, Steins A, et al: [Treatment of venous ulcers with low-frequency pulsed current (Dermapulse): effect on cutaneous microcirculation], *Hautarzt* 48(12):879, 1997.

Kaada B: Vasodilation induced by transcutaneous nerve stimulation in peripheral ischemia (Raynaud's phenomenon and diabetic polyneuropathy), *Eur Heart J* 3(4):303, 1982.

Kaada B: Promoted healing of chronic ulceration by transcutaneous nerve stimulation (TNS), *VASA* 12(3):262, 1983.

Kaada B, Helle K: In search of mediators of skin vasodilation induced by transcutaneous nerve stimulation: IV. In vitro bioassay of the vasoinhibitory activity of sera from patients suffering from peripheral ischaemia, *Gen Pharmacol* 15(2):115, 1984.

Kaada B, Hegland O, Okteldalen O, et al: Failure to influence the VIP level in the cerebrospinal fluid by transcutaneous nerve stimulation in humans, *Gen Pharmacol* 15(6):563, 1984.

Kincaid C, Lavoie K: Inhibition of bacterial growth in vitro following stimulation with high voltage, monophasic, pulsed current, *Phys Ther* 69(8):651, 1989.

Kloth L, Feedar J: Acceleration of wound healing with high voltage, monophasic, pulsed current, *Phys Ther* 68(4):503, 1988.

Lefevre F, Samson D: *Electrical stimulation or electromagnetic therapy as adjunctive treatments for chronic skin wounds*, Chicago, IL, 2005, Blue Cross and Blue Shield Association.

Mertz PM, Davis S, Cazzaniga A, et al: Electrical stimulation: acceleration of soft tissue repair by varying the polarity, *Wounds* 5(3):153, 1993.

National Pressure Ulcer Advisory Panel (NPUAP), European Pressure Ulcer Advisory Panel (EPUAP) and Pan Pacific Pressure Injury Alliance (PPPIA): *Prevention and treatment of pressure ulcers: Clinical Practice Guideline*. In Emily Haesler, editor: Perth, Australia, 2014, Cambridge Media.

Orida N, Feldman J: Directional protrusive pseudopodial activity and motility in macrophages induced by extracellular electric fields, *Cell Motil* 2:243, 1982.

Peters EJG, Armstrong DG, Wunderlich RP, et al: The benefit of electrical stimulation to enhance perfusion in persons with diabetes mellitus, *J Foot Ankle Surg* 37(5):396, 1998.

Robson MC, Cooper DM, Aslam R, et al: Guidelines for the treatment of venous ulcers, *Wound Repair Regen* 14(6):649, 2006.

Steed DL: Guidelines for treatment of diabetic ulcers, *Wound Repair Regen* 14(6):680, 2006.

Stromberg BV: Effects of electrical currents on wound contraction, *Ann Plast Surg* 21(2):121, 1988.

Szuminsky NJ, Albers AC, Unger P, et al: Effect of narrow, pulsed high voltages on bacterial viability, *Phys Ther* 74(7):660, 1994.

Vanable JW Jr: Integumentary potentials and wound healing. In Borgan RB, et al, editors: *Electric fields in vertebrate repair*, New York, 1989, Liss.

Whitney J: Guidelines for treatment of pressure ulcers, *Wound Repair Regen* 14(6):663, 2006.

Wood J, Evans PE, Schallreuter KU, et al: A multicenter study on the use of pulsed low-intensity direct current for healing chronic Stage II and Stage III decubitus ulcers, *Arch Dermatol* 129(8):199, 1993.

Wound, Ostomy and Continence Nurses Society™ (WOCN®): *Guideline for the prevention and management of pressure ulcers (WOCN® clinical practice guideline series no. 2)*, Glenview, IL, 2010, WOCN®.

24

Ultraviolet Light and Ultrasound

Renee Cordrey

OBJECTIVES

1. List at least one indication each for ultraviolet-C, high-frequency ultrasound, and low-frequency ultrasound use.
2. List at least one contraindication for each modality.
3. Explain the mechanism of action for each modality.

The use of physical agents can support wound healing through mechanical action or by their effect on tissue function. Common modalities include ultraviolet (UV) light and ultrasound. Each of these tools offers parameter options that have different effects. Selective use of these devices may reduce wound bioburden, facilitate wound debridement, or speed granulation and reepithelialization.

ULTRAVIOLET LIGHT

Ultraviolet light is a simple-to-use modality that may be a valuable tool in addressing wound bioburden, especially in this era of resistant organisms. Specialized lamps generate UV light. Hot quartz mercury vapor lamps produce UV-A and UV-B light. Cold quartz lamps create UV-C light. These lamps are generally easier to use, and treatment may be started immediately, without a warm-up or cool-down period (Figure 24-1).

Ultraviolet light consists of the portion of the electromagnetic spectrum that is at a higher frequency than visible light. The wavelength ranges from 320 to 400 nm for UV-A, 290 to 320 nm for UV-B, and 185 to 290 nm for UV-C. Ultraviolet light has long been used for treatment of many skin conditions, including psoriasis (Kirke et al, 2007; Lapidoth et al, 2007) and acne vulgaris. In recent decades, usage for those conditions has declined due to the advent of more topical and systemic treatments and the increased awareness of the potential damage from UV radiation. However, UV-C has seen a resurgence in the care of chronic wounds.

Physiologic Effects

Ultraviolet light does not heat tissue. Instead, it is believed to alter cellular function, increase cell wall permeability through altering the shape of proteins, stimulate production of various chemicals such as prostaglandins and arachidonic acid, and increase the production of adenosine triphosphate (Camp et al, 1978). The erythema that results increases local vasodilation, tissue oxygenation, and histamine release. Earlier studies using high doses of UV-C report increases in epithelialization and epithelial cell turnover (Freytes et al, 1965; Wills et al, 1983), increased granulation tissue growth and tissue perfusion at lower doses (Ramsay and Challoner, 1976), stimulated growth factor release (James et al, 1991), and increased autolysis (Kloth, 1995). However, these older studies used a different standard of care for comparison than exists today. Therefore whether UV enhances wound healing in conjunction with advanced wound-healing approaches is not known.

Each form of UV has different effects on tissue. UV-A and UV-B are nonionizing. They are both found environmentally, as they pass through the atmosphere. UV-A produces a mild erythema, whereas UV-B elicits a stronger erythematous response because it penetrates the epidermis. The impact of UV-A can be increased with the use of oral psoralens, a photosensitizing agent, before treatment. UV-A penetrates most deeply—several millimeters into the skin. UV-B produces hyperplasia of the dermis and stratum corneum 3 days after treatment and has been used to toughen scars (Parrish et al, 1981).

UV-C is ionizing and mutagenic but is not linked to skin cancers for several reasons: (1) UV-C only penetrates the most superficial layers of the epidermis; (2) the superficial layers of the epidermis are sloughed often enough to prevent development of neoplasms; and (3) naturally occurring UV-C is blocked by the atmosphere before it reaches the earth's surface. However, as wound treatment exposes the more permanent healing tissue, and not the epidermis, to UV-C radiation, the long-term cancer risk is unknown, although research by Dai et al (2012b) suggests that, in mouse studies, most of the DNA damage is repaired by the body within 48 hours.

UV-C is recognized to be germicidal, which has come to be the primary use for UV treatment. Other evidence suggests that UV-C can increase epithelialization, epithelial cell turnover (Freytes et al, 1965), granulation tissue growth and tissue perfusion at lower doses (Ramsay and Challoner, 1976), growth factor release (James et al, 1991), fibronectin release (Morykwas and Mark, 1998), transforming growth

FIGURE 24-1 Ultraviolet light. (Courtesy National Biological Corporation, Twinsburg, Ohio, USA.)

factor-beta expression (Suo et al, 2002) and autolysis (Kloth, 1995; Spielholz and Kloth, 2000), and speed wound contraction (Morykwas and Mark, 1998).

The bacteriocidal effects of UV light have been recognized for more than a century (Gates, 1928). The mechanism of action is theorized to be inhibition of DNA synthesis (Hall and Mount, 1981). UV-C has been demonstrated to kill methicillin-resistant *Staphylococcus aureus* (MRSA) and vancomycin-resistant enterococcus (VRE) in vitro in 90 seconds (Conner-Kerr et al, 1999). Another in vitro study (Sheldon et al, 2005) found MRSA eradication with use of UV-C, with an even greater impact on *Pseudomonas*. A case series by Thai et al (2002) demonstrated reduced bacterial counts and more wound rapid healing with UV-C use, although treatment was not standardized and there was no control group. Thai et al (2005) later studied the effect of one 180-second UV-C treatment session on semiquantitative swab culture results of 22 patients whose chronic ulcers contained high levels of bacteria and exhibited signs of infection. Types of wounds included pressure, venous, diabetic, and arterial etiologies. Results showed a statistically significant reduction of the predominant bacteria, including *Pseudomonas*, MRSA, and *S. aureus*. UV-C demonstrated nearly complete inactivation of *Candida albicans* after one 15- to 30-second treatment, performing better than the drug nystatin in a mouse trial (Dai et al, 2011). *Aspergillius* was also successfully eradicated after one 15- to 30-second treatment, and prokaryotic organisms such as *Pseudomonas aeruginosa* and *Mycobacterium abscessus* needed only 3 to 5 seconds of exposure to kill the microbes (Sullivan and Conner-Kerr, 2000). *Acinetobacter baumannii* was also shown to be susceptible to UV-C in a mouse study (Dai et al, 2012a). Other work shows multiple-drug resistant organisms needed less exposure time than susceptible ones, as little as 5 to 15 seconds (Rao et al, 2011). Doses needed to damage pathogens have been shown to be nondamaging to keratinocytes and other mammalian cells (Buonanno et al, 2013; Rao et al, 2011).

Data suggest that a higher dose of UV-C may be needed when treating biofilms to overcome the innate resistance of biofilms and because the biofilm matrix may block some of the UV light penetration (Dai et al, 2011, 2012b). Treatment of *P. aeruginosa* biofilms on urinary catheters achieved full disinfection in 30 to 300 minutes, depending on the catheter material, but shorter times were not assessed (Bak et al, 2010). Resistance to UV-C has not been observed but is theoretically possible.

Indications and Use

Because of its antimicrobial effects, UV-C is sometimes used in operating rooms to reduce surgical infections (Buonanno et al, 2013; Ritter et al, 2007). UV-C devices have even been marketed to the consumer to sterilize everything from toothbrushes to drinking water.

Following a systemic review, Reddy et al (2008) did not recommend UV treatment of pressure ulcers. However, an international guideline for treatment of pressure ulcers (EPUAP-NPUAP-PPPIA, 2014) advocates the consideration of UV-C treatment in the short term for pressure ulcers that do not respond to traditional therapies or as adjunctive therapy to reduce bioburden in clean, critically colonized Stage III and IV pressure ulcers. Pressure ulcer guideline recommendations related to UV are based on expert opinion and small in vitro and in vivo studies (Conner-Kerr et al, 1998, 1999; Thai et al, 2005). New evidence has been published in recent years, and the next updates to these guidelines and reviews may reach different conclusions.

There is no standardized way to apply UV-C light to a wound. A common protocol involves the application of petrolatum to the periwound and a towel or sheet drape to the surrounding areas to prevent UV absorption. Some trials have used aluminum foil over the periwound. Limited evidence supports periwound UV treatment for promoting wound closure. The lamp is kept 1 inch from the wound, perpendicular to the skin surface. Treatment has traditionally been for 90 to 120 seconds, although recent research may indicate a shorter time may be effective. Treatment should be applied directly over the wound, without any materials between the wound bed and the light. Plastic transparent films have been shown to block transmission of the UV-C light (Rao et al, 2011). Treatment should be discontinued when the bioburden is adequately reduced. Both the patient and the clinician must wear UV-blocking eye protection. Even if a person does not look directly at the light, the waves may bounce off surfaces and reflect into the eye, causing damage. UV-C is most commonly performed by physical therapists and physical therapist assistants, as ultraviolet therapy is covered in the curriculum, but it may be administered by other trained clinicians.

Contraindications and Precautions

Safe and effective dosage of UV-C may vary based on the distance from the light source, the intensity of the light source, and the size of the treated area. UV-C has a very low risk of causing burns. Contraindications, precautions, and conditions that can be exacerbated by UV treatment (especially with UV-A or UV-B over large areas of the body) vary

BOX 24-1 Contraindications and Conditions Exacerbated by Ultraviolet (UV) Light Therapy

Absolute Contraindications
- History of skin cancer
- Systemic lupus erythematosus
- Fever
- Radiation therapy anywhere on body within previous 3 months
- Sarcoidosis
- Treatment over eye
- Presence of erythema from last UV treatment

Conditions that Can Be Exacerbated by UV Treatment (Especially UV-A or UV-B over Large Areas of Body)
- Pulmonary tuberculosis
- Cardiac disease
- Renal disease
- Hepatic disease
- Human immunodeficiency virus/acquired immunodeficiency syndrome
- Hyperthyroidism
- Diabetes
- Herpes simplex infection

BOX 24-2 Precautions for Ultraviolet (UV) Light Therapy

- Acute eczema or dermatitis
- Radiation therapy more than 3 months earlier
- Photosensitivity
- Human immunodeficiency virus/acquired immunodeficiency syndrome
- Use of photosensitizing medication (may shorten treatment time or preclude treatment altogether)
  - ○ Psoralens (intentionally given to increase susceptibility to UV-A)
  - ○ Tetracycline
  - ○ Sulfonamides
  - ○ Quinolones
  - ○ Gold medications for rheumatoid arthritis
  - ○ Thiazide diuretics
  - ○ Diphenhydramine
  - ○ Oral contraceptives
  - ○ Phenothiazines

according to the source (Box 24-1). Conditions and medications requiring the clinician to use caution when applying UV, usually UV-A and UV-B, treatment are listed in Box 24-2 (Cameron, 2008; Michlovitz and Nolan, 2005).

ULTRASOUND

Ultrasound is a term used to describe sound waves greater than 20,000 Hz, the upper limit of human hearing. Three forms of ultrasound are commonly used: 1 to 3.3 MHz, 40 kHz, and 25 kHz. Each has distinct uses.

Traditional High-Frequency Ultrasound (1.0 to 3.3 MHz)

Traditional clinical therapeutic applications use a frequency of 1 or 3.3 MHz. The user may elect to use a duty cycle. This parameter results in pulsing of the current, with periods of wave production followed by quiet periods. A 20% duty cycle is most commonly used, in which the sound waves are on for 1 ms and then off for 4 ms. Heat is produced but is dispersed so quickly when good perfusion is present that no temperature change occurs in the tissue. Ultrasound has been used to promote soft tissue healing for more than 6 decades, primarily for orthopedic conditions. More recently, that use has extended to wound healing.

An ultrasound device consists of the control unit and the handheld sound head, or *transducer* (Figure 24-2). The user

FIGURE 24-2 A, Ultrasound device. **B,** Close-up of ultrasound parameter settings.(Courtesy Renee Cordrey.)

is able to control the intensity (amount of power used), whether the waves are continuous or pulsed, the duration of treatment, and, on some units, the wavelength. The device runs electricity through a crystal in the sound head, causing the crystal to vibrate through a reverse piezoelectric effect. These vibrations create sound waves that pass through the sound head membrane and into the tissue. These waves elicit both thermal and nonthermal effects.

Physiologic Effects. Nonthermal effects are attributed to cavitation and acoustic microstreaming. Stable cavitation is the vibration of tiny bubbles within the interstitial spaces. With microstreaming, current eddies form around gas bubbles that are near vibrating particles. In addition, streaming stimulates the movement of fluid within and between cells. Some investigators believe that using ultrasound in a water bath stimulates mechanical wound debridement through acoustic streaming of the water itself. These nonthermal effects occur with both pulsed and continuous ultrasound. The resulting forces stimulate an inflammatory response in wounds (Young and Dyson, 1990a), with an increase in histamine release (Demir et al, 2004; Fyfe and Chahl, 1984). Pulsed ultrasound has been shown to stimulate fibroblast proliferation and macrophage phagocytic activity in vitro (Young and Dyson, 1990b; Zhou et al, 2004, 2008). However, peak benefit occurred after 20 minutes of treatment, which is longer than is usually acceptable by the clinician providing the treatment. Other effects of ultrasound include leukocyte adhesion and increased fibrinolysis, permeability of cell membranes and skin, mast cell degranulation, and production of growth factors and nitric oxide (Ennis et al, 2007; Stanisic et al, 2005; Young and Dyson, 1990b).

The thermal effects of continuous ultrasound stimulate an increase in local circulation that disperses heat and increases cell metabolism (Taskan et al, 1997). Increases in macrophage activity, protein synthesis by fibroblasts, and angiogenesis occur (Young and Dyson, 1990a). As a result, wounds may progress through the inflammatory phase more quickly (Demir et al, 2004), or acute inflammation may be reinitiated if healing has stalled. Other work has found increased tensile strength and collagen deposition after ultrasound treatments (Byl et al, 1993; Demir et al, 2004).

Protocol and Clinical Application. Based on theory and in vitro research, high-frequency ultrasound should have a significant impact on wound healing. However, in the more complex in vivo environment, this expectation has not borne out. A common limit of the available research is that treatment time and sound head movement patterns have not always been modified appropriately to accommodate wound size and the effective radiating area of the transducer. Ultrasound treatment is commonly combined with other modalities, which also may influence study results. Robertson and Baker (2001) identified eight randomized clinical trials addressing ultrasound. Seven of the studies were rejected because of inadequate controls, inadequate analysis, inadequate

treatment details, insufficient sample size, or the use of multiple interventions. More current studies continue to omit full descriptions of parameters and technique. Therefore no standard protocol for ultrasound exists and its application to clinical practice is difficult.

In general, low-intensity, high-frequency ultrasound has ranged from 0.1 to 0.3 W/cm², medium-intensity ultrasound from 0.3 to 1.2 W/cm², and high-intensity ultrasound from 1.2 to 3.0 W/cm². Time of treatment varies from 1 to 10 minutes, and transducer frequency has run between 0.3 and 3 MHz. Frequency of treatment has ranged between 1 and 5 days per week, and treatment duration has ranged from 2 weeks through wound closure. Most of these studies used periwound techniques, although Peschen et al (1997) used a water immersion technique. Most studies used pulsed ultrasound, possibly because of the risks of thermal heating in a person with sensory, vascular, or cognitive compromise, common comorbidities in people with chronic wounds.

Indications. International pressure ulcer guidelines recommend considering the use of high-frequency ultrasound as an adjunct for treatment of infected pressure ulcers (EPUAP-NPUAP-PPPIA, 2014). This recommendation is based on expert opinion and a randomized study conducted in 1985 of 40 patients with Stage I and II pressure ulcers (McDiarmid et al, 1985). Pressure ulcer research on high-frequency ultrasound points to a lack of benefit. Two randomized controlled trials demonstrated no difference in healing rates (McDiarmid et al, 1985; ter Reit et al, 1996). A metaanalysis combining the two studies strengthened that conclusion with a stronger sample size (Flemming and Cullum, 2001). Although some trials did show a small improvement in the ultrasound group, the sample sizes were too small to reach statistical significance. Selkowitz et al (2002) conducted a single-subject baseline–ultrasound–sham trial on a Stage III coccyx ulcer using low-intensity pulsed ultrasound. The baseline period had the greatest healing rate and the sham the poorest, although this result may be attributed to natural variation as a wound heals. The Cochrane review of ultrasound for pressure ulcers concluded that there was no evidence supporting the efficacy of high-frequency ultrasound (Baba-Akbari Sari et al, 2006). The WOCN® Society (2010) concurs that there is a lack of evidence about high-frequency ultrasound and pressure ulcers.

Outcomes trials with venous ulcers have been largely inconclusive, often lacking statistical significance (Al-Kurdi et al, 2008; Cullum et al, 2010; Robson et al, 2006; WOCN®, 2010). Other studies using both high-intensity and low-intensity pulsed ultrasound have found no significant difference in the percentage of wounds that closed during the treatment period compared with sham treatment (Ericksson et al, 1991). Studies that showed improvement with ultrasound lacked sufficient description of the baseline data to properly evaluate the results, had poor follow-up, or had significant differences between groups (e.g., wound size) that could lead to the differences in findings (Johannsen, 1998; Peschen et al, 1997). Taradaj et al (2008) found that patients with venous ulcers healed equally well with compression plus venous surgery, pulsed ultrasound, or both compared with compression alone. However, patients had self-selected into the surgery or nonsurgery group, and the ultrasound was delivered in a warm water bath with the leg in a dependent position. Both of these factors could alter the findings.

Contraindications and Precautions. With high-frequency ultrasound, the sound head must be kept in constant motion. If the sound head stays in place for even 0.1 ms, standing waves and banding may occur. A *standing wave* occurs when the sound wave reflects off tissue back onto itself. The resulting interference wave is twice as strong as the original wave, which increases tissue heating and potentially leads to burning. *Banding* is the separation of cells and plasma within the blood vessels. This action causes irreversible damage to the endothelial linings of the vessel walls.

Contraindications are related to the thermal and nonthermal effects of ultrasound. Ultrasound must not be used over the eyes, the heart, the carotid sinuses, a pregnant uterus, or the exposed central nervous system (e.g., over a laminectomy site). The inflammatory, cavitation, and metabolic effects of ultrasound contraindicate its use in situations where it would be harmful, such as areas of active bleeding, active infection, over breast or other silicone implants, over malignancies, and in the presence of thrombophlebitis. Ultrasound should not be used over pacemakers, active epiphyseal plates, the reproductive organs, or orthopedic cement or plastic components because the increased reflection of sound waves overheats local tissue.

A lower-intensity nonthermal setting should be used with wounds on a limb with arterial insufficiency because heat dispersion is compromised and the increased metabolic demands cannot be met. Because of insufficient evidence, the Wound Healing Society stipulates thermal ultrasound is contraindicated in ischemic areas and is not recommended for treatment of arterial ulcers (Hopf et al, 2006).

The clinician must exercise good judgment when deciding whether to use ultrasound. Ultrasound may often be used in the presence of a contraindication if the treatment location is remote to the site of contraindication. For example, ultrasound may be used on a foot wound despite the presence of a cardiac pacemaker, total hip replacement, or pregnancy because of the localized effects of ultrasound. Caution should be used around superficial bones because periosteum heats and burns easily from reflection off the bone. The clinician should be especially vigilant when thermal ultrasound is used in a person with sensory or cognitive deficits who is unable to provide feedback relating to tissue heating. Ultrasound may be used with caution in an area of acute inflammation if the benefits outweigh the risks of increasing inflammation. Because of the risks inherent in the use of high-frequency ultrasound, this intervention should be performed by a physical therapist who has had appropriate training.

Noncontact Low-Frequency Ultrasound (40 kHz)

Noncontact low-frequency ultrasound (NCLFU) is a noncontact method benefiting from the nonthermal effects of ultrasound. At this time, there is one commercially available NCLFU device (MIST, Celleration, Inc., Eden Prairie, MN, USA) (Figures 24-3 and 24-4). Many early studies involving NCLFU were animal trials; however, human trials are becoming more commonplace.

This treatment may be performed by any licensed trained practitioner. A saline vial is attached to the ultrasound transducer handset, which creates a mist. The handset is held close to the wound and is moved in a zigzag pattern across the

FIGURE 24-3 Ultrasound MIST control unit.

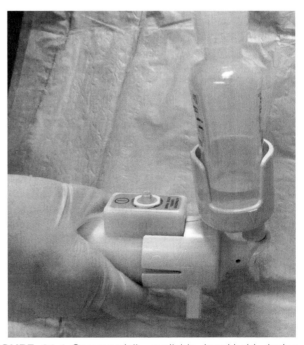

FIGURE 24-4 Commercially available hand-held device is used to vaporize saline into microdroplets that can then be delivered to the wound bed.

wound in each direction. The duration of treatment is based upon wound size. A wound with an area under 10 square centimeters will be treated for 3 minutes, and a wound 170 to 180 square centimeters should receive a 20-minute treatment. If a patient has pain with contact of the handset against the wound, it may be held just off the surface, taking care to maintain cavitation at the wound surface.

Noncontact low-frequency ultrasound has been found to have two primary benefits: wound size reduction and bioburden reduction (Ennis et al, 2007; Kavros and Schenck, 2007; Lai and Pittelkow, 2007). The device vaporizes saline into microdroplets (60 μm), which are then propelled to the wound bed via 40-kHz ultrasonic waves, with an intensity of 1.5 W/cm². Microstreaming and cavitation, which are thought to be the primary sources of any healing effect from ultrasound, are more common with kilohertz ultrasound than with megahertz ultrasound (Ennis et al, 2007; Kavros and Schenck, 2007). Those mechanisms lead to DNA synthesis diminishing for 4 hours after treatment, but then increasing for a 2-day period, stimulating tissue growth (Lai and Pittelkow, 2007). Additionally, a mouse study found that treated wounds had a greater concentration of collagen and blood vessels in the new tissue (Thawer and Houghton, 2004).

A systematic review showed that low-frequency, low-intensity noncontact or low-frequency, high-intensity contact ultrasound improved healing in patients with chronic wounds (venous ulcers and diabetic ulcers), although the authors note that the quality of the data may be threatened by researcher biases (Voigt et al, 2011).

With 12 weeks of NCLFU therapy increased closure rates have been reported with venous insufficiency and Wagner grade 1 and 2 diabetic foot ulcers compared with conventional wound care (Peschen et al, 1997; Weichenthal et al, 1997). In addition, one study noted a reduction in wound size on patents with critical limb ischemia (Kavros et al, 2007, 2008).

Benefits with NCLFU have been observed to include increased granulation tissue, decreased periwound maceration, and decreased volume of exudate (Bell and Cavorsi, 2008). Conversely, the following adverse events were reported with patients with diabetic foot ulcers: pain, erythema, blisters, edema, and ulcer enlargement (Ennis et al, 2005). The Wound, Ostomy and Continence Nurses Society™ (WOCN®) (2008, 2012) gave NCLFU a strength of evidence rating of B for promoting neuropathic ulcer and arterial insufficiency ulcer healing, and recommends considering a trial of NCLFU in wounds with borderline blood flow and without limb-threatening sepsis (strength of evidence C).

International pressure ulcer guidelines do not recommend routine use of NCLFU (40 kHz) for the treatment of pressure ulcers due to insufficient evidence. These recommendations are based on expert opinion and previously reported studies (EPUAP-NPUAP-PPPIA, 2014). An observational study with historical controls using a newly developed, validated suspected deep tissue injury (sDTI) severity scale (Honaker et al, 2014) reported that more wounds resolved spontaneously (18% vs. 2% of control) and those that did open were less severe when treated with NCLFU (Honaker et al, 2013). The effect of this treatment on sDTI remains a hypothesis that needs further investigation.

There is limited evidence that NCLFU may reduce bioburden. In a study by Serena et al (2009), NCLFU was applied to in vitro bacterial samples and to people with pressure ulcers. In this study one treatment of ultrasound reduced *Pseudomonas* by 33%, *Escherichia coli* by 40%, and *Enterococcus faecalis* by 27%. However, MRSA and *S. aureus* were not affected. When treating 11 people with Stage III pressure ulcers for 2 weeks, bioburden reduced from 4×10^7 to 2×10^7 overall, although beta hemolytic streptococcus G was stable and beta hemolytic streptococcus group A increased.

Ultrasonic Low-Frequency Debridement (22.5, 25, 35 kHz)

The third form of ultrasound is ultrasonic debridement. Ultrasonic kilohertz frequencies have been effective at fibrinolysis of the wound surface without causing damage to underlying granulation tissue. Furthermore, softer fibrinous slough is more responsive to ultrasonic debridement than drier, tougher fibrinous tissue (Stanisic et al, 2005; Tan et al, 2007).

The limited number of controlled clinical trials on human chronic ulcers led Ramundo and Gray (2008) to conclude that low-frequency ultrasound may be beneficial at removing necrotic tissue, but the evidence was inconclusive. Currently, international pressure ulcer guidelines recommend considering the use of low-frequency ultrasound for debridement of soft necrotic tissue (not eschar) (EPUAP-NPUAP-PPIA, 2014).

Ultrasonic debridement at 35 kHz may also be effective in reducing bioburden by damaging cell walls. After 30 seconds of treatment, MRSA was reduced from 1 million colony-forming units (CFUs) to 6 CFUs, and MRSA's susceptibility to methicillin improved (Conner-Kerr, 2010). More recently, Attinger and Wolcott (2012) reported that ultrasound is a useful adjunct for debriding biofilm (see Chapter 16).

Saline is used as the transfer media, and the air bubbles in the fluid expand and collapse, causing shockwave formation, cavitation, and erosion and fragmentation of the dead tissue (Wendelken et al, 2006). A variety of probes are available and selected according to the wound surface to be treated. Ultrasound intensity can be adjusted. The treatment is often painless or minimally pain-inducing; some patients may benefit from a topical anesthetic or pain medication before treatment. Ultrasonic debridement may take more time to complete than sharp debridement. Contraindications and precautions are similar to those for sharp debridement. Therefore it should be performed only by practitioners who are qualified in wound debridement. Options for ultrasonic debridement devices are listed in Table 24-1.

TABLE 24-1	**Ultrasonic Debridement Device Options**			
Manufacturer	**Product**	**Transducer Type**	**Frequency**	**Contact**
Arobella Medical, LLC	Qoustic Wound Therapy System	Curette	35 kHz	http://www.arobella.com/products/qoustic-description.htm
Misonix	SonicOne	Probes, with several shape choices	22.5 kHz	http://www.misonix.com/sonicone
Soring	Sonoca 180, Sonoca 185	Probes, with several shape choices	25 kHz	http://www.soering.com/en/products/ultrasound_surgery/surgery_devices/

Please note that products enter and leave the market regularly, so products listed here may no longer be available or may have been updated, and new products may have entered the market since publication.

CLINICAL CONSULT

A: Referral received to consult on a 64-year-old woman with a right lateral leg wound that developed after falling and scraping her leg on a car door 5 months ago. Comorbidities include type 2 diabetes, venous insufficiency in right leg with edema. She is a manager and sits most of the day at work. She walks independently without an assistive device, but does not engage in any exercise program. Past treatment includes dressings, surgical debridement, multilayer compression wraps, negative pressure wound therapy, oral antibiotics, and a cellular/tissue-derived product graft, which failed. Current wound presentation is a full-thickness lesion on right lateral calf, 11.7 × 6.2 × 0.4 cm. Wound base is covered with thick biofilm layer; after debridement, the base is fibrogranular. The copious wound exudate is yellow-green with a sweet odor. Periwound is macerated. Ankle-brachial index (ABI) right leg was 1.05 at the dorsalis pedis and 0.96 at the posterior tibialis. 2+ palpable pulses at both. Right leg with circumferential hemosiderin staining. Hemoglobin A1c from 1 month ago was 6.4. Her reported diet should be adequate, including protein, fruits, and vegetables.

D: Wound presentation is consistent with a traumatic wound, complicated by an edematous limb with venous insufficiency and a history of diabetes under adequate control. The high level of bioburden with biofilm will impair healing, and many past treatments have been unsuccessful.
P: Reduce bioburden in the wound, provide compression and moist wound healing. Consult physical therapy for UV-C to further stimulate cellular activity to promote healing.
I: (1) Routine weekly sharp debridement by wound care as needed to reduce bioburden. Topical cadexomer iodine to manage/treat bioburden. (2) Ultraviolet-C treatments to the right leg wound three times per week initially. Several treatments may be necessary. (3) Consider noncontact, low-frequency ultrasound two to three times per week if wound fails to respond to the UV-C after 4 weeks. (4) Multilayer compression wraps. (5) Therapeutic exercise to improve ankle range of motion improves calf muscle pump strength; instruct patient on a home exercise program.
E: Weekly wound measurements/assessments by PT and notify wound care team if dimensions unchanged after 3 weeks of UV-C. Will modify plan as needed.

SUMMARY

Ultraviolet and ultrasound therapies have long been in existence and used for wound healing, with varying results. Well-controlled human clinical trials are needed to further define the mechanism of action and efficacy of these therapies. As we learn more about how these modalities affect the healing process, these classic tools have the potential to become important additions to the arsenal of wound interventions.

REFERENCES

Al-Kurdi D, Bell-Syer SE, Flemming K: Therapeutic ultrasound for venous leg ulcers, *Cochrane Database Syst Rev* 1:CD001180, 2008.

Attinger C, Wolcott R: Clinically addressing biofilm in chronic wounds, *Adv Wound Care* 1(3):127–132, 2012.

Baba-Akbari Sari A, Flemming K, Cullum NA, et al: Therapeutic ultrasound for pressure ulcers, *Cochrane Database Syst Rev* 3:CD001275, 2006.

Bak J, Ladefoged SD, Tvede M, et al: Disinfection of pseudomonas aeruginosa biofilm contaminated tube lumens with ultraviolet C light emitting diodes, *Biofouling* 26(1):31–38, 2010.

Bell AL, Cavorsi J: Noncontact ultrasound therapy for adjunctive treatment of nonhealing wounds: retrospective analysis, *Phys Ther* 88:1517–1524, 2008.

Buonanno M, Randers-Pehrson G, Bigelow AW, et al: 207-nm UV Light–a promising tool for safe low-cost reduction of surgical site infections. I: In vitro studies, *PLoS One* 8(10):e76968, 2013.

Byl N, McKenzie A, Wong T, et al: Incisional wound healing: a controlled study of low and high dose ultrasound, *J Orthop Sports Ther* 18(5):619–628, 1993.

Cameron MH: *Physical agents in rehabilitation: from research to practice*, ed 3, Philadelphia, 2008, Saunders.

Camp RD, Greaves MW, Hensby CN, et al: Irradiation of human skin by short wavelength ultraviolet radiation (100–290 nm) (u.V.C):

increased concentrations of arachidonic acid and prostaglandines E2 and F2alpha, *Br J Clin Pharmacol* 6(2):145–148, 1978.

Conner-Kerr T, Alston G, Stovall A, et al: The effects of low-frequency ultrasound (35 kHz) on methicillin-resistant Staphylococcus aureus (MRSA) in vitro, *Ostomy Wound Manage* 56(5):32–43, 2010.

Conner-Kerr TA, Sullivan PK, Gaillard J, et al: The effects of ultraviolet radiation on antibiotic-resistant bacteria in vitro, *Ostomy Wound Manage* 44(10):50–56, 1998.

Conner-Kerr TA, Sullivan PK, Keegan A, et al: UVC reduces antibiotic-resistant bacterial numbers in living tissue, *Ostomy Wound Manage* 45(4):84, 1999.

Cullum N, Al-Kurdi D, Bell-Syer SE: Therapeutic ultrasound for venous leg ulcers' *Cochrane Database Syst Rev* 6:CD001180, 2010.

Cullum NA, et al: Therapeutic ultrasound for venous leg ulcers' *Cochrane Database Syst Rev* 6:CD001180, 2010.

Dai T, Kharkwal GB, Zhao J, et al: Ultraviolet-C light for treatment of Candida albicans burn infection in mice, *Photochem Photobiol* 87(2):342–349, 2011.

Dai T, Murray CK, Vrahas MS, et al: Ultraviolet C light for Acinetobacter baumannii wound infections in mice: potential use for battlefield wound decontamination? *J Trauma Acute Care Surg* 73(3):661–667, 2012a.

Dai T, Vrahas MS, Murray CK, et al: Ultraviolet C irradiation: an alternative antimicrobial approach to localized infections? *Expert Rev Anti Infect Ther* 10(2):185–195, 2012b.

Demir H, Yaray S, Kirnap M, et al: Comparison of the effects of laser and ultrasound treatments on experimental wound healing in rats, *J Rehabil Res Dev* 41(5):721–728, 2004.

Ennis WJ, Foremann P, Mozen N, et al: Ultrasound therapy for recalcitrant diabetic foot ulcers: results of a randomized, double-blind, controlled, multicenter study, *Ostomy Wound Manage* 51(8):24–39, 2005.

Ennis WJ, Lee C, Meneses P: A biochemical approach to wound healing through the use of modalities, *Clin Dermatol* 25:63–72, 2007.

Ericksson SV, Lundeberg T, Malm M: A placebo controlled trial of ultrasound therapy in chronic leg ulceration, *Scand J Rehab Med* 23(4):211–213, 1991.

Freytes HA, Fernandez B, Fleming WC: Ultraviolet light in the treatment of indolent ulcers, *South Med J* 58:223–226, 1965.

Fyfe MC, Chahl LA: Mast cell degranulation and increased vascular permeability induced by "therapeutic" ultrasound in the rat ankle joint, *Br J Exp Pathol* 65(6):671–676, 1984.

Gates F: On nuclear derivatives and the lethal action of ultra-violet light, *Science* 68:479–480, 1928.

Hall JD, Mount DW: Mechanisms of DNA replication and mutagenesis in ultraviolet-irradiated bacteria and mammalian cells, *Prog Nucleic Acid Res Mol Biol* 25:53–126, 1981.

Honaker J, et al: Development and psychometric testing of the honaker suspected deep tissue injury severity scale *J Wound Ostomy Continence Nurs* 41(3):238–241, 2014.

Honaker JS, Forston MR, Davis EA, et al: Effects of non contact low-frequency ultrasound on healing of suspected deep tissue injury: a retrospective analysis, *Int Wound J* 10(1):65–72, 2013.

Hopf HW, Ueno C, Aslam R, et al: Guidelines for the treatment of arterial insufficiency ulcers, *Wound Repair Regen* 14:693–710, 2006.

James LC, Moore AM, Wheeler LA, et al: Transforming growth factor alpha: in vivo release by normal human skin following UV irradiation and abrasion, *Skin Pharmacol* 4:61–64, 1991.

Johannsen F, Gam AN, Karlsmark T: Ultrasound therapy in chronic leg ulceration: a meta-analysis, *Wound Repair Regen* 6:121–126, 1998.

Kavros SJ, Liedl DA, Boon AJ, et al: Expedited wound healing with noncontact, low-frequency ultrasound therapy in chronic wounds: a retrospective analysis, *Adv Skin Wound Care* 21(9):416–423, 2008.

Kavros SJ, Miller JL, Hanna SW: Treatment of ischemic wounds with noncontact, low-frequency ultrasound: the Mayo Clinic experience, 2004–2006, *Adv Skin Wound Care* 20(4):221–226, 2007.

Kavros SJ, Schenck EC: Use of noncontact low-frequency ultrasound in the treatment of chronic foot and leg ulcerations: a 51-patient analysis, *J Am Podiatr Med Assoc* 97(2):95–101, 2007.

Kirke SM, Lowder S, Lloyd JJ, et al: A randomized comparison of selective broadband UVB and narrowband UVB in the treatment of psoriasis, *J Invest Dermatol* 127:1641–1646, 2007.

Kloth LC: Physical modalities in wound management: UVC, therapeutic heating and electrical stimulation, *Ostomy Wound Manage* 41(5):18–26, 1995.

Lai JY, Pittelkow MR: Physiological effects of ultrasound mist on fibroblasts, *Int J Dermatol* 46(6):587–593, 2007.

Lapidoth M, Adatto M, David M: Targeted UVB phototherapy for psoriasis: a preliminary study, *Clin Exp Dermatol* 32:642–645, 2007.

McDiarmid T, Burns PN, Lewith GT, et al: Ultrasound and the treatment of pressure sores, *Physiotherapy* 71:66–70, 1985.

Michlovitz SL, Nolan TP Jr: *Modalities for therapeutic intervention*, ed 4, Philadelphia, 2005, FA Davis.

Morykwas MJ, Mark MW: Effects of ultraviolet light on fibroblast fibronectin production and lattice contraction, *Wounds* 10(4):111–117, 1998.

Parrish JA, Zaynoun S, Anderson RR: Cumulative effects of repeated subthreshold doses of ultraviolet radiation, *J Invest Dermatol* 76(5):356–358, 1981.

Peschen M, Weichenthal M, Schöpf E, et al: Low-frequency ultrasound treatment of chronic venous leg ulcers in an outpatient therapy, *Acta Derm Venereol* 77(4):311–314, 1997.

National Pressure Ulcer Advisory Panel (NPUAP), European Pressure Ulcer Advisory Panel (EPUAP) and Pan Pacific Pressure Injury Alliance (PPPIA). Prevention and treatment of pressure ulcers: quick reference guide. In Emily Haesler, editor: Perth, Australia, 2014, Cambridge Media.

Ramsay CA, Challoner AV: Vascular changes in human skin after ultraviolet irradiation, *Br J Dermatol* 94(5):487–493, 1976.

Ramundo J, Gray M: Is ultrasonic mist therapy effective for debriding chronic wounds? *J Wound Ostomy Continence Nurs* 35(6):579–583, 2008.

Rao BK, Kumar P, Rao S, et al: Bactericidal effect of ultraviolet C (UVC), direct and filtered through transparent plastic, on gram-positive cocci: an in vitro study, *Ostomy Wound Manage* 57(7):46–52, 2011.

Reddy M, Gill SS, Kalkar SR, et al: Treatment of pressure ulcers: a systematic review, *JAMA* 300(22):2647–2662, 2008.

Ritter MA, Olberding EM, Malinzak RA: Ultraviolet lighting during orthopaedic surgery and the rate of infection, *J Bone Joint Surg Am* 89:1935–1940, 2007.

Robertson VJ, Baker KG: A review of therapeutic ultrasound: effectiveness studies, *Phys Ther* 81(7):1339–1350, 2001.

Robson MC, Cooper DM, Aslam R, et al: Guidelines for the treatment of venous ulcers, *Wound Repair Regen* 14:649–662, 2006.

Selkowitz DM, Cameron MH, Mainzer A, et al: Efficacy of pulsed low-intensity ultrasound in wound healing: a single-case design, *Ostomy Wound Manage* 48(4):40–50, 2002.

Serena T, Lee SK, Lam K, et al: The impact of noncontact, nonthermal, low-frequency ultrasound on bacterial counts in experimental and chronic wounds, *Ostomy Wound Manage* 55(1): 22–30, 2009.

Sheldon JL, Kokjohn TA, Martin EL: The effects of salt concentration and growth phase on MRSA solar and germicidal ultraviolet radiation resistance, *Ostomy Wound Manage* 51(1):36–38, 2005.

Spielholz NI, Kloth LC: Electrical stimulation and pulsed electromagnetic energy: differences in opinion, *Ostomy Wound Manage* 46(5):8–12, 2000.

Stanisic MM, Provo BJ, Larson DL, et al: Wound debridement with 25 kHz ultrasound, *Adv Skin Wound Care* 18(9):484–490, 2005.

Sullivan PK, Conner-Kerr TA: A comparative study of the effects of UVC irradiation on select procaryotic and eucaryotic wound pathogens, *Ostomy Wound Manage* 46(10):28–34, 2000.

Suo W, Wang X, Wang D: Effect of ultraviolet C irradiation on expression of transforming growth factor-β in wound, *Chinese J Rehabil Theory Pract* 8:5–7, 2002.

Tan J, Abisi S, Smith A, et al: A painless method of ultrasonically assisted debridement of chronic leg ulcers: a pilot study, *Eur J Vasc Endovasc Surg* 33:234–238, 2007.

Taradaj J, Franek A, Brzezinska-Wcislo L, et al: The use of therapeutic ultrasound in venous leg ulcer: a randomized, controlled clinical trial, *Phlebology* 23:178–183, 2008.

Taşkan I, Ozyazgan I, Tercan M, et al: A comparative study of the effect of ultrasound and electrostimulation on wound healing in rats, *Plast Reconstr Surg* 100(4):966–972, 1997.

ter Riet G, Kessels AG, Knipschild P: A randomized clinical trial of ultrasound in the treatment of pressure ulcers, *Phys Ther* 76(12):1301–1311, 1996.

Thai TP, Houghton PE, Campbell KE, et al: Ultraviolet light C in the treatment of chronic wounds with MRSA: a case study, *Ostomy Wound Manage* 48(11):52–60, 2002.

Thai TP, Keast DH, Campbell KE, et al: Effect of ultraviolet light C on bacterial colonization in chronic wounds, *Ostomy Wound Manage* 51(10):32–45, 2005.

Thawer HA, Houghton PE: Effects of ultrasound delivered through a mist of saline to wounds in mice with diabetes mellitus, *J Wound Care* 13(5):171–176, 2004.

Voigt J, Wendelken M, Driver V, et al: Low-frequency ultrasound (20-40 kHz) as an adjunctive therapy for chronic wound healing: a systematic review of the literature and meta-analysis of eight randomized controlled trials, *Int J Low Extrem Wounds* 10(4):190–199, 2011.

Weichenthal M, Mohr P, Stegmann W, et al: Low-frequency ultrasound treatment of chronic venous ulcers, *Wound Repair Regen* 5(1):18–22, 1997.

Wendelken M, et al. Key insights on mapping wounds with ultrasound, *Podiatry Today* 19(7):70–74, 2006.

Wills EE, Anderson TW, Beattie BL, et al: A randomized placebo-controlled trial of ultraviolet light in the treatment of superficial pressure sores, *J Am Geriatr Soc* 31(3):131–133, 1983.

Wound, Ostomy and Continence Nurses Society™ (WOCN®): *Guideline for management of wounds in patients with lower-extremity arterial disease (WOCN® clinical practice guideline series no. 4)*, Mt. Laurel, NJ, 2008, WOCN®.

Wound, Ostomy and Continence Nurses Society™ (WOCN®): *Guideline for the prevention and management of pressure ulcers (WOCN® clinical practice guideline series no. 2)*, Mt. Laurel, NJ, 2010, WOCN®.

Wound, Ostomy and Continence Nurses Society™ (WOCN®): *Guideline for management of wounds in patients with lower-extremity neuropathic disease, (WOCN® clinical practice guideline series, no. 3)*, Mt. Laurel, NJ, 2012, WOCN®.

Young S, Dyson M: Effect of therapeutic ultrasound on the healing of full-thickness excised lesions, *Ultrasonics* 28:175–180, 1990a.

Young S, Dyson M: Macrophage responsiveness to therapeutic ultrasound, *Ultrasound Med Biol* 16:809–816, 1990b.

Zhou S, Bachem MG, Seufferlein T, et al: Low intensity pulsed ultrasound accelerates macrophage phagocytosis by a pathway that requires actin polymerization, Rho, and src/MAPKs activity, *Cell Signal* 20:695–704, 2008.

Zhou S, Schmelz A, Seufferlein T, et al: Molecular mechanisms of low intensity pulsed ultrasound in human skin fibroblasts, *J Biol Chem* 279(52):54463–54469, 2004.

25

Wound Pain: Impact and Assessment

Diane L. Krasner

OBJECTIVES

1. Describe the different types of pain experienced by the patient with a wound.
2. Describe the physiologic effect of pain.
3. List the indicators of pain in the conscious and unconscious patient.
4. Describe ways to interpret pain using verbal and nonverbal tools.
5. Identify the common and unique features of three wound pain models.
6. Discuss the effects of wound pain on quality of life.

General pain concepts, as well as wound pain–specific concepts, guidelines, and research, are essential underpinnings for all wound care clinicians because painful wounds are so ubiquitous. In order to optimize wound-healing outcomes and improve overall quality of life, clinicians and patients must collaborate to manage wound-associated pain. McCaffery first defined pain in 1972 in her pioneering nursing research in this field as "whatever the experiencing person says it is and exists whenever he says it does" (McCaffery and Pasero, 1999). Today this definition poses a clinical dilemma in the case where an individual is unable to communicate (e.g., patient with severe dementia) and is not able to verbalize his or her pain. However, the inability to communicate verbally does not negate the possibility that an individual is experiencing pain and is in need of appropriate pain-relieving treatment (EWMA, 2002; WUWHS, 2004). With McCaffery as cochair, the International Association for the Study of Pain (IASP) and the American Pain Society (APS) subsequently redefined pain as "an unpleasant sensory and emotional experience associated with actual or potential tissue damage, or described in terms of such damage" (McCaffery and Pasero, 1999). The National Advisory Council on Aging (2002) describes pain management as "the elimination or control of pain, with a goal of restoring comfort, quality of life, and the capacity to function as well as possible given individual circumstances and the source of pain."

This chapter discusses pain-related concepts, perception, and consequences of wound pain, as well as physiology, classification, assessment of pain, and an introduction to wound pain models. Chapter 26 provides a detailed discussion of wound pain management.

PERCEPTIONS ABOUT PAIN

A patient's expectation of pain can be largely dependent on his or her cultural and ethnic background, social support system, medical history, and prior pain experience (Morris, 1991). When a patient cannot communicate in the language of the care provider, effective management of his or her pain becomes more difficult and often leads to undertreatment. Improved knowledge and attitudes by health care professionals about wound-associated pain and its management are resulting in improved patient outcomes (Lloyd Jones et al, 2010). Health care providers must be aware of obstacles such as language and cultural barriers and use more care and time in assessing and treating such patients. Interventions that alter a patient's expectation of pain may positively affect the pain experienced by that patient.

A long-held myth in wound care is that venous ulcers and pressure ulcers are not painful. Ironically, in a study of patients with venous ulcers, patients often did not request pain medication because they expected their wounds to be painful (Krasner, 1997). Therefore health care professionals often do not even assess for venous ulcer pain, which then contributes to the undertreatment of venous ulcer pain. In a study conducted by Dallam et al (1995) involving 132 patients with pressure ulcers, 68% reported some type of wound pain, yet only 2% were given analgesics for pressure ulcer pain within 4 hours of pain measurement.

In a 2008 review of the literature on pain with pressure ulcers, reported pain prevalence ranged from 37% to 100%, and ulcer stage was reported to most consistently affect pain (Girouard et al, 2008). In 2009 the National Pressure Ulcer

Advisory Panel (NPUAP) published a systematic literature review and white paper on pressure ulcer pain advocating the importance of pressure ulcer pain and the need for further research in all populations across all settings (Pieper et al, 2009).

In a qualitative study of nurses providing care to patients with a pressure ulcer who experienced pain, nurse generalists and advanced practice nurses were asked to reflect and write a story about the phenomenon of caring for the patient with wound pain (Krasner, 1996). Text analysis of the reflections from the 42 participants revealed three patterns of responses by the caregivers. By examining and understanding these patterns of response and the examples of behaviors relative to each response, valuable insight can be gained into the delivery of more sensitive care that is patient focused rather than wound focused.

The first pattern of response is described as "nursing expertly." With this type of response, the nurse uses a set of skills and behaviors that make a qualitative difference in the patient's care. Skills commonly used include (1) read the pain; (2) attend to the pain; and (3) acknowledge the presence of or potential for pain (i.e., empathize with the patient). "Reading" the pain is a critical aspect of assessing for the presence of pain that extends beyond simply asking patients if they are experiencing pain. It is the recognition of signs associated with pain, such as increased anxiety, sweating, bulging eyes, increased respirations, and exaggerated movement in bed. Unfortunately, these signs are easily overlooked by the caregiver when the patient is nonverbal. Attending to the pain indicates that the nurse has taken steps to control pain with medications, positioning, distraction, and so on. Acknowledging the presence of pain or the potential for an intervention or procedure to trigger pain demonstrates empathy for the patient and creates an opportunity to discuss the nature of the pain and identify strategies to minimize or relieve the pain. Empathic care for the patient with pain is demonstrated by using a slower pace in performing procedures, conducting dressing changes in a gentle fashion, allowing short "breaks" during painful procedures, providing careful explanations for every step of the procedure, providing words of encouragement, and offering a menu of pain control interventions.

The second pattern of caregiver response reported in the study is to actually "deny the pain." In this type of response, the caregiver essentially fails to recognize or treat pain and leaves the patient to deal with the pain alone. Ultimately, to "deny the pain" is associated with the care provider who is trying to cope with personally uncomfortable situations, such as those in which the provider feels powerless, feels as though nothing else can be done to ameliorate the patient's pain, or feels that the situation is "not the best" but is acceptable and somewhat expected. Three key behaviors exhibited by the nurse are typical of this pattern of response. (1) Assuming pain does not exist. This behavior is common, along with the erroneous but previously held belief that venous and pressure ulcers are not painful despite the twinges of pain or other verbal or nonverbal signs the patient would manifest. (2) Ignoring the patient's cries of pain. This behavior could be characteristic of situations where the patient continues to report the presence of pain with a dressing change or sharp debridement despite the analgesic given. (3) Avoidance of personal failure. This behavior is characterized by the nurse who simply avoids interacting with the patient or limits the extent of contact with the patient because the patient continues to experience discomfort and all possible interventions for this patient have been exhausted.

The third and final pattern of response observed by this group of nurses was to "confront the challenge of pain" as exemplified by coping with the frustrations and "being with" the patient. A central benefit to this type of response by the nurse is the insight gained into the meaning of the pain experience to the patient. For example, the challenge of the pain may be triggered more by anxiety, stress, or anticipatory pain (Woo, 2008) rather than pain per se. This insight then can be used to develop a more individualized plan of care. A hermeneutic phenomenologic study by Kohr and Gibson (2008) suggests that although nurses want to do the right thing and protect the patient from physical and psychic wound pain, many barriers to optimal pain management exist.

CONSEQUENCES OF WOUND PAIN

Wound pain negatively affects quality of life and affects physiologic processes, including oxygenation and infection control (Woo et al, 2014a). Unfortunately, many patients with a wound suffer these negative consequences because undertreatment of patients with chronic wound pain is far too common.

Quality of Life

Chronic pain has been well documented to affect a patient's physical, psychological, and spiritual well-being and social concerns. Patients experience lack of sleep, fatigue, anxiety, depression, and fear of future pain. Chronic pain increases caregiver burden and greatly affects roles and relationships (Ferrell, 2005). Patients with wounds are at high risk for acute and chronic pain that tends to be moderately severe to severe in intensity. Uncontrolled wound pain is considered the most significant predictor of impaired quality of life for people with wounds (Dallam et al, 1995; Szor and Bourguignon, 1999). Pressure ulcer pain, specifically, affects activities of daily living because the pain could limit the patient's mobility and ability to reposition, thus increasing the risk for wound deterioration (Popescu and Salcido, 2004).

Specific to venous ulcer pain, Hofman et al (1997) found that for 69% of the patients in their study, pain was "the worst thing about having an ulcer," disrupting sleep and negatively affecting quality of life. Previous studies reported similar findings in patients with venous ulcers (Phillips et al, 1994; Walshe, 1995). Using a Heideggerian hermeneutic phenomenologic approach, Krasner (1997, 1998a, 1998b) described the experience of patients with venous ulcer pain. The common pattern that emerged from the study was "carrying on despite the pain." Eight themes providing a glimpse of the impact of venous ulcer pain on quality of life and activities of daily living were identified (Box 25-1).

People with end-of-life or nonhealable wounds (e.g., Kennedy Terminal Ulcer, skin failure, or Skin Changes At

Life's End [SCALE]) may experience wound-related pain (Edsberg et al, 2014; Sibbald et al, 2009). Careful assessment of each person is warranted, taking into consideration individual risk factors and comorbidities (Brown, 2013; Woo et al, 2014a). Goals, plans of care, and targeted interventions for reducing wound-related pain that are consistent with the individual's palliative/hospice goals and plans of care should be identified and documented in the medical record (Collier et al, 2013). Reducing wound-related pain, promoting comfort and dignity, relieving suffering, and improving quality of life are critical outcomes when the palliative pathway is chosen (Woo et al, 2014b). See Chapter 37 for further information.

Physiologic

Wound pain that is inadequately treated can lead to poor wound healing and increased infection rates. These negative sequelae may occur first because pain may impede the patient's ability to tolerate wound care and second because pain may cause or worsen wound hypoxia. Poor pain control may impede the care provider's ability to cleanse, dress, and debride the wound, all of which are required for healing. When pain is poorly controlled, patients may refuse debridement and cleansing and postpone needed dressing changes. These factors may increase the risk of infection and allow wounds to stagnate.

Acute pain increases circulating catecholamines, including epinephrine, and leads to peripheral vasoconstriction, decreased perfusion of blood to the skin and extremities, and, consequently, reduced oxygen availability in the tissues (Franz et al, 2008). As tissue oxygen decreases, leukocyte activity is progressively impaired so that bacteria have a greater likelihood of remaining viable and causing wound infections (Hopf and Holm, 2008). To function properly (i.e., to remove cellular debris and kill bacteria in the wound), leukocytes require oxygen. A major mechanism by which leukocytes kill bacteria is oxidative bacterial killing. The membrane-bound enzyme phagosomal oxygenase or primary oxidase converts oxygen to superoxide, which itself is bactericidal.

Superoxide is then converted to multiple other bactericidal oxidants within the phagosome, including hydrogen peroxide, hypochlorite (bleach), and hydroxyl radical (Allen et al, 1997). A hypoxic wound environment will further impair wound healing by disrupting fibroblast activity and angiogenesis, thereby negatively affecting collagen synthesis and migration and the delivery of oxygen to the wound cells.

PAIN PHYSIOLOGY

Although pain is a subjective experience, objective physiologic mechanisms control how pain is initiated, transmitted, and perceived. The objective neural response to a painful stimulus (e.g., at the wound) is called *nociception.* Nociception is defined as the detection of impending or actual tissue damage and is accomplished by specialized sensory nerve terminals (nociceptors) derived from $A\delta$ (delta) and C fibers. All nerve endings in the epidermis are considered nociceptors (Popescu and Salcido, 2004). When cells are damaged, chemicals are released, triggering the nerve fibers to transmit the pain impulses along nerve sheaths to the spinal cord. The spinal cord transmits the information to the brain, where it is centrally processed. Synaptic junctions in the spinal cord and brain will either attenuate or amplify the pain signal and thus affect how the intensity of the pain signal will be perceived or interpreted.

In addition to the actual tissue injury that triggers the pain episode, psychological, physical, emotional, and cultural factors, as well as the patient's expectations, collectively define an individual's pain experience. Thus the same type of injury in two different individuals often generates a very different pain experience in terms of severity, quality, and impact. Reported pain may appear to be either less than expected or excessive given the degree of tissue injury. Distress out of proportion to the injury is often ascribed to anxiety, as well as "catastrophizing" (Sullivan and Neish, 1999; Sullivan et al, 1998).

Catastrophizing is significantly correlated with mood and personality variables such as depression, fear of pain, coping strategies, and state and trait anxiety (Rosenstiel and Keefe, 1983; Sullivan et al, 1995). These variables have been shown to be important predictors of the pain experience. Preoperative levels of anxiety and catastrophizing can be predictive of postoperative pain intensity. A study by Granot and Ferber (2005) found that moderately anxious surgical patients are at greater risk for developing greater postoperative pain.

CLASSIFICATIONS

Types of pain may vary by wound type and underlying etiology. For example, pain associated with lower extremity wounds can be related to claudication, to nocturnal or rest pain from ischemia (arterial disease) or increased edema (venous), or to neuropathy (neuropathic) (WOCN®, 2008, 2011, 2012). The types of pain typical of lower extremity ulcers (i.e., arterial, venous, neuropathic) are described in the lower extremity wounds section of this text.

Before initiating pain management interventions (either pharmacologic or nonpharmacologic), the type of wound pain that is being experienced and the source of that pain must be determined. Interventions then can be tailored to the patient's needs and effective outcomes achieved. Pain experts categorize pain into two types: nociceptive and neuropathic.

Nociceptive (Acute) Pain

Nociceptive pain, also referred to as *acute pain,* is the normal processing of the pain impulse. It serves to alert the individual to ongoing or impending injury. Acute pain usually is consistent with the degree of tissue injury; hence, greater tissue injury translates into greater pain sensation. Acute pain can be subclassified as operative, procedural, incident, and background pain (Figure 25-1) (IASP Task Force, 1994; WUWHS, 2004). Nociceptive pain typically is well localized, constant, and time limited (pain resolves when the painful procedure ends) and often has an aching or throbbing quality.

The persistence of severe, inadequately treated acute pain can lead to anatomic and physiologic changes in the nervous system (Woolf and Salter, 2000). The ability of neural tissue to change in response to repeated incoming stimuli, a property known as *neuroplasticity,* can lead to the development of chronic, disabling neuropathic pain (Cohen et al, 2004). Opioids are a commonly used strategy to manage nociceptive pain.

Neuropathic Pain

Neuropathic pain results from damaged or malfunctioning nerve fibers. Nerves can be compressed by a tumor, strangulated by scar tissue, or inflamed by infection. Unlike acute pain, neuropathic pain is not an indication of impending tissue injury; rather, neuropathic pain is an indication that sensory nerves are malfunctioning. Common in chronic wounds, neuropathic pain is often described as burning; it also may have "electric shock-like" qualities.

Neuropathic pain may be visceral or somatic in origin. *Visceral pain* stems from organs or the gastrointestinal tract.

Visceral pain is often described as diffuse and gnawing or cramping and poorly localized (Hader and Guy, 2004). The neural signal crosses into the spinal cord at vagal ganglia and at dorsal root ganglia. This type of pain is commonly seen in conjunction with injuries to internal organs, as occurs with appendicitis, myocardial ischemia, pneumonia, or gastric ulcers (Hader and Guy, 2004). *Somatic pain* originates from the bone, joints, muscles, skin, and connective tissue. As with acute pain, somatic pain is described as a throbbing, well-localized pain. The pain sensation from a wound usually is somatic and can be further subdivided according to the source of the pain.

Numerous pathologic responses to pain may be seen and can result from inadequately treated pain, excessive inflammation, and other pathophysiologic processes. Chronic wound pain, as occurs with a pressure or venous ulcer, is commonly characterized by hyperalgesia (increased response to a normally painful stimulus) and allodynia (pain due to a stimulus that normally does not provoke pain). In the presence of hyperalgesia, any touch to the wound surface or surrounding skin, regardless of how gentle, may be interpreted as painful. Allodynia is present when gentle cleansing of the periwound skin triggers a pain episode. Hyperalgesia and allodynia are responsible for the pain that is "out of proportion" to the stimulus (Popescu and Salcido, 2004). Thus routine dressing changes and periwound skin care become excruciating.

Typically, the pathologic process that initiated the neuropathic pain is not fully reversible. However, with appropriate management of the pathologic process, neuropathic pain can be reduced. Neuropathic pain often responds to antiseizure and antidepressant medications rather than opioids.

Mixed Nociceptive/Neuropathic

Mixed-category pain results from a complex mixture of nociceptive and neuropathic factors. Although the nervous system initially may malfunction, tissue injury resulting from this malfunction triggers the release of inflammatory mediators. Venous ulcer pain has been reported to be a combination of

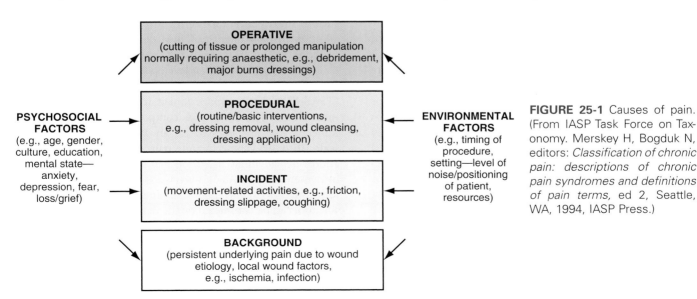

FIGURE 25-1 Causes of pain. (From IASP Task Force on Taxonomy. Merskey H, Bogduk N, editors: *Classification of chronic pain: descriptions of chronic pain syndromes and definitions of pain terms,* ed 2, Seattle, WA, 1994, IASP Press.)

nociceptive and neuropathic pain, a finding that has important ramifications for medicating for pain using polypharmacy (Krasner 1997, 1998a, 1998b).

ASSESSMENT

The goal in controlling wound pain is to reduce or eliminate pain so that patients can resume and perform their activities. In cognitively impaired patients, the goal is to maximize their comfort and enhance their quality of life. A systematic and thorough assessment of wound pain is an essential first step (Kifer, 2012). Most regulatory agencies, such as the Centers for Medicare and Medicaid Services (CMS), state departments of health, and The Joint Commission, require systematic assessment and documentation of pain, pain relief measures, and their efficacy.

The patient's pain experience does not correlate with visible wound manifestations, and there is no direct relationship between pathology and intensity of pain. Although superficial wounds with multiple exposed nerves may be intensely painful (sensory nerve endings are most numerous in the dermis), some patients may not experience intense pain from these wounds. Conversely, subcutaneous tissue contains few sensory nerves, so deep wounds with destruction of dermis would be expected to be less painful. In fact, necrotic and deep subcutaneous tissues can be debrided many times without application of significant analgesia, whereas debridement of wound edges or debridement that disturbs the wound edges (as occurs when pulling adherent eschar) may be extremely painful. Consequently, assessment of pain based upon wound depth is not appropriate and may be flawed. In general, wounds become less painful as they begin active healing. The mechanism is not clear, but probably involves decreased inflammation, covering of exposed nerve endings, and decreased wound ischemia and hypoxia.

In practice, assessment and documentation of pain are inconsistent. Hollinworth (1995) reported inadequate pain management and poor accountability and inadequate or uninformed assessment, management, and documentation of pain at wound dressing changes. Nurses failed to assess pain verbally or to use pain assessment tools. Instead, pain was assessed based on nurses' experience or on nonverbal patient indicators. In a cross-sectional quantitative study of 132 patients with pressure ulcer pain, Dallam et al (1995) found that 59% reported having pain of some type; however, only 2% were given analgesics for the pain (within 4 hours of interview). In a study of venous ulcer healing and pain in current and former users of injected drugs, researchers found many of these patients were denied adequate pain control based upon their history. Researchers concluded that providers need to listen to patient concerns about pain medication and, with the patient, determine the best medication protocol (Pieper, 1994; Pieper et al, 1998).

Many factors must be assessed to adequately manage wound pain: pain history, etiology, condition of the wound, topical wound care, type of pain, and source of wound pain (WOCN®, 2008, 2010, 2011, 2012). Pain assessment should include an assessment of body language and nonverbal cues (e.g., change in activity, loss of appetite, guarding, grimacing, moaning) (Feldt,

2000; NPUAP, EPUAP, PPPIA 2014). Furthermore, because the condition of the wound greatly affects wound pain and the wound condition is frequently changing, pain assessment must be done regularly, with wound manipulations and dressing changes, as well as performed on a routine daily basis. Pain is assessed by its type: nociceptive, neuropathic, or intrinsic (chronic noncyclic); procedural (acute noncyclic); or incident (acute cyclic). With this detailed assessment, appropriate pain control measures can be identified.

Pain History

A pain history should provide sufficient detail to characterize the nature of the pain and factors that affect the patient's pain experience. A pain history may be difficult to obtain when the patient is experiencing referred pain or when the pain is nonspecific.

Self-Report Pain Intensity Scales

Self-report is the most reliable indicator of the existence and intensity of acute pain (APS, 2008). Numerous pain assessment tools are available to quantify the severity of pain and measure the effectiveness of pain control interventions. Intensity-of-pain scales range from simple visual analog scales to complex multidimensional, multipage instruments. For example, visual analog scales measure only one dimension of the pain phenomenon at a time (e.g., intensity, from "no pain" to "worst possible pain"), using words, numbers, faces, or other culturally congruent objects (e.g., coins or poker chips). Examples of these scales are provided in Figure 25-2. Visual analog scales are particularly useful in clinical practice for use with patients who are in active pain and do not have the capacity to complete a long, arduous questionnaire. A systematic review of 164 articles found single-item pain intensity ratings to be valid and reliable (Jensen, 2003).

More complex pain assessment tools, such as the McGill Pain Questionnaire (Melzack, 1975), and its modifications, such as the Dartmouth Pain Questionnaire (Corson and Schneider, 1984), measure a quality of the pain experience, such as functional limitation or impact on quality of life, in addition to pain intensity. These descriptive scales are used primarily in clinical research and specialized pain clinics.

Maida et al (2009) have developed a wound-specific scale called the Toronto Symptom Assessment System for Wounds (TSAS-W). This one-page tool is intended for clinical and research use. The TSAS-W is composed of 10 symptom parameters that are assessed on an 11-point numeric rating scale (0 to 10). These include pain intensity *with* dressings and/or debridement, as well as *between* dressings and/or debridement. The TSAS-W also assesses wound-related symptoms, such as drainage, odor, itching, bleeding, and swelling. The tool can be completed by the patient, the patient assisted by a caregiver, or a caregiver.

A number of general tools have been developed that address psychological stress and pain. These are described and discussed in detail in a review article by Solowiej et al (2010). Nine tools are presented, all of which have utility for assessing stress and pain in people with wounds.

Simple Descriptive Pain Intensity Scale[1]

No	Mild	Moderate	Severe	Very	Worst
pain	pain	pain	pain	severe	possible
				pain	pain

0-10 Numeric Pain Intensity Scale[1]

0 1 2 3 4 5 6 7 8 9 10

No	Moderate	Worst
pain	pain	possible
		pain

Visual Analog Scale (VAS)[2]

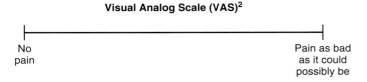

No	Pain as bad
pain	as it could
	possibly be

[1] If used as a graphic rating scale, a 10 cm baseline is recommended.

[2] A 10 cm baseline is recommended for VAS scales.

FIGURE 25-2 Three examples of pain intensity scales as published by the Agency for Healthcare Research and Quality. (From Bergstrom N, Bennett MA, Carlson C, et al: *Treatment of pressure ulcers* [Clinical practice guideline no. 15, AHCPR publication no. 95-0622], Rockville, MD, 1994, U.S. Department of Health and Human Services, Public Health Service.)

Observational Pain Intensity Scales

Nonverbal and cognitively impaired individuals are at risk for poor pain management due to lack of pain assessment. Between 40% and 60% of long-term care residents do not use the analgesics and pain relief medications ordered for them (Horgas and Tsai, 1998; Kaasalainen et al, 1998). Unfortunately, instead of frequently offering *as-needed* pain medications, caregivers tend to interpret *as needed* to mean "when the patient asks for it" (Feldt, 2000). Of course, verbalization of pain or requesting pain medication is unlikely to occur in the nonverbal or cognitively impaired patient.

The cognitively impaired individual has difficulty finding the words to describe discomfort or has impaired executive skills, which limits the ability to correlate a number on a pain scale with the sensation of pain or to interpret the "crying face" of a scale as an indication of "severe" pain (Wynne et al, 2000). However, patients manifest several observational behaviors when they are in pain (Weiner et al, 1999).

The Pain Assessment in Advanced Dementia (PAINAD) scale is presented in Table 25-1. Endorsed for use in long-term care by the American Medical Directors Association (AMDA), the PAINAD scale is an easy-to-use, five-item observational instrument. Items to assess are breathing, negative vocalization, facial expression, body language, and consolability. Each item is rated on a scale from 0 to 2 based on descriptions for each score category. Total scores range from 0 to 10, with a higher score indicating severe pain (Warden et al, 2003).

Another tool developed for use with nonverbal or demented patients is the Checklist of Nonverbal Pain Indicators (CNPI). Like the PAINAD, the CNPI is brief, requires limited time to administer, and does not require extensive knowledge of the patient. The two tools were compared for psychometric properties in a recent study that concluded that both tools "should be used cautiously both in research and clinical settings to minimize floor effects, observation of behaviors using these tools should occur during physical activity and neither instrument should be the sole indicator of pain. Instead they should be only one part of a multidimensional pain assessment program that includes more comprehensive screening tools and other approaches recommended for this population" (Ersek et al, 2010).

TABLE 25-1	**Pain Assessment in Advanced Dementia (PAINAD) Scale**			
Items*	**0**	**1**	**2**	**Score**
Breathing independent of vocalization	Normal	Occasional labored breathing Short period of hyperventilation	Noisy labored breathing Long period of hyperventilation Cheyne-Stokes respirations	
Negative vocalization	None	Occasional moan or groan Low-level speech with a negative or disapproving quality	Repeated troubled calling out Loud moaning or groaning	
Facial expression	Smiling or inexpressive	Sad Frightened Frown	Facial grimacing	
Body language	Relaxed	Tense Distressed pacing Fidgeting	Rigid Fists clenched Knees pulled up Pulling or pushing away Striking out	
Consolability	No need to console	Distracted or reassured	Unable to console, distract, or reassure	
			Total†	

Continued

TABLE 25-1   **Pain Assessment in Advanced Dementia (PAINAD) Scale—cont'd**

Breathing
1. Normal breathing is characterized by effortless, quiet, rhythmic (smooth) respirations.
2. Occasional labored breathing is characterized by episodic bursts of harsh, difficult, or wearing respirations.
3. Short period of hyperventilation is characterized by intervals of rapid, deep breaths lasting a short time.
4. Noisy labored breathing is characterized by negative-sounding respirations on inspiration or expiration. They may be loud, gurgling, or wheezing. They appear strenuous or wearing.
5. Long period of hyperventilation is characterized by an excessive rate and depth of respirations lasting a considerable time.
6. Cheyne-Stokes respirations are characterized by rhythmic waxing and waning of breathing, from very deep to shallow respirations with periods of apnea (cessation of breathing).

Negative Vocalization
1. None is characterized by speech or vocalization that has a neutral or pleasant quality.
2. Occasional moan or groan is characterized by mournful or murmuring sounds, wails, or laments. Groaning is characterized by louder-than-usual inarticulate involuntary sounds, often abruptly beginning and ending.
3. Low-level speech with a negative or disapproving quality is characterized by muttering, mumbling, whining, grumbling, or swearing in a low volume with a complaining, sarcastic, or caustic tone.
4. Repeated troubled calling out is characterized by phrases or words being used over and over in a tone that suggests anxiety, uneasiness, or distress.
5. Loud moaning or groaning is characterized by mournful or murmuring sounds, wails, or laments that are much louder than usual volume. Loud groaning is characterized by louder-than-usual inarticulate involuntary sounds, often abruptly beginning and ending.
6. Crying is characterized by an utterance of emotion accompanied by tears. There may be sobbing or quiet weeping.

Facial Expression
1. Smiling is characterized by upturned corners of the mouth, brightening of the eyes, and a look of pleasure or contentment. Inexpressive refers to a neutral, at ease, relaxed, or blank look.
2. Sad is characterized by an unhappy, lonesome, sorrowful, or dejected look. There may be tears in the eyes.
3. Frightened is characterized by a look of fear, alarm, or heightened anxiety. Eyes appear wide open.
4. Frown is characterized by a downward turn of the corners of the mouth. Increased facial wrinkling in the forehead and around the mouth may appear.
5. Facial grimacing is characterized by a distorted, distressed look. The brow is more wrinkled, as is the area around the mouth. Eyes may be squeezed shut.

Body Language
1. Relaxed is characterized by a calm, restful, mellow appearance. The person seems to be taking it easy.
2. Tense is characterized by a strained, apprehensive, or worried appearance. The jaw may be clenched (exclude any contractures).
3. Distressed pacing is characterized by activity that seems unsettled. A fearful, worried, or disturbed element may be present. The rate may be faster or slower.
4. Fidgeting is characterized by restless movement. Squirming about or wiggling in the chair may occur. The person might be hitching a chair across the room. Repetitive touching, tugging, or rubbing body parts may be observed.
5. Rigid is characterized by stiffening of the body. The arms and/or legs are tight and inflexible. The trunk may appear straight and unyielding (exclude any contractures).
6. Fists clenched is characterized by tightly closed hands. They may be opened and closed repeatedly or held tightly shut.
7. Knees pulled up is characterized by flexing the legs and drawing the knees up toward the chest. An overall troubled appearance may be seen (exclude any contractures).
8. Pulling or pushing away is characterized by resistiveness upon approach or to care. The person may try to escape by yanking or wrenching himself or herself free or shoving you away.
9. Striking out is characterized by hitting, kicking, grabbing, punching, biting, or other forms of personal assault.

Consolability
1. No need to console is characterized by a sense of well-being. The person appears content.
2. Distracted or reassured by voice or touch is characterized by a disruption in the behavior when the person is spoken to or is touched. The behavior stops during the period of interaction, with no indication that the person is distressed.
3. Unable to console, distract, or reassure is characterized by the inability to soothe the person or stop a behavior with words or actions. No amount of comforting, verbal or physical, will alleviate the behavior.

*See the description of each item in the lower part of the table.
†Total scores range from 0 to 10 (based on a scale from 0 to 2 for five items), with a higher score indicating more severe pain (0 = "no pain" to 10 = "severe pain").
From Warden V, Hurley AC, Volicer L: Development and psychometric evaluation of the pain assessment in advanced dementia (PAINAD) scale, *J Am Med Dir Assoc* 4:9–15, 2003, excerpted from Frampton K: Vital sign #5, Caring for the Ages 5(5):26, 2004.

Options for assessing pain in the nonverbal pediatric patient include the FLACC and CRIES observational scales (Tables 25-2 and 25-3). The FLACC (Face, Legs, Activity, Crying, Consolability) scale provides a rating between 0 and 10 and was designed and validated for use with children between the ages of 2 months and 7 years. However, some practitioners have used the FLACC scale with adults who are unable to communicate their pain (Merkel et al, 1997). The CRIES (Crying; Requires O$_2$; Increasing Vital Signs; Expression; Sleepless) pain scale, originally created to assess

TABLE 25-2   FLACC Pain Scale for Children 2 Months to 7 Years

Category	SCORING		
	1	2	3
Face	No particular expression or smile	Occasional grimace or frown, withdrawn, disinterested	Frequent to constant quivering chin, clenched jaw
Legs	Normal position or relaxed	Uneasy, restless, tense	Kicking, or legs drawn up
Activity	Lying quietly, normal position, moves easily	Squirming, shifting back and forth, tense	Arched, rigid or jerking
Cry	No cry (awake or asleep)	Moans or whimpers; occasional complaint	Crying steadily, screams or sobs, frequent complaints
Consolability	Content, relaxed	Reassured by occasional touching, hugging, or being talked to; distractible	Difficult to console or comfort

FLACC, Face, Legs, Activity, Crying, Consolability
From Merkel S, Voepel-Lewis T, Shayevitz JR, et al: The FLACC: a behavioral scale for scoring postoperative pain in young children, *Pediatr Nurse* 23(3):293–297, 1997.

TABLE 25-3   CRIES Pain Scale for Neonates (0 to 6 Months)

Crying
0   No crying, or crying but not high pitched
1   High pitched but infant consolable
2   Inconsolable

Requires O$_2$
Babies experiencing pain manifest decreased oxygenation. Consider other causes of hypoxemia (e.g., oversedation, atelectasis, pneumothorax).
0   No oxygen required; oxygen saturation >95%
1   ≤30% supplemental oxygen required to keep oxygen saturation >95%
2   >30% supplemental oxygen required to keep oxygen saturation >95%

Increased Vital Signs
Take BP last because process may awaken the child, making mean assessments difficult.
0   Both HR and mean BP are unchanged or are less than baseline
1   HR or mean BP is increased ≤20% from baseline level
2   HR or BP is increased >20% over baseline level

Expression
Facial expression most often associated with pain is a grimace, which may be characterized by brow lowering, eyes squeezed shut, deepening nasolabial furrow, or open lips and mouth.
0   No grimace present
1   Grimace alone is present
2   Grimace and noncry vocalization grunt is present

Sleepless
Scored based on infant's state during the hour preceding this recorded score.
0   Child has been continuously asleep
1   Child has awakened at frequent intervals
2   Child has been awake constantly

BP, Blood pressure; *CRIES*, Crying, Requires O$_2$, Increasing Vital Signs, Expression, Sleepless; *HR*, heart rate.
From Krechel SW, Bildner J: CRIES: a new neonatal postoperative pain measurement score-initial testing of validity and reliability, *Paediatr Anaesth* 5:53–61, 1995.

postoperative pain in the neonate, is reportedly effective for use in neonates up to age 6 months (Krechel and Bildner, 1995). Each category is scored on a scale from 0 to 2; total scores range between 0 and 10 (Krechel and Bildner, 1995).

Pain Assessment in Patients with Substance Use Disorders

People with a history of substance use disorders (SUD) can be challenging when it comes to pain assessment, due in part to stigmatization, misconceptions, and provider experience and lack of skills. In 2012 the American Society of Pain Management Nursing (ASPMN) issued an updated position statement on pain management in patients with SUD (Oliver et al, 2012). The document addresses the scope of the problem, barriers to care, and conceptual models and makes ten detailed recommendations. Ethical principles for treating patients with SUD are presented, as well as pediatric risk assessment. The position statement summary concludes, "Patients with substance use disorders can and should be treated with dignity, respect, and the same quality of pain assessment and management as all other patients. Failure to identify and treat the concurrent condition of pain and substance use disorder compromises the ability to treat either condition effectively" (p. 178).

WOUND PAIN CARE MODELS

Wound pain care models assist the clinician in addressing pain through every aspect of wound management. The value of these models is that they go beyond simply listing all possible strategies for controlling wound pain. Rather, these models guide the clinician through a logical, systematic, and thorough assessment of the wound (i.e., etiology and related interventions, topical wound condition and the related interventions, and type of pain) so that interventions can be selected based upon the patient's type and source of pain.

The Chronic Wound Pain Experience (CWPE) model (Krasner, 1995) was empirically and inductively derived. It can be used to assist with establishing a plan of care for pain control (Figure 25-3). The CWPE model introduces a

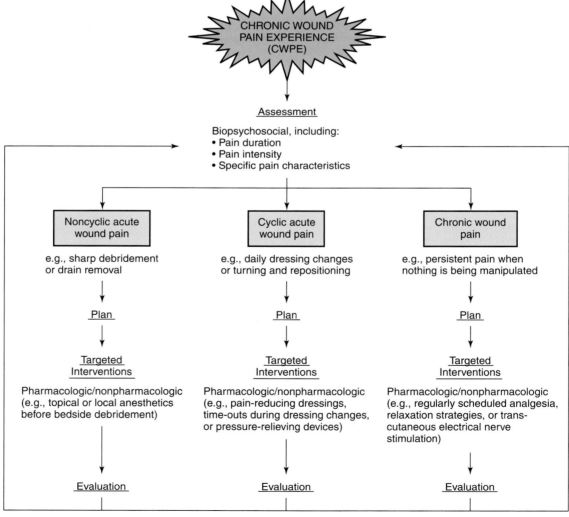

FIGURE 25-3 Chronic wound pain experience (CWPE) model.

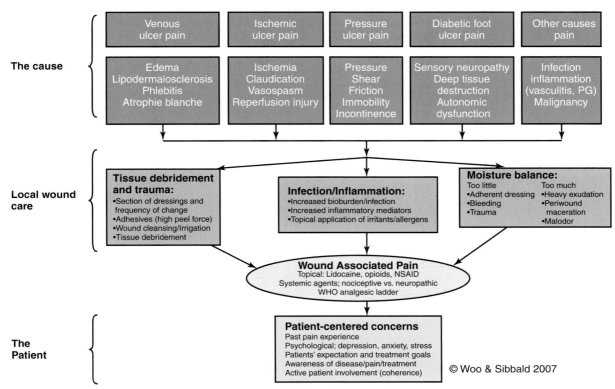

FIGURE 25-4 Wound-associated pain model: the wound, the cause, the patient. (From Woo KY, Sibbald RG: The improvement of wound-associated pain and healing trajectory with a comprehensive foot and leg ulcer care model, *J Wound Ostomy Continence Nurs* 36(2):184–191, 2009.)

classification scheme tailored specifically to pain associated with wounds:

1. Noncyclical acute wound pain: a single episode of pain (e.g., pain that occurs with sharp debridement)
2. Cyclic acute wound pain: acute wound pain that recurs as a result of repeated treatments (e.g., pain that occurs with dressing changes)
3. Chronic wound pain: persistent, continuous pain that occurs without manipulation of the wound

Each type of pain has a menu of appropriate pain control options. The CWPE model assumes that most patients with chronic wounds experience all three types of pain at some time, although not necessarily simultaneously. It also recognizes that some patients may not experience or may not be able to indicate pain. Others may not experience one of the pain types because of the particular course of their treatment or disease (e.g., the patient who has never had sharp debridement may never experience noncyclical acute wound pain). Another assumption is that many commonly held beliefs about wound pain might lack validity (e.g., patients with diabetes do not experience wound pain in the presence of neuropathy).

The Wound Associated Pain (WAP) model (Woo and Sibbald, 2009) guides the clinician through the process of addressing underlying causes of the wound and patient-centered concerns, including anxiety and depression, and providing appropriate local wound care, as well as systemic strategies that address associated pain. The key components are (1) patient-centered concerns; (2) wound etiology; and (3) local wound factors (Figure 25-4). The authors demonstrated pain reduction after the model was used to manage 111 subjects with chronic leg and foot ulcers. Using an 11-point numeric rating scale, the average level of pain was reduced from 6.3 at week 0 to 2.8 at week 4 ($p < .001$).

TRANSLATION TO PRACTICE

An excellent model for how to translate pain assessment into practice is the "Heal Not Hurt" initiative developed by clinicians in the United Kingdom working with an industry partner, Mölnlycke Health Care. This initiative has been described by Trudie Young (2007). The evidence base includes the European Wound Management Association Position Paper on Pain (2002) and the World Union of Wound Healing Societies Consensus Document on Pain (2004). In addition, there is a pocket guide, staff badges, posters on "Heal Not Hurt" for display in the clinical area, and a "Tell us when it hurts" leaflet. This initiative has been successful in raising awareness and stimulating discussion of pain symptoms between patients and providers (Young, 2007).

CLINICAL CONSULT

A: Consulted to recommend treatment options for a 90-year-old, terminally ill patient with end-stage Alzheimer dementia. Patient is on home hospice being cared for by his 88-year-old wife. Two weeks ago he developed a painful Stage II sacral ulcer that has rapidly deteriorated to an unstageable ulcer with hard black eschar, 5 cm × 4 cm. Patient is nonverbal, on bed rest, contracted into a fetal position, doubly incontinent, and taking in minimal oral intake (~25% of meals). He is on a hospital bed with a low air loss mattress replacement. His current turning schedule is q2h from the right side to the left side. The current topical treatment to his sacral ulcer is with a 4″ × 4″ hydrocolloid dressing changed Monday, Wednesday, Friday, and as needed by the hospice nurse or wife. His wound pain is most severe at dressing change and whenever he is turned (he moans and groans).

D: Unstageable pressure ulcer in a hospice patient with goals for nonextension of wound and pain control.

P: Palliative wound care to minimize pain and suffering. Prevent wound deterioration. Wound healing is not anticipated.

I: Nurse and caregiver (wife) understand and consent to the following wound care plan: (1) Continue to use low air loss mattress replacement for pressure redistribution. (2) Change to repositioning schedule as tolerated. (3) Sacral ulcer care: Keep eschar dry. Cover with 4″ × 4″ foam dressing with silicone adhesive and silicone tape border. Change Mondays and Thursdays and as needed. Assess pain daily and at dressing change using the Pain Assessment in Advanced Dementia (PAINAD) scale and premedicate patient as ordered. (4) Incontinence cleanser and moisture barrier for incontinence management.

E: Reconsult if wound exhibits signs of infection, odor with dressing in place, frequent strike through exudate and dressing changes, or if eschar begins to soften or lift.

SUMMARY

Accurately conceptualizing wound pain leads to proficiency in clinical assessment and management of wound pain. Managing wound pain improves patient quality of life and patient satisfaction.

To cure—occasionally.
To relieve—often.
To comfort—always.

— *Hippocrates*

REFERENCES

Allen DB, Maguire JJ, Mahdavian M, et al: Wound hypoxia and acidosis limit neutrophil bacterial killing mechanisms, *Arch Surg* 132(9):991–996, 1997.

American Pain Society (APS): *Principles of analgesic use in the treatment of acute and cancer pain*, ed 5, Glenview, IL, 2008, APS.

Bergstrom N, Bennett MA, Carlson C, et al: *Treatment of pressure ulcers (Clinical practice guideline no. 15, AHCPR publication no. 95-0622)*, Rockville, MD, 1994, U.S. Department of Health and Human Services, Public Health Service.

Brown P: *Quick reference to wound care: palliative, home and clinical practices*, ed 4, Burlington, MA, 2013, Jones & Bartlett.

Cohen SP, Christo PJ, Moroz L: Pain management in trauma patients, *Am J Phys Med Rehabil* 83:142–161, 2004.

Collier KS, Protus BM, Bohn CL, et al: *Wound care at end of life: a guide for hospice professionals*, Montgomery, AL, 2013, HospiScript Services.

Corson J, Schneider M: The Dartmouth pain questionnaire: an adjunct to the McGill pain questionnaire, *Pain* 19:59–69, 1984.

Dallam L, Smyth C, Jackson BS, et al: Pressure ulcer pain: assessment and quantification, *J Wound Ostomy Continence Nurs* 22(5):211–215, 1995.

Edsberg LE, Langemo D, Baharestani MM, et al: Unavoidable pressure injury: state of the science and consensus conference, *J Wound Ostomy Continence Nurs* 41(4):313–334, 2014.

Ersek M, Herr K, Neradilek MB, et al: Comparing the psychometric properties of the Checklist of Nonverbal Pain Indicators (CNPI) and the Pain Assessment in Advanced Dementia (PAIN-AD) instruments, *Pain Medicine* 11:395–404, 2010.

European Wound Management Association (EWMA): *Position document: pain at wound dressing changes*, London, 2002, Medical Education Partnership. http://ewma.org/fileadmin/user_upload/EWMA/pdf/Position_Documents/2002/Spring_2002__English_.pdf. Accessed June 19, 2014.

Feldt KS: Improving assessment and treatment of pain in cognitively impaired nursing home residents, *Ann Longterm Care* 8(9):36–42, 2000.

Ferrell B: Ethical perspectives on pain and suffering, *Pain Manag Nurs* 6(3):83–90, 2005.

Franz MG, Robson MC, Steed DL, et al: Guidelines to aid healing of acute wounds by decreasing impediments of healing, *Wound Repair Regen* 16:723–748, 2008.

Girouard K, Harrison MB, VanDenKerkof E: The symptom of pain with pressure ulcers: a review of the literature, *Ostomy Wound Manage* 54(5):30–40, 42, 2008.

Granot M, Ferber SG: The roles of pain catastrophizing and anxiety in the prediction of postoperative pain intensity: a prospective study, *Clin J Pain* 21:439–445, 2005.

Hader CF, Guy J: Your hand in pain management, *Nurs Manage* 35(11):21–27, 2004.

Hofman D, Ryan TJ, Arnold F, et al: Pain in venous leg ulcers, *J Wound Care* 6(5):222–224, 1997.

Hollinworth H: Nurses' assessment and management of pain at wound dressing changes, *J Wound Care* 4(2):77–83, 1995.

Hopf HW, Holm J: Hyperoxia and infection, *Best Pract Res Clin Anaesthesiol* 22:553–569, 2008.

Horgas AL, Tsai PF: Analgesic drug prescription and use in cognitively impaired nursing home residents, *Nurs Res* 47:235–242, 1998.

IASP Task Force on Taxonomy, Merskey H, Bogduk N, editors: *Classification of chronic pain: descriptions of chronic pain syndromes and definitions of pain terms*, ed 2, Seattle, WA, 1994, IASP Press.

Jensen MP: The validity and reliability of pain measure in adults with cancer, *J Pain* 4(1):2–21, 2003.

Kaasalainen S, Middleton J, Knezacek S, et al: Pain and cognitive status in the institutionalized elderly: perceptions & interventions, *J Gerontol Nurs* 24(8):24–31, 1998.

Kifer ZA: *Fast facts for wound care nursing: practical wound management in a nutshell*, New York, 2012, Springer.

Kohr R, Gibson M: Doing the right thing: using hermeneutic phenomenology to understand management of wound pain, *Ostomy Wound Manage* 54(4):52–60, 2008.

Krasner D: The chronic wound pain experience: a conceptual model, *Ostomy Wound Manage* 41(3):20–25, 1995.

Krasner D: Using a gentler hand: reflections on patients with pressure ulcers who experience pain, *Ostomy Wound Manage* 42(3):20–22, 24, 26, 1996.

Krasner D: *Carrying on despite the pain: living with painful venous ulcers: a Heideggerian hermeneutic analysis* (Doctoral dissertation), Ann Arbor, 1997, University of Michigan.

Krasner D: Painful venous ulcers: themes and stories about living with the pain and suffering, *J Wound Ostomy Continence Nurs* 25(3):158–168, 1998a.

Krasner D: Painful venous ulcers: themes and stories about their impact on quality of life, *Ostomy Wound Manage* 44(9):38–42, 1998b.

Krechel SW, Bildner J: A new neonatal postoperative pain measurement score. Initial testing of validity and reliability, *Paediatr Anaesth* 5:53–61, 1995.

Lloyd Jones M, Greenwood M, Bielby A: Living with wound-associated pain: impact on the patient and what clinicians really think, *J Wound Care* 19(8):340–345, 2010.

Maida V, Ennis M, Kuziemsky C: The Toronto Symptom Assessment System for Wounds: a new clinical and research tool, *Adv Skin Wound Care* 22(10):468–474, 2009.

McCaffery M, Pasero C: *Pain clinical manual*, ed 2, St. Louis, MO, 1999, Mosby.

Melzack R: The McGill pain questionnaire: major properties and scoring methods, *Pain* 1:277–299, 1975.

Merkel SI, Voepel-Lewis T, Shayevitz JR, et al: The FLACC: a behavioral scale for scoring postoperative pain in young children, *Pediatr Nurse* 23(3):293–297, 1997.

Morris DB: *The culture of pain*, Berkeley, 1991, University of California Press.

National Advisory Council on Aging: Stop the pain, *Expression* 15(3), 2002.

National Pressure Ulcer Advisory Panel (NPUAP), European Pressure Ulcer Advisory Panel (EPUAP) and Pan Pacific Pressure Injury Alliance (PPPIA). *Prevention and treatment of pressure ulcers: quick reference guide*. In Emily Haesler, editor: Perth, Australia, 2014, Cambridge Media.

Oliver J, Coggins C, Compton P, et al: American Society for Pain Management nursing (ASPMN) position statement: pain management in patients with substance use disorders, *Pain Manage Nurs* 13(3):169–183, 2012.

Phillips T, Stanton B, Provan A, et al: A study of the impact of leg ulcers on quality of life: financial, social and psychologic implications, *J Am Acad Dermatol* 31(1):49–53, 1994.

Pieper B: A retrospective analysis of venous ulcer healing in current and former drug users of injected drugs, *J Wound Ostomy Continence Nurs* 23(6):291–296, 1994.

Pieper B, Langemo D, Cuddigan J: Pressure ulcer pain: a systematic literature review and National Pressure Ulcer Advisory Panel white paper, *Ostomy Wound Manage* 55(2):16–31, 2009.

Pieper B, Rossi R, Templin T: Pain associated with venous ulcers in injecting drug users, *Ostomy Wound Manage* 44(11):54–58, 60–67, 1998.

Popescu A, Salcido RS: Wound pain: a challenge for the patient and the wound care specialist, *Adv Skin Wound Care* 17(1):14–20, 2004.

Rosenstiel AK, Keefe FJ: The use of coping strategies in chronic low back pain patients: relationship to patient characteristics and current adjustment, *Pain* 17:33–44, 1983.

Sibbald RG, Krasner DL, SCALE Expert Panel: *SCALE: skin changes at life's end: final consensus document*, October 1, 2009. http://www.epuap.org/wp-content/uploads/2012/07/SCALE-Final-Version-2009.pdf. Accessed June 19, 2014.

Solowiej K, Mason V, Upton D, et al: Psychological stress and pain in wound care, part 2: a review of pain and stress assessment tools, *J Wound Care* 19(3):110–115, 2010.

Sullivan MJL, Neish N: The effects of disclosure on pain during dental hygiene treatment: the moderating role of catastrophizing, *Pain* 79:155–163, 1999.

Sullivan MJL, Bishop SR, Pivik J: The pain catastrophizing scale: development and validation, *Psychol Assess* 7:524–532, 1995.

Sullivan MJL, Stanish W, Waite H, et al: Catastrophizing, pain, and disability in patients with soft-tissue injuries, *Pain* 77:253–260, 1998.

Szor JK, Bourguignon C: Description of pressure ulcer pain at rest and at dressing change, *J Wound Ostomy Continence Nurs* 26(3):115–120, 1999.

Walshe C: Living with a venous leg ulcer: a descriptive study of patients' experiences, *J Adv Nurs* 22:1092–1100, 1995.

Warden V, Hurley AC, Volicer L: Development and psychometric evaluation of the pain assessment in advanced dementia (PAINAD) scale, *J Am Med Dir Assoc* 4:9–15, 2003.

Weiner DK, et al: Chronic pain-associated behaviors in the nursing home: resident versus caregiver perception, *Pain* 80:577–588, 1999.

Woo KY: Meeting the challenges of wound-associated pain: anticipatory pain, anxiety, stress and wound healing, *Ostomy Wound Manage* 54(9):10–12, 2008.

Woo KY, et al: Pain in people with chronic wounds: clinical strategies for decreasing pain and improving quality of life. In Krasner DL, editors: *Chronic wound care: the essentials*, Wayne PA, 2014a, HMP Communications, chapter 9.

Woo KY, et al: Palliative wound and pressure ulcer care & SCALE: skin changes at life's end. In Thomas DR, Compton G, editors: *Pressure ulcers in the aging population: a guide for clinicians*, New York, 2014b, Springer, chapter 12.

Woo KY, Sibbald RG: The improvement of wound-associated pain and healing trajectory with a comprehensive foot and leg ulcer care model, *J Wound Ostomy Continence Nurs* 36(2):184–191, 2009.

Woolf CJ, Salter MW: Neuronal plasticity: increasing the gain in pain, *Science* 288:1765–1769, 2000.

World Union of Wound Healing Societies (WUWHS): *Principles of best practice: minimizing pain at wound dressing-related procedures, A consensus document* London, 2004, MEP.

Wound, Ostomy Continence Nurses Society™ (WOCN®): *Guideline for management of wounds in patients with lower-extremity* arterial disease (WOCN® clinical practice guideline series no. 1), Mt. Laurel, NJ, 2008, WOCN®.

Wound, Ostomy Continence Nurses Society™ (WOCN®): *Guideline for prevention and management of pressure ulcers (WOCN® clinical practice guideline series no. 2)*, Mt. Laurel, NJ, 2010, WOCN®.

Wound, Ostomy Continence Nurses Society™ (WOCN®): *Guideline for management of wounds in patients with lower-extremity venous disease (WOCN® clinical practice guideline series no. 4)*, Mt. Laurel, NJ, 2011, WOCN®.

Wound, Ostomy Continence Nurses Society™ (WOCN®): *Guideline for management of wounds in patients with lower-extremity neuropathic disease (WOCN® clinical practice guideline series no. 3)*, Mt. Laurel, NJ, 2012, WOCN®.

Wynne CF, Ling SM, Remsburg R: Comparison of pain assessment instruments in cognitively intact and cognitively impaired nursing home residents, *Geriatr Nurs* 21:20–23, 2000.

Young T: Assessment of wound pain: overview and a new initiative, *Br J Community Nursing* 12(Suppl 12):5–8, 2007.

26

Managing Wound Pain

Harriet W. Hopf, Dag Shapshak, Scott Junkins, and Daniel K. O'Neill

---

OBJECTIVES

1. State three strategies for managing procedural wound pain.
2. State three strategies for managing nonprocedural wound pain.
3. Describe the pharmacologic options for treating wound pain.

Although not all wounds are painful, in general, most acute and chronic wounds cause moderate to severe pain. Management of this pain can be challenging. Given a thoughtful approach and modern pharmacologic and nonpharmacologic interventions, most patients can achieve an acceptable level of pain control. The first step in managing any patient regardless of underlying condition is identifying and measuring the degree, site, and type of pain; a step that guides the appropriate treatment of pain (see Chapter 25). This chapter presents approaches to preventing and managing acute and chronic wound pain.

NONPHARMACOLOGIC PAIN CONTROL

Many nonpharmacologic pain control measures are essential when caring for a patient with a wound. A simple and effective intervention is acknowledging a patient's pain and making a commitment to the patient to address it. Explaining the potential harmful effects of pain on healing, along with a careful explanation of how to manage pain, will help to shape the patient's expectations and increase the individual's sense of control. Both of these strategies may reduce the pain experienced (APMP, 1992). Additional interventions related to pain control begin with controlling and reducing procedural pain or cyclic acute pain through appropriate and conscientious topical care. Active nonpharmacologic pain control measures can include acupuncture, music therapy, a fleece warming boot or a warm blanket, and visualization. Such measures are listed in Box 26-1.

Wound Cleansing

Avoiding cytotoxic topical agents (e.g., antiseptics, antimicrobials), harsh chemicals, and highly concentrated agents for wound cleansing can significantly reduce wound pain. In general, use of these agents should be avoided unless the wound warrants such intervention (e.g., traumatic wound)

and the patient has been adequately anesthetized (Klein et al, 2013; O'Meara et al, 2014).

Periwound Skin Care

Eroded or denuded wound margins can contribute significantly to the pain experienced by the patient with a wound. Use of skin sealants on intact skin can prevent painful denuding of skin or skin stripping. Use of moisture barrier ointments, protective barrier films, or skin barriers on open areas can prevent and/or minimize the pain secondary to damaged wound margins. Chapter 5 provides a detailed description and formulary of products useful for prevention and management of moisture, chemical, and adhesive-related skin damage.

Debridement

Although many factors are considered when a method of debridement is selected, pain is a frequently neglected consideration. Regardless of the method of debridement selected, pain assessment and management must be considered. Wet-to-dry dressing changes for debridement (nonselective and painful) should be avoided. Using autolysis for debridement, when feasible and appropriate, can significantly reduce the pain associated with this procedure (NPUAP-EPUAP, PPPIA, 2014; Robson et al, 2006; Whitney et al, 2006).

Conservative or surgical sharp debridement provokes acute noncyclical pain, which leads patients to ask the clinician to stop the debridement unless they are given additional analgesia or anesthesia (Briggs and Nelson, 2003; Evans and Gray, 2005; Hansson et al, 1993). When sharp debridement is indicated, pharmacologic interventions are an important consideration and are described in detail later in this chapter (O'Neill, 2009, 2012a, 2012b).

Inflammation and Edema

Inflammation and edema contribute to wound pain, so any measures that reduce these likely will provide pain relief. This includes elevation of edematous extremities, appropriate edema-reducing dressings and devices (e.g., compression bandaging and sequential compression pumps), and systemic medications (Robson et al, 2006). Application of ice may be effective if edema is largely related to inflammation. Although it is well established that systemic hypothermia impairs wound healing (Kurz et al, 1996), local application of ice in a normothermic individual may reduce inflammation (Ho et al, 1994) and may transiently improve blood flow to the wound, depending on several factors, including duration (Meeusen et al, 1986).

Support and Positioning

Binders, splints, body positioners, and other devices that stabilize a wound can significantly reduce pain, especially pain related to mobilization. Care must be taken to fit these devices properly so that the wound dressing is appropriately accommodated and increased pressure on the wound does not result. However, certain medical devices, such as immobilizers and negative pressure therapy devices, can become a source of pain. Various methods can be used to reduce that pain, including pressure relief and use of nonadherent dressings at the device–wound interface (NPUAP, EPUAP, PPPIA, 2014).

Positioning patients for comfort and off their wound can reduce pain at the wound site. If this is not possible, judicious use of support surfaces can offer pain relief to bed-bound or chair-bound patients. Individuals should be encouraged to request a "time-out" during any procedure that causes pain. Patients should be premedicated, if needed, before activities that cause or trigger pain. Using lift sheets (to lift and move) instead of draw sheets (that drag) to move patients in bed prevents friction and shear, which can cause painful injuries to the skin and deeper tissues (NPUAP, EPUAP, PPPIA, 2015).

Wound Dressings

Many commercially available moisture-retentive dressings are designed for the care of wounds. The main analgesic efficacy of these products appears to stem from their ability to keep the wound moist and protected from the environment, reduce inflammation, and stimulate healing. Moisture-retentive dressings have at least some capacity to reduce pain associated with wounds (NPUAP, EPUAP, PPPIA, 2014; Steed et al, 2006; Whitney et al, 2006). Thus dressings can be selected with the aim of reducing pain in a particular patient. The most effective dressing will depend on patient factors such as volume of exudate, condition of surrounding skin, wound depth, and necrotic tissue. Dry, wet-to-dry, or wet-to-damp dressings are not moisture retentive and consequently are the most painful. As the gauze dehydrates, it tends to become attached to the wound surface and, along with damaging new granulation tissue, is painful to remove (NPUAP, EPUAP, PPPIA, 2015; Robson et al, 2006; Whitney et al, 2006). The trauma that patients must endure then is multiplied because wet-to-damp or dry dressing must be changed three times per day.

The patient with a wound often dreads the dressing change procedure, which is cyclic in nature. Box 26-1 lists several interventions for nonpharmacologic pain control during dressing changes. Dressings should be selected that will, upon removal, minimize the degree of sensory stimulus to the wound area (EWMA, 2002).

PHARMACOLOGIC INTERVENTIONS

The World Health Organization's (WHO) Pain Clinical Ladder, a three-step analgesic ladder approach for the treatment of cancer pain, can also be used to guide the treatment of nonmalignant pain (Boxes 26-2 and 26-3 and Figure 26-1). This approach uses a combination of pain control medications based on assessment of pain intensity. If pain persists after reassessment, the ladder guides the clinician in adding a medication or combination of medications to effectively control pain (McCaffery and Portenoy, 1999). Pharmacologic interventions can be topical, subcutaneous or perineural injectable, or systemic (McCaffery and Beebe, 1989; McCaffery and Portenoy, 1999).

Topical Medications

Topical analgesics are commonly used before debridement or before manipulation inside the wound margins, which includes wound packing or application of materials that contact the wound. These medications usually are in the form of a jelly, cream, or ointment, although liquid forms and patches are available. They generally include lidocaine or another local anesthetic with sodium channel receptor blockade activity. Topical anesthetics require at least 15 to 30 minutes to reach optimal analgesic states. Although lidocaine preparations have been widely available and safely used for years, topical use of these preparations in open wounds is considered off label in the United States. Topical lidocaine products should be used with caution, taking into consideration toxic doses and levels, especially with large wounds, where systemic

BOX 26-2 World Health Organization Analgesic Ladder (see Figure 26-1)

Step 1

Patients with mild to moderate pain should be treated with a nonopioid analgesic, which should be combined with an adjuvant drug if an indication for one exists.

For example: Nonsteroidal antiinflammatory drugs, acetylsalicylic acid, acetaminophen.

Step 2

Patients who have limited opioid exposure and moderate to severe pain or who fail to achieve adequate relief after a trial of a nonopioid analgesic should be treated with an opioid conventionally used for moderate pain.

For example: Step 1 medications plus codeine, tramadol, and so forth.

Step 3

Patients who have severe pain or who fail to achieve adequate relief after appropriate administration of drugs in step 2 of the analgesic ladder should receive an opioid conventionally used for severe pain.

For example: Step 1 medications and morphine (discontinue step 2 medications).

Note: Unrelieved pain should raise a red flag that attracts the clinician's attention.

These guidelines should be adjusted for elderly patients as described in detail in Kaye et al, 2010.

From McCaffery M, Portenoy RK: Overview of three groups of analgesics. In McCaffrey M, Pasero C, editors: *Pain clinical manual*, ed 2, St. Louis, MO, 1999, Mosby.

BOX 26-3 Examples of Opioid, Nonopioid, and Adjuvant Medications

Opioids
- Codeine
- Dolophine (Methadone)
- Fentanyl
- Hydromorphone (Dilaudid)
- Levorphanol
- Morphine
- Oxycodone
- Tramadol

Combination Medications
- Percocet (oxycodone/acetaminophen)
- Lortab, Vicodin, Norco (hydrocodone/acetaminophen)

Nonopioids
- Aspirin
- Acetaminophen
- Nonsteroidal antiinflammatory drugs (NSAIDs)

Adjuvant Medications
- Tricyclic antidepressants
- Anticonvulsants
- Systemic local anesthetics
- Topical anesthetics

Note that many of these medications should be avoided or given at an adjusted dose in the elderly. Consult the American Geriatric Society Beers List for guidance in elderly patients (Campanelli CM: American Geriatrics Society updated Beers Criteria for potentially inappropriate medication use in older adults: American Geriatrics Society 2012 Beers Criteria Update Expert Panel. *J Am Geriatr Soc* 60(4): 616-631, 2012).

absorption of very large doses could potentially lead to neurologic and/or cardiovascular toxicity.

The most commonly used topical analgesics include 2% and 4% lidocaine jelly, which act on only the superficial layer of tissue and can inactivate exposed wound pain receptors. The strongest evidence base for the effectiveness of topical analgesics in wound care is associated with eutectic mixture of local anesthetics (EMLA) cream, which contains lidocaine and prilocaine. Although manufacturer's instructions indicate EMLA should only be used on intact skin, there is no evidence of harm from application to open wounds, and it is widely used. It is applied 30 to 60 minutes before debridement under occlusion with a film dressing. Instructions for use of EMLA cream are given in Box 26-4 (Evans and Gray, 2005; Hansson et al, 1993). A recent Cochrane review found statistically significant reduction in debridement pain scores with EMLA cream (Briggs et al, 2012).

Topical anesthetic patches also may be useful. Examples include the Synera patch and the Lidoderm (lidocaine) patch. The Synera patch incorporates 70 mg of lidocaine and 70 mg of tetracaine, thus providing fairly rapid onset (20 to 30 minutes) and prolonged duration (up to hours). The patch is self-warmed, which facilitates drug delivery and may improve wound perfusion, although this has not specifically been studied using the Synera patch (Sawyer

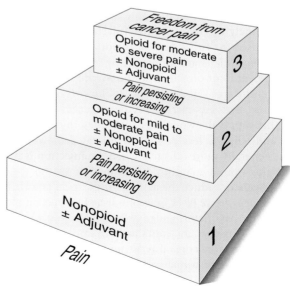

FIGURE 26-1 World Health Organization's analgesic ladder for cancer pain. (From the World Health Organization, 2010.)

et al, 2009). Ibuprofen slow-release foam dressings may also be effective for treatment of painful venous ulcers (Briggs et al, 2012).

Subcutaneous or Perineural Injectable Medications

Injectable medications (subcutaneous or perineural) frequently contain the same type of active drug that is found in the topical analgesic formulations (local anesthetics such as lidocaine). However, these medications are in solution and are designed to be injected into the soft tissue. These medications include lidocaine or longer-acting agents (e.g., bupivacaine, tetracaine). Epinephrine can be added to these medications to cause vasoconstriction, increasing the duration of action, as well as decreasing bleeding. Epinephrine is contraindicated for use in distal areas such as hands and feet because of the risk of necrosis from interruption of blood supply. Epinephrine is generally avoided in wounds due to concern of impairing blood supply, although it may be useful in extremely vascular wounds. Injectable local anesthetics can be used for either field or regional blockade.

A *field blockade* is accomplished by injecting local anesthetic adjacent to or directly into the wound margins, encircling the entire area (Hadzic, 2007). It blocks transmission of pain signals that are carried in the superficial cutaneous nerves that supply the wound area. At times, injection within the wound edges is less painful. If tolerated, however, the block is generally more effective when the injection is made outside the wound margins. Inflammation in the wound may inactivate or reduce the activity of the local anesthetic.

A *regional* or *nerve block* is accomplished by injecting local anesthetic into an often singular, proximal location where the larger nerve bundles are contained. Examples of regional blocks include not only digital, wrist, and ankle blocks, but also other larger, more proximal nerves. Brachial plexus blockade and blockade of lower extremity nerves in the popliteal fossa may provide larger areas of coverage. Regional blocks require more training, but are useful in the management and debridement of wounds that either cross many dermatomes or cover a large area that is supplied by many separate proximal nerves, or

in patients with severe periwound hyperalgesia. Ultrasound or nerve stimulator guidance often is used to improve accuracy and avoid complications of nerve blockade (Hadzic, 2007).

Selective blockade of the sympathetic nervous system may reduce pain and improve healing. Stellate ganglion and lumbar sympathetic blocks can be used for upper and lower extremity sympathetic blockade, respectively. These interventions may optimize blood flow and oxygen delivery while relieving sympathetically mediated pain. Trauma and inflammation may increase sympathetic tone and upregulate α-receptors in the wound, leading to sympathetically maintained pain in lower extremity ulcers (McLachlan et al, 1993). These procedures usually are performed using fluoroscopic x-ray guidance. The goal of these blocks is not temporary relief, but long-term blockade, so they often use an alcohol-based medication to permanently inactivate nerve transmission of the painful area to the spinal cord (Hopf et al, 1997). Spinal cord stimulation is another method for effective long-term sympathetic blockade (Graber and Lifson, 1987; Wu et al, 2008). All nerve blocks can be done safely in an outpatient clinic by properly trained personnel who monitor appropriately for the degree of sedation required.

Use of Regional and General Anesthesia for Debridement

Sharp surgical debridement in patients without complete neuropathy requires anesthesia to protect the patient from the stress response of the painful stimulus (O'Neill, 2009, 2012a, 2012b). Sodium channel blockade with "local anesthetics" such as lidocaine, bupivacaine, or mepivacaine defines the basis of regional anesthesia, which protects the central nervous system from assault of action potentials associated with afferent information. The neuroanatomy and the dermatomal distribution of the surgical stimulus form the basis of selection of the target for drug disposition locally (field block), peripherally (nerve bundle), or centrally (neuroaxial: epidural, spinal). In the absence of sodium channel blockade, some reasonable combination of intravenous and/or inhalational anesthetics in the form of general anesthesia would be required to prevent autonomic or musculoskeletal reflexes. The pharmacology of general anesthetics tends to promote more perturbations of homeostasis such as hemodynamic instability, which would require vigilance and dynamic pharmacologic management. Standard real-time physiologic monitoring as recommended by the American Society of Anesthesiologists (ASA) would be utilized by a qualified anesthesia provider to support homeostasis (ASA, 2014).

Systemic Medications

The goal of systemic medication administration as a pain control strategy is not to stop pain signal transmission from the wound, but to alter the response of the central nervous system (CNS) to that pain signal. Whether the medication is given intravenously, subcutaneously, transcutaneously, or orally, many pain management choices are available when utilizing systemic pain control (Tables 26-1 through 26-3). These include nonsteroidal antiinflammatory drugs (NSAIDs),

TABLE 26-1 Recommended Starting Doses (and Equivalence) for Opioid Treatment of Intrinsic Wound Pain

PO/PR (mg)	Analgesic	IV or IM (mg)
30	Morphine	1 to 5 IV or 5 to 10 IM
6	Hydromorphone (Dilaudid)	0.2 to 0.6 or 1.5
20	Methadone	10 to 20
Not recommended	Meperidine (Demerol)	10 to 30 or 100*
60	Codeine	30 to 60
5 to 10	Oxycodone (Percocet)	N/A

IM, Intramuscular; *IV,* intravenous; *PO,* by mouth; *PR,* per rectum.
*Meperidine should not be used for analgesia because normeperidine, a metabolite, may accumulate. Seizures are common when high doses (1000 mg in 1 day or 600 mg/day for several days) are given. Meperidine is more likely to cause dependence than other clinically used opioids.
Note that many of these medications should be avoided or given at an adjusted dose in the elderly. Consult the American Geriatric Society Beers List for guidance in elderly patients (Campanelli CM: American Geriatrics Society updated Beers Criteria for potentially inappropriate medication use in older adults: American Geriatrics Society 2012 Beers Criteria Update Expert Panel. *J Am Geriatr Soc* 60(4): 616–631, 2012). Acute Pain Management Panel (APMP): *Acute pain management: operative or medical procedures and trauma* (Clinical practice guideline, AHCPR publication no. 92-0032), Rockville, MD, 1992, U.S. Department of Health and Human Services, Public Health Service.

TABLE 26-2 Agents Appropriate for Sedation/Analgesia for Procedures in Adults

Agent	Dose (IV)	Frequency
Diazepam	1 to 2 mg	q3 to 10 min
Lorazepam	0.05 mg/kg (max 4 mg)	One time
Midazolam	0.25 to 1 mg	q1 to 5 min
Fentanyl	Loading dose up 1 μg/kg, then 12.5 to 50 μg	q5 to 10 min
Meperidine	12.5 to 25 mg	q2 to 15 min
Morphine	1 to 3 mg	q2 to 15 min
Droperidol	0.625 to 1.25 mg	q5 to 10 min

Note that many of these medications should be avoided or given at an adjusted dose in the elderly. Consult the American Geriatric Society Beers List for guidance in elderly patients (Campanelli CM: American Geriatrics Society updated Beers Criteria for potentially inappropriate medication use in older adults: American Geriatrics Society 2012 Beers Criteria Update Expert Panel. *J Am Geriatr Soc* 60(4): 616–631, 2012).

opioids (e.g., morphine, methadone, oral lidocaine, acetaminophen, partial mu-receptor agonists (e.g., tramadol, a weak synthetic opioid with a unique mechanism of action that is based on activity at opioid receptors [μ] and reuptake inhibition of serotonin and norepinephrine), anticonvulsants (e.g., gabapentin [Neurontin]), antidepressants, and clonidine (central α2-adrenergic agonist that reduces sympathetic

TABLE 26-3 Pharmacologic Interventions for Neuropathic Pain

Type of Pain	Medication
Dysesthesia	Capsaicin cream topically applied three to four times a day; may take 3 weeks for effect to be seen
	Gabapentin or pregabalin
	Selective serotonin reuptake inhibitor (e.g., fluoxetine, paroxetine)
	Serotonin and noradrenergic reuptake inhibitors (e.g., venlafaxine)
	Dextromethorphan syrup
	Tricyclic antidepressant (e.g., imipramine, amitriptyline)
Paresthesia	Anticonvulsant (e.g., carbamazepine, Tegretol, phenytoin)
	Analgesic (e.g., Tramadol)
Muscular pain	Muscle relaxant (e.g., metaxalone, baclofen [Lioresal], tizanidine by mouth)
General neuropathic pain	Analgesics (e.g., lidocaine [Lidoderm] patch or lidocaine and tetracaine patch [Synera])
	Gabapentin or pregabalin
	Hemorheologic agent (e.g., pentoxifylline [Trental])
	Diuretic (e.g., furosemide, metolazone, bumetanide); may diminish pain with reduction in vasodilation
	Platelet inhibitor, cilostazol (Pletal)
	Bisphosphonate (e.g., pamidronate)
	Aldose reductase inhibitor (e.g., fidarestat, sorbinil)
	Antithromboembolitic therapy (e.g., heparin, warfarin, acetylsalicylic acid, antiinflammatory drugs)
	Clopidogrel (Plavix)

outflow) (Veith et al, 1984). These medications act on different target locations to combat the perception of pain. For example, predominantly neuropathic pain is more responsive to antidepressants and anticonvulsants than to NSAIDs and opioids (WOCN®, 2012). Some medications (e.g., NSAIDs) can also act by secondary means to reduce pain; that is, besides their direct analgesic properties, they reduce inflammation in the wound area, leading to a decrease in pain.

Combining several analgesic agents often is more successful than using a single agent. Drugs may act additively or synergistically. This may allow a reduction in the required dose of each agent, thus potentially reducing side effects while providing equal or even superior analgesia (Hopf and Weitz, 1994). A patient with mixed nociceptive and neuropathic pain will require a combination of analgesics and antidepressants or anticonvulsants.

Because of their potency and reliable analgesic action, opioids are a mainstay of pain management in both acute and chronic settings. One of the actions of opioids is stimulation of receptors in the central and peripheral nervous system that downregulate both the afferent response to pain and central pain perception. Gabapentin (Neurontin) is an excellent drug for treating neuropathic pain, which often occurs in patients with diabetic neuropathy. It is effective for wound pain probably because of the neuropathic nature of much wound pain. The maximum recommended dose is 900 mg by mouth three times daily, but wound pain frequently responds to the lowest dose range of 100 to 200 mg three times daily. Other agents that may be beneficial in the treatment of neuropathic pain include tricyclic antidepressants and pregabalin.

Further research is necessary to confirm which strategies or groups of strategies optimize pain relief and for which type of pain. For example, will applying a topical anesthetic compress before sharp debridement be more effective for this type of acute noncyclical pain than taking an oral pain medication? Around-the-clock medications might be most effective for chronic wound pain. Applying pain-reducing dressings or selecting pressure-reducing devices may prove to reduce acute cyclic pressure ulcer pain more effectively than pharmacologic measures.

Potential Complications of Medical Pain Management

Medications are rarely benign. Almost every drug has an associated set of potential side effects that can be inconvenient or harmful to the patient. The *Physician's Desk Reference* lists every reported side effect for each medication, but certain sets of complications are commonly encountered in the setting of analgesic control. The most powerful systemic analgesic agents are opioids; they have the most acutely serious side effects, including sedation and respiratory depression. Elderly patients may be at greater risk of complications due to comorbid conditions and changes in pharmacokinetics and pharmacodynamics. On the other hand, pain may also be undertreated in the elderly due to underreporting and barriers to pain assessment (Kaye et al, 2010). Careful assessment and management are therefore critical.

Whenever opioids are administered, attention must be given to avoid excess sedation and respiratory depression (O'Neill 2009). This is particularly true when opioids are given to manage procedural pain. Most health care facilities recognize five categories of sedation (Table 26-4). However, these categories are artificially drawn because sedation is a continuum. Sedation is different from simple pain control; sedation implies that the medications are given to specifically facilitate the ability to perform a painful procedure. The use of analgesics or sedatives solely to provide analgesia and/or allay anxiety (as occurs during dressing changes) but with no intention of performing a procedure is not considered sedation. Nonetheless, such drugs must be used with caution because respiratory depression and sedation can be induced whenever these drugs are used. Box 26-5 lists prescribing principles developed by the American Geriatrics Society's Panel on Persistent Pain in Older Persons (2009) for chronic pain management in the long-term care setting.

TABLE 26-4 Categories of Sedation

Level	Category	Definition
1	No sedation	
2	Minimal or light sedation	Patient responds normally to verbal commands. Patient's ventilatory and cardiac functions are unaffected.
3	Moderate or conscious sedation	Patient responds purposefully to verbal commands. Patient's spontaneous ventilation is adequate.
4	Deep sedation	Patient cannot be easily aroused. Patient can respond purposefully following repeated or painful stimulation. Patient has increased probability of respiratory or hemodynamic compromise.
5	Anesthesia	Most often performed in operating room. Patient is not arousable by painful stimulation.

BOX 26-5 Principles that Guide Chronic Wound Pain Management

1. Manage intrinsic (background) pain with medications provided on a routine schedule.
2. Manage break-through pain with fast-acting medications as required (PRN).
3. Consider the following regarding route of administration:
   a. Use the least invasive route first (i.e., administer medications orally, when feasible).
   b. Use topical patches or creams when oral medications are insufficient.
4. Analgesic dose should be titrated to an effective level, starting with a low dose and advancing slowly.
5. Reassessment of background pain, as well as procedural or incident pain, should be ongoing and treatment individualized per patient need.
6. Monitor elderly patients closely for undesirable effects.

American Geriatrics Society Panel on Persistent Pain in Older Persons: The management of persistent pain in older persons, *J Am Geriatr Soc* 50(S6):S205–S224, 2002.

A patient receiving sedation requires constant monitoring, which includes, at a minimum, cardiac monitoring, pulse oximetry, and direct supervision by a provider not involved in performing the procedure (Yoo et al, 2014). When a patient is being managed using sedation, the most serious common complication is respiratory depression. Therefore the sedation should be performed only in a setting where a medical practitioner is available who can provide a definitive airway and handle the complications of ventilatory and/or circulatory collapse. Whenever patients are given analgesics for procedural pain, consideration should be given to monitoring, and facility guidelines should always be followed.

Potential side effects of opioid medications should be discussed at the initiation of therapy. High-dose and/or long-term opioid therapy may place patients at higher risk for hormonal disturbances (decreased testosterone) or sleep disorders. Respiratory depression is the most serious side effect. Other less serious but common side effects include nausea, vomiting, constipation, urinary retention, and pruritus. All patients receiving opioids should be given stool softeners and counseled on ways to prevent constipation, including increased fluid and fiber intake. Antiemetic medications, changing to a different opioid, or limiting opioid dose by using nonopioid analgesics (e.g., NSAIDs) can manage nausea and vomiting. Pruritus can be managed with diphenhydramine or other antihistamines.

Side effects of NSAIDs include stomach pain, ulcers, gastrointestinal bleeding, renal impairment, allergies, and platelet inhibition (Buckley and Brogden, 1990). Side effects of acetaminophen are few, but overdoses (>4 to 6 g/day) can result in acute fulminant liver failure. Care should be exercised when using opioid–acetaminophen combinations, especially those with relatively low-potency opioids and high-dose acetaminophen (500 mg per tablet), such as Vicodin (hydrocodone–acetaminophen). Acetaminophen is a powerful adjunct, so it should be used when possible. For tolerant patients, it should be given separately as an around-the-clock drug to reduce the risk of liver injury. More potent opioids (e.g., oxycodone, hydromorphone [Dilaudid], morphine, methadone) should be selected as well to reduce the number of doses required daily.

Side effects of antiepileptics and antidepressants include sedation, which usually resolves with continued use. These drugs can be started as a bedtime dose for several days to allow acclimatization.

Side effects of clonidine include sedation and dry mouth (acclimatization is rapid). It can decrease blood pressure and heart rate, but at the low doses used to treat wound pain (lower than those commonly used to treat hypertension) rarely causes hypotension or bradycardia. Clonidine is available as a transdermal patch, which allows constant plasma levels and improved compliance. Usually the lowest dose (no. 1 or 2 patch) is sufficient. Clonidine should be used with caution and at the lowest possible dose in the elderly, as side effects are more common. The American Geriatric Society Beers List (Campanelli, 2012) recommends against routine use of clonidine for treatment of hypertension in the elderly due to the potential for orthostatic hypotension and bradycardia (quality of evidence is low), but lower-dose clonidine has been used safely in the elderly for treatment of wound pain. Clonidine may reduce opioid requirements in tolerant patients (Flacke et al, 1987). It often increases perfusion and oxygenation in patients with hypoxic wounds because of their excess sympathetic tone or peripheral vascular disease, which may also reduce pain (Hopf et al, 1996).

Addiction Concerns

The degree of pain that a patient experiences and reports often is influenced by the patient's fear of addiction. A common social and medical problem is drug and alcohol abuse, and treating painful wounds can be especially difficult in patients who abuse these substances. Because patients who are addicted to alcohol or drugs can exhibit tolerance to CNS depressants and opioids, higher dosages of analgesic medications may be required. In addition, liver and kidney disease associated with alcohol or other drug abuse may alter the metabolism and excretion of opioids and other analgesics. Tolerance and altered metabolism, along with variability in recent drug use by the patient and attitudes among health care providers toward addicted patients, are factors that make designing an effective analgesic regimen for these patients difficult.

Furthermore, opioid-addicted patients may exhibit a tendency for hyperalgesia, in which patients experience a greater intensity of pain than expected for a given wound. When treating these individuals, the fundamental principle of pain management is the same as it is for other patients: complaints of pain should be taken seriously and treated aggressively (Cohen et al, 2004). Intravenous drug abusers may require higher doses of analgesics to obtain similar degrees of pain relief because of the development of opioid cross-tolerance. Careful consideration of adjunctive medications or interventions may be useful in this patient population.

The history of opioid prescribing has been particularly variable. Patients have commonly been undertreated with opioid pain medications when opioids were indicated (Owen et al, 1990). However, recent data show some alarming trends in prescription drug misuse and abuse over the past 10 years. In 2009 the American Pain Society detailed the guidelines for opioid prescribing. The risks and benefits of opioid therapy should be carefully weighed and continually assessed in each patient (Chou et al, 2009). Although the fear of becoming addicted is generally unfounded—less than 0.1% of patients receiving opioids for acute pain become addicted—safe prescribing methods and monitoring of therapy are important (APMP, 1992). Medication contracts between patient and prescriber, urine drug screenings, and periodic monitoring of prescriptions filled can be vital in maintaining adherence to medical management.

Because patients frequently take inadequate doses of opioids because of their fear of addiction, they should be reassured and encouraged to use the drugs appropriately. When the doses are inadequate because of side effects, different opioids should be tried and adjunct agents added to reduce the required opioid dose. Referral to a pain medicine specialist may be warranted if pain is poorly controlled or is refractory to appropriate dose escalation; interventions are needed; or comprehensive, multidisciplinary treatment is needed. Pain relief, safety, and active monitoring for medication misuse should be the cornerstones of opioid therapy.

Use of opioids for the treatment of chronic pain has come under recent scrutiny because of long-term consequences of opioid use (CDC, 2013). An important consideration in the treatment of wound pain is the distinction between treating acute and chronic pain. Opioids are appropriate for management of severe acute interventional pain, for example, for debridement. A short course of opioids is appropriate for treatment of chronic wound pain, particularly at the start of treatment, when more procedures and lack of healing lead to more severe wound pain. The goal of therapy should be to transition to nonopioid wound management when feasible and not to routinely continue opioids long term.

CLINICAL CONSULT

A: Consult requested for patient experiencing severe pain at the site of a left shin venous insufficiency ulcer. The patient is an 82-year-old woman who bumped her shin on the dishwasher a month ago, causing a small wound that has increased in size and pain. The wound measures 4.5 × 2.5 × 0.2 cm, is highly exudative and covered in yellow slough. No periwound erythema. Polyurethane foam dressing in place and is changed daily. Both legs are edematous to the knee. Comorbidities include well-controlled hypertension and mild renal insufficiency (creatinine of 1.2 mg/dL). Formerly quite active; now resides in a skilled nursing facility due to leg ulcer. Has taken metoprolol 25 mg PO daily for many years. Recently began furosemide for leg edema and hydromorphone with acetaminophen as needed for pain. Patient states the pain score has remained 8 out of 10 for the past week.

D: Trauma induced venous insufficiency ulcer with severe pain and untreated edema.

P: Improve pain management, edema control, and removal of nonviable wound tissue.

I: (1) Apply EMLA cream or Synera patch 30 minutes prior to dressing change to allow wound irrigation. (2) Honey alginate dressing to the wound bed to stabilize wound pH, provide antimicrobial action, absorb exudate, and promote autolysis. (3) Begin modified compression (25% stretch) initially to accommodate pain. (4) Music therapy or visualization. (5) Discontinue furosemide and hydromorphone/acetaminophen combination and begin acetaminophen, 650 mg orally, four times a day (scheduled doses); not to exceed 3 g per day. (6) Oxycodone, 5 to 10 mg orally every 4 to 6 hours as needed. May apply ice pack over the dressing for up to 20 minutes, four times a day, if it provides relief.

E: Reassessment in 1 week. Patient should receive oxycodone 1 hour prior to scheduled appointment to minimize pain during assessment. Patient understands that she will require compression for life and the degree of compression will be increased as tolerated and converted to compression stockings or a reusable inelastic device for long term use.

SUMMARY

Managing pain associated with the presence of a wound not only enhances the cellular and molecular activities of wound healing, but also enhances the patient's ability to participate in activities essential to healing. Pharmacologic agents need to be selected and titrated to the type and severity of pain. Nonpharmacologic interventions are also important to prevent exacerbation of pain.

REFERENCES

Acute Pain Management Panel (APMP): *Acute pain management: operative or medical procedures and trauma (Clinical practice guideline, AHCPR publication no. 92-0032)*, Rockville, MD, 1992, U.S. Department of Health and Human Services, Public Health Service.

American Geriatrics Society Panel on Persistent Pain in Older Persons: The management of persistent pain in older persons, *J Am Geriatr Soc* 50(Suppl 6):S205–S224, 2002.

American Society of Anesthesiologists (ASA): *Standards, guidelines, and statements and other documents*, 2014. https://www.asahq.org/For-Members/Clinical-Information/Standards-Guidelines-and-Statements.aspx. Accessed December 14, 2014.

Briggs M, Nelson EA: Topical agents or dressings for pain in venous leg ulcers, *Cochrane Database SST Rev* 1:CD001177, 2003.

Briggs M, Nelson EA, Martyn-St James M: Topical agents or dressings for pain in venous leg ulcers, *Cochrane Database SST Rev* 11:CD001177, 2012.

Buckley MM, Brogden RN: Ketorolac: a review of its pharmacodynamic and pharmacokinetic properties, and therapeutic potential, *Drugs* 39(1):86–109, 1990.

Campanelli CM: American Geriatrics Society updated Beers Criteria for potentially inappropriate medication use in older adults: American Geriatrics Society 2012 Beers Criteria Update Expert Panel. *J Am Geriatr Soc* 60(4): 616–631, 2012.

Centers for Disease Control: *Common elements in guidelines for prescribing opioids for chronic pain*, 2013. http://www.cdc.gov/drugoverdose/prescribing/common-elements.html. Accessed Aug 16, 2015.

Chou R, Fancifully GJ, Fine PG, et al: Clinical guidelines for the use of chronic opioid therapy in chronic noncancer pain, *J Pain* 10(2):113–130, 2009.

Cohen SP, Christo PJ, Moroz L: Pain management in trauma patients, *Am J Phys Med Rehabil* 83:142–161, 2004.

European Wound Management Association (EWMA): *Position document: pain at wound dressing changes*, London, 2002, Medical Education Partnership. http://ewma.org/fileadmin/user_

upload/EWMA/pdf/Position_Documents/2002/Spring_2002__English_.pdf. Accessed December 14, 2014.

Evans E, Gray M: Do topical analgesics reduce pain associated with wound dressing changes or debridement of chronic wounds? *J Wound Ostomy Continence Nurs* 32(5):287–290, 2005.

Flacke JW, Bloor BC, Flacke E, et al: Reduced narcotic requirement by clonidine with improved hemodynamic and adrenergic stability in patients undergoing coronary bypass surgery, *Anesthesiology* 67:11–19, 1987.

Graber JN, Lifson A: The use of spinal cord stimulation for severe limb-threatening ischemia: a preliminary report, *Ann Vasc Surg* 1(5):578–582, 1987.

Hadzic A: *Textbook of regional anesthesia and acute pain management*, New York, 2007, McGraw-Hill.

Hansson C, Holm J, Lillieborg S, et al: Repeated treatment with lidocaine/prilocaine cream (EMLA) as a topical anaesthetic for the cleansing of venous leg ulcers. A controlled study, *Acta Derm Venereol* 73(3):231–233, 1993.

Ho SS, Coel MN, Kagawa R, et al: The effects of ice on blood flow and bone metabolism in knees, *Am J Sports Med* 22:537–540, 1994.

Hopf HW, McKay WR, West JM, et al: Percutaneous lumbar sympathetic block increases tissue oxygen in patients with local tissue hypoxia in nonhealing wounds, *Anesth Analg* 84:S305, 1997.

Hopf HW, Weitz S: Postoperative pain management, *Arch Surg* 129(2):128–132, 1994.

Hopf HW, West J, Hunt T: Clonidine increases tissue oxygen in patients with local tissue hypoxia in non-healing wounds, *Wound Repair Regen* 4(1):A129, 1996.

Kaye AD, Baluch A, Scott JT: Pain management in the elderly population: a review, *Ochsner J Fall* 10(3):179–187, 2010.

Klein S, Schreml S, Dolderer J, et al: Evidence-based topical management of chronic wounds according to the T.I.M.E. principle, *J Dtsch Dermatol Ges* 11(9):819–829, 2013.

Kurz A, Sessler DI, Lenhardt R: Perioperative normothermia to reduce the incidence of wound infection and duration of hospitalization, *N Engl J Med* 334(19):1209–1215, 1996.

McCaffery M, Beebe A: *Pain: clinical manual for nursing practice*, St. Louis, MO, 1989, Mosby.

McCaffery M, Portenoy RK: Overview of three groups of analgesics. In McCaffery M, Pasero C, editors: *Pain clinical manual*, ed 2, St. Louis, MO, 1999, Mosby.

McLachlan EM, Jänig W, Devor M, et al: Peripheral nerve injury triggers noradrenergic sprouting within dorsal root ganglia, *Nature* 363(6429):543–546, 1993.

Meeusen R, Lievens P: The use of cryotherapy in sports injuries, *Sports Med* 3:398–414, 1986.

National Pressure Ulcer Advisory Panel (NPUAP), European Pressure Ulcer Advisory Panel (EPUAP) and Pan Pacific Pressure Injury Alliance (PPPIA): Prevention and treatment of pressure ulcers: clinical practice guideline. In Emily Haesler, editor: Perth, Australia, 2014, Cambridge Media.

O'Meara S, Al-Kurdi D, Ologun Y, et al: Antibiotics and antiseptics for venous leg ulcers, *Cochrane Database Syst Rev* 1:CD003557, 2014.

O'Neill DK, Maggi J: Anesthetic care for patients with skin breakdown, *Anesthesiol Clin* 27:599–603, 2009.

O'Neill DK, Robins B, Ayello EA, et al: Regional anaesthesia with sedation protocol to safely debride sacral pressure ulcers, *Int Wound J* 9:525–543, 2012a.

O'Neill DK, Tsui SM, Ayello EA, et al: Anesthesia protocol for heel pressure ulcer debridement, *Adv Skin Wound Care* 25(5):209–219, 2012b.

Owen H, McMillan V, Rogowski D: Postoperative pain therapy: a survey of patients' expectations and their experiences, *Pain* 41:303–307, 1990.

Robson MC, Cooper DM, Aslam R, et al: Guidelines for the treatment of venous ulcers, *Wound Repair Regen* 14(6):649–662, 2006.

Sawyer J, Febbraro S, Masud S, et al: Heated lidocaine/tetracaine patch (Synera, Rapydan) compared with lidocaine/prilocaine cream (EMLA) for topical anaesthesia before vascular access, *Br J Anaesth* 102(2):210–215, 2009.

Steed DL, Attinger C, Colaizzi T, et al: Guidelines for the treatment of diabetic ulcers, *Wound Repair Regen* 14(6):680–692, 2006.

Veith RC, Best JD, Halter JB: Dose-dependent suppression of norepinephrine appearance rate in plasma by clonidine in man, *J Clin Endocrinol Metab* 59:151–155, 1984.

Whitney J, Phillips L, Aslam R, et al: Guidelines for the treatment of pressure ulcers, *Wound Repair Regen* 14(6):663–679, 2006.

Wound, Ostomy and Continence Nurses Society™ (WOCN®): *Guideline for management of wounds in patients with lower-extremity neuropathic disease (WOCN® clinical practice guideline series no. 1)*, Mt. Laurel, NJ, 2012, WOCN®.

Wu M, Linderoth B, Foreman RD: Putative mechanisms behind effects of spinal cord stimulation on vascular diseases: a review of experimental studies, *Auton Neurosci* 138(1–2):9–23, 2008.

Yoo C, Ayello EA, Robins B, et al: Perioperative use of bispectral (BIS) monitor for a pressure ulcer patient with locked-in-syndrome (LIS), *Int Wound J* 11(5):540–545, 2014.

27

Nutritional Assessment and Support

Nancy A. Stotts

OBJECTIVES

1. Compare and contrast the etiology of starvation-related malnutrition, disease-related malnutrition, and acute disease– or injury-related malnutrition.
2. Distinguish between nutrition screening and nutrition assessment, as well as who performs each.
3. Compare and contrast the criteria for malnutrition in the context of starvation, chronic disease, and acute injury.
4. List at least one role for each of the following nutrients in wound healing: protein; carbohydrate; fat; vitamins A, B, C, D, and E; and minerals zinc, copper, and magnesium.
5. Identify the required daily dose for the patient with a wound for calories, protein, zinc, vitamin C, and fluid.

Nutrition is fundamental to normal cellular integrity, as well as tissue repair and regeneration. Carbohydrates, proteins, fat, minerals, vitamins, and fluids are required in sufficient amounts to meet nutritional requirements for these basic processes. Individual needs vary depending on the underlying nutritional status, metabolic rate, and concomitant biologic demands (e.g., diabetes, heart failure, pneumonia, kidney disease).

Wound healing is an anabolic process that requires specific nutrients to fuel the biochemical processes in healing (e.g., vitamin C and zinc are required for hydroxylation of proline in collagen formation) (Arnold and Barbul, 2006; Demling, 2009; Stechmiller, 2010). Although adequate nutrition is important for all patients, it is of particular importance for the patient with a wound to prevent severe or prolonged depletion of nutrients that can affect healing. A patient with a wound may lose as much as 100 g of protein per day through wound exudate (Pompeo, 2007). Furthermore, once malnourished, the tube-fed patient may require 3 to 4 weeks or longer before protein stores normalize.

MALNUTRITION

Nationwide, the prevalence of malnutrition in hospitals is estimated at between 30% and 50% (Jensen et al, 2013), although others report a significantly lower prevalence (Corkins et al, 2014). Some patients are admitted malnourished, and others experience deterioration of nutritional status during their hospitalization. This high prevalence of malnutrition is particularly alarming because malnutrition is associated with increased morbidity and mortality in patients with acute or chronic disease, as well as longer hospitalization

and higher treatment costs, compared with patients without malnutrition (Corkins et al, 2014). Risk factors for malnutrition are listed in Checklist 27-1.

Malnutrition is a state in which nutritional deficiency or an imbalance of energy, protein, and other nutrients causes measurable adverse effects on tissue, body structure, body function, and clinical outcome. Malnutrition is classified as undernutrition or overnutrition and is caused by a deficit or excess of nutrients in the diet, respectively. Historically, the focus of malnutrition has been on the individual's intake, because of the potential for the development of protein malnutrition, or protein-calorie malnutrition. Appreciation of the role of inflammation in malnutrition has turned our thinking about malnutrition upside down. Classic parameters of malnutrition have included weight loss; inadequate intake; and the proteins albumin, prealbumin, and transferrin. Yet shifts in body water, inaccuracies in intake measurement and recording, and inflammatory processes that lower serum protein levels lead to inaccurate diagnoses (Jensen et al, 2009). In fact, the inflammatory response results in reduction of protein levels within 24 hours—even for patients who are not malnourished (Jensen et al, 2012).

Inflammation is an important mediator for nutrition as seen in the new etiologic classifications of malnutrition provided by the International Guideline Committee of the American Society for Parenteral and Enteral Nutrition (A.S.P.E.N.) and the European Society for Clinical Nutrition and Metabolism (Jensen et al, 2013). The three etiologic categories of malnutrition are starvation-related malnutrition, disease-related malnutrition, and acute disease– or injury-related malnutrition (Jensen and Wheeler, 2012). These categories incorporate both undernutrition and overnutrition. Patients can be assigned to more than

CHECKLIST 27-1   Risk Factors for Malnutrition

✓ Hypermetabolism
✓ Weight loss
✓ Decreased appetite
✓ Therapeutic dietary restriction
✓ Inability to buy or prepare food
✓ Lack of teeth or poorly fitting dentures
✓ Inability to feed self
✓ Food intolerance (e.g., as occurs with chemotherapy)
✓ Alterations in ingestion, digestion, absorption, metabolism
✓ Change in pattern or variety of food ingested
✓ Nausea, vomiting, anorexia, diarrhea
✓ Limited income
✓ Social isolation

one of these classifications and may move among them as their situation changes (Jensen et al, 2009, 2013). New diagnostic criteria accompany these etiologic classifications (White et al, 2012).

Starvation-Related Malnutrition

Starvation occurs when caloric intake is inadequate to meet metabolic needs over time. Famine often is the cause in underdeveloped countries, and inadequate intake due to insufficient income or conditions such as depression or anorexia nervosa are seen in developed countries (Jensen and Wheeler, 2012; White et al, 2012). The classic picture of starvation-related malnutrition is the individual with inadequate intake who is in an unstressed state and is hypometabolic (Heimburger, 2008). Initially with inadequate intake, compensatory processes meet the glucose needs of essential tissues (e.g., brain, white blood cells). Glycogen that is stored in the liver is mobilized for energy; however, stores are small and are exhausted in less than 24 hours. Subsequently, glucose needed for cellular activities is formed by the catabolism of protein in muscle and tissues. Protein is not stored in the body, so when protein is used for gluconeogenesis, functional muscle and organs are destroyed and weight loss is rapid. Weight loss occurs from both the breakdown of protein and the osmotic diuresis that allows for excretion of the byproducts of protein metabolism in urine.

If inadequate intake persists, compensatory processes allow fat to become the primary energy source and for protein to be used at a much slower rate (Heimburger, 2008). The brain adapts and uses ketones from fat metabolism for energy, the muscle releases less protein, and the kidneys recycle the end products of protein metabolism for glucose. Over time, the basal metabolic rate decreases and weight loss is slowed. Protein is converted to glucose for use by only a few tissues (e.g., red blood cells, fibroblasts, renal medulla). Serum protein measures decline gradually (Glasgow and Hermann, 2006).

When fat stores are depleted, protein again becomes the primary energy source and is rapidly depleted. Skeletal muscle size rapidly decreases, and serum protein levels fall. If treatment is not prompt, death will ensue.

Disease-Related Malnutrition

This category of malnutrition is seen in persons with chronic diseases where inflammation is chronic and often mild to moderate. Examples include organ failure, rheumatoid arthritis, pancreatic cancer, and sarcopenic obesity (Jensen et al, 2012; White et al, 2012). Here the underlying disease is characterized by a chronic inflammatory response that contributes to the effects of the disease. For example, in end-stage kidney disease, there is a persistent inflammatory response (Tbahriti et al, 2013). Also, obesity is characterized by a chronic inflammatory component that increases activation of kinases, resulting in upregulation of proinflammatory cytokines (Rodriguez-Hernandez et al, 2013).

It is important to recognize that the excess weight of an obese patient does not necessarily reflect adequate nutritional health. Protein deficiency and deficiencies of vitamins and minerals may be present in the obese patient. Unfortunately, nutritional evaluation of the obese person is often incorrectly deferred simply because the individual's weight is so much more than normal (Gallagher and Gates, 2003).

Acute Disease– or Injury-Related Malnutrition

Classically this type of malnutrition is seen with trauma, surgery, or rapid severe onset of a medical condition (e.g., pneumonia) (Jensen and Wheeler, 2012; White et al, 2012). Injury causes stress, catecholamine release, and increased resting energy expenditure. The degree of hypermetabolism is directly related to the severity of injury. For example, severe burns cause a greater increase in metabolic rate than uncomplicated surgery (Demling, 2009). The inflammatory response is elicited concomitantly. Cortisol released from the adrenal cortex enhances protein catabolism, amino acid mobilization, and hepatic glucose production (Heimburger, 2008). Cytokines, including tumor necrosis factor, transforming growth factor-β, and interleukin-1 and interleukin-6, contribute to the stress response. While insulin levels are elevated, insulin resistance prevents anabolism. Positive acute phase proteins increase (e.g., C-reactive protein). Less albumin is synthesized, catabolism increases, and fluids leak into the interstitium and create edema. The low albumin level (<3.5 g/dl) with the elevation of C-reactive protein is an indicator of inflammation (Jensen, 2006). During hypermetabolic periods, caloric needs increase and protein requirements increase disproportionately. Hypermetabolic demands decrease gradually, and, if no additional insult occurs, metabolic needs return to baseline within 10 to 14 days of the acute injury.

In the injured but healthy person, inadequate intake for 5 to 7 days usually is not a problem. Surgical patients are an excellent example. A combination of hypermetabolism and starvation occurs due to inadequate intake. The hypermetabolic response is a physiologic response to injury and results in increased energy needs. At the same time, patients initially are provided with intravenous fluids containing 5% glucose (about 200 calories per liter). The glucose administered spares protein but is not able to meet metabolic needs. As oral intake resumes, caloric intake is less than normal, and auto-catabolism occurs to meet metabolic needs. These patients usually have a brief but rapid decrease in weight. When they return to adequate caloric intake, they regain the lost weight (Heimburger, 2008). If the cause of the stress is not resolved, additional stresses occur (e.g., infection), or the individual's intake does not meet metabolic needs, the patient is set up for a downward spiral.

SCREENING AND ASSESSMENT

Healthy people ingest sufficient carbohydrates, protein, fat, vitamins, minerals, and fluids to meet nutritional needs and maintain a positive nitrogen balance. Wound healing requires additional nutrients, and it is important to evaluate patients with wounds early and at regular intervals. Sample screening and assessment forms discussed in this section are available online (MNA; MST; SNAQ).

Screening for Possible Malnutrition

Nutrition *screening* identifies patients who are (1) not at risk and therefore not in need of a nutritional assessment; (2) at potential risk for malnutrition; or (3) possibly undernourished. The latter two categories indicate the need for a nutritional *assessment* by a registered dietitian (Anthony, 2008; NPUAP, EPUAP, PPPIA, 2014). For the hospitalized patient, nutritional screening provides baseline data on a person's nutritional status and should be done at admission or as early as possible after admission (Green and Watson, 2006; NPUAP, EPUAP, PPPIA, 2014). The nutritional screening tool used should be validated, reliable, relevant to the desired patient group, applicable to different health care settings, able to detect undernutrition and overnutrition, and quick and easy to use (NPUAP, EPUAP, PPPIA, 2014).

The Malnutrition Universal Screening Tool (MUST) and the Short Nutritional Assessment Questionnaire (SNAQ) are recommended by the International Pressure Ulcer Guidelines (NPUAP, EPUAP, PPPIA, 2014) as being the most accurate and readily available nutritional screening tool for the general hospital and inpatient population. Composed of questions that are most predictive of malnutrition, these tools are easy to implement. Each health care setting should have a policy on nutritional screening that acknowledges the need to refer those at risk to a registered dietitian or nutritional support team for a nutritional assessment (NPUAP, EPUAP, PPPIA, 2014).

The Mini Nutritional Assessment (MNA) is an instrument designed for use in older patients that combines screening with assessment. It is a reliable and valid 18-item tool that consists of anthropometric, general, dietary, and subjective assessments; has been used in a variety of health care settings; and has been shown to detect malnutrition before changes in weight or serum protein levels, especially in an elderly population (Bauer et al, 2008). From a cross-sectional study of elderly patients with pressure ulcers, Langkamp-Henken et al (2005) concluded that use of the MNA was advantageous over serum protein levels for screening or assessment.

Recently the new MNA-Short Form has been validated as a standalone screening tool; requiring less time to complete and being more user friendly, the MNA-Short Form has become the preferred form for clinical practice (Kaiser et al, 2009). Furthermore, it has been demonstrated that when body mass index (BMI) is not available, the calf circumference is a valid alternative.

Assessment of Nutritional Status

A nutritional assessment is indicated for the patient who has a wound, is obese, or is screened as being at potential risk for malnutrition. Nutritional assessment is designed to confirm the presence or absence of malnutrition and to measure the extent of existing malnutrition. Although the nurse may be instrumental in gathering the data used in a nutritional assessment, assimilation of the data into an assessment requires a referral to a dietitian or a multidisciplinary nutrition support team (dietitians, nurses, pharmacists, providers). With the implementation of interventions, the patient's response should be monitored closely, often daily. Reassessments are recommended every week, with changes in the patient's condition, and with any significant weight loss. For individuals in home care, it is important to be vigilant to changes in patient status and weight. Significant weight loss is defined as weight loss of 5% or greater within 30 days or 10% or greater within 180 days (NPUAP, EPUAP, PPPIA, 2014).

A systematic approach to nutritional assessment is recommended and includes:
- History and clinical diagnosis
- Clinical signs and physical examination (fever/hypothermia, nonspecific signs of inflammation; e.g., tachycardia)
- Anthropometric data (weight, height, skinfolds)
- Laboratory data
- Dietary information (diet history, 24-hour recall)
- Functional assessment (strength and physical performance) (Jensen et al, 2012)

History and Clinical Diagnosis. No single parameter (e.g., weight, serum protein level) is a valid or reliable marker of nutritional status. Furthermore, many assessment parameters commonly used are affected by other conditions (e.g., kidney disease, dehydration, cancer, and pregnancy). Research is ongoing to determine which parameters provide the most reliable and accurate representation of the malnourished state.

Nutritional status is sometimes evaluated based entirely on data from the patient's history and physical. In these situations, the admission assessment should sequence the history taking so that significant dimensions reflective of nutritional status are clustered. This information can be used to direct the physical examination, laboratory work, and referrals.

Clinical Signs and Physical Examination. The physical examination is performed after the history is taken. Although no single physical finding is diagnostic of malnutrition, many different signs and symptoms are associated with specific nutritional alterations, such as coarse hair or thin skin (Seidel et al, 2008). Signs and symptoms associated with nutritional alterations are listed in Table 27-1. However, these findings correlate with other conditions, such as disease process, medication side effects, metabolic alterations, and age-related changes (Heimburger, 2008). Often the physical assessment findings can be used to confirm concerns or suspicions derived from the data obtained from the patient's history or the laboratory work. For patients at risk of or with early malnutrition, the physical findings for malnutrition may be subtle or absent because some signs do not appear until the malnutrition becomes advanced. With overt malnutrition, anthropometric changes often are key findings. Obese patients are especially difficult to evaluate because their weight may mask the skeletal muscle wasting of malnutrition (Gallagher and Gates, 2003).

Anthropometric Measures. Anthropometric measures are easy to perform and are pivotal in the evaluation of nutritional status. The most commonly used anthropometric parameters are height, weight, and head circumference (children only). Less frequently used are midarm muscle circumference and skinfold measurements (Table 27-2).

TABLE 27-1 Physical Findings Associated with Nutritional Deficiencies

Site	Signs and Symptoms	Nutritional Deficit
Skin	Cracking	Protein
	Petechiae	Vitamin C
	Scaling	Vitamin A
Hair	Corkscrew hairs	Vitamin C
	Easily pluckable hair	Protein
Muscles	Weakness	Protein, calories
Mouth	Bleeding	Vitamins A, C, K
	Atrophic tongue	Protein, iron

TABLE 27-2 Anthropometric Measures

	Measures	Condition Measure Reflects
Common measures	Height and weight (body mass index)	Overnutrition, undernutrition
	Head circumference in children	Undernutrition
Less frequently used measures*	Midarm circumference	Muscle stores
	Skinfold measurements	Fat stores
	Hand-grip strength	Muscle strength Undernutrition

*Measures performed by dietitian.

Weight is the cornerstone in the diagnosis of malnutrition and can be used alone or in relation to height or frame size. Weight is often considered in relation to height. Recent tables for interpretation of these parameters are based on the National Research Council data on weight and height, the dietary guidelines, and BMI. The BMI is calculated by dividing weight (in kilograms) by height (in meters) squared and most often is used to determine whether people are underweight or overweight. Body mass index is a predictor of morbidity and mortality (Gallagher and Gates, 2003; U.S. Preventive Services Task Force, 2003). Body mass index does not evaluate fat distribution; therefore it should be considered in conjunction with other assessment findings (Evans, 2005). Also, the Centers for Disease Control and Prevention (CDC) advise that age and gender can affect the relationship between BMI and body fat, as women and older persons have a greater proportion of fat than do men and younger persons.

Head circumference is used in children to evaluate their growth. Measurements are compared with tables of norms, allowing head size to be classified in percentiles. Chronic undernutrition results in delayed growth of the head, and its identification and treatment are important so that permanent damage does not occur (Mascarenhas et al, 1998). Although the test measures are performed primarily by dietitians, it is important to understand what the test measures mean in order to appreciate the relevance of the findings.

Arm muscle circumference and skinfold measures initially were used in underdeveloped countries and obtained with only the most basic of instruments to evaluate the nutritional status of the population (Jeliffe, 1966). Standards exist in the United States for specific age groups and for a limited number of minority populations (Frisancho, 1984; Gray and Gray, 1979; Marshall et al, 1999). Mid-upper arm circumference is a measure of muscle mass, bones, and skin. It is used to calculate midarm muscle circumference as a measure of lean body mass (Heimburger, 2008). A decrease in arm muscle mass occurs with protein and calorie deficiencies.

Fat stores are measured with a skinfold caliper. The triceps site is most frequently used; other sites include the scapula and waist. Fat stores do not change rapidly, so skinfold thickness is not a sensitive measure of malnutrition. Dietitians, advanced practice nurses, and the nutritional support team may perform arm muscle circumference and skinfold measures.

Laboratory Data. There is no ideal laboratory test for malnutrition. Serum proteins (albumin, prealbumin, transferrin, retinol-binding protein) are synthesized primarily by the liver and vary considerably in their turnover rates. These visceral proteins comprise a small portion of the body's total protein pool. Visceral proteins include erythrocytes, granulocytes, lymphocytes, and other solid tissue organs.

Serum proteins are negative acute phase proteins or reactants during the inflammatory response. Inflammatory processes such as acute or chronic infection, surgery, trauma, and burns trigger a systemic response referred to as the *acute phase response.* The serum levels of most proteins either increase or decrease during the acute phase response. Serum proteins that decrease levels during inflammation are called *negative acute phase reactants* (e.g., albumin and prealbumin) and are expected to return to normal as the inflammatory process resolves. Positive acute phase reactants are proteins that increase levels during times of stress because they are essential for the immune response. C-reactive protein, fibrinogen, protein S, and fibronectin are examples of positive acute phase reactants. Because of its ability to change quickly with changing conditions, the positive acute phase reactant C-reactive protein is a commonly used marker for the presence of inflammation (Banh, 2006; Jensen, 2006).

Historically, albumin was used as a measure of nutritional status and probably is the most frequently measured of the laboratory parameters. Albumin has a long half-life (17 to 21 days) and is not sensitive to rapid changes in nutritional status; albumin levels fall only late during the course of prolonged and premorbid starvation (Demling, 2009; Heimburger, 2008). As a negative acute phase protein influenced by many factors, serum albumin is *not* an appropriate measure for malnutrition; it is a carrier protein and primarily helps to maintain oncotic pressure.

Prealbumin, also known as *thyroxin-binding prealbumin* or *transthyretin*, is a transport protein for thyroxine and vitamin A (Evans et al, 2005). It is affected by many of the same factors that affect albumin. However, because of its short half-life (2 days), prealbumin is expected to reflect decreased intake of protein or calories more rapidly and respond quickly when exogenous nutrients are provided, but the acute phase response limits its capacity.

Transferrin, also an acute phase protein, has a shorter half-life than albumin (8 to 10 days) and a smaller body pool. Its major function is iron transport. Usually about one third of the body's transferrin is bound to iron. Therefore iron status influences transferrin levels such that iron deficiency, which frequently occurs with protein-calorie malnutrition, stimulates

hepatic synthesis, resulting in very high transferrin levels. At the other extreme, certain types of anemia may trigger depressed transferrin levels (Demling, 2009). Transferrin level is not sufficiently sensitive or specific to be a meaningful measurement of nutritional status.

Less commonly measured is retinol-binding protein, a plasma protein with a very short half-life (12 hours) and very low serum levels. It participates in the transport of vitamin A, and its response follows that of prealbumin. Although it has a theoretic advantage over other plasma proteins by virtue of its short half-life, its low normal values and the technical difficulties associated with its measurement limit its usefulness compared with other measures of nutrient status (Evans et al, 2005).

It should be noted that hydration status varies frequently and, if severe, affects serum protein levels. When the patient is dehydrated, serum albumin and prealbumin levels will be falsely elevated. Conversely, when the patient is overhydrated, serum protein levels will be falsely low (Table 27-3). Serum proteins are also affected by a number of other factors (Table 27-4) (Banh, 2006).

TABLE 27-3 Laboratory Measures of Adequate Hydration

Laboratory Test	Underhydration	Normal Values
Serum sodium	>150 mEq/L	130 to 150 mEq/L
Osmolality	>295 mOsm/L	285 to 295 mOsm/L
Blood urea nitrogen (BUN)	Elevated	7 to 23 mg/dl
BUN-creatinine ratio	>25:1	10:1
Urine-specific gravity	>1.028	1.003 to 1.028

TABLE 27-4 Acute Phase Response to Inflammation

Acute Phase Reactants* (Normal Values)	Factors Affecting Reliability (Direction of Response)	Effect of Inflammation	Effect of Recovery from Inflammation
Albumin (3.5 to 5.0 g/dl)	Overhydration (↓) Bed rest (↓) Zinc deficiency (↓)	Negative	Positive (return to normal)
Prealbumin (18 to 45 mg/dl)	Steroid use (↑) Hyperglycemia (↓) Kidney disease (↑)	Negative	Positive (return to normal)
Transferrin (188 to 341 mg/dl)	Iron deficiency (↑) Zinc deficiency (↓) Old age (↓)	Negative	Positive (return to normal)
C-reactive protein (<0.8 mg/L)	Heart disease (↑) Leukemia (no change) Ulcerative colitis (no change)	Positive	Negative (return to normal)

*Values decrease by 25%.

Banh L, *Serum proteins as markers of nutrition: what are we treating?* 2006. http://www.medicine.virginia.edu/clinical/departments/medicine/divisions/digestive-health/nutrition-support-team/nutrition-articles/BanhArticle.pdf/. Accessed April, 2014

Creatinine levels have been used for more than 20 years in nutritional support settings to evaluate lean body mass. Creatinine gives an indirect measure of skeletal muscle mass and is a measure of long-term protein status (Demling, 2009). Creatinine assessment is complex because the patient must have normal renal function and urinary output, have the ability to accurately collect a 24-hour urine sample, be adequately hydrated, and not be on prolonged periods of bed rest or a recent high-protein meal.

Nutritional status also can be evaluated using a 24-hour urine creatinine excretion divided by normal creatinine for height, producing a creatinine height index. An index of 40% to 60% reflects minimal protein depletion, whereas an index less than 40% indicates severe nutrition depletion. Age-specific tables are used to interpret the findings.

Nitrogen balance measures whether sufficient protein is being ingested, absorbed, and metabolized. Nitrogen intake and loss from the body are carefully regulated and, under normal nutritional circumstances, closely approximate each other so that nitrogen turnover is in balance. Anabolism and repair require positive nitrogen balance. Negative nitrogen balance is a reflection of catabolism or inadequate ingestion.

Dietary Intake. A diet history and a 24-hour recall help the dietitian evaluate both recent intake and usual intake patterns. When patients are unable to provide this information due to cognitive status or severity of illness, family members will be called upon to provide recent data.

Functional Assessment. Evaluation of functional ability with hand-grip strength is recommended. Using a simple dynamometer, this evaluation is quick and easy to use. More complex evaluation of stair climbing or time to get out of the chair may be used (Jensen et al, 2012).

Diagnosis of Malnutrition. The diagnosis of malnutrition is made in the context of the patient's overall situation. Six characteristics from the history and physical are evaluated: (1) decreased energy intake; (2) weight loss; (3) fat loss; (4) muscle loss; (5) fluid accumulation; and (6) diminished grip strength (Jensen et al, 2012; White et al, 2012). The criteria for malnutrition in the context of starvation, chronic disease (chronic defined as at least 3 months), and acute illness are listed in Table 27-5. At least two characteristics must be present in order to diagnose malnutrition. Each category of malnutrition is divided into nonsevere and severe. The duration of reduced estimated energy intake is important as a criterion for severity. Also, weight loss has a timeframe to guide the clinician. White et al (2012) recommend that weight and height should be measured, rather than estimated. Clinical judgment is needed in evaluating fat and muscle loss, as well as fluid accumulation; note that the criteria are quite broad in each of these areas. Hand-grip strength has been added as a measure of function. Registered dietitians usually have a dynamometer as part of their equipment and are qualified to perform this measure. Absent from the list are the serum proteins (albumin, prealbumin, etc.) that historically have been an integral part of nutritional assessment.

TABLE 27-5 Criteria for Malnutrition: Starvation-Related, Chronic Disease–Related, and Acute or Injury-Related*

	STARVATION-RELATED MALNUTRITION		CHRONIC DISEASE–RELATED MALNUTRITION**		ACUTE OR INJURY-RELATED MALNUTRITION	
	Nonsevere	**Severe**	**Nonsevere**	**Severe**	**Nonsevere**	**Severe**
Estimated energy intake	<75% for ≥3 months	<50% >1 month	<75% for ≤1 month		<75% for >7 days	≤50% for >5 days
Weight loss	5% in 1 month	>5% in 1 month	5% in 1 month	>5% in 1 month	1–2% in 1 week	>2% in 1 week
	7.5% in 3 months	>7.5% in 3 months	7.5% in 3 months	>7.5% in 3 months	5% in 1 month	>5% in 1 month
	10% in 6 months	>10% in 6 months	10% in 6 months	>10% in 6 months	7.5% in 3 months	>7.5% in 3 months
	20% in 1 year	>20% in 1 year	20% in 1 year	>20% in 1 year		
Body fat reduction	Mild	Severe	Mild	Severe	Mild	Moderate
Muscle mass reduction	Mild	Severe	Mild	Severe	Mild	Moderate
Fluid accumulation	Mild	Severe	Mild	Severe	Mild	Moderate to severe
Hand-grip strength reduction	Not applicable	Measurably	Not applicable	Measurably	Not applicable	Measurably

*Two or more characteristics must be present for malnutrition to be diagnosed.
** Adapted from Table. White JV, Guenter P, Jensen G, et al, Consensus statement of the Academy of Nutrition and Dietetics/American Society for Parenteral and Enteral Nutrition: characteristics recommended for the identification and documentation of adult malnutrition (undernutrition), *J Acad Nutr Diet* 112(5): 730–738, 2012.

NUTRIENT NEEDS FOR HEALING

Body composition is conceptualized as having two components: fat mass and fat-free mass (Demling, 2009). The majority of the body is fat, which acts as a calorie reservoir. Fat is a calorie-dense substrate, with 9 calories per gram of fat. When the body's intake of calories is greater than expenditure, fat deposits form and weight increases. In times of need, fat is catabolized and weight loss occurs.

In contrast, the fat-free compartment, or lean body mass, is composed primarily of protein and water. The protein portion is located predominantly in muscles, red blood cells, connective tissues, and organs, including the skin, which is the largest of the body's organs. Healing requires protein synthesis (Demling, 2009). When energy requirements exceed intake, even for short periods, body protein is broken down to meet metabolic need; the protein in this situation is used for energy rather than for anabolism. Protein has less than half the calories of fat (4 calories per gram); when it is catabolized, weight loss is rapid. Also, because protein is not stored in the body, catabolism of protein results in loss of functional tissue (muscle, organs), which is referred to as *muscle wasting.*

Normal healing requires adequate protein, fat, and carbohydrates, as well as vitamins and minerals (Stechmiller, 2010). When intake, absorption, or metabolism of nutrients does not meet metabolic requirements, biochemical changes occur that have implications for healing (e.g., impaired fibroplasia). However, these changes often occur without clinical manifestations, although they may be detected with appropriate tests (e.g., low zinc levels, below-normal prealbumin levels). Severe changes must occur before signs and symptoms of impaired healing due to malnutrition are manifest (e.g., dehiscence). In part, the wound receives the biologic priority of muscle catabolism, which provides substrates that preferentially allow repair of injured tissues. This protection is tightly tied to the percentage of lean body mass. When more than 15% of lean body mass is lost, impaired healing is seen. At 30% loss of lean body mass, more severe alterations in healing occur (e.g., dehiscence). With 40% loss of lean body mass, death occurs, often due to pneumonia (Demling, 2009).

The best data about nutritional requirements for healing come from the surgical and pressure ulcer literature (Demling, 2009; Heimburger, 2008; NPUAP, EPUAP, PPPIA, 2014; Posthauer, 2006a, 2006b). Energy needs usually are based on a modification of the Harris-Benedict equation, which takes into account the person's age, gender, height, and weight; a portion of the equation considers the individual's stress and activity. This equation provides a good starting point for determining nutritional therapy. The alternative is to perform indirect calorimetry; however, that approach usually is reserved for patients who are hypermetabolic from sepsis or trauma in whom body weight cannot accurately be determined and those who are being weaned from a ventilator (precise prescription in order to avoid excess CO_2 production

and delay weaning) (Heimburger, 2008). Once caloric needs are determined, protein, fat, carbohydrate, and vitamin and mineral distributions are planned.

Calories

The range of normal calories administered is broad and is based on a multitude of factors. Usual caloric needs are 20 to 35 calories per kilogram of body weight. Lower estimates are used for patients with chronic illness who are chronically starved, whereas higher estimates are used for those who are hypermetabolic and have significant injuries (Bistrian and Driscoll, 2008; Posthauer, 2006b). With injury, more calories and substrates are needed for healing than in an uninjured state. About 50% to 60% of an individual's caloric needs are met through carbohydrates, 20% to 25% through protein, and the remainder from fat (Posthauer, 2006b).

Protein

Protein needs are disproportionally increased after injury, and a protein deficiency can prolong a person's healing time (Arnold and Barbul, 2006). In adults, 15% of lean body weight is composed of protein, of which 3% (approximately 300 mg) is turned over daily during normal protein metabolism. Most of this protein is reused in the synthesis of new proteins, and some is lost through excretion. The recommended daily allowance (RDA) of protein for a healthy person is 0.8 g of protein per kilogram per 24 hours; protein needs with injury may increase to 1.25 to 1.5 g per kilogram per day (Demling, 2009; NPUAP, EPUAP, PPPIA, 2014). Older adults often are protein deficient because they have proportionally greater daily protein requirements than younger persons; at the same time, their intake of protein often is inadequate. During times of limited intake, the older adult is at especially high risk for undernutrition (Green and Watson, 2006).

Proteins are made of amino acids, which are necessary to generate acute phase proteins, including collagen and proteoglycans, and are essential for wound healing, hormonal and immune balance, and muscle health. With stress, the amino acids arginine and glutamine become conditional essential amino acids because the body cannot produce these amino acids at a rate adequate to meet the increased need (Posthauer, 2006b).

Arginine

Arginine is converted to ornithine, a precursor to proline and subsequent collagen formation. In animal models, arginine decreases nitrogen loss and stimulates immune function, wound breaking strength, and collagen formation; it also facilitates wound healing by augmenting the release of the anabolic hormones insulin, insulinlike growth factors, glucagon, prolactin, and various growth factors (Posthauer, 2006b; Stechmiller et al, 2005, 2010; Thompson and Fuhrman, 2005). Small clinical studies show the value of arginine in wound healing (Brewer et al, 2010; Desneves et al, 2005; Evans et al, 2014; Leigh et al, 2012). Enteral feeding solutions contain arginine (Stechmiller, 2010) and arginine supplementation is commercially available for clinical use.

Glutamine

As one of the most abundant amino acids in the body, glutamine helps preserve the functional integrity of the intestinal brush border. It is used to synthesize nonessential fatty acids and the nucleotide units of RNA and DNA. With stress, glutamine levels diminish (400 μmol/L), thereby compromising the integrity of the immune system. Replacement is important to reduce the risk of systemic sepsis. By stimulating growth hormone, glutamine enhances immune system function. Normal glutamine levels of 600 μmol/L or higher facilitate intact immunologic function. The patient with a major wound has a glutamine requirement of 0.3 to 0.4 g per kilogram per day (Demling, 2009).

Carbohydrates

Carbohydrates provide a significant portion of nutrients. Carbohydrate is turned to glucose, which is available immediately for adenosine triphosphate (ATP) formation and provides the energy for phagocytosis and collagen development. Glucose levels must be kept within normal limits to facilitate healing; excessive levels result in impaired healing. Glucose also is important to prevent the use of protein as an energy source rather than for anabolism.

Fats

Fats are important for development and stability of cell membranes (both intracellular and cell wall). Fats also participate actively in various aspects of the inflammatory response to injury and thus in healing. The type of fat ingested determines the type of prostaglandins produced. Omega-3 fatty acids favor prostaglandin (PG) E_3 and leukotrienes; they participate in inflammation, vasoconstriction, and platelet aggregation. Omega-6 fatty acids facilitate protection from inflammation and immunosuppression by generating a preponderance of PGE_1 and PGE_2, vasodilators, and antiinflammatory agents (Arnold and Barbul, 2006).

Vitamins

All of the vitamins are needed for tissue repair and regeneration because of their various functions in normal cellular metabolism. Table 27-6 lists the role of various nutrients in healing. Vitamins A and C are especially critical for healing. Vitamin A is fat soluble and is important in various steps of collagen deposition. Collagen is the most important component in scar formation and in maintaining wound closure. In persons treated with corticosteroids, vitamin A is an important antagonist; it reverses all the effects of corticosteroids except for impairment of contracture (Heimburger, 2008).

Vitamin C is a water-soluble vitamin, a cofactor in collagen formation, and is important to fibroplasia. It enables complement to perform its functions. Vitamin C works synergistically with vitamin E to prevent oxidative cell damage. Lack of vitamin C can result in impaired collagen formation.

TABLE 27-6	Role of Nutrients in Wound Healing
Nutrient	**Role in Healing**
Protein	Angiogenesis
	Collagen synthesis/remodeling
	Wound contraction
	Immune function
	Precursor to nitric oxide
Carbohydrate	Energy source
	Protein sparing
	Angiogenesis
Fat	Cell walls
	Intracellular structures
	Inflammation
Vitamin A*	Epithelialization
	Angiogenesis
	Inflammatory response
B vitamins	Cofactor in enzymes
	Immune response
	Synthesis of macronutrients
Vitamin C	Collagen synthesis
	Capillary wall integrity
	Fibroblast function
	Immune function
	Antioxidant
Vitamin D*	Calcium metabolism
Vitamin E*	Antioxidant
Vitamin K*	Coagulation
Copper	Cross-linking collagen
Iron	Collagen formation
	Immune function
	Oxygen transport
Zinc	Collagen formation
	Protein synthesis
	Cell membrane stability
	Immune function

*Fat soluble.

When vitamin C intake ceases, the stores become depleted within 2 to 3 months (Arnold and Barbul, 2006).

Minerals

Among the minerals, zinc, copper, and iron have received the most attention in the context of wound healing. Zinc is important because of its role in protein synthesis, enzyme systems, immune competence, and collagen formation (Heimburger, 2008). Zinc supplementation enhances collagen formation in patients with zinc deficiency. In persons with normal zinc levels, supplementation has not been shown to alter healing (Posthauer, 2006b). Supplementation should be based on serum deficits, and treatment should be limited to 7 to 10 days (220 mg twice per day). Supplementation in those who are not in need may result in disruption of normal phagocytic activity and cause copper deficiency. Copper deficiency may result in weaker scar tissue and decreased tensile strength, predisposing the person to dehiscence. Iron is important in hemoglobin for oxygen transport. Persons with anemia who are not able to compensate for low oxygen with increased circulation rates may experience impaired collagen formation and ineffective phagocytic activity.

Electrolytes

Water and balanced electrolytes are the sea in which the various nutrients function. Adequate hydration and electrolytes provide the physiologic space in which nutrients and oxygen are transported to the site of injury so that healing can occur. The usual rule for fluid is at least 1500 ml per 24 hours, with most individuals receiving fluids based on the equation 30 ml per kilogram body weight (Dwyer, 2008). The exception to this rule is people with heart or kidney disease, for whom the recommendation is 25 ml/kg or replacement of fluid losses; loss of wound fluid or treatment with an air fluidized bed may increase the patient's fluid requirement needs (Posthauer, 2006a, 2006b). Evaluation of hydration status is an integral part of nutritional assessment (Posthauer, 2006a). Table 27-3 lists laboratory measures of hydration.

NUTRITIONAL SUPPORT

Depending on the health care system, the appropriate action to take when a patient is screened as being malnourished or at risk for malnutrition is referring the patient to a dietitian, notifying the provider of the findings, or calling the nutritional support team. A sequence of events for providing nutritional support is summarized in Box 27-1.

Nutritional needs are dependent on many variables, including age, gender, height, weight, presence of severe wasting or obesity, current disease state, and severity of illness. Additional nutrient needs are present when the patient has a wound due to loss of protein and fluid from the wound, as well as the increased demands required to support the wound-healing process. When the patient is at risk for pressure ulcers as identified by the nutrition subscale of the Braden scale, supplementation of dietary intake may be warranted (Whitney et al, 2006).

Most diets are a combination of protein, carbohydrate, fat, vitamins, and minerals, so deficiencies of individual nutrients are uncommon. Increased intake or supplement is needed if the patient is undernourished or at risk for impaired healing (Stechmiller, 2010). Protein intake should be sufficient to support growth of granulation tissue (Whitney et al, 2006; Stechmiller, 2010). Goals of nutritional support for the patient who is at risk or who has an existing wound are to provide a minimum of 30 to 35 kcal per kilogram of body weight per day, with 1.25 to 1.5 g per kilogram per day of protein and 1 ml per kilocalorie per day of fluid intake (NPUAP, EPUAP, PPPIA, 2014; Whitney et al, 2006). Sometimes when patients are ill, they are unable to ingest a balanced diet that provides

---

BOX 27-1 **Sequence of Events for Nutritional Support**

1. Screen nutritional status of all patients upon admission (skip and move to assessment if patient is obese or has a wound)
2. Nutritional assessment of patients at risk for malnutrition:
   - All patients with a wound
   - Obese patients
   - Patients screened to be at risk for malnutrition
3. Estimate nutritional requirements
4. Compare nutrient intake with estimated requirements
5. Provide appropriate nutrition intervention based on nutritional requirements
6. Provide sufficient nutrients
   - 30 to 35 kcal per kilogram of body weight per day
   - 1.25 to 1.5 g of protein per kilogram per day
   - 1 ml of fluid intake per kcal per day
   - 1600 to 2000 retinol equivalents of vitamin A
   - 100 to 1000 mg of vitamin C
   - 15 to 30 mg of zinc
   - 200% of recommended dietary allowance of the B vitamins
   - 20 to 30 mg of iron
   - 0.3 to 0.4 g of glutamine per kilogram per day
   - Daily multivitamin and mineral supplement
7. Monitor intake to ensure patient is meeting nutritional requirements
8. Monitor and evaluate nutritional outcomes, with reassessment of nutritional status at frequent intervals while individual is at risk

---

the needed vitamins and minerals. In that case, a daily multivitamin is recommended, as well as treatment of any detected or suspected deficiencies (NPUAP, EPUAP, PPPIA, 2014). Daily vitamin and mineral needs are increased to 1600 to 2000 retinol equivalents of vitamin A, 100 to 1000 mg of vitamin C, 15 to 30 mg of zinc, 200% of the RDA of the B vitamins, and 20 to 30 mg of iron. Most of these needs can be met with a daily multivitamin and mineral supplement (Bistrian and Driscoll, 2008; NPUAP, EPUAP, PPPIA, 2014; Posthauer, 2006b). Research has demonstrated no acceleration in healing with supplemental vitamin A or C or zinc (Stechmiller, 2010; Whitney et al, 2006). Arginine has been found to have no effect on the rate of healing in patients with a pressure ulcer.

Anabolic steroids have been recommended and demonstrated to be useful in supporting healing in some populations by stimulating increased protein buildup and weight gain (Demling, 2009). Approved by the U.S. Food and Drug Administration in the 1960s for treatment of severe weight loss due to chronic infections, severe trauma, or failure to thrive without a pathophysiologic reason, anabolic steroids have been used to treat severe malnourishment and wasting syndrome typical with human immunodeficiency virus and acquired immunodeficiency syndrome–related conditions and burns. The anabolic steroid oxandrolone (Oxandrin), a testosterone analog, has been shown to decrease catabolism and significantly attenuate lost lean mass with severe wounds. Androgens influence wound healing by increasing collagen deposition and facilitating leukocyte migration and monocyte adhesion to enhance the inflammatory response. Shortened healing times have also been reported with human growth hormone, another anabolic steroid (Oh and Phillips, 2006). Estrogen has been reported to have antiinflammatory properties, decreasing elastase activity so that fibronectin degradation is decreased and collagen content deposition is increased, particularly in estrogen-deficient women. However, estrogen therapy increases the risk of endometrial hyperplasia and cancer and has been observed to adversely affect the quality of scar formation (Oh and Phillips, 2006).

The preferred route of nutritional support is oral, and, whenever possible, the gastrointestinal tract should be used for feeding. A person who is receiving oral feeding should be counseled to select foods that contain protein. Foods high in protein, including milk, eggs, cheese, tuna, and meat, should be encouraged. Supplemental snacks, including pudding, peanut butter and crackers, protein bars, and ice cream, are other sources of protein.

If the patient's intake is not adequate with oral feeding, then one of the various approaches to the gastrointestinal tract used for tube feedings should be considered to supplement or supplant the oral feeding. As with other patient populations, use of specialized nutritional support (tube feeding or parenteral nutrition) is based on the likelihood that prevention or treatment of protein-calorie malnutrition will increase the possibility of recovery, mitigate infection, improve healing, or shorten hospital stay (Bistrian and Driscoll, 2008). For a portion of those who are malnourished, weight loss and debilitation are inevitable consequences of disease that will lead to death, and the outcomes cannot be changed with nutritional support. However, in those in whom nutritional support can enhance outcomes, early nutritional evaluation and initiation of therapy support positive outcomes (Bistrian and Driscoll, 2008). When the gastrointestinal tract cannot be used, parenteral nutrition is the route of choice. At times a combination of peripheral parenteral nutrition and oral intake may be used.

CLINICAL CONSULT

A: 84-year-old Latina woman admitted from a nursing home after a fall that resulted in a fractured hip. Also has abdominal wound from surgery 5 weeks ago for a perforated bowel managed with NPWT. Documentation indicates wound size has not decreased in 2 weeks. She is able to follow directions, has a body mass index (BMI) of 30 (height 5 feet 5 inches, weight 180 pounds). She has a history of glaucoma and dementia. Discussion with the nursing home staff facilitated completion of a Mini Nutritional Assessment, which indicates a decreased appetite, recent 8 pound weight loss, and minimal ability to feed herself. Her complete blood count (CBC) is normal. Her albumin is 2.2 g/dl.

D: Starvation related malnutrition; not compatible with wound healing. At risk for pressure ulcer related to hip fracture and decreased mobility.

P: Control wound bioburden until nutrition improves enough to support wound healing. Prevent further skin breakdown.

I: (1) Immediate referral to dietitian. (2) Assist patient with eating and offer calorie-rich fluid at each visit to the room. (3) C-reactive protein to rule out co-existing inflammation. (4) Continue with NPWT to abdominal wound and silver impregnated hydrocolloid island dressing over hip incision. (5) Reposition every 2 hours and as needed while in bed; use viscoelastic reactive support surface. (6) Continuous passive motion machine on while patient is in bed. (7) Consult with physical therapy for strengthening exercises and ambulation twice daily.

E: Family understands that wound healing cannot be expected until nutrition improves. Plan to revisit in 1 week to review recommendations from dietitian and physical therapy and adjust local wound care as indicated.

SUMMARY

Nutritional assessment and support play important roles in wound healing. All patients with wounds should undergo evaluation of their nutritional status. A thorough nutritional assessment should reveal the risk for or presence of malnutrition and provide the necessary information to develop an individualized nutritional plan of care. The nutritional status should be evaluated at baseline and at regular intervals to determine the effectiveness of the nutritional plan.

REFERENCES

Anthony PS: Nutrition screening tool for hospitalized patients, *Nutra Clin Proct* 23(4):373–382, 2008.

Arnold M, Barbul A: Nutrition and wound healing, *Plast Reconstr Surg* 117(Suppl 7):S42–S58, 2006.

Banh L: Serum proteins as markers of nutrition: what are we treating? *Pract Gastroenterol* 29(10):46–64, 2006.

Bauer JM, Kaiser MJ, Anthony P, et al: The Mini Nutritional Assessment—its history, today's practice, and future perspectives, *Nutr Clin Pract* 23(4):388–396, 2008.

Bistrian BR, Driscoll DF: Enteral and parenteral nutrition therapy. In Fauci AS, Braunwald E, Kasper D, et al, editors: *Harrison's principles of internal medicine*, ed 17, New York, 2008, McGraw-Hill.

Brewer S, Desneves K, Pearce L, et al: Effect of an arginine-containing nutritional supplement on pressure ulcer healing in community spinal patients, *J Wound Care* 19(7):311–316, 2010.

Corkins MR, Guenter P, Dimaria-Ghalili RA, et al: Malnutrition diagnoses in hospitalized patients: United States, 2010, *J Parenter Enteral Nutr* 38(2):186–195, 2014.

Demling RH: Nutrition, anabolism, and the wound healing process: an overview, *Eplasty* 9:e9, 2009.

Desneves KJ, Todorovic BE, Cassar A, et al: Treatment with supplementary arginine, vitamin C and zinc in patients with pressure ulcers: a randomized controlled trial, *Clin Nutr* 24(6):979–987, 2005.

Dwyer J: Nutritional requirements and dietary assessment. In Fauci AS, Braunwald E, Kasper D, et al, editors: *Harrison's principles of internal medicine*, ed 17, New York, 2008, McGraw-Hill.

Evans DC, Martindale RG, Kiraly LN, et al: Nutrition optimization prior to surgery, *Nutr Clin Pract* 29(1):10–21, 2014.

Evans E: Nutritional assessment in chronic wound care, *J Wound Ostomy Continence Nurs* 32(5):317–320, 2005.

Frisancho AR: New standards of weight and body composition by frame size and height for assessment of nutritional status of adults and the elderly, *Am J Clin Nutr* 40(4):808–819, 1984.

Gallagher S, Gates JL: Obesity, panniculitis, panniculectomy, and wound care: understanding the challenges, *J Wound Ostomy Continence Nurs* 30(6):334–341, 2003.

Glasgow SC, Hermann VM: Surgical metabolism and nutrition. In Doherty GM, Way LW, editors: *Current surgical diagnosis and treatment*, ed 12, New York, 2006, McGraw-Hill.

Gray GE, Gray LK: Validity of anthropometric norms used in the assessment of hospitalized patients, *J Parenter Enteral Nutr* 3(5):366–368, 1979.

Green SM, Watson R: Nutritional screening and assessment tools for older adults: literature review, *J Adv Nurs* 54(4):477–490, 2006.

Heimburger DC: Malnutrition and nutritional assessment. In Fauci AS, Braunwald E, Kasper D, et al, editors: *Harrison's principles of internal medicine*, ed 17, New York, 2008, McGraw-Hill.

Jeliffe DB: *The assessment of nutritional status of the community (WHO Monograph no. 53)*, Geneva, Switzerland, 1966, World Health Organization.

Jensen GL: Inflammation as the key interface of the medical and nutrition universes: a provocative examination of the future of clinical nutrition and medicine, *J Parenter Enteral Nutr* 30(5):453–463, 2006.

Jensen GL, Bistrian B, Roubenoff R, et al: Malnutrition syndromes: a conundrum vs continuum, *J Parenter Enteral Nutr* 33(6):710–716, 2009.

Jensen GL, Compher C, Sullivan DH, et al: Recognizing malnutrition in adults: definitions and characteristics, screening, assessment, and team approach, *J Parenter Enteral Nutr* 37(6):802–807, 2013.

Jensen GL, Hsiao PY, Wheeler D: Adult nutrition assessment tutorial, *J Parenter Enteral Nutr* 36(3):267–274, 2012.

Jensen GL, Wheeler D: A new approach to defining and diagnosing malnutrition in adult critical illness, *Curr Opin Crit Care* 18(2):206–211, 2012.

Kaiser MJ, Bauer JM, Ramsch C, et al: Validation of the mini nutritional assessment short-form (MNA-SF): a practical tool for identification of nutritional status, *J Nutr Health Aging* 13(9):782–788, 2009.

Langkamp-Henken B, Hudgens J, Stechmiller JK, et al: Mini nutritional assessment and screening scores are associated with nutritional indicators in elderly people with pressure ulcers, *J Am Diet Assoc* 105(10):1590–1596, 2005.

Leigh B, Desneves K, Rafferty J, et al: The effect of different doses of an arginine-containing supplement on the healing of pressure ulcers, *J Wound Care* 21(3):150–156, 2012.

Malnutrition Screening Tool (MST) http://static.abbottnutrition. com/cms-prod/abbottnutrition.com/img/Malnutrition%20 Screening%20Tool_FINAL.pdf. Accessed August 16, 2015.

Marshall JA, Lopez TK, Shetterly SM, et al: Indicators of nutritional risk in a rural elderly Hispanic and non-Hispanic white population: San Luis Valley health and aging study, *J Am Diet Assoc* 99(3):315–322, 1999.

Mascarenhas MR, Zemel B, Stallings VA: Nutritional assessment in pediatrics, *Nutrition* 14(1):105, 1998.

Mini Nutritional Assessment (MNA) http://mna-elderly.com/. Accessed August 17, 2015.

Myron JA, Merlini G, Sheldon J, et al: Clinical indications for plasma protein assays: transthyretin (prealbumin) in inflammation and malnutrition, *Clin Chem Lab Med* 45(3):419–426, 2007.

National Pressure Ulcer Advisory Panel (NPUAP), European Pressure Ulcer Advisory Panel (EPUAP) and Pan Pacific Pressure Ulcer Alliance (PPPIA): *Prevention and treatment of pressure ulcers: clinical practice guideline*. In Emily Haesler, editor: Osborne Park, Western Australia, 2014, Cambridge Media.

Oh DM, Phillips TJ: Sex hormones and wound healing, *Wounds* 18(1):8–18, 2006.

Pompeo M: Misconceptions about protein requirements for wound healing: results of a prospective study, *Ostomy Wound Manage* 53:30, 2007.

Posthauer ME: Hydration: does it play a role in wound healing? *Adv Skin Wound Care* 19(2):74–76, 2006a.

Posthauer ME: The role of nutrition in wound care, *Adv Skin Wound Care* 19(1):43–52, 2006b.

Rodríguez-Hernández H, Simental-Mendía LE, Rodríguez-Ramírez G, et al: Obesity and inflammation: epidemiology, risk factors, and markers of inflammation, *Int J Endocrinol* 2013:678159.

Seidel HM, Ball JW, Dains JE, et al: *Mosby's guide to physical examination*, ed 7, St. Louis, MO, 2011, Mosby.

Short Nutritional Assessment Questionnaire (SNAQ) http://www. fightmalnutrition.eu/fileadmin/content/malnutrition/Screening_tools/SNAQ_Engels.jpg. Accessed August 16, 2015.

Stechmiller JK: Understanding the role of nutrition and wound healing, *Nutr Clin Pract* 25(1):61–68, 2010.

Stechmiller JK, Childress B, Cowan L: Arginine supplementation and wound healing, *Nutr Clin Pract* 20:52–61, 2005.

Tbahriti HF, Meknassi D, Moussaoui R, et al: Inflammatory status in chronic renal failure: the role of homocysteinemia and pro-inflammatory cytokines, *World J Nephrol* 2(2):31–37, 2013.

Thompson C, Fuhrman MP: Nutrients and wound healing: still searching for the magic bullet, *Nutr Clin Pract* 20(3):331–347, 2005.

U.S. Preventive Services Task Force: *Obesity in adults: screening and management*, Rockville, MD, 2012, Agency for Healthcare Research and Quality. http://www.uspreventiveservicestaskforce. org/Page/Topic/recommendation-summary/obesity-in-adults-screening-and-management. Accessed August 16, 2015.

White JV, Guenter P, Jensen G, et al: Consensus statement of the Academy of Nutrition and Dietetics/American Society for Parenteral and Enteral Nutrition: characteristics recommended for the identification and documentation of adult malnutrition (undernutrition), *J Acad Nutr Diet* 112(5):730–738, 2012.

Whitney J, Phillips L, Aslam R, et al: Guidelines for the treatment of pressure ulcers, *Wound Repair Regen* 14:663–679, 2006.

28

Perfusion and Oxygenation

JoAnne D. Whitney

OBJECTIVES

1. Identify and describe two factors that impair perfusion and related wound repair processes.
2. Describe the microcirculation and tissue oxygen characteristics of the wound environment.
3. Discuss the effects of an activated sympathetic nervous system on the wound repair processes.
4. Differentiate among the roles of wound tissue oxygen and arterial oxygen in wound repair.
5. Describe four interventions to increase tissue oxygen or improve wound healing.

A great deal has been learned over several decades about tissue repair and the importance of perfusion and oxygenation to healing, although much of that information has not been applied widely in daily clinical practice. Recognition is growing that inadequate wound healing and complications of acute wounds, such as surgical site infection, likely have their origins early in the initial inflammatory response and early in the healing process, when tissue breaking strength is low and physiologic responses may not be optimal (Dubay and Franz, 2003).

Classic and recent evidence serves as a guide to understanding the importance of adequate blood flow to peripheral tissues with an adequate oxygen supply so that optimal healing and resistance to infection for acute and chronic wounds may occur. This chapter addresses factors that influence perfusion and local wound oxygenation during wound repair, including autonomic nervous system activation, fluids, supplemental oxygen, pain, stress, hypothermia, obesity, and tobacco use. The efficacy of interventions for modifying these factors to achieve better wound tissue perfusion and healing responses is discussed in light of current evidence.

EFFECT OF OXYGEN AND PERFUSION IN WOUND HEALING

The critical roles of oxygen in healing are summarized in Table 28-1. Oxygen fuels the cellular functions essential to the repair process; therefore the ability to perfuse the tissues and the availability of oxygen (partial pressure of oxygen [Po_2]) to the local wound area are critical to wound healing. The processes of tissue repair that require oxygen include oxidative bacterial killing and resistance to infection, collagen synthesis and fibroplasia, angiogenesis, and epithelialization (Hartmann et al, 1992; Hopf and Rollins, 2007; Hunt et al, 2004; Hunt and Aslam, 2004; Sen, 2003).

Tissue oxygen levels are dependent on both perfusion status and oxygen content of the blood. However, because wounds remove only 1 ml of oxygen per each 100 ml of blood perfusing the tissues, compromised perfusion is more likely to jeopardize wound healing than is compromised oxygenation secondary to pulmonary conditions (Waldorf and Fewkes, 1995). Tissues that are adequately perfused are often able to heal even if the blood is poorly oxygenated or the patient is anemic. In fact, anemia usually does not significantly affect repair unless the hematocrit drops below 20% (Stotts and Wipke-Tevis, 1996). Arterial oxygen levels are not necessarily reflective of tissue oxygen delivery. Although PaO_2 of 90 mm Hg in a healthy volunteer breathing room air maintains a wound Po_2 of 50 mm Hg or greater, the postoperative patient experiencing autonomic nervous system activation or periodic desaturation will exhibit predictably low oxygen levels within the wound. This observation led to an approach of adrenergic activation as an etiology for wound hypoxia (West, 1990).

Wound Tissue Hypoxia

Wound tissue hypoxia occurs to some extent at the time of injury in everyone, regardless of their age or state of health (Silver, 1980). Incisions closed during elective surgery under the best of aseptic conditions appear to have the fewest reparative obstacles to healing. However, any tissue injury disrupts vascular and therefore oxygen supply. All wounds are relatively hypoxic at the center, in the range from 0 to 5 mm Hg (Niinikoski et al, 1972; Silver, 1969). After oxygen leaves the red blood cells in the capillaries, it diffuses into the wound space. The driving force of diffusion is partial pressure. In wounds, damage to the microvasculature, vasoconstriction, and intravascular fluid overload markedly increase intercapillary distances (Hunt and Hopf, 1997).

TABLE 28-1 Important Roles of Oxygen in Wound Healing

Event in Wound Healing	Specific Role of Oxygen
Inflammation: Bacteria control	Oxygen is substrate for enzymatic step for leukocyte production of reactive oxygen species (superoxide and other oxidants) during phagocytosis
Proliferation: Angiogenesis	Local tissue hypoxia and oxidants induce release of growth factors that stimulate angiogenesis
Proliferation: Collagen synthesis and cellular export	Oxygen with adequate vitamin C is required for enzymatic hydroxylation of procollagen to form triple helical, mature collagen structure for export from fibroblasts
	Production and release of collagen are necessary for tissue strength
Proliferation: Epithelialization	Oxygen and growth factors are needed for generation of new epithelium

Local oxygen tension influences wound healing and bacterial control in several ways. Initially injured tissue is hypoxic, a state that acts as a stimulus for repair. The one potentially beneficial effect of moderate hypoxia is enhanced stimulus to neoangiogenesis (Wilson and Clark, 2003; Zamboni et al, 2003). However, prolonged and decreased local wound oxygen (tissue hypoxia) is a major contributor to wound complications (Goodson et al, 1979; Jönsson et al, 1988; Knighton et al, 1984). A main role of oxygen during repair is that of controlling bacteria within the wound site. During repair, production of reactive oxygen species by leukocytes for phagocytosis is needed before rebuilding tissue (Hopf and Rollins, 2007; Hunt et al, 2004). Oxidant production by leukocytes requires molecular oxygen and the presence of tissue oxygen levels of 45 to 80 mm Hg up to 300 mm Hg (Allen et al, 1997). In addition to their role in controlling bacteria, reactive oxygen species serve other roles in healing, which include acting as chemical signals and mitogens for fibroblasts and other cells, inducing cellular adhesion in neutrophils and macrophages, and cellular expression of growth factors that are critical for repair (Sen, 2003). Vascular endothelial growth factor (VEG-f), known to stimulate angiogenesis, is one of the growth factors released in response to (1) hypoxia; (2) increased levels of hypoxia; (3) inducible factor; and (4) reactive oxygen species production (Goldberg and Diegelmann, 2010; Hunt and Aslam, 2004). Through these processes, reactive oxygen species act to help coordinate the tissue repair process.

FACTORS THAT ALTER PERFUSION AND OXYGENATION

Pain and Stress

Cannon (1970) revealed the mechanisms that activate the autonomic nervous system to respond to stress. He directly observed the constriction of blood vessels in peripheral tissues during stress in animals. The mediators of the sympathetic and adrenal response to stress (epinephrine and norepinephrine) induced profound vasoconstriction in subcutaneous and skin blood vessels supplying peripheral tissues (Rowell, 1986). Sympathetic activation in the postoperative period is a function of the severing of afferent nerves, hypovolemia, fear, pain, and cold rather than anesthesia (Halter et al, 1977). Catecholamine levels may remain elevated for days after surgery (Derbyshire and Smith, 1984; Halter et al, 1977), and concentrations vary with the length and severity of surgery (Chernow et al, 1987). Norepinephrine is increased threefold in the early postoperative hours (Derbyshire and Smith, 1984), peaking with the patient's first expression of pain (Niinikoski et al, 1972). Increased levels of circulating catecholamines, including epinephrine, triggered by pain and stress, lead to peripheral vasoconstriction, decreased perfusion of blood to the skin and extremities, and, consequently, reduced oxygen availability in the tissues (Franz et al, 2008; Jensen et al, 1985). Evidence of how stress and pain limit perfusion has been demonstrated by infusion of exogenous epinephrine in healthy subjects. In a study designed to mimic the body's response to stress, increasing levels of epinephrine decreased the level of subcutaneous tissue oxygen 45%, whereas heart rate and arterial Po_2 did not markedly change (Jensen et al, 1985).

Hypothermia

Adverse consequences of perioperative body heat loss are significant and include prolonged hypothermia and postanesthesia recovery, longer postoperative warming time, shivering and thermal discomfort, reduced antibody and cell-mediated responses, reduced tissue oxygen peripherally, and increased incidence of wound infections (Reynolds et al, 2008). The effects of temperature on the amount of vasomotor tone primarily determine cutaneous capillary blood flow. Cooling increases norepinephrine affinity to α-adrenergic receptors on vascular smooth muscle. This augments the response of cutaneous vessels to autonomic activation, which increases constrictive vessel tensions up to fivefold (Vanhoutte et al, 1981).

Hypothermia-induced vasoconstriction has decreased subcutaneous oxygen tension in anesthetized volunteers (FiO_2 0.6 mm Hg) to a mean of 50 mm Hg (Sheffield et al, 1992). Furthermore, a lower blood temperature shifts the oxyhemoglobin curve to the left, thereby increasing the amount of oxygen carried in the blood but decreasing the amount of oxygen released (Severinghaus, 1958). This effect may exacerbate tissue hypoxia induced by peripheral vasoconstriction.

Virtually all anesthetic agents are vasodilators and may cause a rapid initial decrease in core temperature (1°C to 2°C) during the first hour after induction of anesthesia (Sessler, 1993). Internal redistribution of body heat from core to periphery is exacerbated by conductive and evaporative losses as a result of visceral exposure in a cold environment

(Roe, 1971). Rapid initial body heat loss can be limited by heating the operating room and aggressive preoperative warming (Morris, 1971). Preinduction warming may nearly prevent rapid initial body heat loss (Hynson and Sessler, 1992).

Perioperative shivering in the elderly, although rare, is dangerous because oxygen demand may increase by 400% to 500% (Bay et al, 1968). This drastic increase in oxygen demand increases cardiac workload. Increased oxygen consumption has been shown to coincide with core decrements of 0.3°C to 1.2°C (Roe et al, 1966). Prolonged postoperative hypothermia is associated with increased mortality (Slotman et al, 1985) and myocardial ischemia (Frank et al, 1993).

Tobacco

Smoking is associated with poor wound outcomes in part through the catecholamine-mediated vasoconstrictive effects of nicotine, increases in carbon monoxide that reduce blood oxygen content, and effects on immune and proliferative cell function that reduce repair (Gottrup, 2004; Warner, 2005). Vasoconstrictive effects resulting in significant decreases in tissue oxygen tension occur after a single cigarette is smoked, and tissue oxygen requires an hour to return to baseline levels (Jensen et al, 1991). Reductions in tissue oxygen translate clinically into lower amounts of collagen production and reduced wound strength (Jorgensen et al, 1998). A recent systematic review of studies evaluating wound outcomes for smokers and nonsmokers documented increased risk for wound necrosis, healing delay, dehiscence, and complications, including infections associated with smoking (Sørensen, 2012). Based on multiple studies and reviews demonstrating an association between smoking and wound-related problems, including infection and poor wound healing, all patients with wounds should be advised to abstain from smoking.

Smoking is the single most predictive factor of wound complications in patients undergoing elective hip or knee replacement (Møller et al, 2003). Forty-seven percent of patients undergoing abdominoplasty who smoked had wound complications compared with 14.7% of those who did not smoke (Manassa et al, 2003). At least one study has shown that 2 weeks of abstinence is inadequate to limit wound-related problems, whereas a minimum of 3 to 4 weeks of abstinence has been associated with reduced incisional wound infection and improved wound healing (Kuri et al, 2005; Sørensen et al, 2003). Due to the reductions in tissue oxygen supply when a person smokes, the substantial time needed for levels to recover, and the multiple clinical studies documenting the significance of smoking as a factor that impairs healing, the Wound Healing Society recommends that patients stop smoking at least 3 to 4 weeks before elective surgery and that they not resume smoking in the postoperative period (Franz et al, 2008). Abstaining from smoking before surgery decreases surgical wound infections, but has not been shown to reduce other wound-healing problems (Sørensen, 2012).

Obesity

Wound-healing problems are more likely to occur in patients who are overweight, which is a growing national problem. More than 72 million Americans are considered obese (body mass index [BMI] ≥30), representing an obesity rate of 34% in adults older than age 20 years (Ogden et al, 2007). Individuals who are severely obese often suffer from a number of related health problems that potentially affect healing: type 2 diabetes, hypertension, coronary artery disease, sleep apnea, venous stasis disease, lower extremity ulcers, osteoarthritis, urinary incontinence, gastroesophageal reflux disease, fatty liver, cholelithiasis, and depression (Mun et al, 2001).

Obesity as a single factor is an independent predictor of surgical site infection (Harrington et al, 2004). Regardless of the surgical procedure, the incidence of postsurgical wound complications, such as infection and wound dehiscence, are higher in patients with obesity compared with those of normal weight (Franz et al, 2008). Postsurgical wound complication rates of patients with obesity have been reported to be as high as 15% to 22% (Fried et al, 1997; Israelsson and Jönsson, 1997; Myles et al, 2002; Vastine et al, 1999; Winiarsky et al, 1998).

Several studies document low oxygen levels associated with obesity. Abdominal tissue oxygen tension is reported to be negatively associated with the percentage of fat as measured by body composition dual-energy x-ray absorptiometry, with obese subjects found to have lower adipose tissue capillary density (Pasarica et al, 2009). In surgical populations, patients with BMI greater than 30 kg/m^2 who had undergone abdominal surgery had significantly lower tissue oxygen readings compared with those with BMI less than 30 kg/m^2 (Fleishmann et al, 2005; Kabon et al, 2004). Tissue oxygen levels measured in patients with obesity fell below normal, even with administration of supplemental oxygen, and were within a range associated with increased surgical site infection risk. Prolonged administration of supplemental oxygen postoperatively (80% oxygen for 12 to 18 hours) is reported to significantly increase both wound and upper arm tissue oxygen (Kabon et al, 2010).

Because of the increased vulnerability to wound complications, extra vigilance and measures to ensure peripheral perfusion must be taken with patients who are obese, including increased FiO_2 during the perioperative period, unless contraindicated by patient condition, maintenance of normothermia, and adequate fluid resuscitation. Higher oxygen concentrations may be needed in order to maximize tissue levels. In addition, larger doses of prophylactic antibiotics may be needed because of evidence indicating that decreasing serum and tissue concentrations fall below therapeutic levels as BMI increases (Anaya and Dellinger, 2006). Obesity is addressed in greater detail in Chapter 35.

INTERVENTIONS TO IMPROVE PERFUSION AND OXYGEN

Wound tissue oxygen delivery may be impaired unless conditions of diminished peripheral perfusion are anticipated and corrected. Factors most likely to adversely affect perfusion to the wound bed include hypovolemia, hypotension, factors producing vasoconstriction (e.g., cold, sympathetic stimulation), vascular disease, and edema. Correction of adrenergic vasoconstrictive stimuli, particularly cold, pain, and volume loss, elevates tissue Po_2 and leads to fewer postoperative infections (Hopf et al, 1997; Kurz et al, 1996). The degree of regional tissue perfusion regulates the supply of oxygen and therefore is the prime determinant of the competency of wound healing. Strategies for optimizing perfusion by addressing specific sympathetic nervous system activators are described in this section and listed in Table 28-2. As previously described, pain management is a critical strategy for improving perfusion and oxygenation. Techniques for pain control are described in Chapter 26.

TABLE 28-2 Interventions to Reduce Factors that Impair Perfusion and Oxygenation	
Factor	**Examples of Interventions**
Hypothermia	Provide active warming to maintain perioperative normothermia
	Provide postoperative warming and warm blankets
	Prevent heat loss and shivering
	Apply socks, slippers, sweaters, blankets
Pain	Provide analgesia and nonpharmacologic measures (e.g., repositioning, relaxation for pain control) (see Chapter 26)
Fear/stress	Provide patient teaching to reduce fear related to procedures or knowledge deficits
	Administer medications as needed to reduce anxiety and fear
Pharmacologic	If possible, avoid medications that activate the sympathetic nervous system (e.g., beta blockers)
	Avoid high-dose alpha-adrenergic agonists
Smoking	Encourage minimum of 4 weeks' abstinence before surgery until incision is healed
	Refer to tobacco cessation program and encourage successful completion
Obesity	Increase FiO_2 perioperatively unless contraindicated
	Maintain normothermia and fluid balance
	Realize larger doses of prophylactic antibiotics may be needed

Warming

Aggressive intraoperative warming and rapid postoperative warming are effective modalities for minimizing the risks of prolonged hypothermia (Hynson and Sessler, 1992). Sympathetic vasoconstriction can be overcome by warmth to provide uncomplicated healing. In a large study combining intraoperative and postoperative warming, wound infection rates were reduced by 60% (Kurz et al, 1996). Maintenance of normothermia during surgery and in the immediate recovery period is defined as sustaining a minimum core temperature of 36.5°C. In patients undergoing colorectal surgery, a temperature higher than 36°C immediately after surgery is recommended as one of the metrics for documenting optimal care for prevention of surgical infection (Bratzler and Hunt, 2006). Warming before and after surgery may also provide benefit and should be considered. Fewer wound infections (13% vs. 27%) were observed within 8 weeks of elective abdominal surgery in patients who were warmed for 2 hours before and after surgery in addition to the standard warming of all patients during the operation (Wong et al, 2007).

Local Warming. Local wound temperature modification using controlled warming improves blood flow directly to sites of injury and may benefit healing. Multiple small clinical studies examining local warming with chronic wounds (pressure, venous, diabetic, arterial) suggest benefits that include increased transcutaneous wound oxygen, less pain, and fewer infections (Puzziferri et al, 2001; Whitney and Wickline, 2003). Surgical sites with local warming have shown significantly higher tissue oxygen in the immediate recovery period and on the first postoperative day (Plattner et al, 2000) and fewer wound-related complications compared with systemic warming or no warming (Melling et al, 2001; Whitney et al, 2004). Although these studies suggest benefits of local warming, more rigorous research is needed to confirm these benefits, as well as the best methodology (i.e., temperature, duration, frequency) and method of delivery for maximizing them.

Supplemental Oxygen

A growing number of researchers have suggested that increased fraction of inspired oxygen (FiO_2) be routinely prescribed for postoperative patients during the first few days after surgery to increase oxygen delivery to the reparative site. Relatively low levels of supplemental oxygen (28%) in the first 24 to 36 postoperative hours have been shown to increase tissue oxygen tension in patients undergoing below-the-knee amputation and cervical laminectomy procedures (Butler et al, 1987; Whitney et al, 2001). This practice is especially emphasized in patients undergoing lengthy abdominal or pelvic procedures. However, it is important to recognize that correcting tissue hypoxia requires more than simply providing increased FiO_2 to increase arterial saturation (Sao_2) and arterial Po_2. Wound Po_2 may remain unchanged even while the patient is breathing additional oxygen if other important clinical factors are not also addressed. In a study of patients who underwent general surgery, approximately 30% had reduced tissue oxygen tension levels despite adequate urine output and arterial oxygen levels (Chang et al, 1983). This is a result of early postoperative compartmental fluid shifts, in which kidney perfusion is restored at the expense of peripheral vasculature vasoconstriction.

Hyperbaric oxygenation (HBO) is recommended for specific clinical conditions and wound types; however, evidence is insufficient to recommend topical oxygen at the wound surface for wound healing (Hopf et al, 2006; NPUAP, EPUAP, PPPIA, 2015; Robson et al, 2006). Topical oxygen at the wound surface and HBO are discussed in Chapter 22.

Volume Support

Jönsson et al (1987) demonstrated that low tissue oxygen levels in general surgery patients could be raised with infusion of fluids and that a fluid bolus of 250 ml of normal saline was sufficient in most cases. In well-perfused patients, tissue oxygen pressure continues to rise as PaO_2 rises. Findings of subsequent clinical studies in which supplemental fluids were provided perioperatively have produced mixed results of tissue Po_2 change and wound infection related to increasing fluids. In patients undergoing abdominal and colon surgeries, those who received aggressive fluid repletion (defined as maintenance levels of 16 to 18 ml/kg/hr during surgery and 1 hour postoperatively, or for the first 24 postsurgical hours, for an average 1.1-L increase above standard fluids) showed significantly higher wound Po_2 than did patients who received standard fluids (Arkiliç et al, 2003; Hartmann et al, 1992). Higher levels of collagen deposition were associated with the increased fluids and improved wound oxygen status (Hartmann et al, 1992). Testing of fluid supplementation in randomized clinical trials has not shown benefit in terms of reducing surgical site infection. Fewer postsurgical complications, including wound dehiscence, were reported in a randomized clinical trial of 152 cases of elective intraabdominal surgeries in patients randomized to restricted versus liberal fluid repletion protocols (Nisanevich et al, 2005). Kabon et al (2005) reported no significant differences in wound infection rates in their randomized clinical trial comparing small versus large perioperative fluid management in a trial of more than 200 elective colon surgeries. The fluid protocols in each study are not directly comparable, and neither study documented tissue oxygen levels in response to fluid, so interpretation of these differing findings is difficult. Similar lack of benefit associated with higher intraoperative fluids was also shown in a study using a surgical porcine model that measured perianastomotic and anastomotic colon tissue oxygen levels (Kimberger et al, 2007). At present, data suggest that fluid supplementation as a single intervention

is not sufficient to reduce wound infections or improve clinical healing outcomes.

Volume Support Combined with Supplemental Inspired Oxygen

Supporting the critical relationship between vascular volume and tissue oxygen, fluid repletion, along with supplemental oxygen, has been shown to effectively raise wound Po_2. This was demonstrated in a randomized trial of 500 patients, half of whom received 80% oxygen during surgery compared with 30% for the other half. All patients were aggressively hydrated during surgery at a rate of 15 ml/kg/hr and after surgery at a rate of 3.5 ml/kg/hr for the first 24 hours and 2 ml/kg/hr for the subsequent 24 hours. Patients in the higher oxygen group had significantly higher tissue oxygen levels and fewer wound infections (Greif et al, 2000). The clinical findings of the studies on hydration and supplemental oxygen support the practices of ensuring patients are well hydrated and provided oxygen to support wound healing. It is recommended that supplemental oxygen be given in the presence of good peripheral perfusion during surgery and for 24 to 48 hours postoperatively for infection control, as well as for support of collagen synthesis and healing (Chikungwa and Jönsson, 2002; Hopf and Holm, 2008).

The optimal dosage and duration of supplemental oxygen and the optimal fluid replacement rates needed to achieve healing and to prevent complications have yet to be determined. Among 300 patients undergoing colorectal surgery, fewer postoperative wound infections were documented in a trial of 80% versus 30% oxygen provided during surgery and for only 6 hours postoperatively (Belda et al, 2005). Fluids were given at a rate of 15 ml/kg/hr during surgery and then decreased to 3 ml/kg/hr during the first 6 postoperative hours. However, other studies testing 80% versus 30% oxygen given perioperatively to 165 general surgery patients and to women undergoing cesarean delivery did not confirm these findings in terms of wound infection rates (Gardella et al, 2008; Pryor et al, 2004). A number of recent metaanalyses of trials evaluating the effect of increased FiO_2 provided intraoperatively have produced conflicting results on the benefits of this intervention (Hovaguimian et al, 2013; Patel et al, 2013; Togioka et al, 2012). Some benefit was found for patients having colorectal and possibly for abdominal procedures (Hovaguimian et al, 2013; Togioka et al, 2012), whereas another metaanalysis found no benefit with higher oxygen levels during surgery (Patel et al, 2013). Method and protocol differences in the studies (e.g., patient populations, diagnosis of infection, volume of fluid replacement, antibiotic use) may explain the variation in outcomes (Kabon and Kurz, 2006). The conflicting results illustrate the need for additional studies to elucidate dosage (primarily 30% and 80% oxygen concentrations were tested in the studies), timing during the perioperative period that would be most beneficial, standardization of fluid replacement, and the patient populations that are most likely to benefit from this intervention.

Combining More than Two Interventions

Combining the interventions of fluid repletion, oxygen support and warming, and pain control seems warranted given the existing evidence. Hypovolemia is a powerful physiologic vasoconstrictor. Therefore volume replacement and oxygen therapy must coincide with postoperative warming to benefit peripheral perfusion and tissue oxygen supply. Core temperature is not a clinically useful indicator in this equation. Skin surface temperatures do correlate with fingertip blood flow; a forearm-minus-fingertip difference of 4°C defines a state of peripheral vasoconstriction. However, this method is not commonly used in practice (Rubinstein and Sessler, 1990).

The concept of combined interventions received early testing many years ago. In a prospective randomized trial that combined interventions, aggressive postoperative warming and pain control increased the wound Po_2 to 70 mm Hg within 4 to 6 hours, a level nearly equal to that found in normal volunteers (West, 1994). In addition, the actively rewarmed patients who had undergone lengthy abdominal surgeries were given a 1-L fluid bolus to replace fluids lost as urine during the diuresis, which commonly accompanies hypothermia and vasoconstriction. These same interventions have been applied to trauma patients who have demonstrated improved regional perfusion, but only after warming and adequate fluid resuscitation (Knudson et al, 1997). Patients who are warm, well perfused, and oxygenated rarely develop wound infections (Hopf and Holm, 2008; Hopf et al, 1997). In order to test future combined interventions pragmatically, there is need for clinically feasible, reliable, and valid methods to measure the effect of combined interventions on tissue oxygenation (Schreml et al, 2010).

Patient Education

The knowledgeable provider uses theory-based assessment and a coordinated therapeutic plan to optimize wound care within the context of a larger plan, including patient teaching and necessary follow-up. Patients in acute care settings require instruction on wound care, fluid replacement, avoidance of dehydration, cessation of tobacco use, and practical ways to conserve body heat. Unfortunately, this instruction frequently occurs at a time when the patient is fatigued and somewhat overwhelmed by the entire surgical experience. In this case, teaching is best done succinctly and should be reinforced by providing the patient or family member with written guidelines. Follow-up of the patient's understanding and emphasis on healthy postoperative behaviors at clinic appointments reinforce initial teaching.

Cigarette smoking and obesity are particularly deleterious to wound repair because of their effects on both perfusion and oxygenation. Studies indicate a higher incidence of wound infection, dehiscence, and delayed healing among smokers and obese individuals compared with nonsmokers and nonobese individuals. Therefore patients should be counseled regarding the negative effect of smoking and obesity on wound-healing outcomes and should be offered programs and resources as needed to address these lifestyle choices or addictions (Fleishmann et al, 2005; Kabon et al, 2004; Manassa et al, 2003; Sørensen, 2012; Sørensen et al, 2003; Stotts and Wipke-Tevis, 1996). Lifestyle modifications present challenges and may require specialized, targeted interventions that include techniques such as motivational interviewing or other methods to encourage individual willingness and commitment to adopt new behaviors.

MEASURING THE RESPONSE

Although low periwound oxygen is an initial feature of most wounds, continued and unexplained hypoxia is of particular importance. Wound healing is proportional to local oxygen tension. Transcutaneous oxygen tension is a useful, noninvasive way to assess the adequacy of tissue oxygenation near a wound or suture line in relationship to FiO_2 (Figure 28-1). Other technologies for the clinical measurement of tissue oxygen (e.g., luminescence lifetime imaging, near infrared spectroscopy) are under development or testing (Hampton and Schrieber, 2013; Schreml et al, 2010). Defining the contribution of hypoxia in the context of the recent history of the patient and time from wounding clarifies the reason for low wound Po_2. Tests can be conducted to reveal the responsiveness of the wound to factors such as local warming, vasodilating drugs, oxygen therapies, sympathetic blockade, positioning, pain, and anxiety management. For example, during an oxygen challenge (e.g., breathing increased, controlled oxygen via face mask) in the absence of vasoconstriction, significant oxygen diffusion into the capillary-perfused wound edge will occur. Simple, effective, and conservative corrective therapy then can be initiated. Because improved wound Po_2 is a real measure of wound-healing progress, serial measurements of damaged tissue can be obtained during the course of healing.

FIGURE 28-1 Recording transcutaneous oxygen tension near a lower leg wound.

CLINICAL CONSULT

A: 66-year-old Hispanic female patient presents for a preoperative clinic appointment prior to a scheduled colon surgery in 3 weeks for the treatment of colorectal cancer. Patient has reviewed the literature and video related to ostomy management. She verbalized excellent understanding and no concerns related to ostomy management. However, she declines preop marking due to anxiety over wound healing. She has heard that diabetics get infected wounds that never heal. Her history and physical includes obesity, hypertension (controlled) and type 2 diabetes (controlled, HbA1c 5%). She smokes one pack per day and has a body mass index of 33.

D: Appears to accept potential ostomy however declines marking due to anxiety about wound healing.

P: Notify surgeon of patients anxiety, provide reassurance, and teach patient strategies for minimizing risk factors for impaired wound healing.

I: (1) Review impact of smoking on wound healing. Emphasize importance of smoking cessation for 2 weeks prior to surgery. (2) Prescription for nicotine patch obtained and provided to patient. (3) Consult dietitian to continue adequate management of diabetes while receiving information on nutrition to optimize wound healing. (4) Review plans for maximizing oxygenation and perfusion to promote wound healing including oxygen supplementation, pain management, and fluid replacement.

E: Return to clinic in 1 week, plan to meet with surgeon to review wound healing plan, re-eevealuate effectiveness of smoking cessation program, assess and manage anxiety and preop stoma marking. Will also plan to follow closely post op to continue to provide reassurance and education.

SUMMARY

Wound oxygen is a clinically valid and reliable index that responds more rapidly to intravascular fluid shifts than do blood pressure and pulse. When adequate oxygen is available for wound fibroblasts, collagen formation and wound tensile strength can be achieved. Collagen maturation then continues for months after wounding. From the onset of injury, any degree of interference to oxygen delivery will proportionately compromise reparative processes and increase the susceptibility to infection (Hunt and Dunphy, 1979). Therefore supportive care for the patient with a wound must include measures to enhance perfusion. "Standard" interventions to enhance tissue perfusion include measures to prevent hypothermia and hypovolemia, reduce pain and anxiety, and eliminate edema. Approaches requiring further study include routine use of supplemental oxygen, local warming of the wound, use of epidural anesthetic blockade to increase blood flow in the microcirculation, and use of angiogenic growth factors for the management of ischemic wounds (Fakhry and Montgomery, 2012; Murry et al, 2010; Quirinia and Viidik, 1998; Veering and Cousins, 2000; Wu and Mustoe, 1995).

REFERENCES

Allen DB, Maguire JJ, Mahdavian M, et al: Wound hypoxia and acidosis limit neutrophil bacterial killing mechanisms, *Arch Surg* 132(9):991–996, 1997.

Anaya DA, Dellinger EP: The obese surgical patient: a susceptible host for infection, *Surg Infect (Larchmt)* 7(5):473–480, 2006.

Arkiliç CF, Taguchi A, Sharma N, et al: Supplemental perioperative fluid administration increases tissue oxygen pressure, *Surgery* 133(1):49–55, 2003.

Bay J, Nunn JF, Prys-Roberts C: Factors influencing arterial PO2 during recovery from anaesthesia, *Br J Anaesth* 40(6):398–407, 1968.

Belda FJ, Aguilera L, García de la Ascuncón J, et al: Supplemental perioperative oxygen and the risk of surgical wound infection: a randomized controlled trial, *JAMA* 294(16):2035–2042, 2005.

Bratzler DW, Hunt DR: The surgical infection prevention and surgical care improvement projects: national initiatives to improve outcomes for patients having surgery, *Clin Infect Dis* 43(3): 322–330, 2006.

Butler CM, Ham RO, Lafferty K, et al: The effect of adjuvant oxygen therapy on transcutaneous PO2 and healing in the below-knee amputee, *Prosthet Orthot Int* 11(1):10–16, 1987.

Cannon WB: *Bodily changes in pain, hunger, fear and rage: an account of recent researches into the function of emotional excitement,* College Park, MD, 1970, McGrath.

Chang N, Goodson WH 3rd, Gottrup F, et al: Direct measurement of wound and tissue oxygen tension in postoperative patients, *Ann Surg* 197(4):470–478, 1983.

Chernow B, Alexander HR, Smallridge RC, et al: Hormonal responses to graded surgical stress, *Arch Intern Med* 147(7): 1273–1278, 1987.

Chikungwa MT, Jönsson K: The need for perioperative supplemental oxygen, *Cent Afr J Med* 48(5–6):72–74, 2002.

Derbyshire D, Smith G: Sympathoadrenal responses to anaesthesia and surgery, *Br J Anaesth* 56:725–739, 1984.

Dubay DA, Franz MG: Acute wound healing: the biology of acute wound failure, *Surg Clin North Am* 83:463–481, 2003.

Fakhry SM, Montgomery SC: Peri-operative oxygen and the risk of surgical infection, *Surg Infect (Larchmt)* 13(4):228–233, 2012.

Fleischmann E, Kurz A, Niedermayr M, et al: Tissue oxygenation in obese and non-obese patients during laparoscopy, *Obes Surg* 15:813–819, 2005.

Frank SM, Beattie C, Christopherson R, et al: Unintentional hypothermia is associated with postoperative myocardial ischemia: the Perioperative Ischemia Randomized Anesthesia Trial Study Group, *Anesthesiology* 78:468–476, 1993.

Franz MG, Robson RC, Steed DL, et al: Guidelines to aid healing of acute wounds by decreasing impediments of healing, *Wound Repair Regen* 16(6):723–748, 2008.

Fried M, Peskova M, Kasalicky M: Bariatric surgery at the 1st surgical department in Prague: history and some technical aspects, *Obes Surg* 7:22–25, 1997.

Gardella C, Goltra LB, Laschansky E, et al: High-concentration supplemental perioperative oxygen to reduce the incidence of postcesarean surgical site infection: a randomized controlled trial, *Obstet Gynecol* 112(3):545–552, 2008.

Goldberg SR, Diegelmann RF: Wound healing primer, *Surg Clin North Am* 90:1133–1146, 2010.

Goodson WH 3rd, Andrews WS, Thakrai KK, et al: Wound oxygen tension of large vs small wounds in man, *Surg Forum* 30:92–95, 1979.

Gottrup F: Oxygen in wound healing and infection, *World J Surg* 28:312–315, 2004.

Greif R, Akça O, Horn EP, et al: Supplemental perioperative oxygen to reduce the incidence of surgical-wound infection, *N Engl J Med* 342:161–167, 2000.

Halter JB, Pflug AE, Porte D Jr: Mechanism of plasma catecholamine increases during surgical stress in man, *J Clin Endocrinol Metab* 45(5):936–944, 1977.

Hampton DA, Schriber MA: Near infrared spectroscopy: clinical and research uses, *Transfusion* 53:52S–58S, 2013.

Harrington G, Russo P, Spelman D, et al: Surgical-site infection rates and risk factor analysis in coronary artery bypass graft surgery, *Infect Control Hosp Epidemiol* 25(6):472–476, 2004.

Hartmann M, Jönsson K, Zederfeldt B: Effect of tissue perfusion and oxygenation on accumulation of collagen in healing wounds, *Eur J Surg* 158:521–526, 1992.

Hopf HW, Holm J: Hyperoxia and infection, *Best Pract Res Clin Anaesthesiol* 22(3):553–569, 2008.

Hopf HW, Hunt TK, West JM, et al: Wound tissue oxygen tension predicts the risk of wound infection in surgical patients, *Arch Surg* 132:997–1004, 1997.

Hopf HW, Rollins MD: Wounds: an overview of the role of oxygen, *Antioxid Redox Signal* 9(8):1183–1192, 2007.

Hopf HW, Ueno C, Aslam R, et al: Guidelines for the treatment of arterial insufficiency ulcers, *Wound Repair Regen* 14(6):693–710, 2006.

Hovaguimian F, Lysakowski C, Elia N, et al: Effect of intraoperative high inspired oxygen fraction on surgical site infection, postoperative nausea and vomiting, and pulmonary function: systematic review and meta-analysis of randomized controlled trials, *Anesthesiology* 119(2):303–316, 2013.

Hunt TK, Aslam RS: Oxygen 2002: wounds, *Undersea Hyperb Med* 31(1):147–153, 2004.

Hunt TK, Dunphy JE: *Fundamentals of wound management*, New York, 1979, Appleton-Century-Crofts.

Hunt TK, Ellison EC, Sen C: Oxygen: at the foundation of wound healing—introduction, *World J Surg* 28:291–293, 2004.

Hunt TK, Hopf H: Wound healing and wound infection: what surgeons and anesthesiologists can do, *Surg Clin North Am* 77:587–606, 1997.

Hynson JM, Sessler DI: Intraoperative warming therapies: a comparison of three devices, *J Clin Anesth* 4:194–199, 1992.

Israelsson LA, Jönsson T: Overweight and healing of midline incisions: the importance of suture technique, *Eur J Surg* 163:175–180, 1997.

Jensen JA, Goodson WH, Hopf HW, et al: Cigarette smoking decreases tissue oxygen, *Arch Surg* 126:1131–1134, 1991.

Jensen JA, Jönsson K, Goodson WH 3rd, et al: Epinephrine lowers subcutaneous wound oxygen tension, *Curr Surg* 42(6):472–474, 1985.

Jönsson K, Hunt TK, Mathes SJ: Oxygen as an isolated variable influences resistance to infection, *Ann Surg* 208:783–787, 1988.

Jönsson K, Jensen JA, Goodson WH 3rd, et al: Assessment of perfusion in postoperative patients using tissue oxygen measurements, *Br J Surg* 74:263–267, 1987.

Jorgensen LN, Kallehave F, Christensen E, et al: Less collagen production in smokers, *Surgery* 123:450–455, 1998.

Kabon B, Akça O, Taguchi A, et al: Supplemental intravenous crystalloid administration does not reduce the risk of surgical wound infection, *Anesth Analg* 101(5):1546–1553, 2005.

Kabon B, Kurz AL: Optimal perioperative oxygen administration, *Curr Opin Anaesthesiol* 19(1):11–18, 2006.

Kabon B, Nagele A, Reddy D, et al: Obesity decreases perioperative tissue oxygenation, *Anesthesiology* 100(2):274–280, 2004.

Kabon B, Rozum R, Marschalek C, et al: Supplemental postoperative oxygen and tissue oxygen tension in morbidly obese patients, *Obes Surg* 20:885–894, 2010.

Kimberger O, Fleischmann E, Brandt S, et al: Supplemental oxygen, but not supplemental crystalloid fluid, increases tissue oxygen tension in healthy and anastomotic colon in pigs, *Anesth Analg* 105:773–779, 2007.

Knighton DR, Halliday B, Hunt TK: Oxygen as an antibiotic: the effect of inspired oxygen on infection, *Arch Surg* 119:199–204, 1984.

Knudson MM, Bermudez KM, Doyle CA, et al: Use of tissue oxygen tension measurements during resuscitation from hemorrhagic shock, *J Trauma* 42:608–614, 1997.

Kuri M, Nakagawa M, Tanaka H, et al: Determination of the duration of preoperative smoking cessation to improve wound healing after head and neck surgery, *Anesthesiology* 102:892–896, 2005.

Kurz A, Sessler DI, Lenhardt R: Perioperative normothermia to reduce the incidence of surgical-wound infection and shorten hospitalization, *N Engl J Med* 334:1209–1215, 1996.

Manassa EH, Hertl CH, Olbrisch R: Wound healing problems in smokers and nonsmokers after 132 abdominoplasties, *Plast Reconstr Surg* 111:2082–2087, 2003.

Melling AC, Ali B, Scott EM, et al: Effects of preoperative warming on the incidence of wound infection after clean surgery: a randomized controlled trial, *Lancet* 358:876–880, 2001.

Møller AM, Pedersen T, Villebro N, et al: Effect of smoking on early complications after elective orthopaedic surgery, *J Bone Joint Surg Br* 85:178–181, 2003.

Morris RH: Influence of ambient temperature on patient temperature during intraabdominal surgery, *Ann Surg* 173:230–233, 1971.

Mun EC, Blackburn GL, Matthews JB: Current status of medical and surgical therapy for obesity, *Gastroenterology* 120:660–681, 2001.

Murry BW, Huerta S, Dineen S, et al: Surgical site infection in colorectal surgery: a review of the nonpharmacologic tools of prevention, *J Am Coll Surg* 211(6):812–822, 2010.

Myles TD, Gooch J, Santolaya J: Obesity as an independent risk factor for infections morbidity in patients who undergo cesarean delivery, *Obstet Gynecol* 100:959–964, 2002.

National Pressure Ulcer Advisory Panel (NPUAP), European Pressure Ulcer Advisory Panel (EPUAP), Pan Pacific Pressure Injury Alliance (PPPIA): *Prevention and treatment of pressure ulcers, Clinical Practice Guideline.* In Emily Haesler, editor: Perth, Australia, 2014, Cambridge Media.

Niinikoski J, Heughan C, Hunt TK: Oxygen tensions in human wounds, *J Surg Res* 12:77–82, 1972.

Nisanevich V, Felsenstein I, Almogy G, et al: Effect of intraoperative fluid management on outcome after intraabdominal surgery, *Anesthesiology* 103:25–32, 2005.

Ogden CL, Carroll MD, McDowell MA, et al: *Obesity among adults in the United States—no statistically significant change since 2003–2004 (NCHS data brief no. 1)*, Hyattsville, MD, 2007, National Center for Health Statistics.

Pasarica M, Sereda OR, Redman LM, et al: Reduced adipose tissue oxygenation in human obesity: evidence for rarefaction, macrophage chemotaxis, and inflammation without an angiogenic response, *Diabetes* 58(3):718–725, 2009.

Patel SV, Coughlin SC, Malthaner RA: High-concentration oxygen and surgical site infections in abdominal surgery: a meta-analysis, *Can J Surg* 56(4):E82–E90, 2013.

Plattner O, Akça O, Herbst F, et al: The influence of two surgical bandage systems on wound tissue oxygen tension, *Arch Surg* 135(7):818–822, 2000.

Pryor KO, Fahey TJ 3rd, Lien CA, et al: Surgical site infection and the routine use of perioperative hyperoxia in a general surgical population, *JAMA* 291:79–87, 2004.

Puzziferri N, West JM, Hunt TK, et al: Local warming increases oxygenation and decreases pain in ischemic ulcers, *Wound Repair Regen* 9(2):146–147, 2001.

Quirinia A, Viidik A: The effect of recombinant basic fibroblast growth factor (bFGF) in fibrin adhesive vehicle on the healing of ischaemic and normal incisional skin wounds, *Scand J Plast Reconstr Surg Hand Surg* 32:9–18, 1998.

Reynolds L, Beckmann J, Kurz A: Perioperative complications of hypothermia, *Best Pract Res Clin Anaesthesiol* 22:645–657, 2008.

Robson MC, Cooper DM, Aslam R, et al: Guidelines for the treatment of venous ulcers, *Wound Repair Regen* 14(6):649–662, 2006.

Roe CF: Effect of bowel exposure on body temperature during surgical operations, *Am J Surg* 122:13–15, 1971.

Roe CF, Goldberg MJ, Blair CS, et al: The influence of body temperature on early postoperative oxygen consumption, *Surgery* 60:85, 1966.

Rowell LB: *Human circulation: regulation during physical stress*, New York, 1986, Oxford University Press.

Rubinstein EH, Sessler DI: Skin-surface temperature gradients correlate with fingertip blood flow in humans, *Anesthesiology* 73:541–545, 1990.

Schreml S, Szeimies RM, Prantl L, et al: Oxygen in acute and chronic wound healing, *Br J Dermatol* 163:257–268, 2010.

Sen CK: The general case for redox control of wound repair, *Wound Repair Regen* 11:431–438, 2003.

Sessler DI: Perianesthetic thermoregulation and heat balance in humans, *FASEB J* 7(8):638–644, 1993.

Severinghaus J: Oxyhaemoglobin dissociation curve correction for temperature and pH variation in human blood, *J Appl Physiol* 12:485–486, 1958.

Sheffield CW, Hopf HW, Sessler DI, et al: Thermoregulatory vasoconstriction decreases subcutaneous oxygen tension in anesthetized volunteers, *Anesthesiology* 77:A96, 1992.

Silver IA: The measurement of oxygen tension in healing tissue, *Prog Resp Res* 3:124, 1969.

Silver IA: The physiology of wound healing. In Hunt T, editor: *Wound healing and wound infection: theory and surgical practice*, New York, 1980, Appleton-Century-Crofts.

Slotman GJ, Jed EH, Burchard KW: Adverse effects of hypothermia in postoperative patients, *Am J Surg* 49:495–501, 1985.

Sørensen LT: Wound healing and infection in surgery, *Arch Surg* 147:373–383, 2012.

Sørensen LT, Karlsmark T, Gottrup F: Abstinence from smoking reduces incisional wound infection: a randomized controlled trial, *Ann Surg* 238:1–5, 2003.

Stotts NA, Wipke-Tevis D: Co-factors in impaired wound healing, *Ostomy Wound Manage* 42(2):44–46, 48:50–54, 1996.

Togioka B, Galvagno S, Sumida S, et al: The role of perioperative high inspired oxygen therapy in reducing surgical site infection: a meta-analysis, *Anesth Analg* 114:334–342, 2012.

Vanhoutte PM, Verbeuren TJ, Webb RC: Local modulation of adrenergic neuroeffector interaction in the blood vessel well, *Physiol Rev* 61:151–247, 1981.

Vastine VL, Morgan RF, Williams GS, et al: Wound complications of abdominoplasty in obese patients, *Ann Plast Surg* 42:34–39, 1999.

Veering BT, Cousins MJ: Cardiovascular and pulmonary effects of epidural anaesthesia, *Anaesth Intensive Care* 28:620–635, 2000.

Waldorf H, Fewkes J: Wound healing, *Adv Dermatol* 10:77–96, 1995.

Warner DO: Preoperative smoking cessation. How long is long enough? *Anesthesiology* 102:883–884, 2005.

West JM: Wound healing in the surgical patient: influence of the perioperative stress response on perfusion, *AACN Clin Issues Crit Care Nurs* 1(3):595–601, 1990.

West JM: *The effect of postoperative forced-air rewarming on subcutaneous tissue oxygen tension and wound healing in hypothermic abdominal surgery patients*, San Francisco, 1994, University of California, San Francisco.

Whitney JD, Dellinger EP, Wickline M: Warming surgical wounds: effects on healing and wound complications, *Wound Repair Regen* 12:A8, 2004.

Whitney JD, Heiner S, Mygrant BI, et al: Tissue and wound healing effects of short duration postoperative oxygen therapy, *Biol Res Nurs* 2:206–215, 2001.

Whitney JD, Wickline MM: Treating chronic and acute wounds with warming: review of the science and practice implications, *J Wound Ostomy Continence Nurs* 30(4):199–209, 2003.

Wilson JA, Clark JJ: Obesity: impediment to wound healing, *Crit Care Nurs Q* 26(2):119–132, 2003.

Winiarsky R, Barth P, Lotke P: Total knee arthroplasty in morbidly obese patients, *J Bone Joint Surg Am* 80:1770–1774, 1998.

Wong PF, Kumar S, Bohra A, et al: Randomized clinical trial of perioperative systemic warming in major elective abdominal surgery, *Br J Surg* 94:421–426, 2007.

Wu L, Mustoe TA: Effect of ischemia on growth factor enhancement of incisional wound healing, *Surgery* 117:570–576, 1995.

Zamboni WA, Browder LK, Martinez J: Hyperbaric oxygen and wound healing, *Clin Plast Surg* 30:67–75, 2003.

29

Eliminating Noncompliance

Denise P. Nix, Ben Peirce, and Vicki Haugen

OBJECTIVES

1. Identify goals to achieve a sustainable plan of care for skin safety and/or wound management.
2. Describe health change models that affect goal setting and plan of care.
3. Provide examples of unmet patient needs that may be mistaken for patient noncompliance.
4. Summarize The Joint Commission standards related to patient education.
5. Identify strategies to improve education materials and methods.

Historically, the term *noncompliant* has been used to describe the patient who, for whatever reason, does not adopt interventions included in the plan of care. Nurses' descriptions of behaviors from noncompliant patients have ranged from passive resistance and lack of motivation to overt refusal and deliberate interference with care (Hallett et al, 2000). However, patients who have been labeled noncompliant report a lack of understanding of why or what they were supposed to do or an inability to perform prescribed interventions (Edwards et al, 2002).

This gap in perception leads to obvious questions about the noncompliance label, which has been described as an arrogant term suggesting that the patient's job is to do what he or she is told to do by the health care provider (Rappl, 2004; van Rijswijk, 2004). The term *adherence* has been used as an alternative to compliance. It comes closer to describing and emphasizing patient and clinician collaboration in decisions, rather than conveying the idea of obedience (Seley, 2009). Unfortunately many authors have used the term *adherence* interchangeably with *compliance*, so any improvement of meaning has been lost. *Concordance* is a term and model introduced in the United Kingdom that is intended to encompass the idea that the clinician and the patient are equals, there should be an open exchange of beliefs, and that the patient makes informed decisions. The key difference between compliance and concordance is that the former generally focuses on the behavior of one person, the patient, whereas the latter requires the participation of at least two people (Chatterjee, 2006). Regardless of terminology, however, misperceptions remain. The wound specialist's role is to critique the plan of care rather than the patient. This chapter presents important factors to address in order to formulate a sustainable wound management plan designed to achieve mutually agreed upon goals.

SIGNIFICANCE

In the United States more than half of Medicare beneficiaries have five or more chronic conditions reducing quality of life and affecting health care costs. Persons with four or more chronic conditions are 99 times more likely to be hospitalized for care needs that could have been prevented with appropriate primary care (PFCD, 2014). Persons with multiple chronic conditions are more likely to see multiple clinicians and receive care that is fragmented and ineffective. In 2013 U.S. health care spending increased 3.6% to $2.9 trillion, or $9255 per person (CMS, 2014).

Community nurses spend approximately 50% of their time treating leg ulcers (Simon et al, 2004)—the most common wound problem seen in clinical practice. This condition affects approximately 1% to 2% of the population over age 65 years in the United States, United Kingdom, Europe, and Australia (Briggs and Closs, 2003; Finlayson et al, 2009; Takahashi, 2010). In the United States, it is estimated that venous ulcers lead to costs of $2.5 billion and 2 million workdays lost annually (Collins and Seraj, 2010; Morton, 2013). The cornerstone of treatment for venous insufficiency is compression, yet despite provider recommendations, "noncompliance and nonadherence" with use of compression is widely reported (Finlayson et al, 2010; Heinen et al, 2007; Labropoulos et al, 2012; Raju et al, 2007; Weller et al, 2013).

Similar reports of noncompliance and nonadherence are associated with other types of wounds. The Wound, Ostomy and Continence Nurses Society™ (WOCN®) (2010) estimated that $2.2 to $3.6 billion was spent annually for the care of pressure ulcers and cited noncompliance as one of the causes of the 13% to 56% recurrence rate. The Wound Healing Society (Steed et al, 2006) report a 59% recurrence rate of diabetic foot ulcers, and many authors and researchers describe noncompliance and nonadherence with offloading and footwear considered critical to prevent recurrence (Armstrong et al, 2005; Wu et al, 2008).

GOAL SETTING

Goals are set and prioritized into short- and long-term goals. Short-term goals focus on the most pressing issues, such as pain control, infection prevention, and dressing changes. Long-term goals focus on disease management and fostering independence. Discharge goals vary by practice setting. Crucial decisions, such as the patient being able to return to home and live alone, depend on what the patient learns and retains. The minimum performance necessary for the patient to function must be identified, and progress toward this level must be communicated.

Patient, Caregiver, and Clinician as Partners

Outcomes improve when patients are involved in setting goals that affect their lives (Brown, 2014). Patients who can believe in, engage in, cope with, and actively participate in setting goals are more likely to adapt the plan of care (Brown, 2014). Therefore in order to facilitate a sustainable plan of care, health care professionals need a paradigm shift from a directive, paternalistic style to a more collaborative interactive style in which problems, treatment goals, and management strategies are defined together (Chatterjee, 2006; Heisler et al, 2002).

The Family Caregiver Alliance of the National Center on Care Giving data from 2012 state that 52 million people (29% of the population) care for someone who is disabled or ill (FCA, 2015). Hence to achieve a sustainable plan of care, education and goal setting must include families and caregivers. The wound specialist can help the patient and family identify their goals based on what the patient and family are able and willing to do to achieve them. This can be accomplished only if decisions are based on full disclosure and an understanding of relevant information.

Realistic and Evidence Based

The patient and care team together must monitor progress toward the goals of the plan of care to determine whether they are patient centered and realistic, identify actual or potential barriers toward achieving a sustainable plan, and modify the plan accordingly. Ideally, this process should occur while the initial plan of care is being developed so that realistic goals can be set from the onset. Identification and consideration of patient preferences and actions are central to evidence-based decision making (DiCenso et al, 2005). When planned interventions are not completed and goals are not met, the best question is not, "What's wrong with the patient?" Rather, we should be asking, "What's wrong with the plan?" or "Are our goals realistic?"

The goal of wound healing as a standard for all patients is unrealistic and often is inappropriate (Whitney et al, 2006). For example, a patient who is malnourished and does not care to receive enteral or elemental feedings will not achieve the goal of wound healing. Once the patient understands that wound healing is unrealistic, he or she may decide to reconsider supplemental feedings or may aim for a goal that keeps him or her at home, avoids hospital admission, controls symptoms (e.g., odor, exudate), and enhances quality of life as defined by the patient. In other cases, the treatment may produce added discomfort or risk for the patient (Whitney et al, 2006). A patient with an overwhelming disease process, after being informed of all treatment options, may decide to decline supplemental nutrition and set a palliation goal of prevention of pain and wound extension rather than wound healing.

Wound-healing potential must be based on the most current evidence and communicated in such a way that the patient and family understand (e.g., a patient with peripheral vascular disease with an ankle-brachial index <0.5 requires revascularization for healing to occur; venous insufficiency requires compression for wound healing to occur; pressure ulcer healing is not realistic without pressure relief, nutrition support, and management of urinary or fecal incontinence). When healing is no longer realistic, the plan of care should be revised to focus on goals that minimize infection and other complications and that support the patient's comfort and his or her need and desire for socialization.

In order to integrate interventions needed for optimal healing, the patient must face multiple adaptations to accommodate the wound and the underlying disease. To understand the range of adaptations facing the patient, the wound specialist must understand the effect of the wound and interventions on the patient's life. Patient beliefs and perceptions must be revealed in order to dispel any myths or misperceptions and identify teaching/learning needs.

PATIENT PERCEPTIONS AND THE HEALTH BELIEF MODEL

The Health Belief Model (HBM) provides an appropriate framework to guide shared goal setting and development of a sustainable plan of care. Developed nearly a half-century ago by Irwin Rosenstock of the U.S. Public Health Service, the HBM was applied to predict behavioral response to treatment of acutely or chronically ill patients (Rosenstock, 1996). In the decades that followed, the HBM's effectiveness in predicting and explaining health-related actions has been well documented in metaanalyses (Carpenter, 2010; Jones et al, 2014). Core constructs associated with the likelihood of adapting an intervention are listed in Table 29-1 and described in the following sections.

Perceived Threat (Perceived Severity and Susceptibility)

The combination of perceived severity and perceived susceptibility is referred to as *perceived threat*. Perceived severity and susceptibility depend on knowledge about the

TABLE 29-1	Concepts and Application of the Health Belief Model
Perceived susceptibility *Belief about the risk of developing a wound or experiencing negative consequences of a wound (e.g., lost work/income, pain, infection, death)*	• Define population(s) at risk, risk levels • Personalize individualized risk factors • Work toward making perceived susceptibility more consistent with individual's *actual* risk
Perceived severity *Belief about how serious a wound can be*	• Specify consequences of having a wound (e.g., lost work/income, pain, infection, death)
Perceived benefits *Belief in efficacy of interventions to prevent or promote healing of the wound*	• Define each intervention (how, where, when) • Clarify the positive effects to be expected of each
Perceived barriers *Belief about the tangible and psychological costs of the intervention to prevent or promote healing of the wound*	• See Table 29-2
Cues to action	• Help patient identify internal cues to act (erythema, edema, pain, etc.) • Provide information/education • Use reminder systems
Self-efficacy *Confidence in one's ability to adapt/perform intervention*	• Provide training, guidance, and demonstration • Utilize support groups and other venues where vicarious learning from peers can occur • Conduct demonstration returns or "teach backs" • Give verbal reinforcement and encouragement • Help the patient understand that physical symptoms such as change in skin appearance or integrity are not failure, but rather a signal to be more persistent or to revise the plan

condition. The HBM predicts that higher perceived threat leads to higher likelihood of engagement in health-promoting interventions.

Perceived severity encompasses beliefs about the health problem itself, as well as broader effects of the disease on functioning in work and social roles (e.g., whether it is life threatening, life altering, or painful). For example, a patient may perceive that a venous wound is not medically serious. However, learning that venous ulcers lead to an estimated 2 million lost workdays in the United States annually (Collins and Seraj, 2010; Morton, 2013) may help the patient see the wound as serious or severe due to the potential financial consequences.

The HBM predicts that patients who perceive themselves at high risk for a particular health problem such as a wound are more likely to engage in activities that will decrease their risk. Patients with low perceived susceptibility may be in denial, whereas others may acknowledge the possibility but believe it is unlikely to happen to them. This potential range of perceptions underscores the importance of conducting frequent risk assessments together with the patient and family. A discussion with emphasis on each individual risk factor as it applies to the individual patient may help the patient see his or her own vulnerability and need to take action.

Perceived Benefits

Perceived benefits refer to the patient's assessment of the value or effectiveness of various interventions. If the patient believes that a particular action will reduce susceptibility to a health problem or decrease its seriousness, he or she is more likely to embrace the intervention. For example, studies have

shown that patients are significantly more likely to wear compression stockings if they believe the stockings are worthwhile and will prevent wounds (Jull et al, 2004; Van Hecke et al, 2011).

Perceived Barriers

Even if an individual perceives a wound as threatening and believes that a particular action will prevent or eliminate the wound, barriers may prevent implementation. Perceived benefits must outweigh the perceived barriers in order for a change to occur. Barriers to taking action include inconvenience, expense, danger, and discomfort (e.g., pain, emotional upset). For instance, lack of transportation to clinic appointments and significant pain with wound debridement may act as barriers to receiving wound management follow-up. Studies cite cost, appearance, discomfort, and difficulty with application among the reasons for not following recommendations for compression and offloading devices (Armstrong et al, 2004; Coutts and Parslow, 2006; Fierheller et al, 2009). Possible interventions to prevent or minimize various barriers are listed in Table 29-2.

Self-Efficacy

Perceived self-efficacy is an individual's confidence in his or her ability to tackle difficult or novel tasks and to cope with adversity. The patient with high self-efficacy will choose more challenging tasks, and when setbacks occur, he or she will work harder, recover more quickly, and remain committed to his or her goals. Conversely, the patient with low self-efficacy will have a tendency to give up if failure occurs. Self-efficacy is built

TABLE 29-2   Interventions to Prevent or Minimize Barriers to a Sustainable Wound Management Plan

Barrier	Intervention
Inappropriate goals	Collaborate with patient to help him or her articulate goals; make sure goals are mutual
	Set goals based on best evidence
	Ensure goals are clearly written and understood
	Explain interventions needed to accomplish goals before patient commits to the goal
	Provide guidance by breaking goals into intermediate steps with a high likelihood of accomplishment to ensure early success
	Adjust goals as needed for changes in assessment parameters
Depression, pain, anxiety	Be aware that many patients with depression will not ask for help
	Appropriate pain assessment and management (see Chapters 25 and 26)
	Address aspects of wound management that trigger or exacerbate depression, pain, or anxiety
	Collaborate with social services and physician for appropriate referrals
Cognitive impairment, complicated regimens, impaired dexterity	Simplify procedures
	Divide procedures into easier intermediate steps
	Choose dressings that require fewer changes
	Choose products that are easy to use
	Use combination products to minimize steps
	Encourage use of memory aids and assistive devices when indicated
	Clearly label supplies
	Dispense appropriate number of supplies
	Collaborate with occupational therapy
Impaired activity and mobility	Prescribe compression that is compatible with appropriate shoe wear
	Prescribe offloading devices compatible with wheelchair and home environment
	Adapt clinical environment to accommodate patients with mobility impairment (low examination tables, closer parking)
	Be aware of wound management recommendations that may hinder mobility
	Prescribe sitting program compatible with employment and parenting needs
	Facilitate home care when appropriate
Financial barriers, lack of social/ environmental resources	Collaborate with social services
	Identify payer and reimbursement sources
	Learn prices of products and less expensive alternatives
	Learn about resources and available funds available to patients with low income
	Financial guidance for prioritizing
Skepticism	Address concerns immediately
	Be honest about risk versus benefits of recommended interventions
	Respect and incorporate life experiences
	Do not minimize concerns
	Recommend a second opinion
	Provide alternative interventions (and goals as needed)
Knowledge deficit	Develop education plan that matches developmental phase, cognitive and physical abilities, and educational and cultural background (see Boxes 29-1 and 29-2)
	Use multiple methods of educational methods and tools (see Table 29-3)

through (1) verbal encouragement; (2) vicarious learning; (3) perceiving physiologic and affective responses; and (4) performance accomplishment, which is the most powerful of the four sources of self-efficacy. The wound specialist can be a source of self-efficacy through verbal encouragement (Brown, 2014).

Cues to Action

According to the HBM, a cue, or trigger, is necessary for prompting health improvement actions (Glanz et al, 2008). Cues to action can be internal (e.g., pain or wound) or external (e.g., service announcements or educational materials). The intensity of the cues needed to prompt action varies between individuals by perceived susceptibility, seriousness, benefits, and barriers. For example, the patient who believes he or she is at high risk for peripheral vascular disease (PVD) and has an established relationship with a primary care doctor may be easily persuaded to get screened for PVD, whereas the patient who believes he or she is at low risk for PVD and does not have reliable access to health care may require a more intense cue, such as leg pain, in order to get screened.

Modifying Variables

The HBM suggests that modifying variables affect health-related actions indirectly by affecting perceived seriousness, susceptibility, benefits, and barriers (Glanz et al, 2008). Examples of these variables include but are not limited to demographic (e.g., education, culture, economic), psychosocial (e.g., anxiety, depression, social isolation), physical (e.g., cognitive, mobility, dexterity), and structural (e.g., knowledge, experience). Not surprisingly, a number of these variables overlap with the domains of health-related quality of life in older adults (NPUAP, EPUAP, PPPIA, 2014). The following sections provide a discussion related to common modifying variables associated with patients with wounds and factors to consider in order to set appropriate goals, prescribe appropriate intervention, and achieve a sustainable plan of care.

Education and Knowledge. Full disclosure and understanding of relevant information is critical to goal setting and the decision-making process, yet lack of knowledge is one of the most common barriers associated with a failed plan of care. Box 29-1 summarizes The Joint Commission standards for patient education (Canobbio, 2006). Unfortunately, it is estimated that 50% of medical information is lost immediately after a patient speaks with a health professional (So et al, 2003). Therefore education assessment and techniques must take into consideration all the factors that may influence the patient's ability, motivation, and readiness to learn (Checklist 29-1). The educational assessment and plan may require a team approach as described in Chapter 1. For example, speech therapy and occupational therapy can provide vital assessment input for communication, language, and physical and cognitive limitations, as well as techniques to incorporate for successful teaching and learning. The education plan must be age appropriate, taking into account principles of adult learning (Knowles et al, 1998) (Box 29-2) and features of development that affect coping and learning strategies for children as described in Chapter 36. Moreover, structured, culturally appropriate, and patient-specific teachings are found to be better than ad hoc teaching or generalized teaching (Friedman et al, 2011).

Providing ample time for patient teaching has always been a challenge. With shorter hospital stays, the wound specialist

---

BOX 29-1   Summary of The Joint Commission Statements for Patient Education Standards

- Provide patient and family/significant other with information that will enhance their knowledge and skills necessary to promote recovery and improve function.
- Encourage patient participation in decision making, and include family in the teaching process.
- Assess the patient's learning needs, abilities, preferences, and readiness to learn.
- Consider cultural and religious practices, emotional barriers, desire and motivation to learn, physical and cognitive limitations, language barriers, and financial implications of care choices.
- Educate patients about safe and effective use of medications according to the law and their needs.
- Educate patients about safe and effective use of equipment and supplies.
- Educate patients about potential drug–food interactions and provide counseling on nutrition and modified diets.
- Inform patients about access to additional resources in the community.
- Inform patient about when and how to obtain further treatment the patient may need.
- Provide discharge instructions to patient and those responsible for providing continuing care.
- Educate patient regarding self-care activities as appropriate.

From Canobbio MM: *Mosby's handbook of patient teaching*, ed 3, St. Louis, MO, 2006, Mosby.

CHECKLIST 29-1   Educational Assessment

✓ Age and developmental phase
✓ Cognitive abilities
✓ Physical abilities (activity, mobility, dexterity)
✓ Educational background
✓ Life experiences that may influence learning
✓ Cultural and religious practices
✓ Language skills
✓ Occupation
✓ Finances and financial implications of care choices
✓ Type of health care coverage and discharge plan
✓ Support from family and friends
✓ Pain, anxiety, and depression
✓ Learning needs and readiness to learn

BOX 29-2   Principles of Adult Learning

1. Adults want to know why they should learn.
   - Adults are motivated to put time and energy into learning if they know the benefits of learning and the costs of not learning.
2. Adults need to take responsibility.
   - Adult learners perceive themselves as being in charge of their lives and decisions and need to be seen as capable.
3. Adults bring experience to learning.
   - Adults define themselves by their experiences and need to have their experiences valued and respected. Experiences can give deeper meaning to new ideas and skills or may lead to bias.
4. Adults are ready to learn when the need arises.
   - Adults learn when they choose to learn, usually when they perceive a need to learn.
5. Adults are task oriented.
   - Education often is subject centered, and adults need education that is task centered.

Data from Knowles MS, Holton EF III, Swanson RA: *The adult learner*, Houston, TX, 1998, Gulf Publishing.

must take even more care to develop a variety of strategies to ensure the patient's educational needs are identified and that progress toward meeting these needs is communicated to providers in the next care setting. In acute care, the education plan begins at admission and must be incorporated into routine care during frequent daily encounters (Canobbio, 2006). For example, skin inspection can be taught during the patient's bath. Protection of skin surrounding wounds and moist wound healing can be discussed during dressing changes. Each time a patient is repositioned, pressure ulcer prevention strategies can be taught and reinforced. Information may need to be limited to the skills and actions necessary for the patient to learn before discharge.

Complicated regimens present considerable room for error and confusion, especially in the presence of impaired cognition, mobility, or dexterity. Simple procedures and combination products may increase the likelihood of a desired action to take place (Warshaw et al, 2002). Interventions must be described in as few steps as possible. Breaking down steps into smaller segments and having the patient repeat back the steps will lessen the larger task (Price, 2008). Dispensing appropriate amounts of supplies and clearly labeling them simplifies the procedure for the patient. Combining interventions with routines already established (e.g., meal times) will increase the likelihood of success.

Research suggests that combining educational methods leads to better outcomes (Friedman et al, 2011; Redman, 2007). A prospective, randomized study of 28 patients with burn injury compared instructional methods with adherence to dressing changes and hypertrophic scar formation. The standard group received a written handout and verbal rationale for their dressing changes, whereas the enhanced group received a written handout, verbal rationale, and a video presentation. Results revealed that the enhanced group had a statistically significant ($p < .001$) improvement with dressing change consistency and less hypertrophic scar formation (So et al, 2003).

A systematic review conducted by Friedman and colleagues (2011) examined teaching strategies and methods of delivery for patient education. Teaching strategies identified were traditional lectures, discussions, simulated games, computer technology, written material, audiovisual sources, verbal recall, demonstration, and role playing. Results revealed five teaching strategies that increased knowledge, decreased anxiety, and increased patient satisfaction compared with the others: computer technology, audio and videotapes, written materials, demonstrations, and combinations.

Patients can quickly access a plethora of information on the Internet; however, much of the information is inaccurate or incomplete (NPUAP, EPUAP, PPPIA, 2014). Online communities of patients with the same medical condition have emerged and are increasingly being used by consumers as trusted sources of information (Nielson, 2009). However, some Internet sources, if followed, can sabotage the plan of care. Criteria can be applied to assess the credibility of information on the Internet (see Table 1-7). Websites and

e-learnings designed by health professionals and maintained by government and health consumer groups are more likely to contain reputable information (Brace and Schubart, 2010; NPUAP, EPUAP, PPPIA, 2014; Schubart, 2012). The wound specialist should respectfully discuss this information with the patient. Becoming defensive or dismissing the patient's concerns will leave the patient feeling alienated. Such interactions can damage the trust between patient and clinician. The patient should have his or her concerns addressed and should be encouraged to obtain a second opinion, if desired.

Printed materials are an economical use of time if they are well designed and match the learner's reading and literacy levels. Educational methods must be sensitive to the culture of patients who will be using them, addressing their lifestyles and using cultural language and symbols they understand (Redman, 2007). Additionally, tools like the "Teach Back" method have been employed successfully by clinicians when teaching patients with low health literacy (Kripalani and Weiss, 2006). Approximately half of the population in the United States struggles with basic reading skills. For many persons, the materials available are written at a higher level than they can understand—sometimes as many as five grades higher than the school level the patient has completed (Redman, 2007). Techniques that improve readership, comprehension, and memory of printed materials are summarized in Table 29-3 (Buxton, 1999).

Depression, Anxiety, and Pain. A systematic review of the effect of wounds and quality of life underscored the number of problems, such as pain, sleeplessness, social isolation, loneliness, and job loss, that can lead to anxiety and depression (Herber et al, 2007). The National Institute of Mental Health estimates that 14.8 million adults in the United States suffer from depression. This constitutes 6.7% of the population at any given time. Up to 80% of patients with depression are untreated or undiagnosed. Many patients with depression will not ask for help, have difficulty performing activities of daily living, and may be unable to follow through with agreed-upon interventions (Kessler et al, 2005). A quality-of-life survey conducted by Hyland et al (1994) reported that patients spent an average of 1.5 to 2 hours thinking about their wounds. Whether a patient experiences depression before developing a wound or becomes depressed because of the profound challenges the wound presents, the patient's perception related to quality of life should be assessed.

Anxiety and depression affect the ability to objectively assess one's own actions. The patient with anxiety and depression may interpret his or her successes negatively, underestimate his or her achievements, or simply ignore them completely. Verbal encouragement and validation are especially important in these cases to help the patient accurately interpret the experience as successful (Brown, 2014).

It has been reported that over 70% of patients experience pain associated with their wounds. Wound pain and intensity are highly variable. It is not an accurate predicator to make

TABLE 29-3 **Techniques to Improve Health Education Materials**	
Do	**Don't**
Direct Readers to the Message • Use arrows, underlines, bold type, boxes, white space, and bullets to direct readers' eyes to the key messages.	• Use italics, all capital letters, or screens of color over text. • Require reader to look in many directions on the page to read copy and find the message.
Select an Easy-to-Read Typeface • Use 10- to 14-point type size. • Use a typeface with serifs in the body copy (e.g., Times Roman).	• Go below 10-point type size for good readers and 12-point for poor readers. • Mix typefaces or use more than three sizes of print on one page. • Use white letters on black background.
Create Easy-to-Read Copy • Use columns that are 40 to 50 characters wide, left justified. • Use lots of white space. Consider question-and-answer or bullets rather than paragraphs. • Use highly contrasting colors for text and background, such as black on white or cream. • Use the same dark color for headings and body copy or colors with similar intensity.	• Break margins with illustrations or other graphics. If required, break only the right margin. • Use light or unusual ink colors, such as red, green, or orange.
Create Clear Visuals • Convey one key message per visual. Print the message in a caption. • Make the message easy to grasp at a glance. • Show only the "desired" way to act. • Use realistic drawings, photos, or humanlike figures. • Use visuals with which the audience can identify.	• Add any visuals simply to decorate the material. • Include any details or background in the visual that are not required to communicate the message. • Use highly stylized or abstract graphics. • Portray blood cells and other body parts as cartoon characters.

Adapted from Buxton T: Effective ways to improve health education materials, *J Health Educ* 30(1):47–50, 1999. From Redman BK: *The practice of patient education*, ed 10, St. Louis, MO, 2006, Mosby.

clinical assumptions that specific wound types or wound size will define the type of pain the patient is experiencing (Frescos, 2011). Ineffective wound pain management can result in delayed healing and an inability to follow recommended interventions (Briggs and Closs, 2006; Frescos, 2011; Van Hecke et al, 2009). The wound specialist can adjust the wound dressing protocol and the frequency of dressing change in order to diminish pain factors. Offering pain medication before the dressing change addresses both the pain directly and the patient's apprehension about the dressing change. Chapters 25 and 26 provide detailed information related to the assessment and management of wound pain.

Cognitive Ability. Cognitive impairment may be an obvious barrier toward achieving a sustainable treatment plan; however, the presence of cognitive impairment can be subtle. It is important to review past medical records and speak with family members so that cognitive deficits can be identified and the plan of care adjusted accordingly. In many settings, occupational therapy and speech therapy can assist in identifying cognitive deficits and can assist the wound specialist in developing a plan of care that incorporates the unique learning needs of the patient. Patients tend to remember the first

thing they are told. Key factors to enhance learning and retention are to use straightforward language and simple sentences. It is also important to explain why the treatment is needed, simplify the steps in the procedure, use repetition, and ask the patient to repeat back the instructions (Price, 2008).

Dexterity. The wound specialist must have the expertise and resources available to design a plan of care that accommodates the individual with impaired dexterity. For example, many combination dressings and products eliminate the need for cutting tape. The need for long-term use of lower extremity compression stockings requires the patient's ability to apply them. Assisting them or acquiring assistive devices will facilitate routine usage (Brown, 2014). For example, donning household rubber gloves can aid in pulling up compression stockings. Practice and return demonstrations are critical for the patient with impaired dexterity. Impaired dexterity can significantly affect procedure time; selecting dressings that require fewer changes may be more realistic and sustainable.

Activity and Mobility. Impaired activity and mobility affect the patient's ability to accomplish many important activities

---

needed for disease management and wound healing. Unfortunately, these challenges are not always understood by the health care system and lead to inaccurate assumptions about noncompliance (Box 29-3). The extent to which impaired activity and mobility affect a patient's life must be explored thoroughly before realistic goals and interventions can be put in place. For example, the wound specialist must be aware of the many interventions (e.g., sitting restrictions) and devices (e.g., bulky compression and high-profile support surfaces) that actually can create an activity or mobility deficit for the patient (Armstrong et al, 2001, 2003; Furlong, 2001; Phillips, 2001; Rappl, 2004; Wipke-Tevis and Sae-Sia, 2004). Patients have reported losing their jobs or retiring early because of immobility secondary to a wound or treatment for a wound (Ashford et al, 2000; Brod, 1998; Herber et al, 2007; Phillips et al, 1994). Mobility issues can be addressed as a wound team, enlisting physical and occupational therapies early in the plan of care to ensure comprehensive assessment and problem solving for mobility issues. It is unreasonable to expect a patient who is homebound and wheelchair dependent to "comply" with the use of a new support surface if transfer methods from bed to chair and chair to bed were not observed and discussed before selection of the new product.

Finances and Available Resources. The financial impact of a wound on a patient and family ranges from lack of productivity to early retirement and job loss. For persons who are elderly, are chronically ill, or are in a low-income bracket, as much as 31% of their total income may be spent on health care. Patients cut corners with health care in order to afford rent or food (Lantz, 2003). Financial barriers are frequently cited as a reason for failing to fill or pick up medication prescriptions (Durso, 2001). Treatment decisions should be made, bearing in mind what is financially reasonable for the patient, as well as the less expensive alternatives. It is important to be aware of the payer source and the patient's out-of-pocket expenses for noncovered items, transportation, and loss of pay due to time missed from work. Cost is incurred from both the treatment and nontreatment of wounds—the cost of not implementing evidence-based management of wounds is likely to increase from associated complications such as infection, increased hospital admissions, higher expenditure on pharmaceuticals (analgesia, antibiotics), and surgical procedures (AWMA and NZWCS, 2011).

The wound specialist needs to understand the logistics of obtaining equipment and other resources to ensure proper patient care. This is especially important between care settings so that the patient is discharged only after the appropriate equipment and supplies are ready at the next care setting. Resources may not be available due to a lack of funds or support from friends and family for of a variety of reasons (e.g., distance or family dynamics). Although finances are a powerful risk factor, they can be a powerful motivator as well. For example, a family member or patient who is not ready to learn how to do a dressing change may become motivated when he or she learns there will be out-of-pocket expense for another care setting or home care.

Potential or Actual Side Effects. Studies have shown that people are less likely to adopt interventions that have unpleasant side effects (Armstrong et al, 2005; Furlong, 2001; Phillips, 2001; Wipke-Tevis and Sae-Sia, 2004; Wu et al, 2008). People make decisions and agree to interventions based on what they know. If they are uninformed about the side effects or do not understand the impact these side effects may have on their life, they can develop mistrust and skepticism and choose to discontinue an activity. In order to discuss possible side effects and interactions with the patient, it is critical to know how the intervention will affect lifestyle, as well as potential interactions with *all* concurrent medications and therapies. It is important to expect a high potential for discovering multiple concurrent medications and therapies. A 2007 study found that the typical Medicare beneficiary saw two primary care physicians and five specialists annually; pharmacies and diagnostic facilities are not included in these numbers. Patients with several chronic conditions visited as many as 16 physicians in a year (Pham et al, 2007). These data underscore the importance of a holistic assessment that includes concurrent medications and therapies for the patient.

Wound care often requires the introduction of new treatment modalities. Many manufacturers and clinicians facilitate sampling and trialing of products and interventions so the patient can learn by experience before making a full commitment to the interventions. Singh and colleagues (2013) used a protocol for patients undergoing pressure ulcer surgery that involved encouraging prone positioning on a pressure redistribution support surface preoperatively in preparation for the postoperative recovery period. Experts agree that patients should be cared for on a high-specification support surface mattress before pressure ulcer surgery to determine tolerance of the mattress (NPUAP, EPUAP, PPPIA, 2014).

Cultural Factors. Culture refers to patterns of behavior of racial, ethnic, religious, or social groups. The National Quality Forum (NQF) says cultural competence is the ability to meet the needs of diverse patient populations so that delivered health care is safe and equitable. Culturally competent care according to the NQF (2010) tries to eliminate misunderstandings and improve patient adherence with treatments. However, evidence is clear that minorities receive a lower quality of care and suffer disproportionately from higher rates of disease and death even when factors such as access, health insurance, and income are taken into account (Anderson et al, 2003; NQF, 2010).

Improving cultural competence is essential for closing the disparity gap in health care because culture and language can affect someone's beliefs about health, disease, and the behaviors that lead to both. Being respectful of—and responsive to—individuals' cultural needs ensures more effective communication so that a patient's needs can be better met (TJC, 2010).

In The Joint Commission's roadmap to advancing effective communication, cultural competence, and patient- and family-centered care (2010), cultural competence is defined as the ability of the health care provider and health care organizations to understand and respond effectively to the cultural and language needs brought by the patient to the health care encounter. The roadmap further states that cultural competence requires organizations and their personnel to value diversity, assess themselves, manage the dynamics of difference, acquire and institutionalize cultural knowledge, and adapt to diversity and the cultural contexts of individuals and the communities served.

From the first encounter, the wound specialist must openly address the patient's individual cultural factors without stereotyping. Cultural competence is rooted in respect, validation, and openness toward someone with different social and cultural perceptions and expectations than one's own. Because people tend to have an "ethnocentric" view in which they see their own culture as the best, the wound specialist must be aware of his or her own

---

CHECKLIST 29-2 **Examples of Action Steps to Improve Cultural Competence**

✓ Identify what language the patient and health care decision maker prefer to discuss health care.
✓ Provide education materials that are in the patient's preferred language and have translators available.
✓ Ask the patient if there are any cultural, religious, or spiritual beliefs that might influence his or her care.
✓ Identify if the patient has cultural-based modesty issues about care provided by staff of the opposite sex.
✓ Determine whether there are certain garments or items that need to be worn.
✓ Identify any special dietary needs. Provide options that are acceptable to the patient.
✓ Collaborate with patients and families to develop solutions to requests that can't be met.

---

cultural belief system so as not to inflict it on the patient (Jeffs, 2001).

Checklist 29-2 provides examples of action steps to improve cultural competence. The best way to understand a patient's cultural needs is to simply ask, "Are there any cultural, religious, or spiritual beliefs that might influence your care?" Over 24 million people in the United States are considered to have limited English proficiency for health care purposes. It is critical to ask patients what language they prefer to discuss their health care. For patients who are minors or incapacitated, the preferred language of the patient's parent(s), guardian, or surrogate decision maker should also be determined (TJC, 2010).

Care Transitions. Care transitions are defined as patient transfers between either locations or levels of care within the same location. Examples include patients transferring from a hospital to their home after surgery while needing continued wound care, or a patient living at home with a chronic wound and being referred by his or her primary care provider to an outpatient wound clinic. Patients with wounds associated with complex conditions often require care by numerous providers within and between care settings. As previously described, patients with several chronic conditions see up to 16 physicians in a year (Pham et al, 2007). As patients transition between providers, details of the patient's wound management plan can be omitted or communicated incompletely (Bodenheimer, 2008), which then becomes a barrier to effective care. Inefficient care transitions also reduce patient satisfaction and waste valuable resources. Care transitions are most effective when patients understand what to expect in the next location and have input in their wound management plan, when receiving clinicians have complete information from the sending clinicians, and when clinicians in a community work together to understand the requirements and capabilities of each other's care settings (Bodenheimer, 2008).

Patient Refusal Algorithm
Repositioning and/or Heel Offloading

See Repositioning Refusal Care Plan Reference for support on care plan documentation.

Does the patient have the capacity for decision making?
• Demonstrates a general awareness of health situation and the intervention proposed.
• Understands the factual information provided about the recommended intervention.
• Communicates verbally and nonverbally a clear decision regarding intervention based on information.

No — Determine education barriers and document them.

Is patient displaying physically aggressive behavior?

No — Reposition patient and offload heels. Document in EHR.
Update Care Plan with new interventions as appropriate.

Yes — Create/review behavioral care plan and consult Behavioral Analyst.
Follow behavioral care plan. Consult interdisciplinary team members as needed.
Does patient now agree?
No — Staff RN informs Charge RN. Charge RN to approach patient.
Does patient now agree?
No — Inform ANS or Manager to approach patient.
Does patient now agree?
No — Contact Director of unit for next steps (MD, SW, other involvement, etc.).

Yes — Identify and address the reason the patient is refusing (i.e., fan, TV, hot, etc.).
Does patient now agree?
No — If NA, inform staff RN immediately.
Staff RN re-educate patient on importance of intervention.
Further assess for possible causes of refusal.

Yes — Reposition patient and offload heels. Document in EHR.
Update Care Plan with new interventions as appropriate.

FIGURE 29-1 Patient refusal algorithm (From Bethesda Hospital, Member of HealthEast Care System.)

INFORMED REFUSAL

The wound specialist must acknowledge the patient's right to decline care if the decision is based on full comprehension of the consequences. If the decision does not appear to be in the patient's best interest, refusal should be a red flag for the specialist to review all the factors that may be hindering care and seek to offer other potential options more acceptable to the patient. The current plan of care may seem too overwhelming for the patient to cope with, especially when the actions require long-term life changes. For example, the need for lifelong compression stockings may seem overwhelming or confusing if the information received is incomplete or contradictory from one care provider to another (Brown, 2014). Fully informed refusal requires a full reassessment of all the previously mentioned factors in this chapter. Figure 29-1 provides an algorithm for informed patient refusal of positioning for pressure ulcer prevention.

CLINICAL CONSULT

A: Referral for management of pressure ulcer on coccyx of 76-year-old Caucasian gentleman discovered post op day 3. Nurses state the patient keeps refusing to turn on his side. Noted pressure redistribution visco elastic foam mattress with heels slightly floating off bed with use of pillows under the legs. Patient has head of bed at 45 degrees and is watching TV. Indwelling catheter, no reports of fecal incontinence. Discussed reason for reposition refusal. He states it hurts too much to move, does not believe it makes sense to lie on his hip, and can't see the TV if he lies on his side. Wound 3 × 3 cm without measureable depth. Tissue smooth and pink. Peri-wound skin intact. No local signs of infection.

D: Stage II pressure ulcer due to pressure from immobility combined with shear from head of bed elevated above 30 degrees allowing tissue and bone to move in opposite directions.

P: Evaluate if patient is making an informed refusal to repositioning. Educate/reeducate regarding the importance of premedication to control pain, techniques for appropriate positioning for pressure ulcer prevention.

I: (1) Dispel the myth patient must "lie on his hip," 30-degree tilt is sufficient for offloading the coccyx. (2) Discuss the relationship between shear injury and HOB elevation and evaluate if patient can tolerate HOB at 30 degrees or less. (3) Premedicate as needed for effective repositioning. (4) Limit supine positioning as much as possible, position bed so patient can see the TV while he is positioned toward his side. (5) Keep HOB at 30 degrees or less. (6) Continue floating heels while in bed. (7) Provide moist wound healing with hydrocolloid dressing changes 2x/week. (8) Reconsult wound specialist for higher specification support surface if patient is unable to limit supine position or keep HOB at 30 degrees or less.

E: Nurse, patient, and wife understand and agree to plan of care. Will follow up in 1 week to evaluate/monitor effectiveness and adapt plan as needed. Call sooner for questions, concerns, or signs of deterioration.

SUMMARY

The wound management team must be guided by an underlying philosophy that care providers work in partnership with the patient to develop a sustainable plan of care based upon mutually agreed upon goals. Identifying and addressing realistic goals toward achieving a sustainable plan may improve the ability to achieve care plan goals, decrease recurrence rates, and, if appropriate, maximize the potential for wound healing. The wound specialist is in a pivotal position to avoid mislabeling patients as noncompliant. At a very minimum, a complete assessment using the HBM and documentation of interventions addressing the barriers toward achieving a sustainable plan should be completed before such a conclusion can be reached.

REFERENCES

Anderson LM, Scrimshaw SC, Fullilove MT, et al: Culturally competent healthcare systems: a systematic review, *Am J Prev Med* 24(Suppl 3):68–79, 2003.

Armstrong DG, Lavery LA, Kimbriel HR, et al: Activity patterns with diabetic foot ulceration: patients with active ulceration may not adhere to a standard pressure off-loading regimen, *Diabetes Care* 26(9):2595–2597, 2003.

Armstrong DG, Lavery LA, Wu S, et al: Evaluation of removable and irremovable cast walkers in the healing of diabetic foot wounds: a randomized controlled trial, *Diabetes Care* 28(3):551–554, 2005.

Armstrong DG, Nguyen HC, Lavery LA, et al: Off-loading the diabetic foot wound: a randomized clinical trial, *Diabetes Care* 24(6):1019–1022, 2001.

Ashford RL, McGee P, Kinmond K: Perception of quality of life by patients with diabetic foot ulcers, *Diabet Foot* 3:150–155, 2000.

Australian Wound Management Association (AWMA) and the New Zealand Wound Care Society (NZWCS): *Australian and New Zealand clinical practice guideline for prevention and management of venous leg ulcers*, Osborne Park, WA, Australia, 2011, Cambridge Publishing.

Bodenheimer T: Coordinating care—a perilous journey through the health care system, *N Engl J Med* 358(10):1064–1071, 2008.

Brace JA, Schubart JR: A prospective evaluation of a pressure ulcer prevention and management e-learning program for adults with spinal cord injury, *Ostomy Wound Manage* 56(8):40–50, 2010.

Briggs M, Closs SJ: The prevalence of leg ulceration: a review of the literature, *EWMA J* 3(2):14–20, 2003.

Brod M: Quality of life issues in patients with diabetes and lower extremity ulcers: patients and caregivers, *Qual Life Res* 7(4):365–372, 1998.

Brown A: Evaluating the reasons underlying treatment nonadherence in VLU patients: introducing the VeLUSET Part 1 of 2, *J Wound Care* 23(1):37, 40, 42–44, 2014.

Buxton T: Effective ways to improve health education materials, *J Health Educ* 30(1):47, 1999.

Canobbio MM: *Mosby's handbook of patient teaching*, ed 3, St. Louis, MO, 2006, Mosby.

Carpenter CJ: A meta-analysis of the effectiveness of health belief model variables in predicting behavior, *Health Commun* 25(8):661–669, 2010.

Centers for Medicare and Medicaid Services (CMS): National health expenditures 2013 highlights, published 12/09/2014. http://www.cms.gov/Research-Statistics-Data-and-Systems/

Statistics-Trends-and-Reports/NationalHealthExpendData/ downloads/highlights.pdf. Accessed August 16, 2015.

Chatterjee JS: From compliance to concordance in diabetes, *J Med Ethics* 32:507–510, 2006.

Collins L, Seraj S: Diagnosis and treatment of venous ulcers, *Am Fam Physicians* 81(8):989–996, 2010.

Coutts P, Parslow N: Compression stockings: a practical approach to common complaints, *Wound Care Canada* 4(2):20–24, 2006.

DiCenso A, Guyatt G, Ciliska D: *Evidence-based nursing: a guide to clinical practice*, St. Louis, MO, 2005, Mosby.

Durso S: Technological advances for improving medication adherence in the elderly, *Ann Longterm Care* 9(4):43, 2001.

Edwards LM, Moffatt CJ, Franks PJ: An exploration of patients' understanding of leg ulceration, *J Wound Care* 11(1):35–39, 2002.

Family Caregiver Alliance (FCA): *Women and caregiving: facts and figures. Who are the caregivers?* published Feb, 2015 https://caregiver.org/women-and-caregiving-facts-and-figures. Accessed February 25, 2015.

Fierheller M, Anku C, Alavi A: Encouraging patient adherence to therapeutic graduated compression therapy in venous stasis disease: a limited literature review, *Wound Care Canada* 7(1):10–16, 2009.

Finlayson K, Edwards H, Courtney M: Factors associated with recurrence of venous leg ulcers: a survey and retrospective chart review, *Int J Nurs Stud* 46(8):1071–1078, 2009.

Frescos N: What causes wound pain? *J Foot Ankle Res* 4(Suppl 1): 22, 2011.

Friedman AJ, Cosby R, Boyko S, et al: Effective teaching strategies and methods of delivery for patient education: a systematic review and practice guideline recommendations, *J Cancer Educ* 26(1):12–21, 2011.

Furlong W: Venous disease treatment and compliance: the nursing role, *Br J Nurs* 10(Suppl 11):S18–S20, 2001.

Glanz K, Rimer BK, Viswanath K: *Health behavior and health education: theory, research, and practice*, ed 4, San Francisco, CA, 2008, Jossey-Bass, pp 46–49.

Hallett CE, Austin L, Caress A, et al: Community nurses' perceptions of patient "compliance" in wound care: a discourse analysis, *J Adv Nurs* 32(1):115–123, 2000.

Heinen MM, van der Vleuten C, de Rooij MM, et al: Physical activity and adherence to compression therapy in patients with venous leg ulcers, *Arch Dermatol* 143(10):1283–1288, 2007.

Heisler M, Bouknight RR, Hayward RA, et al: The relative importance of physician communication, participatory decision-making, and patient understanding in diabetes self-management, *J Gen Intern Med* 17:243–252, 2002.

Herber OR, Schnepp W, Rieger MA: A systematic review on the impact of leg ulceration on patients' quality of life, *Health Qual Life Outcomes* 5:44, 2007.

Hyland ME, Ley A, Thomson B: Quality of life of leg ulcer patients: questionnaire and preliminary findings, *J Wound Care* 3:294–298, 1994.

Jeffs L: Teaching cultural safety the culturally safe way, *Nurs Prax N Z* 17(3):41–50, 2001.

Jones CJ, Smith H, Llewellyn C: Evaluating the effectiveness of health belief model interventions in improving adherence: a systematic review, *Health Psychol Rev* 8(3):253–269, 2014.

Jull A, Mitchell N, Arroll J, et al: Factors influencing concordance with compression stockings after venous leg ulcer healing, *J Wound Care* 13:90–92, 2004.

Kessler RC, Chiu WT, Demler O, et al: Prevalence, severity, and comorbidity of twelve-month DSM-IV disorders in the National Comorbidity Survey Replication (NCS-R), *Arch Gen Psychiatry* 62(6):617–627, 2005.

Knowles MS, Holton EF III, Swanson RA: *The adult learner*, Houston, TX, 1998, Gulf Publishing.

Kripalani S, Weiss BD: Teaching about health literacy and clear communication, *J Gen Intern Med* 21(8):888–890, 2006.

Labropoulos N, Wang ED, Lanier ST, et al: Factors associated with poor healing and recurrence of venous ulceration, *Plast Reconstr Surg* 129(1):179–186, 2012.

Lantz M: Economic noncompliance in the treatment of depression: when the patient can't afford prescription drugs, *Clin Geriatr* 11(9):18–22, 2003.

Morton LM, Bolton LL, Corbett LQ, et al: An evaluation of the Association for the Advancement of Wound Care venous ulcer guideline and recommendations for future research, *Adv Skin Wound Care* 26(12):553–561, 2013.

National Pressure Ulcer Advisory Panel (NPUAP), European Pressure Ulcer Advisory Panel (EPUAP), and Pan Pacific Pressure Injury Alliance (PPPIA): *Prevention and treatment of pressure ulcers: clinical practice guideline*. In Haesler E, editor, Perth, Australia, 2014, Cambridge Media.

National Quality Forum: *Safe practices for better healthcare–2010* update: A consensus report. Washington, D.C.: NQF available at https://www.qualityforum.org/Publications/2010/04/Safe_ Practices_for_Better_Healthcare_–_2010_Update.aspx, March 2009, National Quality Forum. Accessed August 16, 2015.

Nielson Global Online Consumer Survey: *Global advertising consumers trust real friends and virtual strangers the most*, 2009. http://www.nielsen.com/us/en/newswire/2009/global-advertising-consumers-trust-real-friends-and-virtual-strangers-the-most.html. Accessed August 16, 2015.

Partnership to Fight Chronic Disease (PFCD): *Better care legislation a positive step in fight against the growing epidemic of chronic disease*, 2014. http://www.fightchronicdisease.org/ media-center/releases/better-care-legislation-positive-step-fight-against-growing-epidemic-chronic-d. Accessed February 25, 2014.

Pham HH, Schrag D, O'Malley AS, et al: Care patterns in Medicare and their implications for pay for performance, *N Engl J Med* 356:1130–1139, 2007.

Phillips T: Current approaches to venous ulcers and compression, *Dermatol Surg* 27:611–621, 2001.

Phillips T, Stanton B, Provan A, et al: A study of the impact of leg ulcers on quality of life: financial, social, and psychologic implications, *J Am Acad Dermatol* 31:49–53, 1994.

Price P: Education psychology and compliance, *Diabetes Metab Res Rev* 24:101–105, 2008.

Raju S, Hollis K, Neglen P: Use of compression stockings in CVD: patient compliance and efficacy, *Ann Vasc Surg* 21(6):790–795, 2007.

Rappl L: Non-compliance: adding insult to injury, *Ostomy Wound Manage* 50(5):6, 8, 2004.

Redman BK: *The practice of patient education: a case study approach*, ed 10, St. Louis, MO, 2007, Mosby.

Rosenstock IM: Why people use health services, *Milbank Mem Fund Q* 44(3):94–127, 1996.

Schubart JR: An e-learning program to prevent pressure ulcers in adults with spinal cord injury: a pre- and post- pilot test among rehabilitation patients following discharge to home, *Ostomy Wound Manage* 58(10):38–49, 2012.

Seley JJ: Noncompliance vs. diabetes self care: are we still playing the blame game? *Diabetes Health*, June 19, 2009. https://www.diabeteshealth.com/blog/non-compliance-vs-diabetes-self-care-are-we-still-playing-a-blame-game-2. Accessed February 3, 2010.

Simon DA, Dix FP, McCollum CN: Management of venous leg ulcers, *Br Med J* 328(7452):1358–1362, 2004.

Singh R, Singh R, Rohilla RK, et al: Improvisations in classic and modified techniques of flap surgery to improve the success rate for pressure ulcer healing in patients with spinal cord injury, *Int Wound J* 10(4):455–460, 2013.

So K, Umraw N, Scott J, et al: Effects of enhanced patient education on compliance with silicone gel sheeting and burn scar outcome: a randomized prospective study, *J Burn Care Rehabil* 24(6):411–417, 2003.

Steed DL, Attinger C, Colaizzi T, et al: Guidelines for the treatment of diabetic ulcers, *Wound Repair Regen* 14(6):680–692, 2006.

Takahashi PY, Chandra A, Cha SS, et al: A predictive model for venous ulceration in older adults: results of a retrospective cohort study, *Ostomy Wound Manage* 56(4):60–66, 2010.

The Joint Commission (TJC): *Advancing effective communication, cultural competence, and patient- and family-centered care: a roadmap for hospitals*, Oakbrook Terrace, IL, 2010, TJC.

Van Hecke A, Grypdonck M, Defloor T: A review of why patients with leg ulcers do not adhere to treatment, *J Clin Nurs* 18(3):337–349, 2009.

Van Hecke A, Verhaeghe S, Grypdonck M, et al: Processes underlying adherence to leg ulcer treatment: a qualitative field study, *Int J Nurs Stud* 48:145–155, 2011.

van Rijswijk L: Non-compliance no more, *Ostomy Wound Manage* 50(1):6, 2004.

Warshaw E, Nix D, Kula J, et al: Clinical and cost-effectiveness of a cleanser protectant lotion for treatment of perineal skin breakdown in low-risk patients with incontinence, *Ostomy Wound Manage* 48(6):44–51, 2002.

Weller CD, Buchbinder R, Johnston RV: Interventions for helping people adhere to compression treatments for venous leg ulceration, *Cochrane Database Syst Rev* 9:CD008378, 2013.

Whitney J, Phillips L, Aslam R, et al: Guidelines for the treatment of pressure ulcers, *Wound Repair Regen* 14(6):663–679, 2006.

Wipke-Tevis D, Sae-Sia W: Caring for vascular leg ulcers, *Home Healthc Nurse* 22(4):237–247, 2004.

Wound, Ostomy and Continence Nurses Society™ (WOCN®): *Guideline for prevention and management of pressure ulcers (WOCN® clinical practice guideline series no. 2)*, Glenview IL, 2010, WOCN®.

Wu SC, Jensen JL, Weber AK, et al: Use of pressure offloading devices in diabetic foot ulcers, *Diabetes Care* 31(11):2118–2119, 2008.

Uncommon Wounds and Manifestations of Intrinsic Disease

Ruth A. Bryant

OBJECTIVES

1. Differentiate between staphylococcal scalded skin syndrome and toxic epidermal necrolysis (TEN) and between graft-versus-host disease (GVHD) and pyoderma gangrenosum in terms of manifestations and etiology.
2. Describe the process of tissue damage and treatment options for vasculitis, calciphylaxis, epidermolysis bullosa (EB), GVHD, frostbite, and TEN.
3. Discriminate among the patient populations at risk for calciphylaxis, frostbite, TEN, and extravasation.
4. Compare and contrast the role of debridement in necrotizing fasciitis, TEN, extravasation, and frostbite.
5. Describe the distinguishing features of a chronic wound with malignant transformation.
6. Identify four conditions that require a tissue biopsy for diagnosis.

Wounds commonly referred to as atypical are actually typical manifestations of uncommon conditions. This chapter discusses less common skin pathologies that often are intrinsic to another disease such as infection, inflammatory processes, metabolic disorders, and neoplasms. Although some may be rare, they are often associated with significant morbidity and mortality. When the patient's clinical history or wound progression is inconsistent with common skin lesions or the wound is unresponsive to appropriate treatment, uncommon cutaneous wounds should be considered. The wound specialist should be familiar with the clinical manifestations of these less common conditions to facilitate early detection and prompt referral for appropriate medical management. In many situations, early detection is essential to arrest the underlying pathology and to prevent progression of ulcerations, infection, sepsis, and death.

INFECTIOUS ETIOLOGY

Staphylococcal Scalded Skin Syndrome

Staphylococcal scalded skin syndrome (SSSS) is a superficial blistering skin disorder caused by the exfoliative toxins of some strains of *Staphylococcus aureus*. Initially an infection is present most commonly in the oral or nasal cavities, neck, axillae, groin, or umbilicus (King and de Saint Victor, 2014). The toxins produced by the infecting organism are transferred through the bloodstream to a site remote from the original infection, where significant erythema will develop, followed by separation of the superficial epidermis (i.e., desquamation). The primary lesions are superficial bullae. Secondarily, lesions develop superficial scales. The skin may have a sandpaper feel. Significant pain is unusual for SSSS and, if present, suggests another diagnosis, such as toxic epidermal necrolysis (TEN), a drug-induced necrosis of the epidermis.

Although SSSS has been reported in adults, it most commonly occurs in healthy children 6 years or younger and in neonates (Habif et al, 2005; King and de Saint Victor, 2014). The absence of antibodies to these toxins and an impaired ability to excrete the toxin due to immature renal function are contributing factors for this condition (Jeyakumari et al, 2009). Mortality in children is very low (1% to 5%) unless SSSS is associated with sepsis or a coexisting serious medical condition. Staphylococcal scalded skin syndrome, when it develops in adults, occurs in adults who are chronically ill, immunocompromised, or with renal failure. The mortality rate in adults is substantial (50% to 60%), although this may be attributable to the overall health status of the adults rather than the SSSS (King and de Saint Victor, 2014).

Suspicious sites (nose, eyes, ears, throat, vagina) should be swabbed for microbial cultures to confirm the diagnosis. Bullae from the primary lesion usually yield cultures that are negative for bacteria. A frozen section of sloughing skin is needed to differentiate SSSS from a drug-induced skin reaction (TEN). Full-thickness epidermal necrosis is inconsistent with SSSS and suggests a drug-induced process. Staphylococcal scalded skin syndrome and bullous impetigo also have similar manifestations. Important distinctive features of SSSS include involvement of the face around the mouth, chin, eyes, and nose and absence of mucosal involvement (Jeyakumari et al, 2009).

Once SSSS is diagnosed, treatment consists of supportive care and elimination of the primary infection. Debridement and antibiotics are essential to manage the infection. Topical management of the desquamated skin should address exudate management, pain control, and maintenance of a moist environment. Foam dressings, superabsorbent dressings, sheet hydrogels, and alginates are preferred dressing options; adhesives should be avoided. Steroids may worsen immune function, and nonsteroidal antiinflammatory drugs (NSAIDs) should be avoided because they potentially can reduce renal function (King and de Saint Victor, 2014). When massive tissue loss is apparent, the wound should be managed according to the principles for burn therapy as outlined in Chapter 32.

Toxic Shock Syndrome

Toxic shock syndrome is caused by a toxin produced by certain types of *Staphylococcus* bacterial infections. The most common pathogen for this serious infection is *S. aureus.* Acute onset consists of a widespread macular erythematous eruption (within 1 to 3 days) that extends to include the soles of the feet and the palms of the hands. Desquamation of the skin is highly characteristic of toxic shock syndrome. It occurs 10 days to 3 weeks after onset and primarily includes the fingertips and plantar surfaces of the palms and feet. Additional clinical manifestations include edema of the hands and feet (50%), petechiae (27%), conjunctival infection (85%), oropharyngeal hyperemia (90%), and genital hyperemia (100%) (Habif et al, 2005).

Diagnosis is based on a constellation of symptoms: fever (>102°F), hypotension, rash progressing to desquamation, and mucosal membrane involvement (mouth, eyes, vagina). In addition, the condition must be multisystem as evidenced by impaired functioning of at least three organs (muscular, gastrointestinal, central nervous system, renal, hepatic, hematologic, cardiopulmonary, metabolic) (Habif et al, 2005; Smith, 2008). A skin biopsy is indicated to exclude TEN as a diagnosis.

The goal of treatment of toxic shock syndrome is preventing organ damage through supportive care and aggressive antibiotic therapy; the mortality rate of toxic shock syndrome ranges from 3% to 12% (Habif et al, 2005). Local wound management is based on wound needs (e.g., exudate absorption). Topical dressings should be nonocclusive and nonadhesive.

Necrotizing Fasciitis

Necrotizing fasciitis is an uncommon but serious subcutaneous tissue infection that spreads rapidly along the superficial fascial plane. The overall mortality rate from this very rapidly spreading condition is variable: 20% in pediatric cases and anywhere from 6% to 73% in adults (Anaya and Dellinger, 2007). Necrotizing fasciitis is characterized by widespread necrosis of the fascia and deep subcutaneous tissue, with thrombosis of nutrient vessels and sloughing of overlying tissue (see Plate 59). Although it can occur anywhere in the body, such as the abdomen, perianal area, or inguinal area, it usually occurs in the extremities after a minor operation or injury (Park et al, 2014).

The clinical markers of necrotizing fasciitis are a rapidly spreading erythema in the skin around the wound and subcutaneous crepitus that may be visible on radiograph. Additional signs of necrotizing fasciitis are pain (considered to be out of proportion for the extent of the skin damage), swelling at the site of the wound, chills, fever, and toxemia. The skin may initially appear normal over the cellulitis, but as the infectious process compromises blood supply, the skin becomes erythematous, edematous, and reddish-purple to patchy blue-gray. Bullae form within 3 to 5 days from onset and progress to necrosis of the skin, sloughing, and frank cutaneous gangrene (Anaya and Dellinger, 2007). Tendon sheaths and muscle will liquefy when infected; in the operating room, "dishwater fluid" is the hallmark of liquefactive necrosis.

Necrotizing fasciitis can be detected by its dramatic clinical presentation and by probing the wound. When the affected area is probed with a hemostat through a limited incision, the instrument passes easily along a plane of superficial to deep fascia. This examination helps to distinguish necrotizing fasciitis from cellulitis. This infection is most often polymicrobial with group A streptococci or *S. aureus* predominating. A subset of necrotizing soft tissue infections caused by *Clostridium* species are monomicrobial and associated with a significantly worse prognosis (Anaya and Dellinger, 2007).

The presence of necrotizing fasciitis requires aggressive surgical debridement; any nonviable or questionably viable tissue must be removed. Because the infection spreads subcutaneously, a wound may need to be extended to allow access to and debridement of all necrotic tissue (Attinger et al, 2006). Despite aggressive local control, necrotizing fasciitis has a 24% to 50% mortality rate secondary to persistent wound sepsis or systemic sepsis (Martin et al, 2008). Local wound care consists of close monitoring for further dissection, which indicates progression of the infection. Topical dressing recommendations are largely based on expert opinion or preference. Dressings should be used that meet the needs of the wound (e.g., fill dead space, absorb exudate), allow for frequent monitoring of the wound, deliver topical antimicrobial activity, and are nonadhesive and nonocclusive. Negative pressure wound therapy (NPWT) is an appropriate option for managing the open wound after debridement. Surgical reconstruction of large tissue defects can be achieved with NPWT, skin grafts, and tissue-based products (Mazzone and Schiestl, 2013).

SPIDER BITES

Only 60 of the 20,000 species of spiders in the world are capable of inflicting a bite, and only 4 can cause significant injury; evidence of that tissue damage is documented for only 2 spiders: the brown recluse and the black widow. The brown recluse spider is one of five species of spiders within the genus *Loxosceles*. This spider is about the size of a U.S. quarter, is yellow to brown in color, and has a distinctive fiddle-shaped mark on its back (Rhoads, 2007). The brown recluse spider usually is shy and nocturnal. It tends to avoid humans and seek shelter in abandoned or infrequently used buildings, attics, and basements. Bites generally occur when a person disturbs a pile of wood or rocks, moves boxes that have been stored, or dresses in clothes that have been stored for a long period of time. The most common site for a *Loxosceles* spider bite is on the extremities, but they also can occur on the buttocks or genitalia.

The venom of the brown recluse spider is a mixture of enzymes that destroy cellular membranes, resulting in damage to the surrounding skin, fat, nerves, and blood vessels. Manifestations of a brown recluse spider bite can range from small lesions with erythema to full-thickness necrotic wounds (known as necrotic arachnidism). Fewer than 10% of patients develop severe skin necrosis or other systemic reaction (e.g., loxoscelism, which is characterized by fever, nausea, hemolysis, and thrombocytopenia) (Schwartz, 2009; Zeglin, 2005). Severity of the reaction depends on the amount of venom injected, the site of the bite, and host susceptibility. However, it is the accumulation of activated neutrophils that is responsible for the cutaneous necrosis (Schwartz, 2009). Accumulation of neutrophils occurs 24 to 72 hours before skin necrosis and ulceration. The very young, the elderly, and individuals in poor physical condition are at highest risk for serious illness from a spider bite.

After a spider bite, the person may experience a mild burning sensation or may experience no discomfort at all. Within 6 to 12 hours, itching, pain, a central papule, and erythema may develop. Wounds that progress usually begin to do so within 48 to 72 hours of the bite. As the tissue damage progresses, the characteristic "red, white, and blue" sign of a brown recluse bite develops; the sign consists of a ring of blanched skin (due to vasoconstriction) surrounded by erythema with gray-to-red-purple bullae at the site of the bite (Schwartz, 2009; Zeglin, 2005) (see Plate 62). Severe necrosis is more likely when the bite is located in an area with significant adipose tissue, such as the thighs and buttocks. When the bite remains localized with a central blister, resolution occurs within 3 weeks. Severe bites that develop necrosis heal over a 2- to 3-month time span (Rhoads, 2007).

The standard treatment of spider bite lesions is (1) thorough cleansing; (2) rest; (3) application of ice; (4) compression; and (5) elevation. Oral antiinflammatory medications, an antihistamine, and tetanus vaccine also may be given. If cellulitis appears to be developing, an antibiotic such as erythromycin is indicated (Zeglin, 2005). Treatment of severe necrotic lesions is controversial; however, the goals are to (1) maintain skin integrity; (2) prevent spread of infection; and (3) maintain circulatory status. The following interventions are indicated (Smith et al, 1997): (1) ice pack on the affected area (no heat) to lessen tissue damage; (2) empiric antibiotics to treat cellulitis; (3) NSAIDs to relieve inflammation and pain; (4) tetanus toxoid; and (5) nonocclusive topical dressings to provide a moist environment, fill dead space, and absorb exudate. The site should be monitored for signs of deterioration and cellulitis (Rhoads, 2007).

Patients with severe and rapidly progressing lesions may be given dapsone (Avlosulfon) therapy, which is an inhibitor of neutrophil function. However, it must be administered within hours of a bite to be effective. By inhibiting the spread of neutrophils, dapsone is believed to minimize tissue necrosis (Zeglin, 2005). However, dapsone can have multiple moderate to severe adverse effects. Alternative interventions include hyperbaric oxygenation, nitroglycerin patches, electric shock therapy, and heparin therapy, although no evidence is conclusive for the effectiveness of these treatments. Preliminary research suggests NPWT may be applied promptly after venom exposure to facilitate extraction of the venom and to stimulate granulation tissue formation (Wong et al, 2010). Systemic reactions and complications from the bite of a recluse spider include renal failure and coagulation disorders such as thrombocytopenia and disseminated intravascular coagulopathy (Zeglin, 2005).

PYODERMA GANGRENOSUM

Pyoderma gangrenosum (PG) is a chronic neutrophilic, systemic autoinflammatory, ulcerating skin disease that most likely represents an aberrant immune response to an as-yet-unidentified antigen. It has been characterized by neutrophil dysfunction and over-expression of various leukocytes signaling cytokines such as IL-8, IL-16 and tumor necrosis factor (Ahronowitz et al, 2012; Brooklyn et al, 2006; Reguiaï and Grange, 2007). Histologically, the presence of numerous polymorphonuclear leukocytes creates a dense infiltrate of the dermis that can extend from the superficial dermis to the subcutaneous tissue.

These painful lesions have been associated with underlying systemic diseases, such as inflammatory bowel disease, seropositive rheumatoid arthritis, ankylosing spondylitis, and monoclonal gammopathies (Ahronowitz et al, 2012) (Box 30-1). Almost 50% of cases occur in patients with no known associated systemic disease and are idiopathic (Snyder, 2008; Wollina, 2007). When PG accompanies a systemic disease, it does not necessarily parallel the underlying disease and instead may be triggered by trauma (Paparone et al, 2009).

Pyoderma gangrenosum has several different manifestations, but generally these extremely painful lesions begin with a painful nodule, pustule, or bulla that develops significant induration and erythema and proceeds to ulceration. Five subtypes of PG have been identified: classic (ulcerative), bullous, pustular, vegetative, and peristomal (Ahronowitz et al, 2012). The most common presentation is the classic ulcerative form. With this particular variation, ulcers usually occur on the lower extremities, but may also occur on the abdomen, genitalia, trunk, head, and neck. It is commonly associated with inflammatory bowel disease (particularly Crohn's disease), rheumatoid arthritis, and monoclonal gammopathy and may occur before, during, or after the disease (Aggarwal, 2012; Callen and Jackson, 2007).

Bullous PG is commonly associated with myeloproliferative disease, refractory anemias, and myelogenous leukemia (Callen and Jackson, 2007). These lesions begin as painful, rapidly enlarging vesicles and bullae with central necrosis that evolves into an erosion rather than a necrotic ulcer (Ruocco et al, 2009). The hands, arms, and face are more commonly affected than legs. This particular variation of PG is commonly misdiagnosed as cellulitis. Bullous PG in the patient with acute myeloid leukemia is suggestive of poor prognosis; thus it is important to rule out a hematologic malignancy in the patient who develops bullous PG (Ahronowitz et al, 2012). Treatment of the underlying malignancy results in improvement of the bullous PG.

Vegetative PG is characterized by a single superficial ulcer with a nonpurulent wound bed and the absence of undermining and periwound erythema (Ruocco et al, 2009). This is a nonaggressive form of PG, not associated with systemic disease, and responds well to topical therapy. The most common sites are the head and neck. Pustular PG develops as a painful pustular lesion with erythematous halo and is often associated with irritable bowel disease (IBD) and hepatobiliary disease (Ahronowitz et al, 2012). These lesions are most often found on the legs and upper trunk. Peristomal PG consists of lesions around a stoma commonly associated with IBD, monoclonal gammopathy and connective tissue disease. At onset, the peristomal PG lesion is a painful, erythematous papule with violaceous borders that erodes into ulcers with undermined borders. These lesions are similar in appearance to classic PG.

Common characteristics of the ulcerative PG lesion include irregularly shaped wound edges that are elevated and violaceous (see Plate 63). Ulcers are exudative and extremely tender. The wound base is often filled with yellow slough and/or islands of necrosis; wound edges are undermined. A band of erythema may extend from the wound edge, which defines the direction in which the ulcer will extend. Healing may be present along one edge of the ulcer, whereas enlargement occurs along another edge. Ulcers heal slowly and leave an atrophic, irregular scar. A common and notable characteristic of PG is a phenomenon known as *pathergy*, which is the abnormal and exaggerated inflammatory response to noxious stimuli. Patients often report the lesion developing after minor trauma, such as a bump against a piece of furniture. Minor trauma preceding the development of the ulcer is an important piece of information to obtain during the patient interview (Paparone et al, 2009).

Pyoderma gangrenosum is difficult to diagnose; it is essentially a diagnosis by exclusion. As many as 10% of PG cases are misdiagnosed including vascular disease, vasculitis, malignancies, autoimmune disease, or infection (Box 30-2) thus delaying appropriate treatment. (Ahronowitz et al, 2012). A history and physical examination, skin biopsy for histology and microbiology, and an investigation for an associated illness constitute a complete workup (Box 30-3). Diagnosis is largely based on clinical manifestations (rapidly enlarging, painful ulcer with violaceous, undermined edges and hemorrhagic/necrotic wound bed), a thorough examination in which other ulcerative skin disorders (e.g., vasculitis, Behcet's disease, rheumatoid vasculitis, infections) have been excluded, and pathologic features (Ratnagobal and Sinha,

BOX 30-3   Essential Data in Workup for Suspected Pyoderma Gangrenosum

1. Obtain history of onset of lesions
   - Rapidly enlarging, painful ulcer with violaceous, undermined edges and hemorrhagic/necrotic wound bed
2. Obtain skin biopsy from the erythematous margin of the wound for histology and microbiology
3. Obtain laboratory tests:
   - Routine tests to screen for hematologic, liver, or kidney disorder:
     ○ Complete blood count (CBC) with differential
     ○ Electrolytes
     ○ Urinalysis (UA)
     ○ Liver function
     ○ Erythrocyte sedimentation rate (ESR)
     ○ C-reactive protein (CRP)
   - Rule out systemic disorder
     ○ Antinuclear antibody
     ○ Coagulopathy panel
       ■ Antiphospholipid antibody test
       ■ Cryoglobulins
       ■ Rheumatoid factor
       ■ Antineutrophilic cytoplasmic antibodies (ANCA)
   - Rule out infectious etiology (if risk factors exist):
     ○ Rapid plasma reagin (RPR)
     ○ Hepatitis serologies
     ○ HIV

BOX 30-4   Proposed Diagnostic Criteria for Pyoderma Gangrenosum

Major Criteria (must satisfy both major criteria):
1. Rapid[a] progression of painful,[b] necrolytic, cutaneous ulcer[c] with irregular, violaceous, undermined border
2. Exclusion of other causes of cutaneous ulceration

Minor Criteria (must also satisfy at least two minor criteria):
1. History suggestive of pathergy[d] or clinical finding of cribiform scarring
2. Systemic diseases associated with pyoderma gangrenosum[e]
3. Histopathologic findings (sterile dermal neutrophilia ± mixed inflammation ± lymphocytic vasculitis)
4. Treatment response (rapid response to systemic glucocorticoid treatment)[f]

[a]Characteristic margin expansion of 1 to 2 cm/day, or 50% increase in ulcer size within 1 month.
[b]Pain usually out of proportion to size of ulceration.
[c]Typically preceded by papule, pustule, or bulla.
[d]Ulcer development at sites of minor cutaneous injury.
[e]Inflammatory bowel disease, polyarthritis, myelocytic leukemia, or preleukemia.
[f]Generally responds to dosage of 1 to 2 mg/kg/d, with 50% decrease in size within 1 month.
Adapted from Su WP, Davis MD, Weenig RH, et al: Pyoderma gangrenosum: clinicopathologic correlation and proposed diagnostic criteria, *Int J Dermatol* 43:790–800, 2004.

2013; Tang et al, 2012). Proposed diagnostic criteria are listed in Box 30-4. Even though the ulcer may enlarge due to pathergy, a biopsy (incisional biopsy preferred over punch biopsy) of the ulcer is critical. Although histopathologic findings are not specific for PG, they are supportive of the disease and will exclude malignancy and vasculitic, vasoocclusive, and infectious causes (Ratnagobal and Sinha, 2013). The biopsy must be full thickness and obtained from the erythematous margin of the wound for accurate histopathology. Laboratory tests such as antineutrophilic cytoplasmic antibodies (ANCA), rheumatoid factor (RF), and antiphospholipid antibodies (anticardiolipin antibodies, lupus anticoagulant, rapid plasma reagin [RPR]) are important to exclude other diseases that could account for these lesions (Ratnagobal and Sinha, 2013). Inflammatory markers (erythrocyte sedimentation rate [ESR] and C-reactive protein [CRP]) will also facilitate diagnosis. Because there is no definitive test to confirm the presence of PG, a diagnosis *consistent with* PG is appropriate, but only after a thorough workup is completed (Tang et al, 2012).

Treatment of PG consists of a combination of systemic therapy and local wound care. Table 30-1 summarizes topical medications that have been reported; the most commonly used and effective are corticosteroids, tacrolimus and cyclosporine. Topical corticosteroid medications in the form of cream or tablet (i.e., 5 mg prednisolone) dissolved within sterile water (10 ml) have also been described (Hanley, 2011; Vujnovich, 2005).

Of the various treatments that have been used to manage PG, the most consistent, effective results have been obtained with systemic immunosuppression with corticosteroids and cyclosporine. Large, orally administered doses of prednisolone (60 to 120 mg) are given daily until the disease is under control as demonstrated by the reduction in pain and presence of granulation tissue. Cyclosporine (oral 3 to 10 mg/kg/day and intravenous [IV] 4 mg/kg/day) appears to be particularly effective with PG in the presence of IBD (Ahronowitz et al, 2012). Although PG is not an infectious disease process, it can be complicated by infections. In fact, patients may receive treatment with antibiotics for cellulitis and may not improve because an initial biopsy was not obtained (Callen and Jackson, 2007; Wollina, 2007). Antineutrophillic therapies that interfere with neutrophil chemotaxis such as colchicine, sulfonamides, sulfones, and dapsone have demonstrated improvement in PG in small studies. Dapsone has been used alone or in combination with corticosteroids at doses of 50 to 200 mg/day; topical dapsone has also been effective in improving peristomal PG (Ahronowitz et al, 2012). Biologic agents are also being used to treat PG in very small studies. TNF-α inhibitors have been effective for classic PG, with complete ulcer healing within 7 to 21 days (Reguiaï and Grange, 2007).

Topical wound management should address wound needs, which include exudate management, protection from trauma, a moist wound environment, and pain control. Slough and nonviable tissue present in PG ulcers gradually decrease and transition to a granular wound bed as immunosuppressive medications are implemented and wound exudate is contained.

TABLE 30-1	**Topical Medications for Pyoderma Gangrenosum**		
	Mechanism of Action	**Dose**	**Comments**

Corticosteroids	• Antiinflammatory and immunosuppressive action
	• Reduced neutrophil and macrophage activity
	• Reduced proliferation of T cells
	• Decreased cytokine production
	• Decreased histamine production
	• Decreased IgG production
		Topical:
		• Betamethasone 17 valerate lotion (0.1%)
		• Intralesional injection in combination with systemic corticosteroid:
		  ○ 100 mg triamcinolone acetonide
		  ○ Varying concentrations (up to 40 mg/ml)
		  ○ Varying dosing schedules (i.e., every 4 to 6 weeks)
			Healing occurred with topical in 5 to 8 weeks
			Transparent dressing applied over lotion corticosteroid
			Low level of evidence (case reports of very small number of patients)

Sodium cromoglycate	Inhibits mast cell degranulation, platelet activation, and neutrophil chemotaxis	1-2% aqueous solution applied 3 × per day	Healing in 5-8 weeks Two case series
Topical 5-aminosalicylic acid (5-ASA)	Theorized to inhibit prostaglandin and leukotriene production by scavenging free radicals	10% 5-ASA cream applied daily	Healing in 5 weeks Limited evidence (case reports)
Topical nitrogen mustard	Immunosuppressive and anti-inflammatory agent	Aqueous solution (20%) applied daily	Healing after 3 months Limited evidence (case report)
Topical cyclosporine	Reduced proliferation of T cells by inhibiting interleukin-2 release	35 mg cyclosporine in isotonic saline solution injected intralesionally twice in 1 week	Healing in 3 months
Tacrolumus	Immunosuppressive agent for primary organ transplantation	0.1 to 0.3% (combined with carmellose sodium paste (Orabase)	May cover with thin hydrocolloid or ostomy pouch Reapply daily Healing has been reported in 5 weeks to 4 months More effective in PG lesions larger than 2 cm Highly absorbed through ulcerated tissue; apply to inflamed rim of lesion, not ulcer bed

Typically, management of the wound is necessary before its cause is known. Because of the extreme pain that typifies PG, nonadhesive dressings are preferred. Debridement is achieved only through autolysis and regression of the disease process itself. Aggressive sharp debridement is contraindicated because it will lead to extension of the disease through the process of pathergy. In fact, local care should be delivered with great caution because of the tendency for pathergy to occur. Skin grafts also are to be avoided due to pathergy (Paparone et al, 2009). Antibacterial topical dressings are often warranted to manage the wound bioburden and potential secondary bacterial infections (Callen and Jackson, 2007).

VASCULITIS AND CONNECTIVE TISSUE DISORDERS

Vasculitis comprises a group of disorders that have in common the pathologic features of inflammation of the blood vessels, endothelial swelling, and necrosis. Damage to the blood vessels is attributed to the deposition of circulating immune complexes (Tang et al, 2012). Vessels of any size can be affected, so any organ or system may be involved, resulting in a wide array of symptoms and clinical presentations.

Vasculitis ulcers usually are the sign of a complex process and may indicate a systemic disorder such as rheumatoid arthritis or lupus. However, vasculitis ulcers also can occur as a primary condition (Anderson, 2008; Armitage and Roberts, 2004). Most vasculitic syndromes are believed to have an immunologic etiology.

The size of the vessels involved (large, medium, or small) helps to characterize the skin manifestations. When a small vessel is affected, pinpoint areas of bleeding may develop, and small red or purple spots on the skin (petechiae) may appear, particularly on the legs. Inflammation of larger vessels causes the vessel to swell, producing a nodule that may be palpated. Blood flow will be impaired when the lumen of the blood vessel becomes narrowed or occluded from the edema; thus islands of ischemia or necrosis will develop on the skin, and the tips of digits may become cold or ischemic.

Leukocytoclastic vasculitis, Wegener granulomatosis, and rheumatoid factor are common. Other potential causes include systemic lupus erythematosus, polyarteritis nodosa, hypersensitivity vasculitis, Sjögren syndrome, cryoglobulinemia, scleroderma, and dermatomyositis (Hunter et al, 2002; Rubano and Kerstein, 1998). It is important to point out that leg ulceration has been reported in up to 10% of patients with rheumatoid arthritis (RA) and that the underlying cause is most often vascular (arterial, venous, or mixed) and less commonly RA-specific vasculitis or PG (Seitz et al, 2009).

The general signs and symptoms of vasculitis are fever, myalgias, arthralgias, and malaise. Patients sometimes describe a vague, flulike illness. Peripheral neuropathy may be present. Other symptoms depend on the organ involved, which is determined by the specific disease. For example, cryoglobulinemic vasculitis likely will be associated with renal and skin problems; Wegener granulomatosis may lead to respiratory as well as renal involvement; and the vasculitis associated with Sjögren syndrome attacks the brain, lungs, and skin (Jennette and Falk, 1997).

Cutaneous features of vasculitis can vary depending on the disease, but certain characteristics are common. The lesions can range from erythematous, nonblanching macules and/or nodules to hemorrhagic vesicles and palpable purpura, to necrotic lesions and ulceration. Skin biopsy is critical and is best taken from the margins of early lesions. Two or three sites might be needed to obtain the correct diagnosis (Roenigk and Young, 1996). Caution is warranted when interpreting results because inflammation and infection can mimic vasculitis

(Seitz et al, 2010). Skin ulcers associated with vasculitis are frequently located on the lower extremities in the lateral malleolus or pretibial area, making them difficult to distinguish from venous ulcers (Seitz et al, 2010) (see Plate 64).

The goal of treatment of vasculitis ulcers is control of the underlying disease process. The presence of these painful ulcers necessitates an evaluation for the underlying disease and identification of involved organs, which is then used to guide treatment. Bed rest, nonsteroidal antiinflammatory agents, antihistamines, corticosteroids, and biologic immunosuppressive agents often are necessary (Hunter et al, 2002). Plasmapheresis might be necessary in cases associated with circulating immune complexes. Topical therapy includes removal of necrotic tissue (often through autolysis), prompt identification and treatment of infection, maintenance of a moist wound base, absorption of excess exudate, packing of any dead space, insulation, and protection from further trauma.

The various vasculitis syndromes have many similarities, but also have specific differences unique to some of the diseases. The unique features of RA, systemic lupus erythematosus, and polyarteritis nodosa are listed in Table 30-2.

TABLE 30-2 Characteristics of Skin Lesions with Vasculitis Disorders

Vasculitic Disorder	Description	Ulcer Characteristics
Rheumatoid arthritis	Not well understood Associated with high levels of rheumatoid factor (RF) Evidence of venous insufficiency Limited ankle movement contributes to poor calf muscle pump function and may place patient at risk for venous ulcer development	Begin as palpable purpura and ecchymosis May progress to ulceration Shallow, well demarcated, painful, slow to heal May require addition of compression therapy
Systemic lupus erythematosus (SLE)	Chronic immune disorder Characterized by periods of exacerbation and remission Affects multiple organs (skin, serosal surfaces, central nervous system, kidneys) and red blood cells Circulating immune complexes and autoantibodies cause tissue damage and organ dysfunction No single cause; influenced by environment, host immune responses, hormones Common symptoms include fatigue, weight loss, fever, malaise Butterfly rash (facial edema over cheeks, nose) is typical Potential manifestations include seizures, hemiparesis, pericarditis, pleuritis, renal failure, nausea, vomiting, abdominal pain, arthralgias	Present as palpable purpura Progress to ulceration Occur on malleolar area Present as round lesions with erythematous borders Wound may have atrophy and loss of pigmentation
Polyarteritis nodosa (PAN)	Medium- and small-vessel vasculitis Necrotizing arteritis affecting small- and medium-sized arteries of most organs Involved organs commonly include kidney, liver, intestine, peripheral nerves, skin, muscle Characterized by fresh and healing lesions Clinical manifestations include anorexia, weight loss, fever, fatigue Organ-specific manifestations include abdominal pain, myalgia, arthralgia, paresthesia Subcutaneous painful nodules of lower extremities may develop	Skin involvement occurs in approximately 40% of patients Lesions have "punched out" appearance Painful Lesions may begin as purpura with urticaria before progressing to ulceration May have "starburst" pattern extending from ulcer Painful subcutaneous nodules present

Drug-Induced Vasculitis

In approximately 10% of patients with vasculitis, the cause is a drug reaction rather than a disease process. Drug-induced vasculitis usually is confined to the skin and appears about 1 week after administration of the drug. The drug binds to serum proteins, causing an immune-complex vasculitis (Jennette and Falk, 1997). The typical presentation is purpura and ulceration involving the lower extremities. Once systemic disease has been ruled out, treatment involves removal of the precipitating drug and symptomatic treatment. Antihistamines and NSAIDs are most often prescribed. Corticosteroids may be added for more severe symptoms. Wound care is based on wound needs, and ulcers resolve spontaneously once the drug is removed.

CALCIPHYLAXIS

Calciphylaxis is a type of ischemic subcutaneous arteriolosclerosis and occurs in two forms: calcific uremic arteriolopathy (CUA) and calciphylaxis from nonuremic causes (also known as *calciphylaxis with normal renal and parathyroid function*). Calciphylaxis is an extremely rare metabolic disorder that occurs in 1% to 5% of dialysis-dependent patients (Rogers and Coates, 2008; Wollina, 2013). Clinically, patients with CUA have secondary hyperparathyroidism (secondary to end-stage renal disease) and an elevated calcium-phosphate product level, which leads to vascular, subcutaneous, and cutaneous calcification (Tang et al, 2012). Calcific uremic arteriolopathy is a chronic progressive syndrome of arteriolar media calcification, thrombotic ischemia, and necrotic ulceration (Wollina, 2013). It develops when levels of calcium and phosphate in the blood are no longer solubilized, leading to deposits in the arteriolar wall. Risk factors for calciphylaxis are hyperphosphatemia; decreased serum albumen; elevated sedimentation rate, aluminum, and calcium; and concomitant use of calcium-based phosphate binders, vitamin K antagonists, and heparin (Wollina, 2013).

Calcific uremic arteriolopathy lesions are characterized by induration, necrotic tissue, and a violaceous discoloration (see Plate 65). A significant feature of this condition is severe pain that is refractory to common analgesics. Initially, the lesions are serpiginous, indurated plaques with surrounding pallor or ecchymosis. The lesions progress to subcutaneous nodules and ulcerations that eventually become gangrenous. The distribution of CUA lesions is usually bilateral and symmetric. A proximal distribution pattern (trunk, thighs, upper arms) of CUA and nonuremic CUA is associated with a 50% to 70% mortality rate (Alavi et al, 2010). In contrast, distal calciphylaxis is associated with a 10% mortality rate. A distinctive finding with calciphylaxis is intact peripheral pulses because blood flow distal to or deeper than the necrosis remains intact. This clinical assessment is critical in distinguishing the disease from other forms of peripheral vascular disease. No blood tests are available to confirm the diagnosis of calciphylaxis.

Tissue biopsy is critical for an accurate diagnosis of CUA despite the potential for worsening of the ulcers after biopsy (Tang et al, 2012). Histologically, the smooth muscle cells of the vascular wall develop into osteoidlike cells (Wolliner, 2013). These calcifications precipitate a narrowing of the lumen and hyperplasia. The combination of microvascular calcification of the media layer and hyperplasia within the intima of arterioles with a diameter of approximately 0.04 to 0.1 mm is considered a histologic marker for calciphylaxis. These findings assist in differentiating this disease from peripheral arterial occlusion.

Nonuremic calciphylaxis with a proximal distribution occurs primarily on the upper and inner thighs, abdomen, and breasts (Hafner et al, 2010). It is hypothesized that hypertension, diabetes typical of metabolic syndrome, and morbid obesity are the initiating factors. Additional factors that may precipitate nonuremic calciphylaxis are protein C or S deficiency, antithrombin III deficiency, and systemic corticosteroid therapy (Wollina, 2013).

Treatment of calciphylaxis is neither universally standardized nor necessarily effective (Malabu et al, 2012). The high mortality occurs primarily from multiple end organ disease due to ischemia and infarction. Prompt recognition and treatment yield the best results. Systemically, normalization of abnormal calcium and phosphorus levels is warranted. Therapy includes intensified hemodialysis with noncalcium/nonaluminum phosphate binders, sodium thiosulfate, cinacalcet, hyperbaric oxygen therapy, and parathyroidectomy (Malabu et al, 2012). Sodium thiosulfate (administered by either IV or intraperitoneal infusion) acts as a chelator of cations, converting the insoluble tissue deposits of cations (e.g., calcium) into more soluble cations (Rogers and Coates, 2008). Antibiotics should be given to treat wound infection and prevent sepsis. Historically, most individuals who develop calciphylaxis require limb amputation and reconstructive surgery.

Topical wound management should address specific wound needs: fill dead space, provide a physiologic environment, and absorb exudate. Aggressive debridement and skin grafting are indicated to reduce the potential for wound infection; increased patient survival has been reported with aggressive early debridement (Malabu et al, 2012; Rogers and Coates, 2008; Wallina, 2013). The severity of wound-related pain should be assessed regularly, and control measures for pain should be implemented routinely and during wound procedures.

MARTORELL HYPERTENSIVE ISCHEMIC LEG ULCER

Another type of metabolic ulcer with an ischemic subcutaneous arteriolosclerosis etiology is known as Martorell hypertensive ischemic leg ulcer (HYTILU). Because the manifestations of the HYTILU are quite similar to CUA, nonuremic calciphylaxis, and PG, they may be misdiagnosed as one of these conditions or as necrotizing leukocytoclastic vasculitis. An accurate diagnosis is, however, essential to avoid harmful and detrimental treatments. Table 30-3 presents common differential diagnoses for HYTILU.

TABLE 30-3 Common Differential Diagnoses for Hypertensive Ischemic Leg Ulcer

Cause	Common Location	Clinical Characteristics	Pain	Association	Tests
Venous	Middle malleolus Lateral malleolus/ lower gaiter area	Shallow, granulation tissue base Serpiginous margin Woody fibrosis Venous varicosities Pitting edema Hyperpigmentation	+	Varicose veins Previous surgery Deep vein thrombosis Obesity Multiple pregnancy	Venous Doppler to demonstrate incompetent valves; superficial perforator, or deep Occasionally venous disease is due to clots or occluded vessels
Arterial	Anterior shin or trauma/infection location	Punched-out, fibrous base Deep ulcer	+++	Smoking Coronary artery disease	Arterial Doppler Computed tomography angiography Magnetic resonance angiography
Martorell	Lateral-dorsal of shin	Shallow, necrotic Rapidly enlarging Deep necrosis Palpable pulses	++++	Hypertension Diabetes	Often normal ankle-brachial index unless coexisting arterial disease Deep wedge biopsy to identify small vessel changes and skin necrosis
Pyoderma gangrenosum	Any location	Rapidly enlarging Rolled (metal gray) border that evolves into a central ulcer	+++	Inflammatory bowel disease Rheumatoid arthritis Myeloproliferative disorders 50% idiopathic	Diagnosis of exclusion: clinical picture/ associations with a skin biopsy to rule out other disorders (i.e., infections, vasculitis)
Vasculitis	Often distal with often symmetric lesions	Palpable purpuric lesions Fixed urticarial/blisters Necrosis, ulceration Usually bilateral	++	Hepatitis C/other infections Connective tissue disorders, drugs, malignancy 50% other organ involvement; common to involve joints, liver/kidney (e.g., Henoch-Schnlein purpura)	Biopsy for regular histology and immunofluorescence C-ANCA P-ANCA
Sickle cell	Medial malleolus	May have central necrosis and scarring with frequent coexisting venous disease or infections	++++	Sickle cell anemia Pulmonary hypertension	Sickle prep Hb electrophoresis
Malignant	Any location	Slow expanding Crusted for squamous cell carcinoma Rolled border and telangiectasia for basal cell carcinoma Pigmented lesion with asymmetry, irregular border, color variability (black, blue, red, white) for melanoma	+	Photodamage Previous osteomyelitis sinus Previous radiotherapy edge or a graft or other area of chronic inflammation	Diagnostic biopsy, >1 biopsy may be necessary to ascertain a diagnosis
Calciphylaxis	Any location	Livedo reticularis–like pattern peripherally that evolves into central necrosis bilateral symmetric	+++	Chronic renal failure and renal impairment or on dialysis Secondary hyperparathyroidism	Biopsy
Vasculopathy	Lower leg	Livedo reticularis of the vascular supply leading to local areas of atrophy and necrosis	++	Abnormal circulating proteins: anticoagulant, cryoglobulins, cold agglutinins	Biopsy Appropriate serum factors

From Alavi A, Mayer D, Hafner J, et al: Martorell hypertensive ischemic leg ulcer: an underdiagnosed entity©, *Adv Skin Wound Care* 25(12):563–572, 2012.

Diagnosis of HYTILU is based on history and clinical presentation and then confirmed with biopsy. Patients with HYTILU have a long history of arterial hypertension. Ulcers are characterized with central necrosis and a progressive inflammatory violaceous border. These necrotic skin ulcers develop on the lateral-dorsal aspect of the leg or the Achilles tendon and may be unilateral or bilateral. Necrosis is full thickness extending to the fascia (Hafner et al, 2010). As with PG and calciphylaxis, the HYTILU is extremely painful with either a spontaneous onset or triggered by minor trauma. Confirmation of HYTILU is obtained when a large, elliptical, deep tissue biopsy (extending to fascia) reveals subcutaneous arteriosclerosis. A shallow punch tissue biopsy, however, will be misleading, in that it will yield a dense neutrophil infiltrate in a necrotic dermis suggestive of PG.

Treatment includes addressing underlying pathology (i.e., blood pressure control) and reducing factors that compromise peripheral perfusion (i.e., smoking cessation, blood glucose control, anticoagulants, vasodilators, and graduated compression therapy). Because of the inherent reduced perfusion with this type of ulcer, it is important to monitor and manage wound bioburden with topical antimicrobials and/or systemic antimicrobials. Surgical excision of necrotic tissue, sometimes requiring repeat debridement, followed by autologous split-thickness grafts is considered the most effective treatment, with an overall healing rate of 91% (Alavai et al, 2012; Hafner et al, 2010). Repeat grafting may be necessary due to the ongoing underlying pathology-induced necrosis along the wound margins (Alavi et al, 2012). Wound pain is significantly decreased with the first graft application. Topical wound care before definitive treatment via grafting should include nontraumatic debridement via autolysis. Despite the known tissue toxicity, application of topical antiseptics such as povidone iodine or polyhexamethylene biguanide is recommended to prevent deep and surrounding infection and the risk of limb-threatening infection (Alavi et al, 2012). Nonocclusive, nonadhesive dressings such as hydrogels, honey, alginates, hydrofibers, and foam are appropriate topical dressings.

EPIDERMOLYSIS BULLOSA

Epidermolysis bullosa (EB) is the name given to a group of similar skin conditions with various defects in the epidermal basement membrane. Manifestations include a tendency to develop blisters and erosions in the skin, and sometimes in mucous membranes, after mild mechanical trauma (Ly and Su, 2008). Epidermolysis bullosa is most often inherited, although there is a noninherited form (EB acquisita). There are many types of EB, and symptoms can range from mild, seasonal blistering to life-threatening skin erosions (Schober-Flores, 2003). Epidermolysis bullosa can affect every epithelial structure in the body, including the eyelids, conjunctivae, corneas, bowels, skin, and gums.

BOX 30-5   Characteristics of Epidermolysis Bullosa by Category

Epidermolysis Bullosa Simplex (EBS)
- Intraepidermal blisters
- Heals without scar formation
- Nails and teeth normal
- Occasional cutaneous blistering
- Autosomal-dominant trait

Junctional Epidermolysis Bullosa (JEB)
- Autosomal-recessive trait
- Blisters form at lamina lucida (between epidermis and basement membrane)
- Several subtypes with distinct clinical manifestations

Recessive Dystrophic Epidermolysis Bullosa (RDEB)
- Dystrophic scarring is distinctive feature that serves as clinical marker
- Separation at basement membrane zone deep to basement membrane
- Recessive inheritance
- Blister formation results from even minimal mechanical trauma
- Blisters may be hemorrhagic
- Blisters eventually rupture to form slow-to-heal superficial ulcers that continue to be exposed to minimal mechanical trauma
- Healing always involves scarring, so skin has atrophic and wrinkled appearance
- Elbows, knees, hands, feet are sites of repeated trauma
- Predisposes patient to squamous cell cancer

Dominant Dystrophic Epidermolysis Bullosa (DDEB)
- Formation of blisters below basement membrane
- Autosomal-dominant inheritance
- Trauma-induced blisters form at birth or shortly thereafter
- Blisters heal with scar formation but usually are less extensive than in recessive form
- Predisposes patient to squamous cell cancer

Inherited EB is rare, affecting 100,000 people, mostly children (Pillay, 2008). It is classified as one of three types: EB simplex, junctional EB, or dystrophic EB. At least 23 distinctive phenotypes of EB have been identified. Differences between the three types are based on ultrastructural levels of the skin within which the blisters develop. Immunofluorescence or electron microscopic studies of skin specimens are most reliable in establishing the diagnosis. Distinctive characteristics of EB are listed in Box 30-5.

Extracutaneous manifestations—gastrointestinal, ophthalmologic (corneal abrasions and ulcerations), skeletal (osteoporosis due to decreased weight bearing), genitourinary (obstructive uropathy, immunoglobulin A nephropathy), and cardiac—are common. Chronic anemia may be present due to blood loss from open wounds and poor nutritional intake (Pillay, 2008). The severity of these manifestations varies with the category of EB and the subtype within that category. Gastrointestinal complications are a major source of symptoms and morbidity for all EB patients. The most severe problems are associated with the oropharynx, esophagus, and proximal gut. The simple use of eating utensils and the passage of foods result in the formation of bullae that rupture, erode, and heal with scar formation. Strictures are inevitable, and nutritional problems develop.

Anemia is another major problem with EB and is multifactorial in origin. Poor nutrition resulting from painful oral blisters and esophageal strictures precipitates a deficiency in iron, trace metals, and protein, which contributes to anemia. Protein and blood are also lost through the chronic skin lesions typical of junctional EB and dystrophic EB.

The patient with EB is deprived of an epidermal barrier to bacterial invasion. *S. aureus* and other pathogens often colonize the chronic, nonhealing wound. Sepsis is a serious complication, especially in infants. Judicious use of topical antibiotics is warranted to decrease bacterial flora and minimize the risk of soft tissue infection. Silver sulfadiazine cream is contraindicated in newborns younger than 8 weeks because of the increased risk for kernicterus (Caldwell-Brown et al, 1992). Topical antibiotics should not be used as a lubricating ointment because they are for use with open lesions only. In the presence of cellulitis, systemic antibiotics are required

(Marinkovich and Pham, 2009). Close monitoring of lesions and bacteriologic studies are imperative.

The primary objective in the care of patients with EB is promoting healing and preventing trauma (Pillay, 2008; Schober-Flores, 2003). Nursing considerations include wound care, nutrition, education, pain control, and social support. Wound-healing ability is often compromised in patients due to malnutrition, anemia, increased wound bioburden, and loss of protective functions of the skin (Pillay, 2008). Special precautions to minimize cutaneous trauma during select clinical procedures are listed in Table 30-4. Interventions such as the routine use of convoluted foam on pad rails, sheepskin, an air-fluidized support surface, and joint protectors are important. Low-adherence foam dressings or thin hydrocolloids may be appropriate for protecting the patient's hands or feet. However, if these dressings are used, they should be left in place and allowed to fall off rather than being removed and reapplied on a regular basis.

There is no single approach to wound care for managing EB lesions; rather, interventions should strive to achieve key objectives: containing exudate, avoiding trauma, preventing infection, and maintaining a moist environment (Denyer, 2010; Schober-Flores, 2003). Only nonadherent dressings should be used, and they should be secured with roll gauze, tubular gauze, or a stockinette. Fenestrated, nonadherent

TABLE 30-4 Special Precautions to Minimize Cutaneous Trauma to Patients with Dystrophic Epidermolysis Bullosa During Select Clinical Procedures

Procedure	Suggestions
Blood pressure monitoring	Apply dressing under blood pressure cuff.
Electrocardiogram monitoring	Use nonadhesive plastic film (e.g., Omiderm, which does not interfere with electrical conduction) as a barrier between patient's skin and adhesive of electrode pads.
Urine collections (young children)	Wring out cloth diaper; do not apply urine bags containing adhesives.
Blood drawing	To cleanse skin, allow alcohol or Betadine swab to remain in place for 5 min without rubbing; place tourniquet over padding to protect skin; or apply direct pressure on vein using thumb in parallel position to skin.
Parenteral therapy	Cut piece of extra-thin hydrocolloid dressing into horseshoe shape and put dressing with adhesive backing side in contact with skin. Start intravenous (IV) line between legs of horseshoe bandage and tape tubing onto dressing. Secure IV with roller gauze, or place snug-fitting piece of tube gauze (e.g., Bandnet) on extremity adjacent to IV and secure with tape to tube gauze.
Preoperative preparations (operating room, table, surgical drapes, surgical scrubs)	Operating room table should be well padded. Sheepskin covered by table-sized burn pad (e.g., Exu-Dry, which has double layer of meshed material to minimize friction) is advised. If positioning with pillows is necessary for patient with joint contractures, place Exu-Dry pad between pillow and patient's skin.
	Place sterile sheets of nonadherent mesh (e.g., Exu-Dry Mesh, N-Terface) under sterile drapes to protect exposed skin from friction. Fold mesh over edge of drape and secure with clamps. Adhesive drapes are contraindicated.
	Apply antimicrobial solution to surgical site and allow to remain on skin for 5 minutes, then irrigate to rinse. Repeat this process three times.
Mask-delivered anesthesia	Protect skin on face from possible shearing by using nonadherent foam, which adheres to any damp surface and is easily removed by rewetting; or apply copious amount of petrolatum to face before applying mask.

From Caldwell-Brown D, Gibbons S, Reid M: Nursing aspects of Epidermolysis bullosa: a comprehensive approach. In Lin AN, Carter DM, editors: *Epidermolysis bullosa: basic and clinical aspects,* New York, 1992, Springer Verlag.

dressings can be used so that wound moisture can pass through the fenestrations and be trapped by the cover dressing. Ointments can be applied over the fenestrated layer when trying to reduce wound bioburden. Creative dressing techniques often are necessary for difficult locations, such as the digits or face, particularly to prevent fusion of digits (Denyer, 2010). To avoid sensitization, the use of topical antibiotics is not recommended in the absence of very strong evidence of an infection. When infection is suspected (i.e., presence of increased drainage, odor, or wound pain), antimicrobial dressings (silver or Iodosorb) are appropriate. Vesicles or bullae should be lanced and drained to prevent extension through defectively bound skin layers (Denyer, 2010; Pillay, 2008). Temporary skin substitutes and bioengineered skin hold a great deal of promise for this dangerous disease. Clinical trials also are under way to investigate the therapeutic potential of bone marrow or cord blood transplantation for EB, and results thus far are encouraging (Kiuru et al, 2010; Wagner et al, 2009).

Pruritus is a common problem with EB and is the source of new blister formation and breakdown of healing wounds (Pillay, 2008). Moisturizers (e.g., emollients) and oral antipruritics are often indicated. Atrophic scarring and contractures are common and result in fusion of digits (i.e., mitten deformity or pseudosyndactyly), which requires repeat surgical release of contractures (Fine et al, 2005). Additional complications include squamous cell cancer, which is almost inevitable, so constant monitoring with aggressive skin surveillance is essential (Pillay, 2008). Additional information about this disease is available from the Dystrophic Epidermolysis Bullosa Research Association of America (DebRA, http://www.debra.org).

EXTRAVASATION

The role of the wound care specialist in caring for the patient with an extravasation is to provide consultation in the management of the resulting wound. The initial necessary interventions immediately following extravasation of a chemotherapeutic agent are provided by the oncology staff as guided by best evidence (Sauerland et al, 2006; Wickham et al, 2006). Therefore the wound care specialist is not expected to be familiar with each medication, irritant potential, or immediate postextravasation intervention specific to each medication. However, the wound care specialist may be consulted for wound management once tissue damage is evident. This section will address risk factors, prevention, assessment, and treatment of extravasation injury.

Extravasation is the inadvertent leakage of a drug or solution into surrounding tissue (Sauerland et al, 2006). It generates a reaction in the surrounding tissues that ranges from swelling to an inflammatory reaction and irritation to tissue necrosis (Polovich et al, 2005). In most situations, leakage of IV fluids or medications into surrounding tissues is innocuous. The spectrum of cutaneous reactions depends on whether the

solution that leaked is a nonvesicant, an irritant, or a vesicant. Nonvesicant extravasation creates swelling but no tissue damage. An irritant solution induces an inflammatory reaction but no persistent tissue damage. Nonpharmacologic interventions, such as elevation and applying either cold or warm cloths, are sufficient to reduce swelling and discomfort.

In contrast, extravasation of a vesicant results in blistering and progressive tissue destruction. Vesicants may be nonantineoplastic agents (hyperosmolar solutions, vasopressor agents, antibiotics), but most commonly are antineoplastic agents (Table 30-5). Vesicants cause tissue damage by either binding to DNA within cells or interfering with mitosis. When the vesicant binds with DNA and the cells die, the drug is released into surrounding tissue and binds to more DNA. This process repeats a chain of events such that the area of tissue damage continues to widen. The vesicant then interferes with mitosis, causes tissue damage, and results in cell death but to a lesser degree than expected with DNA-binding chemicals. It is important for the wound specialist to be aware of the potential for significant local reactions caused by nonantineoplastic agents because these medications are administered to many patients in a variety of health care settings.

The incidence of extravasations with antineoplastic infusions ranges from 0.1% to 6% of peripheral infusions and 0.3% to 4.7% of implanted venous access port infusions (Sauerland et al, 2006). This discrepant incidence probably reflects the challenges in measuring the incidence of extravasation. The extent of tissue damage is determined by several factors: drug concentration, amount infiltrated, duration of tissue exposure, extravasation site, and timeliness of post extravasation intervention. Ulcer formation at the extravasation site of a cytotoxic agent may be delayed for several days or weeks as a result of diffusion of the drug into adjacent

TABLE 30-5	Common Vesicants	
DNA-Binding Agents	**Non–DNA-Binding Agents**	**Nonantineoplastic Vesicants**
Anthracycline Agents	**Vinca Alkaloids**	Hyperosmotic solutions
Doxorubicin	Vincristine	Concentrated electrolyte solutions
Daunorubicin	Vinblastine	Agents altering intracellular pH (sodium bicarbonate)
Idarubicin	Vindesine	
Mitoxantrone	Vinorelbine	
Antitumor Antibiotics	**Taxane Agents**	Vasopressors
Mitomycin	Paclitaxel	Phenytoin
Bleomycin	Docetaxel	Aminophylline
Doxorubicin		Mannitol
Alkylating Agents		Chloramphenicol
		Nafcillin
Mechlorethamine		Oxacillin
Platinum analogs		Vancomycin

tissue. Subsequent tissue damage and the formation of slough will progress over several weeks and months (see Plate 66).

Prevention

One of the most important steps in preventing extravasation is patient education so that the patient is aware of the signs and symptoms to report and the risk of extravasation, particularly when receiving antineoplastic medications. With patient education, patients are empowered to help prevent and detect harmful extravasation. Guidelines to prevent extravasation developed by the Oncology Nursing Society further emphasize the value of patient education (Polovich et al, 2005; Smith, 2009).

Recognizing patients at risk for extravasation, along with the risk profile of the medications, can signal the need for precautions that will decrease the occurrence of extravasation injuries. All departments in which vesicants are given must have written guidelines for handling vesicant agents, procedures to detect and treat acute extravasation, and an extravasation kit that contains all the necessary materials and drugs for treating extravasation should it occur (Polovich et al, 2005).

Factors that place a patient at risk for extravasation are patient factors, agent-related factors, clinician factors, and device-related factors (Box 30-6) (Ener et al, 2004; Sauerland et al, 2006). Age, both young and old, is recognized as one of the most significant risk factors because of the condition of blood vessels and skin structure. Any condition that masks inflammation will similarly mask the early warning signs of pending extravasation (e.g., pain and erythema) and therefore make the patient more vulnerable to extravasation (e.g., the patient who is immunosuppressed). In addition, erythema is difficult to identify in darkly pigmented skin, and pain is difficult to identify in infants and individuals with paralysis or impaired communication.

Assessment

Prevention of extravasation injuries includes a thorough assessment of the patient, the venous access, and related risk factors and knowledge of the vesicant potential of the drug. Vesicant agents should be given only through a newly established line. Infusions should be halted at the first sign of discomfort, altered infusion flow, lack of blood return, or local reaction.

During administration of vesicants, the injection site must be monitored closely for sudden swelling, stinging, burning, palpable subcutaneous fluid, bleb formation, pain, and redness. Induration, or obvious ulcer formation, is not an immediate manifestation, and visual inspection cannot determine the potential for or extent of tissue impairment (Polovich et al, 2005). Lack of blood return may suggest extravasation but alone is not always an indicator. Because extravasation can occur without symptoms, periodic reassessment of the injection site after completion of the infusion is warranted. Late indicators of extravasation include localized erythema, inflammation, blanching, induration, vesicle formation, ulceration, and tissue sloughing. However, tissue damage and sloughing may continue for up to 6 months (Froiland, 2007).

Extravasation must be distinguished from other local reactions, such as venous flare and recall. Venous flare is a self-limiting, localized hypersensitivity response that involves the development of an erythematous streak along the course of the vein with pruritus, patchy erythema, and/or urticaria. Venous flare occurs in approximately 3% of antineoplastic agent infusions, does not have the serious sequelae of extravasations, and disappears within 30 minutes (Polovich et al, 2005).

Interventions

Early intervention after extravasation can lessen the severity of tissue injury. It is estimated that one third of all extravasations will produce ulceration in the absence of therapy (Ener et al, 2004). Treatment of extravasation of chemotherapy or biotherapy agents should be guided by best evidence (Polovich et al, 2005; Wickham et al, 2006, 2007). Standard interventions are as follows: (1) disconnect the IV tubing from the IV device; (2) leave the needle in place; (3) attach a 1- to 3-ml syringe to the IV device and aspirate residual drug from the IV; (4) avoid pressure on the site; (5) apply cold or heat (depending on the extravasant) as indicated by published evidence and institutional policy; and (6) elevate the involved extremity for 24 hours (Polovich et al, 2005).

Antidotes for the extravasation of cytotoxic agents are used to neutralize the chemicals in the tissues. The use of

---

BOX 30-6   Risk Factors for Extravasation Injury

Patient Factors
- Impaired ability to communicate pain (confusion, debilitation)
- Age (very young or old)
- Inadequate veins
- Compromised circulation

Agent-Related Factors
- Vesicant potential
- Volume infiltrated
- Concentration
- Repeated use of same vein for administration of vesicant

Device-Related Factors
- Inadequately secured intravenous needle or catheter
- Undesirable intravenous site location (antecubital fossa, dorsum of hand)
- Metal needles and large-gauge catheters for peripheral access sites

Clinician-Related Factors
- Knowledge
- Skill
- Interruptions or distractions

antidotes is largely empirical, although guidelines are available through the Oncology Nursing Society (Polovich et al, 2005; Schulmeister 2009). Manufacturers may be a source of recommendations for the medications they offer. The U.S. Food and Drug Administration (FDA) has approved one drug specifically for extravasations: Totect (dexaroxane), which is administered as an IV infusion into anthracycline extravasations. Hyaluronidase and sodium thiosulfate are often used as antidotes, but are not approved by the FDA for this use (Schulmeister, 2009). Other antidotes have been reported in the literature (topical dimethylsulfoxide, granulocyte-macrophage colony-stimulating factor, dexrazoxane), but evidence is limited (Schulmeister, 2009; Wickham et al, 2006). Hyaluronidase is also an antidote for several antibiotics, total parenteral nutrition, calcium, potassium, and high-concentration dextrose. Additional interventions that have been used include making stab incisions in the involved tissue, flushing with normal saline, and placing drains (Wickham et al, 2006).

Topical Wound Care. During follow-up, the site should be monitored closely for 24 hours, then at 1 week, 2 weeks, and as indicated for pain, redness, swelling, ulceration, and necrosis. Depending on the patient's overall health and immune status, more frequent monitoring of the site may be needed if necrosis and ulceration develop. A referral to a plastic surgeon may be warranted if a large volume of vesicant was extravasated or the area and depth of tissue damage were significant (Polovich et al, 2005). However, routine surgical excision is not warranted because not all vesicant extravasations will cause tissue ulceration (Polovich et al, 2005; Wickham et al, 2006). Surgical debridement may be indicated for extensive tissue damage or overwhelming infection. Surgical intervention, such as skin grafting, often is necessary to achieve wound closure (Polovich et al, 2005; Wickham et al, 2006).

Topical care of extravasation wounds should be dictated by the characteristics of the wound. Key objectives for topical care include absorption of exudate, removal of nonviable tissue, prevention of infection, elimination of dead space, and pain management. As the extent of tissue damage is revealed, the characteristics of the wound will change and the local wound care choices will require modification. The area should be protected from shear and trauma; a transparent dressing can be applied to protect the intact surrounding skin (Froiland, 2007). Hydrogels or hyperosmolar gauze can be used to promote autolysis of slough and necrotic tissue.

Documentation and close follow-up with appropriate consultations are highly recommended. Photographic documentation of the extravasation may be mandated by institutional policy. It is important to record the date and time of the infusion, when extravasation was noted, the size and type of catheter, the drug and amount of drug administered, and the estimated amount of extravasated solution (Polovich et al, 2005; Wickham et al, 2006).

IMMUNE REACTIONS

Toxic Epidermal Necrolysis

Toxic epidermal necrosis is a rare but severe exfoliating disorder characterized by epidermal sloughing at the dermal–epidermal junction. Up to 80% of TEN is caused by a reaction to medication (Poulson et al, 2013) (see Plate 68). Milder variants include erythema multiforme and Stevens-Johnson syndrome (SJS). The Severe Cutaneous Adverse Reaction (SCAR) classification system (Box 30-7) differentiates SJS from TEN based on total body surface area (TBSA) affected. Stevens-Johnson syndrome involves less than 10% of TBSA, whereas TEN involves greater than 30% of TBSA. From 10% to 30% of TBSA affected is described as *SJS/TEN overlap* (French, 2006; Garra and Turner, 2009). Based on seven known adverse prognostic factors, the SCORe of Toxic Epidermal Necrosis (SCORTEN) severity of illness scale (Table 30-6) is used to stratify severity of illness and predict mortality of TEN (Endorf et al, 2008; Harr & French, 2012; Trent et al, 2004). The average mortality of SJS is 1% to 5%, whereas the average mortality of TEN is 25% to 35% (Harr and French, 2012). Death usually results from overwhelming sepsis.

Both SJS and TEN are characterized by epidermal detachment. Mucosal tissue is also affected in greater than 90% of patients with TEN. The lesions affect the mouth, eyes, respiratory tract, and genitourinary tract and tend to be very

---

BOX 30-7 Severe Cutaneous Adverse Reaction (SCAR) Classification System

Erythema Multiforme (EM)
- Typically round targets with three different zones and well-defined borders
- Most prominent on distal portions of extremities (acral distribution)
- Less than 1% of total body surface area involved

Stephens-Johnson Syndrome (SJS)
- Widespread, irregularly shaped, erythematous or purpuric macules
- Blistering occurs on all or part of macule
- Confluence of lesions and epidermal detachment is limited, involving less than 10% of total body surface area

Overlap SJS and Toxic Epidermal Necrolysis (TEN)
- Same as SJS
- 10% to 29% of body surface area involved

TEN "With Spots"
- Blisters become more confluent, resulting in detachment of epidermis and erosions on greater than 30% of total body surface area
- Mucosal surfaces usually involved

TEN "Without Spots"
- Widespread, large, erythematous areas with no discrete lesions (macules or blisters)
- Epidermal detachment involves greater than 10% of total body surface area

TABLE 30-6   SCORTEN Clinical Scoring System for Predicting Outcome in Toxic Epidermal Necrolysis

Clinical–Biologic Parameter	INDIVIDUAL SCORE	
	Yes	No
Age >40 years	1	0
Malignancy	1	0
Tachycardia (>120/min)	1	0
Initial surface of epidermal detachment >10%	1	0
Serum urea >10 mmol/L	1	0
Serum glucose >14mmo/L	1	0
Bicarbonate <20 mmol/L	1	0

SCORTEN (Sum of Individual Scores)	Predicted Mortality (%)
0–1	3.2
2	12.1
3	35.3
4	58.3
≥5	90

From Bastuji-Garin S, Fouchard N, Bertocchi M, et al: SCORTEN: a severity-of-illness score for toxic epidermal necrolysis, *J Invest Dermatol* 115:149–153, 2000.

painful. Mucosal tissue is much less common with SJS. Both SJS and TEN occur in adults and children.

Toxic epidermal necrosis is a T-cell–mediated immune reaction similar to graft-versus-host disease (GVHD) (Endorf et al, 2008). The epidermal necrolysis that occurs appears to be an immune-mediated reaction against epithelial cells involving T cells, cytotoxic reactions, and delayed hypersensitivity (Poulson et al, 2013). The most common medications associated with SJS and TEN are antibiotics and anticonvulsants, but more than 100 drugs, including oxicam, NSAIDs, allopurinol, antiretroviral medications, and corticosteroids, also are associated with this condition (Endorf et al, 2008; Garra and Turner, 2009). Of the antibiotics, sulfonamides are most strongly associated with SJS/TEN; aminopenicillins, quinolones, cephalosporins, tetracyclines, and imidazole antifungals have also been identified (French, 2006). Less commonly, herpes virus, hepatitis A, immunizations, and bone marrow or solid organ transplantation have been associated with TEN (Garra and Turner, 2009). Cutaneous manifestations typically appear within 1 to 4 weeks after starting the medication (Poulson et al, 2013). Within hours the skin becomes painful.

Shortly before clinical skin manifestations (1 to 3 days), the patient may experience a phase of fever and malaise resembling a viral illness. Generalized erythema and macules initially appear on the trunk and then spread to the neck, face, and upper arms. The palms and soles can be affected. An irregularly shaped erythematous, dark-red, or purpuric macular rash typically develops, and the macules gradually coalesce. Mucosal manifestations may include sloughing of stratified epithelium in the upper respiratory tract, mouth, vagina, anal canal, and eyes. These mucosal lesions in conjunction with the macular rash are strongly suspicious of TEN (French, 2006). As epidermal involvement progresses, the macular lesions take on a translucent gray hue that can occur either rapidly (hours) or over several days. As the epidermis necroses, it begins to separate from the dermis, and the macular lesions evolve into flaccid blisters. Slight thumb pressure applied to intact skin next to blisters causes the skin to wrinkle and slide laterally, which indicates a positive Nikolsky sign (top layers of skin slip away from lower layers when slightly rubbed). Although not specific to TEN, a positive Nikolsky sign is a hallmark sign for TEN (Endorf et al, 2008; Garra and Turner, 2009). Large sheets of skin are sloughed, exposing fragile, bleeding dermis.

Punch biopsies from the border of intact epidermis surrounding bullous lesions are needed to make the TEN diagnosis. Necrosis of the epidermis is an essential component in making the definitive diagnosis (Endorf et al, 2008). The differential diagnosis for TEN includes distinction from SSSS, which is distinguished by skin biopsy, and GVHD of the skin, which is distinguished by history.

Treatment of the patient with TEN requires prompt cessation of suspicious medications and supportive care (Endorf et al, 2008). The standard of care for the patient with TEN is transfer to a burn center to best manage the complex and life-threatening complications, such as temperature regulation, electrolyte disturbances, significant nutrition needs, and propensity to wound or skin infections (Endorf et al, 2008; Poulson et al, 2013; Smith, 2007). Delay in transfer of patients to a burn center has been associated with increased mortality (Endorf et al, 2008). In general, systemic corticosteroids are not recommended, enteral rather than parenteral nutrition is recommended, IV administration of immunoglobulin-G may be beneficial but should be sucrose free, empiric prophylactic antibiotics are not recommended, and ophthalmologic consultation to manage ocular manifestations of TEN is recommended (Endorf et al, 2008).

The goal of wound care is preventing infection so that the epithelial cells can resurface the exposed dermis. Sloughed epidermis can be debrided, but a temporary skin substitute (biologic or biosynthetic) or antimicrobial dressings (silver or antibiotic impregnated) should be applied to exfoliated areas; these are discussed in detail in Chapter 19. Sulfa-based topical antibiotics are contraindicated because sulfonamides are strongly associated with TEN.

Graft-versus-Host Disease

After allogeneic bone marrow transplantation (bone marrow from another individual), the transferred immunocompetent cells have the potential to produce a severe reaction in the transplant patient. Clinically, acute GVHD occurs early after transplantation (<100 days). Chronic GVHD occurs 100 days after transplantation. Risk factors that predispose the bone marrow transplantation patient to GVHD include recipient age (>40 years), recipient history of blood transfusions, the conditioning regimen, the prophylaxis protocol, and the number of T cells infused (Alcoser and Burchett, 1999; Sullivan, 1999).

Graft-versus-host disease affects the skin, gut, and liver. It is a clinical diagnosis that cannot be confirmed by laboratory findings (Antin and Deeg, 2005). In the skin, cutaneous manifestations include a maculopapular rash that usually begins on the palms and then spreads to the face, arms, shoulders, and ears (see Plate 69). These manifestations may be asymptomatic, pruritic, or painful. In severe cases, generalized erythema, bullae, and desquamation may be present. Graft-versus-host disease may have the appearance of SSSS, a drug reaction, or TEN. A skin biopsy is beneficial to differentiate among these three possibilities (Antin and Deeg, 2005; Sullivan, 1999).

Treatment of GVHD requires a combination of immunosuppressant and antiviral medications. To stimulate adequate neutrophil levels with these treatment regimens, granulocyte-colony–stimulating factor is also given. Topical wound care requires attention to infection control, maintenance of a physiologic wound environment, and pain management. Adhesive occlusive dressings are seldom desirable. Topical wound management should be determined collaboratively with input and discussion from the marrow transplantation team. More detailed information about this disease is available from additional resources (Ferrara et al, 2005; Ringden, 2005; Thomas et al, 1999). Increasing use of autologous bone marrow stem cells for treatment of cancer patients after lethal irradiation is greatly reducing the incidence of GVHD.

FROSTBITE

Frostbite is a cold-related injury resulting from prolonged exposure to subfreezing temperatures. Skin can freeze at 28°F (−2°C) when no wind is present (Mohr et al, 2009). Wind decreases the amount of time required for skin to freeze. For example, exposed skin freezes within 1 hour when the temperature is 0°F (−18°C) and the wind is 10 mph. However, the skin will freeze in only 30 minutes at the same temperature when the wind is 20 mph. Therefore heat loss is accelerated by wind speed, a concept known as *wind chill temperature.* A wind chill temperature of −40°F will result in tissue freezing within minutes (Mohr et al, 2009). In general, frostbite is a condition of morbidity, not mortality. However, when frostbite is combined with hypothermia or wound-related sepsis, death is possible.

Risk factors for frostbite are listed in Box 30-8. The majority of frostbite patients are male (80%), and 20% have been reported to be homeless (Mohr et al, 2009). Not all cold exposure results in tissue freezing (i.e., frostbite). The spectrum of cold injury is given in Table 30-7.

Extent of tissue damage is influenced by several factors: (1) susceptibility of specific body tissues to cold; (2) rate of cooling; (3) lowest tissue temperature achieved; (4) duration of cold exposure; (5) duration of ischemia; and (6) rewarming condition (Mohr et al, 2009; Twomey et al, 2005). Although skin freezes more quickly with lower temperatures, the speed

---

BOX 30-8 Risk Factors for Frostbite

- Intoxication (alcohol or drugs decrease awareness of cold and impair judgment; alcohol inhibits shivering and causes cutaneous vasodilation)
- Psychiatric illness (e.g., individuals with schizophrenia may have impaired ability to assess tissue cooling or comprehend cold injury)
- Neuropathy
- People who are inexperienced with or new to cold climates
- Homelessness
- Individuals stranded in the cold
- Cold-weather rescuers, soldiers, people who work in the cold
- Winter and high-altitude athletes
- Use of nicotine or other vasoconstrictive drugs
- Inadequate or constrictive clothing
- Underlying conditions (e.g., malnutrition, infection, peripheral vascular disease, atherosclerosis, arthritis, diabetes, thyroid disease, previous cold injury)

TABLE 30-7 Spectrum of Cold Injury

Frostnip	Mild cold injury
	Completely reversible
	Skin pallor, numbness
	Typical on face, hands
	No ice crystal formation, no tissue damage
	Warmed tissue becomes hyperemic; decreased sensation or tingling may persist for weeks
Chilblain (Pernio)	Results from repeated exposure to near-freezing temperatures
	No ice crystal formation
	Skin has violaceous color with plaques or nodules
	May experience pain and pruritus with cold exposure
	Usually located on face, anterior lower leg, hands, feet
Frostbite	Occurs when tissues freeze slowly and form extracellular ice crystals
	Injuries are circumferential and progress distal to proximal
	Potentially reversible
Flash freeze	Extremely rapid cooling and formation of intracellular ice crystals
	Mechanism is contact with cold metals (handles) or volatile liquids
	Rapid onset, almost never circumferential

---

of freezing does not affect the degree of irreversible damage; rather, the extent of damage is related to the length of time the tissue remained frozen. Ultimately, tissue damage occurs as a result of tissue freezing and tissue reperfusion (Mohr et al, 2009; Murphy et al, 2000).

When freezing is slow (as occurs with frostbite), *extra*cellular ice crystals are formed; when freezing is quick (as occurs with flash freeze injury), *intra*cellular and *extra*cellular crystals are formed, and cells lyse. Flash freeze injuries occur after contact with cold surfaces or volatile liquids. Cellular damage, vascular injury, and resulting thrombosis are key mechanisms in the pathophysiologic process of frostbite injury (Twomey et al, 2005).

Rapid rewarming is recommended because it results in less irreversible damage to the tissue. Blood flow is restored quickly, without vasospasm or clot formation. Within 20 minutes, venous stasis develops and progresses retrograde through the capillary bed to the arterioles. When arterial inflow to the capillary bed is unchanged, edema develops. Rapid rewarming results in less irreversible damage to the extremity, despite the inevitable vascular permeability and edema (Mohr et al, 2009). During the ensuing reperfusion, the damaged endothelial lining of the affected blood vessels releases inflammatory mediators (prostaglandins, thromboxanes, bradykinin, histamine) that cause additional edema formation. Ischemic injury to the affected tissue is progressive as a result of (1) capillary compression from increasing edema; (2) stagnation of blood in the vessels; (3) vessel occlusion caused by shedding of damaged endothelium into the blood vessels; and (4) thrombus formation due to the thrombogenic nature of the exposed basement membrane in blood vessels.

Within 6 to 24 hours of rewarming, blisters develop due to the accumulation of extravasated fluid under the detached epidermis. Little or no fluid in the blister implies poor blood flow. Clear blister fluid contains high levels of prostaglandin and thromboxane, which result in vasoconstriction, leukocyte adherence, and platelet aggregation, factors known to intensify dermal ischemia. Blister fluid may also contain blood, which indicates the superficial dermis is damaged and thus more serious tissues damage has occurred than with a clear fluid blister.

Classification of Skin Injury

Initially frozen skin has the same appearance: cold, white, and firm to touch. The digits, ears, nose, and exposed facial skin are the most commonly injured. To classify the severity of the frostbite, the tissue must first thaw, and even then the extent of skin damage will not be apparent for 10 days or more (Mohr et al, 2009). Frostbite injuries can be classified by degree of injury as defined in Table 30-8. Superficial frostbite includes first- and second-degree frostbite injuries, which generally heal. Deep frostbite includes third- and fourth-degree injuries, which are associated with tissue loss and chronic disability. Hemorrhagic bullae located proximally on the limb and distal tissue that remains cold, ischemic, and insensate are indicators of poor prognosis (Mohr et al, 2009).

Management of Frostbite

Similar to burns, treatment of frostbite may occur in a variety of health care settings. The phases or levels of care required

TABLE 30-8	Classification System for Frostbite Injury
Degree of Injury	**Classification**
First	Superficial injury
	Intact sensation
	Normal to hyperemic skin color
	No blister formation on rewarming
	Transient mild burning, stinging, throbbing
	Desquamation but no tissue loss
Second	Superficial injury
	Edema may be substantial
	Blisters filled with clear or milky fluid within 24 hours of injury
Third	Deep injury that results in hemorrhagic blister
	Blood-filled blisters that progress to black eschar over weeks
	Blisters are located deeper in dermis and more proximal
	Skin color is violaceous, soft, or boggy
	Does not blanch to palpation
	Initially no pain, then progresses to shooting, throbbing, and burning pain
Fourth	Results in full-thickness, cyanotic skin appearance
	Full-thickness damage affects muscles, tendons, bone
	Edema forms proximal, not distal, to involved area and becomes line of demarcation between viable tissue and full-thickness infarction
	Distal parts undergo mummification over weeks

for frostbite depend on the severity of the injury. Initial care generally is given at the location at which the injury occurs and addresses life-threatening conditions. Wet clothing should be replaced with dry, soft clothing to minimize further heat loss. The affected area should not be rubbed with warm hands due to risk for further injury. Alcohol or sedatives should not be given because they may enhance heat loss. Rewarming of the affected area should be initiated as soon as possible *unless* there is a danger of refreezing. If refreezing is a risk, get to shelter before attempting to rewarm at the scene. Walking on frostbitten feet can cause tissue chipping or fracture. The affected body part should be wrapped in a blanket for protection during transport.

Emergency department care first addresses life-threatening conditions, such as fluid resuscitation to enhance blood flow and tissue perfusion. Rapid rewarming of the affected body part is attempted using water or wet packs at 40°C to 42°C with a mild antibacterial soap. Warmer temperatures or dry

---

BOX 30-9   Standard Protocol for Frostbite Care

- Rapid rewarming with water at 104°F to 108°F (40°C to 42°C)
- Tetanus prophylaxis
- Narcotic analgesics
- Ibuprofen
- Antibiotics
- Topical aloe vera
- Limb elevation
- No ambulation until edema resolved
- No smoking
- Daily hydrotherapy

Data from Mohr WJ, Jenabzadeh K, Ahrenholz DH: Cold injury, *Hand Clin* 25(4):481–496, 2009.

---

heat should be avoided due to risk for thermal injury. Thawing usually takes 20 to 40 minutes and is complete when the distal tip of the affected area blanches with pressure. Associated dislocations are reduced as soon as thawing is complete. Fractures are managed conservatively until postthaw edema has resolved. The only indication for early surgical intervention is debridement of necrotic tissue and fasciotomy in the case of compartment syndrome. Hemorrhagic blisters are left intact to reduce risk of infection in the injured extremity (Mohr et al, 2009). Once thawed, the injury is kept in sterile nonadherent dressings, elevated, and splinted when possible. Clear fluid blisters usually are aspirated to remove the prostaglandins and thromboxane and thus prevent further dermal damage.

Weeks can pass before frostbitten tissue demarcates to reveal viable and nonviable tissue. Therefore any decision about amputation should be delayed as long as possible. The goals of management for frostbite include salvaging as much tissue as possible, achieving maximal return of function, optimizing nutrition for healing, and preventing sepsis. Box 30-9 gives the standard protocol for frostbite care. Thrombolytic therapy is also used within 24 hours postwarming to correct the underlying pathology (thrombi formation) leading to delayed tissue necrosis. The goals of topical wound care are maintaining a moist wound environment, protecting the skin from further cold-related damage, and reducing bacterial bioburden (Varnado, 2008). Light compression may be used to manage edema. Splints are indicated to maintain proper immobilization of limbs, and range-of-motion exercises prevent long-term contractures. Neuropathic pain is common and challenging to alleviate.

PRIMARY MALIGNANCY AND MALIGNANT TRANSFORMATION WOUNDS (MARJOLIN ULCER)

Malignancies can develop on the skin as a primary malignancy (e.g., an existing malignancy such as lymphoma, sarcoma, squamous cell cancer, ulcerates) or as a malignant transformation in a long-standing wound. In general, malignancies that present as ulcers often go misdiagnosed for a long time because practitioners mistake them for nonmalignant ulcers. An increase in the frequency of skin cancers and the malignant transformation of wounds is anticipated as the population of people who have received a transplant and/or who are immunosuppressed increases (Alexander, 2009; Snyder et al, 2003).

Examples of primary malignant wounds include Kaposi sarcoma, lymphoma, melanoma, basal cell carcinoma (BCC), and SCC. Primary malignant wounds have a rapid onset and develop in many locations of the skin, frequently on sun-exposed areas that have not undergone radiotherapy (Snyder et al, 2003). Basal cell carcinoma arises from the epidermal basal cells and has a very low metastatic potential. Primary squamous cell cancer arises from the keratinizing epidermal cells and can metastasize and grow very quickly.

Conversion of a chronic wound to a malignancy is a slow process; the risk of malignancy increases with the length of time the ulcer has been present. Ulcers present for 20 plus years are susceptible to developing SCC or BCC. Of chronic wounds, 1.7% will undergo malignant degeneration, most commonly SCC. Marjolin originally reported the problem in chronic burn wounds; however, this malignant transformation has also been observed in venous ulcers, pressure ulcers, sinus tracts secondary to osteomyelitis and fistulas, and scar tissue. Among trauma patients, burn patients are at the highest risk for malignant transformation of chronic wounds. Marjolin ulcers present as flat, indolent, white/pearly lesions with indurated and elevated margins (Ethridge et al, 2007). They have a malodorous exudate and can be mistaken for infection. Marjolin ulcers with SCC have a high metastatic potential and require expedient diagnosis and treatment (Tang et al, 2012).

Any clinical cause for suspicion, such as raised borders, unusual wound base, unexplained pain, changes in shape or color, previous history, or family history of skin cancer, requires referral for biopsy. Ulcers or lesions that do not respond to optimal therapy also warrant a referral for biopsy (Snyder et al, 2003). Biopsy technique is critical to cancer detection. It is recommended that wounds be biopsied from multiple sites (i.e., at 12, 6, 3, and 9 o'clock positions) and from multiple depths (e.g., 2, 4, and 6 mm). The biopsy sites should be recorded because rebiopsy is indicated if the wound does not respond as expected to treatment (Snyder, 2006).

BLOOD DYSCRASIAS

Two types of blood dyscrasias may lead to chronic leg ulceration: sickle cell anemia and thalassemia. Their etiologies, ulcer characteristics, and treatments are summarized in Table 30-9.

TABLE 30-9   Characteristics of Skin Lesions with Blood Dyscrasias

Blood Dyscrasia	Pathology	Ulcer Characteristics	Treatment
Sickle cell anemia	Sickled blood cells are rigid May clump together, occluding microcirculation Damage to endothelium leads to thrombus formation Altered vasomotor response can lead to rise in capillary pressure and edema formation	Exact etiology of ulceration is unclear Located on lower leg near malleolus May be single or multiple Can range significantly in size Ulcers are well defined, vary in depth, have raised borders Tend to heal slowly High recurrence rate	Control of edema (compression therapy and/or bed rest) Systemic management of underlying disease process (address anemia either pharmacologically or by transfusion) Debridement Prevention of infection Protection from trauma Pain management Moist wound healing (e.g., with hydrocolloids)
Thalassemia	Microcytic anemia common in people of Mediterranean descent	Etiology related to decreased hemoglobin and increased iron loading, making patients more susceptible to trauma	Blood transfusions and iron chelation therapy Topical care based on wound needs and moist wound healing principles Emphasis on insulating wound to prevent hypothermia Protect wound from further trauma

CLINICAL CONSULT

A: A wound consult is received for a 36-year-old female breast cancer patient with a chemotherapy extravasation of Adriamycin that occurred 5 days earlier. Intravenous administration was immediately stopped when the patient reported stinging and pain in the IV site followed by an inability to obtain a blood return in the IV tubing. Initial care consisted of withdrawing residual chemotherapy, applying ice to the site, and site monitoring. A soft, boggy, necrotic tissue area began developing at the site during the first week. Currently extravasation site on right forearm is erythematous extending 5 cm from puncture site with central island of soft adherent gray-black necrosis measuring 4 cm × 3 cm. Lower arm slightly edematous. Recent WBC in normal limits. Patient reports she has good appetite and is meeting her protein intake needs.

D: Vesicant extravasation resulting from Adriamycin.

P: Implement moist wound therapy with hydrogel to wound bed to aid in autolysis. Monitor closely to reassess erythema and effectiveness of autolysis. Call clinic if erythema increases in intensity or dimension. Will consider adding antimicrobial if erythema persists. Revise topical dressing as wound conditions change following autolysis and consider CTPs as needed for closure.

I: (1) Apply skin protectant around wound bed. (2) Trim hydrogel sheet to size of wound and place over wound. Cover with a nonadherent dressing and secure with roll gauze or nonadherent wrap. (3) Patient instructed to keep arm at chest level to reduce edema and protect wound from pressure, trauma, and extremes in temperature.

E: Return to monitor autolysis in 4 days.

SUMMARY

Although the wound specialist is not expected to be proficient in the overall care of patients with the unusual pathologies described in this chapter, the management of the resulting complex cutaneous wounds requires astute observation, close monitoring, and adherence to the principles of wound healing. As with other chronic wounds, the goals of treatment for these types of wounds range from healing to palliation to symptom management. Collaboration with the multidisciplinary team (medical staff, surgeons, nursing staff, physical therapy, dietitians) is essential to identify these rare complications early during onset and implement interventions that are timely and appropriate to minimize tissue damage and maximize healing.

REFERENCES

Aggarwal S: Recognition and management of pyoderma gangrenosum, *Dermatology* 22(5):26–30, 2012.

Ahronowitz I, Harp J, Shinkai K: Etiology and management of pyoderma gangrenosum: a comprehensive review, *Am J Clin Dermatol* 13(3):191–211, 2012.

Alavi A, Mayer D, Hafner J, et al: Martorell hypertensive ischemic leg ulcer: an underdiagnosed entity, *Adv Skin Wound Care* 25(12):563–572, 2012.

Alcoser PW, Burchett S: Bone marrow transplantation: immune system suppression and reconstitution, *Am J Nurs* 99(6):26–31, 1999.

Alexander S: Malignant fungating wounds: key symptoms and psychosocial issues, *J Wound Care* 18(8):325–329, 2009.

Anaya DA, Dellinger EP: Surgical infections and choice of antibiotics. In Townsend CM Jr, Beauchamp RD, Evers BM, et al, editors: *Sabiston textbook of surgery*, ed 18, Philadelphia, 2007, Saunders, p. 2152.

Anderson I: Mixed aetiology: complexity and comorbidity in leg ulceration, *Br J Nurs* 17(15):S17–S23, 2008.

Antin JH, Deeg HJ: Clinical spectrum of acute graft-vs-host disease. In Ferrara JF, Cooke KR, Deeg HJ, editors: *Graft-vs-host disease*, ed 3, New York, 2005, Marcel Dekker.

Armitage M, Roberts J: Caring for patients with leg ulcers and an underlying vasculitic condition, *Br J Community Nurse Suppl*, S16–S22, 2004.

Attinger CE, Janis JE, Steinberg J, et al: Clinical approach to wounds: debridement and wound bed preparation including the use of dressings and wound-healing adjuvants, *Plast Reconstr Surg* 117(Suppl 7):S72– S109, 2006.

Bastuji-Garin S, Fouchard N, Bertocchi M, et al: SCORTEN: a severity-of-illness score for toxic epidermal necrolysis, *J Invest Dermatol* 115:149–153, 2000.

Brooklyn T, Dunnill G, Probert C: Diagnosis and treatment of pyoderma gangrenosum, *BMJ* 333(7560):181–184, 2006.

Cackovic M, Chung C, Bolton LL, et al: Leg ulceration in the sickle cell patient, *J Am Coll Surg* 187(3):307–309, 1998.

Caldwell-Brown D, Gibbons S, Reid M: Nursing aspects of Epidermolysis bullosa: a comprehensive approach. In Lin AN, Carter DM, editors: *Epidermolysis bullosa: basic and clinical aspects*, New York, 1992, Springer Verlag.

Callen JP, Jackson JM: Pyoderma gangrenosum: an update, *Rheum Dis Clin North Am* 33:787–802, 2007.

Chung C, Cackovic M, Kerstein MD: Leg ulcers in patients with sickle cell disease, *Adv Wound Care* 9(5):46–50, 1996.

Denyer JE: Wound management for children with epidermolysis bullosa, *Dermatol Clin* 28(1):257–264, 2010.

Endorf FE, Cancio LC, Gibran NS: Toxic epidermal necrolysis clinical guidelines, *J Burn Care Res* 29(5):706–712, 2008.

Ener RA, Meglathery SB, Styler M: Extravasation of systemic hemato-oncological therapies, *Ann Oncol* 15:858–862, 2004.

Ethridge RT, et al: Wound healing. In Townsend CM Jr, Beauchamp RD, Evers BM, et al, editors: *Sabiston textbook of surgery*, ed 18, Philadelphia, 2007, Saunders.

Ferrara JF, et al, editors: *Graft-vs-host disease*, ed 3, New York, 2005, Marcel Dekker.

Fine JD, Johnson LB, Weiner M: Pseudosyndactyly and musculoskeletal contractures in inherited epidermolysis bullosa: experience of the National Epidermolysis Bullosa Registry, 1986–2002, *J Hand Surg Br* 30(1):14–22, 2005.

French LE: Toxic epidermal necrolysis and Stevens Johnson syndrome: our current understanding, *Allergol Int* 55(1):9–16, 2006.

Froiland K: Extravasation injuries: implications for WOC nursing, *J Wound Ostomy Continence Nurs* 34(3):299–302, 2007.

Garra GP, Turner ED: *Toxic epidermal necrolysis*, 2009. http://emedicine.medscape.com/article/787323-overview. Accessed January 29, 2010.

Habif TP, Campbell JL Jr, Chapman MS, et al: *Skin disease: diagnosis and treatment*, ed 2, St. Louis, MO, 2005, Mosby.

Hafner J, Keusch G, Wahl C, et al: Uremic small artery disease with medial calcification and intimal hyperplasia (so-called calciphylaxis): a complication of chronic renal failure and benefit from parathyroidectomy, *J Am Acad Dermatol* 33: 954–962, 1995.

Hanley J: Effective management of peristomal pyoderma gangrenosum, *Br J Nurs* 20(7):S12–S17, 2011.

Harr T, French LE: Stevens-Johnson syndrome and toxic epidermal necrolysis, *Chem Immunol Allergy* 97:149–166, 2012.

Hunter JAA, et al: *Clinical dermatology*, Oxford, 2002, Blackwell Science.

Jennette J, Falk R: Small-vessel vasculitis, *N Engl J Med* 337(21): 1512–1523, 1997.

Jeyakumari D, Gopal R, Eswaran M, et al: Staphylococcal scalded skin syndrome in a newborn, *J Glob Infect Dis* 1(1):45–47, 2009.

King RW, de Saint Victor PR: *Staphylococcal scalded skin syndrome*, 2014. http://emedicine.medscape.com/article/788199-overview. Accessed August 18, 2015.

Kiuru M, Itoh M, Cairo MS, et al: Bone marrow stem cell therapy for recessive dystrophic epidermolysis bullosa, *Dermatol Clin* 28(2):371–382, 2010.

Ly L, Su JC: Dressings used in epidermolysis bullosa blister wounds: a review, *J Wound Care* 17(11):482–492, 2008.

Malabu UH, Manickam V, Kan G, et al: Calcific uremic arteriolopathy on multimodal combination therapy: still unmet goal, *Int J Nephrol*, 2012:390768, 2012.

Marinkovich MP, Pham N: *Epidermolysis bullosa*, 2009. http://emedicine.medscape.com/article/1062939-overview. Accessed February 8, 2010.

Martin DA, Nanci GN, Marlowe SI, et al: Necrotizing fasciitis with no mortality or limb loss, *Am Surg* 74(9):809–812, 2008.

Mazzone L, Schiestl C: Management of septic skin necroses, *Eur J Peditar Surg* 23(5):349–358, 2013.

Mohr WJ, Jenabzadeh K, Ahrenholz DH: Cold injury, *Hand Clin* 25(4):481–496, 2009.

Murphy JV, Banwell PE, Roberts AH, et al: Frostbite: pathogenesis and treatment, *J Trauma* 48:171–178, 2000.

Paparone PP, Paparone PW, Paparone P: Post-traumatic pyoderma gangrenosum, *Wounds* 21(4):89–94, 2009.

Park JRC, Choi JR, Song JY, et al: Necrotizing fasciitis of the thigh secondary to radiation colitis in a rectal cancer patient, *J Korean Soc Coloproctol* 28(6):325–329, 2014.

Pillay E: Epidermolysis bullosa. Part 1: causes, presentation and complications, *Br J Nurs* 17(5):292–296, 2008.

Polovich M, White J, Kelleher L: *Chemotherapy and biotherapy guidelines and recommendations for practice*, ed 2, Philadelphia, 2005, Hanley and Belfus.

Poulsen VOB, Nielsen J, Poulsen TD: Rapidly developing toxic epidermal necrolysis, *Case Rep Emerg Med* 2013:985951, 2013.

Ratnagobal S, Sinha S: Pyoderma gangrenosum: guideline for wound practitioners, *J Wound Care* 22(2):68–73, 2013.

Reguiaï A, Grange F: Therapy in pyoderma gangrenosum associated with inflammatory bowel disease, *Am J Clin Dermatol* 8(2): 67–77, 2007.

Rhoads J: Epidemiology of the brown recluse spider bite, *J Am Acad Nurse Pract* 19(2):79–85, 2007.

Ringden O: Introduction to graft-versus-host disease, *Biol Blood Marrow Transplant* 11(Suppl 2):17–20, 2005.

Roenigk H, Young J: Leg ulcers. In Young J, Olin J, Bartholomew J, editors: *Peripheral vascular diseases*, ed 2, St. Louis, MO, 1996, Mosby.

Rogers NM, Coates PTH: Calcific uraemic arteriolopathy: an update, *Curr Opin Nephrol Hypertens* 17:629–634, 2008.

Rubano J, Kerstein M: Arterial insufficiency and vasculitides, *J Wound Ostomy Continence Nurs* 25(3):147, 1998.

Ruocco E, Sangiuliano S, Gravina AG, et al: Pyoderma gangrenosum: an updated review, *J Eur Acad Dermatol Venereol* 23: 1008–1017, 2009.

Sauerland C, Engelking C, Wickham R, et al: Vesicant extravasation part I: mechanisms, pathogenesis, and nursing care to reduce risk, *Oncol Nurs Forum* 33(6):1134–1141, 2006.

Schober-Flores C: Epidermolysis bullosa: the challenges of wound care, *Dermatol Nurse* 15(2):135–138, 141–144, 2003.

Schulmeister L: Vesicant chemotherapy extravasation antidotes and treatments, *Clin J Oncol Nurs* 13(4):395–398, 2009.

Schwartz RA: *Spider envenomation, brown recluse*, 2009. http://www.emedicine.com/DERM/topic598.htm. Accessed June 29, 2009.

Seitz CS, Berens N, Bröcker EB, et al: Leg ulceration in rheumatoid arthritis–an underreported multicausal complication with considerable morbidity: analysis of thirty-six patients and review of the literature, *Dermatology* 220:268–273, 2010.

Smith DB, Ickstadt J, Kucera J: Brown recluse spider bite: a case study, *J Wound Ostomy Continence Nurs* 24(3):137–143, 1997.

Smith DS: *Toxic shock syndrome*, 2008. http://www.nlm.nih.gov/medlineplus/ency/article/000653.htm. Accessed January 29, 2010.

Smith LH: Toxic epidermal necrolysis, *Clin J Oncol Nurs* 11(3):333–336, 2007.

Smith LH: National patient safety goal #13: patients' active involvement in their own care: preventing chemotherapy extravasation, *Clin J Oncol Nurs* 13(2):233–234, 2009.

Snyder R: Skin cancers and chronic wounds. In Norman R, editor: *Handbook of geriatric dermatology*, New York, 2006, Cambridge University Press.

Snyder RJ: "Immunopathic" ulcers, *Podiatr Manage* 185–188, 2008.

Snyder RJ, Stillman RM, Weiss SD: Epidermoid cancers that masquerade as venous ulcer disease, *Ostomy Wound Manage* 49(4):63–66, 2003.

Sullivan KM: Graft-versus-host disease. In Thomas ED, et al, editors: *Hematopoietic cell transplantation*, ed 2, Malden, MA, 1999, Blackwell Science.

Tang JC, Vivas A, Rey A, et al: Atypical ulcers: wound biopsy results from a university wound pathology service, *Ostomy Wound Manage* 58(6):20–29, 2012.

Thomas ED, et al: *Hematopoietic cell transplantation*, ed 2, Malden, Mass, 1999, Blackwell Science.

Trent JT, Kirsner RS, Romanelli P, et al: Use of SCORTEN to accurately predict mortality in patients with toxic epidermal necrolysis in the United States, *Arch Dermatol* 140:890–892, 2004.

Twomey JA, Peltier GL, Zera RT: An open-label study to evaluate the safety and efficacy of tissue plasminogen activator in treatment of severe frostbite, *J Trauma* 59:1350–1355, 2005.

Varnado M: Frostbite, *J Wound Ostomy Continence Nurs* 35(3): 341–346, 2008.

Vujinovich A: Clinical treatment options for peristomal pyoderma gangrenosum, *Br J Nurs* 14(16):S4–S8, 2005.

Wagner JE, Ishida-Yamamoto A, Macgrath JA, et al: Adult stem cells for treatment of recessive dystrophic epidermolysis bullosa (RDEB), *J Invest Dermatol* 129(Suppl 1):S55, 2009.

Wickham R, Engelking C, Sauerland C, et al: Vesicant extravasation part II: evidence-based management and continuing controversies, *Oncol Nurs Forum* 33(6):1143–1150, 2006.

Wickham R, et al: Letters to the editor. Readers share comments and questions about extravasation management, *Oncol Nurs Forum* 34(2):275–280, 2007.

Wollina U: Pyoderma gangrenosum—a review, *Orphanet J Rare Dis* 2:19, 2007.

Wollina U: Update on cutaneous calciphylaxis, *Indian Dermatol* 58(2):87–92, 2013.

Wong SL, Schneider AM, Argenta LC, et al: Loxoscelism and negative pressure wound therapy (vacuum-assisted closure): an experimental study, *Int Wound J* 7:488–492, 2010.

Zeglin D: Brown recluse spider bites, *Am J Nurs* 105(2):64–68, 2005.

Traumatic Wounds: Bullets, Blasts, and Vehicle Crashes

Vincente S. Nelson, David R. Crumbley, and Eric Elster

OBJECTIVES

1. Identify the five most common war wounds.
2. Describe critical components of acute management of traumatic wounds.
3. List three initial assessments of a traumatic wound.
4. Define compartment syndrome.

Traumatic wounds result from any foreign body impact that results in tissue damage. Their etiology can vary widely: bullet or projectile wounds, blasts, industrial accidents, falls, and car crashes. Modern care for the trauma patient has its origins in military medicine. Practices developed to treat war injuries have been modified and refined to address civilian trauma. War injuries tend to be exaggerations of civilian injuries. For example, an M16 or AK-47 round causes significantly more damage than a 22 and 45 round, even though the mechanism is largely the same. For this reason, this chapter emphasizes treatment of war wounds. Although the severity of injury may be different, the principles guiding wound care remain the same. Box 31-1 lists the components of traumatic wound care.

ETIOLOGY OF WAR WOUNDS

Weapon-related injuries are of two basic types: those resulting from small arms fire and those resulting from explosive munitions. Small arms fire includes pistols, rifles, and machine guns. Explosive munitions include mines, grenades, mortars, missiles, bombs, and improvised explosive devices (IEDs). The primary mechanism of injury among U.S. troops has changed dramatically over the years. Gunshot wounds, which comprised nearly 30% of injuries in Vietnam, now only account for 25% (Champion et al, 2010). In comparison, blasts, which accounted for 60% in Vietnam, comprised the lion's share in Operation Enduring Freedom, accounting for nearly three quarters of the injuries (Kelly et al, 2008). Regardless of the mechanism of injury, extremity wounds have comprised the majority of wounds among U.S. and UK soldiers since World War I, followed by head and neck, thoracic, and abdominal injuries (Burris et al, 2004). Blast injuries characteristically injure multiple organ systems, resulting in elevated Injury Severity Scores (ISS). The ISS

was developed in 1974 as a way to quantify the injury burden in patients with multiple injury sites (Baker et al, 1974). Injury Severity Score calculators are available on the Internet (Trauma .org, 2014). The formula breaks the body down into six areas and assigns a score of 1 to 6 to each of the sites. The scores from the three most injured sites are then squared and summed to provide the total ISS. Interestingly, the Case Fatality Rate (CFR), a measure of the overall lethality of a conflict, has fallen over subsequent conflicts despite increasingly more powerful firepower (Holcomb et al, 2006). The mortality rate has fallen from its peak in World War II at 30%, down to 25% in Vietnam, to barely 10% in Iraq and Afghanistan (Gawande, 2004).

Bullet Wounds

Small arms fire a projectile (aka, a bullet) at an object. When in motion, a projectile compresses the air in front of it and creates a shockwave. The shockwave contacts an object before the projectile. The shockwave can injure hollow viscera, such as the lungs, bowel, and eardrums. The shockwave also can knock a victim against surrounding objects. However, the shockwave is not known to cause direct injury to solid tissue.

Upon contact with tissue, a projectile creates two cavities: a permanent cavity and a temporary cavity. The temporary cavity is much larger than the permanent cavity. Elastic tissue such as muscle, fat, and connective tissue will expand and rebound, leaving only the permanent cavity. Nonelastic tissue, such as bone, will fracture secondary to the temporary cavity (Burris et al, 2004).

Further damage is caused by two additional aspects of bullets. When traveling through tissue, bullets fragment after several centimeters. This increases the diameter of the injured tissue beyond the diameter of the bullet. Bullets also yaw, or tumble. When in contact with tissue, bullets rotate 180 degrees. This tumbling greatly increases the damage by a round. Bullets

BOX 31-1 Components of Traumatic Wound Care

- Stabilization of injured patient via Advanced Trauma Life Support (ATLS) protocol is first step in traumatic wound care.
- Wound treatment is same regardless of etiology, although etiology may help practitioner discover concurrent occult injuries.
- Blood vessels, nerves, and bones must be covered with soft tissue if exposed in a wound to prevent further injury.
- Surgical debridement, low-to-intermediate pressure pulsatile lavage irrigation, and negative pressure therapy using vacuum-assisted closure repeated every 48 to 72 hours until wound closure or coverage are the hallmarks of traumatic wound care.
- Negative pressure dressings facilitate healing, decrease patient stress, and reduce provider time commitments.
- Optimizing the wound base includes reducing bacterial load and improving blood supply.
- Wound closure may occur through a variety of techniques based on size and location. Techniques for soft tissue wounds include primary closure, secondary intention, muscle and fasciocutaneous flaps, skin grafting, and skin substitutes.
- Techniques to close open abdominal wounds (used alone or in combination) include primary fascial closure, delayed fascial closure, component separation, planned ventral hernia, and serial abdominal closure.
- Systemic disease, the inflammatory response, and poor nutrition adversely affect wound closure; normalization of physiology, provision of adequate nutrition, and treatment of local or systemic infection are integral parts of wound healing.
- Chronic wounds are treated by converting the wound to an acute wound and treating it accordingly.
- Amputation is necessary for limb injuries when limb salvage is impossible, treatment of life-threatening injuries precludes prompt treatment of severe limb injuries, and limb ischemia time exceeds 6 hours.
- Tetanus vaccination should be standard practice for all patients with traumatic wounds.

that yaw earlier cause more damage. Higher-velocity bullets cause more damage than lower-velocity rounds, but yaw and fragmentation more heavily influence the amount of damage inflicted (Burris et al, 2004). Common misconceptions regarding bullets are that bullets yaw in flight, that bullets with a full metal jacket do not fragment, and that exit wounds are larger than entrance wounds.

Explosive Munitions (Ballistic, Blast, and Thermal)

Explosive munitions come in a large variety and inflict damage in multiple ways. The three types of damage inflicted by most explosive munitions are ballistic, blast, and thermal. Depending on a person's distance from an explosion, they can be exposed to any or all of these elements.

Ballistic injuries can be sustained far away from the blast. They are caused by flying fragments, whether it is the shell casing of a grenade, the ball bearings in an antipersonnel bomb, or the random dirt and debris from the area near an explosion. Different weapons are designed to propel fragments of different masses and velocities. Most explosive munitions have been designed to disperse fragments evenly. However, some weapons are shaped to fire fragments in a particular direction.

Blast injuries are caused by the sonic shockwave produced by the explosion. The shockwave typically has a much smaller range than ballistic damage. As with bullets, the shockwave can inflict damage to hollow organs. Explosions produce a much larger shockwave than bullets. Therefore injuries resulting from a body being thrown against an object are much more common. Thermobaric devices are designed to cause much larger shockwaves. During the initial explosion, these devices disperse a volatile substance such as fuel vapor. The fuel vapor then ignites and produces a longer and more powerful secondary explosion. This technology is frequently used in "bunker-busting" devices (Buchanon, 2006).

Thermal injuries of varying thickness are the third type of injury inflicted by a blast. This damage is done only at the site of the explosion. Different types of explosive munitions have been developed for different uses. There are a wide variety of grenades. Fragmentary grenades are antipersonnel tools that inflict injuries primarily through ballistic damage. Concussion grenades are designed to inflict blast damage. An incendiary grenade disperses hot chemicals to cause thermal injuries.

Three types of antipersonnel land mines predominate. *Static* land mines are planted and activated when stepped on. These mines commonly result in single, double, and even triple traumatic amputations, creating the so-called *dismounted IED injury pattern* that has characterized the conflicts in Iraq and Afghanistan (Singleton, 2013). Further injury is caused by the fragments that are driven up between fascial planes. This results in treatment regimens that center on serial operative debridements; a practice that brings substantial discomfort to both patient and family, and significantly increases overall morbidity and hospital length of stay. *Bounding* land mines bounce 1 to 2 m after being stepped upon. They then spray fragments, which enable them to injure multiple targets simultaneously. *Horizontal spray* land mines propel fragments in one direction and typically are remotely or tripwire activated.

Several types of antiarmor devices exist. A shaped charge is designed to direct an explosion at a target. Two types of fragments can injure people in an armored vehicle: fragments from the charge and spall, which is debris knocked off the armor plating. Some vehicle interiors are coated with Teflon as an antispall liner. Teflon can burn and produce toxic fumes if the thermal damage from the explosion is significant. Rocket-propelled grenades (RPGs) and tube-launched, optically tracked, wire-guided (TOW) missiles are two types of shaped charges. An explosively formed projectile (EFP) is a specialized shaped charge that is commonly used by insurgents in Iraq. Kinetic energy rounds are aerodynamically shaped pieces of metal, usually depleted uranium or tungsten. Depleted uranium has a hypothetical risk of heavy metal toxicity, but the risks surrounding fragment removal exceed the risk of heavy metal toxicity, so removal is not recommended (Buchanon, 2006). Two common types of kinetic energy rounds are armor-piercing, fin-stabilized, discarding sabots (APFSDS) and high-explosive, antitank (HEAT) shells. Antitank mines are similar to land mines except the former are more powerful and are designed to disable vehicles. In Iraq and Afghanistan, the most common antitank mine is the IED or roadside bomb. These blasts transfer large amounts of energy through the floor to the occupants, resulting in characteristic injuries to the lower extremities, spine, and head (Ramasamy et al, 2011). Coalition forces have mitigated these effects through several vehicular improvements, such as addition of a V-shaped hull, reinforcing floor boards, and adding passenger restraints.

Vehicle Crashes

Vehicle crashes are yet another type of injury. Although some soft tissue injury may be due to penetrating trauma, much of the damage sustained is due to blunt trauma. Closed head injuries, fractures, cardiac contusions, pneumothoraces, spinal cord injuries, and spleen and liver injuries typically result from blunt trauma. Most of these blunt injuries are deceleration injuries. Organs in hollow cavities (brain, heart, abdominal viscera) are injured by contacting soft tissue or shearing off of ligaments and vessels. Traumatic brain injury and traumatic aortic rupture are two frequently fatal deceleration injuries. Crush injuries may result when a patient is trapped in a vehicle after a crash. The lower extremities and pelvis are particularly vulnerable in car crashes.

ACUTE MANAGEMENT OF TRAUMATIC WOUNDS

Advanced Trauma Life Support

The acute management of traumatic wounds is a component of the Advanced Trauma Life Support (ATLS) guidelines. Treatment of any wounded patient should follow these guidelines. Failure to recognize and correct life-threatening problems early postinjury will make wound care meaningless. Advanced Trauma Life Support guidelines emphasize an organized and methodical approach to trauma. A brief overview of the guidelines is given here, but a more comprehensive review can be found in most general surgery texts. Anyone caring for acutely traumatized patients should take the ATLS course offered by the American College of Surgeons.

Any trauma can be managed using the ABCDE method: airway, breathing, circulation, disability, and exposure. The airway and breathing components of the ATLS guidelines emphasize that a person who is not able to breathe cannot oxygenate his or her tissues. This situation quickly leads to tissue ischemia, organ failure, and death. Priority should be given toward securing the patient's airway. If the patient is unconscious, has an altered consciousness, or has injuries that compromise the airway, a temporary airway (e.g., nasopharyngeal tube, oropharyngeal tube, cricothyroidotomy) should be established until a definitive airway (e.g., endotracheal tube or tracheostomy tube) can be placed. Next, any injuries that prevent respiration should be addressed immediately. This includes simple or tension pneumothorax or hemothorax. All are addressed with a tube thoracostomy (chest tube).

Once a person is able to oxygenate and ventilate, attention should be given to circulation. Organs and tissue that are not perfused will become ischemic. Beyond the obvious risk of death, ischemia has profound negative effects on wound healing. Ischemia results in larger wounds, longer healing times, and higher incidences of wound failure and infection. Some of the problems that can compromise circulation include cardiac tamponade, shock, and bleeding. Cardiac tamponade can be treated emergently by pericardiocentesis. In trauma, shock (the inability to maintain end organ perfusion) is predominantly secondary to hemorrhage, but a patient also may present with neurogenic shock, septic shock, cardiogenic shock, or adrenal insufficiency.

Control of Bleeding. Hemorrhage remains the number-one cause of preventable death on the battlefield, accounting for over 90% of such injuries (Eastridge et al, 2012). Hemorrhagic shock is treated by first resuscitating the patient with crystalloid solutions (e.g., 0.9% NaCl or lactated Ringer's solution) and then blood products. Trauma patients are notoriously challenging to treat because their injuries make them susceptible to multiple coagulopathies (Hess et al, 2008). A new generation of diagnostic adjuncts, like rapid thrombelastography (r-TEG), is helpful in guiding resuscitation (Holcolmb et al, 2012). Thrombelastography and other diagnostic tests of the same family are bedside diagnostics that rely on blood's tendency to coagulate under shear conditions to calculate various coagulation profiles (Hagemo et al, 2013). It is composed of a pin and cup whose oscillations through the sample lead to fibrin formation. These times are representative of specific components of the clotting cascade (Johansson et al, 2009). Using this technology, a provider can determine exactly what component is deficient and can replete it accordingly. Second, the source of bleeding is identified and controlled. A significant portion of trauma-related bleeding is internal. Fatal internal bleeding can occur in the thorax, abdomen, pelvis, and long bones (e.g., femur). Identifying the bleeding source requires knowledge of the mechanism of injury and the use of various imaging modalities or surgical exploration. If a patient is hemodynamically unstable, surgical correction of the bleeding is necessary. Once bleeding control has been established, the patient can be assessed for neurologic disability and treated accordingly. The patient's clothing should be removed to ensure that no injury has been overlooked. The management of trauma is team oriented and multidisciplinary, and several steps of the ATLS guidelines may progress simultaneously depending on the resources of the hospital.

To control hemorrhage, direct pressure should be the initial therapy. Direct pressure is noninvasive, requires no supplies other than a hand, and prevents further damage to the injured vessel and other tissue. When a wound is too large or the bleeding is too brisk, control of bleeding can be attempted with a tourniquet. A tourniquet circumferentially applies pressure proximal to damaged, bleeding tissue. The pressure is transferred to the underlying vessels, causing occlusion of the arteries and veins. Tourniquets are more effective than direct pressure in stopping hemorrhage. They can be purchased or constructed out of something as simple as a belt or a bed sheet.

Tourniquet use comes at a price, however. When applied, hypoperfusion and subsequent ischemia occur to all tissue distal to the point of compression. Prolonged tourniquet use (as short as 90 minutes) can result in ischemia, compartment syndrome, and nerve damage. Use for more than 6 hours can result in limb loss (Beekley et al, 2008; Kam et al, 2001). Therefore tourniquet use is traditionally not recommended for civilian extremity trauma in the United States. Traumatic hemorrhage typically requires definitive surgical correction.

However, in a combat theater, multiple factors may lead to delayed casualty evacuation. Environmental (e.g., sandstorms), geographic (e.g., mountain ranges), and tactical (e.g., ongoing combat) factors can delay evacuation for hours, if not days. Among combat fatalities, 30% to 40% result from hemorrhage (Perkins et al, 2008). In patients who are not killed immediately, hemorrhage is the most preventable cause of death. Advanced Trauma Life Support protocol should be followed as strictly as field capabilities

allow. Placement of a tourniquet can temporarily halt bleeding, allowing perfusion of crucial organs and survival until an adequate surgical facility can be reached. Recent research derived from U.S. experiences in Iraq and Afghanistan suggests tourniquets are safe and limb loss is low when tourniquets are applied judiciously (Beekley et al, 2008; Kragh et al, 2009).

Upon the patient's arrival to an operating room, tourniquets should be removed and the patient's wounds explored for sites of bleeding. Blind clamping of vessels can lead to ischemia of healthy tissue and therefore should be avoided. Damaged vessels can be addressed with ligation or graft repair, depending on the structure and degree of collateral flow. If external bleeding occurs where a tourniquet cannot be applied (e.g., axial areas) or if a tourniquet inadequately stops hemorrhage, a hemostatic dressing can be applied. Table 31-1 lists examples and descriptions of hemostatic agents and dressings (Kozen et al, 2008; Neuffer et al, 2004; Perkins et al, 2008; Pusateri et al, 2003; Rhee et al, 2008). Recent evidence from the CRASH-2 trial suggests that tranexamic acid (TXA) significantly reduces death due to hemorrhage and improves 28-day all-cause mortality if administered within 3 hours of injury; administration of the antifibrinolytic outside of this window is associated with decreased survival due to bleeding (Roberts et al, 2013). Further research is necessary before the drug is considered a standard of care, especially in the prehospital setting; however, the U.S. military and several prominent U.S. trauma centers have already secured a place for it in their formularies.

Immunization

Once a patient has been stabilized, tetanus prophylaxis should be administered. Tetanus, a disease characterized by intense

TABLE 31-1 Examples of Hemostatic Agents and Dressings

Component	Brand Name	Manufacturer	Formulation
Zeolite	QuikClot	Z-Medica	Powders and beads
			Zeolite is a mineral
Gelatins	Gelfoam	Pharmacia Upjohn	Absorbable foam dressing
	FloSeal	Baxter Health Care	Absorptive granules
Collagen	Avitene	CR Bard	Sponge
Microporous polysaccharides	TraumaDEX	Bleed-X	Plant-based powder
	BioHemostat	Hemodyne	Absorptive granules in a dressing
			Derived of volcanic rock
Chitosan derived from shrimp shells	Celox	SAM Medical	Granular powder or gauze dressing
	HemCon	HemCon Medical Technologies	Patch or bandage
	ChitoFlex		Impregnated packing
	ChitoGauze		Impregnated gauze
Fibrin sealant	Tisseel VH Crosseal	Baxter Health Care	Tissue adhesive
Polyethylene glycol	CoSeal		Tissue adhesive
Cyanoacrylate	Dermabond	Ethicon	Tissue adhesive

muscle contractions and autonomic dysfunction, is caused by a toxin produced by the anaerobic bacteria *Clostridium tetani*. These contractions can be fatal if they affect the diaphragm (Wood, 2004). Wounds necessitating tetanus prophylaxis include wounds older than 6 hours, those with significant contamination or associated necrotic or ischemic tissue, puncture wounds, stab and gunshot wounds, and wounds resulting from burns or frostbite (Wood, 2004). Patients who were immunized within the past 5 years or who have received a tetanus booster during this period may be exempt. Due to the significant contamination of war wounds and the difficulties in verifying medical records in a combat environment, many trauma surgeons recommend immunizing all wounded patients (Anaya and Dellinger, 2007).

Irrigation and Assessment

Once a patient's life- and limb-threatening injuries have been addressed, it is appropriate to start wound care. Regardless of the etiology, traumatic wounds almost always occur in a non-sterile environment. Therefore, by definition, traumatic wounds are contaminated by debris and foreign objects from the surrounding environment. Many weapons are designed to embed foreign objects in their targets. Explosive munitions displace large volumes of dirt and debris upon detonation. To treat a traumatic wound, you must first assess the nature and extent of wounding, including size; depth; and nerve, bone, or blood vessel exposure. Irrigation of the wound with sterile saline or water facilitates proper assessment and removes gross debris and contaminants and chemicals that could lead to further tissue injury (NPUAP, EPUAP, PPPIA, 2014).

Coverage and Repair of Vital Structures

There are three types of nerve injury. *Neuropraxia,* the most minor nerve injury, is a conduction block of the nerve. These injuries are common in blunt trauma and compartment syndrome. Function lost secondary to neuropraxia usually returns in 3 months. *Axonotmesis* is an intermediate injury to the nerve that results from damage to the axon. The surrounding endoneurium and perineurium remain intact. The damaged axon will undergo wallerian degeneration (degeneration of the axon distal to the injury) but then slowly grow back (about 1 cm/month). Most function will return after this type of injury. Both neuropraxia and axonotmesis will heal without specific intervention. The most severe type of nerve injury is *neurotmesis,* or complete transaction of the nerve. If the injury is secondary to penetrating trauma, it usually can be repaired. Neurotmesis secondary to gunshot wounds has a less favorable outcome. The gunshot wound results in thermal and shockwave injuries in addition to the penetrating injury, making functional recovery after surgical repair less likely. Optimally, a nerve should be repaired with a tension-free anastomosis. If this cannot be done because of a substantial defect in the nerve, grafting can be attempted. Autologous nerve grafting, usually using a patient's sural nerve as the donor, is the most common technique. Autologous vein grafts also can be used to guide regenerating nerves over defects. The timing of nerve repair depends on the degree of contamination and the need for subsequent operations to the same wound. Regardless of the degree of injury, an exposed nerve should be covered with soft tissue (Peterson and Lehman, 2008). The exposed nerve is at higher risk for infection and iatrogenic injury during subsequent surgery. A nerve that is allowed to heal without soft tissue coverage becomes highly susceptible to even minor blunt trauma.

Traumatic wounds may contain open fractures that need to be reduced and stabilized. Open fractures are at risk for infection, bleeding, increased soft tissue damage, delayed union, and nonunion. Bone infections (osteomyelitis) are difficult to treat because of the density of the bone and the paucity of adjacent blood vessels supplying the cortical bone. After the wound is irrigated and debrided, open fractures are stabilized, either temporarily or definitively. Depending on the fractured bone, fixation can be achieved by a variety of methods, most commonly screw and/or plate fixation for periarticular fractures and intramedullary nails or external fixators for diaphyseal fractures. After fixation, open fractures require soft tissue coverage with either local tissue or transferred flaps. This typically is performed at a subsequent, definitive operation. Because coverage often cannot be performed at the initial operation due to contamination, infection, or physiologic reasons, a sterile dressing is placed over the bone until a later time when surgery can be performed under more favorable conditions (Smith et al, 2008).

A wound should be explored for exposed traumatized blood vessels. Similar to nerves, exposed vessels are at risk for infection and iatrogenic injury during subsequent operations. Furthermore, any compromise to the blood supply compromises all the tissue it supplies. Medium and large arteries that supply an area of soft tissue without adequate collateral flow require repair around the time of injury. Examples include the superficial femoral, common femoral, and brachial arteries. Due to the presence of collateral veins, most major veins can be ligated following injury. If needed, repair can be performed using a variety of techniques, depending on the vessel and degree of injury. Most exposed vessels in open wounds will occur in the extremities. Repair of these vessels is by autologous or prosthetic graft. In the acute setting, a patient may be too unstable to tolerate a long operation. If this is the case and the patient has a large defect to a vessel supplying a limb, a temporary vascular shunt can be placed to maintain blood flow to the limb until definitive vascular repair can be achieved. Once a patient is able to tolerate a longer operation, the injured vessel should be repaired with an autologous vein graft, typically the saphenous vein, or an artificial conduit such as polytetrafluoroethylene. In most cases an autologous vein graft is preferred over an artificial graft because of superior patency rates. Next, consideration should be given to coverage of the exposed vessel. In addition to the risks of infection and iatrogenic injury, vessel walls will desiccate, erode, and possibly disrupt if wounds are allowed to heal without coverage. Coverage of a blood vessel can be provided by myocutaneous flap or fasciocutaneous flap. When the wound is too large for flap coverage or is too contaminated for a viable flap, an extraanatomic bypass of the injured vessel should be performed, directing a graft to route the blood vessel around the wound in an uninjured tissue plane. When an injured vessel is being repaired, the graft should be similarly routed through uninjured, well-perfused tissue planes (Frykberg and Schinco, 2008).

Debridement

Once a wound has been irrigated copiously and assessed, all nonviable tissue should be debrided to prevent its negative effects to the wound bed (see Chapter 17). For the patient with a traumatic wound, the continued presence of nonviable tissue poses significant threats systemically by releasing toxic oxygen radicals, chemokines, cytokines, electrolytes, myoglobin, and other muscle breakdown products. These molecules lead to deleterious inflammatory responses that are exacerbated by resuscitation, leading to systemic inflammatory responses such as systemic inflammatory response syndrome (SIRS), compensatory antiinflammatory response syndrome (CARS), and multiorgan dysfunction syndrome (MODS) (Table 31-2) (Drago, 2007). The SIRS response can become a maladaptive and hypermetabolic physiologic state that leads to prolonged healing times, poor wound healing, and various other complications. Compensatory antiinflammatory response syndrome is the body's attempt at compensating for SIRS. This compensation also is maladaptive, leading to increased infectious morbidity. Multiorgan dysfunction syndrome is the end result of an exaggerated or prolonged SIRS response, which is characterized by multisystem organ failure and high morbidity and mortality rates. Further injury caused by necrotic tissue includes kidney damage secondary to myoglobin released by necrotic muscle. Lysis of cells releases a large volume of electrolytes and metabolic products. Of particular concern is hyperkalemia, which can lead to fatal cardiac dysrhythmias.

Although some surgeons advocate the use of bedside wound exploration for smaller wounds, most traumatic wounds should be irrigated and debrided in the operating room to minimize patient discomfort and allow for adequate exploration. If the patient requires an operation for a traumatic injury, irrigation and debridement of the wound can take place during the operation once the patient is stable and all life-threatening injuries have been addressed.

Fasciotomy

Fasciotomies are performed for compartment syndrome or prophylactically for patients at risk for compartment syndrome. Compartment syndrome occurs after a crush injury or vascular injury with subsequent reperfusion in a closed fascial space, usually an extremity, although the abdomen and pelvis also can be involved. Tissue edema following injury places increased pressure directly on capillaries, resulting in decreased perfusion and ischemia. Additionally, external pressure on veins reduces capillary flow and further diminishes perfusion (Clayton et al, 1977). If ischemia continues, permanent nerve damage, renal failure, and loss of limb can ensue. Unlike open wounds, compartment syndrome has a more occult presentation. Symptoms include pain, paresthesias, paresis, poikilothermia, and pallor of the affected extremity. An absence of pulses may be noted in an affected limb but typically is a late finding. Compartment pressure can be measured using a needle attached to a Stryker Intracompartmental Pressure Monitor System or a modified arterial line kit that is inserted through the fascia. Normal compartment pressures range from 0 to 15 mm Hg, whereas an elevated pressure mandating treatment is either a compartment pressure greater than 30 mm Hg or compartment pressure 35 mm Hg less than arterial diastolic pressure (Browner and DeAngelis, 2007; Losken and Schaefer, 2008). Treatment involves surgical decompression of compartments by incising the surrounding deep investing muscular fascia (fasciotomy). In trauma, fasciotomies are performed prophylactically in patients at risk for compartment syndrome (e.g., those with severe crush injuries with or without prolonged ischemia). Once the fasciotomy

TABLE 31-2	Criteria for Definition of SIRS, Sepsis, MODS, CARS				
SIRS	**Sepsis**	**Severe Sepsis**	**Septic Shock**	**MODS**	**CARS**
Two or more of the following criteria: • Temperature>38° or <35° • Heart rate >90/min • Respiration rate >20/min or apical pulse CO_2 <32 mm Hg • Leukocytes >12,000,<4,000 mm³ or more than 10% of immature forms	With documented infection	Sepsis associated with organic dysfunction, hypoperfusion, or hypotension	Sepsis with refractory hypotension to appropriate reanimation and hyperperfusion manifestations	Failure of two or more organs so homeostasis cannot be sustained without support	• Cutaneous anergy • Hypothermia • Leukopenia • Susceptibility to infection • Failure to clear infection

Adapted from: Drago A: *Systemic inflammatory response syndrome (S.I.R.S) after cardiac surgery,* Federación Argentina de Cardiología, 5th International Congress of Cardiology on the Internet, 2007. http://www.fac.org.ar/qcvc/llave/c130i/dragoa.php. Accessed August 21, 2014; Ward N, Casserly B, Ayala A: The compensatory anti-inflammatory response syndrome (CARS) in critically ill patients, *Clin Chest Med* 29(4):617–625, 2008.

is performed, subacute management of the open wound begins.

SUBACUTE MANAGEMENT OF TRAUMATIC WOUNDS

Usually, the degree of contamination, the severity of the wound, and the local and systemic inflammatory response to the critically ill state of the wounded patient do not allow for wound closure after initial evaluation, irrigation, and debridement because care must be focused on lifesaving procedures, ensuring adequate airway and ventilation, stopping blood loss, and preventing further organ injury. Therefore wound bed preparation and wound closure are planned during the subacute phase of traumatic wound management.

Serial Irrigation and Debridement

Although a wound bed may appear to be free of necrotic tissue after initial debridement, repeat evaluation during subacute management may reveal additional necrosis. Patients with traumatic wounds tend to have physiologic, immunologic, and nutritional derangements that predispose them to infection. On a local level, wounds are predisposed to colonization. Therefore traumatic wounds typically require serial irrigation, evaluation, and debridement. Traditionally, open traumatic wounds are evaluated on a daily or twice-daily basis.

Debridement should be performed using an atraumatic surgical technique (Attinger et al, 2006). Examples include sharp dissection and bipolar cautery, which allow for minimal destruction of underlying, healthy tissue. Healthy tissue is well vascularized and bleeds. Other hallmarks of viable tissue depend on the tissue type (Table 31-3). Healthy fascia appears white and glistens. Fat is bright yellow. Viable muscle can be recognized by the 4 Cs: red Color, Contraction upon stimulation with forceps or electrocautery, strong Consistency, and Capacity to bleed (Volgas, 2007). Most bleeding resulting from surgical debridement can be stopped with direct pressure. If direct pressure is inadequate, suture ligation or pinpoint electrocautery can be used.

Reevaluation of a traumatic wound with repeat irrigation and debridement should occur at least twice per week even if no grossly necrotic or nonviable tissue is noted in the wound

TABLE 31-3	Characteristics of Healthy Tissue
Tissue	**Characteristics**
Skin	Compressible, blanching, sensate, noncongested
Fascia	Glistening white
Adipose	Bright yellow, nondusky, capacity to bleed
Muscle	Beefy red, contractile when stimulated with electrocautery, capacity to bleed, firm consistency

bed (Attinger et al, 2006). As wound healing progresses, the extent of debridement needed decreases. Once a bed of granulation tissue is present throughout the wound, debridement may no longer be needed. At this point, wound irrigation and the use of negative pressure dressings can maintain the bacterial load at sufficiently low levels.

Many traumatic wounds have exposed bone. Although radiographs and magnetic resonance imaging are the standard techniques for diagnosing osteomyelitis, the presence of exposed bone in a wound is associated with up to a 66% chance of osteomyelitis (Brothers et al, 1998; Grayson et al, 1995). Infected or nonviable bone is friable and should be debrided. Curettes, Cobb elevators, and rongeurs are sharp surgical instruments typically used for bone debridement. Once bone has been adequately debrided, it should be covered with soft tissue (Attinger et al, 2006). Occasionally, adjacent tissue can be sutured over the defect. Otherwise, a rotational or free myocutaneous flap is needed. In cases where anatomic or physiologic restrictions contraindicate a flap procedure or ongoing infection is suspected, bone will granulate. Secondary intention is suboptimal because granulation is slow and takes several weeks. Early flap reconstruction is associated with shorter hospital stays for patients with traumatic wounds (Stanec et al, 1993).

Should a traumatic wound become infected, the infection can travel very quickly along fascial planes, a condition known as *necrotizing fasciitis*. Tendon necrosis or infection can be difficult to manage. Overzealous debridement of a tendon can lead to loss of muscle function. Care should be taken to preserve as much healthy tissue as possible. If the paratenon surrounding the tendon requires debridement, the tendon must be kept moist to prevent desiccation and necrosis. Because infection can quickly spread along tendons, small incisions should be made in the healthy tendon or muscle proximal and distal to the infected or necrotic tissue. Small tendons may require sacrifice if they become infected. Larger tendons should be preserved as much as possible. Reconstruction of certain large tendons (e.g., Achilles tendon) is possible using pedicle or free flaps (Attinger et al, 2006).

Following debridement, irrigation or pulse lavage (see Chapter 17) should be performed to remove bacteria and loose debris. Tangential hydrosurgery is a technique that combines irrigation and debridement. A device called the Versajet debrides tissue by shooting a stream of water across a small gap. The stream is very high pressure, up to 15,000 psi. The high-pressure stream creates a vacuum that pulverizes surrounding necrotic tissue, removes it from the wound bed, and preserves adjacent healthy tissue (Granick et al, 2007; Klein et al, 2005). Due to the high pressure generated by the device, the procedure is associated with a significant amount of discomfort and anxiety to the patient. Subsequently, adequate anesthesia in the form of conscious sedation, spinal, or general anesthesia is recommended. Recent literature has argued against the use of high-pressure systems due to its high rate of tissue damage and bacterial rebound. Because of this, low-tech systems, like the bulb syringe, have returned to favor (Tintle et al, 2010).

Dressings

After the wound is irrigated and debrided, it should be covered with a sterile dressing. Different types of dressings perform different functions (Stojadinovic et al, 2008). In acute traumatic wounds, wet to dry dressings are no longer the standard of care. In wounds that are heavily colonized, dressings moistened with sodium hypochlorite (i.e., Dakin's solution) instead of water or saline may still be utilized. Sodium hypochlorite is a bleach that is bactericidal but has cytotoxic effects on healthy cells (Wilson et al, 2005). Depending on the degree of colonization, either half-strength or quarter-strength Dakin's solution can be used until the level of contamination decreases.

Negative pressure wound therapy (NPWT) between 75 and 150 mm Hg is the most commonly used dressing for traumatic wounds following debridement of necrotic tissue and all eschar. Negative pressure wound therapy is described in detail in Chapter 21. It removes effluent from the wound. Less effluent results in less wound edema and faster healing. Negative pressure dressings are occlusive, preventing contamination of the wound by additional bacteria or debris. The therapy is believed to stimulate granulation tissue by promoting capillary growth. Intermittent instead of continuous negative pressure has been shown to further increase the rate of granulation tissue formation (Lindstedt et al, 2008; Ubbink et al, 2008).

Different variants of wound filler dressings can be used for NPWT. A silver-impregnated sponge is available for infected wounds or for wounds with a heavy bacterial load. Silver ions are bacteriocidal and have potency against multidrug-resistant bacteria, such as methicillin-resistant *Staphylococcus aureus,* vancomycin-resistant *Enterococcus,* and *Pseudomonas aeruginosa* (Tredget et al, 1998; Yin et al, 1999). Because the standard sponge adheres to the wound base, a nonadherent sponge was developed. The nonadherent sponge is moist and works like the standard sponge, except that it does not microdebride. Use of the nonadherent sponge is reserved for wounds that contain structures such as tendons, where adherence is detrimental and moisture is required. Due to the high expense of the nonadherent sponge, an alternative method involves placing a nonadherent contact layer, such as Xeroform, Mepitel, or Adaptic over the top of the vulnerable structure such as bone, tendon, nerves, and blood vessels to protect the tissues from the foam. Some surgeons use this technique over the top of skin grafts to take advantage of increased capillary growth while preventing graft removal. Two randomized control trials demonstrated decreased graft loss (Llanos et al, 2006) and improved cosmetic outcome (Moisidis et al, 2004) when negative pressure dressings were placed over grafts.

For small, shallow wounds not amenable to NPWT, numerous alternative dressings may be used (see Chapters 16, 18, and 19). Dressings that reduce bacterial load and microdebride are generally preferred for traumatic wounds.

Antibiotic Beads

An additional adjunct that has been used for treatment of traumatic wounds with open fractures has been antibiotic cement or beads. Osteomyelitis is hard to treat due to the difficulty in achieving therapeutic levels of antibiotics in bone. Treatment generally requires 6 or more weeks of intravenous antibiotics. As an adjunct to systemic antibiotics, several German orthopedic surgeons placed antibiotics in bone cement used for hip arthroplasty (Buchholz and Engelbrecht, 1970). A reduction in postoperative arthroplasty infections was noted, leading to more widespread use of antibiotic-impregnated bone cement. Antibiotic-impregnated beads subsequently were developed for temporary placement at sites of bone debrided for osteomyelitis. The beads are created by mixing bone cement powder, typically polymerized polymethylmethacrylate (PMMA), with powdered antibiotics before adding liquid methylmethacrylate to make the adhesive cement. Before hardening, the beads can be threaded on a permanent suture to facilitate removal. Only a few antibiotics are available in powdered form, limiting the choice to aminoglycosides, vancomycin, and β-lactams (Wininger and Fass, 1996).

In traumatic wounds with open fractures, antibiotic beads have been used to decrease the bacterial load of the wound. In a study of 1085 patients with compound limb fractures requiring debridement and stabilization, 845 received gentamicin-impregnated antibiotic beads plus systemic antibiotics versus 240 treated with systemic antibiotics alone. The rate of infection decreased from 12% to 3.7% in the group that received the beads (Ostermann et al, 1995). Due to the high incidence of multidrug-resistant Acinetobacter infections in U.S. soldiers with traumatic wounds sustained in Iraq and Afghanistan, antibiotic beads have become a frequently used method for treating and preventing osteomyelitis.

Wound Closure

The timing of wound closure is an important clinical decision. The goal of closure is to protect the underlying tissue, restore the innate immunologic barrier of skin, and provide a cosmetically acceptable outcome. Although most healthy wounds will granulate and close by secondary intention, surgical closure reduces the duration of closure, produces a cosmetically superior appearance, decreases the need for wound care resources, and decreases the time burden on the patient. Improper timing of closure leads to dehiscence and failure. Dehiscence results when a closed wound reopens. Failure includes dehiscence, but also may include failure of a wound to accept a graft (e.g., skin graft). Currently, no laboratory tests or imaging modalities can predict the optimal time for wound closure. Providers are forced to rely on clinical factors, including wound appearance and patient physiology, as well as their own clinical experience. Due to the large number of traumatic wounds cared for by the U.S. Navy and Army Medical Corps, work is being done to describe the molecular mechanisms dictating wound failure.

Current criteria used to determine timing of wound closure include the patient's general condition, injury location, adequacy of perfusion, and gross appearance of the wound bed. Factors related to the patient's general condition include nutritional and nonspecific systemic inflammatory parameters. Relevance of injury location and visual assessment of the wound, such as the appearance of granulation tissue, are subjectively determined by the surgeon. However, considerable interobserver variability exists in wound assessment.

Once a wound has a base of healthy granulation tissue without evidence of infection, the wound can be closed. Several techniques are used to close traumatic wounds. As previously stated, secondary intention is one method. Secondary intention involves the growth of skin over the top of a granulated wound from the wound edge. No surgical intervention is necessary for secondary intention; however, the long duration (several months), resources needed (wound dressings), and cosmetic outcome do not favor its use, especially for large traumatic wounds.

For wounds with healthy skin edges, primary or delayed primary closure can be attempted. The term *delayed* refers to the time lapse between initial wound care and the time of closure. Delayed primary closure involves approximating the edges of a wound and fixating them together. Multiple methods for fixating skin exist, including skin adhesives, sutures, and staples. Each method, along with selection, application, removal, and incision care considerations, is described in Chapter 34. Regardless of the mechanism used, skin closures should be under low tension. High-tension closures result in failure and dehiscence.

Occasionally, larger wounds cannot be surgically closed due to unacceptably high tension, so a skin graft must be considered. As previously discussed, the provider must first analyze a wound for exposed bone, nerve, or blood vessel. If one of these structures appears in the wound base, a muscle, myocutaneous, or fasciocutaneous flap should be used for cover. Coverage protects nerves and vessels from subsequent trauma and bone from skin erosion. As described in Chapter 33, many types of tissue flaps exist, including pedicle flaps, rotational flaps, and free flaps. Choice of flap type and procedure usually requires an experienced plastic surgeon. Flaps, especially free flaps, require frequent monitoring in the first 48 hours to ensure adequate perfusion. Most flaps also contain a segment of skin. If the flap does not, a skin graft may be performed once the flap is viable and secure. Skin grafts are described in Chapter 32.

Several artificial skin substitutes have been developed (see Chapter 19). Although none of these substitutes can replace an autograft, they can promote graft acceptance. These products, in combination with NPWT, have proven useful in wounds with exposed tendon, allowing for granulation over tendon and eventual skin grafting (Helgeson et al, 2007).

Open Abdomen

Visceral swelling results secondary to trauma and is caused by massive cytokine release, increased vascular permeability, and loss of fluid to the interstitial space, most notably following resuscitation. Although the swelling typically resolves in 1 to 2 weeks, the bowel becomes so large that the abdominal wall cannot be reapproximated. Closure of the abdominal wall also can be difficult if a trauma results directly in a large soft tissue defect, or a "loss of domain."

Regardless of the cause, closure of the abdomen is necessary to contain and protect the viscera, prevent desiccation of the bowel, and prevent peritonitis. Multiple techniques have been developed to close the abdomen. The simplest method is primary fascial closure. To close an abdomen by primary fascial closure, a component separation is performed. Component separation dissects skin off the anterior rectus sheath and incises the external oblique fascia, allowing for increased mobilization of the fascia and closure (Ramirez et al, 1990). To reduce the amount of dissection needed and resultant large soft tissue flaps, laparoscopic versions of this procedure have been developed (Milburn et al, 2007; Rosen et al, 2007). A serious shortcoming of these techniques is the limited mobilization obtained by component separation, usually 10 to 16 cm (Shestak et al, 2000). The other major drawback is the high rate of ventral hernia formation, typically 5% to 10% (Lowe et al, 2000; Shestak et al, 2000). For these reasons, other techniques have been developed to close the abdomen.

One technique is the planned ventral hernia. In this technique, an absorbable mesh is used to close the fascial defect. Once the mesh granulates, a split-thickness skin graft is placed over the wound. Over time, the mesh is absorbed and a ventral hernia results. The ventral hernia is then surgically repaired 6 to 12 months after the trauma (Fabian et al, 1994; Jernigan et al, 2003; Weinberg et al, 2008). Due to the high rate of enterocutaneous fistula formation (approximately 8% of patients) and the need for future major abdominal surgeries, this technique is less popular than delayed fascial closure.

Delayed fascial closure involves placement of an NPWT, dressing such as an ABThera dressing over the open abdomen until bowel swelling reduces enough to allow closure by component separation and/or a mesh. Decreased adhesions between the abdominal wall and bowel have been noted. A negative pressure dressing is created by placing a plastic sheet or towel over the viscera and under the abdominal wall. The dressing is placed over the towel and is covered by an occlusive dressing. The dressing is connected to negative pressure. Every 2 to 3 days, the patient returns to the operating room and the dressing is changed under sterile conditions until abdominal closure is reasonable (Argenta et al, 2006; Bee et al, 2008; Morykwas et al, 1997; Schecter et al, 2006). Complications are decreased with this method and include fistula (5%), bowel obstruction (2%), and abscess formation (4%) (Barker et al, 2007).

Another technique used to close open abdomens is serial abdominal closure (Kafie et al, 2003). Serial abdominal closure requires placement of a temporary mesh in the open abdomen. As bowel edema lessens, the mesh loosens. During serial operations, the central portion of the loose mesh is cut and the edges are sewn together. Eventually, the residual mesh is removed and the abdomen is closed (Barker et al, 2007; Vertrees et al, 2008).

A variety of rotational and free muscle flaps have been used to cover large abdominal wounds. Muscle flaps typically are used when ostomies, drain sites, and multiple prior procedures have distorted or destroyed the normal anatomic planes. The rectus abdominis and tensor fascia lata are the two most commonly used muscles for flaps (Mathes et al, 2000).

Combination techniques have been attempted. For soldiers with large abdominal wounds resulting from blast injuries in Iraq and Afghanistan, a combined technique called *early-delayed fascial closure* has been described. The method combines delayed fascial closure, serial abdominal closure, and use of temporary and permanent meshes (Vertrees et al, 2008).

Choice of closure technique is largely based on anatomic factors, complication rates, and surgeon's experience and preference. Technique choice should emphasize protecting the bowel, closing the abdominal wall in a timely manner to allow rehabilitation, and preventing complications such as enterocutaneous fistulas and recurrent hernias.

Amputation

Extremely severe blast and crush injuries may result in mangled extremities with unsalvageable wounds. In these situations, amputation may be the only viable option. The decision to amputate can be extremely difficult due to the resulting cosmetic, functional, and psychological defects. Reasons to amputate include prolonged limb ischemia, irreparable peripheral nerve injury with no hope of meaningful limb rehabilitation, and presence of concurrent life-threatening injuries. Usually, the need to amputate is fairly straightforward. However, in a subset of trauma patients the duration of limb ischemia or degree of nerve injury may cause a surgeon to attempt limb salvage when amputation is warranted. Due to increased patient mortality rates and high hospital costs associated with failed efforts at limb salvage, a series of different limb injury scoring systems have been developed. One system is the Mangled Extremity Severity Score (MESS). The MESS ranks the degree of soft tissue/skeletal injury, limb ischemia, shock, and age; a score of 7 correlates with a need to amputate (Johansen et al, 1990). Other scoring systems include the Limb Salvage Index (LSI); Predictive Salvage Index (PSI); Hannover Fracture Scale-97 (HFS-97); and Nerve Injury, Ischemia, Soft Tissue Injury, Skeletal Injury, Shock, and Age of Patient Score (NISSSA). Two large studies evaluated the utility of these scoring systems. In a large prospective study, Bosse et al (2001) found that none of these scores could accurately predict limb salvage potential. A retrospective study by Ly et al (2008) found that no available scoring system was predictive of functional recovery of patients undergoing limb salvage.

The results of the Lower Extremity Assessment Project (LEAP) have been released. The LEAP is a prospective, observational study conducted over 2 years in eight level 1 trauma centers. Although patients undergoing either limb salvage or amputation experienced a high number of complications, a significantly increased incidence of complications was noted in the limb salvage group (37.7% vs. 24.8%) (Harris et al, 2009).

Over the past 7 years in U.S. military medical facilities, we have cared for more than 850 service members with amputation returning from Operations Iraqi Freedom and Enduring Freedom. Among the amputees, 88% have sustained blast injuries. Other amputations are sustained secondary to multiple gunshot wound and motor vehicle crash–related wounds, which can be nearly as bad. Approximately 20% of amputees have lost more than one limb. About 60% have sustained significant soft tissue wounds over other areas of the body. In prior conflicts, a significant number of these patients would have died, but improvements in medical knowledge and evacuation time have resulted in better outcomes. As a result, substantial improvements have been made in limb prostheses and physical rehabilitation.

Approximately 80% of combat-related amputations are performed within the zone of injury and therefore typically require delayed closure and result in frequent wound-healing problems. Over the past year we have seen an increasing number of individuals returning after 1 or more years of living with a limb that went through multiple salvage procedures but just was not functioning at the level desired by the individuals, so they were presenting for an elective amputation (n = 51).

Due to increasing progress in prosthesis design and limb reconstruction (including areas such as hand transplantation) and faster patient evacuation times, limb salvage will continue to be a complex decision. Patients should be made aware, however, that they can have meaningful recoveries following amputation.

Heterotopic Ossification

Heterotopic ossification is the formation of lamellar bone in nonosseous tissue. Multiple events have been associated with its formation, including traumatic amputation, spinal cord trauma, severe head injuries, total hip arthroplasty, thermal or electrical burns, acetabular or elbow fractures, familial disorders, and neoplasm. Heterotopic ossification is a source of pain, causes breakdown of overlying skin, and interferes with prosthesis fitting and use (Potter et al, 2006).

Heterotopic ossification in the extremities remains a common complication in the setting of high-energy wartime extremity trauma. Recent literature suggests that the incidence may be higher than previously reported, particularly in blast-injured amputees and in those in whom the definitive amputation was performed within the zone of injury. A 63% incidence has been noted in the residual limbs of U.S. soldiers injured in Iraq and Afghanistan (Potter et al, 2007).

An area of concern regarding heterotopic ossification and high-energy long bone fractures is the method of definitive fixation. Heterotopic ossification is a known complication of both external fixation and internal fixation. Because heterotopic ossification formation may result following muscle injury that occurs during surgical fixation, it is possible that in the patient with multiple injuries, internal fixation carries an increased risk of developing heterotopic ossification compared with definitive external fixation, especially when definitive internal fixation is delayed.

Prophylaxis against ectopic bone formation is well established in patients undergoing arthroplasty and operative treatment of acetabular fractures. Local radiation therapy and nonsteroidal antiinflammatory drugs (NSAIDs) have been found to reduce the incidence of heterotopic ossification. After a severe trauma, many patients are too unstable to undergo radiation therapy and have contraindications against NSAID use, including renal failure and increased bleeding risks. In a combat zone, providing radiation is logistically difficult (Potter et al, 2006, 2007).

Surgical excision is a mainstay of treatment. However, in amputees, excision may require limb revision. In most patients with heterotopic ossification, ectopic bone is removed once it has matured and become symptomatic. Orthopedic surgeons in the U.S. military have found that early excision results in faster recovery times and quicker prosthesis rehabilitation (Forsberg et al, 2008; Potter et al, 2006, 2007).

CLINICAL CONSULT

A: Consulted for ileostomy pouch leakage into abdominal wound. 23-year-old male hospitalized for abdominal injury from a gang fight and bullet injury necessitating an exploratory surgery, repair of ruptured bowel, and construction of new ileostomy. Ileostomy 3 inches from abdominal wound, 1 inch round, moist, red protruding lumen at the apex. Producing liquid stool. Abdominal wound, predominantly granulation tissue 10 × 4 × 2 cm, periwound skin with moisture-associated dermatitis due to excess wound exudate and stool. Moist gauze dressings changed 3 times daily and as needed for soiled dressings.
D: Potential for infection and inaccurate output measurement due to ineffective pouching and excessive wound moisture.

P: Negative pressure wound therapy (NPWT) to promote wound contraction, manage wound exudate, decrease frequency of dressing changes, and protect the wound (via transparent dressing/drape seal). Resize ostomy pattern to offset opening to better accommodate limited adhesive surface adjacent to wound.
I: (1) Patient taught to empty pouch when ⅓ to ½ full to prevent leakage and disruption of the dressing. Will reinforce.
E: Plan to revisit next dressing change day to evaluate effectiveness of NPWT and new pouching technique. Patient understands he will demonstrate ability to empty, remove, prepare and apply his ostomy pouch in preparation for possible discharge next week.

SUMMARY

When a wound occurs as a result of trauma, numerous patient care issues must be addressed emergently, such as airway stabilization, adequacy of cardiovascular function, and hemostasis. Tourniquets or hemostatic dressings are often needed to arrest bleeding. Once the patient is stabilized, the wound cleansing can begin so that a complete wound assessment can be obtained. Traumatic wounds are contaminated with environmental debris and may contain open fractures. Aggressive, prompt surgical debridement is generally needed to remove nonviable tissue and prevent extension of necrosis. Due to the life-threatening nature of most traumatic wounds, wound closure may not take place until the patient is stabilized. Many options exist for wound closure, and it is desirable to close the wound as soon as possible once clean granulation tissue is present.

REFERENCES

Anaya DA, Dellinger EP: Surgical infections and choice of antibiotics. In Townsend CM Jr, et al, editors: *Sabiston textbook of surgery*, Philadelphia, 2007, Saunders.

Argenta LC, Morykwas MJ, Marks MW, et al: Vacuum-assisted closure: state of clinic art, *Plast Reconstr Surg* 117(Suppl 7): 127S–142S, 2006.

Attinger CE, Janis JE, Steinberg J, et al: Clinical approach to wounds: debridement and wound bed preparation including the use of dressings and wound-healing adjuvants, *Plast Reconstr Surg* 117(Suppl 7):72S–109S, 2006.

Baker SP, O'Neill B, Haddon W Jr, et al: The injury severity score: A method for describing patients with multiple injuries and evaluating emergency care, *J Trauma* 14(3):187–196, 1974.

Barker DE, Green JM, Maxwell RA, et al: Experience with vacuum-pack temporary abdominal wound closure in 258 trauma and general and vascular surgical patients, *J Am Coll Surg* 204(5):784–792, 2007.

Bee TK, Croce MA, Magnotti LJ, et al: Temporary abdominal closure techniques: a prospective randomized trial comparing polyglactin 910 mesh and vacuum-assisted closure, *J Trauma* 65(2):337–342, 2008.

Beekley AC, Sebesta JA, Blackbourne LH, et al: Prehospital tourniquet use in Operation Iraqi Freedom: effect on hemorrhage control and outcomes, *J Trauma* 64(Suppl 2): S28–S37, 2008.

Bosse MJ, MacKenzie EJ, Kellam JF, et al: A prospective evaluation of the clinical utility of the lower-extremity injury-severity scores, *J Bone Joint Surg Am* 83A(1):3–14, 2001.

Brothers TE, Tagge DU, Stutley JE, et al: Magnetic resonance imaging differentiates between necrotizing and non-necrotizing fasciitis of the lower extremity, *J Am Coll Surg* 187(4):416–421, 1998.

Browner BD, DeAngelis JP: Emergency care of musculoskeletal injuries. In Townsend CM Jr, et al, editors: *Sabiston textbook of surgery*, Philadelphia, 2007, Saunders.

Buchanon BJ: *Gunpowder, explosives, and the state: a technological history*, Aldershot, UK, 2006, Ashgate.

Buchholz HW, Engelbrecht H: [Depot effects of various antibiotics mixed with Palacos resins], *Chirurg* 41(11):511–515, 1970.

Burris DG, Dougherty PJ, Elliot DC, et al: *Emergency war surgery*, ed 3, Washington, DC, 2004, Borden Institute.

Champion HR, Holcomb JB, Lawnick MM, et al: Improved characterization of combat injury, *J Trauma* 68(5):1139–1150, 2010.

Clayton JM, Hayes AC, Barnes RW: Tissue pressure and perfusion in the compartment syndrome, *J Surg Res* 22(4):333–339, 1977.

Drago A: *Systemic inflammatory response syndrome (S.I.R.S) after cardiac surgery, Federación Argentina de Cardiología, 5th International Congress of Cardiology on the Internet*, 2007. http://www.fac.org.ar/qcvc/llave/c130i/dragoa.php. Accessed June 1, 2014.

Eastridge BJ, Mabry RL, Seguin P, et al: Death on the battlefield (2001–2011): implications for the future of combat casualty care, *J Trauma Acute Care Surg* 73(6 Suppl 5):S431–S437, 2012.

Fabian TC, Croce MA, Pritchard FE, et al: Planned ventral hernia. Staged management for acute abdominal wall defects, *Ann Surg* 219(6):643–650, 1994.

Forsberg JA, Elster EA, Andersen RC, et al: Correlation of procalcitonin and cytokine expression with dehiscence of wartime extremity wounds, *J Bone Joint Surg Am* 90(3):580–588, 2008.

Frykberg ER, Schinco MA: *Peripheral vascular injury*. In Feliciano DV, et al, editors: *Trauma*, New York, 2008, McGraw-Hill.

Gawande A: Casualties of war–military care for the wounded from Iraq and Afghanistan, *N Engl J Med* 351(24):2471–2475, 2004.

Granick MS, Tenenhaus M, Knox KR, et al: Comparison of wound irrigation and tangential hydrodissection in bacterial clearance of contaminated wounds: results of a randomized, controlled clinical study, *Ostomy Wound Manage* 53(4):64–66, 68–70, 72, 2007.

Grayson ML, Gibbons GW, Balogh K, et al: Probing to bone in infected pedal ulcers. A clinical sign of underlying osteomyelitis in diabetic patients, *JAMA* 273(9):721–723, 1995.

Hagemo JS, Næss PA, Johansson P, et al: Evaluation of TEG(®) and RoTEM(®) inter-changeability in trauma patients, *Injury* 44:600–605, 2013.

Harris AM, Althausen PL, Kellam J, et al: Complications following limb-threatening lower extremity trauma, *J Orthop Trauma* 23(1):1–6, 2009.

Helgeson MD, Potter BK, Evans KN, et al: Bioartificial dermal substitute: a preliminary report on its use for the management of complex combat-related soft tissue wounds, *J Orthop Trauma* 21(6):394–399, 2007.

Hess JR, Brohi K, Dutton RP, et al: The coagulopathy of trauma: a review of mechanisms, *J Trauma* 65(4):748–754, 2008.

Holcomb JB, Minei KM, Scerbo ML, et al: Admission rapid thrombelastography can replace conventional coagulation tests in the emergency department: experience with 1974 consecutive trauma patients, *Ann Surg* 256(3):476–486, 2012.

Holcomb JB, Stansbury LG, Champion HR, et al: Understanding combat casualty care statistics, *J Trauma* 60(2):397–401, 2006.

Jernigan TW, Fabian TC, Croce MA, et al: Staged management of giant abdominal wall defects: acute and long-term results, *Ann Surg* 238(3):349–355, 2003.

Johansen K, Daines M, Howey T, et al: Objective criteria accurately predict amputation following lower extremity trauma, *J Trauma* 30(5):568–572, 1990.

Johansson PI, Stissing T, Bochsen L, et al: Thrombelastography and thromboelastometry in assessing coagulopathy in trauma, *Scand J Trauma Resusc Emerg Med* 17:45, 2009.

Kafie FE, Tessier DJ, Williams RA, et al: Serial abdominal closure technique (the "SAC" procedure): a novel method for delayed closure of the abdominal wall, *Am Surg* 69(2):102–105, 2003.

Kam PC, Kavanagh R, Yoong FF: The arterial tourniquet: pathophysiological consequences and anaesthetic implications, *Anaesthesia* 56(6):534–545, 2001.

Kelly JF, Ritenour AE, McLaughlin DF, et al: Injury severity and causes of death from Operation Iraqi Freedom and Operation Enduring Freedom: 2003-2004 versus 2006, *J Trauma* 64(Suppl 2):S21–S26; discussion S26–S27, 2008.

Klein MB, Hunter S, Heimbach DM, et al: The Versajet water dissector: a new tool for tangential excision, *J Burn Care Rehabil* 26(6):483–487, 2005.

Kozen BG, Kircher SJ, Henao J, et al: An alternative hemostatic dressing: comparison of CELOX, HemCon, and QuikClot, *Acad Emerg Med* 15(1):74–81, 2008.

Kragh JF Jr, Walters TJ, Baer DG, et al: Survival with emergency tourniquet use to stop bleeding in major limb trauma, *Ann Surg* 249(1):1–7, 2009.

Lindstedt S, Malmsjö M, Gesslein B, et al: Evaluation of continuous and intermittent myocardial topical negative pressure, *J Cardiovasc Med* 9(8):813–819, 2008.

Llanos S, Danilla S, Barraza C, et al: Effectiveness of negative pressure closure in the integration of split thickness skin grafts: a randomized, double-masked, controlled trial, *Ann Surg* 244(5):700–705, 2006.

Losken A, Schaefer TG: Reconstructive surgery after trauma. In Feliciano DV, et al, editors: *Trauma*, New York, 2008, McGraw-Hill.

Lowe JB, Garza JR, Bowman JL, et al: Endoscopically assisted "components separation" for closure of abdominal wall defects, *Plast Reconstr Surg* 105(2):720–729, 2000.

Ly TV, Travison TG, Castillo RC, et al: Ability of lower-extremity injury severity scores to predict functional outcome after limb salvage, *J Bone Joint Surg Am* 90(8):1738–1743, 2008.

Mathes SJ, Steinwald PM, Foster RD, et al: Complex abdominal wall reconstruction: a comparison of flap and mesh closure, *Ann Surg* 232(4):586–596, 2000.

Milburn ML, Shah PK, Friedman EB, et al: Laparoscopically assisted components separation technique for ventral incisional hernia repair, *Hernia* 11(2):157–161, 2007.

Moisidis E, Heath T, Boorer C, et al: A prospective, blinded, randomized, controlled clinical trial of topical negative pressure use in skin grafting, *Plast Reconstr Surg* 114(4):917–922, 2004.

Morykwas MJ, Argenta LC, Shelton-Brown EI, et al: Vacuum-assisted closure: a new method for wound control and treatment: animal studies and basic foundation, *Ann Plast Surg* 38(6):553–562, 1997.

National Pressure Ulcer Advisory Panel (NPUAP), European Pressure Ulcer Advisory Panel (EPUAP), Pan Pacific Pressure Injury Alliance (PPPIA): *Prevention and treatment of pressure ulcer: Clinical Practice Guideline*. In Haesler E, editor: Perth, Australia, 2014, Cambridge Media.

Neuffer MC, McDivitt J, Rose D, et al: Hemostatic dressings for the first responder: a review, *Mil Med* 169(9):716–720, 2004.

Ostermann P, Seligson D, Henry SL: Local antibiotic therapy for severe open fractures. A review of 1085 consecutive cases, *J Bone Joint Surg Br* 77(1):93–97, 1995.

Perkins JG, Cap AP, Weiss BM, et al: Massive transfusion and nonsurgical hemostatic agents, *Crit Care Med* 36(Suppl 7): S325–S339, 2008.

Peterson SL, Lehman TP: Upper extremity injury. In Feliciano DV, et al, editors: *Trauma*, New York, 2008, McGraw-Hill.

Potter BK, Burns TC, Lacap AP, et al: Heterotopic ossification in the residual limbs of traumatic and combat-related amputees, *J Am Acad Orthop Surg* 14(Spec No. 10):S191–S197, 2006.

Potter BK, Burns TC, Lacap AP, et al: Heterotopic ossification following traumatic and combat-related amputations. Prevalence, risk factors, and preliminary results of excision, *J Bone Joint Surg Am* 89(3):476–486, 2007.

Pusateri AE, Modrow HE, Harris RA, et al: Advanced hemostatic dressing development program: animal model selection criteria and results of a study of nine hemostatic dressings in a model of severe large venous hemorrhage and hepatic injury in swine, *J Trauma* 55(3):518–526, 2003.

Ramasamy A, Hill AM, Phillip R, et al: The modern "deck-slap" injury—calcaneal blast fractures from vehicle explosions, *J Trauma* 71(6):1694–1698, 2011.

Ramirez OM, Ruas E, Dellon AL: "Components separation" method for closure of abdominal-wall defects: an anatomic and clinical study, *Plast Reconstr Surg* 86(3):519–526, 1990.

Rhee P, Brown C, Martin M, et al: QuikClot use in trauma for hemorrhage control: case series of 103 documented uses, *J Trauma* 64(4):1093–1099, 2008.

Roberts I, Shakur H, Coats T, et al: The CRASH-2 trial: a randomised controlled trial and economic evaluation of the effects of tranexamic acid on death, vascular occlusive events and transfusion requirement in bleeding trauma patients, *Health Technol Assess* 17(10):1–79, 2013.

Rosen MJ, Williams C, Jin J, et al: Laparoscopic versus open-component separation: a comparative analysis in a porcine model, *Am J Surg* 194(3):385–389, 2007.

Schecter WP, Ivatury RR, Rotondo MF, et al: Open abdomen after trauma and abdominal sepsis: a strategy for management, *J Am Coll Surg* 203(3):390–396, 2006.

Shestak KC, Edington HJ, Johnson RR, et al: The separation of anatomic components technique for the reconstruction of massive midline abdominal wall defects: anatomy, surgical technique, applications, and limitations revisited, *Plast Reconstr Surg* 105(2):731–738, 2000.

Singleton JA, Gibb IE, Hunt NC, et al: Identifying future "unexpected" survivors: a retrospective cohort study of fatal injury patterns in victims of improvised explosive devices, *BMJ Open* 3(8):1–8, 2013.

Smith WR, et al: Lower extremity. In Feliciano DV, et al, editors: *Trauma*, New York, 2008, McGraw-Hill.

Stanec Z, Skrbić S, Dzepina I, et al: High-energy war wounds: flap reconstruction, *Ann Plast Surg* 31(2):97–102, 1993.

Stojadinovic A, Carlson JW, Schultz GS, et al: Topical advances in wound care, *Gynecol Oncol* 111(Suppl 2):S70–S80, 2008.

Tintle SM, Keeling JJ, Shawen SB, et al: Traumatic and trauma-related amputations: part I: general principles and lower-extremity amputations, *J Bone Joint Surg Am* 92(17):2852–2868, 2010.

Trauma.org. *Trauma scoring: injury severity score calculator.* http:// www.trauma.org/archive/scores/iss.html. Accessed August 25, 2015.

Tredget EE, Shankowsky HA, Groeneveld A, et al: A matched-pair, randomized study evaluating the efficacy and safety of Acticoat silver-coated dressing for the treatment of burn wounds, *J Burn Care Rehabil* 19(6):531–537, 1998.

Ubbink DT, Westerbos SJ, Nelson EA, et al: A systematic review of topical negative pressure therapy for acute and chronic wounds, *Br J Surg* 95(6):685–692, 2008.

Vertrees A, Greer L, Pickett C, et al: Modern management of complex open abdominal wounds of war: a 5-year experience, *J Am Coll Surg* 207(6):801–809, 2008.

Volgas DA: Care of the soft tissue envelope. In Stannard JP, et al, editors: *Surgical treatment of orthopaedic trauma*, New York, 2007, Thieme Medical Publishers, p 976.

Ward N, Casserly B, Ayala A: The compensatory anti-inflammatory response syndrome (CARS) in critically ill patients, *Clin Chest Med* 29(4):617–625, 2008.

Weinberg JA, George RL, Griffin RL, et al: Closing the open abdomen: improved success with Wittmann Patch staged abdominal closure, *J Trauma* 65(2):345–348, 2008.

Wilson JR, Mills JG, Prather ID, et al: A toxicity index of skin and wound cleansers used on in vitro fibroblasts and keratinocytes, *Adv Skin Wound Care* 18(7):373–378, 2005.

Wininger DA, Fass RJ: Antibiotic-impregnated cement and beads for orthopedic infections, *Antimicrob Agents Chemother* 40(12):2675–2679, 1996.

Wood MJ: Toxin-mediated disorders: tetanus, botulism, and diphtheria. In Cohen J, et al, editors: *Infectious diseases*, Philadelphia, 2004, Mosby.

Yin HQ, Langford R, Burrell RE: Comparative evaluation of the antimicrobial activity of ACTICOAT antimicrobial barrier dressing, *J Burn Care Rehabil* 20(3):195–200, 1999.

Burns

Jill Evans

1. Identify the three phases of burn care and discuss the goals of each phase.
2. Discuss the causes of burns, including thermal, chemical, and electrical injuries.
3. Identify how the three zones of tissue damage relate to the depth of the burn wound.
4. Compare and contrast the severity of burn trauma using the following terminology: superficial, superficial partial-thickness, deep partial-thickness, and full-thickness burns.
5. Describe three methods commonly used to calculate the total body surface area of a burn.
6. Describe the advantages and disadvantages of at least four topical burn care products or dressings.
7. Describe the indications and techniques for escharotomy, fasciotomy, tangential excision, and skin grafting.
8. Distinguish among indicators for managing the patient with a burn in the outpatient setting, the inpatient setting, and a specialized burn care facility.
9. Identify three principles of managing burn wounds in an outpatient setting.

Patients with burn injuries present with unique, complex care needs that require the collaboration and expertise of a multidisciplinary team consisting of providers, nurses, physical and occupational therapists, a pharmacist, nutrition specialist, case manager, and social worker. In addition to topical wound care needs, the patient is at risk for systemic complications associated with the absence of large amounts of epidermis and/or dermis (e.g., edema, wound infection).

Beyond the patient's physical needs, all burn team members must be aware of the psychological impact of acute injury, the phases of recovery from a burn injury, and the long-term rehabilitation needs of the patient. Throughout the United States, a number of specialized burn centers are dedicated to the management of the patient with a burn and other conditions that require care similar to burn care. In a facility that does not provide this type of specialized care, it is crucial that the wound specialist facilitate referral immediately. Box 32-1 lists the criteria for burn center referral.

EPIDEMIOLOGY

It is estimated that more than one million burn injuries occur each year in the United States, with more than 450,000 annual emergency department visits and more than 40,000 hospital admissions (American Burn Association, 2012). The majority of these injuries involve burns of less than 10% of the total body surface area (TBSA). Flame burns and scalds from hot liquids account for almost 80% of reported cases; over 70% of these injuries occur in the home (American Burn Association, 2013). The National Burn Repository 2013 Report (American Burn Association, 2013), which includes data from 2003 to 2012 on more than 175,000 inpatient burn cases from 91 U.S. burn centers, further identifies characteristics of burn-injured patients. Nearly 70% of all burn victims are male; the mean age of all reported cases is 32 years; 20% of all burn injuries occur in children younger than 5 years and 12% in patients 60 years and older. The mortality rate for all reported cases is 3.4%.

TYPES OF BURN INJURY

Burns result from thermal, electrical, and chemical injuries. Inhalation injury occurs frequently and is the most common accompanying injury seen in patients with burns.

Thermal (Flame, Scald, and Contact)
Flame. Thermal burns are the most common cause of burn injuries. They result from exposure to flames, scalds from hot liquids, and contact with hot objects. The severity of injury is related to the temperature and duration of contact. *Flame* burns commonly involve exposure to fire with ignition of clothing. Outdoor trash and brush fires frequently involve use of an accelerant (Wibbenmeyer et al, 2003).

BOX 32-1 Criteria for Burn Center Referral

- Partial-thickness burns >10% of total body surface area
- All full-thickness burns
- Burns that involve the face, hands, feet, genitalia, perineum, major joints
- Electrical burns, including lightning injury
- Chemical burns
- Inhalation injury
- Presence of preexisting medical disorders that could complicate management, prolong recovery, or affect mortality
- Patients with concomitant trauma in whom the burn poses the greatest risk of morbidity or mortality
- Burned children in hospitals without qualified personnel or equipment to care for children
- Patients who require special social, emotional, or long-term rehabilitative intervention

Adapted from American Burn Association: Guidelines for the operations of burn centers, *J Burn Care Res* 28(1):134–141, 2007.

House fires are a significant cause of flame burn injury and are associated with the additional risk of smoke inhalation injury. Smoke inhalation injury is present in approximately 10% to 20% of patients admitted to burn centers (Palmieri, 2007). In 2012, fire departments in the United States responded to 480,500 home and structure fires, which resulted in 2855 nonfirefighter deaths and 16,500 injuries. Direct property damage is estimated at $12.4 billion (Karter, 2013). Most fatalities at fire scenes are caused by inhalation of smoke with toxic compounds (Palmieri, 2007). The combustion of most substances generates materials, such as carbon monoxide, hydrogen cyanide, ammonia, and aldehydes, that are toxic to the respiratory tract (McCall and Cahill, 2005). Carboxyhemoglobin levels of 50% to 70% are often found in patients with such exposure. Administration of 100% humidified oxygen through a nonrebreather mask should be initiated as soon as possible (American Burn Association, 2011).

Inhaled hot air (temperatures >150°C) causes heat injury to respiratory epithelia (Palmieri, 2007). Tissue edema can occur rapidly to the upper airway and may cause airway obstruction. The patient with burns to the face, singed nasal and facial hair, edema of the tongue or pharynx, increased respiratory rate, and a history of injury within an enclosed space should be monitored closely for airway obstruction due to edema (McCall and Cahill, 2005). Intubation with mechanical ventilation may be necessary to provide adequate oxygenation until the edema resolves.

Scald. Most *scald* injuries occur in the kitchen or bathroom of the home and are associated with hot water exposure and cooking (food and grease spills) (Evans et al, 2006; Lowell et al, 2008). The severity of a scald burn injury is related to the temperature of the exposing liquid and length of time of exposure. The most common standard for the maximum temperature of hot tap water delivered by residential water heaters is 120°F/48°C. At this temperature, the skin of adults requires an average of 5 minutes' exposure for a full-thickness burn to occur; infants and small children may sustain second-degree burns in 1 minute or less of exposure at this temperature. Safe bathing temperature for infants and small children is 100°F/37°C (American Burn Association, 2014).

Contact. *Contact* burns can occur in the home or in the workplace. They frequently occur on the hands, face, and upper body as the object is touched. Common causes of contact burns include oven doors, fireplace screens, space heaters, clothing and curling irons, cookware, and hot machinery and containers (Alden et al, 2006; Hunt et al, 2000; Wibbenmeyer et al, 2003). Children younger than 5 years are at particular risk for scald and contact injuries due to a limited ability to recognize and respond appropriately to danger. The elderly have predisposing factors associated with age that put them at risk for burn injury, including reduced reaction times, decreased dexterity, decreased mobility, inaccurate risk assessment, and impaired senses (Redlick et al, 2002). Working adults are at risk for scald and contact burns; exposure to hot objects or substances is the second-leading cause of burn injury in the workplace (Hunt et al, 2000).

Electrical

Electrical injuries account for approximately 4% of burn center admissions (American Burn Association, 2013). It is estimated that as many as 50,000 injuries and 1000 deaths from electrical causes occur each year in the United States. The American Burn Association (2011) estimates that the risk of being struck by lightning in the United States is approximately one per million per year; lightning strikes kill 80 to 100 people each year and injure another 300. Tissue injury results when electrical energy is converted into thermal or heat energy. The extent of injury to the body when it becomes part of an electrical current is determined by the (1) strength and type of current, (2) pathway of flow, (3) local tissue resistance, and (4) duration of exposure (American Burn Association, 2011).

Classification of electrical injuries is divided into four categories: high voltage (>1000 V), low voltage (<1000 V), lightning strikes, and electric arc without passage of current through the body. The highest incidence of injuries is work related and high voltage, with the primary victims being young men (Arnoldo et al, 2004). Electrical injuries in children are generally low voltage, occur in the home, and involve contact with electrical appliances or frayed cords or placement of objects into electrical outlets. Because of the mechanism of injury, electrically injured patients are at risk for concomitant blunt trauma, soft tissue injuries, and thermal (flame or flash) burns (American Burn Association, 2011). Electrical injuries may also result in potentially fatal cardiac dysrhythmias. Practice guidelines for the management of electrical injuries recommend an electrocardiogram be performed on all patients who sustain either high- or low-voltage electrical injuries (Arnoldo et al, 2006).

Chemical (Alkalis, Acids, and Organic Compounds)

Chemical burns account for about 3% of burn unit admissions (American Burn Association, 2013), with approximately 60,000 people seeking medical treatment each year. Chemical injuries are progressive in nature, and it is often difficult to determine the severity of the injury early in the course of treatment; the burn may initially appear superficial but in reality be quite deep (American Burn Association, 2011).

The severity of chemical burns is related to the agent of exposure; duration of contact; and agent's concentration, volume, and mechanism of action. Tissue damage continues after initial exposure until the chemical is removed or inactivated (diluted) with irrigation. In general, neutralization of the agent with another chemical is not recommended unless the exact mechanism is known because the reaction may generate more heat and result in further tissue destruction (American Burn Association, 2011). Health care providers must protect themselves from exposure by using universal precautions and eye protection while caring for the chemical-injured patient. The American Burn Association (2011) identifies the common causes of chemical injury as alkalis, acids, and organic compounds.

Alkalis are commonly found in oven and drain cleaners, fertilizers, industrial cleaners, and cement and concrete. Alkalis damage tissue by liquefaction necrosis and protein denaturation, which allows for deeper spread of the chemical into tissues and a more severe injury. *Acids* are found in bathroom cleansers, rust removers, acidifiers for home swimming pools, and industrial drain cleaners. Acids damage tissue by coagulation necrosis and protein precipitation, causing a thick leathery eschar. *Organic compounds,* such as phenols and petroleum products (gasoline, diesel fuel, and creosote), can be responsible for systemic toxicity and contact chemical burns. Organic compounds cause cutaneous damage as a result of their fat solvent action and, once absorbed, can produce toxic effects on the renal and hepatic systems (American Burn Association, 2011).

Health care providers must have a high degree of suspicion of lower airway injury related to inhalation of noxious chemicals in patients who were injured in an enclosed space or have a history of loss of consciousness at the scene of a fire (American Burn Association, 2011). Chemical inhalation may cause sloughing of the airway-lining epithelium, mucus secretion, inflammation, atelectasis, and airway obstruction. Clinical evolution is delayed from 1 to 3 days after exposure (Palmieri, 2007). Treatment requires ventilatory support, meticulous pulmonary toilet, and general critical care management.

EVALUATION OF BURN INJURY
Zones of Tissue Damage

Determining burn depth can be difficult for even the most experienced burn care provider. Immediately following injury, burns may appear superficial but declare themselves to be deeper by postburn day 3 (Gibran and Heimbach, 2000). The phrase "zones of tissue damage" describes the extent of the injury from the deepest or most severely damaged area to the superficial or outermost area. The three zones of tissue damage are zone of coagulation, zone of stasis, and zone of hyperemia (Jackson, 1953). The *zone of coagulation* is the area of greatest damage, is closest to the heat source, and is characterized by coagulation of cells. The *zone of stasis* surrounds the zone of coagulation and involves the vascular system in the area. Thrombosis and vasoconstriction cause transient dermal ischemia. Circulation will return if the area is adequately perfused and protected from further damage from infection, desiccation, and mechanical stress during transfers and repositioning. The *zone of hyperemia* is the outermost area. Usually no cellular death occurs because this area is only minimally damaged. Cells in this zone recover in 7 to 10 days. The area is reddened because of vasodilation and inflammation. The zone of hyperemia is similar to a superficial partial-thickness burn.

Severity of the Burn Wound

Treatment of the burn wound is based on the depth, extent, and severity of the injury. The depth of the injury is based on the number of cells injured or destroyed. With the exception of the fourth degree, the traditional classification of burns as first, second, and third degree has largely been replaced by the more descriptive designations of superficial, superficial partial-thickness, deep partial-thickness, and full-thickness injury (Figure 32-1). Most burns are not uniform in depth; the edges may be shallower than the central aspect. The severity of the burn can deteriorate in certain circumstances and become more severe, a process known as *wound conversion.* Risk factors for wound conversion are similar to factors that impair other acute and chronic wounds (e.g., oxygenation, infection, mechanical trauma, malnutrition).

Calculation of Body Surface Area Burned

Three methods are used to determine the extent of a burn injury: (1) Lund-Browder chart (Figure 32-2), (2) rule of nines (Figure 32-3), and (3) hand method. The Lund-Browder chart is the most accurate method for estimating burn extent in patients of all ages, as it takes into account changes in percentage of body surface area for specific body parts that occur in different developmental stages (Lund and Browder, 1944). The Lund-Browder chart is completed at admission to determine fluid requirements and is repeated after 72 hours to recalculate any areas of burn injury that may have extended. The rule of nines (EMT, 2014) is based on 11 anatomic regions of the body representing 9% (or multiples of 9%) of TBSA (Knaysi et al, 1968). The rule of nines must be modified for use in children because it does not accurately reflect body surface area in children younger than 15 years (Deitch and Rutan, 2000). Neither the Lund-Browder chart nor rule of nines may accurately reflect TBSA in morbidly obese patients (Williams and Wohlgemuth, 2013). The hand method of determining the extent of a burn injury is

		WOUND APPEARANCE	WOUND SENSATION	COURSE OF HEALING
EPIDERMIS Sweat duct Capillary	PARTIAL-THICKNESS BURN — 1st-degree	Epidermis remains intact and without blisters Erythema; skin blanches with pressure	Painful	Discomfort lasts 48-72 hours. Desquamation occurs in 3-7 days.
Sebaceous gland Nerve endings DERMIS Hair follicle	PARTIAL-THICKNESS BURN — 2nd-degree	Wet, shiny, weeping surface Blisters Wound blanches with pressure	Painful Very sensitive to touch, air currents	Superficial partial-thickness burn heals in <21 days. Deep partial-thickness burn requires >21 days for healing. Healing rates vary with burn depth and presence/absence of infection.
Sweat gland Fat Blood vessels	FULL-THICKNESS BURN — 3rd-degree	Color variable (i.e., deep red, white, black, brown) Surface dry Thrombosed vessels visible No blanching	Insensate (↓ pinprick sensation)	Autografting is required for healing.
Bone	FULL-THICKNESS BURN — 4th-degree	Color variable Charring visible in deepest areas Extremity movement limited	Insensate	Amputation of extremities is likely. Autografting is required for healing.

FIGURE 32-1 Burn injury classification according to depth of injury. (Adapted from Black JM, Hawks JH: *Medical-surgical nursing: clinical management for positive outcomes,* ed 8, St. Louis, MO, 2009, Saunders.)

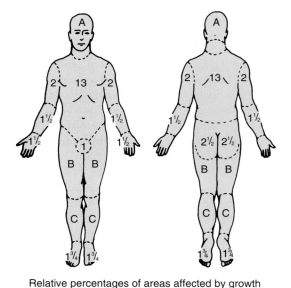

Relative percentages of areas affected by growth (age in years)

	0	1	5	10	15	Adult
A: Half of head	9½	8½	6½	5½	4½	3½
B: Half of thigh	2¾	3¼	4	4¼	4½	4¾
C: Half of leg	2½	2½	2¾	3	3¼	3½

Second degree _____ and
Third degree _____ =
Total percent burned _____

FIGURE 32-2 The Lund-Browder chart for estimating burn extent. Areas represent percentages of body surface area that vary according to age. The accompanying table indicates the relative percentages of these areas in various stages of life. (From Sabeston DC Jr, editor: *Textbook of surgery: the biographical basis of modern surgical practice,* ed 11, Philadelphia, PA, 1977, Saunders.)

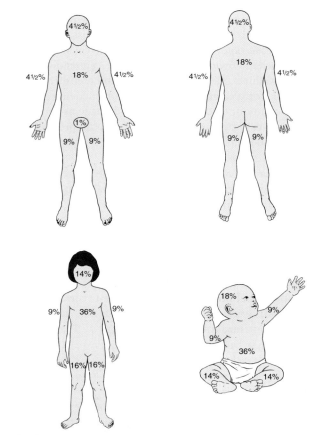

FIGURE 32-3 Rule of nines (From Mosby: *Mosby's dictionary of medicine, nursing and health professions,* ed 9, St. Louis, 2013, Mosby.)

TABLE 32-1 American Burn Association Categories of Burn Injury		
Minor Burns	**Moderate Burns**	**Major Burns**
Adults: 15% TBSA Children and elderly: 10% TBSA <2% TBSA full-thickness burns not involving cosmetic or functional risk or impairment of face, ears, eyes, feet, hands, perineum	Adults: 15% to 25% TBSA, mixed partial/full thickness Children <10 years or adults >40 years: 10% to 20% TBSA < 10% TBSA full-thickness burns not involving cosmetic or functional risk or impairment of the face, ears, eyes, feet, hands, perineum	All patients: >25% TBSA Children <10 years or adults >40 years: 20% TBSA >10% TBSA full-thickness burns All burns of face, eyes, ears, hands, or perineum, especially if functional or cosmetic impairment exists All high-voltage electrical burns All burns with inhalation injury or major trauma Poor-risk patients

TBSA, Total body surface area.

useful for estimating small, scattered burns. The patient's hand, including the fingers, represents approximately 1% of TBSA (American Burn Association, 2011). The TBSA burned is expressed as a percentage and helps estimate the extent of the injury for diagnosis, treatment, prognosis, and statistical analysis.

Referral Criteria

The American Burn Association has categorized burns as minor, moderate, and major (Table 32-1) and has defined the criteria for burn center referral (see Box 32-1). Patients with major burn injuries or those who meet the criteria identified in Box 32-1 require treatment in a specialized center. A burn center is a facility with a burn provider as director and a highly trained, multidisciplinary staff dedicated to caring for the patient with burns (American Burn Association, 2007).

PATHOPHYSIOLOGY OF BURN INJURY ON THE BODY

Inflammatory mediators released from the damaged cells at the site of the burn (e.g., arachidonic acid metabolites, oxidants, histamine, serotonin, kinins, other vasoactive amines) cause increased capillary permeability not only at the site of injury, but also throughout the body (Ahrns, 2004). In patients with a burn wound greater than 20% to 25%, this response is most severe in the first 24 hours. Although capillary permeability returns to normal roughly 18 to 24 hours after injury, the initial body response is a dramatic outpouring of fluids, electrolytes, and protein into the interstitial space, which creates intravascular volume deficits. The release of fluids through the hyperpermeable capillaries and the increased capillary pressure combine to create local or systemic edema. The body responds with a classic hemodynamic response: an almost immediate fall in cardiac output, metabolic rate, oxygen consumption, and blood pressure, along with ongoing fluid imbalance and cellular shock, for 3 to 7 days (Pham et al, 2008).

The fluid and electrolyte imbalance that immediately results after a burn injury dominates postburn care priorities and poses potential complications to the pulmonary, cardiovascular, and renal systems. The shift of protein from the intracellular space and vascular compartment into the interstitial space causes numerous potential complications, such as edema, pulmonary edema, blister formation, weeping of fluid, hypovolemia, hypoproteinemia, tachycardia, increased capillary pressure, vasoconstriction of the microcirculation, decreased central venous pressure, and decreased urinary output. Sodium, magnesium, calcium, and phosphorus loss can occur directly through open burn wounds (Supple, 2004). Potassium is released from damaged cells, triggering hyperkalemia and metabolic acidosis.

Restoration and maintenance of intravascular volume with fluid similar to that which is lost in the tissues are essential aspects of burn management. Loss of skin integrity causes increased fluid and heat loss through the wound. Evaporative fluid loss caused by loss of skin integrity is 4 to 20 times the normal rate, which contributes to hypovolemia; this fluid loss continues until all the wounds are closed. Hypothermia should be prevented rigorously throughout the phases of recovery. Localized hypothermia causes vasoconstriction to the burn-injured area, decreasing blood flow and tissue oxygenation, which may lead to deepening of the injury. Systemic hypothermia induces peripheral vasoconstriction that may similarly increase the depth of the burn injury, decrease enzymatic activity, depress muscle reflexes, interfere with clotting mechanisms and respiration, and cause cardiac arrhythmias (American Burn Association, 2011).

The hypermetabolic response post–burn injury is characterized by increased levels of inflammatory mediators, catecholamines, and corticosteroids. The increase in the metabolic rate results in insulin resistance, increased gluconeogenesis, lipolysis, and proteolysis. Provision of adequate and early nutrition support with the correct balance of nutrients is essential to mitigating this hypermetabolic and hypercatabolic response (Hall, 2012). The severity and duration of hypermetabolic activity are directly proportional to the extent of injury. The peak occurs in the first 2 weeks and slowly returns to normal with closure of the wound. Elevated catecholamines, decreased bowel perfusion, and increased gastric secretions place the burn patient at risk for paralytic ileus, intestinal mucosal atrophy, decreased nutrient absorption, Curling stress ulcer, and impaired ability to function as a bacterial barrier (Supple, 2004).

PHASES OF BURN CARE

Burn care is divided into three overlapping phases of recovery: emergent, acute/wound care, and rehabilitation. The emergent phase is the first 72 hours after injury, focusing on assessment and initial management. The acute/wound care phase begins when the patient has been stabilized. Goals of this period include healing partial-thickness wounds, grafting full-thickness wounds, and preventing complications. Wound management during the acute phase consists of debridement, daily wound care, and surgical interventions for wound closure. The rehabilitation phase begins when wound healing is complete and focuses on restoring or maximizing the patient's functional capacity. This phase may last several years and deals with functional and cosmetic problems associated with contractures and scar tissue formation.

Emergent Phase

As with any trauma victim, the initial assessment of the patient with a burn injury includes the primary and secondary surveys. The primary survey (conducted out in the field) includes advanced burn life support (ABLS) as outlined by the American College of Surgeons Committee on Trauma (American Burn Association, 2011). The guidelines include the ABCDE assessment: airway, breathing, circulation, disability, and exposure and evaluation.

The secondary survey is initiated after immediate resuscitative measures are established and includes a complete physical assessment and medical history. Because care is based on the mechanism, location, and severity of the injury, as much information as possible regarding the incident should be obtained, such as whether the injury occurred in an enclosed space, chemicals were involved, and the victim lost consciousness. Aspects of the patient's medical history (e.g., preexisting disease, medications, allergies, alcohol or drug use, immunization status) influence management decisions (American Burn Association, 2011).

Care during the emergent phase centers on emergency management and stabilization and on wound assessment/diagnosis. The first 24 hours are devoted to fluid resuscitation, ventilatory management, and establishing the hemodynamic stability of the patient. During this phase, the depth and extent of the wound are estimated in order to calculate the severity of the injury and fluid resuscitation needs.

Large burns reach maximum edema within 12 to 24 hours postinjury. The goal of fluid resuscitation is to maintain adequate tissue and vital organ perfusion while preventing complications associated with inadequate or excessive fluid therapy (American Burn Association, 2011). If fluid resuscitation is inadequate, hypovolemia will progress

and acute renal failure will occur. The amount of fluid for replacement depends on the extent and depth of the burn and the patient's age and medical history. Many fluid resuscitation formulas exist, and most are based on the percentage of TBSA burned, body weight, or a combination of both. According to the American Burn Association, fluid resuscitation, regardless of solution type or estimated need, should be titrated to maintain urine output of approximately 0.5 to 1.0 ml/kg/hr in adults and 1.0 to 1.5 ml/kg/hr in children. Increased volume requirements can be anticipated in patients with full-thickness injury, inhalation injury, and delay in resuscitation (Pham et al, 2008). Adequacy of resuscitation is determined by urinary output, mental status, peripheral temperature, systolic blood pressure, heart rate, and base deficit (Sheridan, 2002).

For a small partial-thickness burn (see Table 32-1), the development of edema is immediate and rapid (within 4 hours), limited to the wound site, and peaks within 12 hours (Demling et al, 1978). Oral resuscitation is appropriate for burns less than 20% TBSA, as these burns are not associated with severe systemic inflammation and vasodilation in nonburned tissues (Pham et al, 2008). Intravenous supplementation can be used if the patient has difficulties meeting the oral intake goal.

Aggressive nutrition support is recommended after severe burn injury. The American Burn Association practice guidelines recommend enteral nutritional support should be implemented as soon as possible to prevent stress ulcers, increase intestinal blood flow, preserve gastrointestinal function, and minimize bacterial translocation from the gut as a result of mucosal atrophy (Mosier et al, 2011; Rodriguez et al, 2011). Initiation within 24 hours has also been found to decrease the rate of wound infection and intensive care unit (ICU) length of stay without a significant difference in rates of hyperglycemia, abdominal compartment syndrome, and gastrointestinal bleeding (Mosier et al, 2011). The parenteral route may be used in select patients whose caloric requirements cannot be supplied enterally, such as with prolonged ileus (Rodriguez et al, 2011).

Nearly all burn centers report supplementing vitamins and/or minerals (Graves et al, 2009). Dosage guidelines established by the National Advisory Group/American Medical Association are appropriate for burn-injured patients unless symptoms of deficiency occur. Because zinc deficiencies are well documented in burn-injured patients, supplemental zinc and vitamin C are often required (Sicoutris and Holmes, 2006). Nutrition assessment and support are discussed in great detail in Chapter 27.

This phase ends when capillary permeability begins to normalize and the patient begins to diurese the large volume of fluid given for resuscitation, usually around postburn day 4.

Wound Stabilization. Wound intervention during the emergent phase involves cleansing, debridement, and prevention of obstructed blood flow from edema and eschar formation. The usual burn wound care given during this period follows patient stabilization and involves cleansing the areas with a nonirritating detergent and rinsing with warm water. The environment should be warmed to prevent hypothermia. Loose necrotic or devitalized tissue is lightly debrided, and large intact bullae (>2 cm) are opened. Full-thickness wounds usually are dressed with a topical antimicrobial agent; systemic prophylactic antibiotics are not routinely used unless specific organisms have been identified (American Burn Association, 2001).

Escharotomy. Deep partial-thickness or full-thickness burns that are circumferential, or nearly circumferential, to an extremity may require an escharotomy to relieve pressure. Edema and eschar formation can obstruct venous return and lead to decreased arterial blood flow. Early identification of extremities at risk and serial examination are essential; monitoring should include skin temperature, sensation, motion, pain with passive motion, changes in the quality of peripheral pulses, and capillary refill. The escharotomy is a linear incision through the full-thickness wound dividing the eschar. Full-thickness eschar lacks nerve endings, so pain is minimal, although small doses of narcotics and anxiolytics are given intravenously to control background pain and anxiety. This procedure can be done at the bedside with a sterile field and scalpel or electrocautery to control the small amount of bleeding that occurs (American Burn Association, 2011; Orgill and Piccolo, 2009). Midmedial and midlateral incisions are designed to completely section the eschar while preventing injury to underlying superficial structures. The structures most at risk during escharotomy are the brachial artery in the upper arm, the ulnar nerve at the elbow, the superficial peroneal nerve at the knee, and the neurovascular bundles and extensors of the digits (Sheridan, 2002). Monitoring of the previous parameters should be continued to determine whether the escharotomy was successful in returning blood flow.

Similarly, deep circumferential burns to the chest and/or abdomen may restrict the expansion needed for breathing and adequate ventilation. Frequent assessment of the adequacy of chest expansion, quality of respirations, oxygenation, and mental status of the patient is essential. Circumferential chest burns require an escharotomy placed in the anterior axillary line bilaterally. If there is significant extension of the burn onto the adjacent abdominal wall, the incisions should be extended to this area and connected by a transverse incision along the costal margin (American Burn Association, 2011).

Fasciotomy. In contrast to the decreased blood flow seen in circumferential burns requiring escharotomy, extremity compartment syndrome involves edema within the deep fascia of the muscles, and may occur in both burned and nonburned limbs. Causes of acute compartment syndrome include massive fluid resuscitation, high-voltage electrical injury damaging the muscle, crush injuries, and delay in escharotomy (ischemia-reperfusion injury). A fasciotomy, or surgical incision of the fascia, then is necessary (American Burn Association, 2011). See Chapter 31 for further information about fasciotomy and postoperative management.

Emergent Phase Pain Control and Emotional Support. During each of the phases of burn recovery, the patient with a burn faces numerous sources of anxiety and types of pain: exposure of nerve endings, inflammation, edema, dressing changes, debridement, insertion of intravenous lines, blood draws, invasive monitoring procedures, physical and occupational therapy, and surgical procedures (Byers et al, 2001). The burn patient's needs change over the course of each day and in each phase of recovery and include two distinct components: continuous background pain and severe pain experienced with treatment. Both pharmacologic and nonpharmacologic interventions are used to manage burn pain (Connor-Ballard, 2009).

Assessment of the patient's pain must include identifying the cause of the pain, a reliable pain rating tool, and interventions appropriate to the phase of care. During the emergent hypermetabolic phase, opioids such as morphine sulfate (considered the gold standard for moderate to severe acute pain) are best administered in small, frequent doses. Moderate sedation with analgesia, under appropriate supervision and monitoring, may be used during the initial assessment and management while stabilization is ongoing. Severe background pain can be managed with morphine sulfate through continuous infusion or patient-controlled analgesia (PCA). Mild to moderate background pain can be managed with short-acting oral opioids such as oxycodone and acetaminophen combinations (Connor-Ballard, 2009).

Emotional support in the emergent phase focuses on reducing the patient's and family's anxiety. Anxiety reduces the patient's ability to tolerate and cope with painful experiences (Connor-Ballard, 2009) and is a source of frustration and stress for family members (Smith et al, 2011). Communication regarding purpose of procedures, nonpharmacologic pain interventions such as elevation of burned extremities or properly fitted splints, and facilitating involvement of the family in the plan of care have proven successful in terms of the patient and family experience (American Academy of Pediatrics, 2014; Connor-Ballard, 2009). Interventions for the acute/wound care and rehabilitation phases are discussed later in this chapter.

Acute/Wound Care Phase

Care of the burn wound is a priority of the acute/wound care phase. Goals of this phase are to heal partial-thickness wounds, graft full-thickness wounds, and prevent complications such as infection. Wound cleansing and debridement, in conjunction with the appropriate topical agent, dressing, or skin replacement, are required to prevent infection and promote wound healing.

Initially, wound care is dependent on the location, extent, and depth of the wound. The management of burn injuries can differ significantly based on injury location, joint involvement, small body surface area (BSA) burns as opposed to large BSA burns, and partial as opposed to full-thickness burns (see Figure 32-1 and Table 32-1). Factors that influence the care plan may include age of the patient, pain and anxiety management, and ability of the patient and/or caregiver to participate in daily care.

Hydrotherapy. Team members in the burn unit perform gentle cleansing, debridement, and wound assessments during daily hydrotherapy (treatment using water). Hydrotherapy for burn care may be accomplished by tub immersion or, more commonly, by shower cart (Davison et al, 2010). The patient is medicated for pain and anxiety before the procedure, so this is an ideal time for physical and occupational therapists to perform range-of-motion (ROM) exercises and functional evaluations. Diversionary activities such as music or videos are often used to assist with patient coping during painful dressing changes and procedures (Tan et al, 2010). For the pediatric patient, the child life specialist (CLS) is invaluable in providing developmentally appropriate activities while role modeling supportive behaviors to caregivers.

Bioburden Management. Upon stabilization of the burn-injured patient, deep partial-thickness and full-thickness burn wounds undergo excision and temporary or permanent closure of the wound. The aims of this early surgical excision are removal of dead tissue to halt the overwhelming inflammatory response and to prevent infection. A more conservative approach is required for those patients who remain hemodynamically unstable, have a severe inhalation injury, or have existing medical conditions that increase the risk of operative intervention (Church et al, 2006). Burn wound surfaces are sterile immediately after injury but eventually become colonized with microorganisms. The risk of invasive wound infection is related to the cause and extent of the burn injury and the type and amount of microorganisms colonizing the wound (Church et al, 2006). Gram-positive bacteria, such as staphylococci, heavily colonize the burn wound surface within 48 hours if topical antimicrobials are not used. Within 5 to 7 days, other microbes, including gram-positive bacteria, gram-negative bacteria, yeasts, fungi, and virus, are present on the wound. Gram-negative bacteria have emerged as the most common cause of invasive wound infection (Coban, 2012; Church et al, 2006). Local signs of invasive burn wound infection include the conversion of partial-thickness to full-thickness injury, rapidly extending cellulitis of noninjured tissue around the wound, and rapid eschar separation (Church et al, 2006). During the acute phase, frequent and regular (one to two times daily) assessment of the burn wound is essential for early detection of a potential burn wound infection.

Nonbacterial sources of infection include yeast, fungus, and virus (e.g., herpes). Fungi can be found throughout the environment, including the air, nonsterile wound supplies, and laundry items. Although fungi, particularly Candida species, are commonly found on burn wounds, candida wound infections are not common in burn patients. When a fungal infection does occur, it is most frequently caused by Candida in patients with large burns who receive broad-spectrum antibiotics for treatment of other infections. Fungal infections are treated with topical and systemic antifungal agents

only if systemic infection is confirmed (Struck and Gille, 2013). A viral infection in the patient with a burn injury usually is localized. Herpetic infections most commonly occur in healing or recently healed partial-thickness burns. Assessment and management of bacterial bioburden, including descriptions and indications for topical antimicrobials, are described in Chapter 16.

Topical antimicrobials. Topical antimicrobials are indicated for deep burns that cannot undergo early excision and wound closure but are not proved necessary for shallow burns, donor sites, and meshed skin grafts (Franz et al, 2008). The ideal topical antimicrobial for the patient with the burn should (1) have a broad spectrum of activity; (2) have minimal systemic absorption; (3) not delay wound healing; (4) penetrate eschar well; (5) be painless upon application; and (6) be inexpensive (Patel et al, 2008). Silver sulfadiazine is the most commonly used *prophylactic* topical antimicrobial for burn care. However, a metaanalysis of 14 randomized controlled trials (RCTs) involving 877 participants compared silver dressings or topical silver (used with dressings) with nonsilver dressings. The results led Aziz and colleagues (2011) to suggest that silver-containing dressings and topical silver were no better or worse than a variety of control dressings in the prevention of wound infection or wound healing. Because no single product meets all of these criteria, an antimicrobial should be chosen based on the individual patient and the wound needs. The next section briefly discusses the topical antimicrobials most commonly used with burns.

Silver sulfadiazine. Silver is active against both gram-positive and gram-negative organisms and fungus. Silver sulfadiazine, which is available as a 1% cream, is easy to apply without pain on application and has a relatively low toxicity (Church et al, 2006; Honari, 2004). Several cases of transient leukopenia have been reported in patients receiving silver sulfadiazine therapy (Hosseini et al, 2007). Leukopenia associated with silver sulfadiazine administration is primarily characterized by decreased neutrophil count. Maximal white blood cell depression occurs within 2 to 4 days of initiation of therapy. Rebound to normal leukocyte levels follows onset within 2 to 3 days. Recovery is not influenced by continuation of silver sulfadiazine therapy.

Silver antimicrobial dressings. Silver antimicrobial dressings provide a broad spectrum of antimicrobial and bactericidal coverage, including vancomycin-resistant enterococcus, methicillin-resistant *Staphylococcus aureus, Pseudomonas aeruginosa,* and Candida. Ionic silver dressings are available in many forms and are discussed in Chapters 16 and 18. Some of these dressings are contraindicated for particular burn injuries, so it is essential to check the manufacturer's information for indications and contraindications.

Mafenide acetate. Mafenide acetate (Sulfamylon) is a suspension cream with broad-spectrum activity against gram-positive and gram-negative organisms, including *P. aeruginosa.* Mafenide penetrates burn eschar well, so it is useful when infection is suspected or vascular supply is minimal (Honari, 2004). Mafenide is a potent carbonic anhydrase inhibitor.

Metabolic acidosis is a frequent side effect when mafenide is used on burns greater than 25% TBSA. Other adverse effects include pain on application to partial-thickness burns and a maculopapular rash. A 5% solution also is available and is approved for use as a prophylactic agent applied as a soak to fresh autografts (Honori, 2004).

Bacitracin/neomycin/polymyxin. Bacitracin/neomycin/polymyxin is nontoxic and moisturizing and can be reapplied one to five times daily, so they are useful for facial and perineal burns. Bacitracin alone has mild antimicrobial activity against gram-positive bacteria, so the addition of neomycin and polymyxin B bolsters gram-negative coverage (Patel, et al, 2008).

Cellular- and/or Tissue-Based Products.
Cellular- and/or tissue-based products (CTPs), often referred to as temporary skin substitutes or biologic, synthetic, biosynthetic, or bioengineered dressings, are effective with partial-thickness burns while the patient is awaiting epithelialization and with excised full-thickness burns while the patient is awaiting skin graft closure. As explained in Chapter 19, when skin is replaced by a material from a source other than the patient, the material will not provide permanent wound closure and eventually will be rejected. However, the product can maintain a wound free of infection until epithelialization or permanent wound closure occurs (Franz et al, 2008). Additional benefits include a reduction of heat and water loss from the wound, less pain as sensory nerve terminals are covered, fewer dressing changes required, and increased patient participation with therapies and activities critical to recovery (Delatte et al, 2001; Lesher et al, 2011). Ideally, the product will not be rejected until after the host has established a healthy epithelial wound bed. Descriptions, components, indications, and contraindications of each of the skin substitutes are given in Chapter 19. The next section briefly discusses the types of CTPs most appropriate for burns based on severity and location.

Extracellular matrix scaffolds. Extracellular matrix scaffolds, also referred to as dermal replacements, are used to promote rapid dermis production with minimal scar tissue formation. These products are useful for treatment of large, full-thickness BSA burns. Examples include Integra and Alloderm. When used in conjunction with thin autografts, dermal replacements may decrease the amount of scar tissue formation, which improves the elasticity and flexibility of healed burns by allowing more normal ingrowth of the body's own vascular cells and tissues (Paul, 2008).

Biobrane, a biosynthetic extracellular matrix scaffold, is used for the management of superficial partial-thickness wounds, as a donor site dressing, and on excised burns that do not have eschar. Biobrane readily conforms to surface irregularities, so it can be placed on the joints, face, and trunk, thus promoting an early return to activities of daily living. Biobrane is also available as a preformed glove for use on partial-thickness burns to the hand.

BGC Matrix wound dressing is an extracellular wound matrix useful for the management of partial-thickness burns and donor sites. As the BGC Matrix dressing becomes dry and well adhered to the wound, the dressing becomes quite stiff, which limits its use over joints and on the face and neck; these same properties make it ideal as a donor site dressing because it does not easily become dislodged from the donor site as the patient resumes activity (Delatte et al, 2001).

Allograft. Allograft, cadaveric human skin harvested from human donors, is considered to be the gold standard for excised burns when no donor sites are available. Allografts applied to excised burn wounds prepare the area for definitive closure by preventing desiccation of the wound, promoting reepithelialization, and suppressing bacterial proliferation (Calota et al, 2012). However, supply may be limited and, as with any human donor situation, there is a potential for disease transmission.

Xenograft. Xenograft (heterograft, split-thickness pigskin) is a non-human skin graft and is used primarily as a dressing for partial-thickness burns that are not expected to require skin grafting. As a true biologic dressing containing growth factors, xenograft is applied to wounds to create an optimal environment for reepithelialization, and may be left on the wound to dry as healing occurs underneath (Honori, 2004). Xenograft is easier to obtain, but is not as effective as allograft when used as a temporary dressing with excised wounds because it does not establish vessel-to-vessel connections (Pruitt, 1997).

Surgical Excision and Autograft Closure.
Early eschar excision and graft closure are recommended for deep burn wounds to decrease risk of infection, improve survival, and initiate healing. Exceptions include (1) special areas such as the hands and face where improved outcomes from early excision and closure have not been demonstrated and (2) patients at the extremes of age or with comorbid conditions for whom early excision and grafting would impose significant insult (i.e., inhalation injury) (Franz et al, 2008).

In general, if the burn is greater than 30% TBSA, graft closure is done in stages because the operative process of excision and harvesting skin involves blood loss and is physiologically stressful, and donor sites need time to heal before they are reused. When an excised burn is so large that donor sites for split-thickness skin grafts are insufficient, nonimmunogenic cultured epidermal autograft (Epicell) can serve as a permanent skin replacement without fear of rejection (Franz et al, 2008). A temporary skin graft can be used to cover the wound and protect it from infection while awaiting the cultured epidermal autograft.

Split-thickness skin grafts are the most commonly used autografts. The skin is harvested using a guarded dermatome, which controls the thickness of the graft (usually 0.008 to 0.0012 inch thick), and includes the epidermis and a thin layer of dermis. Split-thickness skin grafts may be used as sheets or meshed to provide expansion (Mozingo, 1998). Sheet grafts provide a better functional and cosmetic result and are commonly used on the face, hands, feet, neck, and joints. Postoperatively, sheet grafts may collect serous drainage or blood, which can lift the graft from the wound bed, causing graft loss. Frequent assessment identifies the presence of excess fluid or hematoma, which can be removed by aspiration or rolling of a cotton-tipped applicator to the surface of the graft to remove collected fluid.

For large BSA burns or patients with limited donor sites, the harvested skin is guided through a mechanical meshing/expansion device (Kagan et al, 2013) to allow the skin to be expanded for more wound coverage. The meshed graft is secured with staples or sutures and then covered with a nonadherent inner layer to prevent shearing. Fluff gauze moistened with a topical antimicrobial, such as 5% Sulfamylon or triple antibiotic solution, is placed to prevent desiccation. If the graft is applied to an extremity or joint, splints are fitted at this time to maintain a position of function while engraftment occurs. The dressing usually is left in place for 4 to 7 days before changing, at which time the graft is inspected and redressed. The dressing is changed daily until the graft is sufficiently stable to remain open to air, usually in about 2 weeks. Physical and occupational therapy can be resumed after 5 to 7 days, starting with ROM exercises and progressing at an individual rate depending on the area grafted and the patient's condition. Splinting continues to areas at risk for contracture.

Split-thickness skin graft donor sites heal by epithelialization, which is facilitated in a moist environment. The ideal donor site dressing also prevents infection, minimizes patient discomfort, and promotes a quality cosmetic outcome (Bailey et al, 2011). Advanced wound care dressings may be more effective than simple impregnated gauze dressings at accelerating healing and decreasing pain in skin graft donor sites. The small differences in improvement must be balanced with the differences in cost and patient comfort (Franz et al, 2008). As with most wounds, dressing selection is dependent on the characteristics of the wound (donor site location, size, proximity to other wounds). Healing of donor sites in a timely manner is especially important in patients with large BSA burns who will need reharvesting to obtain full wound coverage. It may be prudent to consider the administration of human growth hormone or the testosterone analog oxandrolone to enhance healing of the donor site because both of these agents have been shown to significantly decrease weight and nitrogen loss and increase healing rates (Wolf et al, 2006).

Full-thickness skin grafts are obtained by surgically excising the entire thickness of the donor skin to the level of the subcutaneous tissue, resulting in grafts 0.025 to 0.030 inch thick. Transfer of the entire dermal layer is accomplished, which makes the graft durable and less prone to contracture. Full-thickness skin grafts are limited to use for small full-thickness burns and are frequently used in reconstructive surgery. The full-thickness skin graft donor site is a full-thickness wound, which usually is closed by primary suturing or split-thickness grafting (Mozingo, 1998).

Acute/Wound Care Phase Pain and Emotional Support.

Pain and anxiety may lead to prolongation of the stress response after injury, which could potentially delay wound healing and lengthen recovery time (Monafo,1995). During the acute/wound care phase, supplemental pain and anxiety control measures such as morphine, benzodiazepines, acetaminophen with codeine, acetaminophen, and nonnarcotic medications such as nonsteroidal antiinflammatory drugs continue to be necessary to control background or procedural pain (Davis and Sheely-Adolphson, 1997). Anxiolytic agents are commonly given to augment pain medications and assist the patient's ability to cope. Pharmacologic agents to promote sleep may play a role in overall burn pain management, as poor sleep can reduce pain tolerance (Connor-Ballard, 2009).

Nonpharmacologic measures play a large role in pain management in this phase of care. Positioning, relaxation techniques, cognitive strategies, and the presence of significant others for emotional support have proven beneficial as adjuncts to pharmacologic pain control (Connor-Ballard, 2009). Chapters 25 and 26 discuss pain as a critical cofactor in wound healing and provide valuable information related to understanding, assessing, and managing pain.

Pediatrics. Although children experience the same physical stress as adults during burn recovery, their behavioral responses can be quite different and are related to their stage of development. Behavioral responses typically include anxiety, agitation, anger, conditioned fear, and regression. Causes of psychological and emotional distress include separation anxiety, repeated painful procedures, and loss of control and independence (Adcock et al, 1998). Specific suggestions and interventions are listed in Box 32-2 and described in Chapter 36.

The American Academy of Pediatrics 2014 Policy Statement states that the inclusion of a CLS on the multidisciplinary care team is a quality benchmark of integrated family-centered care and an indicator of excellence in pediatric care. The CLS focuses on the optimal well-being and development

---

BOX 32-2   Interventions for Psychological Support of the Pediatric Burn Patient

- Encourage parents and family to be present during hospitalization.
- Include a child developmental specialist as a member of the care team.
- Consider the child's developmental stage when planning and implementing care.
- Model supportive behaviors.
- Isolate painful procedures to a particular place and identify the child's room as a "safe zone."
- Allow older children some control and choices regarding wound care and therapy.
- Provide preparation before and assistance with coping during painful procedures.
- Make appropriate resources available to children who may show long-term adjustment issues.

See also Chapter 36.

of children while promoting coping skills and minimizing the adverse effects of hospitalization and health care. The CLS on the burn team uses therapeutic play, nonpharmacologic pain control interventions, and procedural preparation adapted to the child's developmental stage to support the injured child and family throughout their recovery and serves as the team's expert in developmentally appropriate care (American Academy of Pediatrics, 2014).

The incidence of attention deficit hyperactivity disorder is estimated to be as high as 20% in children admitted to burn centers (Mangus et al, 2004). This should be addressed throughout the phases of burn recovery to optimize participation in the recovery process (Sheridan, 2007). Acute stress syndrome and posttraumatic stress syndrome also should be assessed for and anticipated, as up to 30% of burn-injured children may develop significant symptoms (Ehde et al, 2000; Stoddard et al, 2006).

Abuse and Neglect. Approximately 10% of child abuse cases involve burning, and up to 20% of pediatric burn admissions involve abuse or neglect (Ruth et al, 2003). Burn care providers must understand the assessment and interventional processes related to suspected abuse and neglect cases. Knowledge of individual institutions' protocols governing the management of these cases is key to maintaining patient safety and obtaining optimal outcomes. Primary responsibility for initial assessments, communications with law enforcement, and initiation of specific interventions may involve nursing or medical staff, specialized teams for abuse and neglect, and social services (Doctor, 1998). Similar considerations are applicable to adult patients who have been deliberately injured. Stone et al (1970) identified criteria for burn injuries that are suspicious for abuse or neglect (Box 32-3).

BOX 32-3 Nonaccidental Burn Criteria

- Multiple hematomas or scars in various stages of healing
- Concurrent injuries or evidence of neglect (e.g., malnutrition)
- History of prior hospitalization for "accidental" trauma
- Unexplained delay between time of injury and first attempt to obtain medical attention
- Burns appear older than the alleged time of the accident
- Account of accident not compatible with age and ability of patient
- Adults in charge allege that there are no witnesses to the "accident" and that the child was merely discovered to have been burned
- Relatives other than parents bring injured child to the hospital
- Burn is attributed to the action of a sibling or other child (this can, in fact, happen)
- Injured child is excessively withdrawn, submissive, or overly polite or does not cry during painful procedures
- Scalds on hands or feet, often symmetric, appear to be full thickness in depth, suggesting extremities were forcibly immersed and held in hot liquid
- Isolated burns of buttocks that could hardly be produced by accidental means in children

---

Rehabilitation Phase

The goal of the rehabilitation phase is to restore or maximize the patient's functional capacity. This rehabilitation phase begins once wound healing is complete and may last several weeks to several years, depending on the extent and severity of the burn injury. Skin- and wound-related complications that manifest after healing, such as scarring, contractures, and itching, require management during the rehabilitation phase.

Excessive Scarring, Contractures, and Itch. Excessive scarring is rare in burn injuries that heal within 21 days (Franz et al, 2008). Patients with deep burns, children, young adults, and patients with darkly pigmented skin are at particular risk (Engrav et al, 2007). Two types of scarring are seen postburn injury. *Hypertrophic* scars are red, raised, painful, itchy, and lack elasticity. Hypertrophic scars remain within the boundary of the original injury, regress with time, and are more frequently seen after burn injury. *Keloids* are firm, fibrous nodules that extend beyond the original wound margin and are often hyperpigmented (Berman et al, 2008; Mafong and Ashinoff, 2000).

Excessive scar formation and treatment modalities are described in Chapter 4 and Table 4-3. The exact pathophysiology of scar formation and the mechanism of action of these treatment modalities are not known. Treatments most frequently used with burn scars, alone or in combination, include pressure garments (Endorf and Ahrenholz, 2011), hydrogel or silicone sheeting (Li-Tsang et al, 2010), corticosteroid injections, surgical excision, and laser.

Scar contracture is the primary cause of functional deficits in the patient with a burn. A contracture is essentially a shortening of a scar over a joint surface that limits joint mobility. A study by Schneider et al (2006) identified contractures as developing in more than one third of hospitalized burn-injured patients by the time of discharge. The shoulder was the most frequently affected joint (38%), followed by the elbow (34%) and the knee (22%). Patients at risk for contracture development included those with longer lengths of stay, higher percentage BSA burns, and inhalation injury. To prevent limited ROM, scarring, and contractures, rehabilitation begins shortly after the patient is injured and includes positioning, splinting, and the use of physical agents such as hydrotherapy, paraffin, ultrasound, and electrical stimulation. Therapeutic exercise may include active and/or passive ROM, stretching, and strengthening to increase the elasticity of healing skin and maintain full ROM and function (Carrougher et al, 2009).

Treatment of postburn injury scarring can last several months to years. Compliance with the treatment plan may be difficult to achieve because patients find pressure garments uncomfortable and confining. It is important to instruct patients and caregivers that any treatment of hypertrophic or keloid scars is aimed at minimizing the scars. Complete normalization of the skin to preburn appearance and texture may not be possible. In a metaanalysis of excessive scarring treatments, the mean amount of improvement to be expected was only 60% (Franz et al, 2008).

Patients recovering from burn injuries experience itching from a variety of sources. Histamines released during the inflammatory phase of healing cause itch, particularly in large BSA burns that take longer to heal. Infection also prolongs healing time and causes excess production of collagen in the wound, which leads to hypertrophic scarring and an increased amount of itch. Itching can be a side effect of the morphine used to manage burn pain (Matheson et al, 2001). Itching in a burn wound usually begins within 2 weeks of the injury and may last for an extended period. Carrougher et al (2012) found that more than 73% of adult burn survivors were still affected by itch 2 years postinjury. Current treatment of itching includes a combination of oral or topical antihistamines; topical doxepin hydrochloride, a potent histamine receptor antagonist (Gibran et al, 2007); skin moisturizers; and pressure garments (Bell and Gabriel, 2009).

Discharge Planning. The main goal of treatment throughout all phases of recovery is functional return of the patient to preburn lifestyle or as close to that lifestyle as is reasonably possible. The patient with a burn injury is identified as a candidate for discharge when wound healing is progressing; nutritional intake is adequate to support continued healing; pain, itching, and infection are controlled with medications by mouth; and the patient and/or caregiver have demonstrated competence in wound care and exercises. The discharge process is similar for major and minor burns and should incorporate five major areas of patient/caregiver education: (1) wound management, (2) pain and itch relief, (3) exercises, (4) scar maturation, and (5) emotional support for the patient and family.

An individualized plan of care that addresses age-specific needs is necessary for each patient with a burn injury. The discharge goal for pediatric patients is social reintegration. Appropriate objectives to be met before discharge include the following:
1. The child will achieve an age-appropriate level of functioning.
2. The child and caregiver will understand the processes of injury and recovery.
3. The child will begin to integrate a new body image.

Many burn centers offer school reentry programs that provide psychosocial support for the child and education about the burn recovery process for teachers and classmates. Camps for children with a history of severe burn injury, staffed by burn care professionals, provide the opportunity for the child to meet and socialize with other children with burns. Burn camp participants have reported that the experience has helped them with identity formation and reflection, improved their social interactions, and increased their initiative, all positive developmental outcomes for adolescents (Rimmer et al, 2012).

Goals for discharge planning for the adult patient with a burn injury often focus on return to work. Employment equates with life satisfaction, provides an identity, and allows for financial independence. Dyster-Aas et al (2007) has shown an association between failing to return to work after burn injury and poor outcomes on quality of life relating to health, including both physical and psychological health changes. Planning for discharge of the elderly patient must begin at admission and involve the multidisciplinary team. Comorbidities are more common in this population, and social issues may prolong hospitalization. Early assessment, both medical and psychosocial, may decrease length of stay and more accurately identify ongoing management concerns and needs (Solanki et al, 2011).

OUTPATIENT BURN MANAGEMENT

The American Burn Association injury severity grading system classifies burn injuries as minor, moderate, or severe. Many minor and moderate burn injuries now are treated on an outpatient basis only. Over the 10-year period from 2003 to 2012, the average length of hospital stay for burn-injured patients has decreased from 10 days to 8 days (American Burn Association, 2013). Factors that may influence the shift to outpatient care include a desire to decrease health care costs, reduction in the risk of nosocomial infections, psychological benefits of home care, increasing numbers of outpatient surgical procedures, direct referrals to burn clinics for care (Moss, 2004), and new developments in wound dressings. It is estimated that 90% of burn-injured patients who receive medical care do so on an outpatient basis (Peck et al, 2007).

Assessment of the outpatient includes history of injury; medical history; psychosocial and economic assessments; and evaluation of the location, extent, depth, and severity of the burn injury. Although most minor and some moderate burn injuries can receive appropriate care on an outpatient basis, hospital admission should be considered if factors that influence the patient's safety or the patient's ability to heal are identified in the assessment. Inpatient care may be required if the cause of injury is suspected of being not accidental, the presence of chronic disease would prolong wound healing, resources are lacking to provide daily care or return to clinic, the location of the burn impairs ability to provide self-care and perform activities of daily living, or wound care/therapy needs are such that pain cannot adequately be controlled with oral medication (Moss, 2004).

The goals for the patient with a burn who is treated in the outpatient setting include wound protection, timely wound healing, adequate pain control, and rapid rehabilitation with return to school or work (Moss, 2004). Wound care in the outpatient setting begins with gentle cleansing with mild soap and water to remove devitalized skin and debris. Appropriate pain medication by mouth is generally used for small burns seen in the clinic setting. If extensive debridement is required, additional medications for pain and anxiety will be needed, and this is best performed in the more controlled setting of the emergency department or inpatient burn unit. Controversy exists as to whether to shave the hair surrounding a wound or to unroof intact blisters (Moss, 2004). Often, small blisters to the palms, fingers, or soles of the feet are left intact if they do not limit ROM, whereas larger blisters (>2 cm) are debrided (Honari, 2004).

Individual assessments of the extent and depth of the wound and the size, location, and fragility of the blisters will dictate treatment. Wound care and dressings should be kept as simple as possible, and the wound is kept clean, moist, and protected. In addition to selecting a dressing that meets the needs of the wound, priorities include patient comfort, mobility, and activity. Evaluation of the risk for functional impairment is performed at this time by the physical or occupational therapist, and the appropriate splinting or exercises are implemented.

Patient and/or caregiver education is vital to successful outpatient management. Explanations regarding the depth of the wound and demonstration of appropriate wound care techniques and dressing application should be given in conjunction with written instructions. Instructions should include information specific to the wound, signs and symptoms of infection, therapy schedule, activity restrictions, nutrition, pain management, and how to contact the burn team for assistance (Moss, 2004).

Initial follow-up visits may range in frequency from daily to weekly, based on factors identified in the initial assessment and including the extent and depth of the burn and the ability of the patient or caregiver to adequately perform daily care and monitor the wound. Once healing occurs, intermittent visits continue until the scar maturation process has ended, as evidenced by a mature scar that is soft, supple, of normal color, and without contractures (Moss, 2004). As the wound heals, patients are instructed on side effects of burn injury that may occur: excessive scarring; itching; sleep disturbances; discomfort associated with pressure garments, splinting, and exercise; and color and texture changes to the skin. Newly healed burn wounds are more sensitive to ultraviolet light, so the need for protection in the form of a sunscreen with a sun protection factor (SPF) of 30 and for covering the area with clothing should be incorporated into the teaching plan. Appropriate referrals for support and counseling should be made in a timely manner for patients experiencing distress related to psychological symptoms.

CLINICAL CONSULT

A: KC is a 14-month-old female who was burned less than 1 hour ago when she pulled a pot of boiling water off the stove. She has deep partial and shallow full thickness burns to her face, upper body, bilateral upper extremities, left hand, and left leg. The left arm and left hand are burned circumferentially; there is no stocking/glove distribution. KC is a direct admit to the burn intensive care unit (ICU). She weighs 13 kg on admission, has no past medical history, and is up to date on immunizations. Initial assessment and stabilization have been completed. Fluid resuscitation and maintenance fluids initiated, indwelling urinary catheter and oxygen saturation monitor placed, vital signs (VS) every hour, admission labs done. Parents are at the bedside; no other family members were injured.

D: 35% total body surface area (TBSA) accidental scald burn injury; 20% partial thickness to face, chest, back; and 15% full thickness to left arm, left hand, left leg.

P: Burn wound assessment and dressing application at bedside per pediatric burn team under moderate sedation. Initiate supportive care for patient and family.

I: (1) Partial-thickness burns debrided and Biobrane placed; full-thickness wounds debrided and silver sulfadiazine placed; bacitracin ointment to face after cleansing. (2) Position with head of bed (HOB) elevated on pressure redistribution support surface and burned extremities elevated. (3) Circulation checks every hour to areas of full-thickness circumferential burns to left arm, hand, and leg. (4) Feeding tube placed and enteral feeds initiated per protocol. (5) Pain and anxiety management per continuous morphine and midazolam infusion with bolus during procedures. (6) Stress ulcer prophylaxis and nutritional supplementation began. (7) Consults: physical therapy (PT), occupational therapy (OT), social work, child life, pediatric intensive care, ophthalmology. (8) Plan for operating room (OR) for debridement; possible skin grafting of full-thickness wounds in 2 to 3 days.

E: Daily wound assessment per burn team. Strict I and O. Follow-up labs: comprehensive metabolic panel (CMP), Mg, Phos every morning, and complete blood count (CBC) with differential every morning (if silver sulfadiazine used on >20% TBSA). Plan of care has been reviewed with parents.

SUMMARY

Whether involved in the care of a patient with massive tissue loss or a minor burn, the wound care specialist must be familiar with the principles of initial assessment, management based on the type and severity of injury, and prevention of complications. Knowledge of the phases of recovery and the associated therapeutic and psychosocial needs of the patient contributes to optimal outcomes.

REFERENCES

Adcock RJ, et al: Psychologic and emotional recovery. In Carrougher GJ, editor: *Burn care and therapy*, St. Louis, MO, 1998, Mosby.

Ahrns KS: Trends in burn resuscitation: shifting the focus from fluids to adequate endpoint monitoring, edema control, and adjuvant therapies, *Crit Care Nurs Clin North Am* 16(1):75–98, 2004.

Alden NE, Rabbitts A, Yurt RW: Contact burns: is further prevention necessary? *J Burn Care Res* 27(4):472–475, 2006.

American Academy of Pediatrics: Policy statement: Child life services, *Pediatrics* 133(5):e1471–e1479, 2014.

American Burn Association: Guidelines for the operations of burn centers, *J Burn Care Res* 28(1):134–141, 2007.

American Burn Association: *Advanced burn life support course*, Chicago, 2011, American Burn Association.

American Burn Association: *Burn incidence and treatment in the United States: 2012 fact sheet*, Chicago, 2012, American Burn Association.

American Burn Association: *National burn repository 2013 report*, Chicago, 2013, American Burn Association.

American Burn Association: *Scald injury prevention educator's guide*, 2014. http://www.ameriburn.org/Preven/ ScaldInjuryEducator'sGuide.pdf. Accessed June 2, 2014.

Arnoldo B, Klein M, Gibran NS: Practice guidelines for the management of electrical injuries, *J Burn Care Res* 27(4):439–447, 2006.

Arnoldo BD, Purdue GF, Kowalske K, et al: Electrical injuries: a 20-year review, *J Burn Care Rehabil* 25(6):479–484, 2004.

Bailey S, Carmean M, Cinat M, et al: A randomized comparison study of Aquacel Ag and Glucan II as donor site dressings with regard to healing time, cosmesis, infection rate, and patient's perceived pain: a pilot study, *J Burn Care Res* 32(6):627–632, 2011.

Bell PL, Gabriel V: Evidence based review for the treatment of post-burn pruritus, *J Burn Care Res* 30(1):55–61, 2009.

Berman B, Viera MH, Amini S, et al: Prevention and management of hypertrophic scars and keloids after burns in children, *J Craniofac Surg* 19(4):989–1006, 2008.

Byers JF, Bridges F, Kijek J, et al: Burn patients' pain and anxiety experiences, *J Burn Care Rehabil* 22(2):144–149, 2001.

Calota DR, Nitescu C, Florescu IP, et al: Surgical management of extensive burns treatment using allografts, *J Med Life* 5(4): 486–490, 2012.

Carrougher GJ, Hoffman HG, Nakmura D, et al: The effect of virtual reality on pain and range of motion in adults with burn injuries, *J Burn Care Res* 30(5):785–791, 2009.

Carrougher GJ, Martinez EM, McMullen KS, et al: Pruritus in adult burn survivors: post burn prevalence and risk factors associated with increased intensity, *J Burn Care Res* 34(1):94–101, 2012.

Church D, Elsayad S, Reid O, et al: Burn wound infections, *Clin Microbiol Rev* 19(2):403–434, 2006.

Coban YK: Infection control in severely burned patients, *World J Crit Care Med* 1(4):94–101, 2012.

Connor-Ballard PA: Understanding and managing burn pain: part 2, *Am J Nurs* 109(5):54–62, 2009.

Davis ST, Sheely-Adolphson P: Burn management. Psychosocial interventions: pharmacologic and psychologic modalities, *Nurs Clin North Am* 32(2):331–342, 1997.

Davison PG, Loiselle FB, Nickerson D: Survey on current hydrotherapy use among North American burn centers, *J Burn Care Res* 31(3):393–399, 2010.

Deitch EA, Rutan RL: The challenges of children: the first 48 hours, *J Burn Care Rehabil* 21(5):424–430, 2000.

Delatte SJ, Evans J, Hebra A, et al: Effectiveness of beta-glucan collagen for treatment of partial-thickness burns in children, *J Pediatr Surg* 36(1):113–118, 2001.

Demling R, Mazzess R, Witt R, et al: The study of burn edema using dichromatic absorptiometry, *J Trauma* 18:124–124, 1978.

Doctor M: Abuse through burns. In Carrougher GJ, editor: *Burn care and therapy*, St. Louis, MO, 1998, Mosby.

Dyster-Aas J, Kildal M, Willebrand M: Return to work and health-related quality of life after burn injury, *J Rehabil Med* 39:49–55, 2007.

Ehde DM, Patterson DR, Wiechman SA, et al: Post-traumatic stress symptoms and distress 1 year after burn injury, *J Burn Care Rehabil* 21(2):105–511, 2000.

Emergency Medical Technician (EMT): *Rule of nines*, April 27, 2014. http://www.emtresource.com/emergencies/burns/rule-of-nines. Accessed June 2, 2014.

Endorf FW, Ahrenholz D: Burn management, *Curr Opin Crit Care* 17:601–605, 2011.

Engrav LH, Garner WL, Tredget EE: Hypertrophic scar, wound contraction and hyper-hypopigmentation, *J Burn Care Res* 28(4):593–597, 2007.

Evans J, Dobos C, Tagge EP: Your patients may be at risk: preventing pediatric burn injuries, *J S C Med Assoc* 102:17–18, 2006.

Franz MG, Robson MC, Steed DL, et al: Guidelines to aid healing of acute wounds by decreasing impediments of healing, *Wound Repair Regen* 16(6):723–748, 2008.

Gibran NS, Boyce S, Greenhalgh DG: Cutaneous wound healing, *J Burn Care Res* 28(4):577–579, 2007.

Gibran NS, Heimbach DM: Current status of burn wound pathophysiology, *Clin Plast Surg* 27(1):11–22, 2000.

Graves C, Saffle J, Cochran A: Actual burn nutrition care practices: an update, *J Burn Care Res* 30(1):77–82, 2009.

Hall KL, Shahrokhi S, Jeschke MG: Enteral nutrition support in burn care: a review of current recommendations as instituted in the Ross Tilley Burn Centre, *Nutrients* 4(11): 1554–1566, 2012.

Honari S: Topical therapies and antimicrobials in the management of burn wounds, *Crit Care Nurs Clin North Am* 16(1):1–11, 2004.

Hosseini SV, Tanideh N, Kohanteb J, et al: Comparison between alpha and silver sulfadiazine ointments in treatment of pseudomonas infections in 3rd degree burns, *Int J Surg* 5(1):23–26, 2007.

Hunt JP, Calvert CT, Peck MD, et al: Occupation-related burn injuries, *J Burn Care Rehabil* 21(4):327–332, 2000.

Jackson D: The diagnosis of the depth of burning, *J Br Surg* 40:588–596, 1953.

Kagan RJ, Peck MD, Ahrenholz DH, et al: Surgical management of the burn wound and use of skin substitutes: an expert white panel paper, *J Burn Care Res* 34(2):e60–e79, 2013.

Karter MJ: *Fire loss in the United States series (1982, 1992, 2002, 2011, and 2012)*, Quincy, MA, 2013, National Fire Protection Association.

Knaysi GA, Crikelair GF, Cosman B: The rule of nines: its history and accuracy, *Plast Reconstr Surg* 41:560–563, 1968.

Lesher AP, Curry RH, Evans J, et al: Effectiveness of Biobrane for treatment of partial-thickness burns in children, *J Pediatr Surg* 46:1759–1763, 2011.

Li-Tsang CWP, Zheng YP, Lai JC: A randomized clinical trial to study the effect of silicone gel dressings and pressure support on posttraumatic hypertrophic scars, *J Burn Care Res* 31(3):448–457, 2010.

Lowell G, Quinlan K, Gottlieb LJ: Preventing unintentional scald burns: moving beyond tap water, *Pediatrics* 122(4):799–804, 2008.

Lund C, Browder N: The estimation of area of burns, *Surg Gynecol Obstet* 79:352–358, 1944.

Mafong EA, Ashinoff R: Treatment of hypertrophic scars and keloids: a review, *Aesthet Surg J* 20(2):114–121, 2000.

Mangus RS, Bergman D, Zieger M, et al: Burn injuries in children with attention deficit/hyperactivity disorder, *Burns* 30(2): 148–150, 2004.

Matheson JD, Clayton J, Muller MJ: The reduction of itch during burn wound healing, *J Burn Care Rehabil* 22(1):76–81, 2001.

McCall JE, Cahill TJ: Respiratory care of the burn patient, *J Burn Care Rehabil* 26(3):200–206, 2005.

Monafo WW: Physiology of pain, *J Burn Care Rehabil* 16(3 Pt 2): 345–347, 1995.

Mosier MJ, Pham TN, Klein MB, et al: Early enteral nutrition in burns: compliance with guidelines and associated outcomes in a multicenter study, *J Burn Care Res* 32:104–109, 2011.

Moss LS: Outpatient management of the burn patient, *Crit Care Nurs Clin North Am* 16(1):109–117, 2004.

Mozingo DW: Surgical management. In Carrougher GJ, editor: *Burn care and therapy*, St. Louis, MO, 1998, Mosby.

Orgill DP, Piccolo N: Escharotomy and decompressive therapies in burns, *J Burn Care Res* 30(5):759–768, 2009.

Palmieri TL: Inhalation injury: research progress and needs, *J Burn Care Res* 28(4):549–554, 2007.

Patel PP, Vasquez SA, Granick MS, et al: Topical antimicrobials in pediatric burn wound management, *J Craniofac Surg* 19(4):913–922, 2008.

Paul CN: Skin substitutes in burn care, *Wounds* 20(7):203–205, 2008.

Peck MD, Brigham P, Patterson D: Invited critique: national study of emergency department visits for burn injuries, 1993 to 2004, *J Burn Care Res* 28(5):691–693, 2007.

Pham TN, Cancio LC, Gibran NS: American Burn Association practice guidelines burn shock resuscitation, *J Burn Care Res* 29(1):257–266, 2008.

Pruitt BA Jr: The evolutionary development of biologic dressings and skin substitutes, *J Burn Care Rehabil* 18(1 Pt 2):S2–S5, 1997.

Redlick F, Cooke A, Gomez M, et al: A survey of risk factors for burns in the elderly and prevention strategies, *J Burn Care Rehabil* 23(5):351–356, 2002.

Rimmer RB, Pressman MS, Takach OP, et al: Burn injured adolescents report gaining multiple developmental benefits and improved life skills as a result of burn camp attendance, *J Burn Care Res* 33(4):552–560, 2012.

Rodriguez NA, Jeschke MG, Williams FN, et al: Nutrition in burns: Galveston contributions, *J Parenter Enteral Nutr* 35(6):704–714, 2011.

Ruth GD, Smith S, Bronson M, et al: Outcomes related to burn-related child abuse: a case series, *J Burn Care Rehabil* 24(5): 318–321, 2003.

Schneider JC, Holavanahalli R, Helm P, et al: Contractures in burn injury: defining the problem, *J Burn Care Res* 27(4):508–514, 2006.

Sheridan RL: Burns, *Crit Care Med* 30(Suppl 11):S500–S514, 2002.

Sheridan RL: Burns at the extremes of age, *J Burn Care Rehabil* 28(4):580–585, 2007.

Sicoutris CP, Holmes JH: Fire and smoke injuries, *Crit Care Nurs Clin North Am* 18(3):403–417, xi, 2006.

Smith AL, Murray DA, McBride CJ: A comparison of nurses' and parents' or caregivers' perceptions during pediatric burn dressing changes: an exploratory study, *J Burn Care Res* 32(2): 185–199, 2011.

Solanki NS, Greenwood JE, Mackie IP, et al: Social issues prolong elderly burn patient hospitalization, *J Burn Care* 32(3):387–391, 2011.

Stoddard FJ, Saxe G, Ronfeldt H, et al: Acute stress symptoms in young children with burns, *J Am Acad Child Adolesc Psychiatry* 45:87–93, 2006.

Stone NH, Rinaldo L, Humphrey CR, et al: Child abuse by burning, *Surg Clin North Am* 50:1419–1424, 1970.

Struck MF, Gille J: Fugal infections in burns: a comprehensive review, *Ann Burns and Fire Disasters* 26(3):147–153, 2013.

Supple KG: Physiologic response to burn injury, *Crit Care Nurs Clin North Am* 16(1):119–126, 2004.

Tan X, Yowlder CJ, Super DM, et al: The efficacy of music therapy protocols for decreasing pain, anxiety, and muscle tension during burn dressing changes: a prospective randomized crossover trial, *J Burn Care Res* 31(4):590–597, 2010.

Wibbenmeyer LA, Amelon MJ, Torner JC, et al: Population-based assessment of burn injury in southern Iowa: identification of children and young-adult at-risk groups and behaviors, *J Burn Care Rehabil* 24(4):192–202, 2003.

Williams RY, Wohlgemuth SD: Does the "rule of nines" apply to morbidly obese burn victims? *J Burn Care Res* 34(4):447–452, 2013.

Wolf SE, Edelman LS, Kemalyan N, et al: Effects of oxandrolone on outcome measures in the severely burned: a multicenter prospective randomized double-blind trial, *J Burn Care Res* 27(2):131–139, 2006.

33

Reconstructive Surgery

Joyce M. Black and Jonathan S. Black

OBJECTIVES

1. List three factors considered in surgical decision making.
2. Discuss four methods of wound closure.
3. Identify urgent operative conditions.
4. Describe preoperative and postoperative interventions for patients undergoing surgical flaps.

Surgical intervention for chronic wounds is seldom the first choice. In general, much local care of the wound has preceded any decision for surgery. However, some chronic wounds deteriorate and require emergent operative management, and some wounds reach a point in the healing trajectory where surgery is indicated to aid wound closure. This chapter addresses the wounds that benefit from operative treatment, decisions about operative care, and care of the patient and the wound before and after surgery.

HISTORY OF SURGERY FOR WOUNDS

Wounds, mostly resulting from trauma, have existed since the beginning of man. The Edwin Smith Papyrus, which was written more than 5000 years ago, is the oldest known surgical treatise. It contains 142 different references to the management of sores and wounds. Surgical management of wounds is nearly as old. Hippocrates said, "He who wishes to be a surgeon should go to war." His words highlight the relationship between surgical advances and war-related injury. Modern reconstructive surgery had its beginnings with traumatic injury, at a time when the nose was cut off as a form of punishment. In Italy during the sixteenth century, noses were reconstructed using the skin of the inner upper aspect of the arm. This flap is known as the Tagliacozzi flap and even today is the emblem for the American Association of Plastic Surgeons. Modern plastic surgery came into its own during World War II when the sulfa antibiotic allowed many wounded soldiers to survive their injuries, and consequently they required reconstructive surgery. Today, surgery remains an important aspect of wound care and advances in surgical options continue to be made.

SURGICAL DECISION MAKING

Assessment of the Patient

A comprehensive patient assessment is required to determine the risk-to-benefit ratio and the type of surgical procedure indicated. The patient's condition forms the primary aspect of the risk portion of the risk-to-benefit ratio. Although it is always ideal to have a closed wound, the patient must be able to tolerate anesthesia, surgery, blood loss, and postoperative restrictions. An estimation of anesthetic risk, such as the American Society of Anesthesiologists (ASA) classification, provides an objective measure of relative risk for surgery. The patient must also be able to tolerate the pain and immobility after surgery, and the facility must be willing to keep the patient as long as the surgeon deems necessary for safe healing. Finally, the consequences of leaving a wound open must also be identified and considered as a potential benefit to operative intervention.

Assessment of the Wound

Planning surgery requires an understanding of the wound in terms of causative factors and missing or needed tissue. Information concerning these two issues guides the selection of the most appropriate surgical option.

Causative Factors. What caused the wound? Is the wound acute or chronic? Acute traumatic wounds may be missing fragments of skin, but with removal of these devitalized tissues and mobilization of surrounding skin, the laceration may be closed primarily. If the wound is chronic, can the factors contributing to the chronic nature of the wound be corrected? The underlying etiology of the wound must be corrected or minimized (e.g., pressure) and cofactors treated (e.g., infection, ischemia, malnutrition) before healing can ensue. For example, the wound complicated by an ischemic process will require improvement of blood flow in order to heal. Likewise, an ischial pressure ulcer will not heal if the patient continues to sit on the ulcer. Surgical reconstruction of wounds in which the causative factor has not been addressed is not likely to succeed (Franz et al, 2008; NPUAP, EPUAP, PPPIA, 2014; WOCN®, 2010).

Missing/Needed Tissue. When planning surgical reconstruction of a wound, a full understanding of exactly what tissues are missing is needed in order to reconstruct the area for restoration of both form and function. If a wound lacks only skin, replacing the skin (skin graft) may be a reasonable option, provided other patient conditions are well managed. However, simply putting skin on a wound without controlling infection, ischemia, or pressure is a doomed enterprise. Frequently, tissue padding (e.g., subcutaneous tissue and muscle) is needed to protect a bony prominence from recurrent breakdown, so a flap containing these elements would be necessary.

SELECTION OF WOUND CLOSURE METHOD

Selecting a method of closure depends on a holistic assessment that considers the needs and goals of the patient. A common set of decision-making steps (e.g., the reconstructive ladder) serves as a guide for plastic and reconstructive surgery (Figure 33-1). The simplest method that accomplishes the patient's goals usually is the first choice. In addition to the complexity of the surgery, consideration is given to the morbidity that would be created for the donor site. For example, if a person lost a thumb, transplantation of the great toe to replace the thumb would be considered; however, the thumb would not be used to replace a great toe.

When considering donor site morbidity for pressure ulcer surgery, it is important to keep in mind that tissues usually

can be moved or donated only once. Therefore the choice of which tissue to use is important. Surgeons try to select donor areas that will not interfere with future potential flap donor sites, especially in patients with paraplegia or quadriplegia because this patient population often requires more than one operation during their lifetime. Large wounds of the entire perineum in patients with paralysis may require removal of the femur and filleting of the remaining lower extremity tissues to form an adequately sized flap of muscle and skin that will sufficiently close the wound. This situation is a dramatic example of donor site morbidity.

Surgical wound closure can be achieved using a number of techniques, such as linear closure, secondary healing, skin grafts, skin substitutes, and tissue flaps. Many factors are considered when determining the optimum wound closure technique. When little tissue is missing, the skin is sufficiently pliable, and the wound is considered to be clean, a linear closure (i.e., approximating the wound edges and securing with suture) is a reasonable choice.

Secondary healing (i.e., letting a wound heal by scar tissue formation and contracture) is the simplest method of healing and a logical selection for a clean Stage II pressure ulcer. The ongoing risk of infection in the deeper open wound, however, may prompt a decision for surgical closure to speed healing. Similarly, some partial-thickness wounds (e.g., burn on the hand) create significant morbidity due to the contractile scars that form during healing. In these situations, skin grafting could be warranted to minimize contracture with the added benefit of closing the wound more quickly.

Skin grafts (i.e., sections of intact epidermis and upper layer of the dermis) can be removed from the patient's donor site and transferred to cover shallow, vascularized wounds. Split-thickness skin grafts can be placed as entire pieces of skin or meshed to promote drainage of wound exudate and contouring to the skin surface. Skin grafts also can be full thickness, but only where vascularity in the donor site is sufficient to heal full-thickness grafts.

Skin grafts provide superficial coverage but do not replace deeper tissue layers, such as subcutaneous tissue and muscle; thus they are unable to provide the padding needed to protect bony prominences from recurrent breakdown. Therefore skin grafts are rarely used in the surgical management of pressure ulcers, except to close donor sites from flaps containing multiple layers of tissue. Skin grafts are commonly used to manage burn wounds and are described in greater detail in Chapter 32. Skin grafts have also been used in the management of venous ulcers (AAWC, 2010).

Cellular- and/or tissue-based products (CTPs), often referred to as skin substitutes, can be used to close a wound. The CTP can be epidermis only, dermis only, or both. Epidermal CTPs are composed of keratinocytes, take 2 to 3 weeks to "grow," and are generally used when the patient does not have sufficient healthy skin graft donor sites available. Dermal CTPs are composed of fibroblasts embedded in a "matrix" material that provides a scaffolding for cellular and capillaries migration. Additional CTPs such as

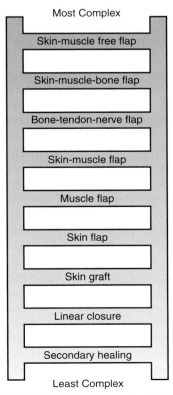

Most Complex

Skin-muscle free flap

Skin-muscle-bone flap

Bone-tendon-nerve flap

Skin-muscle flap

Muscle flap

Skin flap

Skin graft

Linear closure

Secondary healing

Least Complex

FIGURE 33-1 Reconstructive ladder.

epidermal CTPs and extracellular matrix CTPs are discussed in Chapter 19.

Tissue Flaps

Tissue flaps involve the transfer of skin and underlying structures (e.g., subcutaneous tissue, fascia, muscle) to fill a defect, pad prominent bone, or protect underlying vital structures (e.g., major vessel). Flaps differ from skin grafts in that they carry their own blood supply with them. The native nutrient vessels are moved along with the flap or are reestablished (microsurgery) once the flap is transferred. Maintaining this blood supply is the crucial aspect of flap survival. Tissue flaps are either local or distant (free).

Local flaps are most commonly used for pressure ulcers (Hansen, 2013; NPUAP, EPUAP, PPPIA, 2014). They are categorized by the anatomic structures they encompass, the method used to move the flap, or the method used to perfuse the flap (Box 33-1).

Anatomic Structures. Skin flaps are portions of skin moved from their usual location to cover a defect. Skin flaps are used to surgically close defects from skin cancer excision. Fasciocutaneous flaps include portions of the epidermis, dermis, and subcutaneous tissue supported by the underlying fascia. Fasciocutaneous flaps do provide padding and superficial coverage. Recently, this flap type is more often considered equivalent to flaps involving muscle for use in pressure sore reconstruction not complicated by infection (Hansen, 2013).

Myocutaneous (also called musculocutaneous) flaps involve rotation of all soft tissue layers (skin, subcutaneous tissue, fascia, muscle). These flaps provide optimal coverage for bony prominences and therefore are frequently used in the surgical reconstruction of chest wall defects, cancer excision defects, complex leg wounds, pressure ulcers, and other full-thickness wounds. Myocutaneous flaps carry along with them the native arterial and venous blood supplies to the muscle and the overlying skin. Because these flaps must survive on their original blood flow, their reach is limited by

their nutrient vessel(s). When the flaps are pulled or stretched beyond their limits, the blood vessels also are stretched and are not able to perfuse the flaps. Therefore postoperative monitoring of arterial inflow and venous outflow is crucial for flap survival.

The area of potential reach for each muscle flap is known. For example, the biceps femoris muscle (one of the lateral hamstring muscles) is supplied with blood via arteries from the profunda femoris. The flap has an arc of rotation that can cover defects of the ischium and groin.

Methods Used to Move the Flap

Flaps can be classified according to the surgical technique used to transport them to the recipient site as advancement flaps and rotation flaps. *Advancement* flaps involve elevation of the tissue to be transferred, undermining of the wound edges, and advancement of the tissue into the defect. Advancement flaps are useful in areas with significant redundant skin that can stretch. *Rotation* flaps are used to fill defects adjacent to the donor tissue. A flap is outlined on three sides, the tissue is elevated, and the flap is rotated into the defect. The donor site may be closed surgically or may require a split-thickness skin graft for closure. *Transposition* flaps are rotation flaps that are moved across normal skin to fill a defect (as opposed to being directly adjacent to the defect).

Methods of Retaining Perfusion

The perfusion of the flap is important in the design of the flap. All flaps of tissue carry with them a blood supply (unlike a skin graft). *Random flaps* depend on the dermal and subdermal vessels for their blood supply. Because these vessels are small, the blood supply to these flaps is tenuous. *Axial flaps* are designed to include an artery, which increases vascularity and the chances for flap survival. These vessels nourish the flap until new collateral capillary systems are established between the flap and the wound bed. Common axial flaps include the pectoralis flap to reconstruct the neck after radical neck surgery and the tensor fasciae latae flap used to close ischial pressure ulcers. When tissue is not available locally, it can sometimes be brought in using a free flap. This type of operation is more technically challenging because it requires microvascular surgical techniques. In this approach, the donor tissue, along with its blood supply, is completely removed from the donor site and transferred to the recipient site. The artery and vein that supply the flap are attached by microvascular techniques to vessels near the wound. These types of flaps can be used to repair wounds of the head and neck, breast, or lower third of the leg. For example, recalcitrant venous ulcers with severe lipodermatosclerosis may benefit from free flap transfer by allowing wide excision of diseased tissue and replacing it with healthy tissue with its own microvasculature and uninjured venous valves (Robson et al, 2006).

Tissue Expansion

An additional surgical option for wound closure is tissue expansion to stretch tissue, including skin near the wound,

---

BOX 33-1 | **Categories of Surgical Tissue Flaps**

Local Flaps

Classified by anatomic structures:
- Skin flap
- Fasciocutaneous
- Myocutaneous or musculocutaneous flap

Classified by method used to move flap:
- Advancement flap
- Rotation flap
- Transposition flap

Classified by methods of retaining perfusion:
- Random flap
- Axial flap

Distant (Free) Flaps

which then can be moved into the wound bed. The oldest example of this principle is the growing abdomen in pregnancy. Silicone expanders, or hollow pouches, are placed surgically into the subcutaneous or submuscular tissue layer in an area adjacent to the defect. Sterile fluid is injected into the expander at routine intervals until the pouch is fully expanded. This process induces expansion of the overlying tissue layers. When there is sufficient tissue to provide coverage of the defect, the expander is removed and the wound is closed. The stretched tissue then can be closed primarily or moved to cover the defect. For example, a scalp wound with alopecia may be treated with tissue expanders placed alongside the bare area to expand the hair-bearing scalp. Once fully expanded, the bare area is excised and the expanded hair-bearing tissue is moved to cover the defect.

NONOPERATIVE CONDITIONS

Although it is important to know how to perform any given operation, it is equally important to know when not to operate. This discussion centers on the most common problems that rule out the use of surgical intervention; other conditions also may exist.

A pressure ulcer in a malnourished patient should not be repaired until the underlying malnutrition is controlled and the patient is anabolic again (NPUAP, EPUAP, PPPIA, 2014). If malnutrition is a volitional decision, then surgery should not be an option. If the pressure ulcer did not heal due to malnutrition, then the surgical wound will not heal for the same reason. A typical flap doubles or triples the surface area of the wound the body must heal (the donor site wound also must heal now).

Recalcitrant venous insufficiency ulcers require a bed of well-oxygenated granulation tissue to nourish a skin graft. If the edema cannot be controlled or the patient is unable to wear an external compression device, a skin graft will not survive.

Calciphylaxis is due to ischemia in the skin from vascular calcification. It is most commonly seen in patients with renal failure, hypercalcemia, and hyperphosphatemia. Lesions usually develop on the legs and begin as areas of mottled skin that progress into painful, firm areas of necrosis. Surgery, if considered, usually consists of debridement of the lesion to prevent sepsis. However, until the underlying problems are controlled, the wounds often reappear.

Stable eschar on the heel frequently presents as a nonoperative condition. Stable eschar is dry, hard, and firmly attached to the underlying skin; indications of an infection (induration, erythema, pain) are absent. Stable eschar on the heels should be left intact, not debrided and not softened. Slowly, the eschar will release at the edges as the underlying tissue heals while the eschar forms a barrier to protect underlying relatively ischemic tendon and bone. The loose eschar then can be trimmed. Moistening or softening the eschar encourages invasion of bacteria. Removal of the eschar exposes the fat pad, which can desiccate and expose the calcaneus.

A retrospective review of 263 pressure ulcers on the heels with stable eschar that were not debrided reported healing in all but one patient. It required 11 weeks to heal eschar and 6 weeks to heal blisters with offloading. This data review had 41% lost to follow-up (Shannon, 2013).

Operative closure of the ischemic wound is contraindicated. Despite long-standing recommendations for serial debridement, debridements on ischemic lower extremity wounds often will make the wound larger, and eventually more necrotic, with little hope of healing. Unless arterial inflow can be reestablished, the wound is best left alone. Local wound care for ischemic wounds, such as arterial wounds, includes pain control, protection, and coverage with dressing material that is easily removed.

Inability to adhere to postoperative care requirements can be a significant deterrent to healing of a surgical wound. If the patient cannot remain off the flap, consume adequate calories, and control fecal and/or urinary contamination of the incision, the skin graft or flap likely will fail. It is important to keep in mind that only a given number of flap options can be used in a lifetime. Once a muscle is used, it cannot be used again. Therefore the decision to operate should be made only after the patient is adequately educated regarding the interventions necessary postoperatively to reduce complications and prevent recurrence. A review of 227 flaps to close ischial pressure ulcers reported 88 recurrences (39%). Recurrence was highest in patients who were younger than 45 years, had low albumin, and had elevated hemoglobin A1c (Keys et al, 2010).

Pyoderma gangrenosum is a rare condition that causes painful wounds on the lower extremities. Its cause is unknown and thought to be immune related. It is associated with other immunologic disorders, including rheumatoid arthritis and inflammatory bowel disease. It evolves from a small wound and is often confused by patients as a spider bite. These wounds often have a characteristic purple discoloration. A skin biopsy is typically performed showing a dense infiltration of neutrophils. Corticosteroids and other immunologic therapies are used for treatment. These ulcers are not treated surgically, as this tends to enlarge the ulcers.

URGENT OPERATIVE CONDITIONS
Traumatic Wounds

Patients with traumatic wounds must undergo a thorough assessment to be certain they do not have major vessel, nerve, or tendon injury; therefore the examination must be completed before the administration of local anesthetics. The wound is closed primarily when possible, without creating donor site morbidity; for example, pulling the lower eyelid down and exposing the eye because the lid cannot close. Facial wounds require small sutures to avoid excess scar formation. The timing of suture removal is dependent on the anatomic location and method of closure. For example, sutures on the face are generally removed sooner than sutures on the lower leg or buttocks. Linear wound closure, as well as suture removal method, timing, and technique are described in Chapter 34.

When patients are severely injured, their wound issues may become the second priority to airway, breathing, and circulation. Clean wounds should be dressed with normal saline gauze and, if possible, closed within 12 to 24 hours. After that time, they are considered contaminated. Operative closure should be a delayed primary closure, or the wound should be allowed to heal secondarily, with scar revision at a later date. Chapter 31 further discusses the care of patients with traumatic wounds.

Abscess

An abscess is a local collection of pus and sometimes blood. Abscesses are incised and drained. The remaining cavity may require packing to prevent healing from occurring at the surface before healing occurs in the deeper tissues.

Gangrene

Wet gangrene develops from a sudden interruption in blood supply, as occurs with burns, freezing, hematoma, or injury that becomes infected, or from primary infection of tissues from certain bacteria. Wet gangrene from any organism can quickly spread into surrounding tissues as a result of the bacteria and destroy muscle and other tissues. The patient has pain and fever. Malodor is often the most obvious sign. The tissue becomes discolored, blistered, and boggy and may have crepitus if the wound is infected with gas-forming organisms such as *Clostridium perfringens* (formerly known as *Clostridium welchii*). Frequently no line of demarcation exists between normal and infected tissue. Anaerobic infections can develop into gas gangrene within 1 to 2 days, and if the patient develops bacteremia, the mortality rate increases. If the gangrene is recognized and treated early and aggressively, mortality rates range from 25% to 35% (Mills et al, 2013). Surgery for wet gangrene includes radical removal of infected tissues or amputation. Hyperbaric oxygen therapy (HBOT) may also be used. Spreading gangrene is a surgical emergency. The wounds from these operations can be large and deep, with extensive areas of tissue loss.

In contrast, *dry* gangrene develops slowly from progressive loss of arterial supply, commonly in the extremities. A coagulative necrosis develops, and the tissue becomes black, dry, scaly, and greasy. A clear line of demarcation exists between viable and gangrenous tissue. The body will slowly slough the gangrenous tissue at the line of demarcation. Surgery may not be needed unless the area becomes infected. Although the gangrene is not painful at this stage, it likely was painful earlier in the process because of ischemia, and adjacent compromised tissue may exhibit ischemic pain. Dry gangrene should be covered with dry dressings and the tissue not moistened to prevent conversion to wet gangrene. An area of dry gangrene should never be soaked.

Necrotizing Fasciitis

Necrotizing fasciitis is a rapidly spreading, inflammatory infection of the deep fascia, with secondary necrosis of the subcutaneous tissues. The causative bacteria may be aerobic or anaerobic. Frequently, the cause is two synergistic bacteria that thrive in the hypoxic tissues. Because of the common presence of gas-forming organisms, subcutaneous air is classically described in necrotizing fasciitis and readily seen on radiograph. Pain out of proportion to the physical findings is a hallmark sign. The infection spreads rapidly along the fascial plane. These infections can be difficult to recognize in their early stages, but they rapidly progress to septic shock and organ failure. Emergency aggressive surgical debridement is required to remove all the necrotic tissue. Empiric broad-spectrum intravenous antibiotics are used until culture findings are known; however, the shock does not improve until the involved tissue is debrided.

Hyperbaric oxygen therapy is an important adjunct to treatment where available. Wang (2003) conducted a systematic review of HBOT and reported that it may be helpful for some wounds, but there is insufficient evidence to ascertain the appropriate time to initiate therapy and to establish criteria that determine whether patients will benefit.

PREOPERATIVE MANAGEMENT

Reducing Cofactors

When the health care team has the luxury of time, improving the patient's underlying condition will improve surgical wound healing (Franz et al, 2008). Many comorbid conditions can delay healing of both chronic and acute surgical wounds. Some of the most common conditions that require correction in this patient population (perfusion, oxygenation, bioburden, corticosteroids, diabetes, malnutrition, nicotine) are discussed in detail within chapters throughout this text. Permanent or temporary fecal and urinary diversions are sometimes needed to obtain a healed wound. Use of a bowel program or catheterization can divert urine and fecal material without the need for additional surgery (Whitney et al, 2006).

Spasms and Contractures. Patients with paraplegia, quadriplegia, or other neurologic diseases have spasms that can lead to friction damage or traction on the incision, which can cause dehiscence. Spasms and fixed contractures also may limit postoperative positioning and leave patients at risk for development of new pressure ulcers. Management of muscle spasm and contractures should begin preoperatively and continue until the wound is completely healed (NPUAP, EPUAP, PPPIA, 2014).

Social Support. Closure of pressure ulcers with flaps is technically possible in many cases. However, maintaining a closed wound is difficult unless the patient has a social network that can encourage adherence to postoperative restrictions and promote a lifetime of self-care (NPUAP, EPUAP, PPPIA, 2014). A retrospective review by Schryvers et al (2000) of 168 patients with pressure ulcers revealed that the majority of patients were paraplegic, unemployed men who had a low level of education. Most lived alone or with family but were independent in self-care. They concluded that securing a safe home for placement after rehabilitation is crucial to the outcome. Therefore the ability of the individual to return home safely should be known before surgery. Kierney et al (1998) achieved a very low 19% ulcer recurrence rate by combining efforts of plastic surgery and physical medicine. In their experience, social service assistance is provided to each individual. The individual's wheelchair, wheelchair cushion, and other mechanical devices are assessed before surgery.

Wound Bed Preparation

Successful closure of any wound requires a clean, perfusing wound bed. Excisional debridement helps prepare the wound bed that is likely to heal either by acute wound-healing methods or by attachment of surgically transferred tissues. A recurring criticism of sharp and surgical debridement is that it is nonselective so viable and nonviable tissues are removed. Although this statement is true from a broad-brush perspective, most surgical debridements are done until the wound bed is clean and bleeding. Even though some layers of viable tissue may be sacrificed, there is a greater likelihood of removing all nonviable tissue, senescent cells, and avascular biofilm protective to bacteria (see Chapter 16). Failure to remove these wound factors often leads to failure of the surgical effort. Newer debridement instruments can actually debride in thin layers less than 1 mm thick. Techniques for wound debridement are discussed in Chapter 17.

Although the exact mechanism of action is unproven, it appears that negative pressure applied to the wound bed reduces surrounding tissue edema, allowing new, enriched blood to flow into the wound. The pull on the tissues also stimulates granulation tissue growth, allowing definitive closure to occur earlier than usual. This is analogous to tissue expansion using negative pressure rather than positive. The removal of wound exudate reduces the colonization on the wound surface. Negative pressure wound therapy (NPWT) is especially useful for accelerating the process of wound bed preparation for flaps, treating dehisced wounds, and preparing wounds for delayed linear closure (Fife et al, 2004; Robson et al, 2006). Negative

pressure wound therapy may be used as a bridge between wound preparation and surgery, which allows time for the health care team to optimize the patient's condition for success of the reconstruction. It should be noted, however, that wounds healed with just NPWT and allowed to close via contracture may create unstable scarring over time, seen as scar tissue ulceration and pain with any stretching of the scar.

OPERATIVE MANAGEMENT

International pressure ulcer guidelines recommend surgical consultation for operative repair in individuals with Stage III or IV pressure ulcers that are not closing with conservative treatment and for individuals who desire more rapid closure of the ulcer (NPUAP, EPUAP, PPPIA, 2014). Pressure ulcer excision and closure are commonly completed with patients under general anesthesia, even in those with paralysis, to reduce spastic and reflexic muscle movement and to control their vasomotor instability. Blood loss is anticipated, and patients should have blood typed and cross-matched for intraoperative administration.

Sacral Ulcers

The sacrum is the most common location for pressure ulcers. Large skin defects in the sacral area are not uncommon and can be associated with even larger areas of undermining. Fortunately, these ulcers rarely are deep. Ostectomy of the sacral prominence is necessary if bone is infected. Coverage is most commonly obtained with a large gluteal myocutaneous or fasciocutaneous flap (Figure 33-2).

Greater Trochanteric Ulcers

Ulcers on the greater trochanter are seen in patients, many of whom have severe contractures and can only lie on their sides. The tensor fasciae latae myocutaneous flap is the workhorse of ulcer covering in this region. It is most commonly designed as a transposition flap with a large resultant dog-ear (Figure 33-3). V-Y advancement (see the next section on

FIGURE 33-2 Sacral ulcers can be closed with a gluteus maximus myocutaneous flap. **A,** Gluteus muscle is identified using landmarks guided by the ischial tuberosity and the posterior iliac spine. **B,** Segment of the muscle is rotated into the wound and is fed by the superior gluteal artery. **C,** Muscle is divided and moved into the wound. The wound is closed primarily with a long incision to avoid tension. (From Song DH, *Lower extremity, trunk, and burns*, vol 4. In Neligan PC: *Plastic surgery*, ed 3, Philadelphia, 2013, Elsevier.)

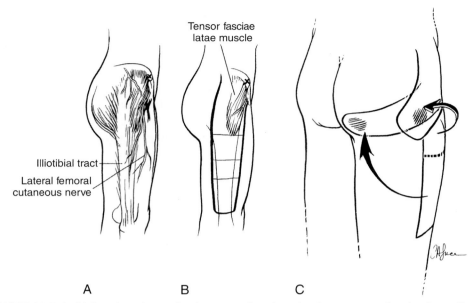

FIGURE 33-3 Ischial and trochanteric ulcers can be closed using a tensor fasciae latae flap. **A,** Muscle is found on the lateral thigh and fed by the femoral circumflex artery, which enters at the superior anterior iliac spine. **B,** Advantage of the flap is the long muscle and skin cover. **C,** Arc of rotation can provide coverage for both ischial and trochanteric ulcers. (From Cohen S: Pressure sores. In McCarthy J, editor: *Plastic surgery*, Philadelphia, 1990, Saunders.)

ischial ulcers for description of the V-Y flap) and rotation of the tensor fasciae latae flap often give an excellent functional and better aesthetic result. Other flaps include the rectus femoris myocutaneous flap and random bipedicle or unipedicle fasciocutaneous flaps.

Ischial Ulcers

Ischial ulcers occur from prolonged erect sitting without changes in position and are most common in patients with lower limb paralysis. Usually, a small skin wound with a large cavity beneath the surface is present. The ischial tuberosity is the pressure point and is always involved. Ischial ostectomy is avoided if the bone is not infected because this procedure distributes the body weight onto the perineum, and the resulting ulcers are very difficult to manage.

Many options for flaps to cover ischial ulcers exist, including the tensor fasciae latae (see Figure 33-3). The hamstring V-Y myocutaneous flap can be used for patients with recurrent ulcerations in extremely large defects. This flap is particularly valuable for layer defects because thorough dissection yields 10 to 12 cm of advancement. It is called a *V-Y flap* because the flap is raised with V-shaped incisions and then closed as a Y. This flap is well vascularized by segmental perforators from the hamstrings originating from the deep femoral artery. However, because the origins and insertions of the muscles are severed, this flap cannot be used in an ambulatory patient. Additional myocutaneous flaps for ischial ulcer closure include the rectus abdominis flap and the gracilis flap.

The gluteus maximus muscle flap offers a large amount of well-vascularized tissue with which to fill the defect. Even in the patient with a spinal cord injury, significant muscle mass still exists. Skin closure of the donor site can be obtained by linear closure in some cases or by a separate, inferiorly based fasciocutaneous rotation flap. It can be designed as a split muscle flap preserving donor-site function in the ambulatory patient.

Ischial ulcers in paralyzed patients are difficult wounds. The recurrence of ulcers in this population can be high. The acute surgical wound can be delayed in healing, and the psychosocial components in the patient can lead to recurrence. Krause and Broderick (2004) reported that the odds of having a recurrent pressure ulcer were reduced with a healthy lifestyle, being employed, and having a positive social network.

Multiple Pressure Ulcers

Extensive ulcerations of the sacrum, trochanters, and ischium are not uncommon, particularly in paralyzed patients. Removal of the femur combined with amputation of the leg allows the use of the skin and muscle from the thigh, called a *total thigh flap*, and has sometimes been necessary to provide enough tissue to close these extensive multiple wounds. Before surgery, urologic evaluation is completed because of the frequency of urinary infection. Urinary diversion may be required. Fecal diversion (temporary colostomy) also may be necessary. Common complications after surgery include hemorrhage and infection. Prolonged immobilization on special pressure redistribution beds is needed postoperatively, or these flaps will fail.

POSTOPERATIVE MANAGEMENT

Skin Grafts

Survival of skin grafts depends on revascularization of the grafted skin. Initially the skin survives because of the plasma on the wound surface. Within 72 hours, new vessels should traverse the graft and change it to a pink color. The change in color of the grafted skin signifies what is called a *take* and often is expressed as a percentage of take or adherence to the wound bed that occurs through the ingrowth of new capillaries and fibrin bands. For example, a split-thickness skin graft is reported to have a 90% take after 72 hours when the first dressing is changed.

The two factors most commonly associated with skin graft failure are (1) failure to adequately immobilize the graft, which is critical to revascularization; and (2) inadequate wound bed preparation (debridement). One of the most common clinical problems after lower extremity skin grafting is failure to prevent edema in the wound bed. The patient must keep the skin graft site elevated for at least 72 hours. All too often, the patient tries to get to the bathroom quickly or to sit briefly on the edge of the bed, and the grafted site becomes engorged with blood despite stented dressings and wraps. Clear instructions are imperative.

Negative pressure wound therapy is sometimes used over skin grafts to promote adherence. Although the actual mechanism of action is not known, it is likely that NPWT immobilizes the graft and reduces edema in the wound bed. The graft may be meshed for NPWT to be more effective, especially in large surface area grafts. The NPWT sponge should not be placed directly on the graft, so nonadherent wound contact dressings are usually placed directly on the graft site. Constant suction must be applied for 72 hours. If NPWT fails to function, the surgeon should be notified before the vacuum on the device is reestablished.

Once the graft has taken, the site is dry and prone to pruritus, dermatitis, or folliculitis. These conditions occur because sweat and oil glands are located in the deep dermis and are not transferred with partial-thickness skin grafts. Patients must be taught to develop lifelong strategies to protect and moisturize the skin.

The donor site for the split-thickness skin graft is a partial-thickness wound, which heals by reepithelialization. Donor sites require protection for healing. Usual covers for donor sites include transparent films; fine mesh gauze; Xeroform; and an ointment containing castor oil, balsam of Peru, and trypsin. A small study of 36 patients showed that the ointment led to healing in an average of 11 days (Carson et al, 2003). Two trials of donor site healing in burned patients comparing film, foam, hydrofiber, or alginate showed faster healing with alginates (Brenner et al, 2014; Fernandes de Carvalho et al, 2013).

Flaps

After flap surgery the patient is placed on a specialty bed that provides pressure redistribution and eliminates shear (e.g., low air-loss bed or air-fluidized bed). A minimum requirement is 10 days on a specialty bed; however, the time a patient is on the specialty bed varies by surgeon and the take of the flap. There are few studies examining the outcomes of one bed to another after flap surgery (Finnegan et al, 2008). Taking the patient off the bed and having the patient sit too early are common causes of flap injury or failure. The flap should not be pulled while the patient is being turned or is being slid to the edge of the bed because the edges of the flap can be pulled apart. Therefore the use of turning sheets is imperative. The patient should not be allowed to move from the bed without permission of the surgeon, for example, onto a cart for a diagnostic test. Closed suction drainage devices are used in the wound and undermined areas until drainage is minimal to reduce the risk of hematoma and infection.

Mobility and exposure to pressure are gradually increased, beginning 3 to 5 weeks after the procedure, with careful monitoring of skin and suture lines (Ahluwalia et al, 2010; Keys et al, 2010). Padding for the seating surface (chair or wheelchair) should be provided after surgery to reduce the risk of ischemia. If the patient is wheelchair dependent, the seat cushion should be assessed before use. Inadequate pressure redistribution might have been the cause of the ulceration and will recur if the seat cushion is not revised or replaced. The patient should be reeducated on methods for reducing skin pressure and for monitoring skin daily for early signs of breakdown. Methods used by paraplegics to transfer from bed to chair (e.g., slide boards) should be discouraged until the flap is fully healed due to the shearing from the lateral movement.

Complications include flap necrosis due to spasm or stretch of the feeding blood vessels to the flap. The tissue appears pale and is cool or cold. Assessment of the vascular status of a flap can be improved by having two nurses examine the flap together at shift change to establish a baseline appearance.

Separation of the suture line can occur. Suture line tension often is aggravated by moving or pulling forces. Seldom is surgery performed to close the dehisced area; most often the open area is allowed to heal secondarily.

The most common complication is recurrence of the ulcer. Early recurrences are due to mobilizing the patient too much and too early, which frequently is done in an effort to reduce hospital length of stay. Late recurrences are often due to failure to change the previous lifestyle behaviors that caused the first ulcer. Support, equipment, and educational needs must be addressed and in place before patient discharge to facilitate adaptation (see Chapter 29) and prevent reoccurrence. Flaps are not as resilient as native tissue, and periods of time sitting on the flaps must be limited in duration for the patient's lifetime. Remember that only a few flap sites are available for reconstruction of any given area; once they are all used, the prognosis is grim.

CLINICAL CONSULT

A: Patient seen in wound clinic with plastic surgeon. 34-year-old male paraplegic asking for surgical closure of nonhealing sacral pressure ulcer of 3 months' duration. Wound 5 × 6 × 2 cm, wound base primarily nonviable adherent yellow slough, with moderate exudate and mild periwound erythema. Patient is currently afebrile with no other local signs of infection. Followed by home care. Patient is sitting slumped in his chair on a foam cushion but demonstrates ability to raise himself off of the chair effectively.

D: Unstageable sacral pressure ulcer related to limited mobility.

P: Optimize local wound care, nutrition, and offloading prior to evaluation for surgical closure.

I: (1) Sharp debridement followed by alginate dressing covered with foam to promote autolysis and manage exudate. (2) Instructions provided to home care to change daily initially then every other day as exudate decreases. (3) Sent for nutrition evaluation and recommendations. (4) Patient declined low air loss bed due to difficulties with transferring. He states he can and will stay off his back; on foam viscoelastic mattress at home. (5) An appointment with physical therapy was made for a seating evaluation. (6) Surgeon explained flap surgery process in detail including need to commit postoperatively to bed rest on an advanced therapy support surface for several weeks followed by short seating trials on a specialized seating surface with slow incremental increases.

E: Return to clinic in 1 week for sharp debridement if needed, discuss RD and PT evaluations, and evaluate effectiveness of local wound care. Consider trial of specialty mattress prior to considering surgical wound closure.

SUMMARY

Many surgical wound closure techniques are available. However, surgical closure of wounds is not a panacea and is not appropriate for all wounds or all patients. The success of surgical wound closures is contingent upon management of several issues, such as the causative factors of the wound, the type of tissue missing and needed, the patient's general physiologic condition, the type of wound closure technique selected, preoperative nutritional status, postoperative care, and lifestyle behaviors.

REFERENCES

Ahluwalia R, Martin D, Mahoney JL: The operative treatment of pressure wounds: a 10-year experience in flap selection, *Int Wound J* 7(2):103–106, 2010.

Association for the Advancement of Wound Care (AAWC): *Venous ulcer guideline*, Malvern, PA, 2010, AAWC. http://aawconline. org/wp-content/uploads/2014/02/AAWC-Venous-Ulcer-Guideline-Update+Algorithm-v28-updated-11Feb2014.pdf.

Brenner M, Hilliard C, Peel G, et al: Management of pediatric skin-graft donor sites: a randomized controlled trial of three wound care products, *J Burn Care Res.* 2015 Jan-Feb;36(1):159–166, 2015.

Carson SN, Wiggins C, Overall K, et al: Using a castor oil-balsam of Peru-trypsin ointment to assist in healing skin graft donor sites, *Ostomy Wound Manage* 49(6):60–64, 2003.

Fernandes de Carvalho V, Paggiaro AO, Isaac C, et al: Clinical trial comparing 3 different wound dressings for the management of partial-thickness skin graft donor sites, *J Wound Ostomy Continence Nurs* 38(6):643–647, 2011.

Fife CE, Otto G, Walker D, et al: Healing dehisced surgical wounds with negative pressure wound therapy, *Ostomy Wound Manage* 50(Suppl 4A):28–31, 2004.

Finnegan M, Gazzerro L, Finnegan JO, et al: Comparing the effectiveness of a specialized alternating air pressure mattress replacement system and an air-fluidized integrated bed in the management of post-operative flap patients: a randomized control pilot study, *J Tissue Viability* 17(1):2–9, 2008.

Franz MG, Robson MC, Steed DL, et al: Guidelines to aid healing of acute wounds by decreasing impediments of healing, *Wound Repair Regen* 16:723–748, 2008.

Hansen SL, Young DM, Lang P, et al: Flap classification and applications. In Neligan P, editor: *Plastic surgery*, ed 3, St. Louis, MO, 2013, Elsevier.

Keys KA, Daniali LN, Warner KJ, et al: Multivariate predictors of failure after flap coverage of pressure ulcers, *Plast Reconstr Surg* 125:1725–1734, 2010.

Kierney PC, Engrav LH, Isik FF, et al: Results of 268 pressure sores in 158 patients managed jointly by plastic surgery and rehabilitation medicine, *Plast Reconstr Surg* 102(3):765–772, 1998.

Krause J, Broderick L: Patterns of recurrent pressure ulcers after spinal cord injury: identification of risk and protective factors 5 years or more after onset, *Arch Phys Med Rehabil* 85(8):1257–1264, 2004.

Mills MK, Faraklas I, Davis C, et al: Outcomes from treatment of necrotizing soft-tissue infections: results from the National Surgical Quality Improvement Program database, *Am J Surg* 200(6):790–794, 2010.

National Pressure Ulcer Advisory Panel (NPUAP), European Pressure Ulcer Advisory Panel (EPUAP), Pan Pacific Pressure Injury Alliance (PPPIA): *Prevention and treatment of pressure ulcers; clinical practice guideline.* In Haesler E, editor: Perth, Australia, 2014, Cambridge Media.

Robson MC, Cooper DM, Aslam R, et al: Guidelines for the treatment of venous ulcers, *Wound Repair Regen* 14(6):649–662, 2006.

Schryvers OI, Stranc MF, Nance PW: Surgical treatment of pressure ulcers: 20-year experience, *Arch Phys Med Rehabil* 81(12):1556–1562, 2000.

Shannon MM: A retrospective descriptive study of nursing home residents with heel eschar or blisters, *Ostomy Wound Manage* 59(1):20–27, 2013.

Wang C, Schwaitzberg S, Berliner E, et al: Hyperbaric oxygen for treating wounds: a systematic review of the literature, *Arch Surg* 138(3):272–280, 2003.

Whitney J, Phillips L, Aslam R, et al: Guidelines for the treatment of pressure ulcers, *Wound Repair Regen* 14(6):663–679, 2006.

Wound, Ostomy and Continence Nurses Society™ (WOCN®): *Guideline for prevention and management of pressure ulcers (WOCN® clinical practice guideline series no. 2)*, Glenview, IL, 2010, WOCN®.

34

Surgical Wounds and Incision Care

JoAnne D. Whitney

OBJECTIVES

1. Discuss current issues related to surgical wound infection and recommendations made by national collaboratives or evidence-based guidelines to address these problems and improve outcomes.
2. Compare intrinsic and extrinsic (modifiable) patient characteristics associated with surgical wound-healing complications or infection.
3. Identify wound assessment characteristics comparing the ASEPSIS method of evaluating wounds with Centers for Disease Control and Prevention–defined characteristics for surgical site infection.
4. Identify evidence-based measures for surgical wounds, including dressings; topical treatment; and care of sutures, staples, and tissue adhesives.
5. Discuss three aspects of care or evaluation for patients with surgical wounds and how they can help to promote healing and prevent complications of healing.

Approximately 54 million surgeries are performed each year in the United States (CDC, 2010). Although surgical procedures have become less invasive through the development and use of arthroscopic and laparoscopic techniques, many surgeries still are performed through open incisions. Even the less invasive surgical approaches create an incision and an acute wound requiring a normal physiologic wound-healing response (see Chapter 4). Surgical wounds that heal within an expected timeframe and without complications are considered acute wounds (Franz et al, 2008). In caring for the patient with a surgical wound, a major goal is preventing complications such as surgical site infection (SSI) and wound-healing failure through careful surveillance and interventions. Surveillance is largely accomplished through patient evaluation for risk factors and assessment of the surgical wound for signs of disruption in healing. Interventions are targeted toward reducing modifiable risk factors associated with healing complications and providing systemic and environmental support to facilitate healing to the greatest extent possible. Box 34-1 lists the 11 impediments to surgical wound healing addressed in the guidelines (Franz et al, 2008), many of which are addressed in detail in chapters throughout this text.

SURGICAL WOUND CLOSURE

The goal of wound healing is to reestablish tissue integrity and function with a cosmetically acceptable result and to prevent infection. These are also the goals of wound closure. Surgical wounds are closed primarily or are left open for either delayed primary closure or healing by secondary intention (see Figure 4-2). Primary wound closure is the fastest method for facilitating wound healing (Hollander, 2003). However, wounds with greater than 10^5 bacteria per gram of tissue should not be closed (Franz et al, 2008). In these cases, wounds are often left open and then closed on a delayed schedule, but ideally within a few days, once bacterial load is reduced below critical levels and the wound bed is healthy and can support healing. Primary repair should approximate (see Plate 70), but not strangulate, the incision (Franz et al, 2008). Incisions are approximated with sutures, staples, adhesive tapes, and skin adhesives to provide support and stability to tissues until healing has progressed and an acceptable degree of wound tensile tissue strength is reestablished.

Sutures and Staples

Multiple techniques and suture materials are available for closing an incision. National guidelines state that the type of suture material used does not matter in terms of SSI or post-surgery wound complications, as long as the primary repair is anatomic and perfused (Franz et al, 2008; Hemming et al, 2013). The choice of suture technique depends on the type and anatomic location of the wound, the thickness of the skin, the degree of tension, and the desired cosmetic result. For example, absorbable sutures are used to close tissues deeper than the epidermis and to provide tissue support, relieve skin tension, and reduce wound dead space (Hollander, 2003). Continuous sutures are recommended for closure of laparotomy fascial incisions; however, the type of suture does not affect healing. Surgical site infection in wounds after saphenous vein graft harvesting are problematic, but current evidence does not favor staples or sutures in terms of

BOX 34-1 **Impediments to Surgical Wound Healing**

- Inadequate wound perfusion
- Presence of nonviable tissue
- Wound hematoma or seroma
- Infection or increased tissue bioburden
- Mechanical factors during wound repair
- Systemic immunodeficiencies
- Cancer and cancer treatment factors
- Systemic conditions, diabetes mellitus, obesity, malnutrition
- Burn injuries
- External agents (e.g., tobacco, drugs)
- Excessive scar formation

infection risk (Biancari and Tiozzo, 2010). Current evidence also indicates that external or internal retention sutures do not prevent dehiscence and that dehiscence is more likely associated with other factors such as comorbidities (e.g., trauma and wound contamination) (Franz et al, 2008). Staples are commonly used to close the epidermis with acceptable healing and cosmetic result and no increase in infection (Hollander, 2003).

Sutures should be removed within 1 to 2 weeks of their placement, depending on the anatomic location: 3 to 5 days for the face; 7 to 10 days for scalp, chest, fingers, hand, and lower extremity; and 10 to 14 days for the back, forearm, and foot (Hollander, 2003; Wu, 2006). Sutures left in too long can lead to suture marks, local tissue reaction, and scarring. Premature suture removal places the wound at risk for reopening (Hollander, 2003; Wu, 2006). With the appropriate equipment, suture and staple removal is not difficult. The suture should be gently grasped by the knot and elevated slightly with forceps. One side of the suture is cut at skin level. With the forceps still grasping the knot, the suture is gently pulled toward the wound or suture line until the suture material is completely removed (Wilson et al, 2000).

Skin Adhesives

Tissue adhesives and derivatives of cyanoacrylate and other materials that add strength and flexibility have been used for several years for lacerations and other types of wound closure. An updated Cochrane review compared adhesives to sutures (ten trials) or adhesives to staples used for incision closure. The review identified a difference in rate of dehiscence between adhesives and sutures, favoring the use of sutures to reduce dehiscence; faster time to closure was found for staples in comparison to adhesives, but this was based on a single trial (Coulthard et al, 2010). The overall conclusion was that there is no evidence that SSI rates differ based on wound closure with tissue adhesives, sutures, tapes, or staples or between types of tissue adhesives. The authors also noted that evaluation of adhesives in patients with healing risk factors and for wounds with high tension requires additional study because these subpopulations were excluded from the

trials that were reviewed; therefore the comparative effectiveness is not known. Skin adhesives are not recommended for use with complex lacerations with wound edges that are difficult to approximate (Hollander, 2003). No removal is required for adhesives, although some cannot be exposed to water. Ointments should be avoided because they may loosen the adhesive and cause wound dehiscence (Hollander, 2003). Tissue adhesives slough off 5 to 10 days after they are applied.

Steri-Strips. Wound closure tapes, or Steri-Strips, are reinforced microporous surgical adhesive tape. Steri-Strips are used to provide extra support to a suture line when running subcuticular sutures are used or after sutures are removed. Wound closure tapes may reduce spreading of the scar if they are kept in place for several weeks after suture removal. Often they are used with a tissue adhesive. These tapes are rarely used for primary wound closure (Wilson et al, 2000). There is very little evidence of use for primary closure. However, a randomized trial of 51 patients comparing Steri-Strips to suture closure of wounds after breast reduction or abdominal surgery found scar quality (patient and surgeon assessment) and comfort (patient report) indicated similar outcomes in abdominal wounds but poorer outcomes when used for breast wound closure (Kerrigan and Homa, 2010).

SURGICAL WOUND ASSESSMENT

Clinically, there is no single, standard, widely accepted method for assessing healing of acute wounds. Additional issues arise because assessment parameters that are documented and descriptions of surgical incision healing by care providers vary and in some cases are not recorded. This concern is illustrated by a retrospective chart audit of surgical cases that documented 59.6% (89/152) did not have complete wound assessments (Gillespie et al, 2014).

Physiologically, deposition of collagen in the wound begins immediately in the inflammatory phase and peaks during the proliferative phase, approximately 4 to 21 days after wounding. Sufficient synthesis of collagen early during the healing process is critical to successful repair. Wound dehiscence is most likely to occur fairly early after surgery (by postoperative day 5 to 8) in patients in whom normal physiologic healing responses, such as collagen synthesis, lag. However, a method for direct observation of collagen production in acute wounds has not been validated; thus the term *healing ridge* is not mentioned in the acute wound guidelines and has been deleted from Outcome and Assessment Information Set (OASIS) documentation requirements (Franz et al, 2008; WOCN®, 2014).

ASEPSIS Scoring Tool

Acute wound complications can be evaluated on the basis of specific parameters using the ASEPSIS scoring tool. ASEPSIS is an acronym for seven wound assessment parameters that

BOX 34-2 ASEPSIS Scoring Tool for Evaluating Acute Wound Complications

Instructions for use: The surgical wound site is observed (if possible for the first 5 postoperative days) and the wound characteristics scored according to the proportion of the wound affected and the presence of the characteristic. Additional points are added based on factors such as antibiotic treatment specifically for wound infection. Daily points for characteristics and any additional factors are added for the final wound score and are interpreted according to the category of infection as shown in the table.

TOTAL SCORE: CATEGORY OF INFECTION

0 to 10: Satisfactory healing
11 to 20: Disturbance of healing
21 to 30: Minor wound infection
31 to 40: Moderate wound infection
>40: Severe wound infection

ASEPSIS WOUND SCORE

Wound Characteristic	Proportion of Wound Affected (%)					
	0	<20	20 to 39	40 to 59	60 to 79	≥80
Serous exudate*	0	1	2	3	4	5
Erythema*	0	1	2	3	4	5
Purulent exudate*	0	2	4	6	8	10
Separation of deep tissue*	0	2	4	6	8	10

	Criteria and Points		Score
A	**A**dditional treatments†		
	Antibiotics = 10	Drainage of pus (local anesthesia) = 5	Debridement of wound (general anesthesia) = 10	
S	**S**erous discharge = sum of daily scores (0 to 5 points possible each day)		
E	**E**rythema = sum of daily scores (0 to 5 points possible each day)		
P	**P**urulent exudate = sum of daily scores (0 to 10 points possible each day)		
S	**S**eparation of deep tissue = sum of daily scores (0 to 10 points possible each day)		
I	**I**solation of bacteria† = 10		
S	**S**tay as inpatient prolonged over 14 days† = 5		
		Total Score	

*Indicates factors that are scored only on days 0 to 5 of the first 7 postoperative days.
†Indicates factors that are scored and added to the total score once.

are described within the tool and presented in Box 34-2. The ASEPSIS tool, although primarily used in research, may also be used as a quantitative tool for surgical wound evaluation clinically. When used, it offers a scale for evaluating surgical wounds with greater objectivity and ability to be reproduced than clinician assessment. The ASEPSIS method was originally developed in cardiac surgery patients to evaluate characteristics of the surgical incision associated with infection (Wilson et al, 1986a). In a validation study, ASEPSIS was reported to be as sensitive and significantly more specific compared with other clinical indicators of wound problems or to wound assessments made using standard definitions of wound infections (Wilson et al, 1990). Interrater reliability of 0.96 has been reported in patients undergoing general surgery (Byrne et al, 1989). Similar reliability has been shown for sternal and leg wounds of patients after cardiac surgery (Wilson et al, 1986b). Topaloglu et al (2008) noted statistically significant correlations between preoperative wound infection risk indices and ASEPSIS scores. The authors of this study reported ASEPSIS was easy to use, repeatable, and effective as an infection surveillance method. Summed scores over wound assessments performed each day for the first 5 postoperative days indicate severity of infection or complication.

Impediments to Surgical Wound Healing

Although ongoing assessment of the surgical wound is critical, identifying impediments to healing is important so that they may be minimized or eliminated when possible. Box 34-1 lists impediments to surgical wound healing (Franz et al, 2008). Most of these (perfusion and smoking, nonviable tissue, infection, mechanical factors, obesity, diabetes, malnutrition, and burn injuries) are discussed in greater detail in chapters throughout this text.

Hematoma or Seroma. The occurrence of hematoma or seroma in surgical wounds has increased because of greater clinical use of anticoagulants and prophylactic treatments now recommended and implemented for deep vein thrombosis (Franz et al, 2007). When detected, hematoma or seroma requires intervention for removal by needle aspiration or prophylactic drainage (Franz et al, 2008). The presence of fluid collections, seromas, or hematomas delays healing in acute wounds through mechanisms of pressure and ischemia to the wound edges and adjacent tissues (Franz et al, 2008).

Surgical Wound Infection. Infections in surgical wounds are a concern, with 290,000 reported each year and high associated costs in terms of mortality, morbidity, and economic expenditures (Anderson et al, 2008). Surgical site infection is among the top three hospital-acquired conditions, with an estimated cost of $34,000 per infection (Lucado et al, 2006-2010; Scott, 2009; Stone et al, 2005). Surgical wound infection is termed SSI. Many definitions of SSI exist, and much data on how SSI is measured and monitored are available. In the United States recent updated data on health care–associated infections, including SSI, are collected through a prevalence survey that included a large number of U.S. acute care hospitals (Magill et al, 2014). Results are published and are also available on the Centers for Disease Control and Prevention (CDC) website. The CDC criteria established in 1999 (Mangram et al, 1999) for diagnosing various types of SSIs are widely accepted; the criteria are listed in Table 34-1. Infections of episiotomies, newborn circumcision sites, burns, and stitch abscesses are not classified as SSIs.

Surgical site infections occur within 30 days of surgery or within 1 year if an implant has been inserted and the infection involves the site of surgery. Surgical site infection is an incision infection or an organ/space infection (Mangram et al, 1999). *Superficial incision infection* involves only skin and subcutaneous tissue at the incision. *Deep incision infection* involves the deep tissues, including the muscles and fascia. *Infection of the organ/spaces* involves organs or body cavities that were manipulated during surgery.

In 2002 the Centers for Medicare & Medicaid Services commissioned the Surgical Infection Prevention Collaborative. Through intensive work efforts, the Surgical Infection Prevention Collaborative and then the Surgical Care Improvement Project (consisting of several multiagency cooperatives) produced guidelines for preventing surgical wound infection (Bratzler and Houck, 2004; Bratzler and Hunt, 2006). Surgical site infection prevention targets the perioperative period and has led to specific, evidence-supported guidelines for antibiotic choice and administration, hair removal, glucose control, and normothermia (for colon surgeries). For surgical wounds for which prophylactic antibiotics are used, administration within 60 minutes of surgery and choice of antibiotic consistent with published guidelines are recommended to attain effective tissue concentration (Anderson et al, 2008; Mangram et al, 1999).

Table 34-2 lists both intrinsic and extrinsic risk factors for SSI that have been identified in several studies. Risk factors that occurred in more than one study include diabetes, age extremes, obesity, malnutrition, ascites, low hematocrit, steroid use, smoking, and remote infection (Anderson et al, 2008; Barie, 2002; Haridas and Malangoni, 2008; Kompatscher et al, 2003; Malone et al, 2002; Mangram et al, 1999; Smith et al, 2004; Sørensen et al, 2005).

Further analysis shows that important factors were different for superficial infections (previous operation, prolonged duration of surgery, low albumin, chronic obstructive pulmonary disease) compared with deep and organ space infections (low albumin, previous operation). These data highlight some new factors that convey risk and emphasize that risk profiles are likely to vary for superficial versus deeper surgical infections (Haridas and Malangoni, 2008).

A number of risk factors are irreversible, but several may be modified through patient advisement and modification of aspects of perioperative care. Understanding who is at risk for SSI provides an opportunity for both preventive measures and to increase surveillance so that early detection can occur and timely intervention can be initiated.

Systemic Conditions. Perhaps the single most advantageous action that can be taken to minimize SSI risk is to prevent hyperglycemia. Hyperglycemia, with whole blood glucose level greater than 200 mg/dl in the 48 hours after surgery, is associated with diminished wound strength and significant reduction in the phagocytic ability of neutrophils (Goodson and Hunt, 1979; Latham et al, 2001). Perioperatively, elevated blood glucose levels are associated with complications for patients who undergo many types of general surgical procedures (Kwon et al, 2013).

TABLE 34-1 CDC Criteria for Incisional and Deep/Organ Space Infection

Superficial SSI	Deep Incisional SSI	Organ/Space SSI
Purulent damage	Purulent damage	Purulent damage
Positive wound culture	Incision dehisces or is opened by physician when patient has one of the following: fever, local pain, tenderness (unless site is culture negative)	Positive wound culture
At least one of the following: signs or symptoms of infection, pain, or tenderness; local swelling; redness; heat	Abscess or other evidence of infection found on examination, x-ray study, histopathology	Abscess or other evidence of infection found on examination, x-ray study, histopathology
Superficial incision is deliberately opened by a surgeon unless incision culture is negative		
Diagnosis by surgeon or attending physician	Diagnosis by surgeon or attending physician	Diagnosis by surgeon or attending physician

CDC, Centers for Disease Control and Prevention; *SSI,* surgical site infection.
Modified from Mangram AJ, Horan TC, Pearson ML, et al: Guideline for prevention of surgical site infection, *Infect Control Hosp Epidemiol* 20(4):252, 1999. http://www.cdc.gov/hicpac/SSI/001_SSI.html. Accessed June 5, 2014.

TABLE 34-2   Risk Factors for Surgical Site Infection

Intrinsic		Extrinsic	
Existing disease	Chronic obstructive pulmonary disease Congestive cardiac failure Diabetes Peripheral vascular disease Skin disease in surgical area	Presurgical factors	Current surgery through previous incision Emergency surgery Previous surgery Hair removal
Additional factors	Age Ascites Chronic inflammation Excessive alcohol use Hypercholesterolemia Hyperglycemia Hypoxemia Low albumin Low hemoglobin or hematocrit Malnutrition Nicotine use Prior surgical site radiation Remote infection Skin carrier of staphylococcus Steroid or other immunosuppressive medications	Perioperative factors	Estimated blood loss ≥500 mL Hypothermia Blood products Surgery ≥2 hours

Recommendations for patients with cardiovascular disease and for wound healing of acute wounds advocate for protocol-based glycemic control to achieve individualized target blood glucose levels, generally in the range from 80 to 180 mg/dl (Franz et al, 2008). Some research has suggested a narrower range from 80 to 120 mg/dl, maintained by insulin infusion protocol, as the ideal target in order to reduce deep sternal wound infections (Kramer et al, 2008), but this has been debated in recent literature because of the occurrence of hypoglycemic complications under conditions of very stringent control (Russo, 2012). Although an ideal target is not entirely certain, a range of 140 to 160 mg/dl is suggested for surgeries such as hernia repair (Martindale and Deveney, 2013). Consistent themes for best care are careful monitoring including glucose checks preoperatively, with and without a history of diabetes in certain groups, such as bariatric and colon procedures (Kwon et al, 2013) and control of diabetes, both preoperatively and perioperatively and extending well into the postoperative period, to optimize the healing environment during the months of collagen remodeling.

Obesity is an independent predictor of SSI (Harrington et al, 2004). Increased body mass index, intraabdominal fat, and subcutaneous fat are significantly associated with surgery-related complications, including wound infection (Tsukada et al, 2004). A number of retrospective and prospective studies in cardiac, general, and gynecologic surgery populations have documented an increased risk for SSI in patients who are obese (Israelsson and Jonsson 1997; Myles et al, 2002; Vastine et al, 1999; Winiarsky et al, 1998). Regardless of the type of surgical procedure performed, the incidence of postsurgical wound complications in patients who are overweight, obese, or morbidly obese compared with those of normal weight is high, with reported rates of 15% to 22%.

In an observational study of 1211 patients undergoing total hip replacement, morbid obesity was significantly associated with prolonged wound drainage and, in turn, with higher risk for (42%) and rates of SSI (Patel et al, 2007).

Factors that can be clinically evaluated and optimized in patients with obesity have been identified. In patients with obesity, perfusion and oxygenation of the surgical wound is more likely to be compromised. Therefore interventions that ensure adequate blood flow and oxygen delivery, such as increased perioperative FiO_2 (80% oxygen) and systemic warming to maintain normothermia, are important (see Chapter 28). Control of hyperglycemia in the perioperative period, provision of adequate doses of prophylactic antibiotics to maintain therapeutic serum and tissue levels (double the standard dose if weight is greater than 220 lb or body mass index is 35 or higher), closure of the subcutaneous tissue layer when its depth is greater than 2 cm, and laparoscopic surgery when possible are additional recommendations to decrease SSI in obese patients (Anaya and Dellinger, 2006; Walsh et al, 2009).

TOPICAL INCISION CARE

Regardless of their origin, wounds progress through the same phases of the reparative process in order to heal: inflammation, angiogenesis, fibroplasia and matrix deposition, and epithelialization. Knowledgeable assessment of the patient's surgical incision site includes evaluation of the primary dressing, epithelial resurfacing, wound closure, and local changes at the wound site that may signal infection. All healing incisions should be protected from sun exposure to prevent permanent hyperpigmentation (Ship and Weiss, 1985). General components of topical incision care are listed in Box 34-3 and described in this section.

BOX 34-3 Topical Incision Care

1. Keep incisions dry without prolonged exposure to moisture (including topical antibiotics and moisture).
2. Maintain original postoperative dressing for 48 to 72 hours (cleanse incision with sterile saline and use aseptic technique for changing dressings if needed in first 48 hours).
3. After 48 to 72 hours, patient may shower if suture line is closed with no drainage.
4. Timing of suture or staple removal depends on wound location:
   - 3 to 5 days face
   - 7 to 10 days for scalp, chest, fingers, hand, lower extremity
   - 10 to 14 days for the back
5. Protect surgical wound incision from exposure to sun.

Dressings provide initial protection, exudate absorption, and thermal insulation for acute wounds. Studies evaluating dressings that provide a moist, occlusive, or semiocclusive environment compared with standard dry absorbent gauze postsurgical dressings find no difference in the incidence of SSI for wounds after cardiac, vascular, or gastrointestinal surgeries; in patient comfort; or in cost (Shinohara et al, 2008; Vogt et al, 2007; Wynne et al, 2004). A recent systematic review and metaanalysis of 16 randomized controlled trials (RCTs) (n = 2594 patients) (Dumville et al, 2011; Walter et al, 2012) included comparisons of basic contact dressings with no dressing; different types of basic contact dressings; or basic contact dressings with film, hydrocolloid/matrix hydrocolloid, or hydrofiber. The 16 studies in the review included children or adults with surgical incisions healing by primary intention, wounds of all contamination levels (clean, clean-contaminated, contaminated), and dressings applied immediately after surgery. The metaanalysis found no statistically significant differences in rates of SSI for any of the comparisons, and the authors concluded there is insufficient evidence to suggest the type of surgical wound dressing reduces SSI (Walter et al, 2012). However, the results should be viewed cautiously, as studies were small and assessed as having either unclear or high risk of bias.

Additional outcomes relevant to surgical incision beyond SSI include patient satisfaction, comfort, pain, convenience, and cost. In terms of the outcome of cost, the data are mixed. Dry absorbent dressings are reported to be less expensive (Vogt et al, 2007; Wynne et al, 2004), although Shinohara et al (2008) found hydrocolloid dressings were less costly. None of the studies or the metaanalysis found differences in comfort between dressing types, and it is noted that meaningful data on pain are lacking (Walters et al, 2012). Further research on the impact of various dressings on meaningful outcomes with quality measurement methods is needed.

Incisional negative pressure wound therapy (INPWT) is also used in some cases and applied to closed surgical incisions. The effectiveness of INPWT to decrease instances of infection or dehiscence or to improve the rate of healing in primarily closed wounds is unclear. A Cochrane systematic review of five trials that included studies of INPWT treatment of skin grafts (n = 3) and acute wound incisions (n = 2) did not demonstrate any benefits (Webster et al, 2012). A subsequent systematic review of ten studies evaluated the effect of INPWT on wound complications, including infection, dehiscence, seroma or hematoma formation, skin necrosis/blistering, time to dry wound, or reoperation (Ingargiola et al, 2013). Results indicate INPWT may decrease infection rates, but also highlighted the need for larger, well-controlled trials and the inclusion of not only clinical outcomes but also cost-efficacy analysis. More detailed information on NPWT is presented in Chapter 21.

Of interest, some data suggest that dressings that provide some level of pressure or compression may actually impede local tissue perfusion (Plattner et al, 2000). This finding was based on the observation that wounds covered with dressings that provide some level of pressure had tissue oxygen levels 12 mm Hg lower than wounds with less constrictive covers. In the interest of supporting oxygen delivery to acute wounds, avoiding extra pressure over the wound seems prudent unless required for hemostasis.

Surgical dressings usually are removed 48 to 72 hours after injury, which is consistent with CDC guidelines for prevention of SSIs (Mangram et al, 1999), with guidelines from the United Kingdom (Leaper et al, 2008), and with recent systematic review (Toon et al, 2013). Aseptic technique for dressing changes and use of sterile saline if needed for cleansing are recommended within the 48-hour timeframe (Leaper et al, 2008). If the wound is closed and dry after 48 hours, patients may shower.

Use of topical antibiotics on closed surgical incisions is not supported by current evidence and is not recommended by recent guidelines (Franz et al, 2008; Leaper et al, 2008). A trial comparing no ointment, paraffin, and mupirocin ointment on excised and sutured skin lesions (n = 562 wounds) reported no differences in wound infection rate and, interestingly, significantly fewer scar complications in patients treated without any ointment (Dixon et al, 2006).

Resurfacing of the wound closed by primary intention occurs within 2 to 3 days after wounding because of the presence of intact epithelial appendages, such as hair follicles, and the relatively short distance that cells in the interrupted epithelial tissue must traverse. Although the incisional wound does not have the structural integrity (tensile strength) to withstand force at this time, by postoperative day 2 or 3, the incision is "sealed" and impenetrable to bacteria. However, many patients prefer that the wound remain covered. As healing evolves, some incisions begin to itch as a result of wound contraction or simply dry skin. Desire to view the surgical scar is personal. The presence of a dressing allows patients to gradually incorporate changes in body image. Although an incisional dressing may no longer be necessary once epithelial cells have resurfaced the wound, a soft dressing placed over the suture line often limits local irritation and provides additional comfort and support, particularly as the patient begins to wear regular clothing.

CLINICAL CONSULT

Memorandum
To: Dr. Johnson, MD, Chief of Surgery
From: WOC Nursing Staff
S: Recent increase in SSI rates.
B: Per your request we met to discuss, review the literature, audit and propose a plan to decrease SSI rates at General Hospital. We conducted an audit of a sample of 15-perioperative patients.
A: This small sample size revealed inconstant practices with the management of postoperative incisions ranging from leaving incisions open to air, applying a dry gauze dressing changed daily, or a composite dressing changed every 3 days or sooner for strike through exudate or increased pain, edema, erythema, or warm to touch around the dressing. We also noted many practice variations related to smoking cessation, nutrition, hair removal, decolonization, and warming.

R: In the short term (this month), we recommend implementing a standard dressing for incisions; a sterile composite dressing with a waterproof bacterial barrier that consists of a non-adherent absorbent pad bonded to a larger thin film transparent dressing to be applied in the OR and changed every 3 days or sooner for strike through exudate or increased pain, edema, erythema, or warmth around the dressing. Three examples on our purchasing contract have been sent to your office for your review. We would also like to audit the medical records of the last 20 patients for SSI (proposed audit form attached). Once we have the data, we will look for trends in risk factors we might be able to better control or minimize. Our time line for audits, analysis, and recommendations is 6 weeks.

SUMMARY

A significant number of surgeries are performed annually in the United States and globally. Surgical wound complications include failure to heal, as occurs with dehiscence or hernia, and SSI. Wound assessment for indications of healing complication and infection surveillance are important in the first 3 to 4 weeks postsurgery in order to detect problems quickly and provide therapy, as well as to capture accurate rates and level of severity of SSIs. A number of factors contribute to surgical wound complications, and some of these factors can be modified in advance of surgery. Other interventions are critical to monitor and modify during the perioperative procedure. National safety initiatives, quality reporting measures, and evidence-based guidelines for acute wounds offer new insights into risk and strategies to decrease wound-healing failure after surgery.

REFERENCES

Anaya DA, Dellinger EP: The obese surgical patient: a susceptible host for infection, *Surg Infect (Larchmt)* 7:473–480, 2006.

Anderson DJ, Kaye KS, Classen D, et al: Strategies to prevent surgical site infections in acute care hospitals, *Infect Control Hosp Epidemiol* 29:S51–S61, 2008.

Barie PS: Surgical site infections: epidemiology and prevention, *Surg Infect (Larchmt)* 3(Suppl 1):S9–S21, 2002.

Biancari F, Tiozzo V: Staples versus sutures for closing leg wounds after vein graft harvesting for coronary artery bypass surgery, *Cochrane Database Syst Rev* 5:CD008057, 2010.

Bratzler DW, Houck PM: Antimicrobial prophylaxis for surgery: an advisory statement from the National Surgical Infection Prevention Project, *Clin Infect Dis* 38:1706–1715, 2004.

Bratzler DW, Hunt DR: The surgical infection prevention and surgical care improvement projects: national initiatives to improve outcomes for patients having surgery, *Clin Infect Dis* 43:322–330, 2006.

Byrne D, Malek MM, Davey PG, et al: Postoperative wound scoring, *Biomed Pharmacother* 43:669–673, 1989.

Centers for Disease Control (CDC): *Inpatient surgery*, National Hospital Discharge Survey, 2010. http://www.cdc.gov/nchs/fastats/inpatient-surgery.htm. Accessed May 26, 2014.

Coulthard P, Esposito M, Worthington HV, et al: Tissue adhesive for closure of surgical incisions, *Cochrane Database Syst Rev* 5:CD004287, 2010.

Dixon AJ, Dixon MP, Dixon JB: Randomized clinical trial of the effect of applying ointment to surgical wounds before occlusive dressing, *Br J Surg* 93:937–943, 2006.

Dumville JC, Walter CJ, Sharp CA, et al: Dressings for the prevention of surgical site infection, *Cochrane Database Syst Rev* 7:CD003091, 2011.

Franz MG, Robson MC, Steed DL: Guidelines to aid healing of acute wounds by decreasing impediments of healing, *Wound Repair Regen* 16:723–748, 2008.

Franz MG, Steed DL, Robson MC: Optimizing healing of the acute wound by minimizing complications, *Curr Prob Surg* 44:679–763, 2007.

Gillespie BM, Chaboyer W, Kang E, et al: Postsurgery wound assessment and management practices: a chart audit, *J Clin Nurs* 23:3250–3261, 2014.

Goodson WH 3rd, Hunt TK: Wound healing and the diabetic patient, *Surg Gynecol Obstet* 149:600–608, 1979.

Haridas M, Malangoni MA: Predictive factors for surgical site infection in general surgery, *Surgery* 144:496–501, 2008.

Harrington G, Russo P, Spelman D, et al: Surgical-site infection rates and risk factor analysis in coronary artery bypass graft surgery, *Infect Control Hosp Epidemiol* 25:472–476, 2004.

Hemming K, Pinkney T, Futaba K, et al: A systematic review of systematic reviews and panoramic meta-analysis: staples versus sutures for surgical procedures, *PLoS One* 8(10):e75132, 2013.

Hollander JE: Wound closure options. In Singer AJ, Hollander JE, editors: *Lacerations and acute wounds: an evidence-based guide*, Philadelphia, 2003, FA Davis.

Ingargiola MJ, Daniali LN, Lee ES: Does the application of incisional negative pressure therapy to high-risk wounds prevent surgical site complications? A systematic review, *ePlasty* 13:e49, 2013.

Israelsson LA, Jonsson T: Overweight and healing of midline incisions: the importance of suture technique, *Eur J Surg* 163:175–180, 1997.

Kerrigan CL, Homa K: Evaluation of a new wound closure device for linear surgical incisions: 3M Steri-Strip S surgical skin closure versus subcuticular closure, *Plast Reconstr Surg* 125(1):186–192, 2010.

Kompatscher P, von Planta A, Spicher I, et al: Comparison of the incidence and predicted risk of surgical site infection after breast reconstruction, *Anesthetic Plast Surg* 27(4):308–314, 2003.

Kramer R, Groom R, Weldner D, et al: Glycemic control and reduction of deep sternal wound infection rates: a multidisciplinary approach, *Arch Surg* 143:451–456, 2008.

Kwon S, Thompson R, Dellinger P, et al: Importance of perioperative glycemic control in general surgery: a report from the Surgical Care and Outcomes Assessment Program, *Ann Surg* 257:8–14, 2013.

Latham RL, Lancaster AD, Covington JF, et al: The association of diabetes and glucose control with surgical-site infections among cardiothoracic surgery patients, *Infect Control Hosp Epidemiol* 22:607–612, 2001.

Leaper D, Burman-Roy S, Palanca A, et al: Prevention and treatment of surgical site infection: summary of NICE guidance, *BMJ* 337:a1924, 2008.

Lucado J, Paez K, Andrews R, et al: *Adult hospital stays with infections due to medical care, 2007 (Healthcare Cost and Utilization Project [HCUP] Statistical brief no. 94)*, Rockville, MD, 2006–2010, Agency for Healthcare Policy and Research.

Malone DL, Genuit T, Tracy JK, et al: Surgical site infections: reanalysis of risk factors, *J Surg Res* 103(1):89–95, 2002.

Mangram AJ, Horan TC, Pearson ML, et al: Guideline for prevention of surgical site infection, *Infect Control Hosp Epidemiol* 20:250–278, 1999.

Martindale RG, Deveney CW: Abdominal wall reconstruction preoperative risk reduction, *Surg Clin North Am* 93:1041–1055, 2013.

Magill SS, Edwards JR, Bamberg W, et al: Multistate point-prevalence survey of health care-associated infections, *N Engl J Med* 370: 1198–1208, 2014.

Myles TD, Gooch J, Santolaya J: Obesity as an independent risk factor for infections morbidity in patients who undergo cesarean delivery, *Obstet Gynecol* 100:959–964, 2002.

Patel VP, Walsh M, Sehgal B, et al: Factors associated with prolonged wound drainage after primary total hip and knee arthroplasty, *J Bone Joint Surg Am* 89:33–38, 2007.

Plattner O, Akça O, Herbst F, et al: The influence of two surgical bandage systems on wound tissue oxygen tension, *Arch Surg* 135:818–822, 2000.

Russo N: Postanesthesia care unit perioperative glycemic control, *Anesthesiol Clin* 3:445–466, 2012.

Scott R: *The direct medical costs of healthcare-associated infections in U.S. hospitals and the benefits of prevention*, 2009. http://www.cdc.gov/hai/pdfs/hai/scott_costpaper.pdf. Accessed June 5, 2014.

Shinohara T, Yamashita Y, Satoh K, et al: Prospective evaluation of occlusive hydrocolloid dressing versus conventional gauze dressing regarding the healing effect after abdominal operations: randomized controlled trial, *Asian J Surg* 31(1):1–5, 2008.

Ship AG, Weiss PR: Pigmentation after dermabrasion: an avoidable complication, *Plast Reconstr Surg* 75:528–532, 1985.

Smith RL, Bohl JK, McElearney ST, et al: Wound infection after elective colorectal resection, *Ann Surg* 239(5):599–605, 2004.

Sørensen LT, Hemmingsen U, Kallehave F, et al: Risk factors for tissue and wound complications in gastrointestinal surgery, *Ann Surg* 241:654–658, 2005.

Stone PW, Braccia D, Larson E: Systematic review of economic analyses of health care-associated infections, *Am J Infect Control* 33(9):501–509, 2005.

Topaloglu S, Akin M, Avsar FM, et al: Correlation of risk and post-operative assessment methods in wound surveillance, *J Surg Res* 146:211–217, 2008.

Toon CD, Ramamoorthy R, Davidson BR, et al: Early versus delayed dressing removal after primary closure of clean and clean-contaminated surgical wounds, *Cochrane Database Syst Rev* 9:CD010259, 2013.

Tsukada K, Miyazaki T, Kato H, et al: Body fat accumulation and postoperative complications after abdominal surgery, *Am Surg* 70:347–351, 2004.

Vastine VL, Morgan RF, Williams GS, et al: Wound complications of abdominoplasty in obese patients, *Ann Plast Surg* 42:34–39, 1999.

Vogt DC, Uhlyarik M, Schroeder TV: Moist wound healing compared with standard care of treatment of primary closed vascular surgical wound: a prospective randomized controlled study, *Wound Repair Regen* 15:624–627, 2007.

Walsh C, Scaife C, Hopf H: Prevention and management of surgical site infections in morbidly obese women, *Obstet Gynecol* 113:411–415, 2009.

Walter CJ, Dumville JC, Sharp CA, et al: Systematic review and meta-analysis of wound dressings in the prevention of surgical-site infections in surgical wounds healing by primary intention, *Br J Surg* 99:1185–1194, 2012.

Webster J, Scuffham P, Sherriff KL, et al: Negative pressure wound therapy for skin grafts and surgical wounds healing by primary intention, *Cochrane Database Syst Rev* 4:CD009261, 2012.

Wilson APR, Treasure T, Sturridge MF, et al: A scoring method (ASEPSIS) for postoperative wound infections for use in clinical trials of antibiotic prophylaxis, *Lancet* 1(8476):311–313, 1986a.

Wilson APR, Webster A, Gruneberg RN, et al: Repeatability of ASEPSIS wound scoring method, *Lancet* 1(8491):1208–1209, 1986b.

Wilson APR, Weavill C, Burridge J, et al: The use of the wound scoring method "ASEPSIS" in postoperative wound surveillance, *J Hosp Infect* 16(4):297–309, 1990.

Wilson JL, Kocurek K, Doty BJ: A systematic approach to laceration repair. Tricks to ensure the desired cosmetic result, *Postgrad Med* 107(4):77–83, 87–88, 2000.

Winiarsky R, Barth P, Lotke P: Total knee arthroplasty in morbidly obese patients, *J Bone Joint Surg Am* 80(12):1770–1774, 1998.

Wound, Ostomy and Continence Nurses Society™ (WOCN®): *Guidance on OASIS-C1/ICD-9 Changed Items & Data Collection* published sept 3, 2014 http://c.ymcdn.com/sites/www.wocn.org/resource/resmgr/Publications/WOCN_Guidance_on_OASIS-C1_In.pdf. Accessed June 4, 2015.

Wu TL: Plastic surgery made easy. Simple techniques for closing skin defects and improving cosmetic results, *Aust Fam Physician* 35:492–496, 2006.

Wynne R, Botti M, Stedman H, et al: Effect of three wound dressings on infection, healing comfort, and cost in patients with sternotomy wounds: a randomized trial, *Chest* 125(1):43–49, 2004.

35

Skin Care Needs of the Obese Patient

Susan Gallagher

OBJECTIVES

1. Define obesity.
2. Describe necessary accommodations in the physical environment for the obese patient.
3. Identify risk factors for three common skin complications in the obese patient population.

4. Discuss two common pulmonary complications in the obese patient population.

Sixty-seven percent of Americans are overweight, more than one third of all Americans are obese, and 3% to 10% (at least 8 million) are morbidly obese (Flegal et al, 2012). Morbid obesity, once a rare occurrence in America, has essentially quadrupled since the 1980s (Gallagher, 2014). Research also shows that the heaviest Americans have become even heavier in the past decade (Beydoun and Wang, 2009). Studies suggest a substantial increase in obesity among all age, ethnic, racial, and socioeconomic groups (Lanz et al, 1998). In the early 1960s, only one fourth of Americans were overweight; today more than two thirds of U.S. adults are overweight, as are 31% of U.S. children (Flegal et al, 2012; Ogden et al, 2012).

Worldwide, the number of individuals who are overweight or obese, which totals nearly 2 billion, now exceeds the number of those suffering from starvation (Barrios and Jones, 2007; World Health Organization, 2015).

Obesity has an economic, physical, and emotional impact on our patients. Americans spend close to $117 billion on obesity-related health problems, and $33 billion is spent annually in attempts to control or lose weight. The medical costs of obesity-related illnesses in the United States have been estimated at $209.7 billion annually (in 2008 dollars). For example, with regard to impact on pharmaceutical costs, obesity is associated with a more than 13-fold increase in the cost of antidiabetic medications. The cost of absenteeism to employers has been estimated to exceed $4.3 billion annually (Apovian, 2013; Cawley et al, 2012). Despite efforts at weight loss, Americans continue to gain weight, with obesity reaching epidemic proportions. Obesity is a factor in five of the ten leading causes of death and is considered the second most common cause of preventable death in the United States (West Virginia Department of Health and Human Resources, 2014). In addition to the physiologic costs, some authors argue that obesity is associated with emotional conditions such as situational depression, altered self-esteem, and social isolation (Gallagher, 2012; Pull, 2010). However, others argue that society's response to the obese person (i.e., prejudice and discrimination) leads to these emotional conditions (Puhl et al, 2014). Major comorbidities associated with obesity include type 2 diabetes, cardiovascular disease, hypertension, sleep apnea or obesity hypoventilation syndrome, and lipid disorders, including metabolic syndrome. Other associated conditions include malnutrition, immobility, and depression. These comorbidities affect the morbidly obese patient disproportionately and at a younger age. Diagnosis in the obese patient is difficult, and procedures are technically more complicated, which ultimately places the obese patient at a disadvantage (Gallagher, 2012). In addition, many hospitals, clinics, and home care settings are not prepared to meet the needs of the obese patient group because of inadequate equipment and insufficient personnel to accommodate the needs of the larger patient, factors known to contribute to the patient's risk of mechanical skin damage due to pressure, shear, or taping. However, advances in information, intervention, equipment, and education have helped reduce some of these risks (Gallagher, 2014).

DEFINING OBESITY

Obesity is defined as a body mass index (BMI) of 30 or greater; morbid obesity is defined as BMI greater than 40 (Box 35-1). *Bariatrics* is a term derived from the Greek word *baros* and refers to the practice of health care relating to the treatment of obesity and associated conditions. The American Society for Metabolic and Bariatric Surgery (2014) defines obesity as a lifelong, progressive, life-threatening, genetically related, multifactorial disease of excess fat storage with multiple comorbidities. Others describe obesity simply as the excessive accumulation of body fat, which manifests as slow, steady, progressive increase in body weight. However, recent discoveries suggest that obesity is more than simply overeating or lack of control. Genetics; gender; physiology; biochemistry; neuroscience; and cultural, environmental, and psychosocial factors influence weight and its regulation (Ludwig and Pollack, 2009). As far back as 1994, the National Institutes of Health regarded obesity simply as a diagnostic category that represents a complex and multifactorial disease. However, obesity is most recently viewed as a chronic, multifactorial condition (NIH, 2012).

Misunderstandings about the etiologies of obesity are common among health care providers. For example, obesity has long been perceived as a problem of self-discipline. Such misunderstandings can fuel prejudice and discrimination. In a culture that worships thinness, obese patients experience discrimination in schools, the workplace, and health care settings (Puhl and Heuer, 2009). As early as 1997, health care clinicians were often noted as biased against the larger patient (Thone, 1997).

Prejudice and discrimination pose barriers to care, regardless of practice setting or professional discipline. The overwhelming misunderstanding of obesity likely interferes with preplanning efforts, access to services, and resource allocation. This misunderstanding is not universal, but is pervasive enough to pose obstacles, and clinicians interested in making changes will need to recognize these barriers (Camden et al, 2008; Gallagher, 2011).

ALTERED SKIN FUNCTION

In the obese person, a greater percentage of centralized and cutaneous adiposity is responsible for a number of changes in skin physiology and comorbidities that directly affect the skin. For example, the obese individual must perspire more efficiently when overheated in order to cool the body adequately due to the difference in the weight-to-skin ratio of the obese. Thus the barrier function of the skin is altered to have increased transepidermal water loss than in skin with less adiposity. Dry skin is characteristic of obesity as a consequence of a fundamentally altered epidermal barrier. Levels of androgens, insulin, growth hormone, and insulinlike growth factors frequently are elevated, triggering sebaceous gland activity, altered skin pH, and an increased prevalence of inflammatory or noninflammatory papules, pustules, nodules, or cystonodules over the head, face, neck, back, or arms (Pokorny, 2008).

UNIQUE NEEDS

Common problems associated with the obese patient that interfere, at least potentially, with skin integrity include pressure ulcers, intertrigo, incontinence-associated dermatitis (IAD), and foot dysfunction. Risk factors, manifestations, and prevention and management are described in Chapters 5, 7, 14, and 15; however, unique aspects occur in the obese patient population.

Pressure Management

Pressure ulcers are considered areas of localized injury to the skin and/or underlying tissue as a result of pressure, or pressure in combination with shear (NPUAP, EPUAP, PPPIA, 2014). Pressure ulcers typically occur over a bony prominence and develop because of the inability to adequately offload the pressure; this is particularly true among very heavy patients. To compound this problem, friction and pressure can exist in locations unique to the obese person (Gallagher, 2011; Pokorny, 2008). Atypical or unusual pressure ulcers can result from tubes or catheters, an ill-fitting chair or wheelchair, or pressure within skin folds or over a point of contact not typically observed among nonobese patients (Gallagher, 2011; WOCN®, 2010).

Tubes and catheters can burrow into skin folds and ulcerate the skin surface. Pressure from side rails and armrests not designed to accommodate a larger person can cause pressure ulcers on the patient's hips (WOCN®, 2010). Patients often develop pressure injury over the buttocks rather than over the sacrum, an area that frequently is the point of maximum contact with the surface, because of the obese patient's atypical body configuration. Shearing/pressure damage can develop lateral to the gluteal cleft over the fleshy part of the buttocks due to insufficient repositioning or transfer onto a stretcher or the operating room table. Interventions to prevent these types of mechanical injuries are listed in Table 35-1.

Bariatric beds with a pressure redistribution mattress will reduce the risk of pressure ulcers, promote patient independence, improve clinical outcomes, decrease staff workload, and help control unnecessary costs (Gallagher, 2012). As described in Chapter 9, bariatric support surfaces are available in foam, air, gel, and water. They offer features with or without microclimate and moisture control that include low-friction covers. These devices are extremely useful for reducing friction and

BOX 35-1	**Body Mass Index Categories**
Underweight	<18.5
Normal weight	18.5 to 24.9
Overweight	25 to 29.9
Obesity	≥30
Morbid obesity	≥40

Source: National Heart, Lung, and Blood Institute, Bethesda, MD.

TABLE 35-1 Management of Skin Damage in the Obese Patient

Type of Skin Damage	Causative Factor	Prevention Intervention
Pressure	Tubes and catheters burrow into skin folds	Reposition tubes and catheters every 2 hours Place tubes so that patient does not rest on them Use tube and catheter holders
	Pressure between skin folds or under large breasts	Reposition large abdominal panniculus every 2 hours to prevent pressure injury beneath panniculus Physically reposition pannus off suprapubic area every 2 hours Use side-lying position with pannus lifted away from underlying skin surface, allowing air flow to regions Reposition breasts every 2 hours
	Pressure ulcer on hips or lateral thighs from side rails and armrests	Use properly sized bariatric equipment
	Pressure injury occurs in slightly lateral fleshy areas of the buttocks rather than midline (directly over the sacrum) because it is difficult to prevent excess skin on buttocks from being folded and compressed when repositioning the patient	Bariatric support surface Proper repositioning Trapeze Establish, communicate, and implement safest transfer and positioning method to prevent shear that can be used during handoffs
Moisture-associated skin damage (e.g., intertrigo)	Excess perspiration to more efficiently cool the body when overheated Redundant skin creating skin folds Severe pruritus, burning, local pain between skin folds	Use cotton clothing (particularly undergarments) Maintain weight Avoid tight clothing Avoid corticosteroids and antibiotics Burow's solution (aluminum acetate) soak applied for 15 to 20 minutes twice per day to soothe and dry affected area

shear and dissipating moisture. In addition to benefiting the patient, bariatric beds provide specific features that affect the staff and facility, as listed in Table 35-2 (Gallagher, 2011; Kramer and Gallagher, 2004). The support surface with lateral rotation therapy, often used for select pulmonary situations, has been used to help with repositioning a very large patient whose need for frequent turning may otherwise pose a realistic challenge (Camden, 2008). Additional precautions during lateral rotation to prevent friction and shear are well advised. The patient should be fitted to the appropriately sized surface with correct pressure settings, and frequent assessments for skin changes must be implemented (Gallagher, 2012; NPUAP, EPUAP, PPPIA, 2014).

Skin Fold Management

Moisture-associated skin damage (MASD), pressure, and intertrigo can develop between skin folds of the obese patient. Common sites include the inner thighs, axilla, underside of breasts, and panniculus. Pressure from the weight of the pannus over the suprapubic area or breasts against the chest wall and upper abdomen are sufficient to cause skin breakdown (see Plate 71).

Because the obese patient experiences increased perspiration and sebum production and a change in skin pH, the barrier function of the skin is compromised. In addition, coexisting conditions in the obese patient that will further increase the risk of MASD and intertrigo include diabetes mellitus, immunosuppression, infection, and chronic corticosteroid

and antibiotic use. Intertrigo (inflammation within cutaneous folds) can become an intertriginous infection with bacterial, viral, or fungal organisms alone or in combination (WOCN®, 2010). Clinical manifestations of intertrigo in this patient population include scaling, erythema, and small pustules. Patients often complain of itching or burning that can progress to fissures and maceration. In the face of associated pruritus, patients may scratch the skin surface, further compromising skin integrity and leading to a secondary bacterial invasion. Not surprisingly, many obese patients indicate they are constantly battling some degree of intertrigo in skin folds. When an individual is hospitalized, moisture from urine, perspiration, or wound drainage exacerbates this chronic but otherwise mild condition (Beitz, 2014).

Knowing the obese patient is at risk for MASD and intertrigo, preventive interventions should be implemented upon admission (WOCN®, 2010). In addition to the interventions presented in Box 5-4, management strategies unique to the obese patient are presented in Table 35-1.

Not all intertrigo is a fungal infection. As with all wound and skin care interventions, the area must be reassessed within a reasonable amount of time after the treatment plan is implemented to determine the effectiveness of that intervention. If the condition does not improve within 24 hours or the skin condition continues to deteriorate, a bacterial, viral, or fungal infection may develop, particularly when the skin is broken or denuded. This could progress to cellulitis or

TABLE 35-2	Benefits of Bariatric Bed Features for Patient, Care Staff, and Facility		
Feature	**Patient Benefit**	**Staff Benefit**	**Cost Benefit/Risk Reduction**
600- to 1000-lb capacity	Safely supports weight Eliminates fear of bed breaking	Reduces risk of injury during care	Reduces risk of patient injury (and possible litigation) if bed breaks Reduces risk of worker's compensation injury
Integrated scale	Safety Retained dignity More accurate than portable, under-mattress scales	Less time consuming than using a loading dock More accurate	Reduces risk of inappropriate treatment due to inaccurate weights
Expandable	Enhances patient participation by providing sufficient room in bed for proper repositioning	Bed width is a safe surface distance to prevent back injuries from overreaching Reduces risk of nosocomial pressure ulcer development from railings, skin fold pressure	Reduces risk of worker's compensation injury Reduces risk for litigation and citations from regulating agencies for nosocomial pressure ulcers
Trendelenburg/ reverse Trendelenburg	Decreases friction on back when "boosting"	Helps with gravity-assisted "boosting" for fewer lifting injuries	Reduces risk of worker's compensation injury
Cardio-Chair	Increases mobility Decreases cardiac and pulmonary decomposition Facilitates faster recovery	Facilitates patient mobility Decreases staff lifting Simplifies transfers	Reduces risk of worker's compensation injury Reduces length of stay by decreasing effects of immobility
Trapeze	Increases mobility Facilitates patient independence Decreases friction on skin Facilitates deep breathing and pulmonary hygiene	Decreases staff lifting Facilitates mobility Reduces risk for nosocomial pressure ulcer development	Reduces risk of worker's compensation injury Reduces length of stay by decreasing effects of immobility or staff injury Reduces risk for litigation and citations from regulating agencies for nosocomial pressure ulcers
Therapeutic mattress with microclimate control	Redistributes pressure appropriately to reduce risk of mechanical trauma (pressure, shear, friction) Facilitates moisture evaporation to reduce moisture entrapment in skin folds and sweating	Eases transfers and turning of patients Saves additional linen changes due to adequate control of perspiration Reduces risk for nosocomial pressure ulcer development	Reduces risk of worker's compensation injury Reduces risk for litigation and citations from regulating agencies for effects of immobility Reduces length of stay by decreasing nosocomial pressure ulcers

Data from Kramer K: WOC nurses as advocates for patients who are morbidly obese: a case study promoting use of bariatric beds, *J Wound Ostomy Continence Nurs* 31(6):379-384, 2004; Gallagher SM: Special patient populations. In Charney W, editor: *Epidemic of medical errors and hospital-acquired infections,* Boca Raton, FL, 2012, CRC Press; Gallagher SM: The intersection of ostomy and wound management, obesity, and associated science, *Ostomy Wound Manage* 60(1):6–7, 2014.

sepsis if left untreated, so further evaluation is necessary and the primary care provider should be notified. Topical antimicrobial dressings, such as silver-impregnated textile products, may be appropriate at this point.

Incontinence-Associated Dermatitis

Increased BMI has a direct association with urinary incontinence and is a risk factor for urinary incontinence independent of age (Osborne et al, 2013). Sleep apnea, another condition associated with obesity, can lead to decreases in oxygen tension and relative central nervous system hypoxia, both of which cause increased excitability of autonomic neurons and thus trigger urgency. Continuous positive pressure ventilation has been

reported to improve symptoms associated with urinary incontinence, such as urgency and enuresis (Steers and Suratt, 1997).

Many otherwise continent persons develop short-term acute incontinence when they are physically dependent in a health care setting. This condition may occur because of medication, delays in locating a caregiver to place the patient on the bedpan, or simply because the patient cannot access a commode in time to prevent an incontinent episode. Additional barriers to maintaining continence include inadequate staffing, negative attitudes by the staff (American Nurses Association, 2013; Rose, 2006), and reluctance on the part of the patient to ask for assistance. It is critical that health care providers collaborate with the patient and family to address and minimize these barriers. Maintaining clean, dry skin is the objective, and if the patient needs assistance in this effort, caregivers are available to help.

After each incontinent episode, the entire affected area should be cleansed with a no-rinse incontinence cleanser, dried, and appropriate skin sealant or moisture barrier applied. Perineal skin cleansers have been more effective than traditional soap and water and have become the standard of care because bar soap tends to dry the skin and create an alkaline pH on the epidermal skin surface, increasing the risk for skin injury (WOCN®, 2010). Table 5-4 and Box 5-4 list strategies and products used for the prevention and management of IAD. Patients report that drying the buttocks and the perineal area and between folds with an institutionally approved blow dryer on the cool setting is more comfortable than towel drying. This technique may be less traumatic to the outermost layer of skin (Blackett et al, 2011). An important potential barrier to the staff's ability to provide adequate perineal care is the lack of properly fitting gloves; health care facilities must provide elbow-length gloves for the staff caring for the bariatric patient (Blackett et al, 2011). If IAD develops despite preventive efforts, the skin care protocol must be reassessed and updated to include a moisture barrier ointment, skin barrier paste or barrier strip, external fecal pouch, or internal fecal device, all of which are described in Chapter 5.

Foot and Lower Leg Pathology

Because the feet carry a person's entire weight, heavier individuals are prone to wear-and-tear injuries. Some activities can create loads on the feet as much as four times the body's weight. In addition, foot pain could signal other serious medical conditions, such as arthritis, nerve and circulatory disorders, and diabetes. Among the obese population, foot discomfort or dysfunction requires prompt attention. Foot pain can discourage an obese patient from seeking outpatient wound care or ongoing diabetes follow-up due to ambulation and transportation difficulties. Accommodations in the physical environment that promote patient safety and comfort may overcome some of these obstacles (Checklist 35-1); however, a podiatry consultation is also warranted when foot discomfort is reported. As described in Chapters 14 and 15, when the joints of the feet are involved, medication, physical therapy, exercise, orthotics, braces, specially designed shoes, and surgery are among the tools that can be used to restore feet to as near-normal function as possible.

A number of factors place the individual at risk for lower extremity venous disease (LEVD), one of which is obesity. Further, having a BMI greater than 30 places the person at risk for poor healing once an ulcer develops. Patients with LEVD are encouraged to stay mobile, exercise, and get plenty of physical activity. In addition to local interventions, the Wound, Ostomy, and Continence Nurses Society™ (WOCN®) Guidelines (2011) suggest that obese patients have tailored programs that address functional limitations.

Lower extremity arterial disease (LEAD) is considered common among the obese individual. Characteristics of the

---

CHECKLIST 35-1 Accommodations in Physical Environment for the Obese Patient

✓ Larger, wider blood pressure cuff
✓ Long needles
✓ Larger tracheostomy ties
✓ Longer abdominal binders
✓ Large gowns/drapes
✓ Elbow-length gloves for incontinence cleanup
✓ Bed frame wide enough for effective repositioning
✓ Pressure redistribution support surface
✓ Overhead trapeze to facilitate repositioning when appropriate
✓ Bariatric ceiling or floor-based lift for safely moving the patient (e.g., ceiling lifts)
✓ Bedside commode (appropriate size)
✓ Wide wheelchair with specialized cushion
✓ Walker with proper support
✓ Size-friendly art and magazines
✓ Larger clinic examination tables anchored to floor with adequate step
✓ Sturdy, armless chair for clinic waiting rooms
✓ Air displacement lateral transfer devices
✓ Mechanical lifts with provisions for limb band, pannus sling, turning band, lithotomy band, repositioning sling

---

middle-aged adult suffering with LEAD are multiple comorbid conditions that coincide with metabolic syndrome, which is associated with obesity. These comorbid conditions include hypertension, coronary artery disease, diabetes, and chronic renal insufficiency. Further, the obese person with LEAD is at increased risk for associated mortality. Obesity has been associated with an increase in functional decline with LEAD, and no studies to date have addressed the effects of weight loss on LEAD (WOCN®, 2008). See Chapter 11 for additional reading on LEAD.

Regardless of the foot or leg pathology, self-assessment and professional assessment and treatment can be challenging. Obesity and/or decreased flexibility can prevent a patient from seeing his or her feet. Self-inspection can be difficult, with these limitations often requiring family or outside help (WOCN®, 2012). Physical inspection can be a real life challenge because positioning larger, heavier individuals poses threats to caregiver safety (Gallagher, 2014). Arnold (2014) describes trends in the emerging science of safe patient handling and mobility that serve the wound care provider either in the clinic or at the bedside. Specially designed slings, bands, and devices to position heavier patients safely are available and serve as an adjunct to dignified, comprehensive care (Gallagher, 2011).

THE SURGICAL EXPERIENCE

The surgical experience predisposes the patient to skin injury due to intraoperative mechanical factors (shear, friction, and pressure) and postoperative factors (immobility, pain, sedation, fear of falling, and inadequate staffing). In addition, the obese patient is at increased risk for impaired healing of the surgical incision and complications from the anesthesia and from the surgical procedure itself (e.g., cardiovascular, respiratory complications) that can further jeopardize wound healing (Martindale and Deveney, 2013).

Addressing Mechanical Threats to Skin Integrity

Although the patient may be awake and alert shortly after surgery, extra personnel and supportive equipment are required to transfer the patient, particularly to prevent shearing injury or placing undue stress on the incision. Early activity is encouraged to decrease the chances of immobility-related complications (Gallagher, 2011). Using bariatric equipment that will convert into a chair will facilitate achieving early mobilization. Deconditioning can occur very rapidly in the obese patient when mobilization after surgery is delayed, thus increasing the risk for skin- and wound-related complications. A physical therapy consultation within 24 hours of an intensive care unit admission may be valuable to (1) evaluate for and demonstrate immobility-related equipment and (2) provide passive and active exercises to slow deconditioning (Gallagher, 2010). The larger patient typically has several comorbid conditions, so postoperative recovery can be complicated and require close monitoring. However, it is important to assess and reassess the skin frequently (at least every 8 hours) so that potential complications can be prevented or identified and interventions applied early (Gallagher, 2012). This can be challenging due to the patient's size and postoperative slumber, but in today's environment of best-practice zero tolerance for nosocomial pressure ulcers, cannot be overlooked or postponed. Preplanning for the obese patient by having proper bariatric equipment and appropriate staffing available is essential to providing competent, safe postoperative care.

After surgery, the obese patient seems to breathe more easily when the bed is at 30 degrees because this position reduces the weight of the abdominal adipose tissue pressing against the diaphragm (Lasater-Erhard, 1995). The challenge in terms of skin care is that the patient who fears shortness of breath may refuse repositioning from the 30-degree, semi-Fowler's position, thus placing the patient at risk for sacral pressure injury. Introducing pressure redistribution early in the admission may reduce some of this risk, along with patient and clinical education designed to improve awareness about the risk. An appropriate bariatric support surface and trapeze should be in place to reduce shear on the sacrum and adequately redistribute pressure. The patient should be encouraged to offload and shift his or her weight at regular intervals, including reducing the head of the bed when possible, to prevent prolonged pressure to the sacrum. Similarly, the lower back should be monitored frequently for signs of friction or shear.

Incisions and Sutured Wounds

Obesity is associated with a higher incidence of wound complications, such as surgical site infection and wound dehiscence (Franz et al, 2008; Glance et al, 2010; Martindale and Deveney, 2013). A significant contributing factor is hypoperfusion of adipose tissue due to the higher ratio of tissue mass to capillaries in adipose tissue. The resulting decreased

oxygen tension in adipose tissue is essentially inadequate to meet the oxygen needs of the healing surgical incision (Anaya and Dellinger, 2006). Additional factors that contribute to the increased rate of surgical site infections in the obese patient include perioperative hyperglycemia (obesity is associated with insulin resistance and hyperglycemia), prolonged operative time (operative time is an independent predictor of surgical site infection), and suboptimal doses of prophylactic antibiotics to achieve therapeutic tissue concentrations (Anaya and Dellinger, 2006). In addition to optimizing tissue oxygen tension, as discussed in Chapters 28 and 34, Anaya and Dellinger (2006) recommend tight perioperative glucose control, larger doses of prophylactic antibiotics to maximize serum and tissue concentrations intraoperatively, and performance of laparoscopic operations whenever feasible.

Incised and sutured wounds are expected to create a watertight seal within 48 hours; however, wound healing can be delayed in some obese patients due to malnutrition if the patient has a diet that lacks essential vitamins and nutrients. When the incision is within a skin fold, wound healing can be delayed due to moisture entrapment and bioburden in the skin fold. A well-placed and well-constructed stoma will be critical to prevent postoperative peristomal and stoma complications that can be aggravated by irregularities in abdominal topography (Colwell, 2014).

To reduce the occurrence of abdominal wound separation, a surgical binder can be used to support the surgical incision. The binder should rest no higher than 4 cm below the xiphoid process and should allow 2.5 cm of space between the skin and binder to avoid constricting the chest wall and hampering ventilation. Binders are especially important when the patient ambulates. Some patients find the binders so comfortable that they ask to leave the binder on at all times. Regular and routine skin assessments of the area under the binder are important to monitor for signs of early pressure-related breakdown.

Hypoventilation Syndrome and Sleep Apnea

Morbidly obese patients tend to have pulmonary problems, two in particular: obesity hypoventilation syndrome and sleep apnea. Obesity hypoventilation syndrome is an acute respiratory condition in which the weight of fatty tissue on the rib cage and chest prevents the chest wall from expanding fully. Because patients are unable to breathe in and out fully, ventilatory insufficiency can occur (Gallagher, 2012).

Sleep apnea usually occurs when the patient is asleep in the supine position. The weight of the excess fatty tissue in the neck causes the throat to narrow, severely restricting or even cutting off breathing for seconds or even minutes at a time. Breathing can be made easier by keeping the patient in the semi-Fowler's position, which takes some of the pressure off the diaphragm. Mobilizing the patient as early as possible also will help. At home, many patients manage the problems of nighttime sleep apnea by using a continuous positive airway pressure machine (Casale et al, 2009; Shinohara et al, 1997). However, in the health care setting, some patients use bilevel positive airway pressure for a short time after extubation.

Tracheostomy Care

If long-term ventilatory support becomes necessary, performing a tracheostomy can be especially challenging if the trachea is buried deep within fatty tissue. A large wound may be needed in order to locate the trachea. This larger wound can lead to complications such as bleeding, infection, or damage to the surrounding tissue. Postoperative tracheostomy care, therefore, must include steps to protect the peristomal skin, manage the tracheostomy, and contain wound drainage. Locally, a non-adhesive absorptive wound dressing is appropriate. Compounding the potential skin-related problems associated with a tracheostomy in the obese patient is the inadequacy of standard-sized tracheostomy tubes for use in patients with larger necks. In addition, narrow cloth tracheostomy ties can burrow deep within the folds of the neck, further damaging the skin. Wider tracheostomy tie material should be used to accommodate the obese patient. When additional pressure relief is needed under the tracheostomy tie, padding such as a gauze or foam dressing can be applied between the skin and the tie.

NUTRITIONAL CONSIDERATIONS

Research suggests that 7% to 12% of the obese population in general is malnourished (Moize et al, 2003). Macronutrients and micronutrients have long been recognized as essential in skin integrity and wound healing among all individuals, but especially in those at risk, such as obese patients, whose nutritional status may be compromised because of repeated dieting and weight cycling, simple misunderstanding of proper nutrition, or weight loss surgery (Bal et al, 2012). Weight loss surgery is a metabolic surgery designed to produce malnutrition. Energy deficit occurs due to decreased food intake, food intolerance, and nutrient malabsorption. The goal in weight loss surgery or any weight loss program is to achieve monitored weight loss without adverse complications (Valentino et al, 2010). However, nutritional deficiencies and their consequences can develop if additional unforeseen events occur, such as injury to the skin and wound development. Critically ill obese individuals are already at risk for inflammatory issues that predispose them to sepsis at a rate greater than that of their lean peers. This becomes especially problematic in the face of protein deficiencies because protein malnutrition leads to even more severe inflammation and increased overall morbidity.

The malabsorptive procedures performed for purposes of weight loss carry the risk of interfering with absorption of iron, calcium, and the fat-soluble vitamins, such as vitamins A, D, E, and K (Strohmayer et al, 2010). Chapter 27 discusses the role and dietary sources of these nutrients; Table 27-6 lists their specific relevance to the wound repair process.

QUALITY IMPROVEMENT

Even with good education, clinical skills, and motivation, the delivery of safe, effective skin and wound care still can be extremely challenging. In managing the skin care needs of the obese patient, preplanning for equipment is an essential first step (see Checklist 35-1). However, it simply is not sufficient to adequately prevent the costly, predictable complications that occur in caring for obese patients and their skin. A comprehensive, interdisciplinary patient care approach is necessary to provide safe patient care in a timely, cost-effective manner but also to prevent caregiver injury. This approach should include (1) a bariatric task force; (2) a criteria-based protocol, which includes preplanning equipment; (3) competencies/skill set; and (4) outcome measurement efforts (Gallagher, 2012).

Bariatric Task Force

The bariatric task force is an interdisciplinary quality improvement effort designed to address ongoing issues and ideas. The value of an interdisciplinary approach cannot be overlooked. Pharmacists, physical/occupational and respiratory therapists, providers, clinical nurse specialists, the wound specialist, and others are essential in planning care. Each member of the team brings a unique and important perspective and should attend sensitivity training by a nationally accredited body. The entire health care team must be diligent in caring for the morbidly obese patient.

Criteria-Based Protocol

Health care facilities, regardless of where care is delivered, should have a plan in place for the special skin care needs of the morbidly obese patient. This could include resources such as equipment or clinical experts. A criteria-based protocol is simply preplanning based on specifically designated criteria. The patient's weight, BMI, body width, and clinical condition serve as such criteria (Gallagher, 2011). Actual weight is particularly useful because breakage, failure to function properly, or patient or caregiver injury can occur if the weight limit of equipment is exceeded. Body width is described as the patient's body at his or her widest point, which could be at the hips, the shoulders, across the belly when side-lying, or ankle-to-ankle. Furthermore, any clinical condition that interferes with mobility, such as pain, sedation, fear, or resistance to participating in care, places the patient at risk. Criteria-based protocols should be designed to meet the needs of the patient by ensuring access to resources, such as specialty equipment and clinical experts, in a timely, cost-effective manner (Blackett et al, 2011; Gallagher et al, 2012).

Communication and timing are critical to prevent the costly, predictable, and often preventable complications associated with caring for very complex patients. Although sometimes difficult to arrange, a face-to-face interdisciplinary conference, which is planned within 24 hours of admission or service, may prevent costly intervention later. Consider including the patient's significant other because this person may offer insight into the patient's special needs. Documentation of meetings, individual goals, and corresponding intervention may protect the institution from risk. This level of accountability also outlines more fully each clinician's responsibilities and, when the timing is right, smooths the transition from one health care setting to another.

Competency Skill Sets

Minimizing the challenges that basic care of the obese patient can present is simple. Typically straightforward tasks such as patient repositioning and urinal placement can require several staff members and various skills to accomplish these tasks safely and effectively. Education to ensure basic skills or competencies is imperative. In creating the bariatric care program, initially a survey to the staff can be used to determine their actual learning needs. Members of the bariatric task force can serve as a pool of experts to develop lesson plans and education addressing identified clinical needs. For example, when clinicians are seeking information on caregiver safety, a physical/occupational therapist, nurse expert, risk manager, and patient member of the task force could develop a 1-hour module to teach these skills.

Outcomes Measurement

In order to ensure the success of a comprehensive bariatric program, it is essential to monitor and collect relevant and appropriate outcomes. Patient and staff satisfaction, safety, and unexpected or adverse outcomes are among the issues that should be monitored.

CLINICAL CONSULT

A: Wound specialist referral for nonhealing abdominal pressure ulcer. Patient is 55-year-old female with obesity, 250 pounds, admitted to the EC for pancreatitis. Family practitioner notes state that the patient works full time as a teacher, is quite active, and has no pressure ulcers anywhere but her abdomen. The patient has been applying bacitracin and gauze every day after her shower. She has been doing her best to lose weight in hopes to reduce the pressure from her pannus. She has lost 30 pounds in the past 2 weeks by drastically cutting calories. The patient consented to a wound assessment despite her obvious discomfort. She is currently on an appropriately sized foam pressure redistribution mattress. Skin inspection under pannus revealed 10 × 4 cm of erythema and both dry and moist desquamation, satellite lesions noted, patient complains of intense itch/burn sensation.

D: Pannus intertrigo dermatitis (ITD) secondary to moisture and friction on opposing skin surfaces. Satellite lesions are indicative of secondary candidiasis. Possible malnutrition despite obesity.

P: Optimize nutrition, minimize moisture and friction at apposing skin folds, treat candidiasis, and teach the patient how to manage skin folds to prevent future recurrences.

I: (1) Consult nutrition services. (2) Discontinue bacitracin to help restore normal flora. (3) Initiate one time application of burrows solution for 20 minutes. (4) Twice daily, gently rinse with saline and dry completely, apply antifungal moisture barrier to clean dry skin followed by soft moisture wicking soft textile or cloth to keep opposing skin free from friction and moisture.

E: Nurse and patient understand and agree to plan of care. Nurses will manage skin folds until pancreatitis improves and patient is better able to participate with care. Plan to return in 3 days to evaluate effectiveness of interventions and discuss realistic management strategies for the home and work environment, which will most likely include daily pH balanced cleansing, moisture wicking soft textile or cloth, and dietician guided weight loss.

SUMMARY

Bariatric patients do not need more care or better care than any other patient. What this special population needs are resources to level the playing field, so all patients receive the same quality of care, regardless of size, weight, or body habitus. In order to fully understand the risk for skin injury and wound infection, it is imperative to have a collaborative partnership with the patient. Insensitivity threatens this. Both the caregiver and patient must feel at ease with communication. Patients must be willing to allow a comprehensive physical assessment in order to ensure early identification of skin and wound changes. To that same extent, patients should feel comfortable drawing attention to themselves if they believe there is a change in an existing wound or a change in the intact skin.

With obesity on the rise, wound care providers are increasingly responsible for managing the needs of this complex patient population. Although equipment is a helpful adjunct to care, it is never a substitute for care. Numerous resources are available. Compiling these resources in the form of a comprehensive bariatric care plan may ensure the most favorable outcome. The obese patient poses many care challenges, and it is in the interest of health care organizations to meet these skin and wound care challenges in a clinically, ethically, and legally sound manner.

REFERENCES

American Nurses Association: *ANA principles for nurse staffing*, ed 2, Silver Spring, MD, 2013, ANA.

American Society for Metabolic and Bariatric Surgery: *The disease of obesity*, https://asmbs.org/patients/disease-of-obesity. Accessed August 25, 2015.

Anaya DA, Dellinger EP: The obese surgical patient: a susceptible host for infection, *Surg Infect (Larchmt)* 7:473–480, 2006.

Apovian CM: The clinical and economic consequences of obesity, *Am J Manag Care* 19(Suppl 10):S219–S228, 2013.

Arnold M: Maximizing mobility, preserving skin integrity and preventing complications during the care of the obese patient. One hospital's solutions for patient and caregiver safety. A pictorial narrative of care tasks, *Ostomy Wound Manage* 60(1):24–29, 2014.

Bal BS, Finelli FC, Shope TR, et al: Nutritional deficiencies after bariatric surgery, *Nat Rev Endocrinol* 8(9):544–556, 2012.

Barrios L, Jones DB: Healthcare economics of weight loss surgery, *Bariatr Times* 4(8):1, 16–17, 20–21, 2007.

Beitz J: Providing quality skin and wound care for the bariatric patient: an overview of clinical challenges, *Ostomy Wound Manage* 60(1):12–21, 2014.

Beydoun MA, Wang Y: Gender-ethnic disparity in BMI and waist circumference distribution shifts in U.S. adults, *Obesity* 17(1):169–176, 2009.

Blackett A, Gallagher S, Dugan S, et al: Caring for persons with bariatric health care issues, *J Wound Ostomy Continence Nurs* 38(2):133–138, 2011.

Camden SG: Pressure ulcers, CMS and patients of size, *Bariatr Times* 5(12):1, 8–13, 2008.

Camden SG, Brannan S, Davis P: Best practices for sensitive care and the obese patient: task report, *Bariatr Nurs Surg Patient Care* 3(3):189–196, 2008.

Casale M, Pappacena M, Rinaldi V, et al: Obstructive sleep apnea syndrome: from phenotype to genetic basis, *Curr Genomics* 10(2):119–126, 2009.

Cawley J, Meyerhoefer C: The medical care costs of obesity: an instrumental variables approach, *J Health Econ* 31(1):219–230, 2012.

Colwell J: The role of obesity in the patient undergoing colorectal surgery and fecal diversion: a review of the literature, *Ostomy Wound Manage* 60(1):24–28, 2014.

Flegal KM, Carroll MD, Kit BK, et al: Prevalence of obesity and trends in the distribution of body mass index among U.S. adults, 1999–2010, *JAMA* 307(5):491–497, 2012.

Franz MG, Robson MC, Steed DL, et al: Guidelines to aid healing of acute wounds by decreasing impediments of healing, *Wound Repair Regen* 16(6):723–748, 2008.

Gallagher SM: Exploring the relationship between obesity, patient safety, and caregiver injury, *Am J SPHM* 1(2):8–12, 2011.

Gallagher SM: Special patient populations. In Charney W, editor: *Epidemic of medical errors and hospital-acquired infections*, Boca Raton, FL, 2012, CRC Press, pp 225–238.

Gallagher SM: *American Nurses Association implementation guide to safe patient handling and mobility*, Silver Springs, MD, 2013, Nursing World.

Gallagher SM: The intersection of ostomy and wound management, obesity, and associated science, *Ostomy Wound Manage* 60(1):6–7, 2014.

Glance LG, Wissler R, Mukamel DB, et al: Perioperative outcomes among patients with the modified metabolic syndrome who are undergoing noncardiac surgery, *Anesthesiology* 113(4):859–872, 2010.

Kramer K: WOC nurses as advocates for patients who are morbidly obese: a case study promoting use of bariatric beds, *J Wound Ostomy Continence Nurs* 31(6):379–384, 2004.

Lanz P, House JS, Lepkowski JM, et al: Socioeconomic factors, health behaviors, and mortality, *JAMA* 279(2):1703–1708, 1998.

Lasater-Erhard M: The effect of patient position of arterial oxygen saturation, *Crit Care Nurs* 15:31–36, 1995.

Ludwig DS, Pollack HA: Obesity and the economy, *JAMA* 301(5):533–535, 2009.

Martindale RG, Deveney CW: Preoperative risk reduction: strategies to optimize outcomes, *Surg Clin North Am* 93(5):1041–1055, 2013.

Moize V, Geliebter A, Gluck ME, et al: Obese patients have inadequate protein intake related to protein status up to 1 year following Roux-en-Y gastric bypass, *Obes Surg* 13:23–28, 2003.

National Institutes of Health: *What causes overweight and obesity?* 2012. http://www.nhlbi.nih.gov/health/health-topics/topics/obe/causes.html. Accessed June 1, 2014.

National Pressure Ulcer Advisory Panel (NPUAP), European Pressure Ulcer Advisory Panel (EPUAP), Pan Pacific Pressure Injury Alliance (PPPIA): In Haesler E, editor: *Prevention and treatment of pressure ulcers: clinical practice guideline*, Perth, Australia, 2014, Cambridge Media.

Ogden CL, Carroll MD, Kit BK, et al: Prevalence of obesity and trends in body mass index among U.S. children and adolescents, 1999–2010, *JAMA* 307(5):483–490, 2012.

Osborn DJ, Strain M, Gomelsky A, et al: Obesity and female stress urinary incontinence, *Urology* 82(4):759–763, 2013.

Pokorny ME: Lead in: skin physiology and disease in the obese patient, *Bariatr Nurs Surg Patient Care* 3(2):125–128, 2008.

Puhl RM, Heuer CA: The stigma of obesity: a review and update, *Obesity* 17(5):941–964, 2009.

Puhl RM, Luedicke J, Grilo CM: Obesity bias in training: attitudes, beliefs, and observations among advanced trainees in professional health disciplines, *Obesity* 22(4):1008–1015, 2014.

Pull C: Current psychological assessment practices in obesity surgery programs: what to assess and why, *Curr Opin Psychiatry* 23(1):30–36, 2010.

Rose M: Nurse staffing requirements for care of morbidly obese patients in the acute care setting, *Bariatr Nurs Surg Patient Care* 1:115–120, 2006.

Shinohara E, Kihara S, Yamashita S, et al: Visceral fat accumulation as an important risk factor for obstructive sleep apnea syndrome in obese subjects, *J Intern Med* 241:11–18, 1997.

Strohmayer E, Via MA, Yanagisawa R: Metabolic management following bariatric surgery, *Mt Sinai J Med* 77(5):431–445, 2010.

Steers WD, Suratt PM: Sleep apnea as a cause of daytime and nocturnal enuresis, *Lancet* 349(9069):1604, 1997.

Thone RR: *Fat: a fate worse than death*, New York, 1997, Harrington Park Press.

Valentino D, Sriram K, Shankar P: Update on micronutrients in bariatric surgery, *Curr Opin Clin Nutr Metab Care* 14(6):635–641, 2011.

West Virginia Department of Health and Human Resources: *Obesity and mortality*, 2014. http://www.wvdhhr.org/bph/oehp/obesity/mortality.htm. Accessed February 1, 2014.

World Health Organization: *Obesity and overweight*, http://www.who.int/mediacentre/factsheets/fs311/en/. Accessed August 25, 2015.

Wound, Ostomy and Continence Nurses Society™ (WOCN®): *Guideline for management of patients with lower extremity arterial disease (WOCN® clinical practice guidelines series no. 1)*, Mt. Laurel, NJ, 2008, WOCN®.

Wound, Ostomy and Continence Nurses Society™ (WOCN®): *Prevention and management of pressure ulcers (WOCN® clinical practice guidelines series no. 2)*, Glenview, IL, 2010, WOCN®.

Wound, Ostomy and Continence Nurses Society™ (WOCN®): *Guideline for management of patients with lower extremity venous ulcers (WOCN® clinical practice guidelines series no. 4)*, Glenview, IL, 2011, WOCN®.

Wound, Ostomy and Continence Nurses Society™ (WOCN®): *Guideline for management of patients with lower extremity neuropathic disease (WOCN® clinical practice guidelines series no. 3)*, Glenview, IL, 2012, WOCN®.

36

Skin Care Needs of the Neonatal and Pediatric Patient

Denise P. Nix, Michelle Best, and Ruth A. Bryant

OBJECTIVES

1. Define the terms *infancy, neonate, premature, preterm* and *late preterm*.
2. Identify skin, risk, and pain assessment tools designed for neonatal pediatric patients.
3. Discuss special considerations for premature and neonatal skin care, including bathing and use of cleansers, antiseptics, and emollients.

4. List risk factors for skin breakdown for pediatric patients.
5. Describe common pediatric skin conditions and age-related, developmentally sensitive interventions.
6. Identify wound care products that are safe for use in pediatric patients.

The physiology of wound repair, principles of wound care, and common skin conditions are the same for pediatric and adult patients. However, there are significant differences in morphologic and functional skin characteristics as well as developmental phases that influence assessment and intervention strategies. This chapter focuses on *unique* considerations for neonatal and pediatric skin care and should not be read in isolation of related chapters throughout the text that detail critical information applicable to both adults and children.

NEONATAL TERMINOLOGY AND SKIN CHARACTERISTICS

Many terms are used to describe stages of infant development (Table 36-1). *Infancy* refers to the first year of life. During the first 28 days of life, an infant may be referred to as a *neonate*. If born before 37 weeks of gestational age, the infant or neonate is *premature* or *preterm*. Developmental and structural differences in neonatal skin are significant compared with adult skin. Variations in neonatal skin and environmental influences that shape caregiving practices are described in Tables 3-1 and 3-2 and include underdevelopment of the stratum corneum, diminished cohesion between the epidermis and dermis, dermal instability, and skin surface pH (AWHONN, 2013).

Premature neonatal skin is thin and poorly keratinized and functions weakly as a barrier. Infants born at the limits of viability are more suited to the "aquatic environment" in utero than to atmospheric conditions. Transepidermal water loss (TEWL) is high; application and removal of adhesives to

the outer immature epidermal layer can leave behind damaged skin prone to infection and occasional scarring. At 24 weeks' gestation, TEWL can be 10 times greater compared with an infant born at term (Darmstadt and Dinulos, 2000; Ness et al, 2013). Interestingly, exposure of the premature infant's skin to air seems to accelerate skin maturation. Infants born at 23 to 25 weeks' gestation may require as long as 8 weeks to develop a functional skin barrier. Late preterm infants develop more mature barrier function 2 to 3 weeks after birth. Barrier function and skin maturation continue to evolve throughout the first year of life (Kalia et al, 1998).

Due to their greater ratio of surface area to volume and immature barrier function compared with the full-term infant, percutaneous absorption of topically applied agents (soaps, lotions, antiseptics, alcohol, etc.) place the premature infant at greater risk for skin complications and systemic toxicities (Mancini, 2004). Risk may also be increased due to the premature infant's own alterations in metabolism, excretion, distribution, and protein binding of chemical agents and drugs (AWHONN, 2013; Darmstadt and Dinulos, 2000).

Bathing and Moisturizing

Bathing newborns with water alone is equally as effective as mild cleansers in decreasing bacteria on the skin. Less frequent bathing and strict attention to heat loss and avoidance of cold stress minimizes behavioral and physiologic instability in infants. Infants immersed in water at the correct temperature (between 100° and 104°F) are calmer, quieter, and experience less heat loss than infants receiving a sponge bath. The infant bath should be in a draft-free, warm room

TABLE 36-1	Definition of Terms
Infancy	First year of life
Neonate	Newborn infant less than 28 days of life (from birth to 4 weeks of age)
Premature or preterm infant	Infant born before 37 weeks' gestation
Late preterm infant	Infant born between 34 and 37 weeks' gestation

TABLE 36-2	Examples of Transcutaneous Absorption of Topical Products in Neonates, Infants, and Children (Examples not Inclusive)	
Compound	**Toxicity**
Aniline (dye used in laundry)	Methemoglobinemia
Pentachlorophenol (laundry disinfectant)	Tachycardia, sweating, hepatomegaly, metabolic acidosis
Hexachlorophene (topical antiseptic)	Vacuolar encephalopathy
Boric acid (baby powder)	Vomiting, diarrhea, erythroderma, seizures
Salicylic acid	Metabolic acidosis
Isopropyl alcohol under occlusion	Hemorrhagic skin necrosis
Urea (exfoliating, emollient ingredient)	Uremia
Povidone-iodine (topical antiseptic)	Hypothyroidism, goiter
Benzocaine and prilocaine (topical anesthetics)	Methemoglobinemia
Methylene blue (dye)	Methemoglobinemia

Data from Fernandes JD, Machado MCR, de Oliveira ZNP: Children and newborn skin care and prevention, *An Bras Dermatol* 86(1): 102–110, 2011.

(between 79° and 81°F). Warm towels should be used for drying. Procedures for bathing and drying should be as brief as possible to facilitate thermoregulation (Loring et al, 2012). When skin cleansers are indicated (e.g., heavy soiling), a mild liquid baby cleanser used sparingly with a neutral pH (5.5 to 7.0) is recommended (AWHONN, 2013; Blume-Peytavi et al, 2009). Neonatal bathing equipment must be properly used and cleaned according to institutional guidelines (AWHONN, 2013).

Due to immature barrier function and thermoregulation, the preterm infant less than 32 weeks' gestation is generally not bathed daily or immersed for bathing during the first week of life. Instead, it is recommended to wrap the baby in a warm towel with one body part exposed at a time, and soft cotton cloths or cotton balls are squeezed to run warm water over the skin so friction (rubbing) does not occur. If skin breakdown is present, warm sterile water is recommended (AWHONN, 2013).

Bathing introduces changes to the stratum corneum that can dry the skin. Moisturizing creams or ointments may be indicated for dry, flaking, or fissured skin. Petrolatum-based products without preservatives, perfumes, or dyes have been recommended (Lund and Osborne, 2004). However, an association between infection and a petrolatum-based emollient has been reported with preemies less than 750 g who may also be referred to as micropreemies (Visscher, 2009b). Therefore the benefits of emollient use to prevent skin breakdown and/or treat dryness in the micropreemie should be weighed against the risk of infection, and every effort should be made to prevent contamination of the emollient container and surrounding treatment surfaces (AWHONN, 2013; Visscher, 2009b).

Topical Antiseptics and Antimicrobial Agents

Topical application of antiseptics and antimicrobial agents has been known to create irritant contact dermatitis, sensitization, and systemic toxicity in the infant population. Examples of topical products (including some antimicrobials) at risk for transcutaneous absorption and toxicity in neonates, infants, and children are included in Table 36-2. Hemorrhagic necrosis of the dermis from the absorption of isopropyl alcohol under occlusion has been reported; the resulting necrosis is sometimes mistaken for bruising or pressure. Povidone-iodine has been associated with skin injury and carries the risk of systemic toxicity

involving thyroid function (Fernandes et al, 2011). Another irritant source for the infant patient population is the use of disinfectants such as chlorhexidine gluconate (CHG). A disinfectant application is recommended before invasive procedures in neonatal and premature populations. Due to the risk of chemical contact dermatitis, the Food and Drug Administration (FDA) recommends using CHG skin antiseptics with caution in premature infants or infants less than 2 months of age. To limit exposure to disinfectants, water or saline can be used to remove the disinfectant after the procedure (AWHONN, 2013). As always, manufacturer's recommendations for safe product use should be reviewed.

Organic, Natural, and Herbal Products

"Natural" products are often considered harmless; however, because of the poor regulations that exist in monitoring them, adverse reactions do occur. There is little incentive for pharmaceutical companies to investigate or standardize these preparations because it is unlikely patents would be applicable. Herbs that are known for causing this condition include aloe, arnica, bromelain, calendula, chamomile, goldenseal, tea tree oil, and yarrow. The most common dermatologic reaction from herbal therapies is allergic contact dermatitis. However, more serious events such as Stevens-Johnson syndrome have occurred when combination preparations were used. Therefore experts recommend avoiding their use with infants and children because of the uncertainty of adverse reactions that could occur (AWHONN, 2013; Vender, 2003). Natural fragrances such as essential oils may also be allergens and irritants and are not necessarily safer than synthetic fragrances. Interestingly, a product can be labeled "fragrance free" if the scented ingredient is added for a purpose other than fragrance. Likewise, products labeled "unscented" may contain a fragrance if it is added to mask the odor of a product (AWHONN, 2013).

SKIN INSPECTION AND RISK ASSESSMENT

Preventing skin complications always starts with understanding the potential etiologies and conditions that place an individual at risk. Evidence-based guidelines recommend conducting a head-to-toe skin inspection at least daily (AWHONN, 2013; NPUAP, EPUAP, PPPIA, 2014; WOCN®, 2010). An assessment of risk for skin breakdown should occur in conjunction with the skin inspection. The use of assessment tools tested for validity and reliability designed for the pediatric and neonate population should be considered to provide objective measurements. Examples are provided in Table 36-3 and Box 36-1.

PEDIATRIC CONDITIONS THAT AFFECT THE SKIN

As previously stated, related chapters throughout the text discuss types of skin damage and important considerations applicable to both adults and children. The following sections provide additional considerations specific for neonates and children affected by pressure ulcers, diaper dermatitis, gastrostomies, fecal and urinary diversions, medical adhesive–related skin damage, burns, and extravasation.

Pressure Ulcers

All components for creating and maintaining a quality pressure ulcer prevention program (PUPP), including medical device–related pressure ulcer prevention, are described in Chapter 8 and should be thoroughly reviewed for pressure ulcer prevention in any patient population. Information specific to pediatric pressure ulcer prevalence, incidence, risk assessment, support surface selection, and repositioning for the small yet rapidly growing neonate and pediatric patient are included in this section.

As with adults, significant variability of methodologies exists for pressure ulcer prevalence and incidence data collection among the pediatric population. However, it is clear that pressure ulcers present a clinically significant problem. International pressure ulcer guidelines (NPUAP, EPUAP, PPPIA, 2014) report aggregated international pressure ulcer data from multiple pediatric care settings between 2000 and 2012 range from 0.47% to 72.5% prevalence to 0.25% to 27% incidence.

Although the etiology and classification for pressure ulcers is the same for adults and children (see Chapter 7), it is the distribution and causative factors that are unique for this specific population. Pressure ulcers on infants and toddlers occur primarily on the head/occipital region (31%), and more than 50% are related to equipment (see Plate 30b-d) and devices, particularly respiratory equipment (Baharestani and Ratliff, 2007; Murray et al, 2013; Willock et al, 2005). The preponderance of pressure ulcers on the occipital region is due to the proportionately larger size/weight of the head compared with the rest of the body (NPUAP, EPUAP, PPPIA, 2014).

Pediatric populations with the highest risk for pressure ulcer development include the critically, chronically, or terminally ill patient, as well as those with spinal cord injuries and medical devices (Curley et al, 2003a; Dixon and Ratliff, 2005; Hickey et al, 2000; Kottner 2010; McLane et al, 2004; Noonan et al, 2006; Schindler et al, 2011; Schluer et al, 2012). Factors found to be significantly associated with pressure ulcer development ($p < .05$) are low birth weight, skin texture immaturity, incubator temperature and humidity, support surface, and limited position changes (Fuji et al, 2010). All children with medical devices (most frequently respiratory equipment) are at risk for pressure ulcer development (Fuji et al, 2010; NPUAP, EPUAP, PPPIA, 2014; Schindler et al, 2011; Schluer et al, 2012). As emphasized in Chapter 8, interdisciplinary involvement is a key component of prevention and management of device-related pressure ulcers.

Skin inspection must include adequate lighting and palpation, especially in the presence of darkly pigmented skin or hair on the occipital region. Skin folds need to be gently separated, and medical devices may require careful repositioning for an adequate assessment. Age-appropriate pressure ulcer risk and skin assessments should be performed and documented at least on admission; daily; and with procedures that may alter pressure, friction, shear, and/or moisture. Inspection around and under medical devices should occur at least twice daily according to international pressure ulcer guidelines (NPUAP, EPUAP, PPPIA, 2014) and every 1 to 4 hours according to the Association of Women's Health, Obstetric and Neonatal Nurses (AWHONN, 2013). Both guidelines recommend considering the use of a reliable and valid pediatric risk assessment tool to facilitate a structured assessment.

Table 36-1 and Box 36-1 summarize several neonatal and pediatric pressure ulcer risk assessment scales that have undergone reliability and validity studies for their use in neonatal and pediatric populations. The Braden Q and the Glamorgan scales predict immobility-related pressure ulcers. The Glamorgan scale, however, also includes medical device–related pressure ulcers. The Starkid Skin Scale is based on the Braden Q. Neonatal skin assessment scales include the Neonatal Skin Risk Assessment Scale (Dolack et al, 2013) and the Neonatal Skin Condition scale (Lund and Osborne, 2004). The Braden Q & P is an example of a setting-specific risk scale tailored to the perioperative area. With the Braden Q & P, the activity category is eliminated

TABLE 36-3 Pediatric and Neonatal Skin Condition Scales/Tools

Tool Name	Measurement	Intended Age	Brief Description	Validity	Reliability	Reference
Braden Q	Pediatric PU Risk	21 days to 8 years	Adapted from Braden pressure scale, all 6 Braden subscales plus 7th Tissue Perfusion and Oxygenation. Score <16 at risk for skin breakdown. Subscale scores 1 (least favorable) to 4 (most favorable). More applicable to acute pediatric population than neonates Other: no cost, no modifications allowed, translations available Research populations: pediatric: neonates, home, ICU	+	+	Curley et al, 2003b Kelechi et al, 2013 Noonan et al, 2011 Available at http://www.marthaaqcurley.com/braden-q.html (accessed March 9, 2015)
Braden Q + P	Pediatric Perioperative PU Risk and Intervention					Galvin and Curley, 2012 Available at http://www.marthaaqcurley.com/braden-q.html (accessed March 9, 2015)
Glamorgan	Pediatric PU Risk	Birth to 18 years	Developed using expert opinion of relevant factors from a literature review and statistical analysis of collected inpatient data. The higher the score, the greater the risk: 0 not at risk 10+ at risk, 15+ high risk, 20+ very high risk Scale publically available, permission to reprint requested	+ sensitivity 98% specificity 67%	+	Willock et al, 2008 Anthony et al, 2010 Available at http://img.docstoccdn.com/thumb/orig/4467445.png (accessed March 9, 2015)
AWHONN/NANN Neonatal Skin Condition Score Association of Women's Health, Obstetric and Neonatal Nurses and National Association of Neonatal Nurses (NANN)	Skin condition	Birth to 28 days	Observation of dryness, erythema and breakdown on a 1–9 scale; higher the skin score = greater potential for systemic infection, breakdown, and longer hospitalization Sample size 2,820 infants from 51 NICU and well-baby nurseries in 27 states in the United States More applicable to infants >1000 g Pressure ulcer risk not measured directly, breakdown not specific to pressure ulcer			Lund and Osborne, 2004 Box 36-1
NSRAS	NICU PU Risk	26 to 40 weeks' gestation	Specific for neonatal population at risk for skin breakdown, based on the Braden Scale for Predicting Pressure Sore Risk and includes gestational age category. Developed in 1997; subscale descriptor revision at later date. 6 subscales lower scores = higher risk, higher scores = lower risk. Piloted on 32 neonates.	+ sensitivity 83% specificity at 81%	+ reliable for general physical condition, activity and nutrition	Dolack et al, 2013
Starkid Skin Scale	Skin Condition	Hospitalized children	Adapted from the Braden Q: 6 subscales rated on scale 1 to 4 with lower scores representing higher risk: mobility/activity, sensory perception, moisture, friction/shear, nutrition and tissue perfusion/oxygenation. Request permission to reprint	Sensitivity low at 17.5%, high specificity of 98.5%	Internal reliability 0.71, inter-rater reliability is 0.85	Suddaby et al, 2005

and the mobility and sensory categories of the Braden Q are replaced with length of surgical time and decreased, respectively, because that is the common operative/procedural patient experience. The Braden Q & P was trialed on patients undergoing cardiac surgery and results reported for 2010 and 2011 for a total of 356 procedures (Galvin and Curley, 2012).

It is critical to consider size and weight when selecting products that are safe to use in the chairs; beds; cribs; and under head, elbows, and heels of pediatric patients. For example, a child below the manufacturer's minimum weight requirement may sink in between cushions of a low-air-loss surface, lodge between alternating air cells, or slide through the oversized side rails, creating the potential for entrapment and other safety concerns (McLane et al, 2002; NPUAP, EPUAP, PPPIA, 2014).

When selecting a pressure redistribution support surface for children, consideration should be given to the bony prominence most at risk. Due to the greater size and weight of the head, a high-specification pressure redistribution support surface should be utilized to prevent occipital pressure ulcers with premature infants and younger children (NPUAP, EPUAP, PPPIA, 2014). A variety of media have been trialed and used for pressure redistribution with pediatric patients, including fluid, gel, and foam (García-Molina et al, 2012; McInnes et al, 2013; McLane et al, 2002; Turnage-Carrier et al, 2008). Chapter 9 provides a detailed overview of pressure redistribution surfaces and how to identify a higher-specification support surface.

Parents and caregivers should be taught that pressure redistribution is one of the many benefits to holding infants (Fuji et al, 2010; Razmus et al, 2008; Schinder et al, 2011; Turnage-Carrier et al, 2008). While in bed, experts recommend floating the heels off the bed surface and diligent repositioning of the head, even for neonates and small children on higher-specification support surfaces, due to the very small surface areas of pediatric heels and very large surface area of pediatric heads (NPUAP, EPUAP, PPPIA,

2014). Progressive mobility techniques, including slow incremental turning as discussed in Chapter 8, should be used whenever possible for pressure ulcer prevention in children and adults (Janowski, 2010).

Diaper Dermatitis/Incontinence-Associated Dermatitis

As described in Chapter 5, diaper dermatitis, also known as *perineal dermatitis, diaper rash,* and many other names, is included within a broader group of skin conditions that are referred to as *moisture-associated skin damage* (MASD), which includes incontinence-associated dermatitis (IAD). Recently the term *IAD* has replaced diaper, perineal, and nappy dermatitis in a number of clinical settings and populations to acknowledge dermatitis from contact with urine and/or feces that may affect more than the perineal and diaper area and apply to people of any age. The World Health Organization's (WHO) *International Classification of Diseases* (ICD-10, in use since 1994) contains coding for diaper dermatitis, but does not contain a separate classification or code for IAD (WHO, 2014). Experts recommend coding that differentiates between the terms *IAD* and *diaper dermatitis* (age being an important distinction) to facilitate consistent terminology to improve and clarify education and research. (For the purposes of this chapter, the AWHONN [2013] and WHO [2014] term *diaper dermatitis* will be used to describe this condition in the neonate and young child where continence is not developmentally anticipated or expected.)

Diaper dermatitis among hospitalized pediatric patients has been reported to be 16% to 42% (McLane et al, 2004; Noonan et al, 2006). Diaper dermatitis in children (see Plate 15) generally affects the skin in greatest contact with the diaper, including the buttocks, perianal, medial thighs, mons pubis, labia majora, and scrotum (Shin, 2005). As discussed in Chapter 5, candidiasis frequently coexists with diaper dermatitis. Table 5-3 provides guidance for differentiating between IAD/diaper dermatitis, candidiasis, and other skin conditions that can develop near the perineal region.

Common risk factors for diaper dermatitis include frequent stooling, antibiotic use, malabsorption, opiate withdrawal, and abnormal rectal sphincter tone. Pediatric populations especially at risk include those born with congenital anomalies that result in impaired sphincter tone such as spina bifida, corrective colorectal surgery such as Hirschsprung disease, or genitourinary and/or pelvic surgeries such as imperforate anus. Also at risk are children with diseases that affect the digestive tract such as malabsorption syndromes, inflammatory bowel disease, or short bowel disease associated with prematurity. Children exposed to conditions and medications that cause diarrhea such as with antibiotics, chemotherapy, opiate withdrawal, or neonatal abstinence syndrome are also at great risk for diaper dermatitis as a result of diarrhea (Visscher 2009a).

Prevention and management of diaper dermatitis/IAD require appropriate cleaning, protection, and containment as described in Chapter 5. Table 5-4 provides examples and descriptions of products commonly available for cleansing and protecting perineal skin to prevent and manage diaper dermatitis. Although commonly used for adults and children, many of these products are not appropriate for young and premature neonates.

Cleansing must be gentle and limited to the removal of the soiled layer of the skin protectant only. Vigorously rubbing off the skin protectant moisture barrier product is not necessary and should be avoided. Appropriate methods to cleanse the diaper area should consider products that have been tested on neonates such as soft cloths, water, disposable diaper wipes, and gentle cleansers designed for use in the pediatric/neonate population in the perineal area (AWHONN, 2013). Odio et al (2001) compared 100% cotton premium brand children's washcloths to disposable baby wipes and found the wipe superior to washcloths on both healthy and damaged skin. In the perianal area, where wiping is generally more vigorous, the wipes showed a statistically significant advantage over the washcloths in terms of skin gentleness. Repetitive wiping with cotton washcloths produced detectable disruption of the skin barrier, whereas similar cleansing with wipes did not. The addition of soap to the washcloth resulted in the highest degree of skin barrier disruption (Visscher, 2009a). As discussed previously, temperature control during cleansing and bathing is critical with the neonate, and perineal cleansing is no exception.

A moisture barrier skin protectant should be applied at every diaper change of infants and children with actual or potential diaper dermatitis. In neonates, preference should be given to formulations with fewer additives and chemicals that are potentially absorbed through the skin, such as those containing topical vitamin A (AWHONN, 2013; Davies et al, 2006).

Skin protectants are formulated as creams, pastes, lotions, or films and packaged into wipes, wands, packets, sprays, and tubes. To function as a skin protectant, it must contain a known barrier as an active ingredient (e.g., petrolatum, zinc oxide, dimethicone) alone or in combination (Beekman et al, 2015). The active ingredients in FDA-approved topical moisture barrier skin protectants must be present in certain concentrations to be designated as an over-the-counter moisture barrier skin protectant, including those marketed for pediatric use. Active ingredients frequently found in products labeled for pediatric use and their FDA-specified concentrations include zinc oxide (1% to 25% minimum concentration), petrolatum and white petrolatum (30% to 100%), and dimethicone (minimum 1% to 30%). Other ingredients must be listed in order of their amount unless they are 1% or less. In that case, they can be listed in any order (FDA, 2003).

Moisture barrier skin protectant pastes are a mixture of absorbent material (e.g., carboxymethylcellulose) and ointments to increase the consistency so they adhere to moist denuded skin. As stated previously, it is appropriate to remove only the soiled layer of the barrier during cleansing. Moisture barrier skin protectant films are liquids that contain a polymer (e.g., acrylate based) dissolved in a solvent. Upon application, films form a transparent protective coating on the skin. They are not labeled as having an active ingredient (Beekman et al, 2015). The FDA has approved alcohol-free barrier films as treatment of diaper dermatitis in neonates older than 28 days old. They can be applied every 24 hours (AWHONN, 2013).

Treatment of diaper dermatitis complicated by a yeast or bacterial infection is discussed in Chapter 5. Antifungal powders kept away from the child's airway are safely used in the treatment of candidiasis. Several powder-free options are also available. Baby powder and cornstarch should not be used, as they can actually increase yeast or bacterial growth and cause respiratory irritation. Application of topical antibiotics and corticosteroid in the diaper area should be avoided, except in unique circumstances, used short term, and directed by a health care provider. Overuse of topical corticosteroids has been linked to Cushing syndrome, systemic toxicity, and dermal atrophy in infants (AWHONN, 2013; Darmstadt and Dinulos, 2000; Nield and Kamat, 2007). If diaper dermatitis does not improve with appropriate evidence-based care, allergic contact dermatitis should be considered due to enhanced sensitizations to allergens in the moist environment and increasing reports of diaper dye dermatitis. For diaper dye dermatitis, the preferred treatment is the use of dye-free diapers. Occasionally topical corticosteroids are used (AWHONN, 2013; Jackson, 2010; Smith and Jacob, 2009).

Association of Women's Health, Obstetric and Neonatal Nurses clinical practice guidelines (2013) recommend diaper changes every 1 to 3 hours during the day and at least once at night. Obviously more changes may be required to limit exposure of urine and feces to the skin. Tight-fitting diapers hold irritants against the skin and should be avoided. Advances in the design and manufacturing process of both reusable and disposable diapers provide consumers with more choice of effective products to contain urine and stool while eliminating some of the negative effects associated with diapering such as diaper dermatitis and environmental impact. The quality of diapers varies and should be considered in product selection. A synthetic material next to the skin should promote passage of liquid through to the next layer to keep the skin dry. Plastic-back products to prevent leaking can cause overhydration, leading to diaper dermatitis. Therefore disposable diapers with a microporous membrane permeable to air and vapor keep the skin drier and are preferred (Akin et al, 2001; Shin, 2005). As previously mentioned, ointments and pastes should be applied as directed by the manufacturer, never to the diaper itself, and not so thick that it might block or limit fluid uptake of diapers causing overhydration of the stratum corneum, leakage, and increased risk of diaper dermatitis (Zehrer, 2005).

As directed by the health care provider, oral or topical cholestyramine may be considered to prevent loose stools in infants that excrete high amounts of bile acids in their stool. Cholestyramine when given enterally is thought to provide a barrier function by binding with bile salts excreted in the stool, for example, in children with short gut syndrome (White et al, 1996). Finally, experts encourage and support breastfeeding when possible through infancy because stool and urine of breastfed infants have a lower pH than that in formula-fed infants. The stool of breastfed infants also contains lower levels of enzymes, resulting in less perineal irritation (AWHONN, 2013; Lin et al, 2005).

Medical Adhesive–Related Skin Injury

Medical adhesive–related skin injury (MARSI) is found in all ages and patient care settings. Because neonates have diminished cohesion between the epidermal and dermal layers, MARSI is reported as the primary cause of skin breakdown in neonatal intensive care units (AWHONN, 2013). Silicone tape and a paper tape have been demonstrated to cause minimal skin damage when used with healthy children ages 9 to 47 months (Grove et al, 2014). Unfortunately, they are not appropriate in all situations, for example, securing tubes and catheters considered critical such as endotracheal tubes, chest, or extracorporeal membrane oxygenation (ECMO) catheters (McNichol et al, 2013). Chapter 5 provides a comprehensive review of prevention and management of MARSI. Box 5-5 lists strategies for the prevention of MARSI.

Although a nonalcohol-based protective barrier film may be applied to the skin before tape application to protect the epidermis from stripping with tape removal, the use of these products with the infant younger than 28 days has not been studied (McNichol et al, 2013). Due to reports of toxicity and skin reaction solvents, bonding agents and adhesive removers should not be used with neonates. Instead, mineral oil, petrolatum, or water can be used to loosen adhesives as needed (AWHONN, 2013).

Gastrostomies

Gastrostomy tubes are placed in children for a variety of feeding disorders that may include central nervous system disorders, gastrointestinal (GI) conditions, cerebral palsy, failure to thrive, cardiac conditions, and esophageal anomalies (Borkowski, 2005). Enteral nutrition is indicated when the pediatric patient has insufficient normal oral intake and at least a partially functional gut (Braegger et al, 2010). The majority of children treated at pediatric facilities will have a low-profile feeding tube with a balloon. Gastrostomy tubes are removed when children can take all their nutrition by mouth. In some cases, surgical closure is required; however, most gastrostomies will close without intervention.

Gastric secretions are caustic to the skin and require very little time to erode the epidermis, leading to dermatitis, candidiasis, hypergranulation, or ulceration (see Plate 72).

Chapter 37 is dedicated to patients with percutaneous tubes and describes strategies for prevention and management of peritube skin conditions. Emphasis is placed on interventions to prevent leakage such as appropriate tube selection (type and size), accurate placement and replacement when indicated, effective size appropriate stabilization, and age-appropriate moisture barrier skin protectants (as described earlier) to keep moisture and enzymes from penetrating the epidermis.

Pediatric gastrostomy tube considerations include filling balloons with the correct volume. Underinflation increases the risk for dislodgement and backflow, and overinflation may block the gastric outlet, resulting in poor emptying of the stomach and vomiting. For very tiny infants, a 5-mL balloon of a 14Fr low-profile tube may be too large. Decreasing the volume in the balloon is recommended, as the balloon may become soft, fail to form into the correct shape, and easily migrate or become dislodged. Low-profile tubes that require 2 mL minimum of fluid to inflate the balloon are available for tiny infants.

Children may also develop leakage due to the inability to tolerate the volume or the rate of the feeding. Infants and children are generally fed by nasogastric tubes before gastrostomy placement. After surgery, children may return to their presurgical feeding rates within a few days. Others, however, may take 2 to 3 weeks before they tolerate the same rate without leaking. Generally these are children who have always had difficulty tolerating feedings, such as those with complex cardiac anomalies, gastroesophageal reflux, or short bowel syndrome. It is critically important to lengthen the time over which the feedings are given in order to allow the tract to heal and prevent peristomal skin breakdown. A child receiving feedings over 45 minutes may need to have feedings given over 1.5 hours. Some children need a period of continuous feedings. The onset of an acute illness such a respiratory infection and cough or intestinal infection and diarrhea may require adjustments in standard tube-feeding regimens until the illness resolves. Constipation is another, sometimes overlooked, cause of peritube leakage (Axelrod et al, 2006; Braegger et al, 2010; Mills et al, 2013).

Tube stabilization can be challenging, depending on gastrostomy type (skin level vs. long tube), new versus established placement, feeding schedule/administration, the patient's age, size of the abdomen, and development. Tube stabilizing devices manufactured for adult patients are often too large and may be unsafe. Whenever possible, adult stabilization devices should not be modified for children. Even if they are modified to fit a smaller abdomen, the adhesive backing is too strong for the underdeveloped skin of infants and young children. Stabilization using an H tape or "goal post"–like taping pattern can hold the newly placed long tube in a straight vertical position. Braegger et al (2010) provides a detailed clinical practice guideline to enteral nutrition in the pediatric patient based on available evidence and expert opinion.

Urinary and Fecal Diversions

The most common conditions that typically require the creation of an ostomy include congenital malformations and medical conditions such as Hirschsprung disease, imperforate anus and urogenital malformations, familial adenomatous polyposis (FAP), and necrotizing enterocolitis (NEC).

Pouching is recommended for containment of stool and urine in all pediatric populations. Referral to a certified ostomy nurse (www.wocn.org) for preop marking, teaching, and ongoing assessment and assessment management recommendations will facilitate patient and family satisfaction, cost-effective utilization of pouching supplies, and follow-up for ongoing needs and changes as the patient grows.

The benefits of stoma site marking before surgery for adults to identify body contours that might prevent pouch adhesion are recognized. Stoma preoperative site marking, although recommended in pediatric practice, is typically limited by the nature of the surgery itself. Stoma placement, particularly in newborns, is usually emergent and the patient is critically ill. Planned stoma surgeries should be marked. Depending on the type of stoma placed and the surgeon's preference, wound, ostomy, and continence (WOC) nurses should be requested to mark for other stoma sites such as gastrostomy or antegrade continence enema (ACE) sites or continent fecal or urinary diversions. In rare cases, diapering may be the only option to contain the urine and/or stool output.

Factors that influence pouch effectiveness, wear time, and peristomal skin breakdown in infants and children include:

1. Nature of the surgical procedure: Depending on the age of the child, stoma placement in children is rarely a planned event done when the child's clinical status and nutrition have been optimized. In fact, the majority of infants who receive stomas undergo surgery emergently when they are critically ill.
2. Stoma placement: An ostomy may be created through an incision due to limited abdominal space or a desire to minimize scarring. Infants with NEC can have multiple stomas brought through the incision.
3. Characteristics of the infant's abdomen: Limited surface area for a stoma placement, lack of muscular development, proximity to additional monitoring devices, and changes in abdominal contours when crying.

Pouching. In order to protect peristomal skin, promote a reliable wear time, and prevent leakage, the following must occur:

- Selection of an appropriate ostomy pouching system with features that will accommodate the specific needs of the patient's body
- Competent and consistent technique for preparation (both the pouch and skin), application, and removal of the pouching system
- Timely pouch emptying when one third to one half full of flatus, liquid, or stool

When cleansing peristomal skin, only water should be used. A cleansing product such as a wipe containing an emollient will impair the adhesion of the pouch. The same considerations for cleansing and protecting neonatal perineal skin also apply to neonatal peristomal skin.

For an optimal seal, a syringe filled with alcohol-free skin barrier paste may be used for a more precise application to clean, dry peristomal skin around the mucocutaneous junction and into uneven skin surfaces such as a healed incision. Many skin barrier pastes contain alcohol and may irritate young skin. In the absence of alcohol-free skin barrier paste, strip pastes and barrier rings can be used. They are alcohol free, easier to remove from the skin, can be cut or molded to the shape needed, and can be used to create convexity if needed. Pouches must be changed *before* leakage occurs, preferably on a schedule (i.e., ranging from every 24 to 72 hours for infants and twice a week for older pediatric patients). Examining the integrity of the pouch barrier upon removal can help determine whether a pouch wear time (change schedule) needs to be adjusted. As with any procedure involving medical adhesives, precisions should be taken to prevent MARSI.

Box 36-2 contains pouching tips for infant/pediatric ostomies. Box 36-3 contains a list of organizations that provide free educational tools, many of them online (for health care

---

BOX 36-2 Pouching Tips for Infant/Pediatric Stomas

- Avoid use of pastes that contain alcohol, which can irritate skin. A syringe can be filled with skin barrier paste to ease the application of a thin bead of paste to the wafer or skin.
- Barrier strips and rings have gentle adhesives and can be cut or molded to specific shape.
- Apply pouch to clean, dry skin absent of wrinkles and creases.
- Change pouch on routine basis (do not wait for it to leak).
- Teach caregivers to assess skin barrier for signs of erosion upon removal.
- Inform parents that another pouch size may be necessary as child grows.
- Cotton balls can be put in pouch to wick effluent off wafer, extending wear time.
- Position pouch so that tail of pouch empties toward infant's side to facilitate emptying into diaper.
- Urinary pouch with antireflux will increase wear time when used to contain liquid output from ileostomy.
- Do not rinse pouch.

BOX 36-3 Ostomy Online Resources

- Wound, Ostomy and Continence Nurses Society™ http://www.wocn.org/
- American College of Surgeons Surgical Patient Education Program https://www.facs.org/education/patient-education
- United Ostomy Association of America (UOAA) www.uoaa.org
- American Society of Colon and Rectal Surgeons (ASCRS) www.ascrs.org

providers and patients and families), that contain pouch-changing procedures and nonbiased education related to the numerous accessories and options in equipment that may be needed at any point in time while living with an ostomy. Again, the importance of involving a board-certified ostomy nurse to prevent and manage these complications throughout the lifespan cannot be understated.

Unsuccessful pouching can lead to many of the complications seen with leaking gastrostomies such as painful dermatitis and hyperplasia (see Plate 72). If pouching is unsatisfactory, absorptive products and moisture barrier skin protectants (see Table 5-4) are used with the same considerations and precautions for neonates as previously discussed in the diaper dermatitis section of this chapter.

Burn/Thermal Injury

The most common types of burns in the infant and toddler are scalds or contact burns. Toddlers are at high risk for sustaining burns to their chest, arms, face, hands, and abdomen as they begin to walk and explore their environment, grabbing onto tables, tablecloths, and radiators to pull themselves up to standing. Hot liquids pulled down from tables result in burns to the head, face, and chest. Burns to the hands are common, especially in cold climates and homes with radiator heat. Hot water tanks set above 120 degrees put children at risk during bathing. As discussed in Chapter 32, approximately 10% of child abuse cases involve burning, and up to 20% of pediatric burn admissions involve abuse or neglect. Criteria for those burn injuries that are suspicious for abuse or neglect are listed in Box 32-3.

Chapter 32 provides a detailed discussion related to burn care. Keeping dressings in place when children are burned is particularly challenging because of their location and because children are so active. Unaffected thumbs should be kept out of the dressing whenever possible. Flexible tube net dressing or socks over the hand can also be used to keep the dressings in place.

Intravenous Extravasation Injury

Extravasation injury (formally called *infiltration injury*) is the inadvertent leaking or infusing of vesicant or nonvesicant solution into the surrounding tissue instead of into the vascular pathway (AWHONN, 2013). Neonates, especially premature infants, are at very high risk for serious skin damage from extravasation due to immature skin structures, lack of subcutaneous tissue, and the small size of their blood vessels.

Careful and frequent assessment of site (at least every hour according to AWHONN, 2013) is vital for prevention. Infusion pumps alone are not reliable for detecting an infiltrate; in fact, severe consequences have been reported to progress unnoticed for up to 72 hours. Injuries range from cosmetic to functional and from ischemia to compartment syndrome requiring surgery, prolonged hospitalization, and significant morbidity (Amjad et al, 2011).

CHECKLIST 36-1 Extravasation Prevention Strategies

✓ Use small enough plastic/silicone catheter to avoid restriction of blood flow.
✓ Avoid repeated use of a vein.
✓ Avoid placing an IV in an area difficult to immobilize.
✓ Use transparent tape to secure.
✓ Cover the site with a sterile semipermeable transparent dressing that will permit ongoing visualization of the insertion site.
✓ Upper extremities less likely to infiltrate or leak compared with peripheral IV in lower extremities or scalp veins.
✓ Place tape loosely over bony prominences to avoid restricting blood flow to the extremity. Do not circle around the arm.
✓ Limit IV glucose to 12.5%.
✓ Dilute medications as much as possible before administration of other solutions to prevent extravasation.

Checklist 36-1 contains a list of extravasation prevention strategies. Risk is minimized with the use of vascular access devices made of plastic instead of steel in places that are easier to immobilize. If an arm board is used, it should be secured without completely circling tape around the extremity. Correct fluid concentrations and diluents before IV medicines should be administered. Securing the IV site with a transparent adhesive dressing is preferred so that the site can be frequently monitored (Beall et al, 2013).

In children, negative blood return in the tubing does not confirm infiltration because small catheters can prevent withdraw of blood even when patent. Likewise, blood return into the tubing does not rule out extravasation (AWHONN, 2013). Signs and symptoms of extravasation include swelling, pain, blanching or coolness, inability to flush, leakage, erythema, or blister. Several infiltration grading scales have been developed and mentioned in the guidelines, including one developed by the Infusion Nurses Society, the Milliam Scale that refers to joints involved rather than inches, thus reflecting the degree of severity relative to the size of the patient; another is the Thigpen Grading Scale, which delineates treatment options (Amjad et al, 2011; AWHONN, 2013; Thigpen, 2007).

Once symptoms are noted, swift action may minimize adverse outcomes and the degree of skin damage: (1) disconnect the tubing from the IV device; (2) leave the needle in place; (3) attach a 1- to 3-ml syringe to the IV device and aspirate residual drug from the IV; (4) avoid pressure on the site; (5) elevate the involved extremity as soon as possible.

If applicable, knowledgeable and competent providers may administer an appropriate antidote (e.g., hyaluronidase), subcutaneous not IV, to neutralize chemicals as soon as possible. Aseptic puncture techniques have been used by qualified providers to remove fluid and toxic agents from under the skin. These techniques have been reported to dramatically decrease swelling and complications; however, risk for infection and further tissue damage will need to be carefully considered. Unlike adults, topical application of heat or cold is not recommended for neonates due to risk of thermal injury in already immature, compromised, and perhaps hypoperfused skin (AWHONN, 2013).

Ongoing local wound care will depend on the characteristics of the wound and maintaining a physiologic environment (moist but not too moist, free from nonviable tissue and infection, elimination of dead space). Often, extravasation wounds evolve to reveal the extent of the tissue damage, changing the characteristics of the wound and requiring a change in the local wound care protocol. Therefore a variety of dressings may be needed over time for successful management of pediatric extravasation wounds (Lehr et al, 2004; Sawatzky-Dickson et al, 2006).

Support for Healing

Chapters 16 to 18 provide details for wound bed preparation and principles of wound management, including infection, debridement, and topical management, to create a physiologic wound environment. Maximizing nutrition and reducing or eliminating other cofactors such as pain, nutrition, perfusion, and oxygenation are presented in Chapters 25 to 27. Additional pediatric-specific considerations are provided in this section.

Nutritional Support

Nutritional assessment and monitoring, as well as diet, supplements, and feeding strategies, are vital components of any skin integrity care plan. Neonates and children, however, are generally at higher risk for nutritional deficiencies than adults due to the greater demands generated during the phase of life that the body grows most rapidly, while at the same time having smaller appetites and less ability for food and supplement intake. Premature infants have even greater nutritional requirements than term infants due to their diminished nutrient stores at birth (Ditzenberger, 2010). Additionally, children with actual or potential skin breakdown tend to have coexisting conditions and illnesses that increase nutritional needs while further compromising the ability to meet nutritional needs. A pediatrician, dietitian, or other qualified health professional should perform an age-appropriate nutritional assessment, which may include strategies discussed in Chapter 27, such as anthropometric (with head circumference) measurements; growth charts; nutritional screening tools; and consideration of hydration, fluid shifts, and needs associated with any existing comorbidities and skin conditions (Mehta and Compher, 2009; Ranade and Collins, 2011; Skillman and Wischmeyer, 2008). Nutrition subscores found in pressure ulcer risk or skin assessment tools should only be used to supplement comprehensive nutritional assessments conducted by trained and qualified health professionals.

Address Anxiety and Discomfort

Any condition that affects the skin of a child will most likely involve procedures and interventions that create anxiety and/or discomfort. Examples range from changing dressings, pouches, and tube/device stabilizers to debridement, intubation, or surgery. Skin assessment alone, especially in the presence of skin breakdown, can also be painful and frightening to a child. Regardless of the type of assessment or procedure, age-appropriate and developmentally appropriate assessment and management of pain and discomfort must be accomplished.

Features of development, such as how a child of a particular age thinks, what he or she fears, and how he or she learns, are pertinent to helping children cope with health-related activities (Tables 36-4 and 36-5). Developmentally focused preprocedure preparation, caregiver/parent presence and participation during the procedure, and the use of cognitive-based interventions during the procedure and postprocedure follow-up are recognized strategies to facilitate child coping and mastery, both physically and emotionally, for any procedures but especially painful procedures (Baharenstani, 2007; Hockenberry et al, 2011). Options for assessing pain in neonatal and infant patients include the CRIES, FLACC, and Faces Pain Scale, which are described in Chapter 25, Tables 25-2 and 25-3, and Figure 25-2.

Pain management in preemies, neonates, and infants can include nonpharmacologic analgesia such as 24% sucrose given orally directly on the tongue by syringe, if the infant is intubated according to postconceptual age, or by pacifier dipped in the sucrose solution and repeated as needed for pain. Sucrose alone is recommended for minor procedures such as heelstick, venipuncture, venous catheterization, nasogastric insertion, bladder catheterizations, intramuscular or subcutaneous injections, eye examinations, dressing changes, and tape removal. Sucrose may be combined with other analgesic agents for moderately painful procedures, such as lumbar puncture, circumcision, chest tube insertion, percutaneous central venous catheter insertion, or intraosseous access (Stevens et al, 2010).

Eutectic mixture of local anesthetics (EMLA) (lidocaine and prilocaine) for topical anesthesia (described in Chapter 26) has been safely used on *intact* skin of neonates and children before painful procedures. For neonates (minimum gestation age 37 weeks) and children weighing less than 20 kg, the area and duration of application should be limited. Table 36-6 shows the FDA's maximum recommended doses, application areas, and application times for EMLA Cream based on a child's age and weight. EMLA Cream applied to larger areas or for longer times than those recommended could result in sufficient absorption of lidocaine and prilocaine resulting in serious adverse effects. Practitioners should carefully instruct caregivers to avoid application of excessive amounts of EMLA

TABLE 36-4 **Features of Development that Are Pertinent to Helping Children Cope with Procedures**

	Birth to 2 Years	2 to 7 Years	7 to 12 Years	Adolescence
How the child thinks and solves problems	Sensory motor experience develops schema (well-defined and repeated sequences of actions and perceptions) Memory is obvious by 3 to 4 months Begins using symbols for thought reasoning between 18 and 24 months	Thinking is dominated by perceptions rather than logic Verbal communication important for learning Exploratory manipulations helps child learn Child watches, listens, asks questions (Why? How?) Classifies similar things Perceptions limited to single salient feature, so difficult for child to differentiate unessential from essential properties of an experience Uses memory to reconstruct past events Uses imagination to cope Egocentric point of view	Learns from interacting with peers and own experiences Able to understand viewpoints of others Able to see relative nature of things (e.g., this hurts a little; that hurts a lot) Uses deductive logic with respect to tangible (concrete) experiences (if this, then that) Able to view things in context (e.g., "the shot hurt, but it will make me better") Evaluates painful intensive actions in terms of logical function rather than punishment Understands unseen body mechanics/functions Makes use of sensory and procedural information	Uses reason and logical thinking Interested in theoretically possible problems and questions Able to engage in self-reflection Learns from verbally presented ideas and arguments
Major fears and worries	Separation from parents Anything unfamiliar, especially when not with a parent	Separation from parents Harm to body Punishment for wrongdoing	Body injury Loss of body functions Loss of control	Uncertain about self as person Concerned if body, thoughts, feelings are "normal"
Understanding cause and effect	By about 3 months, may associate an action with a result In second year: magical thinking; believes that what is wished for happens	Everything happens by intention Misbehavior is followed by punishment Interprets unrelated events to be related	Before about 9 years, views illness as a consequence of transgressions of rules At about 9 years, begins to understand that illness may have multiple causes	Uses formal rules of logic and evidence to assess cause and effect

From Pridham K, Adelson F, Hansen MF: Helping children deal with procedures in a clinic setting: a developmental approach, *J Pediatr Nurs* 2:13–22, 1987.

TABLE 36-5 **Distraction Techniques for the Neonate and Child**

Age	Distraction Techniques
Infant 0 to 12 months	Parent's voice (e.g., talking, singing on tape) touching (e.g., holding and rocking) pacifier, music, swaddling, massage
Toddler 12 to 36 months	Same as infants: pinwheels, storytelling, peek-a-boo, busy box
Preschool age 3 to 5 years	Pinwheels, feathers, pop-up books Noise makers, storytelling, music, singing, comfort item (stuffed animals, blankies)
School age 6 to 12 years	Electronic toys, computer and TV games pop-up books, I Spy books, storytelling imagery, breathing techniques, muscle relaxation Participation in procedure

Data from Hockenberry MJ, McCarthy K, Taylor O, et al: Managing painful procedures in children with cancer, *J Pediatr Hematol Oncol* 33(2):119–127, 2011.

Cream. As always, follow manufacturer's instructions for use (FDA, 2015).

Liposomal lidocaine is an over-the-counter option for children over 2 years of age. Liposomal lidocaine offers a more rapid onset and less expensive alternative to EMLA. Unlike EMLA, it has not been found to induce methemoglobinemia. However, safety data are lacking for liposomal lidocaine use in infants and children younger than 2 years of age (Eidelman et al, 2005).

Dressing Selection

There are even fewer studies comparing the effectiveness and safety of dressings with children than there are with adults. If approved by the FDA for use with children, they all have the same indications and reimbursement parameters for children as described for adults in Chapter 18. Primarily, dressings should be selected based on the characteristics of the wound (size, depth, location, exudate, periwound skin).

TABLE 36-6 EMLA Maximum Recommended Doses for Neonates and Pediatric Intact Skin

Age and Body Weight Requirements	Maximum Total Dose of EMLA Cream	Maximum Application Area	Maximum Application Time
0 up to 3 months or <5 kg	1 g	10 cm^2	1 hour
3 up to 12 months and >5 kg	2 g	20 cm^2	4 hours
1 to 6 years and >10 kg	10 g	100 cm^2	4 hours
7 to 12 years and >20 kg	20 g	300 cm^2	4 hours

Note: If a patient older than 3 months does not meet the minimum weight requirement, the maximum total dose of EMLA Cream should be restricted to that which corresponds to the patient's weight.
Source: Food and Drug Administration (FDA): *EMLA Cream* (NDA 19-941/S-018) 2006. http://www.accessdata.fda.gov/drugsatfda_docs/label/2006/019941s018lbl.pdf. Accessed March 25, 2015.

Dressings commonly used for pediatric patients with a variety of wounds include transparent, hydrocolloids, foams, silicones, and hydrofibers (King et al, 2013; Morris et al, 2009). Hydrogels are commonly used and reported to be effective in neonatal and pediatric case studies describing the management of toxic epidermal necrolysis, wound dehiscence, extravasation injuries, pressure ulcers, fungating lesions, and burns (AWHONN, 2013; Caniano et al, 2005; Cisler-Cahill, 2006; McCord and Levy; 2006).

The use of dressings that contain calcium, enzymes, silver, iodine, or other antimicromials in children and neonates must take into account concerns for toxicity. For example, elevated serum silver levels have been documented in children with burns treated with silver-containing dressings (Wang et al, 2009). There have been a few studies in pediatric oncology documenting the safety and efficacy of medical-grade honey in children (Biglari et al, 2012; Simon et al, 2006). With neonates, however, most reports have been positive, but either anecdotal or case studies (Bell, 2007). As with all wound dressings, appropriate measures must be taken to prevent MARSI.

Safety and efficacy have not been established by the FDA to approve negative pressure wound therapy (NPWT) for use with neonates, infants, and children. However, guidelines have been proposed for its use with the pediatric population and include age- and wound-specific recommendations for negative pressure settings (Table 36-7) and choice of foam dressing (Baharestani et al, 2009).

TABLE 36-7 Recommended Negative Pressure Settings for Children

Newborn (birth to 1 month)	50 to 75 mm Hg
Infants (>1 month to 2 years)	50 to 75 mm Hg
Children (>2 to 12 years)	75 to 125 mm Hg
Adolescents (>12 years)	75 to 125 mm Hg

Adapted from Baharestani MM: Use of negative pressure wound therapy in the treatment of neonatal and pediatric wounds: a retrospective examination of clinical outcomes, *Ostomy Wound Manage* 53(6): 75–83, 2007.

Several retrospective case series using NPWT off-label provide some evidence of safe and effective use in the pediatric population for a variety of acute and chronic wounds, including infected wounds, those with exposed orthopedic hardware, and surgical wound dehiscence (Baharestani, 2007; Bütter et al, 2006; McCord et al, 2007; Mooney et al, 2000; Rentea et al, 2013).

Chapter 21 is a must-read for serious considerations before NPWT application, including mechanism of action, indications and contraindications for use (including FDA alerts), and clinical application including important issues with transferring care. Safe use of NPWT is paramount. Serious safety events in adults have included injury and death related to bleeding and infection secondary to retained foam dressing particles left in the wound.

CLINICAL CONSULT

A: Consulted for 4-year-old boy in the emergency department after falling off his tricycle. Immunizations current. No known allergies. Patient was crying and agitated until his parents were brought into the treatment room, encouraged to stay and assist in age-appropriate distraction techniques. Tightly secured dry gauze was soaked off with warm saline (to avoid painful removal). Bilateral knees with large 5 × 5 cm irregularly shaped abrasions. Initial cleanse with hypochlorous solution. No foreign body (dirt/gravel) noted in the wounds. Moderate dried exudate. Periwound skin without erythema. No local signs of infection. No other signs of injury.

D: Road abrasions.
P: Cleanse with normal saline or shower per patient and parent preference. Dress wound with gentle silicone foam dressing to promote moist wound healing while minimizing periwound exudate and pain. Change every 5 days, sooner if strike through exudate.
I: (1) Parent teaching with demonstration return using adequate technique for removal and application of dressings. (2) Parents verbalize signs and symptoms of infection.
E: Follow up planned with the patient's pediatrician in 7-10 days or sooner if wound shows signs of infection or deterioration.

SUMMARY

Infants and children suffer many skin-related problems. Research into all areas of pediatric wound care and prevention is needed. Ongoing education of staff and parents related to wound healing is essential. Nurses experienced in wound care can improve the lives of sick children with their knowledge of skin health, skin maintenance, wound healing, and expertise using advanced wound care products.

REFERENCES

Akin F, Spraker M, Aly R, et al: Effects of breathable disposable diapers: reduced prevalence of Candida and common diaper dermatitis, *Pediatr Dermatol* 18(4):282–290, 2001.

Amjad I, Murphy T, Nylander-Housholder L, et al: A new approach to management of intravenous infiltration in pediatric patients: pathophysiology, classification, and treatment, *J Infus Nurs* 34(4):242–249, 2011.

Anthony D, Willock J, Baharestani M: A comparison of Braden Q, Garvin and Glamorgan risk assessment scales in paediatrics, *J Tissue Viability* 19(3):98–105, 2010.

Association of Women's Health, Obstetric and Neonatal Nurses (AWHONN) and National Association of Neonatal Nurses: *Neonatal skin care evidence-based clinical practice guideline*, ed 3, Washington, DC, 2013, AWHONN.

Axelrod D, Kazmerski K, Iyer K: Pediatric enteral nutrition, *JPEN J Parenter Enteral Nutr* 30(Suppl 1):S21–S26, 2006.

Baharestani M, Amjad I, Bookout K, et al: V.A.C. therapy in the management of paediatric wounds: clinical review and experience, *Int Wound J* 6(Suppl 1):1–26, 2009.

Baharestani MM: Use of negative pressure wound therapy in the treatment of neonatal and pediatric wounds: a retrospective examination of clinical outcomes, *Ostomy Wound Manage* 53(6):75–83, 2007.

Baharestani MM, Ratliff CR: Pressure ulcers in neonates and children: an NPUAP white paper, *Adv Skin Wound Care* 20(4): 208–220, 2007.

Beall V, Hall B, Mulholland JT, et al: Neonatal extravasation. Overview and algorithm for evidence-based treatment, *NAINR* 13(4):189–195, 2013.

Beeckman D, Campbell J, Campbell K, et al: *Proceedings from the Global IAD Expert Panel*. Incontinence associated dermatitis: moving prevention forward, London, 2015, Wounds International.

Bell SG: The therapeutic use of honey, *Neonatal Netw* 26(4): 247–251, 2007.

Biglari B, Moghaddam A, Santos K, et al: Multicentre prospective observational study on professional wound care using honey (Medihoney), *Int Wound J* 10(3):252–259, 2012.

Blume-Peytavi U, Cork M, Faergemann J, et al: Bathing and cleansing in newborns from day 1 to first year of life: recommendations from a European round table meeting, *J Eur Acad Dermatol Venereol* 23(7):751–759, 2009.

Borkowski S: Similar gastrostomy peristomal skin irritations in three pediatric patients, *J Wound Ostomy Continence Nurs* 31(4):201–205, 2005.

Braegger C, Decsi T, Dias JA, et al: Practical approach to paediatric enteral nutrition: a comment by the ESPGHAN committee on nutrition, *J Pediatr Gastroenterol Nutr* 51(1):110–122, 2010.

Bütter A, Emran M, Al-Jazaeri A, et al: Vacuum-assisted closure for wound management in the pediatric population, *J Pediatr Surg* 41(5):940–942, 2006.

Caniano DA, Ruth B, Teich S: Wound management with vacuum-assisted closure: experience in 51 pediatric patients, *J Pediatr Surg* 40:128–132, 2005.

Cisler-Cahill L: A protocol for the use of amorphous hydrogel to support wound healing in neonatal patients, *Neonatal Netw* 25(4):267–273, 2006.

Curley MA, Quigley SM, Lin M: Pressure ulcers in pediatric intensive care: incidence and associated factors, *Pediatr Crit Care Med* 4(3):284–290, 2003a.

Curley MA, Razmus IS, Roberts KE, et al: Predicting pressure ulcer risk in pediatric patients: the Braden Q Scale, *Nurs Res* 52(1):22–33, 2003b.

Darmstadt GL, Dinulos JG: Neonatal skin care, *Pediatr Clin North Am* 47(4):757–782, 2000.

Davies MW, Dore AJ, Perissinotto KL: Topical vitamin A, or its derivatives, for treating and preventing napkin dermatitis in infants, *Cochrane Database Syst Rev* 4:CD004300, 2005.

Ditzenberger GR: Nutritional management. In Verklan MT, Walden M, editors: *Core curriculum for neonatal intensive care nursing*, ed 4, St. Louis, MO, 2010, Elsevier, pp 182–207.

Dixon M, Ratliff C: Pediatric pressure ulcer prevalence—one hospital's experience, *Ostomy Wound Manage* 51(6):44–50, 2005.

Dolack M, Huffines B, Stikes R, et al: Updated neonatal skin risk assessment scale (NSRAS), *Ky Nurse* 61(4):6, 2013.

Eidelman A, Weiss JM, Lau J, et al: Topical anesthetics for dermal instrumentation: a systematic review of randomized, controlled trials, *Ann Emerg Med* 46(4):343–351, 2005.

Fernandes JD, Machado MCR, de Oliveira ZNP: Children and newborn skin care and prevention, *An Bras Dermatol* 86(1):102–110, 2011.

Food and Drug Administration (FDA): *EMLA cream (NDA 19-941/S-018)*, 2006. http://www.accessdata.fda.gov/drugsatfda_docs/label/2006/019941s018lbl.pdf. Accessed March 25, 2015.

Food and Drug Administration (FDA): Skin protectant drug products for over-the-counter human use; final monograph. Final rule, *Fed Regist* 68(107):33362–33381, 2003. http://www.accessdata.fda.gov/scripts/cdrh/cfdocs/cfcfr/CFRSearch.cfm?CFRPart=347. Accessed June 5, 2015.

Fujii K, Sugama J, Okuwa M: Incidence and risk factors of pressure ulcers in seven neonatal intensive care units in Japan: a multisite prospective cohort study, *Int Wound J* 7(5):323–328, 2010.

Galvin PA, Curley MAQ: The Braden Q+P: a pediatric perioperative pressure ulcer risk assessment and intervention tool, *AORN J* 96(3):261–270, 2012.

García-Molina P, Balaquer-López E, Torra I, et al: A prospective longitudinal study to assess use of continuous and reactive low-pressure mattresses to reduce pressure ulcer incidence in a pediatric intensive care unit, *Ostomy Wound Manage* 58(7):32–39, 2012.

Grove GL, Zerweck CR, Ekholm BP, et al: Randomized comparison of a silicone tape and a paper tape for gentleness in healthy children, *J Wound Ostomy Continence Nurs* 41(1): 40–48, 2014.

Heimall LM, Storey B, Stellar JJ, et al: Beginning at the bottom: evidence-based care of diaper dermatitis, *MCN Am J Matern Child Nurs* 37(1):10–16, 2012.

Hickey KJ, Anderson CJ, Vogel LC: Pressure ulcers in pediatric spinal cord injury, *Top Spinal Cord Inj Rehabil* 6(Suppl):85–90, 2000.

Hockenberry MJ, McCarthy K, Taylor O, et al: Managing painful procedures in children with cancer, *J Pediatr Hematol Oncol* 33(2):119–127, 2011.

Jackson PD: Diaper dermatitis: protecting the bottom line, *Adv Nurse Pract* 18(3):35–36, 38–41, 2010.

Janowski IM: Tips for protecting critically ill patients from pressure ulcer, *Crit Care Nurse* 30(2):7–9, 2010.

Jaryszak EM, Shah RK, Amling J, et al: Pediatric tracheotomy wound complications: incidence and significance, *Arch Otolaryngol Head Neck Surg* 137(4):363–366, 2011.

Kalia YN, Nonato LB, Lund CH, et al: Development of skin barrier function in premature infants, *J Invest Dermatol* 111(2): 320–326, 1998.

Kelechi TJ, Arndt JV, Dove A: Review of pressure ulcer risk assessment scales, *J Wound Ostomy Continence Nurs* 40(3):232–236, 2013.

King A, Stellar J J, Blevins A, et al: Dressings and products in pediatric wound care, *Adv Wound Care* 3(4):324–334, 2014.

Kottner J, Hauss A, Schlüer AB, et al: Validation and clinical impact of pediatric pressure ulcer risk assessment scales: a systematic review, *Int J Nurs Stud* 50(6):807–818, 2013.

Lehr VT, Lulic-Botica M, Lindblad WJ, et al: Management of infiltration injury in neonates using duoderm hydroactive gel, *Am J Perinatol* 21(7):409–414, 2004.

Lin RL, Tinkle LL, Janniger CK: Skin care of the healthy newborn, *Cutis* 75(1):25–30, 2005.

Loring C, Gregory K, Gargan B, et al: Tub bathing improves thermoregulation of the late preterm infant, *J Obstet Gynecol Neonatal Nurs* 41(2):171–179, 2012.

Lund CH, Osborne JW: Validity and reliability of the neonatal skin condition score, *J Obstet Gynecol Neonatal Nurs* 33(3):320–327, 2004.

Mancini AJ: Skin, *Pediatrics* 113(Suppl 4):1114–1119, 2004.

Markham T, Kennedy F, Collins P: Topical sucralfate for erosive irritant diaper dermatitis, *Arch Dermatol* 136(10):1199–1200, 2000.

McCord S, Levy ML: Practical guide to pediatric wound care, *Semin Plast Surg* 20(3):192–199, 2006.

McCord S, Naik-Mathuria BJ, Murphy KM, et al: Negative pressure wound therapy is effective to manage a variety of wounds in infants and children, *Wound Repair Regen* 15(3):296–301, 2007.

McInnes E, Jammali-Blasi A, Cullum N, et al: Support surfaces for treating pressure injury: a Cochrane systematic review, *Int J Nurs Stud* 50(3):419–430, 2013.

McLane K, Bookout K, McCord S, et al: The 2003 national pediatric pressure ulcer and skin breakdown prevalence survey: a multisite study, *J Wound Ostomy Continence Nurs* 31(4): 168–178, 2004.

McLane K, Krouskip T, McCord S, et al: Comparison of interface pressures in the pediatric population among various support surfaces, *J Wound Ostomy Continence Nurs* 29: 243–251, 2002.

McNichol L, Lund C, Osborne C, et al: Medical adhesives and patient safety: state of the science: consensus statements for the assessment, prevention, and treatment of adhesive-related skin injuries, *J Wound Ostomy Continence Nurs* 40(4):365–380, 2013.

Mehta NM, Compher C, A.S.P.E.N. Board of Directors: A.S.P.E.N. clinical guidelines: nutrition support of the critically ill child, *JPEN J Parenter Enteral Nutr* 33(3):260–276, 2009.

Mills J, Ramsey E, Rich S, et al, editors: *Texas Children's Hospital pediatric nutrition reference guide*, ed 10, Houston, TX, 2013, Texas Children's Hospital.

Mooney JF 3rd, Argenta LC, Marks MW, et al: Treatment of soft tissue defects in pediatric patients using the V.A.C. system, *Clin Orthop Relat Res* 376:26–31, 2000.

Morris C, Emsley P, Marland E, et al: Use of wound dressings with soft silicone adhesive technology, *Paediatr Nurs* 21(3):38–43, 2009.

Murray JS, Noonan C, Quigley S, et al: Medical device-related hospital-acquired pressure ulcers in children: an integrative review, *J Pediatr Nurs* 28(6):585–595, 2013.

National Pressure Ulcer Advisory Panel (NPUAP), European Pressure Ulcer Advisory Panel (EPUAP), Pan Pacific Pressure Injury Alliance (PPPIA): In Haesler E, editor: *Prevention and treatment of pressure ulcers: clinical practice guideline*, Perth, Australia, 2014, Cambridge Media.

Ness MJ, Davis DM, Carey WA: Neonatal skin care: a concise review, *Int J Dermatol* 52(1):14–22, 2013.

Nield LS, Kamat D: Prevention, diagnosis, and management of diaper dermatitis, *Clin Pediatr (Phila)* 46(6):480–486, 2007.

Noonan C, Quigley S, Curley M: Skin integrity in hospitalized infants and children: a prevalence survey, *J Pediatr Nurs* 21(6):445–453, 2006.

Noonan C, Quigley S, Curley M: Using the Braden Q Scale to predict pressure ulcer risk in pediatric patients, *J Pediatr Nurs* 26(6):566–575, 2011.

Odio M, Streicher-Scott J, Hansen R: Disposable baby wipes: efficacy and skin mildness, *Dermatol Nurs* 13(2):107–121, 2001.

Rana AR, Michalsky MP, Teich S, et al: Childhood obesity: a risk factor for injuries observed at a level-1 trauma center, *J Pediatr Surg* 44(8):1601–1605, 2009.

Ranade D, Collins N: Children with wounds: the importance of nutrition, *Ostomy Wound Manage* 57(10):14–24, 2011.

Razmus I, Lewis L, Wilson D: Pressure ulcer development in infants: state of the science, *J Healthc Qual* 30(5):36–42, 2008.

Rentea RM, Somers KK, Cassidy L, et al: Negative pressure wound therapy in infants and children: a single-institution experience, *J Surg Res* 184(1):658–864, 2013.

Sawatzky-Dickson D, Bodnaryk K: Neonatal intravenous extravasation injuries: evaluation of a wound care protocol, *Neonatal Netw* 25(1):13–19, 2006.

Schindler C, Mikhailov TA, Kuhn EM, et al: Protecting fragile skin: nursing interventions to decrease development of pressure ulcers in pediatric intensive care, *Am J Crit Care* 20(1):26–34, 2011.

Schlüer AB, Halfens RJ, Schols JM: Pediatric pressure ulcer prevalence: a multicenter, cross-sectional, point prevalence study in Switzerland, *Ostomy Wound Manage* 58(7):18–31, 2012.

Shin HT: Diaper dermatitis that does not quit, *Dermatol Ther* 18:124–135, 2005.

Simon A, Sofka K, Wiszniewsky G, et al: Wound care with antibacterial honey (Medihoney) in pediatric hematology-oncology, *Support Care Cancer* 14(1):91–97, 2006.

Skillman HE, Wischmeyer PE: Nutrition therapy in critically ill infants and children, *JPEN J Parenter Enteral Nutr* 32(5):520–534, 2008.

Smith WJ, Jacob SE: The role of allergic contact dermatitis in diaper dermatitis, *Pediatr Dermatol* 26(3):369–370, 2009.

Stevens B, Yamada J, Ohlsson A: Sucrose for analgesia in newborn infants undergoing painful procedures, *Cochrane Database Syst Rev* 1:CD001069, 2010.

Suddaby EC, Barnett S, Facteau L: Skin breakdown in acute care pediatrics, *Pediatr Nurs* 31(2):132–138, 2005.

Thigpen JL: Peripheral intravenous extravasation: nursing procedure for initial treatment, *Neonatal Netw* 26(6):379–384, 2007.

Turnage-Carrier C, McLane KM, Gregurich MA: Interface pressure comparison of healthy premature infants with various neonatal bed surfaces, *Adv Neonatal Care* 8(3):176–184, 2008.

Vender RB: Adverse reactions to herbal therapy in dermatology, *Skin Therapy Lett* 8(3):5–8, 2003.

Visscher MO: Recent advances in diaper dermatitis: etiology and treatment, *Pediatr Health* 3(1):81–98, 2009a.

Visscher MO: Update on the use of topical agents in neonates, *Newborn Infant Nurs Rev* 9(1):31–47, 2009b.

Wang XQ, Kempf M, Mott J, et al: Silver absorption on burns after the application of Acticoat: data from pediatric patients and a porcine burn model, *J Burn Care Res* 30(2):341–348, 2009.

White CM, Gailey RA, Lippe S: Cholestyramine ointment to treat buttocks rash and anal excoriation in an infant, *Ann Pharmacother* 30(9):954–956, 1996.

Willock J, Anthony D, Richardson J: Inter-rater reliability of the Glamorgan Paediatric Pressure Ulcer Risk Assessment Scale, *Paediatr Nurs* 20(7):14–19, 2008.

Willock J, Harris C, Harrison J, et al: Identifying the characteristics of children with pressure ulcers, *Nurs Times* 101(11):40–43, 2005.

World Health Organization: *International classification of diseases, 2010.* http://www.who.int/classifications/icd/en/. Accessed June 4, 2015.

Wound, Ostomy and Continence Nurses Society™ (WOCN®): *Guideline for management of pressure ulcers (WOCN® clinical practice guideline series no. 2)*, Mt. Laurel, NJ, 2010, WOCN®.

Zehrer CL, Newman DK, Grove GL, et al: Assessment of diaper-clogging potential of petrolatum moisture barriers, *Ostomy Wound Manage* 51:54–58, 2005.

37

Managing Wounds in Palliative Care

Ruth A. Bryant*

OBJECTIVES

1. Distinguish between palliative and hospice care.
2. List types of wounds common to palliative care
3. Describe the possible etiologies of a malignant cutaneous wound and clinical manifestations.
4. Define Marjolin ulcer.
5. List at least four goals in the management of a fungating wound in palliative care.
6. Describe at least four interventions used to achieve the goals associated with palliative wound care.
7. Explain the difference in debridement of a nonmalignant necrotic wound compared with debridement of a malignant cutaneous wound.
8. Identify at least four categories of dressings common in the care of the malignant cutaneous wound.

Palliative care is a concept associated with end of life and with goals such as relief from distressing symptoms, easing of pain, and enhanced quality of life. When healing the wound is not an appropriate or realistic goal, the goal is palliation or maintenance. Many factors influence whether the goal is wound healing or palliation. This chapter describes the patient situations in which palliative wound care would be appropriate, the types of wounds that may be associated with palliation, and the principles of palliative wound care. Among the many challenges facing patients in palliative or hospice care are the issues surrounding skin and wound care. Because untreated wounds can lead to physical discomfort and impair quality of life, it is appropriate that they receive attention.

DEFINITION OF TERMS

Palliative care is an approach to care that is patient and family centered, focused on symptom management, relief of suffering, and improved quality of life rather than cure or lengthening life (Resnick, 2012). Physical, intellectual, psychosocial, and spiritual needs are addressed in palliative care to facilitate patient autonomy, informed decision making, and choice (NQF, 2006; WHO, 2008). Palliative care is not synonymous with the abandonment of hope or treatment options. No specific therapies are excluded if they can improve the patient's quality of life (Alvarez et al, 2002; Stephen-Haynes, 2008). In fact, palliative care is ideally a general approach to

patient care that should be routinely integrated into primary care and should occur concurrently with other treatments. Palliative care is not limited to end-of-life situations. Although it is indicated for patients with a life-threatening condition, it is also relevant for those with a debilitating illness that encompasses a broad range of diagnoses, including people who are living with a persistent or recurring illness that adversely affects their daily functioning or will predictably reduce life expectancy (Dahlin, 20013; Resnick, 2012). Palliative care focuses on the palliative journey from diagnosis onward rather than focusing on the last days of life (Stephen-Haynes, 2008; Westwood, 2014). Therefore palliative care services are indicated across the trajectory of a patient's illness and are not restricted to the end-of-life phase (NQF, 2006). Specialists in palliative care, those who have received formal education in palliative care and are credentialed in the field, may be consulted to provide specialty-level palliative care when the complexity of the situation warrants (Dahlin, 2013).

Hospice care is similar to palliative care in that the goals are to alleviate symptoms and improve quality of life. However, hospice is appropriate for patients who have a limited life expectancy of 6 months or less (Resnick, 2012). When the patient enters the terminal stage of an illness or condition, curative treatments are no longer effective, and/or the patient no longer desires to continue them, hospice becomes the care of choice. Hospice provides comprehensive biomedical, psychosocial, and spiritual support as patients face the end of life (AAHPM 2008; NQF, 2006). The key difference between palliative care and hospice is that palliative care is appropriate, regardless of the stage of the disease or the need for other therapies and can be rendered along

*The author acknowledges Margaret Goldberg for her work on developing content of this chapter in the fourth edition of *Acute and Chronic Wounds: Current Management Concepts*.

with life-prolonging treatment as the main focus of care (Westwood, 2014).

PALLIATIVE WOUND CARE

Palliative wound care has been defined as the "incorporation of strategies that prioritize symptomatic relief and wound improvement ahead of wound healing" (Alvarez et al, 2007). In a concept analysis, Emmons and Lachman (2010) described palliative wound care as a holistic and integrated approach to care that addresses symptom management and psychosocial well-being, is multidisciplinary, is driven by patient/family goals, and is integrated into everyday wound care principles and practice. An important aspect of palliative wound care is the management of symptoms such as odor, exudate, bleeding, pain, and infection and maintenance of skin integrity. Prevention of wound deterioration is desirable but is not always realistic, as with a fungating wound (Maund, 2008; Naylor, 2005; Stanley et al, 2008). Palliative care is elected care rather than care that is forced upon the patient; the focus is on physical, psychosocial, and spiritual issues during end of life (Hughes et al, 2005).

Indications

Palliative wound care as a goal of wound management is often related to end of life, when healing interventions are inconsistent with the patient's end-of-life goals. However, palliative wound care may also be indicated when the underlying etiology or existing cofactors cannot be overcome as a result of advanced illness and poor physical state. Although malignancies and metastases are commonly associated with palliative wound care, the patient's condition and situation will also dictate the need for palliative wound care. Palliation as a goal for wound management may be indicated in the following situations:

1. *The patient is terminally ill.* Most often this is a patient who has cancer, but it could just as well be a patient who has end-stage renal disease or significant congestive heart failure. The wound could be an open surgical wound, pressure ulcer, a burn, radiation dermatitis, etc.
2. *Overwhelming comorbidities are present.* As an example, a patient may have significant hypotension after a massive cardiac arrest and require high doses of a vasopressor medication to achieve an adequate blood pressure. The resulting vasoconstriction may be sufficient enough to cause a gradual transition in the fingertips or toes to cyanosis and then necrosis. Clearly the comorbidities dictate that the priority is sustaining adequate blood pressure.
3. *Patient choice.* This is the situation where a patient does not have overwhelming comorbidities or a terminal illness yet simply chooses palliation as a goal. Possible reasons may include a preference to continue a certain lifestyle that jeopardizes wound healing, a realization that the modifications needed for treatment are not feasible or

consistent with other priorities, a financial burden, or a decision based on the patient's age.

Types of Wounds Common to Palliative Care

The etiology of wounds in the patient receiving palliative care can be nonmalignancy or malignancy related. The nonmalignant wound common in palliative care is the wound that develops from mechanical trauma (e.g., unrelieved pressure, shear, friction, skin stripping), moisture-associated skin damage (MASD) (urinary incontinence, fecal incontinence, etc.), or infection (e.g., candidiasis or herpes). These nonmalignant wounds are prevented and managed with the same interventions, resources, and tools described throughout this textbook. Malignancy-related wounds may be a primary tumor, metastasis, or malignant transformation. Malignancy-related wounds have common wound characteristics that warrant unique kinds of care.

NONMALIGNANCY-RELATED WOUNDS

Any type of wound can be observed in a patient receiving palliative or hospice care. Some of the most common include pressure ulcers, skin stripping, and chemical dermatitis with coexisting pressure ulcers, which is perhaps the most common (Naylor, 2005; Richards et al, 2007; Stephen-Haynes, 2008). Galvin (2002) reports that of all the ulcers that developed in the palliative care unit, 78.4% were sacral pressure ulcers.

The frequency of pressure ulcers in the patient receiving palliative care is varied, with an incidence reported as high as 43% (Walding, 2005). Galvin (2002) found 26.1% of patients admitted to a palliative care program over a 2-year timeframe had a pressure ulcer, and 12% of all patients admitted to the palliative care setting developed a pressure ulcer during the stay. Within hospice programs, the literature reports an incidence of pressure ulcers ranging from 10% to 17.5%; prevalence is reported at 27% (Reifsnyder and Magee, 2005; Tippett, 2005). In a small study of a hospice program, a total of 35% of patients had some type of skin issue, 50% of them being pressure ulcers (Tippett, 2005).

Pressure Ulcer Prevention

While skin deterioration or "failure" may occur at the end of life, pressure ulcer prevention and skin care are critically important components of palliative care (Beldon, 2011; McGill and Chaplin, 2002; Sibbald et al, 2009; Westwood, 2014). As many as 10% of patients develop a new pressure ulcer within the first 3 months of admission to a hospice program (Reifsnyder and Magee, 2005). Of interest, however, in a survey of inpatient palliative care units, only 61% had a written policy for pressure ulcer prevention, 17.6% indicated their policy was under development, and 19.6% reported they did not have a policy. A pressure ulcer prevention program has been presented in detail in Chapters 8 and 9. In the palliative care setting, risk assessment and prevention have a few unique considerations.

Risk Assessment. International guidelines recommend pressure ulcer risk assessment for palliative care patients on a regular basis using a structured, consistent approach (NPUAP, EPUAP, PPPIA, 2014). Rather than assessing pressure ulcer risk solely by completing a risk assessment tool, they also recommend using a validated risk assessment tool, a comprehensive skin assessment, *and* clinical judgment with regard to key risk factors. The Marie Curie Centre's Hunters Hill Risk Assessment tool (recommended by the NPUAP, EPUAP, and PPPIA guideline), Palliative Performance Scale, the F.R.A.I.L. Healing Probability Assessment Tool and the Hospice Pressure Ulcer Risk Assessment Scale (HoRT) were designed and tested specifically for the individual at or near the end of life (Chaplin, 2000; Chrisman, 2010; Henoch and Gustaffson, 2003; NPUAP, EPUAP, PPPIA, 2014; Woo et al, 2015). In contrast, many experts suggest that *every* palliative care patient should be considered at "high risk" for pressure ulcer development (Richards et al, 2007; Walding, 2005). Risk assessment should be obtained within 6 to 12 hours of admission and should be reassessed on a daily basis because of the speed with which the palliative patient's condition can change (McGill and Chaplin, 1999).

Factors that contribute to pressure ulcer formation in palliative care patients include fragile skin condition, older age, decreasing food and fluid intake, altered sensation, poor general physical condition, decreased mobility, pain, compromised immunity, poor oxygenation, and lean body type (Naylor and McGill, 2005; Woo, Krasner, Kennedy et al, 2015). Of interest, Brink et al (2006) found that patients who used an indwelling urinary catheter or had an ostomy were more than four times more likely to develop one or more ulcers. Additional unique variables associated with pressure ulcer formation included new pain site, shortness of breath, and inability to lie flat (Brink et al, 2006). One fourth of all palliative home care patients experienced the inability to lie flat because of shortness of breath, which increased the patient's risk of pressure ulcer formation. Thus repositioning may exacerbate shortness of breath and require a modification in the standard of care to utilize a higher level of support surface so that repositioning can be less frequent.

Prevention. Pressure ulcer prevention interventions are vital for the palliative care patient population, particularly because the development and resulting treatment often are painful (Eisenberger and Zeleznik, 2004). At the same time, the pressure ulcer prevention plan of care must be reflective of and consistent with the patient's clinical picture and end-of-life goals. Reducing or eliminating some risk factors may not be achievable or in accordance with the comfort-focused goals of palliative care (Reifsnyder and Magee, 2005). For example, maintaining the head of the bed lower than 30 degrees or turning the patient every 2 hours may not be realistic or consistent with the patient's wishes. In these instances, complete patient and family education becomes more critical than ever

so that the patient and family are fully informed before they make decisions that may lead to pressure ulcer development. At the same time, it is the responsibility of the wound care provider to recommend the support surface that would best redistribute coccyx pressure while accommodating the patient's need for an elevated head of bed. The international pressure ulcer treatment guidelines (NPUAP, EPUAP, PPPIA, 2014) instruct the care provider to consider changing the support surface to improve pressure redistribution and comfort.

Prevention measures that are most universally appropriate in palliative care include (1) adequate and appropriate offloading with a support surface; (2) adequate pain control for optimal positioning; and (3) incontinence management (containment and skin protection). However, good pain management is critical to being able to provide these basic prevention interventions (Liao and Arnold, 2007). The international guidelines stipulate the patient should be premedicated 20 to 30 minutes before a scheduled position change when he or she experiences significant pain with movement (NPUAP, EPUAP, PPPIA, 2014).

Whether all pressure ulcers that occur in palliative care patients are preventable or whether some are inevitable is not clear (Chaplin, 2004). Debate is growing about the possibility that as death approaches the skin begins to fail, primarily because of altered perfusion, which puts the patient at risk for further breakdown (Stanley et al, 2008). Richards et al (2007) reported that among a group of 61 end-of-life patients in palliative care, 8 of 13 new ulcers developed within 2 weeks of the patient's death. In another study of palliative care wounds, nearly half of the pressure ulcers healed despite short treatment periods, underscoring the point that palliative wound care measures resulted in significant healing. However, regardless of the outcome of this debate, it is incumbent upon the wound specialist to provide care that is compliant with national guidelines for the prevention of pressure ulcers and to not withhold preventive interventions based on the designation of palliative or end-of-life care. Furthermore, documentation should record the implementation of assessments and interventions reflective of the guidelines, as well as when interventions were withheld and why. A nosocomial pressure ulcer then can be considered inevitable when it develops even though the care provided met the standard of care for pressure ulcer prevention.

Pressure Ulcer Care

Pressure ulcer care in the palliative care patient should closely follow the international guidelines on pressure ulcer treatment and deviate from that standard only as needed and indicated by the international guidelines (NPUAP, EPUAP, PPPIA, 2014). Overall, the palliative care guidelines encourage comfort, prompt symptom management, consistency between care provided and the patient's goals, and change guided by the values and goals of the patient and family. Specific and unique issues relative to exudate control, pain control, odor control, debridement, assessment and monitoring of healing, and dressing selection are discussed later in this chapter.

MALIGNANCY-RELATED WOUNDS

Malignancy-related wounds can be a primary cutaneous tumor, a metastasis, or a malignant transformation of an existing ulcer. The common primary cutaneous tumors that can present as a wound are untreated basal cell cancer (see Plate 73), squamous cell cancer (see Plate 74a), and malignant melanoma (Gerlach, 2005). A primary tumor also can invade up into the skin and erode through the skin to form a malignant wound (Hampton, 2008). Although any tumor left untreated can cause a malignant wound, the most common cancers are breast and soft tissue sarcoma (Naylor, 2002). A tumor can metastasize to the skin when it has invaded blood or lymph vessels; consequently, circulating malignant cells become trapped in the tiny skin capillaries. Seeding of malignant cells can occur during surgery to the abdominal wall, for example. Cancer of the ovary, cecum, and rectum can infiltrate the anterior wall of the abdomen (Grocott, 2007).

Malignant Cutaneous Wounds

Collectively, any wound that is a primary or metastatic skin lesion is referred to as a *malignant cutaneous wound,* also commonly known as a *fungating malignant wound* (see Plate 74b). These malignant cutaneous wounds usually are chronic, ulcerating, open, and draining (Bauer and Gerlach, 2000; Recka et al, 2012).

A malignant cutaneous wound begins as a small, firm nodule under the surface of the skin that may be flesh colored, pink, red, violet, or brown (Gerlach, 2005; Naylor, 2002). As the malignant cells proliferate, they interfere with the capillaries and lymph vessels. Although the tumor develops its own microcirculation, it is disorganized and has impaired blood-clotting abilities (Naylor, 2002). These lesions can develop into necrotic "cauliflowerlike" eruptions on the skin that progress to exudative and hemorrhagic wounds. Anaerobic organisms (usually *Bacteroides*) flourish on the necrotic tissue and produce volatile fatty acids as metabolic end-products that are responsible for the characteristic pungent and penetrating odor; this odor is a source of great embarrassment and distress to the patient, family, and caregivers (Draper, 2005; Piggin, 2003). One in ten patients with a metastatic disease has cutaneous metastases (Recka et al, 2012). The patient with a malignant cutaneous wound may have no symptoms or may experience pruritus, pain, stinging, exudate, odor, and thickening and hardening of the skin (Alexander, 2010; Moore, 2002; Seaman, 2006).

Malignant cutaneous wounds have a poor outcome. Treatment options for these fungating malignant wounds are aimed at the underlying pathology and include radiotherapy, chemotherapy, hormone therapy, surgery, cryotherapy, or laser therapy. External beam radiation therapy may be used to control local metastases, which in turn may help control malignant cutaneous wound symptoms.

Malignant cutaneous wounds are often misinterpreted initially as an ulcer with an etiology of pressure, arterial insufficiency, or pyoderma. When the wound fails to progress despite appropriate topical therapy, cancer should be suspected and biopsies obtained from at least four different locations in the base of the wound. These kinds of wounds will appear abnormal (e.g., thickened, rolled wound edges) and should be thoroughly assessed (Gerlach, 2005).

Marjolin Ulcer

Malignant transformation of an existing ulcer occurs in approximately 2% of all chronic wounds (e.g., pressure ulcer, sinus tract, irradiated skin, burn wound, venous ulcer). The site of chronic irritation and inflammation is a common location for this malignant transformation, otherwise called a *Marjolin ulcer,* which tends to be an aggressive tumor. Treatment is based upon the size and extent of the wound and the condition of the patient (Gerlach, 2005).

OBJECTIVES IN THE CARE OF THE MALIGNANT CUTANEOUS WOUND

Wound management decisions are a balance of meeting the patient's priorities and achieving the identified aims arising from the comprehensive assessment (Chaplin, 2004; Woo et al, 2015). Goals of care and treatment priorities are negotiated with each patient based on the stage of the underlying disease process and the potential for available therapeutic options to be beneficial and meet personal preferences (Ferris et al, 2007). Above all, quality of life is the guiding principle when planning patient care (British Columbia Cancer Agency, 2011).

In most situations, the quality of care given to patients with malignant fungating wounds is the most important factor in determining their quality of life (Williams, 1997). The priorities of topical care address the common symptoms of a malignant wound: odor, exudate, pain, bleeding, and pruritus. Interventions include control of bioburden, debridement, exudate-absorbent dressings, wound cleansing, and protection of the surrounding skin, as summarized in Table 37-1 and described in the following sections.

Control Pain and Pruritus

Causes of pain in the malignant wound may be multiple and include emotional factors, neuropathic pain (due to nerve damage from the tumor), and procedural pain, as occurs with dressing removal (Grocott, 2007) (see Chapters 25 and 26 for detailed information related to pain assessment and management). When pain is related to underlying disease, practitioners, including interventional radiologists, anesthesiology pain specialists, radiation oncologists, surgical oncologists, and pharmacists, should be part of the team helping to manage complex pain issues (Krouse,

TABLE 37-1 Interventions for Palliative Wound Care

Pain Management	Odor Management	Exudate Control
Nontraumatic Dressing Changes Contact layer Gauzes, nonadherent or coated Foam Protective barrier films Nontraumatic tapes	**Wound Cleansing** Ionic cleansers Sodium-impregnated gauze Antimicrobials	**Exudate Collection and Containment** Foam, alginates, hydrofiber dressings, absorptive powders Wound drainage pouch
Periwound Skin Management Nontraumatic tapes Skin sealants (alcohol free) Barrier ointment/cream Hydrocolloid wafer	**Deodorizers** Charcoal dressings Chloromycetin solution Metronidazole gel	**Indicators for Dressing Changes** When pooling on intact skin occurs When strikethrough occurs
	Debridement Dry, hard, necrotic tissue (hydrogel, enzymatic debriders) Wet sloughy tissue (polysaccharide beads, starch, copolymer dressing)	**Control of Bleeding** Hemostatic dressings Nonadherent gauze Alginates Sliver nitrate sticks Monsel's solution
	Reduction of Bacterial Burden Irrigation with ionic cleansers Antimicrobial dressings and creams Absorptive dressings Sodium-impregnated gauze Oral antimicrobials	

2008). In addition to systemic analgesia and rapid-onset, short-acting analgesics administered before beginning dressing changes, topical anesthetics can be used to control pain (Tice, 2006). Topical lidocaine or benzocaine or ice packs applied before or after wound care may be beneficial (Seaman, 2006; Woo et al, 2015). Topical eutectic mixture of local anesthetic cream (EMLA 5%) (containing lidocaine with prilocaine) has been used to reduce pain intensity (Evans and Gray, 2005). EMLA should be applied in a thick layer and covered with plastic film, then allowed to wait from 30 to 45 minutes for anesthetic effects to develop (Chrisman, 2010). Diligence is required in the use of EMLA cream because it has a pH of 9.4 and can penetrate damaged skin. Daily application of a topical opioid-infused amorphous hydrogel (10 mg morphine sulfate in 8 g of hydrogel) has been used anecdotally to manage painful pressure ulcers and malignant wounds (Ashfield, 2005; Back and Findlay, 1995), as well as in randomized controlled studies (Zeppetella and Ribeiro, 2005; Zeppetella et al, 2003), with significantly improved pain control compared with pretreatment medications. Similar results have been reported with use of either crushed oxycodone or meperidine topically in two patients with sickle cell ulcers (Ballas, 2002). Nociceptive pain should also be managed with nonsteroidal anti-inflammatory medications (Woo et al, 2015). Nonpharmacologic measures for pain management include heat or cold, energy therapies (Reiki, healing touch), relaxation and deep breathing, mindfulness meditation, hypnosis, and the use of "time-outs" (Woo et al, 2015).

Although a malignant or fungating wound is characteristically painful, a key source of pain is the trauma associated with dressing changes. Consequently, controlling or minimizing pain requires attention to the reduction or elimination of mechanical trauma and preventing medical adhesive–related skin injury (MARSI). Two primary interventions are (1) minimization of trauma associated with dressing changes by using nonadhesive dressings and (2) infrequent dressing changes. The malignant or fungating wound site has an increased tendency to bleed when disturbed, which may aggravate the presence of pain. Infrequent dressing changes reduce the potential for bleeding. When bleeding is a concern, appropriate dressings that reduce the potential for a bleeding episode must be selected.

The malignant wound often triggers pruritus at the wound site as the skin tissues stretch in response to the growing tumor. Diphenhydramine or hydroxyzine may be warranted to manage the pruritus and moisturizers applied to keep the periwound skin supple (Gerlach, 2005).

Atraumatic Dressing Changes

Nonadhesive but absorbent dressings are recommended to achieve atraumatic dressing removal. Dressing selection options include a contact-layer dressing, nonadherent gauze, impregnated gauze (e.g., hydrogel- or petrolatum-impregnated gauze), and semipermeable foam dressings. To eliminate unnecessary dressing changes, dressings that have a long wearing time should be selected and preferably changed no more often than every 3 days (Schim and Cullen,

2005). However, once-daily dressing changes may be necessary for the highly exudative wound. Protective barrier films, particularly those without alcohol, can be applied to the surrounding skin to further decrease trauma to periwound skin. Atraumatic tapes and mesh netting can be used to affix dressings, thereby avoiding trauma to the surrounding skin upon removal.

Control or Prevent Bleeding

Erosion of capillaries can lead to significant spontaneous bleeding. Atraumatic dressing removal is critical to avoid precipitating a bleeding episode. If bleeding occurs even with the use of atraumatic dressing removal techniques, direct pressure and an ice pack can be applied initially. If these are ineffective, many different types of dressings and products are available that assist in the control of bleeding (see Table 31-1). Monsel's solution (ferric subsulfate) has been shown to be an effective adjunct to compression for hemostasis (Alvarez et al, 2007). A comprehensive wound assessment should direct the choice of which dressing is most appropriate. Absorbable hemostatic dressings and silver nitrate cautery sticks can be used to specifically control small bleeding points. Alginates have been demonstrated to exhibit hemostatic effects and have been useful for heavily exudative wounds. Nonadherent gauze is an option that will absorb exudate without adhering to the wound bed. Significant bleeding events may require oral antifibrinolytics, radiotherapy, and embolization. Although vasoconstrictive effects can result in ischemia and consequently necrosis, gauze saturated with topical adrenaline 1:1000 may be applied for emergent situations; however, the patient should be monitored for systemic absorption of the medications (Grocott, 1999; Seaman, 2006). These more aggressive options are appropriate if they will improve the quality of life in patients with a malignant wound (Seaman, 2006).

Manage Periwound Skin

The nature of wounds occurring in palliative care predisposes toward maceration and denudement, and care should focus on preventing epidermal stripping, maceration, contact dermatitis, infection, and moisture associated skin damage (Stephen-Haynes, 2008; Woo et al, 2015). Routine skin assessments should be obtained to monitor for signs and symptoms of bacterial infection (induration, localized erythema, heat, pain) and fungal infection (erythematous, papular rash). Interventions to protect the fragile periwound skin include nonadhesive dressings, alcohol-free protective barrier films, and bracketing the wound bed with skin barrier strips to serve as a barrier to exudate and an anchor for adhesives. Additional measures to protect periwound skin are described in Chapter 5.

Control Odor

Malodor is recognized as having a physical and psychological impact by reducing appetite, affecting well-being, causing social isolation, and distorting body image (Fletcher, 2008; Piggin, 2003; West, 2007). Odor can be caused by necrotic tissue, bacterial burden, infection, or saturated dressings. Objective assessment for the presence of odor is difficult, so subjective reporting by the patient should guide interventions (Collier, 1997).

Interventions appropriate for control of odor include wound cleansing, use of wound deodorizers, debridement, and treatment of infection. Many of these interventions can be used simultaneously to aggressively attack the problem of odor. Approaches for the management of odor include wound cleansing, topical deodorizers, room deodorizers, topical and oral antimicrobials, debridement, carbon dressings, and manuka honey (Chrisman, 2010). Topical metronidazole gel (0.75% to 0.80%) is associated with control of anaerobic bacteria and protozoal infections. It is applied directly to the wound once daily for 5 to 7 days or more as needed. Metronidazole tables may also be crushed and placed on the wound bed (Chrisman, 2010; NPUAP, EPUAP, PPPIA, 2014). In a systematic review of the literature examining topical agents to reduce odor in malignant wounds, da Costa Santos and colleagues (2010) found that topical metronidazole, sodium-impregnated gauze, charcoal or activated charcoal dressings, and curcumin ointment yielded a grade B (moderate level) recommendation. Grades C and D recommendations, the lowest level of evidence that are mostly based on case studies and expert opinion, included the use of topical arsenic trioxide, essential oils, green tea extract, hydropolymer dressings, antiseptic solutions, hydrogels, and debridement enzymes. Despite the volume of literature on managing odor, there is still a lack of high-quality rigorous studies to provide high-level recommendations.

Wound Cleansing. Gentle removal of exudate and debris from the wound base can aid in odor management (NPUAP, EPUAP, PPPIA, 2014). Wound cleansing with gentle irrigations rather than swabbing of the surface while minimizing trauma is recommended. Normal saline, ionic irrigants, and commercial wound cleansers with surfactants can be used (Seaman, 2006). A daily shower with the water aimed slightly above the wound may be an effective method for cleansing the wound.

Deodorizers. Deodorizers can be used topically as well as within the room to control odor. Strategies such as use of aromatherapy oils, expensive aftershave lotions, room deodorizers, and scented candles tend to mask the odor of the malignant wound and overall yield unsatisfactory results (West, 2007; Wilson, 2005). Use of a "sugar paste" has been reported in the literature as an effective deodorizing preparation by reducing bioburden and necrotic tissue. However, the commercially available manuka honey is preferred because its processing is standardized so that the product is sterilized, thus eliminating the risk of botulism, and it is safe from toxins that are present in certain nectars (Wilson, 2005).

Although not appropriate when the objective is wound healing, Chloromycetin solution has been reported to be an effective wound deodorant. Gauze is moistened with the Chloromycetin solution and applied to the wound surface; it is generally changed twice daily so that the dressing will remain moist. Skin protection should be implemented to keep the solution from contacting the surrounding skin because Chloromycetin will cause an irritant reaction to intact skin. Puri-Clens has also been applied to wounds for odor control.

Antimicrobials. Antimicrobial creams and sodium-impregnated gauze both may assist in reducing bacterial numbers, thereby reducing odor. Dressings with an antimicrobial component that assist in controlling the wound bioburden include those that contain silver, iodine, or honey (White and Cutting, 2006). Exudate can increase and become viscous and malodorous when a wound becomes infected (Steven-Haynes, 2008). Infections are treated systemically, locally, or both.

Oral (systemic) metronidazole can be given as 200-mg tablets twice per day to reduce the anaerobic bacterial load in the wound. Although this treatment has been reported to be quite successful, notable adverse effects are metallic taste in mouth, furred tongue, nausea and vomiting, and intolerance to alcohol, in addition to development of resistance to the bacteria (West, 2007).

In contrast, topical metronidazole decreases bacterial load at the wound site but without the nausea and vomiting that sometimes accompanies oral metronidazole (Finlay et al, 1996; Kalinski et al, 2005). Metronidazole has been applied directly to the wound or on petrolatum gauze and can be used in combination with calcium alginate, hydrofiber, or foam dressings (Alvarez et al, 2007). Seaman (2006) described crushing metronidazole tablets in sterile water and creating either a 0.5% solution (5 mg/1 cc) or a 1% solution (10 mg/1 cc). The solution can then be used as a wound irrigant or used to saturate gauze and pack on the wound bed, including any tunnels or undermining.

Metronidazole gel (0.75%) is commercially available and can be applied to the wound bed and then covered with a saline-soaked gauze or hydrogel. Topical metronidazole is changed daily, and odor should be eradicated or greatly diminished between 3 and 7 days (Chrisman, 2010). Contact layers are often used in combination with antimicrobials (e.g., metronidazole gel or crushed tablets), which significantly reduce the bacteria that cause the odor and drainage.

Debridement. Necrotic tissue can be extremely pungent and malodorous, so removing nonviable tissue is beneficial to controlling odor. Only loose necrotic tissue should be removed by sharp debridement; it should only be performed by a clinician trained in sharp debridement and only if the process is not painful to the patient (Seaman,

2006). Surgical debridement of these wounds should be avoided because of the risk of bleeding (Wilson, 2005). However, when extensive necrotic tissue is present or the size of the fungating wound affects quality of life, surgical debridement (i.e., debulking) may be warranted if it is compatible with the patient's palliative goals of care (Seaman, 2006). As discussed in Chapter 17, mechanical debridement is not recommended because of the tendency for wounds to bleed and because of the pain that is triggered by wet-to-dry dressings.

Conservative debridement (e.g., with autolysis or enzymes) is preferred. Hydrogel dressings are a gentle method of debridement because they soften the necrotic tissue (see Plates 52–54) and facilitate its separation from the wound bed (Young, 1997) (see Chapters 17 and 18 for further discussion of debridement and contraindications). These dressings have the additional benefit of providing a soothing effect and providing pain control. Realistically, the malignant cutaneous wound is quite exudative, however, so a hydrogel dressing (a dressing designed to donate, not absorb, moisture) often is inappropriate. Absorptive dressings (polysaccharide beads, sodium-impregnated gauze, starch copolymer beads, alginates, hydrofibers) are most appropriate and can be combined with superabsorbent dressings to increase the absorptive capacity of the dressing and extend the time between dressing changes.

Charcoal Dressings. Charcoal dressings can reduce odor by filtering out the chemicals that cause the odor and by absorbing bacteria (Naylor, 2002); these dressings do not address contributing factors such as odor-causing bacteria. Odor with each dressing change will continue. Therefore carbon dressings are typically used as an adjunctive method of odor reduction along with treatments such as topical antimicrobials that address the cause of bacterial overload.

As an outer covering, charcoal-impregnated dressings can be used either as a primary dressing (when the wound is not exudative) or as a secondary dressing (over a primary absorptive dressing) to suppress odor. These dressings are changed when they become moist (moisture inactivates the charcoal) and when the charcoal is saturated so that it is no longer effective. Charcoal dressings are effective only when they are "sealed" around all four edges so that odor is forced to pass through the charcoal filter. Because some wounds are so irregularly shaped and the topography is so varied, securing the charcoal dressing may be too difficult to attain. Charcoal dressings may require changes ranging from daily to every 2 or 3 days depending on the extent of the odor. Charcoal dressings combined with an antimicrobial are available and serve the dual purpose of reducing bioburden and odor.

Collect and Contain Exudate

High levels of exudate from the malignant cutaneous wound are the result of abnormal capillary permeability within the wound (due to disorganized tumor vasculature), secretion of vascular permeability factor by tumor cells, and autolysis of necrotic tissue by bacterial proteases (Draper, 2005). The surrounding tissue of a malignant or fungating wound often is edematous such that even a small ulcer or nodule can produce prolific amounts of exudate. In addition to topical antimicrobials, interventions that aid in exudate control include (1) absorptive atraumatic dressings and (2) containment devices.

Moderately or highly exudative wounds require dressings that are capable of absorbing high volumes of exudate. Moderate to large amounts of exudate can be contained with semipermeable foam dressings and alginates. Very heavily exudative wounds may require a superabsorbent pad in conjunction with an alginate dressing, a hydrofiber dressing, or maltodextrin powder (see product formulary in Table 18-2). If further protection of the wound bed is necessary to control pain, a contact-layer dressing can be used to line the wound. Two-layer permeable vented dressings also may be used. With these dressings, the perforated nonadherent layer protects the wound surface and permits passage of exudate to an absorbent and permeable layer (Chrisman, 2015; Grocott, 1999).

Dressing change frequency is primarily a function of the volume of exudate produced, the volume of necrotic tissue present, and the patient's hydration status and activity level. As with other wounds, dressings for malignant or fungating wounds should be changed when exudate is pooling over intact skin or when "strikethrough" occurs. Ideally, dressings should not require changing more often than once per day.

Wound drainage pouches are available from most ostomy manufacturers. These pouches are indicated when the volume of exudate produced exceeds the capabilities of the dressings. Pouching should be considered when dressings must be changed more often than two to three times daily, when the skin begins to show early signs of damage, when the patient's ability to ambulate is hampered, or when odor is uncontrolled. These products have various desirable features, such as attached skin barriers, flexible adhesive surfaces, and an access window over the wound site. Many wound pouches also have an attached tubular drain spout that facilitates connecting the pouch to a drainage container so that the fluid does not pool over the wound site or over fill the pouch, a common source of leakage. Chapter 38 describes various techniques for pouching the draining wound.

Negative pressure wound therapy (NPWT) devices have been reported in palliative wound care to contain exudate, control odor, and decrease the number of painful dressing changes (Alvarez et al, 2007; Ford-Dunn, 2006). However, reimbursement for these devices when used in the palliative care wound is seldom approved and therefore not affordable. Manufacturer's recommendations for use of NPWT in *malignant* wounds should be carefully reviewed before use in palliative wounds. More information regarding the use of NPWT can be found in Chapter 21.

EVALUATION

Reviewing wound management decisions regularly is essential because the condition of any wound is dynamic, especially in palliative care (Chaplin, 2000). Toward this end, care is targeted to the areas of most concern to the patient and family while maximizing the effects of the intervention (Benbow, 2008). It is useful to begin the assessment by asking the patient what aspects of the wound or wound care interventions are of greatest concern. It may be surprising to learn that dressing changes as often as two to three times daily do not upset the patient as much as the odor from the wound or the constant drainage.

CLINICAL CONSULT

A: Wound consult ordered to the home of an 88-year-old female who is in hospice and accepting of dying, but has a large metastatic fungating cutaneous wound over the right breast. The family—a daughter, son-in-law, and granddaughter—are caring for the patient in her home. The wound measures 10 X 6 cm, cauliflower appearance of mixed gray/yellow and white exudative tissue. The surrounding skin has MARSI with skin stripping. Currently dressings are being changed twice daily to control odor and exudate and the family is using gauze and ABD pads with microporous tape. The patient and family acknowledge the dressing changes are extremely painful.
D: Patient with a fungating malignant wound at end of life.
P: Goals for this patient and family are to contain odor and exudate and reduce pain at the site.
I: (1) Apply topical mixture of lidocaine 2.5% and prilocaine 2.5% to wound, cover with nonadherent pad solution 30 minutes prior to dressing change. (2) Rinse off wound with NS or hypochlorous solution and dab very lightly to dry. (3) Apply no-sting skin sealant to entire periwound skin. (4) Sprinkle crushed metronidazole over wound surface to reduce anaerobic bacteria load and control odor. (5) Apply nonadherent silicone-based wound liner. (6) Cover with alginate or hydrofiber dressings to contain exudate. (7) Place super absorbent wound dressing over alginate/hydrofiber. (8) Secure with tubular stockinette applied around chest if patient is able to raise both arms; may need to use "Montgomery straps" to secure dressings if stockinette not feasible.
E: Consider adding charcoal cover dressing over super absorbent wound dressing if odor continues to permeate. Change dressings once per day if exudate saturating cover dressing; goal is to change dressing every other day. The hospice team notified of the change in plan of care and will reconsult if new plan fails to improve comfort for patient and family.

SUMMARY

The American Academy of Hospice and Palliative Medicine (AAHPM, 2008) position statement maintains that all seriously ill patients who have symptoms that are difficult to treat or who face challenging decisions about goals of care should have access to palliative care consultation and/or hospice. Efforts to enhance quality of life should be offered alongside curative and or restorative medical care, with palliative care a fundamental component of excellent medical care and not an alternative after other approaches have been pursued.

The potential skin complications associated with palliative wounds are amenable to the application of wound-healing principles. As with other chronic wounds, the goals for these types of wounds range from healing to palliation and symptom management.

Practitioners must advocate for changes in policy, regulations, and reimbursement guidelines that may limit palliative wound care practice (Ferris et al, 2007). Furthermore, the wound care community should highlight nonclosure endpoints for wound care, such as wound stabilization and improvement (Alvarez, 2005).

REFERENCES

Alexander SJ: An intense and unforgettable experience: the lived experience of malignant wounds from the perspectives of patients, caregivers and nurses, *Int Wound J* 7(6):456–465, 2010.

Alvarez OM: Editorial message, *Wounds* 17(4), 2005.

Alvarez OM, Kalinski C, Nusbaum J, et al: Incorporating wound healing strategies to improve palliation (symptom management) in patients with chronic wounds, *J Palliat Med* 10(5):1161–1189, 2007.

Alvarez OM, Meehan M, Ennis W, et al: Chronic wounds: palliative management for the frail population—Part II–III, *Wounds* 14(Suppl 8):S5–S27, 2002.

American Academy of Hospice and Palliative Medicine (AAHPM): *Position statement on access to palliative care and hospice,* Glenview, IL, 2008, AAHPM.

Ashfield T: The use of topical opioids to relieve pressure ulcer pain, *Nurs Stand* 19(45):90–92, 2005.

Back IN, Finlay I: Analgesic effects of topical opioids on painful skin ulcers, *J Pain Symptom Manage* 10(7):493, 1995.

Ballas SK: Treatment of painful sickle cell leg ulcers with topical opioids, *Blood* 99:1096, 2002.

Bauer C, Gerlach MA: Care of metastatic skin lesions, *J Wound Ostomy Continence Nurs* 27(4):247–251, 2000.

Beldon P: Managing skin changes at life's end, *Wound Essentials* 6:76–79, 2011.

Benbow M: Exuding wounds, *J Commun Nurs* 22(11):20, 23–24, 26, 2008.

Brink P, Smith TF, Linkewich B: Factors associated with pressure ulcers in palliative home care, *J Palliat Med* 9(6):1369–1375, 2006.

British Columbia Cancer Agency: *Cancer management guidelines: supportive care: chronic ulcerating malignant skin lesions; care of malignant wounds,* May 2011. http://www.bccancer.bc.ca/HPI/CancerManagementGuidelines/SupportiveCare/Chronic UlceratingMalignantSkinLesions/default.htm. Accessed March 1, 2015.

Chaplin J: Pressure sore risk assessment in palliative care, *J Tissue Viability* 10(1):27–31, 2000.

Chaplin J: Wound management in palliative care, *Nurs Stand* 19(1):39–42, 2004.

Chaplin J, McGill M: Pressure sore prevention, *Palliative Care Today* 8(3):38–39, 1999.

Chrisman CA: Care of chronic wounds in palliative care and end-of life patients, *Int Wound J* 7(4):214–235, 2010.

Collier M: The assessment of patients with malignant fungating wounds: a holistic approach, part 1, *Nurs Times* 93(44):1–4, 1997.

da Costa Santos CM, de Mattos Pimenta CA, Nobre MR: A systematic review of topical treatments to control the odor of malignant fungating wounds, *J Pain Symptom Manage* 39(6):1065–1076, 2010.

Dahlin, C: *National Consensus Project for Quality Palliative Care: clinical practice guidelines for quality palliative care,* ed 3, 2013. http://www.nationalconsensusproject.org/guidelines_download2.aspx. Accessed June 25, 2015.

Draper C: The management of malodour and exudates in fungating wounds, *Br J Nurs* 14(11):S4–S12, 2005.

Eisenberger A, Zeleznik J: Care planning for pressure ulcers in hospice. The team effect, *Palliat Support Care* 2:283–289, 2004.

Emmons KR, Lachman VD: Palliative wound care: a concept analysis, *J Wound Ostomy Continence Nurs* 37(6):639–644, 2010.

Evans E, Gray M: Do topical analgesics reduce pain associated with wound dressing changes or debridement of chronic wounds? *J Wound Ostomy Continence Nurs* 32(5):287–290, 2005.

Ferris FD, Al Khateib AA, Fromantin I, et al: Palliative wound care: managing chronic wounds across life's continuum: a consensus statement from the International Palliative Wound Care Initiative, *J Palliat Med* 10(1):37–39, 2007.

Finlay IG, Bowszyc J, Ramlau C, et al: The effect of topical 0.75% metronidazole gel on malodorous cutaneous ulcers, *J Pain Symptom Manage* 11(3):158–162, 1996.

Fletcher J: Malodorous wounds, assessment and management, *Wound Essent* 3:14–17, 2008.

Ford-Dunn S: Use of vacuum assisted closure therapy in the palliation of a malignant wound, *Palliat Med* 20:477–478, 2006.

Galvin J: An audit of pressure ulcer incidence in a palliative care setting, *Int J Palliat Nurs* 8(5):214–221, 2002.

Gerlach MA: Wound care issues in the patient with cancer, *Nurs Clin North Am* 40(2):295–323, 2005.

Grocott P: The management of fungating malignant wounds, *J Wound Care* 8(5):232–234, 1999.

Grocott P: Care of patients with fungating malignant wounds, *Nurs Stand* 21(24):57–58, 60, 2007, 62 passim.

Hampton S: Malodorous fungating wounds: how dressings alleviate symptoms, *Br J Community Nurs* 13(6):S31–S32, S34, 2008, S36 passim.

Henoch I, Gustaffson M: Pressure ulcers in palliative care: development of a hospice pressure ulcer risk assessment scale, *Int J Palliat Nurs* 9(11):474–484, 2003.

Hughes RG, Bakos AD, O'Mara A, et al: Palliative wound are at the end of life, *Home Health Care Manag Pract* 17(3):196–202, 2005.

Kalinski C, Schnepf M, Laboy D, et al: Effectiveness of a topical formulation containing metronidazole for wound odor and exudate control, *Wounds* 17:84–90, 2005.

Krouse RS: Palliative care for cancer patients: an interdisciplinary approach, *Cancer Chemother Rev* 3(4):152–160, 2008.

Liao S, Arnold RM: Wound care in advanced illness: application of palliative care principles, *J Palliat Med* 10(5):1159–1160, 2007.

Maund M: Use of an ionic sheet hydrogel dressing on fungating wounds: two case studies, *J Wound Care* 17(2):65–68, 2008.

McGill M, Chaplin J: Pressure ulcer prevention in palliative care 1: results of a UK survey, *Int J Palliat Nurs* 8(3):110–119, 2002.

Moore S: Cutaneous metastatic breast cancer, *Clin J Oncol Nurs* 6(5):255–260, 2002.

National Pressure Ulcer Advisory Panel (NPUAP), European Pressure Ulcer Advisory Panel (EPUAP), Pan Pacific Pressure Injury Alliance: *Prevention and treatment of pressure ulcers: clinical practice guideline*. In Haesler E, editor: Perth, Australia, 2014, Cambridge Media.

National Quality Forum (NQF): *A national framework and preferred practices for palliative and hospice care*, 2006. http://www.qualityforum.org/Publications/2006/12/A_National_Framework_and_Preferred_Practices_for_Palliative_and_Hospice_Care_Quality.aspx. Accessed March 10, 2015.

Naylor W: *Part 1: symptom control in the management of fungating wounds*, 2002. http://www.worldwidewounds.com/2002/march/Naylor/Symptom-Control-Fungating-Wounds.html. Accessed March 10, 2015.

Naylor WA: A guide to wound management in palliative care, *Int J Palliat Nurs* 11(11):572–579, 2005.

Piggin C: Malodorous fungating wounds: uncertain concepts underlying the management of social isolation, *Int J Palliat Nurs* 9(5):216–221, 2003.

Recka K, Montagnini M, Vitale CA: Management of bleeding associated with malignant wounds, *J Palliat Med* 15(8):952–954, 2012.

Reifsnyder J, Magee HS: Development of pressure ulcers in patients receiving home hospice care, *Wounds* 17(4):74–79, 2005.

Resnick B: Differentiating programs versus philosophies of care: palliative care and hospice are not equal, *Geriatr Nurs* 33(6):427–429, 2012.

Richards A, Lelechi TJ, Hennessy W, et al: Risk factors and wound management for palliative care patients, *J Hospice Palliat Nurs* 9(4):179–181, 2007.

Schim SM, Cullen B: Wound care at the end of life, *Nurs Clin North Am* 40(2):281–294, 2005.

Seaman S: Management of malignant fungating wounds in advanced cancer, *Semin Oncol Nurs* 22(3):185–193, 2006.

Sibbald RG, Krasner DL, Lutz JB: SCALE: Skin changes at life's end: final consensus statement, *Adv Skin Wound Care* 23(5):225–236, 2010.

Stanley KJ, Sawrun D, Treantafilos M: Ethical issues and clinical expertise at the end of life, *Nurs Clin North Am* 43(2):259–275, 2008.

Stephen-Haynes J: An overview of caring for those with palliative wounds, *Br J Community Nurs* 13(12):S2–S4, 2008.

Tice M: Wound care in the face of life-limiting illness, *Home Health Nurse* 24(2):115–118, 2006.

Tippett A: Wounds at the end of life, *Wounds* 17(4):91–98, 2005.

Walding M: Pressure area care and the management of fungating wounds. In Faull C, Carter Y, Daniels L, editors: *Handbook of palliative care*, ed 2, Oxford, 2005, Blackwell.

West D: A palliative approach to the management of malodour from malignant fungating tumours, *Int J Palliat Nurs* 13(3):137–142, 2007.

Westwood R: The principles behind end of life care and the implications for patients' skin, *J Clin Nursing* 28(3):58–64, 2014.

White R, Cutting K: *Modern exudate management: a review of wound treatments*, 2006. http://www.worldwidewounds.com/2006/september/White/Modern-Exudate-Mgt.html. Accessed June 25, 2015.

Williams C: Management of fungating wounds, *Br J Community Nurs* 2(9):423, 1997.

Wilson V: Assessment and management of fungating wounds: a review, *Br J Community Nurs* 10(3):S28–S34, 2005.

Woo KY, Krasner DL, Kennedy B, et al: Palliative wound care management strategies for palliative patients and their circles of care. *Advances in Skin & Wound Care* 28(3):130–140, 2015.

World Health Organization (WHO): *WHO definition of palliative care*, 2008. http://www.who.int/cancer/palliative/definition/en. Accessed June 25, 2015.

Zeppetella G, Paul J, Ribeiro MD: Analgesic efficacy of morphine applied topically to painful ulcers, *J Pain Symptom Manage* 25:555–558, 2003.

Zeppetella G, Ribeiro MD: Morphine in intrasite gel applied topically to painful ulcers, *J Pain Symptom Manage* 29:118–119, 2005.

38

Management of Draining Wounds and Fistulas

Ruth A. Bryant and Michelle Best

OBJECTIVES

1. Identify medical conditions associated with fistula formation.
2. Distinguish between a draining wound and a fistula, and distinguish between an enteric fistula and an enteroatmospheric fistula.
3. List three complications that contribute to mortality from fistulas.
4. Identify proper terminology of a fistula according to involved structures.
5. Describe three ways to classify fistulas.
6. List the risk factors for postoperative fistula development and for irradiation-induced fistulas.
7. Identify the six objectives of medical management for the patient with a fistula.
8. List factors known to correlate with spontaneous closure and known to impede spontaneous closure of fistula tracts.
9. Describe surgical procedures commonly used to close or bypass fistula tracts.
10. List eight nursing management goals for the patient with a fistula.
11. Describe four essential assessments that guide the management of the patient with a fistula.
12. Explain the role of four different types of skin barriers and their indications for use.
13. Identify features to be considered when selecting a fistula pouching system.
14. Briefly describe the "bridging" technique and identify indications for its use.
15. Identify options for odor control in a wound managed with dressings and in a wound managed with pouching.
16. Describe the role of negative pressure wound therapy (NPWT) and closed wound suction in the management of enterocutaneous and enteratmospheric fistulae.

The presence of a draining wound or fistula can be a frustrating and disheartening experience for the patient and family because it typically represents a major complication. It can also be a difficult experience for caregivers. However, management can be quite rewarding when effluent is successfully contained, odor is controlled, the patient is comfortable, and realistic resolution is attained. Management for this patient population requires astute assessment skills, knowledge of pathophysiology, competent technical skills, diligent follow-up, persistence, and knowledge of management alternatives.

Fistula management is more than skin protection and containment. In this chapter the pathophysiology of fistula formation, the medical and surgical aspects of managing a patient with a fistula, and the nursing management (i.e., skin protection, odor control, containment techniques) of the patient with a fistula will be presented. The techniques discussed in this chapter also are applicable to other types of wounds and drain sites that are not adequately contained by dressings.

EPIDEMIOLOGY AND ETIOLOGY

Gastrointestinal (GI) fistulas are serious complications associated with high morbidity, high mortality (5% to 20%), extended hospital stays, and increased costs (Dudrick and Panait, 2011; Kassis and Makary, 2008). Mortality rates increase to as high as 40% when the fistula occurs in middle of an open abdominal wound (Marinis et al, 2013). Malnutrition, sepsis, and electrolyte imbalance are the predominate causes of death. Fistulas develop in a wide array of complex patient conditions and often are concentrated in large medical centers. Frequency data (i.e., incidence and prevalence) therefore tend to be skewed and difficult to interpret. Factors affecting the prognosis of the patient with a fistula, however, are well known, although largely based on expert opinion and case series.

Causative factors and conditions for fistula formation include unintended operative injury to the intestine; disruption of an anastomotic leak; technical difficulties with anastomosis; abscess at the site of the anastomosis; and coexisting disease such as inflammatory bowel disease, cancer, or diverticulitis

(Dudrick and Panait, 2011). The following are risk factors that increase the likelihood of fistula formation when these medical conditions are present: severe malnutrition, sepsis, hypotension, vasopressor therapy, and steroid therapy. Enterocutaneous fistulas develop either spontaneously or postoperatively. In many reports, 75% to 85% of enterocutaneous fistulas are iatrogenic, occur postoperatively, and represent a leak in the anastomosis (Nussbaum and Fischer, 2006). Ischemia; tension; poor surgical technique; extensive lysis of adhesives; inadequate bowel prep such as with emergency surgery or trauma surgery; and preexisting conditions such as morbid obesity, systemic hypotension, local sepsis, and prior radiation therapy contribute to the risk of anastomotic complications (Kassis and Makary, 2008; Pfeifer et al, 2011). Maykel and Fischer (2003) advocate specific prevention strategies when faced with emergency surgery: provide adequate intravenous fluids, ensure adequate circulatory support, keep the patient warm, and provide appropriately timed broad-spectrum antibiotics. In addition, when surgery is planned, they consider adequate nutritional preparation to be the most important step in preventing an anastomotic breakdown. The patients at highest risk for an anastomotic breakdown are the severely malnourished patients as manifested by a hydrated serum albumin level less than 3 g/dl and weight loss of 10% to 15% over a 4- to 6-month period (Kassis and Makary, 2008).

Approximately 25% of fistulas are acquired, that is, they develop spontaneously and are associated with an intrinsic intestinal disease (cancer, radiation, diverticulitis, inflammatory bowel disease, appendicitis) or external trauma. Spontaneous fistulas are generally resistant to spontaneous closure. Patients who have been treated for a pelvic malignancy are particularly vulnerable to fistula formation because of radiation damage to the rectum, anal canal, and gynecologic organs (Saclarides, 2002; Tran and Thorson, 2008). Irradiation triggers occlusive vasculitis, fibrosis, and impaired collagen synthesis, a process termed *radiation-induced endarteritis.* Because the endarteritis persists, complications may develop immediately after radiation (within 6 months) or years later (as much as 30 years), although the majority will develop within 1 to 5 years (Pfeifer et al, 2011). Additional risk factors for irradiation-induced fistulas include coexisting processes such as atherosclerosis, hypertension, diabetes mellitus, advanced age, cigarette smoking, pelvic inflammatory disease, and previous pelvic surgery. Pelvic radiation doses exceeding 5000 cGy increase the incidence of bowel injury (Hollington et al, 2004; Saclarides, 2002; Tran and Thorson, 2008).

The three most common and highly significant complications associated with fistulas are sepsis, malnutrition, and fluid and electrolyte imbalance (Berry and Fischer, 1996). The loss of hypertonic protein-rich fistula effluent contributes to fluid and electrolyte depletion and malnutrition because of the loss of sodium bicarbonate and amino acids (Nussbaum and Fischer, 2006). Sepsis occurs as a result of abscess formation and compromised immune response due to poor nutritional status (Makhdoom et al, 2000). Uncontrolled sepsis and coexisting malnutrition are primarily responsible for the mortality in patients with enterocutaneous fistulas (Hollington et al, 2004; Nussbaum and Fischer, 2006; Yaner and Yaner, 2011).

TERMINOLOGY

Definitions

Fistula is a Latin word meaning "pipe" or "flute." A fistula is an abnormal passage between two or more epithelialized surfaces so that a communication tract develops from one hollow organ to another hollow organ or to the external environment allowing the loss of nutrients, fluids, and/or secretions (Dudrik and Panait, 2011) (Figures 38-1 and 38-2). An enterocutaneous fistula communicates specifically between the lumen of the GI tract and the skin. A fistula that develops in the base of an open abdominal wound bed is referred to as an *enteroatmospheric fistula* (EAF) (Figure 38-3) (Marinis et al, 2013).

It is important to distinguish between a fistula and a drain site or draining wound. Not all wounds that drain are fistulas. The term *draining wound* may refer to a surgical site that is draining, a tube site that is draining, or a puncture site (e.g., paracentesis, needle-guided intervention). Drain tubes may be placed either surgically or by interventional radiology to drain a pocket of fluid (e.g., abscess or seroma). For example, a drain tube, such as a Penrose, sump catheter, or Jackson Pratt, may be placed in a surgical incision or through a stab wound to facilitate drainage of pooled fluid. A draining wound, surgically placed drain site, or wound dehiscence should not be misinterpreted as a fistula.

Classification

Several methods are used to classify fistulas. These classification schemes are useful in predicting the morbidity rate, mortality rate, and potential for spontaneous closure (Wong et al, 2004).

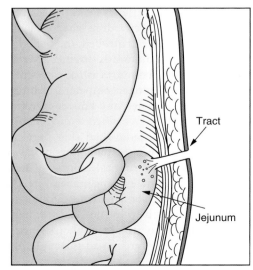

FIGURE 38-1 Simple enterocutaneous fistula.

FIGURE 38-2 Complex type 1 fistula with associated abscess.

FIGURE 38-3 Complex type 2 fistula with multiple openings associated with large abdominal wall defect.

BOX 38-1 Classification of Fistulas by Complexity

Simple
- Short, direct tract
- No associated abscess
- No other organ involvement

Complex
- Type 1
  - Associated with abscess
  - Multiple organ involvement
- Type 2 (also known as enteroatmospheric fistula or EAF)
  - Opens into base of disrupted wound

TABLE 38-1 Fistula Terminology

From	To	Name	Internal/External
Pancreas	Colon	Pancreatico-colonic	Internal
Jejunum	Rectum	Jejunorectal	External
Intestine	Skin	Enterocutaneous	External
Intestine	Colon	Enterocolonic	Internal
Intestine	Bladder	Enterovesical	Internal
Intestine	Vagina	Enterovaginal	External
Intestine	Wound bed or surface	Enteroatmospheric	External
Colon	Skin	Colocutaneous	External
Colon	Colon	Colocolonic	Internal
Colon	Bladder	Colovesical	Internal
Rectum	Vagina	Rectovaginal	External
Bladder	Skin	Vesicocutaneous	External
Bladder	Vagina	Vesicovaginal	External

Modified from Irrgang S, Bryant R: Management of the enterocutaneous fistula, *J Enterostomal Ther* 11:211–228, 1984.

From an anatomic perspective, the fistula may be simple or complex (Box 38-1). The simple fistula has a short, direct tract; no abscess; and no other organ involved, whereas the complex fistula is associated with an abscess, has multiple organ involvement, or may open into the base of a wound. As previously stated, the fistula that opens into the base of an open abdominal wound is known as the *EAF*, which requires specific and unique management techniques.

A fistula may be classified according to location. The internal fistula exists between internal structures, whereas the external fistula communicates between an internal organ and the skin, vagina, or rectum. This classification system is more specific in that the site of origin and site of termination are identified. Examples of such terminology are listed in Table 38-1.

A fistula may be classified according to volume of output (Table 38-2). A high-output fistula is most commonly defined as producing more than 500 ml per 24 hours, a moderate-output fistula is associated with output of 200 to 500 ml per 24 hours, and a low-output fistula produces less than 200 ml per 24 hours (Maykel and Fischer, 2003; Nussbaum and Fischer, 2006). The frequencies of sepsis, malnutrition, and fluid and electrolyte imbalance are directly related to fistula output. Fistula output is a direct reflection of the fistula's site of origin. Distal large-bowel fistulas typically have low output (<200 ml per 24 hours), whereas most proximal small-bowel fistulas are considered high output because they may produce from 1000 to as much as 3000 ml per 24 hours, at least initially. The high-output fistula is associated with severe malnutrition, significant fluid and electrolyte disturbance, higher morbidity and mortality rates, and lower spontaneous closure rate (Kassis and Makary, 2008; Wong et al, 2004). However, regardless of volume of output, the EAF will not close spontaneously and requires surgical intervention (Marinis et al, 2013; Whelan and Ivatury, 2011).

TABLE 38-2 Fistula Classification

	Designation	Characteristics
Location	Internal	Tract contained within body
	External	Tract exits through skin or wound bed
Involved structures	Colon	Colon
	Entero-	Small bowel
	Vesico-	Bladder
	Vaginal	Vagina
	Cutaneous	Skin
	Recto-	Rectum
Volume	High output	>500 ml per 24 hours
	Moderate output	200 to 500 ml per 24 hours
	Low output	<200 ml per 24 hours

Modified from Boarini J, Bryant RA, Irrgang SJ: Fistula management, *Semin Oncol Nurs* 2(4):287–292, 1986.

MANIFESTATIONS

Fever and abdominal pain are the initial indicators of a possible fistula (Nussbaum and Fischer, 2006). The passage of GI secretions or urine through an unintentional opening onto the skin heralds the development of a cutaneous fistula. Manifestations of a fistula exiting through the vagina (i.e., rectovaginal or vesicovaginal) include passage of gas, feces, purulent material, or urine through the vagina and discharge that is extremely malodorous. Irradiation-induced rectovaginal fistulas often are preceded by diarrhea, passage of mucus and blood rectally, a sensation of rectal pressure, and a constant urge to defecate (Saclarides, 2002). An initial manifestation of a fistula between the intestinal tract and the urinary bladder (e.g., colovesical fistula) is the passage of gas or stool-stained urine through the urethra.

MEDICAL MANAGEMENT

The desired endpoint of the medical management of a fistula is spontaneous closure. Approximately 19% to 40% of all fistulas will close spontaneously with conservative medical management, but only when sepsis is controlled and nutrition support is adequate and appropriate (Kassis and Makary, 2008). Of the fistulas that do heal spontaneously, 80% to 90% do so within 5 weeks, provided the patient is adequately nourished (Kassis and Makary, 2008; Maykel and Fischer, 2003). Factors known to correlate with spontaneous fistula closure include absence of sepsis, adequate nutritional support, low output, and classification as a postoperative fistula (Campos et al, 1999; Nussbaum and Fischer, 2006).

Approximately 90% of simple type 1 fistulas close spontaneously, whereas the complex type 2 fistulas (EAF) will always require some type of surgical intervention to achieve closure (Shecter, 2011; Wong et al, 2004).

Achievement of the medical management goals requires patience, astute assessment skills, and the cooperation of many health care specialists. Medical management can be divided into nonsurgical treatment and surgical treatment. A comprehensive and effective interdisciplinary and multidisciplinary team approach is vital to achieve closure and reduce mortality and morbidity.

Nonsurgical Treatment

The nonsurgical treatment of fistulas requires a comprehensive plan of care with attention to six specific objectives.

Objective 1: Fluid and Electrolyte Replacement. From 5 to 9 L of fluid rich in sodium, potassium, chloride, and bicarbonate is secreted into the GI tract daily. The loss of fluid and electrolytes that accompanies the presentation of a high-output fistula may result in hypovolemia and circulatory failure. Such blood volume imbalances must be corrected before initiating nutritional support or definition of the fistula tract. Adequate tissue perfusion and urine output must be maintained. Potential electrolyte imbalances should be anticipated and can be inferred from an understanding of the usual electrolyte composition of GI secretions. Electrolyte replacement can also be guided by measuring the electrolyte composition of the fistula output and serum (Schecter, 2011).

Objective 2: Control of Infection. Sepsis is the major cause of death in patients with enteric fistulas. The bacteria proliferate rapidly in the poorly vascularized tissue typically surrounding a fistula tract (Kassis and Makary, 2008). Pooling of bowel contents as a result of the dehiscence of a suture line precipitates localized and then diffuse abdominal pain, ileus, fever, and, ultimately, septic shock. The presence of systemic or local sepsis must be evaluated, typically with computed tomographic scanning or ultrasound. Effective drainage can be accomplished by use of percutaneous radiographic techniques or surgery. The specific approach depends on abscess location, patient status, and available resources. Surgical laparotomy for control of sepsis should be limited to proximal diversion and drainage of the abscess. Definitive repair of the fistula is undertaken at a later time only after inflammation has receded and nutrition is restored. Abscess contents should be cultured (aerobic and anaerobic) and Gram stained to identify the causative organisms and sensitivities. Organisms are most commonly of bowel origin: coliform, *Bacteroides*, and enterococci. Staphylococci also may be present. Antibiotics are only appropriate in the presence of an infection and in conjunction with adequate drainage of the abscess (Wong et al, 2004).

Objective 3: Control of Fistula Output and Skin Protection. Drainage of intestinal contents onto the skin will result in epidermal erosion and pain within only a few hours. Aggressive skin protection is essential and should be initiated at once. This is discussed specifically in the "Nursing Management" section.

Intestinal output must be minimized. Conventional methods for achieving this goal are giving the patient nothing by mouth (NPO) and administering proton pump inhibitors (H_2 antagonists or PPIs) and medications to slow intestinal transit. NPO status decreases luminal contents, GI stimulation, and pancreaticobiliary secretion. Administering PPIs reduces stress ulcerations and decreases gastric, biliary, and pancreatic secretions. The dose is titrated to achieve a fistula output less than 1 L per day and effluent pH greater than 6 (Bleier and Hedrick, 2010). Despite reducing GI secretions, H_2 receptors have not been shown to speed closure of the enterocutaneous fistula (Maykel and Fischer, 2003). Medications that slow intestinal transit are the priority in reducing fistula output (Table 38-3). Of these, loperamide is the most effective and should be taken 30 minutes before meals when the patient is eating (Bleier and Hedrick, 2010).

Octreotide may be used as an adjunct when other medications have failed. It is a synthetic analog of somatostatin, which is a naturally occurring hormone present throughout the body. More than two thirds of somatostatin is derived from the GI tract, especially the distal portion of the stomach, duodenum, jejunum, and pancreas. In the presence of fat, protein, and carbohydrates with a meal, somatostatin secretion significantly increases. Somatostatin release is inhibited by the release of acetylcholine from cholinergic neurons (Nussbaum and Fischer, 2006). It has extensive, well-known biologic effects that include inhibition of gastric, biliary, pancreatic, and salivary secretions and reduced GI motility, gastric emptying, and gallbladder emptying. When used in combination with total parenteral nutrition (TPN), a synergistic effect on reduced GI secretions can be expected. The short half-life of 1 to 2 minutes requires that somatostatin be administered through continuous intravenous infusion (250 mcg/hr). The analog octreotide has a half-life of almost 2 hours, so it can be administered three times daily subcutaneously (300 mcg/day).

Results from available prospective controlled studies and randomized controlled studies of octreotide have been mixed. The most encouraging results of octreotide are seen with postoperative, high-output, small-bowel fistulas in which fluid-, electrolyte-, and protein-store depletion is prevented. Fistula output reductions of 40% to 90% after 48 hours and reduced time to closure (50 days to 5–10 days) have been reported (Fagniez and Yahchouchy, 1999; Hesse et al, 2001; Schecter, 2011). These medications are less effective with fistulas associated with intrinsic bowel diseases, such as ulcerative colitis or Crohn's disease (Hild et al, 1986; Schecter, 2011). Somatostatin or octreotide administration should be stopped if fistula output does not decrease in the first 48 hours of treatment or if no response is seen after 2 to 3 weeks of treatment, respectively. Octreotide should be used with caution due to reports of villous atrophy, interruption of intestinal adaptation, acute cholecystitis, and inhibition of growth hormone thereby potentially inhibiting immune function (Maykel and Fischer, 2003; Schecter, 2011).

Objective 4: Nutritional Support. Malnutrition is a significant complication experienced by most patients with a fistula. Several factors contribute to the fistula patient's poor nutritional status. Often the patient is malnourished before the fistula develops. Additional factors contributing to negative nitrogen balance include reduced protein intake, inefficient nutrient use, excessive losses of protein-rich fluids (especially from pancreatic and proximal jejunal fistulas), and muscle protein breakdown (hypercatabolism) that occurs with sepsis. Daily small-bowel secretions contain as much as 75 g of protein (12 g of nitrogen); desquamated cells; and pancreatic, biliary tract, small-bowel, and gastric secretions, all of which are normally reabsorbed by the bowel (Yaner and Yaner, 2011).

Adequate nutritional support is achieved when the patient is maintained in a state of positive nitrogen balance and receives adequate vitamin and trace mineral replacement. The amount of calories and protein required will depend on the patient's preexisting status, sepsis, and fistula output. Nutritional recommendations for calories and protein are provided in Table 38-4.

It is important to initiate nutritional support without delay because lean body mass is lost at a rate of 300 to 900 g per 24 hours depending on the degree of stress (Maykel and Fischer, 2003). Trace elements (e.g., copper, zinc, magnesium), multivitamins, and vitamins (B, C, K) must be supplemented (Maykel and Fischer, 2003; Wong et al, 2004). González-Pinto and Gónzález (2001) recommend twice the recommended daily allowance (RDA) for vitamins and trace minerals and up to 10 times the RDA for vitamin C.

The route of nutritional support is contingent upon the patient's ability to ingest sufficient quantities, the location of the fistula tract, the absorptive capacity of the bowel mucosa, and the patient's tolerance. At first, TPN is often initiated in the second or third day of fistula management. This is often associated with a decreased fistula output (by as much as 30%

TABLE 38-3 Antimotility Medications for High-Output Fistulas

Medication	Dose
Loperamide	Up to 4 mg four times daily
Diphenoxylate	2.5 to 5 mg up to four times daily
Tincture of opium	0.3 to 1.0 ml up to four times daily
Codeine	15 to 100 mg up to four times daily
Paregoric	5 to 10 ml two to four times daily
Proton pump inhibitors	Dosage varies by agent
Octreotide	50 to 500 micrograms (µg) subcutaneously up to three times daily

(Bleier JIS and Hedrick T, 2010.)

TABLE 38-4	Nutritional Recommendations in the Patient with a Fistula		
	Baseline	**Low Output**	**High Output**
Calories (carbohydrates and fat)*	20 kcal/kg/24 hour	25 to 30 kcal/kg/24 hours	Up to two times daily overall daily requirements
Proteins	0.8 to 1.0 g/kg 24 hours	1.5 to 2 g/kg/24 hours	2 to 2.5 times baseline protein requirements

*No more than 30% of daily caloric needs should be provided as lipids.
(Bleier JIS and Hedrick T, 2010.)

to 50%), as well as modification of the composition of GI and pancreatic sections (Yaner and Yaner, 2011). Unfortunately, there are serious complications associated with TPN, such as bacterial translocation, access site infections, and metabolic disorders. The oral route of nutritional support is appropriate for colonic fistulas, whereas the preferred route for distal ileal fistulas is enteral nutrition accompanied by simultaneous "bowel rest." This may not be feasible in the presence of feeding intolerance, inability to access the GI tract, or high fistula output, all of which may require TPN to improve spontaneous closure rates (Schecter, 2011). In general, TPN is indicated for patients with duodenal, pancreatic, or jejunoileal fistulas (Yaner and Yaner, 2011).

Enteral nutrition is the preferred route of nutritional support in recognition that even small amounts will maintain the normal structural, immunologic, and hormonal integrity of the GI tract and prevent translocation of bacteria. However, enteral nutrition requires approximately 4 feet of small intestine between the ligament of Treitz and the fistula orifice (Dudrick et al, 1999; Knechtges and Zimmermann, 2009; Maykel and Fischer, 2003). When the GI tract is functional and the patient is cooperative, enteral nutrition may also be achieved when fistulas are located in the most proximal bowel by placing the feeding tube distal to the fistula orifice (Yaner and Yaner, 2011). Many types of enteral solutions are available, and a dietitian should be consulted to recommend the most appropriate solution and administration procedure so that GI intolerance (e.g., diarrhea, abdominal distention) can be avoided.

Objective 5: Definition of Fistula Tract. After the patient is stabilized (fluid and electrolytes balanced and infection controlled), the fistula must be examined to ascertain (1) the origin of the fistula tract; (2) the condition of adjacent bowel; (3) the presence of additional abscess pockets; and (4) the presence of distal obstruction or bowel discontinuity. Water-soluble contrast agents (e.g., Renografin, Hypaque, Gastrografin) are preferred to visualize the fistula tract and are administered through the fistula orifice using a soft-tip catheter. A computed tomographic scan is indicated only when the patient is not responding to conservative treatment. If other organs are involved, additional tests (e.g., cystoscopy or intravenous pyelogram) should be pursued (Wong et al, 2004).

Objective 6: Conservative Management. As already described, the majority of fistulas will heal spontaneously with

patience, time, and conservative management (positive nitrogen balance with nutritional support, sepsis-free state). The challenge is trying to shorten the time to spontaneous healing and increasing the number of fistulas that heal spontaneously.

Fistula closure is sometimes successful with the insertion of clotting substances into the fistula tract. The concept of using fibrin for anastomosis of tissue was first used for hemostasis in 1909 (Migaly and Rolandelli, 2006). Fibrin sealants (also referred to as *fibrin glue*) are composed of a concentrated allotment of fibrinogen/factor XIII/fibronectin and thrombin that congeals to form an insoluble fibrin clot when mixed with calcium chloride, a process that essentially replicates the last step of the coagulation cascade (Kassis and Makary, 2008; Tran and Thorson, 2008). The mechanism of action consists of fibrin glue providing a "matrix" for the influx of various cells and collagen formation (Buchanan et al, 2003).

Fibrin sealant products can be created from the patient's own plasma (autologous) or from human plasma that has been collected and pooled from many donors (heterologous) after screening and viral testing. The fibrin glue is applied endoscopically at the origin of the fistula to seal the fistula (Migaly and Rolandelli, 2006). Although fibrin sealant products appear to have a role in the management of low-output fistulas (e.g., perirectal), the role of fibrin glue relative to the complexity of the fistula and timing of the procedure has yet to be determined.

Surgical Treatment

Immediate surgery is imperative when (1) a septic focus has been identified; (2) uncontrolled hemorrhage has developed; (3) bowel necrosis has developed; or (4) an evisceration is present. However, closure of the fistula or excision of the fistula tract should *not* be attempted under these circumstances.

Surgical intervention to close the fistula will be required when impediments to spontaneous closure have been identified. Factors known to prevent spontaneous closure are listed in Box 38-2 (Nussbaum and Fischer, 2006). If any of these factors are present and closure of the fistula is the ultimate goal for the patient, surgical intervention will eventually be necessary. Surgical procedures may also be indicated for palliation.

The exact timing for surgical intervention is variable, depending on the patient's status. In general, operative interventions to close the fistula tract should be delayed until the patient is in a positive nitrogen balance and control of infection is established. Corrective surgery for a simple or complex type 1 fistula that continues to produce effluent is commonly undertaken within 4 to 6 weeks when the patient is nutritionally and metabolically stable and in a sepsis-free environment (Redden et al, 2013). However it is important that definitive surgery such as this be delayed until the abdominal wall is soft and supple; tissues should return to a normal soft, pliable state, particularly in the presence of irradiated tissue (Schecter, 2011; Wong et al, 2004).

Complex type 2 fistulas invariably require definitive surgery; however, the timing of surgery is not well defined. Nutritional status, metabolic status, and immunocompetence should be normalized, and the obliterative peritonitis and inflammation associated with chronic peritoneal contamination should be resolved (Marinis et al, 2013; Schecter, 2011; Wong et al, 2004). Judicious timing of surgery for complex type 2 fistulas is warranted. The most often reported timing ranges from 3 to 6 months.

The surgical interventions available for management of enterocutaneous fistulas will either divert the GI tract (without resection of the fistula) or provide definitive resection of the fistula tract (Nussbaum and Fischer, 2006). Factors such as location, size, and cause of the fistula; the patient's overall status; and the presence of irradiated tissue will influence the approach selected. However, Maykel and Fischer (2003) warn that the best results occur with resection of the fistula and end-to-end anastomosis and that other surgical procedures represent a compromise.

Diversion techniques divert the fecal stream away from the fistula site; removal of the fistula is not accomplished. Resection of the fistula is not always appropriate or possible in the presence of extensive or recurrent malignancy or when tissue perfusion is inadequate in the vicinity of the fistula (secondary to numerous surgical resections, scar formation, uncontrolled diabetes, or prior irradiation).

Diversion can be achieved by creating a stoma proximal to the fistula or by anastomosing (end to end or side to side) the two segments of bowel on both sides of the fistula (e.g., ileotransverse anastomosis when the fistula communicates with the right colon). This latter procedure may be referred to as an *intestinal bypass* in which the segment of bowel containing the fistula is completely isolated and separated from the fecal stream.

When closure of the fistula is the goal, resection will be necessary. The advantage of this technique is that the diseased tissue is removed. An end-to-end anastomosis of the intestine with resection of the fistula tract is performed. To protect the anastomosis, diversion of the fecal stream through a temporary stoma may be indicated. If the distal part of the rectum is not suitable for anastomosis or the anal sphincters are not competent, a permanent stoma with a Hartmann's pouch may be the safest procedure.

Enteric fistulas communicating with the urinary tract will always require diversion of the fecal stream proximal to the fistula site to prevent urinary tract infections and pyelonephritis.

NURSING MANAGEMENT

The occurrence of a fistula lengthens recovery time, whether closure is spontaneous or occurs with surgical repair. This section focuses on the technical management of the patient with a fistula. The principles and techniques presented are applicable to all types of draining wounds and drain sites. Principles are presented so that management can be tailored to achieve effective solutions. However, the care plan must also include detailed attention to patient and family needs, involvement, education, and emotional support.

Technically, the patient with a fistula is one of the most challenging patients encountered by wound and ostomy care providers. Critical thinking skills are necessary to synthesize assessment data, product knowledge (advantages, disadvantages, effectiveness, and guidelines for use), patient needs, and physiology into realistic goals. Principles of wound care and principles of ostomy management are applied to the management of these clinical problems. There is also an art involved in the techniques presented in this chapter.

Goals

Effective nursing management of the enterocutaneous fistula strives to achieve eight goals, as listed in Box 38-3. The primary goal of fistula management is containment of effluent.

By doing that, the remaining goals are often also achieved. Interventions to achieve the goals begin as soon as the patient is noted to have a fistula; they are not contingent upon medical diagnosis.

Four general principles should guide the care of the patient with a fistula (Rolstad and Wong, 2004):

1. Assess the pouching system and seal frequently; expect changes.
2. Build flexibility into the care plan.
3. Innovate, using the easiest, most practical approach first.
4. Recognize that care of the patient is frequently provided by inexperienced caregivers.

Assessment

The method selected to manage a fistula is guided by the assessment of the four key fistula characteristics outlined in Box 38-4 and described next. Because fistulas change in shape and contour over time, repeat assessment and monitoring are necessary. Modifications to the initial containment system are invariably necessary (Scardillo and Folkedahl, 1998; Wiltshire, 1996; Zwanziger, 1999).

Source. Initially, little information may be available regarding the origin of the fistula or the involved organs (if diagnostic studies have not yet been conducted). However, it may be possible to identify the probable origin of the fistula based on assessment of fistula output (volume, odor, consistency, composition) (Table 38-5). This information provides insight into the patient's risk for altered skin integrity and provides

---

BOX 38-4   Fistula Assessment and Documentation Guide

1. Source (e.g., small bowel, bladder, esophagus)
2. Characteristics of effluent
   a. Volume
   b. Odor? (If yes, describe)
   c. Consistency (e.g., liquid, semiformed, formed, gas)
   d. Composition
      I. Color (e.g., clear, yellow, green, brown)
      II. Active enzymes
      III. Extremes in pH
3. Topography and size
   a. Number of sites
   b. Location(s)
   c. Length and width of each (include patterns)
   d. Openings (e.g., below skin level, at skin level, above skin level)
   e. Proximity to bony prominences, scars, abdominal creases, incision, drain(s), stoma
   f. Muscle tone surrounding opening (e.g., firm, soft, flaccid)
   g. Contours at the fistula opening (e.g., flat, shallow depth [$<\frac{1}{16}$ inch], moderate depth [$\frac{1}{16}$ to $\frac{1}{4}$ inch], or deep [$>\frac{1}{4}$ inch])
4. Perifistular skin integrity at each location (e.g., intact, macerated, erythematous, denuded or eroded, ulcerated, infected)

---

decision points for selection of the management approach. For example, a fistula producing semiformed, odorous effluent likely is communicating with the left transverse or descending colon. Effluent from the transverse or descending colon will be less damaging to the skin than the output from the ileum. Therefore in this situation, the primary goals of nursing management will be containment of effluent and odor control.

Characteristics of Effluent. Characteristics of effluent that must be considered in fistula management include volume, odor, consistency, and composition. In general, the fistula with output volumes greater than 100 ml over 24 hours requires containment using a pouch or suction.

Odor is another factor when selecting a management method. The patient with a malodorous output of only 10 to 20 ml per 24 hours may require a pouching system, even if just to contain odor. Odor may originate from numerous sources, including exudate, necrotic or infected tissue, soiled dressings, dressing materials, and chemicals used during treatment.

Consistency of effluent is particularly important when pouching because it affects the type of drainage spout needed and subsequently the type of pouch selected. It also influences the need for additional skin barriers. Liquid effluent is much more corrosive than thick effluent and results in premature erosion of the skin barrier.

The color of effluent acts as an indicator of fistula source (see Table 38-5). In the presence of effluent with active enzymes or extremes in pH, the perifistular skin will require aggressive protection. However, all perifistular skin should be monitored and protected from moisture, even when effluent composition does not include active enzymes. Until radiographic studies are performed, the enzymatic and pH composition of the effluent can be inferred from the volume and consistency of the drainage.

Fistula Opening. The size of the fistula opening is determined by measuring the length and width in centimeters. A pattern is always useful because the fistula orifice is usually irregularly shaped. The pattern should be kept in the patient's room with supplies. The fistula opening may occur in a wound bed (the EAF) or directly on the skin surface.

Abdominal Topography. Assessment is performed with the patient in a supine and semi-Fowler's position. The cutaneous fistula locations are identified and documented. The area is assessed for the presence of irregular skin surfaces that are created by scars or creases. This assessment indicates how flexible the adhesive in contact with the skin must be and whether filling agents, such as skin barrier paste or strips, are needed to level irregular surfaces (see Plates 75 and 76). In addition, the number of cutaneous fistula openings, the location of each, and the proximity to a bony prominence or other obstacles (e.g., retention sutures or stoma) are assessed and documented. These characteristics will help to determine

TABLE 38-5   Characteristics of Gastrointestinal Secretions

Source	Secretions	pH	24-Hour Volume (cc)	Color	ELECTROLYTE CONCENTRATION			
					Na (mg)	K (mEq)	Cl (mg)	HCO₃ (mg)
Saliva	Ptyalin, maltase	6 to 7	1000 to 1200	Clear	20 to 80	16 to 23	24 to 44	20 to 60
Gastric juice	Pepsin, rennin (chymosin) lipase, hydrochloric acid	1 to 3.5	2000 to 3000	Clear/green	20 to 100	4 to 12	52 to 124	0
Pancreatic juice	Amylase, trypsin, chymotrypsin, lipase, sodium bicarbonate	8 to 8.3	700 to 1200	Clear/milky	120 to 150	2 to 7	54 to 95	70 to 110
Bile	Bile salts, phospholipids	7.8	500 to 700	Golden brown to greenish yellow	120 to 200	3 to 12	80 to 120	30 to 50
Duodenum, jejunum, ileum	Peptidase, trypsin, lipase, maltase, sucrase, lactase	7.8 to 8	2000 to 3000	Gold to dark gold	80 to 130	11 to 21	48 to 116	20 to 30
Colon		7.5 to 8.9	50 to 200	Brown	4	9	2	—

Cl, Chloride; *HCO₃,* bicarbonate; *Na,* sodium; *K,* potassium.

the size and shape of the adhesive surface needed to secure the sites but not impinge on the prominence or protrusion. If two cutaneous sites are too far apart to be pouched in one system, two pouches may be necessary.

Muscle tone in the area and skin contours should be assessed. Decreased abdominal muscle tone can be expected in the patient who lacks exercise or is overweight, in the elderly, and in the infant. Aging affects subcutaneous tissue support. Muscle tone may be characterized as firm, soft, or flaccid.

It is important to assess the level at which the fistula opening exits onto the skin. Contours of the skin surrounding the fistula opening may be classified as flat, shallow (<¹⁄₁₆ inch), moderate depth (¹⁄₁₆ to ¼ inch), or deep (>¼) (Rolstad and Boarini, 1996). The EAF requires assessment of both the fistula opening and the surrounding wound bed.

Protection of Perifistula Skin or Healing of Surrounding Wound Bed. Perifistular skin condition should be assessed and documented at each dressing or pouch change. Constant exposure of the epidermis to moisture, active enzymes, extremes in pH of fluids, and mechanical trauma frequently lead to breaks in skin integrity. Denudation of perifistular skin is a common complication in fistula patients and often is present when the patient is first seen with the fistula. Skin constantly bathed in fluid causes maceration, whereas effluent with enzymatic drainage or extremes in pH levels creates erythema and denuded or eroded perifistular skin. The perifistular skin may also develop an infection as a consequence

of moisture entrapment against the skin and antibiotic-precipitated changes in the normal skin flora. Candidiasis is a common secondary complication as depicted in Plate 16. Chapter 5 provides additional information to facilitate delineation of fungal infection from irritant, chemical, or contact dermatitis.

Although visual inspection of the skin is best, data can also be obtained from the nursing staff and patient to aid assessment. For example, when frequent dressing changes (every 4 hours) are reported, skin will deteriorate quickly as a result of moisture, chemical, and mechanical injury. Patient reports of burning or stinging sensations around the fistula or wound commonly indicate denudation of the epidermis.

The ideal management of the EAF is isolation of the effluent from the surrounding wound bed. However, this is not always possible. Various methods of effluent containment are described later in this chapter.

Planning and Implementation

Four key questions should be asked when planning the technical management of a fistula:
1. Is the output volume more than 100 ml in 24 hours?
2. Is odor a problem?
3. Is the fistula opening less than 3 inches?
4. Is an access cap needed?

Figure 38-4 shows an algorithm that incorporates these four questions to guide decision making for managing a fistula.

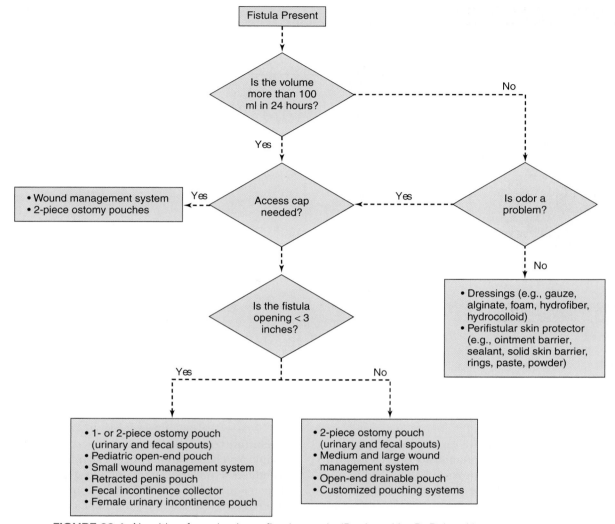

FIGURE 38-4 Algorithm for selecting a fistula pouch. (Designed by B. Rolstad.)

Fistulas can be managed with pouches, dressings, suction, or all three. When planning the specific fistula management approach, the four key questions and the goals that have been identified by the health care team and patient must be considered. In most situations, the priority goals are containment of effluent, odor control, and perifistular skin protection. Initially some goals may be compromised, such as ease of care, patient mobility, and cost containment because of the acuteness of the situation. This section presents nursing interventions that facilitate attainment of each goal for the nursing management of fistulas.

Skin Protection. The potential for skin breakdown (either perifistular in the cutaneous fistula or periwound in the EAF) is always present when a fistula exists. Preventive strategies should be implemented early and be accompanied by frequent monitoring. Strategies include atraumatic adhesive removal and protection of the skin from exposure to effluent. Dressings alone do not offer skin protection, so concurrent use of a skin barrier often is necessary. Skin barriers are

available in various forms (Figure 38-5). Table 38-6 summarizes the characteristics and indications of each type of skin barrier.

If pouching is selected as the management approach, pectin-based skin barriers usually are integrated into the pouching system during manufacturing. Additional pectin-based skin barriers may be required to caulk edges, fill creases, and/or add convexity. Skin protectants may also be used to protect the periwound and perifistula skin from effluent and adhesives. All of these products can be used alone or in conjunction with one another.

At times, skin barrier wafers and pastes need to be applied over an intact incision as part of the management system. This is done to secure the system and prevent leakage of effluent from the fistula onto the incision.

Skin barrier powders are used to absorb moisture from denuded skin and to create a dry surface. Adhesives or ointments then can be applied to the dry surface. Severely denuded skin may require the creation of an "artificial scab" with the skin barrier powder by alternating layers of the skin barrier powder and a skin sealant or skin cement. The pouching system then may be applied directly over the artificial scab. Applying either skin cement or spray adhesive to the artificial scab and pouch adhesive surface is often needed to enhance adherence. Skin barrier powders should not be confused with talc or cornstarch, which do not provide skin protection.

In nonpouching management approaches, petroleum-, dimethicone-, or zinc-based ointments are used to provide skin protection. These products are particularly useful for low-volume, odorless fistulas and usually are inexpensive. They are applied to perifistular skin, particularly the edges, and covered with dressings. Ointments are not intended for use under adhesives. Frequency of application is indicated on the product and may differ depending on the product formulation and use.

FIGURE 38-5 Examples of skin barriers: wafer, paste, ring, powder, sealant.

Containment of Effluent. Containment of effluent is accomplished with nonpouching and pouching approaches. The

TABLE 38-6   Guide to Use of Skin Barriers in Fistula Management

Type of Skin Barrier	Characteristics	Indications
Solid wafers (4 inch × 4 inch or 8 inch × 8 inch)	• Pectin-based wafers with adhesive surface • Available as wafers or rings • Have moist tack • Have varied flexibility • May be cut into wedges, rings, or strips • Have varied durability to effluent • Changed only when they loosen from perifistular edges or once every 7 days	• Provide skin protection, referred to as laying down a protective platform • Level irregular skin surfaces • Protect perifistular skin from effluent when dressings are used or skin is exposed • Gauze dressings are applied over the skin barrier wafer and taped to wafer rather to skin
Skin barrier rings	• Available in hydrocolloid and karaya formulations • Have moist tack • Have varied flexibility • Have varied durability to effluent • Hydrocolloid formulations • Recommended for fistula management	• Level irregular skin surfaces • Protect perifistular skin from effluent when dressings are used or skin is exposed
Paste (tube or strip)	• Commercial preparations contain alcohol, which can create burning sensation if skin is denuded • Extremely tacky; should be applied as thin bead and smoothed into place with damp gloved finger or tongue blade • Contains solvents; allow to dry briefly so that solvents can escape before other products are applied	• Level irregular skin surfaces • Protect exposed skin from effluent (i.e., with pouching) • Extend duration of solid-wafer barrier when pouching
Powder	• Must be used lightly; can be used in combination with sealants to create artificial scab • Residual powder alters adhesion	• Absorb moisture from superficial denudement before applying ointments or adhesives
Skin protectant	• Liquid, nonalcohol, and alcohol preparations • Nonalcohol skin protectants are indicated for use on denuded skin • Must be allowed to dry to permit solvents to dissipate • Available in various forms (wipes, gel, wands, roll-ons, pump spray)	• Can be used under adhesives to protect fragile skin during adhesive removal (i.e., skin stripping) • Improve adherence of adhesives to skin (particularly oily skin) • Protect perifistular and periwound skin from effluent or maceration when dressings are used • Used in combination with skin barrier powders; creates artificial scab

choice of effluent containment is influenced by volume of effluent, presence of odor, abdominal contours, and care setting.

Nonpouching options. Nonpouching options include dressings and barriers, drains, and suction techniques. The method chosen is greatly influenced by the volume of output.

Dressings and barriers. Nonpouching options are indicated when (1) fistula output is low (<100 ml per 24 hours); (2) odor is not present; and (3) skin contours or location of the fistula makes pouching impossible. Containment of effluent can be achieved with dressings intended for absorption, which include gauze (sponges or strip packing), alginates, foam, and combinations of dressings. Packing should be done only with dressing materials that can be retrieved from the wound. For example, a strip packing material may be gently packed into a low-volume drain site. A 2-inch tail of dressing material is left outside the wound and is used to retrieve the packing at dressing changes. Entrapment of effluent against the skin may cause maceration and breakdown; therefore skin barriers must be used in conjunction with the dressings to protect the skin (see Table 38-6).

If, despite best efforts, the skin becomes compromised or output volume exceeds 100 ml in 24 hours, dressings become less effective and more time intensive to manage. The application of additional dressings will not increase the absorbency of the dressing or lengthen the time between dressing changes. As a rule, a pouching system should be used when dressings must be changed more often than every 4 hours. Conversely, when a fistula site has low volume, a small pouching system may be used so that the patient does not have to change the pouch more than once every 7 days.

This approach provides convenience and protects the surrounding skin.

Vaginal fistula management options. Vaginal fistulas (Figure 38-6) occasionally develop secondary to pelvic irradiation or obstetric trauma; as a result the patient is incontinent of feces or urine through the vagina. The uncontrolled passage of feces or urine vaginally results in severe perivaginal skin denudation and discomfort. Aggressive nursing care is essential to prevent these complications.

Skin protection can be achieved with barrier ointments, pastes, and pads. Frequent dressing changes are necessary to prevent entrapment of caustic drainage contents against the skin. These options for vaginal fistulas are less than optimal because they are labor intensive, do not promote patient mobility, do not adequately contain the fecal contents, and fail to control odor. A female urinary incontinence pouch may be useful in these situations and may be connected to straight drainage. However, the difficult location and moist surface surrounding the vaginal orifice make application of an adhesive pouching system challenging.

Containment of vaginal drainage is challenging. One option that does not require adhesives is to create a vaginal drain device modified from the procedure initially described by Adrien (1983). A vaginal/menstrual cup can be inserted a short distance into the vagina to contain low-output fistula drainage. To allow continuous drainage of a higher fistula output, a cruciate incision can be made through a reusable vaginal cup, through which a catheter is threaded. Because the vaginal cup occludes the vagina, the drainage is either collected and contained by the cup or directed down the catheter.

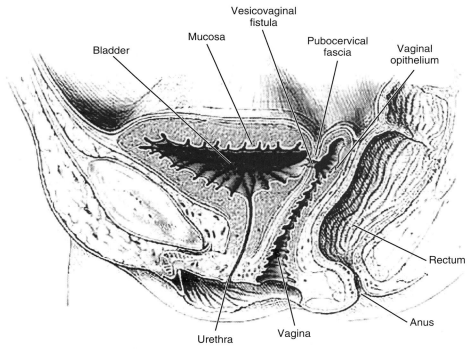

FIGURE 38-6 Vaginal fistula between vagina and bladder.

The discomfort to the patient created by such manipulation of the labia and vagina can be minimized by lubricating the device with lidocaine jelly (Xylocaine). Tubing is attached to the device to channel the fistula contents into a straight drainage collection bag. The drainage tubing can be anchored to the patient's inner thigh.

A vaginal drain device will remain in place effectively while the patient is reclining. As the patient becomes more ambulatory, the device may have a tendency to become dislodged; however, because the procedure is so easy, the patient can reinsert the vaginal cup as needed. Gentle irrigation of the tubing may be indicated if the tubing becomes occluded by fistula material. A vaginal drain device may be a temporary or permanent management technique depending on the patient's status.

Closed suction systems. Closed suction systems continue to be a viable, reliable, and cost-effective method for managing high-output fistulas, especially with EAF (Davis et al, 2000; Jones et al, 2003; Kordasiewicz, 2004). Catheters attached to low intermittent suction may be used when routine pouching is ineffective or overwhelmed by the volume of output (Beitz and Caldwell, 1998; Lange et al, 1989). However, suction does not provide complete containment of effluent; dressings and skin protection still are necessary. Effluent must be liquid for suction to be effective; thick or particulate drainage will occlude the catheter. The wound is cleansed, and a layer of saline-moistened gauze is placed in the wound bed. The catheter is laid in the wound and directed toward the bottom of the setup. Another layer of moist gauze may be applied over the catheter, and a large transparent dressing may be applied as a secondary dressing (Hollis and Reyna, 1985; Jeter et al, 1990). Skin barrier paste, strips, or rings are sometimes necessary to fill in irregular skin surfaces and to seal around the catheter as it exits from the transparent dressing. Suction tubing is then attached to the suction catheter and set at a low level of continuous suction. A Hemovac can provide the suction for short periods to increase the patient's mobility. This dressing usually is changed every 1 to 2 days.

A catheter that is inserted into the fistula tract will act as a foreign body and may interfere with healing and even increase fistula output (Welch, 1997). On the other hand, a catheter coiled in a defect above the orifice or in the open wound surrounding the fistula opening will not inhibit closure. Because firm tubes can injure fragile tissue, only soft, flexible suction catheters should be used with fistulas (Welch, 1997). Suction catheters should be considered a short-term intervention because of the limitations placed on patient mobility and the time-intensive nature of the care.

Negative pressure wound therapy. The evolution of the closed suction system is negative pressure wound therapy (NPWT). This technique has demonstrated clinical wound-healing benefits. The system incorporates a sponge and subatmospheric pressure, which results in reduced periwound edema and mechanical stretching of cells. Mechanical stretching of cells is believed to stimulate the wound repair process. Negative pressure wound therapy is used with an EAF to facilitate healing of the wound bed. However, NPWT should not be used over the fistula itself. Isolation of the fistulized bowel from the negative pressure system is critical. Thus it is appropriate only for the surrounding wound, as demonstrated in Plate 77. Further information about the application and use of NPWT is presented in Chapter 21.

Pouching system options and features. Volume and odor are the primary indications for pouching. Dressings are contraindicated when odor is problematic or the volume of effluent exceeds 100 ml in 24 hours. However, patients with low-volume, nonodorous output may choose a pouch for convenience. The pouch may be changed once per week and is less expensive than dressings.

Numerous techniques for managing fistulas have been reported in the literature (Boarini et al, 1986; Davis et al, 2000; Irrgang and Bryant, 1984; Jones et al, 2003; Kordasiewicz, 2004; O'Brien et al, 1998; Rolstad and Wong, 2004; Skingley, 1998; Smith, 1982, 1986). Ostomy pouches (fecal or urinary; adult or pediatric) can be used, as well as pouches specifically designed for managing complex wounds. Pouching preserves patient dignity by containing embarrassing odor and drainage. Pouching is an effective strategy for pain control because it requires less manipulation of the wound and protects the surrounding skin from painful denudement caused by caustic drainage. An effective pouching system also offers a sense of control to the nursing staff because effluent is contained and emptied at specific intervals. Pouch changes are scheduled at convenient times before leakage occurs. Intervening to prevent the embarrassment of odor and leaking dressings can protect a patient's dignity. A routine pouch change procedure and fistula pouching tips are listed in Boxes 38-5 and 38-6, respectively.

Historically, frequent modifications of skin barriers, adhesives, and/or pouches were required to effectively manage the

---

BOX 38-5 Sizable Pouch Change Procedure: Fistula

1. Assemble equipment: pouch with attached skin barrier, pattern, skin barrier strip, paste or ring, scissors, paper tape, closure clip, water, gauze, or tissue.
2. Prepare pouch.
   a. Trace pattern onto skin barrier surface of pouch.
   b. Cut skin barrier pouch to size of pattern.
   c. Remove protective backing(s) from pouch.
3. Remove and apply pouch.
   a. Remove pouch, using one hand to gently push skin away from adhesive.
   b. Discard pouch and save closure clip.
   c. Control any discharge with gauze or tissue.
   d. Clean skin with water and dry thoroughly.
   e. Apply paste, strip, or ring around fistula or stoma. Fill in any uneven skin surfaces with paste or skin barrier strips. Use damp finger or tongue blade to apply paste.
   f. Apply new pouch, centering wound site in opening.
   g. Tape edges of adhesive surface in picture frame effect with paper tape.
   h. Close bottom of pouch with clip.

1. Schedule the procedure, if possible, to allow education and participation from nursing staff and other caregivers.
2. Set up all equipment before starting procedure. Fistula function is unpredictable and may otherwise occur when adhesives are not completely set up.
3. Cut opening in pouch adhesive approximately ⅛ inch larger than fistula cutaneous opening.
4. Protect exposed periwound skin with skin barrier paste (see Plate 76).
5. Apertures much larger than actual fistula opening may be necessary with severe, deep depressions that create irregular skin surfaces.
6. Follow universal precautions with clean technique during procedures. Sterile products are an unnecessary expense and are not shown to control infection.
7. To remove adhesives from skin, gently roll off adherent material with dry gauze. Solvents may be used, but must be cleansed thoroughly from skin before adhesive application. Do not scrub or abrade skin. It may be necessary to leave small amounts of residual paste or cement on skin but should not hinder pouch adhesion.
8. Cleanse skin with tap water or commercially available skin cleanser and gauze. Cleansers will emulsify fecal material and are primarily indicated when fistula drainage is adherent to surrounding skin. Cleansers should be nongreasy and rinsed thoroughly; use on denuded skin is discouraged. Dry thoroughly.
9. Minimize pooling of corrosive effluent over skin barrier by angling tail of pouch off to reclining patient's side, or attach drainage tubing to enable continuous drainage.
10. Empty pouch when one third to half full. Encourage patient to monitor.

Knowledge of available features of products is essential to make appropriate choices. Features include adhesive skin barrier surface, pouch capacity, pouch material (film and outlet), and wound access (Box 38-7 and Figure 38-7).

Adhesive skin barrier surface. When the cutaneous opening is less than 3 inches, a one- or two-piece ostomy pouch may be used. For fistulas larger than 3 inches, commercially available wound management systems or modifications of larger pouches are warranted. In either case, the adhesive skin barrier surface must be large enough to accommodate the fistula opening and generally allow for 1 to 2 inches of adhesive contact around the fistula. The adhesive surface should be applied in such a fashion as to avoid obstacles in the perifistular skin area, such as a bony prominence or drain site. If this is not possible, a pouch with a smaller adhesive surface may be needed.

Conversely, a large amount of adhesive contact (over 4 to 5 inches) with the surrounding skin is generally not necessary and may be detrimental. Movement-induced skin changes under the adhesive surface will precipitate leakage and disruption of the pouch seal.

Pouching systems may have a starter hole for cutting the opening into irregular shapes or may be presized (e.g., for round, regular shapes). Although starter holes are convenient for cutting, they restrict the positioning of the opening in the adhesive because the opening includes the starter hole. In some situations, the opening may have to be covered with a skin barrier so that other locations on the adhesive may be cut to fit the size of the fistula.

A few pouches are available without an integrated skin barrier wafer. In these situations, the fistula pattern must be used to cut a hole in the skin barrier wafer and the pouch.

complicated fistula. Few alternatives were available to manage the fistula with a large cutaneous opening, irregular contours of the skin, and other unique situations. Materials used for pouches included garbage bags, colostomy irrigation sleeves, and sandwich bags. Today, manufactured wound management systems are designed for the difficult-to-manage site. Solid-wafer skin barriers with durable formulations that provide longer wear time are integrated into most pouching systems. Cutting surfaces of the skin barriers are available to manage a broad range of fistula opening sizes, ranging from the small opening of a starter hole to 9½ × 6 inches. However, it remains essential to fill irregular skin surfaces so that a flat, stable surface is attained for the pouching system.

Selecting a pouching system that supports the perifistular tissue and stabilizes soft skin may be necessary. In general, if the skin is soft or flaccid, a firm skin barrier adhesive and possibly a belt may be indicated. In contrast, firm skin surrounding the fistula site is best managed with a flexible, soft adhesive surface. Examples of soft, pliable materials include powder, skin barrier paste, wafers, strips, and rings. Methods for achieving firm support include firm rings, convexity in ostomy pouching systems, and belts.

Adhesive Surface
- Integrated skin barrier
- Size and shape of cutting surface
- Sizable versus presized adhesive surface
- Presence or absence of starter hole
- Degree of flexibility of skin barrier wafer

Pouch Capacity
- Volume (3- to 4-hour capacity preferred)

Pouch Material
- Odorproof or odor-resistant pouch film
- Transparent versus opaque film
- Fecal outlet (clamp closure)
- Spout for liquids (urinary outlet)
- Wide drain for viscous material
- Wide tubular outlet can be converted to open-end drain

Wound Access
- Two-piece pouch
- Access window on wound management system
- Wide tubular outlet can be converted to open-end drain

FIGURE 38-7 Examples of pouches. Note variety of sizes of the adhesive surface, outlet spouts, and access windows.

The skin barrier is then attached to the pouch, and the system is applied directly to the skin.

Pouch capacity. The capacity of the pouch is predetermined by the size of the adhesive surface; typically pouches with larger adhesive surfaces have larger pouch capacities. Generally, a pouch with the capacity to contain 3 to 4 hours' worth of effluent is recommended so that the risk of leakage is minimized. A smaller-capacity pouch may be used if the caregiver or patient is willing to empty the pouch more frequently or if the pouch can be connected to straight drainage. Small-volume, closed-end pouches may also be indicated for the patient with minimal malodorous output. This pouch can be changed and discarded once or twice per week.

Pouch outlet. Effluent consistency and volume dictate the best type of outlet spout for pouch management. Pouches are designed with either urinary (or liquid) outlets or fecal outlets (see Figure 38-7). The urinary outlet is indicated for liquid effluent. It is convenient because it may be connected to straight drainage. When a urinary pouch is used for fistula care, the antireflux mechanism will obstruct flow; therefore the antireflux mechanism must be pulled apart. Fecal outlets (or open-end drains) are appropriate for thick, mushy effluent and are secured with a clamp.

The two-piece ostomy system, fecal incontinence collectors, and wound management systems offer the benefit of having a urinary outlet that can be attached to a bedside bag. As the effluent thickens, the outlet can be trimmed off and secured with a clamp, transforming the pouch from a urinary to a fecal pouch without having to remove the pouch from the skin.

Two-piece high-output pouching systems are available that combine the desirable features of an ostomy system (e.g., presized adhesive surface and convexity) with outlets that can accommodate the varying consistency of effluent typical of a fistula.

Adaptations can be made to pouches to accommodate fistula consistency. For example, when formed output becomes liquid, urinary pouch–adapter latex drainage tubing can be attached to a fecal pouch. If the output begins to thicken or form particulate matter, wider respiratory tubing can be attached to the tail of an open-end drain (Box 38-8).

Wound access. At times, access to the fistula site may be desirable so that tubes can be advanced, the fistula can be assessed easily, or skin barrier pastes can be reinforced. Access to the site without disruption of the pouch adhesive can be achieved with a two-piece pouch or with a pouch that has an attached "access window." When such access features are not available or have an inadequate adhesive surface size, wide open-end drains can be used. Cuffing the pouch film back can facilitate limited access to the fistula site.

Pouch film. Urinary drainage equipment and some fecal pouches may be more odor resistant than odorproof. More frequent pouch changes may be necessary to prevent the odor from permeating the pouch film, or more aggressive odor management techniques (e.g., oral deodorizers) may be required. Pouching systems marketed as wound management systems are transparent to allow for visual inspection. Ostomy pouches adapted for fistula care provide choices in film color (transparent, opaque, beige tone).

BOX 38-8   Addition of Continuous Drainage Tube to Fecal Outlet Pouch

Equipment
- Fecal pouch or open-end drain
- Connector to fit tubing and bedside system
- Five inches of wide-lumen tubing or respiratory tubing
- Rubber band
- Bedside drainage system

Procedure
1. Cut desired size for fistula in skin barrier adhesive of fecal pouch or open-end drain.
2. Insert wide-lumen tubing or respiratory tubing into drain spout.
3. Working at adhesive surface, reach inside pouch and pull drain spout and tubing through opening cut in skin barrier adhesive.
4. Wrap rubber band securely around tubing to secure.
5. From bottom of pouch, pull tubing through so that outlet spout is in its normal location. Tail of pouch now is cuffed around tubing inside pouch.
6. Attach to bedside drainage system.

Note: If wide respiratory tubing is used, a condom catheter can be used to connect the pouch to bedside drainage.

Pouching system adaptations

Adhesives. Additional adhesive is available as cement, medical adhesive spray forms, and sheet forms. Cements and sprays are applied according to the manufacturer's instructions; most require time to become tacky. They are used to enhance the tack of an existing adhesive and to extend the adhesive surface on a pouch. Adhesives may also be warranted to improve the tack when several applications of skin barrier powder are required in the presence of severe denudation. Occasionally, liquid adhesive is used in combination with skin barrier powders to protect exposed skin from caustic effluent. This procedure is similar to the artificial scab discussed previously.

Because fistulas vary in size and shape and abdominal contours can be dramatic, large and unusually shaped pouch apertures may be necessary. Sheets of adhesives (or double-faced adhesive disks) can be used to increase the adhesive surface on a pouch. Box 38-9 describes the procedure for adding an adhesive sheet to a pouch.

Another option is simply to create a pouch (Box 38-10). The advantage to this technique is that it offers immediate skin protection and containment of affluent using readily available supplies. Although this is a temporary intervention, it allows the care provider time to design a management system and to obtain commercially available products with the desirable features identified in the plan of care.

Another method that can be used to acquire a large adhesive surface is to attach two open-end drainable pouches, a technique called *saddlebagging* (Figure 38-8). Pouch features that facilitate saddlebagging include no attached solid-wafer skin barrier, no floating collar, and no starter hole. A large

BOX 38-9   Procedure for Adding Adhesive Sheets to Enlarge Pouch Adhesive Surface

Equipment
- Pouch without floating collar
- Double-faced adhesive sheet or disk

Procedure
1. Remove protective paper from one side of adhesive sheet.
2. Attach this adhesive sheet adjacent to existing adhesive on pouch (edges may overlap slightly).
3. Trace desired opening size on protective paper, covering adhesive surface.
4. Cut to desired size.
5. Prepare solid-wafer skin barrier (usually 8 × 8 inches), attach to adhesive surface on pouch, and continue in usual fashion.

BOX 38-10   Procedure for Making Temporary Fistula Pouch

Equipment
- Plastic bag
- Skin barrier wafer
- Double-faced adhesive sheet or double-faced tape

Procedure
1. Remove protective paper from one side of adhesive sheet and apply to area of pouch where adhesive and barrier are intended to be (in absence of adhesive sheets, substitute with overlapping strips of double-sided tape).
2. Remove other side of adhesive sheet or tape.
3. Attach skin barrier wafer (top side toward exposed adhesive on pouch).
4. Cut barrier of pouch to desired size.
5. Remove skin barrier wafer protective paper backing.
6. Continue in usual fashion.

FIGURE 38-8 Saddlebagging technique in which two open-ended drainable pouches are connected along the adhesive surface to create a large adhesive surface.

BOX 38-11   Saddlebagging Technique

Equipment
- Two open-end drains (without floating collar or attached skin barrier or starter hole)
- Solid-wafer skin barrier (8 × 8 inches)
- Skin barrier paste

Procedure
1. Align pouches as final product is intended to appear on abdomen.
2. Peel protective backing away from adhesive along common edges of pouches approximately ½ to 1 inch.
3. Attach two pouches along this ½- to 1-inch margin only.
4. Trace pattern of wound onto new adhesive surface (combined pouch adhesive surfaces).
5. Cut out pouch opening; do not cut into "seam" created by combining pouches.
6. Trace pattern onto solid-wafer skin barrier and cut out.
7. Remove protective paper backing from pouch adhesive surface and attach to solid-wafer skin barrier.
8. Prepare skin as indicated by wound contours and continue pouching procedure.

Note: Both pouches will fill with drainage and will require emptying.

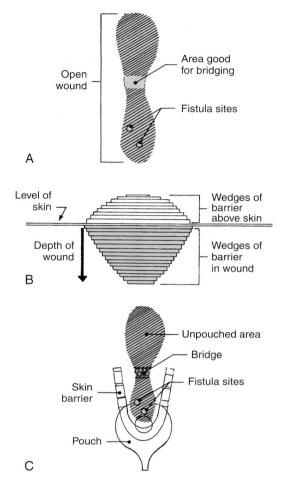

FIGURE 38-9 Bridging technique. **A,** Area of wound where fistula sites are located and identified can be separated from remainder of wound. **B,** Cross-sectional view of tapered skin barrier wedges used to fill wound defect and to extend slightly above level of skin. **C,** Demonstration of how a pouch is applied over a bridge and fistula, leaving the area of the wound that is not draining available for more appropriate wound care.

solid-wafer skin barrier is then attached to the new combined adhesive surface, and the pouch is prepared in the usual fashion. Box 38-11 describes the saddlebagging technique.

Bridging technique. The bridging technique is a procedure that can be used to isolate the EAF from the wound bed. This technique may be achieved in a variety of ways. Solid-wafer skin barriers or convex barrier rings can be applied in layers to isolate the fistula opening (Figure 38-9). A routine pouch or more complicated pouching system can then be applied over this to contain the fistula and allow independent wound care and fistula management. This procedure is very successful when used in conjunction with NPWT (see Plate 77). Box 38-12 describes the steps involved in the bridging technique.

Catheter Ports. When a catheter or tube is in place at a fistula site, leakage onto perifistular skin may occur. A pouching system with an attached catheter port may be used to collect the drainage. A catheter port is a nipple-shaped device that attaches to the external wall of a pouch. The catheter is disconnected, threaded through the pouch opening on the adhesive surface, and then threaded through the catheter port itself so that the catheter can be reconnected to drainage. The pouch is then secured to the skin in the usual fashion. Detailed instructions from the manufacturer accompany the catheter port. With this technique, drainage around the catheter is collected in the pouch while the catheter continues to drain by suction or gravity (see Figure 39-16).

Silicone molding. A silicone molding technique using a dental mold material to fashion an impression of the fistula opening and perifistular area in an attempt to create a smooth surface to which a pouch can be applied has been

reported (Strega, 1977). When used, this procedure was reserved for the recessed fistula located in an open wound or the fistula surrounded by numerous irregular skin surfaces. However, the silicone mold procedure is less commonly used now because of the advances in wound management products (Box 38-13).

Trough procedure. When fistulas are contained within the depressions of a wound such that a routine pouching system fails, the trough procedure may be useful. With this procedure, one or several strips of a transparent dressing are used to occlude the wound and trap effluent in the wound depression (Figure 38-10). A small opening is made in the transparent dressing at the most dependent aspect of the wound, and an ostomy pouch is applied over this opening. No pattern is required.

To enhance adherence of the transparent dressing to the skin peripheral to the fistula or wound (and to protect

---

BOX 38-12   Bridging Technique

1. Assess wound and determine most appropriate location for "bridge." Be sure all sites from which drainage is produced are included on the side of wound to be pouched. For simplification of bridging procedure, areas that are narrower or shallower should be selected.
2. Apply layered wedges of solid-wafer skin barrier and paste to create bridge. Wedges must be custom cut to fit dimensions of wound at that level; usually the bottom wedge is narrowest because the deepest part of the wound typically is the narrowest area. Each successive wedge is a little wider until the skin barrier wafer wedges reach skin level.
3. Continue to layer solid-wafer barrier wedges above skin level, using progressively smaller and narrower wedges (to create pressure dressing effect).
4. Apply solid-wafer skin barrier to cover newly created bridge and extend onto intact skin. Paste may be needed to smooth "seams."
5. Continue with routine or complex pouching procedure as indicated.

Note: Skin barrier paste, adhesive spray, or cement can be used between wedges but is not routinely necessary.

BOX 38-13   Silicone Mold

Equipment
- Emesis basin
- Tongue blade
- Dow Corning medical grade elastomer 382
- Dow Corning Catalyst M and eye dropper
- Red rubber catheter (optional)
- Skin barrier paste
- Ostomy pouch with belt
- Adhesives (silicone spray necessary to adhere to mold)

Preparation
1. Cleanse skin around wound with water and pat dry.
2. Pour elastomer into dry emesis basin; usually 1 or 1½ ounces is enough for moderate-sized cast.
3. Add 10 to 12 drops of Catalyst M for each ounce of elastomer.
4. Stir thoroughly with tongue blade.
5. If necessary, place suction catheter into fistula opening to contain drainage while cast is setting.
6. When elastomer has slightly thickened, pour on patient's abdomen or in open wound around fistula orifice to a ¼-inch thickness.
7. Allow mold to harden for 3 to 5 minutes in wound.
8. Gently lift mold out of wound.
9. Remove catheter from cast.
10. Trim edges of cast to form gently rounded surfaces.
11. Trim fistula opening in cast to be sure opening is adequate.

Application
1. Spread smooth layer of skin barrier paste on back of mold using tongue blade and allow to set until it is firm to touch. *Note:* Silicone spray can be applied to the surface to increase adherence with or without the paste.
2. Place mold into wound. Seal edges with skin barrier paste.
3. Apply tape on all edges of mold.
4. Apply ostomy pouch with belt tabs over opening in the mold; attach belt.

---

perifistular skin), strips of a solid-wafer skin barrier should be applied. Directions for the trough procedure are given in Box 38-14.

Odor control. In general, odor control measures are indicated any time the patient and/or family perceive an odor to be objectionable, even if the odor seems almost imperceptible.

The method of odor control depends on whether dressings or pouches are being used. Gauze dressings do not control odor; therefore charcoal-impregnated dressings may be needed over the gauze dressings. However, charcoal becomes inactivated with moisture, so these dressings should not come into contact with wound drainage. Charcoal dressings are most cost effective with low-output fistulas, for which the dressings remain intact for 24 to 48 hours. These dressings are effective only when all edges of the dressing are taped to the skin. Pouches provide odor control. However, when the pouch is emptied, odor may be noticeable. Therefore odor management must be a component of the care plan.

Odor is best controlled by use of a pouch to contain the effluent. A pouch may be the preferred management technique simply to contain the odor, regardless of the volume of output. Although most pouches have an odorproof film, the film's ability to contain odor varies. For example, many urinary pouches and urinary drainable systems are not odorproof and may become saturated with odor quickly.

To control odor, (1) dispose of soiled linens and dressings from the room promptly; (2) use care in emptying pouches to prevent splashing effluent on the patient or on linens; (3) cleanse the tail of drainable fecal pouches after emptying; and (4) use deodorants appropriately.

Deodorants can be taken internally (orally) or used externally (in the pouch or as a room spray). Internal deodorants are available in tablet form but are generally discouraged in the presence of a pathologic condition such as a fistula. External deodorants are available in liquids, powders, and tablets and are placed in the pouch after each emptying. Room deodorants are particularly useful when emptying the pouch, changing the pouch, or changing dressings. The room deodorant selected should eliminate rather than mask odor. With the many types of deodorants now available, patients, families, and caregivers should not have to tolerate the odor that often accompanies fistulas.

Patient Comfort. Areas to address to promote patient comfort include prevention and early treatment of perifistular skin irritation, pain control, and education to decrease anxiety. Leaking pouches, wet dressings on the skin, and odor in the patient's room all negatively affect morale. Medicating the patient before dressing or pouch changes may be indicated.

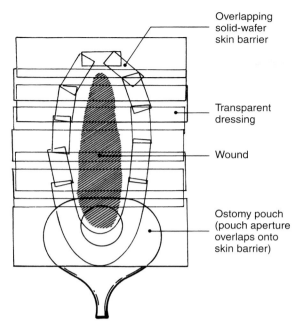

Overlapping
solid-wafer
skin barrier

Transparent
dressing

Wound

Ostomy pouch
(pouch aperture
overlaps onto
skin barrier)

FIGURE 38-10 Trough procedure. Note overlapping skin barrier wafers and transparent dressing strips. Pouch opening must overlap onto skin barrier wafer at inferior aspect of wound.

BOX 38-14 Trough Procedure

1. Prepare skin and fill irregular skin surface as usual.
2. Apply overlapping strips of solid-wafer barrier along wound edges.
3. Apply skin barrier paste to smooth "seams" (between barrier edges and along skin edges). *Note:* Inferior aspect of wound should be bordered with a solid piece of barrier instead of overlapping strips to prevent leakage.
4. Cut strips of transparent dressing wide enough to cover wound and skin barrier strips. Calculate length of strips so that strips overlap intact skin with 1- to 2-inch margins.
5. Reserve one strip of transparent dressing to be applied to the most inferior aspect of wound.
6. Attach a drainable pouch (can be urinary or fecal) to this one strip of transparent dressing.
7. Cut hole in pouch or transparent dressing adhesive surface so that it is lower than inferior wound margins (should clear wound edges to provide adequate drainage).
8. Beginning at top of wound, apply transparent dressing in overlapping strips.
9. Attach final strip of transparent dressing (with attached pouch) so that bottom of pouch opening is secured onto skin barrier wafer.

Factors contributing to skin irritation include damp dressings, presence of caustic effluent in contact with the skin, and frequent tape application and removal. When selecting and evaluating a management technique, interventions appropriate to prevent unnecessary patient discomfort should be considered.

Accurate Measurement of Effluent. Accurate measurement of effluent from a fistula or drain site is critical to the success of fluid and electrolyte resuscitation and nutritional support. As the patient becomes stabilized, accurate measurement of the effluent is less important. Pouching offers the most objective method for monitoring output, and suction is accurate only if the effluent does not leak around the catheters. Dressings can provide an estimate of volume if the dressings are weighed; however, this method is time consuming, messy, and inconsistent from caregiver to caregiver.

Patient Mobility. Consideration for optimizing the patient's activity should be of paramount importance when a fistula management method is being selected. Restrictions on physical activity predispose the patient to physical complications such as pneumonia, pressure ulcers, and thrombophlebitis, as well as to psychosocial complications such as depression and withdrawal. Because limitations on a patient's physical activity are sometimes necessary when suction or dressings are used to contain effluent, these interventions should be used only on a temporary basis. Pouches are less likely to restrict mobility. When wound suction is used with the fistula, temporary suction can be maintained with the portable devices such as a Hemovac, or the suction tubing can be clamped off for a very short period. The drawback, however, to clamping off the suction tubing is that effluent production by the fistula is unpredictable and can occur suddenly, causing the pouching system adhesive to fail.

Ease of Use. Complex patient situations may necessitate unique pouching systems that may be expensive and labor intensive. These unique adaptations often set up hurdles to the successful participation of care providers. These complicated systems increase the chance of error in application and the time required of the caregiver. Therefore management may be complex initially and require the expertise of a certified ostomy care nurse (COCN). As care progresses, the method of pouching should be simplified as much as possible to a more user-friendly system so that its care can be delegated. Several conveniences are available and should be considered as long as effectiveness is not compromised (Box 38-15).

BOX 38-15 User-Friendly Considerations in Fistula Care

1. Use presized pouch rather than sizable pouch whenever possible.
2. Avoid suction when pouching is effective.
3. Fill skin defects with strip paste rather than tube paste in patients with manual dexterity problems.
4. Use pouching systems with convexity rather than creating convexity with layers of skin barriers.
5. Use one-piece rather than two-piece pouches.
6. Select equipment that is easy to access in the community. Mail order of products is a convenience as long as orders are placed before patient's supplies are depleted.

Cost Containment. Accountable, appropriate fistula management requires selection of treatment options that are cost effective. For example, a fistula pouch with a wound access window is more costly than a sizable ostomy pouch, which probably would yield the same wear time. However, if use of a pouch with an access window prolongs wear time by providing access for wound care and paste application, it may be the most cost-effective option, even if the pouch is changed every other day. Cost containment implies attention not only to products and materials, but also to labor and time.

Evaluation

Accomplishment of Goals. The nurse should take time to reflect on the eight nursing management goals and evaluate how well they have been accomplished. Can steps be omitted? Is the skin intact? Is odor controlled? As the fistula stabilizes, the technical approach should be reevaluated and simplified as much as possible. One management system is seldom effective from the onset of the fistula until closure. For example, one fistula may be managed over its course with a pouch, dressings, suction, or all three. While the patient is in the hospital, suction may be a workable option; however, mobility is compromised, and plans for home care are complicated. Therefore developing a pouching system that does not require suction would be an important simplification. Similarly, using products that are difficult to obtain is a complicating step and may be expensive. Planning to use an effective system that is easy and readily available is essential to facilitate the delivery of care.

Making Changes. It is important to expect changes in fistula care and to modify interventions as needed. Seldom will the first pouch applied to a complex fistula be effective. Generally, modifications are necessary in the pouch pattern, size of adhesive surface, and use of skin barrier pastes or wafer strips. Changes are best made one at a time so that the effect of each modification can be accurately assessed. The addition of a belt may be warranted to add security to the pouch system, particularly on obese patients or when the perifistular skin is mobile.

The nurse must provide close monitoring for the duration of the fistula, regardless of the health care setting. An inquisitive, analytic approach will facilitate identifying steps to improve the duration of the pouching system. For example, if the pouch leaks, is the leak between the skin and the barrier or between the barrier and the pouch? Is the pouch being emptied when it is one third to one half full to prevent overfilling?

CLINICAL CONSULT

A: A 36-year-old female patient is seen in consult for recommendations to address three enterocutaneous fistulas on her abdomen from metastatic cervical cancer. The patient is terminal and wants to go home for her last days. However, in spite of multiple trials of pouching the draining abdominal fistulas, all attempts have failed and leaked caustic stool on her skin.
D: Metastatic cervical cancer resulting in small-bowel fistula.
P: The goal for care is to contain the fistula output and protect her skin. After meeting the patient, a simple plan was developed that the patient and caregivers could handle: apply extra thin skin barrier wafer to encircle fistulas. She then will layer super-absorbent nonadherent dressings over the site to wick effluent away from her skin and secure them in place with mesh panties. A full incontinence brief can be used over the mesh panties to add security for drainage containment.
I: The patient is given the dressings and instructions for care. She is instructed she can shower off the dressings at any time.
E: The patient will be given phone contact for any added support or changes in plan of care.

SUMMARY

Successful management of a patient with a fistula requires close monitoring and a plan of care that addresses the technical, educational, and emotional needs of the patient. Care often crosses many health care settings with varying levels of expertise in the unique containment and skin protection vital to the patient's well-being. In these situations, special arrangements must be made for appropriate follow-up of these complex patients.

REFERENCES

Adrien L: Vaginal fistulas: adaptation of management method for patients with radiation damage, *J Enterostomal Ther* 10(6):229–230, 1983.

Beitz JM, Caldwell D: Abdominal wound with enterocutaneous fistula: a case study, *J Wound Ostomy Continence Nurs* 25(2):102–106, 1998.

Berry SM, Fischer JE: Classification and pathophysiology of enterocutaneous fistulas, *Surg Clin North Am* 76(5):1009–1018, 1996.

Bleier JI, Hedrick T: Metabolic support of the enterocutaneous fistula patient, *Clin Colon Rectal Surg* 23(3):142–148, 2010.

Boarini J, Bryant RA, Irrgang SJ: Fistula management, *Semin Oncol Nurs* 2(4):287–292, 1986.

Buchanan GN, Bartram CI, Phillips RK, et al: Efficacy of fibrin sealant in the management of complex anal fistula: a prospective trial, *Dis Colon Rectum* 46(9):1167–1174, 2003.

Campos AC, Andrade DF, Campos GM, et al: A multivariate model to determine prognostic factors in gastrointestinal fistulas, *J Am Coll Surg* 188(5):483–490, 1999.

Davis M, Dere K, Hadley G: Options for managing an open wound with draining enterocutaneous fistula, *J Wound Ostomy Continence Nurs* 27(2):118–123, 2000.

Dudrick SJ, Maharaj AR, McKelvey AA: Artificial nutritional support in patients with gastrointestinal fistulas, *World J Surg* 23(6):570–576, 1999.

Dudrick SJ, Panait L: Metabolic consequences of patients with gastrointestinal fistulas, *Eur J Trauma Emerg Surg* 37(3):215–225, 2011.

Fagniez PL, Yahchouchy E: Use of somatostatin in the treatment of digestive fistulas. Pharmacoeconomic issues, *Digestion* 60(Suppl 3):65–70, 1999.

González-Pinto I, González EM: Optimizing the treatment of upper gastrointestinal fistula, *Gut* 49(Suppl 4):22–31, 2001.

Hesse U, Ysebaert D, de Hemptinne B: Role of somatostatin-14 and its analogues in the management of gastrointestinal fistulae: clinical data, *Gut* 49(Suppl 4):11–21, 2001.

Hild P, Dobroschke J, Henneking K, et al: Treatment of enterocutaneous fistulas and somatostatin, *Lancet* 2(8507): 626, 1986.

Hollington P, Mawdsley J, Lim W, et al: An 11-year experience of enterocutaneous fistulas, *Br J Surg* 91(12):1646–1651, 2004.

Hollis HW, Reyna TM: A practical approach to wound care in patients with complex enterocutaneous fistulas, *Surg Gynecol Obstet* 161(2):179–180, 1985.

Irrgang S, Bryant R: Management of the enterocutaneous fistula, *J Enterostomal Ther* 11:211–228, 1984.

Jeter KF, Tintte T, Chariker M: Managing draining wounds and fistulae: new and established methods. In Krasner D, editor: *Chronic wound care: a clinical source book for healthcare professionals*, King of Prussia, PA, 1990, Health Management, pp 240–246.

Jones EG, Harbit M, Anderson R: Management of an ileostomy and mucous fistula located in a dehisced wound in a patient with morbid obesity, *J Wound Ostomy Continence Nurs* 30(6):351–356, 2003.

Kassis ES, Makary MA: Enterocutaneous fistula. In Cameron JS, editor: *Current surgical therapy*, ed 9, St. Louis, MO, 2008, Mosby.

Knechtges P, Zimmermann EM: Intra-abdominal abscesses and fistulae. In Yamada T, Alpers DH, Laine L, et al, editors: *Textbook of gastroenterology*, vol II, ed 6, Philadelphia, 2015, Lippincott Williams & Wilkins.

Kordasiewicz LM: Abdominal wound with fistula and large amount of drainage status after incarcerated hernia repair, *J Wound Ostomy Continence Nurs* 31(3):150–152, 2004.

Lange MP, Thebo LM, Tiede SM, et al: Management of multiple enterocutaneous fistulas, *Heart Lung* 18(4):386–390, 1989.

Makhdoom ZA, Komar MJ, Still CD: Nutrition and enterocutaneous fistulas, *J Clin Gastroenterol* 31(3):195–204, 2000.

Marinis A, Gkiokas G, Argyra E, et al: "Enteroatmospheric fistulae"—gastrointestinal openings in the open abdomen: a review and recent proposal of a surgical technique, *Scand J Surg* 102(2):61–68, 2013.

Maykel JA, Fischer JE: Current management of intestinal fistulas. In Cameron JL, editor: *Advances in surgery*, St. Louis, MO, 2003, Mosby.

Migaly J, Rolandelli RH: Suturing stapling and tissue adhesives. In Yeo CJ, Dempsey DT, Klein AS, et al, editors: *Shackelford's surgery of the alimentary tract*, ed 6, St. Louis, MO, 2006, Saunders.

Nussbaum MS, Fischer DR: Gastric, duodenal and small intestinal fistulas. In Yeo CJ, Dempsey DT, Klein AS, et al, editors: *Shackelford's surgery of the alimentary tract*, ed 6, St. Louis, MO, 2006, Saunders.

O'Brien B, Landis-Erdman J, Erwin-Toth P: Nursing management of multiple enterocutaneous fistulae located in the center of a large open abdominal wound: a case study, *Ostomy Wound Manage* 44(1):20–24, 1998.

Pfeifer J, Tomasch G, Uranues S: The surgical anatomy and etiology of gastrointestinal fistulas, *Eur J Trauma Emerg Surg* 37:209–213, 2011.

Redden MH, Ramsay P, Humphries T, et al: The etiology of Enterocutaneous fistula predicts outcome, *Ochsner J* 13: 507–511, 2013.

Rolstad B, Boarini J: Principles and techniques in the use of convexity, *Ostomy Wound Manage* 42(1):24–26, 28–32, 1996.

Rolstad B, Wong WD: Nursing management of cutaneous intestinal fistulas. In Cataldo PA, MacKeigan JM, editors: *Intestinal stomas: principles, techniques and management*, ed 2, New York, 2004, Marcel Dekker.

Saclarides TJ: Rectovaginal fistula, *Surg Clin North Am* 82(6): 1261–1272, 2002.

Scardillo J, Folkedahl B: Management of a complex high-output fistula, *J Wound Ostomy Continence Nurs* 25(4):217–220, 1998.

Shecter WP: Management of enterocutaneous fistulas, *Surg Clin North Am* 91(3):481–491, 2011.

Skingley S: The management of a faecal fistula, *Nurs Times* 94(16):64–66, 68, 1998.

Smith DB: Fistulas of the head and neck, *J Enterostomal Ther* 9(5):20–24, 1982.

Smith DB: Multiple stomas, fistulas and draining wounds. In Smith DB, Johnson DR, editors: *Ostomy care and the cancer patient: surgical and clinical considerations*, New York, 1986, Grune & Stratton.

Streza GA, Laing BJ, Gilsdorf RB: Management of enterocutaneous fistulas and problem stomas with silicone casting of the abdominal wall defect, *Am J Surg* 134(6):772-776, Dec 1977.

Tran NA, Thorson AG: Rectovaginal fistula. In Cameron JL, editor: *Current surgical therapy*, ed 9, St. Louis, MO, 2008, Mosby.

Welch JP: Duodenal, gastric, and biliary fistulas. In Zinner MJ, et al, editors: *Maingot's abdominal operations*, vol 1, ed 10, Stamford, CT, 1997, Appleton & Lange.

Whelan JF Jr, Ivatury RR: Enterocutaneous fistulas: an overview, *Eur J Trauma Emerg Surg* 37:251–258, 2011.

Wiltshire BL: Challenging enterocutaneous fistula: a case presentation, *J Wound Ostomy Continence Nurs* 23(6):297–301, 1996.

Wong WD, Buie WD, Annamaneni RK: Management of intestinal fistulas. In Cataldo PA, MacKeigan JM, editors: *Intestinal stomas: principles, techniques, and management*, ed 2, New York, 2004, Marcel Dekker.

Yanar F, Yanar H: Nutritional support in patients with gastrointestinal fistula, *Eur J Trauma Emerg Surg* 37:227–231, 2011.

Zwanziger PJ: Pouching a draining duodenal cutaneous fistula: a case study, *J Wound Ostomy Continence Nurs* 26(1):25–29, 1999.

39

Percutaneous Tube Management

Ruth A. Bryant

OBJECTIVES

1. Identify two primary reasons for using percutaneous tubes.
2. Distinguish among the placement approaches for gastrostomy and jejunostomy, including indications and overview of technique.
3. Explain the rationale for tube stabilization.
4. Describe at least two options for stabilizing gastrostomy or jejunostomy tubes.

5. For each complication listed, identify a prevention and management approach: peritubular leakage, tube migration, candidiasis, and tube occlusion.
6. Identify percutaneous tubes that can be irrigated and those that cannot be irrigated.
7. Describe routine site care for the patient with a percutaneous tube.

Although described in the thirteenth century, planned surgical gastrostomy as a procedure was first proposed in 1837 and performed 12 years later in 1849, with the first reported survival of the procedure performed by S. Jones in 1876 (Wu and Soper, 2004). Today the use of tubes is commonplace within the gastrointestinal (GI) tract, as well as other organs and spaces, on a temporary or a long-term basis. Percutaneous tubes are placed for a variety of purposes, including feeding, decompression, and drainage. Although feeding tubes can be placed by the gastroenterologist, surgeon, and interventional radiologist, most percutaneous drainage tubes are inserted into the desired body part by an interventional radiologist using computed tomographic or fluoroscopic guidance (Simons and Remington, 2013; Yarmus et al, 2013). This indicates the need for the wound care specialist to network with these specialties to facilitate positive patient outcomes and optimal patient care.

Malfunction of these tubes can result in skin erosion, denudement, inflammation, and pain such that referral to the wound care specialist becomes necessary. This chapter reviews the different types of percutaneous tubes; their purpose; and procedures for placement, nursing management, and potential complications.

Effective nursing management of the patient with a percutaneous tube requires an understanding of the anatomy and physiology of the affected body system, the pathology involved, the rationale for tube placement, the method of tube insertion, and the anticipated length of time that the tube will be necessary. Although specific care procedures vary depending on the body system involved and the purpose of tube placement, management should always include routine care designed to maintain tube function and prevent peritubular

complications, patient/caregiver education, and routine surveillance for tube dysfunction or complications. Comprehensive care is best provided with a collaborative team approach involving, but not limited to, the interventional radiologist, interventional radiology nurse, gastroenterologist, surgeon or internist, and nurse.

GASTROSTOMY AND JEJUNOSTOMY DEVICES

A *gastrostomy* is an opening into the stomach, and a *jejunostomy* is an opening into the jejunum. Such procedures may be used to provide decompression or enteral support for a patient unable to ingest adequate nutrients orally (DeChicco and Matarese, 2003). Enteral nutrition offers many potential advantages over parenteral nutrition, including lower rates of infectious and metabolic complications, decreased hospital length of stay, and reduced cost. Many of the benefits of enteral feeding are in part due to preservation of gut integrity (histologic structure and physical viability) better than parenteral feeding (Harbison, 2007). Enteral support is generally appropriate through a nasogastric or nasoenteric feeding tube for short-term access (i.e., less than 3 to 4 weeks) in the patient who is at low risk for aspiration (Bloch and Mueller, 2004; DeChicco and Matarese, 2003; Wu and Soper, 2004). When the risk of aspiration exists, placement of a nasogastric feeding tube, however, is discouraged and endoscopically placed tubes are preferred. The patient's history and results of physical examination, barium studies, fluoroscopy, and manometry are useful when evaluating the patient's risk for aspiration. Consultation with the neurologist and speech pathologist also is beneficial. Box 39-1 lists the risk factors for aspiration.

PLACEMENT APPROACHES

For more than a century, gastrostomy placement required surgical intervention involving anesthesia and the traditional preoperative preparation for abdominal surgery. Historically, a suture was placed around the base of the tube at skin level and then through the skin to immobilize the gastrostomy tube. Gastrostomy tubes usually were connected to suction for 12 to 24 hours to reduce tension on the suture line. Feedings were delayed until bowel sounds, tube patency, and proper placement of the tube were confirmed.

Today, a gastrostomy or jejunostomy is created by one of three approaches: surgical, endoscopic, or interventional radiologic. Open laparotomy is rarely performed due to the success of the much less invasive endoscopic and laparoscopic techniques (Duh and McQuaid, 2000). Figure 39-1 presents an algorithm for determining the most appropriate means of enteral access.

Surgical Approaches

A surgically placed gastrostomy or jejunostomy tube can be accomplished through an open surgical procedure or a laparoscopic procedure. Surgical placement is relatively expensive, requires anesthesia and the use of sterile dressings, and exposes the patient to many potential complications. The surgical approach is reserved for the patient with pharyngeal, esophageal, or gastric obstructions or upper GI tumors, or for the patient in whom abdominal surgery is already being performed for other purposes. Surgical placement is also performed when endoscopic placement has failed (Beyers, 2003). Although these procedures are less common today, they may still be placed in unique situations and therefore it is important to have an understanding of their purpose.

Open Surgical Procedure. The most common open surgical procedures for gastrostomy tube placement are the Stamm, the Witzel, and the Janeway. The Stamm and the Witzel are the simplest procedures and are considered temporary; the Janeway is more of a long-term or permanent procedure (Bloch and Mueller, 2004; Gincherman and Torosian, 1996).

Stamm gastrostomy. Stamm gastrostomy is the standard open gastrostomy, the gold standard for transabdominal gastric access (Harbison, 2007). Creation of a Stamm gastrostomy begins by making a small incision in the left upper quadrant of the abdomen. Another small incision is made over and through the body of the stomach, through which a catheter (Foley, mushroom, Malecot, or gastrostomy replacement tube) is inserted (Figure 39-2). Several purse-string sutures are used to invaginate the stomach around the tube. The stomach is then fixed to the abdominal wall at the catheter site, and traditionally a nonabsorbable suture is used to secure the catheter to the skin. Although the Stamm gastrostomy is the simplest surgical technique to perform and remove, it is frequently difficult to manage and is plagued with

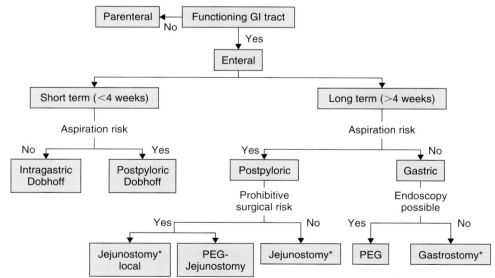

FIGURE 39-1 Enteral access algorithm for selecting the most appropriate technique for an individual patient. (From Gorman RC, Morris JB: Minimally invasive access to the gastrointestinal tract. In Rombeau JL, Rolandelli RH: *Clinical nutrition: enteral and tube feeding,* ed 3, Philadelphia, 1997, Saunders.)

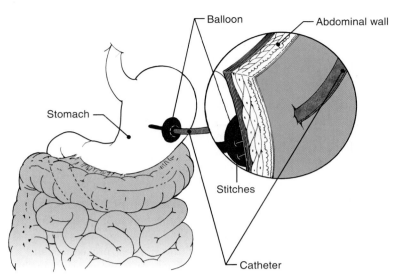

FIGURE 39-2 Stamm gastrostomy tube technique, oblique view. An incision is placed through the abdominal wall into the stomach, through which a catheter is passed.

FIGURE 39-3 Witzel gastrostomy. This is similar to the Stamm gastrostomy with the addition of a 4- to 6-cm seromuscular tunnel of the stomach wall, through which the gastrostomy tube is placed. (From Patterson RS: Enteral nutrition delivery systems. In Grant JA, Kennedy-Caldwell C, editors: *Nutritional support nursing*, Philadelphia, 1988, Grune & Stratton.)

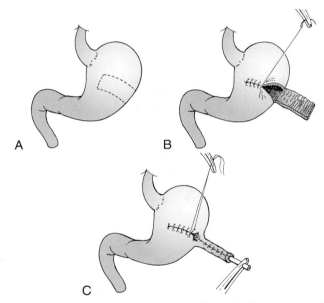

FIGURE 39-4 Janeway gastrostomy. A surgically constructed, mucosa-lined gastric passageway is brought out onto the abdominal surface as a permanent mucocutaneous stoma.

complications such as peritubular leakage, wound infection, peritonitis, and tube dislodgment (Beyers, 2003).

Witzel gastrostomy. Witzel gastrostomy is created similarly to the Stamm gastrostomy, with the additional construction of a 4- to 6-cm seromuscular tunnel of the stomach wall through which the gastrostomy tube is placed (Figure 39-3). The seromuscular tunnel is designed to reduce the risk of peritubular leakage, particularly when the stomach is distended or the tube is removed.

Janeway gastrostomy. Janeway gastrostomy is a surgically constructed, mucosa-lined gastric passageway that is brought out onto the abdominal surface as a permanent mucocutaneous stoma. Figure 39-4 illustrates how the Janeway gastrostomy

is constructed. Postoperatively, an inflated balloon-tip catheter is placed in the tract. Once the tract has matured (7 to 10 days), the tube is removed. A tube is inserted into the Janeway gastrostomy during each feeding and then removed. This type of permanent gastrostomy requires more operative time than the Stamm gastrostomy and results in many similar complications (Gorman et al, 1995).

Witzel jejunostomy. The Witzel technique is the most common technique for surgically placed jejunostomy. The Witzel technique can be used to create a jejunostomy either at the conclusion of a surgical procedure or as an isolated procedure. The usual site is the left upper quadrant. A loop of jejunum 15 to 20 cm from the ligament of Treitz is brought up to the wound, and a circular purse-string suture is placed in the antimesenteric border. An incision through the center of the pursestring suture is made, and a 14-French (14Fr) feeding catheter is inserted into the jejunal lumen and advanced. A serosal tunnel is constructed at the exit site in the jejunal wall, extending approximately 5 to 6 cm proximally. The catheter is brought to the skin through a separate incision and secured, typically with sutures. The loop of intestine is anchored to the anterior abdominal wall (Wu and Soper, 2004).

Needle catheter jejunostomy. The needle catheter jejunostomy is a simple procedure that is most often done at the conclusion of a surgical procedure when prolonged enteral support is anticipated. At approximately 30 to 40 cm distal to the ligament of Treitz, a 14- to 16-gauge needle is inserted into the jejunal wall. A feeding catheter is advanced through the needle 30 to 40 cm distally, and the needle is withdrawn. A purse-string suture is made around the tube to close the jejunal opening around the catheter. The loop of bowel is anchored to the anterior abdominal wall, and the catheter is secured to the skin (Figure 39-5) (Harbison, 2007).

Laparoscopic Surgical Approach. The laparoscopic approach for insertion of the gastrostomy or jejunostomy has been possible since the introduction of high-resolution video cameras and has the advantages of minimal invasion

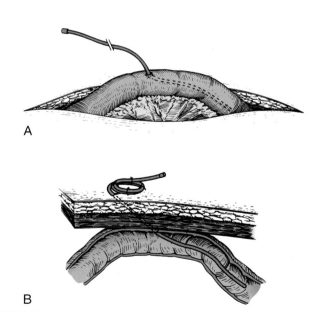

A

B

FIGURE 39-5 Technique for placement of a needle catheter jejunostomy. **A,** The catheter is inserted into the lumen of the jejunum for a distance of 40 to 50 cm and secured into place with a purse-string suture. **B,** The jejunum is secured to the anterior abdominal wall. The feeding catheter is removed postoperatively when the patient can tolerate oral feedings. (From Bland KI et al: *Atlas of surgical oncology,* Philadelphia, 1995, Saunders.)

and few surgical side effects (Georgeson, 1997). This approach also provides the opportunity to selectively determine the site of the tube within the stomach (e.g., lesser-curvature gastrostomy rather than the more commonly selected greater-curvature), which may be important in the patient who is at high risk for reflux or aspiration. In addition, biopsy specimens can be obtained if necessary or malignancy staging can be conducted (Coates and MacFadyen, 1996). This technique requires a smaller incision than the open surgical approach, but local or general anesthesia is still needed.

Laparoscopic gastrostomy. The indication for laparoscopic gastrostomy for feeding is the inability to perform percutaneous endoscopic gastrostomy, such as with a morbidly obese patient. A small supraumbilical incision is made through which the camera port is placed, and a 5-mm port is placed in the epigastrium. An atraumatic instrument is used to grasp the stomach, and the site for the proposed gastrostomy is identified. An 18-gauge angiocatheter is passed through the anterior abdomen, at the site chosen for the gastrostomy, and into the stomach. The needle is removed, and a soft J-wire is passed into the stomach. Dilators (12Fr and 14Fr) are placed over this J-wire. A 16Fr peel-away catheter is placed over the dilator, and a 16Fr catheter is inserted through the sheath. The catheter is positioned against the stomach wall by inflating the balloon or securing the internal bumper. This particular type of gastrostomy is less commonly used than the Stamm due to technical requirements and pneumoperitoneum (Harbison, 2007).

Laparoscopic jejunostomy. Specific indications for laparoscopic jejunostomy include concomitant laparoscopy for other problems and difficult laparoscopic gastrostomy. It is a minimally invasive procedure with desirable advantages of reduced postoperative pain and shortened recuperative time; general anesthesia is required. The procedure is more expensive than percutaneous or surgical placement. Two methods described by Wu and Soper (2004) are briefly discussed in this section.

The laparoscope is inserted through a small incision above the umbilicus. The proximal small bowel is identified and traced 25 cm distal to the ligament of Treitz, and the antimesenteric border is withdrawn into the umbilical wound. At this location in the small bowel, a Witzel tunnel is created or concentric purse-string sutures are placed, and a 12Fr catheter is inserted into the bowel. The bowel is secured to the fascia around the tube and returned to the abdominal cavity, and the fascia and skin are closed. The catheter is tunneled subcutaneously to exit the skin at the site previously selected on the abdomen.

In another technique, T-fasteners (or tacks) are inserted through the skin into the bowel lumen to anchor and retract the bowel against the abdominal wall (Duh and McQuaid, 2000; Wu and Soper 2004). Once the bowel is anchored, a percutaneous jejunostomy tube can be placed directly through the abdominal wall (Figure 39-6).

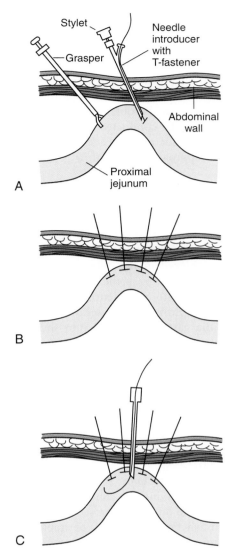

FIGURE 39-6 Laparoscopic jejunostomy with T-fasteners, which are inserted through the skin into the bowel lumen to anchor and retract the bowel against the abdominal wall before a percutaneous jejunostomy tube is inserted directly through the abdominal wall.

Endoscopic Approach

The endoscopic approach to gastrostomy tube placement, known as *percutaneous endoscopic gastrostomy* (PEG), was first described by Gauderer et al (1980) and is the procedure of choice. These devices can be placed under local anesthesia and conscious sedation outside the operating room, thus avoiding the complications associated with surgical procedures.

Contraindications to PEG include inability to perform upper endoscopy, inability to illuminate the abdominal wall, ascites, esophageal obstruction, hepatomegaly, previous gastric resection, and uncorrectable coagulopathy (Bankhead and Rolandell, 2005). Morbid obesity has traditionally presented an obstacle to PEG placement, due to the difficulty in transillumination through the thickness of the overlying adipose

tissue. A recent report, however, described the use of an 8-inch-long spinal needle and 240-cm-long guidewire commonly used in endoscopic retrograde cholangiopancreatography (ERCP) procedures to overcome the problem of transillumination (Senadhi et al, 2012).

Variations to the original technique exist; all involve a complete esophagogastroduodenoscopy, insufflation of air into the stomach, and transillumination of the stomach. After application of a topical pharyngeal anesthetic and sedation, an endoscope is passed into the stomach. Air is insufflated into the stomach, which distends the stomach against the anterior abdominal wall. The proposed gastrostomy site is then transilluminated. The endoscopy assistant indents the abdomen at the proposed gastrostomy site, which should be at least 2 cm below the costal margin. At this point, several different techniques have been described to insert the PEG.

"Pull" (Ponsky) Technique. A small incision is made over the illuminated site, and a large-gauge angiocatheter is inserted into the stomach. The needle is withdrawn, and 60 inches of suture are passed through the catheter into the stomach. With a biopsy snare, the endoscopist grasps the suture and pulls so that the endoscope is removed with the suture attached (Figure 39-7). The gastrostomy tube is attached to the suture. By pulling on the suture at the abdominal gastrostomy site, the endoscopist draws the tube through the esophagus into the stomach and positions it snugly against the anterior stomach wall. To verify proper position of the PEG, an endoscope is passed again. Once placement is confirmed, the endoscope is removed, and the PEG secured at the skin level (Harbison, 2007).

"Over the Wire" (Sachs-Vine) Technique. With this technique, a long, flexible guidewire is inserted through the angiocatheter into the stomach. With use of the biopsy snare and endoscope, the wire is snared and pulled up through the esophagus and out the patient's mouth (Figure 39-8). The PEG tube is pushed over the guidewire and advanced through the esophagus to the stomach and positioned against the anterior stomach wall. As with the "pull" technique, PEG placement is checked with the endoscope, which is then removed, and the PEG is secured.

"Push" (Russell) Technique. Modifications to the Ponsky or Sachs-Vine technique in which the second passage of the endoscope is obviated have been described. Another technique is a modification of the push technique that involves passing a dilator with a peel-away introducer over the guidewire. The endoscopist confirms the position of the dilator, the dilator is removed, and a well-lubricated catheter is placed through the introducer as the introducer is peeled away. The endoscopist verifies adequate placement of the catheter against the anterior stomach wall, and the endoscope is removed (Bankhead and Rolandell, 2005).

Percutaneous Endoscopic Jejunostomy. Several innovative techniques to obtain postpyloric enteral access through

A

B

C

D

E — Endoscope

FIGURE 39-7 Ponsky (pull) percutaneous endoscopic gastrostomy (PEG) technique. **A,** After local anesthesia is instilled, a 10-mm transverse incision is made, through which a tapered cannula needle is introduced under direct endoscopic vision. A looped heavy suture is directed through the catheter into the stomach, secured with a polypectomy snare, and withdrawn from the patient's mouth. **B,** The well-lubricated PEG catheter is now secured to the suture, and steady traction is directed down the posterior pharynx into the esophagus. **C,** The endoscope is reintroduced (see **E**), and under direct vision the catheter is pulled across the gastroesophageal junction and then approximated to the anterior gastric wall. It is imperative that the inner cross-bar gently approximates the mucosa without excess tension to avoid ischemic necrosis. The stomach is decompressed by aspiration, and the gastroscope is withdrawn. **D,** The outer cross-bar is gently approximated to the skin level and secured with two 0-0 Prolene sutures. (From Gorman RC, Morris JB: Minimally invasive access to the gastrointestinal tract. In Rombeau JL, Rolandelli RH: *Clinical nutrition: enteral and tube feeding,* ed 3, Philadelphia, 1997, Saunders.)

endoscopic placement of the percutaneous endoscopic jejunostomy (PEJ) have been described. The two basic approaches—transpyloric PEJ and directed PEJ—are briefly described.

Transpyloric PEJ. A small feeding tube with a weighted tip and an attached heavy suture tie are passed through a previously established gastrostomy. Under endoscopic visualization,

the suture is grasped with a biopsy forceps, and the suture and attached feeding tube are guided into the duodenum (Figure 39-9). The endoscope is withdrawn. An excess amount of tubing is left within the stomach to allow peristalsis to pull the weighted tip past the ligament of Treitz.

Transpyloric PEJ is associated with considerable long-term complications, including (1) separation of the inner PEJ

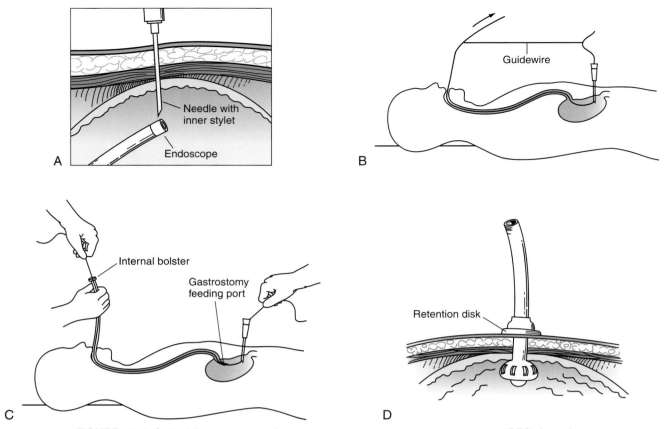

FIGURE 39-8 Sachs-Vine technique for percutaneous endoscopic gastrostomy (PEG) insertion. **A,** Needle is inserted through abdomen into the stomach under visualization by endoscopist. **B,** Endoscope is withdrawn, pulling guidewire up through the esophagus, out the patient's mouth. **C,** PEG tube is pushed over the guidewire and advanced through the esophagus to the stomach. **D,** PEG is positioned against the anterior stomach wall.

FIGURE 39-9 Transpyloric percutaneous endoscopic jejunostomy. Endoscopist guides the weighted tip of the feeding tube into the duodenum.

tube from the outer gastrostomy tube; (2) clogging of the small-diameter PEJ; and (3) kinking of the PEJ. Furthermore, the goal of reduced aspiration pneumonia has not been achieved, possibly as a result of retrograde migration of the tube back into the stomach or impaired pyloric sphincter function triggered by the presence of the tube (Gorman and Morris, 1997).

Directed PEJ. A PEJ can be placed directly through the abdominal wall into the jejunum using a modification of the Ponsky PEG procedure. In this approach, the endoscope is advanced past the pylorus approximately 20 cm distal to the ligament of Treitz, and the abdominal wall is transilluminated. Using a small-gauge needle, the jejunum is cannulated through the abdominal wall, a heavy thread is inserted, a biopsy forceps is used to grasp the thread, and the thread is withdrawn through the mouth. The thread is tied to a feeding tube (typically mushroom tipped), which is pulled into position under endoscopic observation.

Another directed PEJ technique involves a small incision in the upper quadrant. The endoscope is inserted beyond the ligament of Treitz, and the proximal end of the jejunum is clamped. In the small incision, a short segment of jejunum is eviscerated using the Witzel technique. The feeding tube is placed into the jejunum, the jejunum is returned to the abdominal cavity, and the proximal and distal ends of the jejunum are secured to the abdominal wall. The directed PEJ seems to alleviate the problems associated with transpyloric placement (tube migration, clogging, and aspiration). Evidence for the long-term benefits, efficacy, and use of this procedure is inconclusive.

Interventional Radiologic Approach

Percutaneous Gastrostomy via Radiologic Intervention. Recent advances have led to the development of a radiographic approach to percutaneous gastrostomy tube placement. Percutaneous tubes placed by the interventional radiologist are an alternative when surgical or endoscopic procedures are not feasible. In many hospitals, it is the preferred method of tube placement. The interventional radiology nurse takes the lead in preparing the patient for the procedure, providing patient education, and monitoring the patient's recovery.

In the radiographic approach, the stomach is dilated with air, and a needle is percutaneously inserted into the stomach. A J-wire is threaded into the stomach under fluoroscopic guidance, and the needle is withdrawn. A 1-cm-long incision is made into the skin at the exit site of the wire. When entry into the stomach has been determined, the tract is slowly dilated and the permanent catheter inserted. These catheters usually have a balloon that is inflated and positioned snugly against the gastric wall. Stabilization at the skin surface is achieved using a suture or a tube stabilization device.

- T-tacks are small anchors that are deployed into the stomach during the beginning phase of gastrostomy or gastrostomy-jejunostomy tube placement.
- T-tacks pull and hold the stomach firmly against the abdominal wall. This helps the radiologists so that they do not have to work through "dead" space when placing the tube into the stomach.
- T-tacks *must* be cut within 7 to 10 days of placement to prevent reverse crater ulcerations in the stomach mucosal lining.
- Metal "T"s simply pass through the patient's GI tract.

Percutaneous Jejunostomy via Radiologic Intervention. This technique first requires radiologic access to the stomach as is done for percutaneous gastrostomy placement via radiology. A guidewire is passed through the duodenum and into the jejunum. A balloon occluder catheter is inserted over the guidewire and placed in the jejunum. The balloon is inflated with air and water-soluble contrast so that the position can be checked by fluoroscopy. Still under fluoroscopic surveillance, an 18-gauge needle is inserted into the jejunum, and the balloon is punctured. A guidewire is passed into the tract, and the tract is dilated to approximately 10Fr size so that a feeding catheter can be inserted. The balloon occluder catheter is removed, and the feeding catheter is secured to the skin.

Conversion of Gastrostomy to Gastrostomy-Jejunostomy Tube. Repeat aspirations may necessitate conversion of an existing gastrostomy tube to a gastrostomy-jejunostomy tube. This can be done using endoscopy or radiology with a combined gastrostomy-jejunostomy tube, or by inserting a smaller-diameter feeding tube through the gastrostomy tube. When a combined gastrostomy-jejunostomy tube is used, the gastrostomy tube is removed, and an angiocatheter and guidewire are inserted and advanced through the pylorus. The guidewire is further advanced distal to the ligament of Treitz, and the angiocatheter is removed. A gastrostomy-jejunostomy tube is inserted over the guidewire and advanced into the jejunum, and the guidewire is removed. The gastrostomy internal bumper or balloon is secured snugly against the stomach mucosa. An external securing device (bumper, flange, or commercial device) is used to secure the tube against the skin. Three ports will be apparent: gastric (proximal) port, duodenal or jejunal (distal) port, and balloon port (Figure 39-10).

FIGURE 39-10 Transgastric jejunal tube. This dual-lumen tube is placed surgically and allows for jejunal feedings while providing gastric decompression. (From Rombeau JL, Rolandelli RH: *Clinical nutrition: enteral and tube feeding*, ed 3, Philadelphia, 1997, Saunders.)

When a combined gastrostomy-jejunostomy tube is not available, a jejunal tube can be placed, and the external end of the jejunal tube can be threaded into a gastrostomy tube. The gastrostomy tube is advanced over the jejunal tube, and the internal gastrostomy bumper is positioned against the anterior stomach wall. External stabilization of the tube to the skin is necessary.

Summary of Placement Techniques

The type of patient who typically requires these tubes is a major reason for the high morbidity rate. Patients commonly have multiple medical problems and are malnourished. For these reasons, the surgical approach to tube placement has quickly been replaced by the endoscopic or radiographic approach. Endoscopic techniques for enteral tube placement have a lower complication rate, are more cost effective than surgical methods, and can be performed on an outpatient basis. Performance of these techniques requires the ability to insert an endoscope. Laparoscopic and radiologic techniques are used less frequently but are options when endoscopy is not anatomically feasible or when surgery is too risky.

A key consideration for the type of tube placed is whether prepyloric or postpyloric delivery of enteral feedings is preferred (Harbison, 2007). Percutaneous endoscopic gastrostomy tube placement into the stomach preserves the integrity of the cardiac sphincter, decreasing the risk of gastroesophageal reflux and pulmonary aspiration (Jung et al, 2011). However, in the presence of significant gastroesophageal reflux, impaired gastric emptying, or primary disease of the stomach, postpyloric placement (i.e., in the proximal duodenum or jejunum) is often preferred.

FEEDING TUBE FEATURES

The type of tube used for gastrostomy or jejunostomy depends in part on the anatomic site in which the tube is placed and the reason for tube placement. Features of the tube to consider include material composition, tube diameter, tip configurations, and number of ports.

Material Composition

Historically, gastrostomy and jejunostomy tubes were made from rubber, polyvinyl chloride, and latex, which are very stiff and uncomfortable. The softer and more pliable polyurethane and silicone tubes have been used most frequently because these materials are associated with less soft tissue reaction and longer wear time. These features are particularly advantageous in older patients because of the increased fragility of the GI mucosa in this population (Lysen, 2003). Polyurethane tubes are often preferred to silicone tubes, however, because polyurethane tubes are more resilient and less likely to deteriorate (Naik et al, 2009). In addition, aspiration of intestinal or gastric contents from silicone tubes is difficult because the walls of the tube collapse (Lysen, 2003).

Tube Diameter

The outer diameter (OD) of the lumen is referred to in French (Fr) units. A 1Fr tube is 0.33 mm across. However, the internal diameter (ID) can vary for any OD French size depending on the material used. For example, silicone tubes have thicker walls than polyurethane tubes, so their internal diameter will be smaller even though they are labeled with the same French size.

The risk of the tube becoming clogged decreases as ID increases. However, for the patient's comfort, the smallest ID nasogastric tube possible that allows unimpeded flow of formula should be used. When enteral formulas containing fiber or viscous formulas will be administered, an 8Fr or larger tube is recommended. Gastrostomy tubes most often are 12Fr, jejunostomy tubes should be 6Fr, and needle catheter jejunostomy tubes should be smaller than 8Fr (Lysen, 2003).

Tip Configurations

Several tip configurations are illustrated in Figure 39-11. Foley catheters are not designed for use as gastrostomy tubes and should not be used because the balloon of the Foley catheter is subject to decay from gastric acid, necessitating periodic and regular replacement. In addition, Foley catheters do not have an external bumper and will migrate if an external tube stabilization device is not applied. Migration can cause gastric outlet obstruction by blocking the pylorus. Specifically designed gastrostomy tubes, many silicone based, commonly known as a *G-tube* or *replacement gastrostomy tube,* are essential to use.

Another tip configuration (and one used to a great extent on the PEG) is the disk. This tip cannot be removed by simple extraction through the skin; it must be cut off. The tip is passed through the GI tract or retrieved endoscopically. The PEG tip may also have a cross-bar or bulb tip, which cannot be extracted through the skin.

Tubes may have a type of mushroom catheter known as a *Pezzer tip.* These rubber tubes have stiff, round, pointed tips. The Pezzer tip has only minimal tiny holes and becomes easily plugged. This type of tip cannot be removed easily. The Malecot tube, also considered a mushroom catheter, has a bulbous tip with much larger openings. This type of tube can be removed more easily and is less likely to become obstructed than the Pezzer tip.

Ports

Tubes with multiple ports are available. Some gastrostomy tubes have three ports: balloon, feeding, and medication. A triple-lumen tube may be used when patients require both proximal decompression and enteral feeding. This tube has four outlets or ports: a gastric lumen for gastric suction, a proximal duodenal lumen for duodenal suction, a distal duodenal lumen for feeding, and a gastric balloon. To maintain proper tube placement, the gastric balloon is inflated with sterile water or air (depending on the manufacturer's specific recommendation), and a retaining disk or tube stabilization device is applied at skin level. These tubes may be confusing to the staff because the tubes are placed in the anticipated

FIGURE 39-11 Tip configuration of enteral tubes. Note that the Foley with balloon tip is included to provide comparison in tip designs; it is not an appropriate tube for enteral feedings.

location for a gastrostomy tube but deliver feedings to the jejunum. Ports should be clearly labeled, and a diagram of the tube should be available in the patient's care plan to provide clarity.

LOW-PROFILE GASTROSTOMY DEVICE (BUTTON)

A skin-level gastric conduit that is flush with the abdominal surface is known as a *gastrostomy button* (Foutch et al,

1989; Gauderer and Stellato, 1986; Gauderer et al, 1988). The button was first developed for use in children who require long-term gastrostomy feedings. It is a short silicone tube with a flip-top opening, a one-way antireflux valve (to prevent leakage of stomach contents around the tube), and a radiopaque dome that fits snugly against the stomach wall (Figure 39-12). Some devices have special tubing that opens the reflux valve to permit decompression of the stomach.

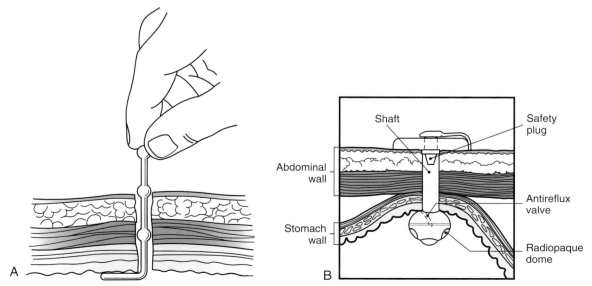

FIGURE 39-12 Gastrostomy button. **A,** Correct gastrostomy button size is determined by using a device to measure the width of the abdominal wall. **B,** Gastrostomy feeding button in place.

To administer feedings, an adapter is passed through the one-way valve and connected to a feeding catheter. When the feeding is completed, the tube is flushed with water, the adapter is removed, and the flip-top opening is closed.

A button can be inserted in a clinic setting in an established gastrostomy tract and does not require patient anesthesia. It may also be placed as the initial device in a one-step procedure (Georgeson, 1999). The device is available in different shaft lengths and diameters. Correct shaft length is critical to ensure proper positioning of the dome of the button against the anterior stomach wall and prevent gastric reflux around the button. The appropriate shaft length is determined by inserting a special measuring device into the tract. An obturator is inserted into the button to straighten the dome of the button, making insertion of the button into the tract possible. The button should be lubricated to facilitate insertion. Once the button is in place, the obturator is removed and the flip-top opening closed. The device may have to be resized if the patient's weight changes.

Disadvantages of the button include the potential for dysfunction of the antireflux valve with subsequent leakage and the need for replacement every 3 to 4 months. Studies and refinements of the device are ongoing. Current reports demonstrate good success, few complications, and high user satisfaction.

NURSING MANAGEMENT OF ENTERIC TUBES

Any patient who is malnourished or expected to have inadequate oral intake for 5 to 7 days should be considered for enteral access for nutritional support. The GI tract should be used whenever possible when nutritional supplementation is required (Harbison, 2007). Short-term support can be delivered through a small-bore nasoenteric tube. When supplementation for more than 7 to 14 days is anticipated, GI intubation through a gastrostomy or jejunostomy should be considered. The patient with moderate to severe malnourishment who is undergoing an open laparotomy should be considered for a low jejunostomy or gastrostomy placed at the same time (Harbison, 2007).

Optimal management of patients requiring long-term gastrostomy or jejunostomy tubes begins in the preplacement phase. Assessment of each patient should include the reason for each tube alternative, the risks and benefits associated with various treatment options, and the commitment of the patient or caregiver to long-term management. Preplacement information and instructions are critical to adequately prepare the patient and family for what they will be expected to do.

Nursing staff must be prepared to care for the patient with an enteric tube. Much of the success of these tubes depends on proper care. Topics that must be addressed include preplacement site selection, site care, tube patency, tube stabilization, and management of complications. It is advisable to develop a competency checklist for the nursing staff who care for a significant number of patients with feeding tubes.

Preplacement Site Selection

Tube exit sites should be selected preoperatively to reduce the potential for complications and to facilitate self-care. Site selection is commonly based on vague guidelines such as "3 to 5 cm below the costal margin" and "avoidance of the costal margin." However, in the patient who has a protuberant hernia or is malnourished or confined to a wheelchair, this location may present a substantial problem such that it affects the integrity of the skin. Two techniques can be used to select a preplacement site, depending on whether the tube will be placed endoscopically or surgically (Hanlon, 1998). Preplacement site selection is even more important in the infant and particularly when an ostomy is present.

Endoscopic Placement. When the tube is placed by the endoscopic approach, the location of the tube depends on transillumination. Therefore the specific site for the tube cannot be determined before the procedure. Nonetheless, by marking important abdominal landmarks (e.g., skin crease, fold, or scar; costal margin; belt line; prosthetic equipment; hernia), the endoscopist can attempt to place the tube in a site that will avoid these landmarks. An indelible marker should be sufficient for these markings.

Surgical Placement. When the tube will be placed surgically, the technique used for preplacement site selection is the same as that used to mark a stoma site. The patient should be assessed while he or she is standing, sitting, bending, and in the supine position. The objective is to find 1 inch of smooth skin surface that is free of creases, folds, and scars and avoids the belt line and bony structures. Again, a surgical marking pen can be used to place an "X" at the desired location. A transparent dressing can be applied over the marking when surgery is not scheduled for several days.

Site Care

Nationally accepted evidence-based guidelines on site care with PEG tubes do not exist and therefore much of the care is based on clinical expertise and local preference. The information presented in this section and Box 39-2 is drawn from clinical experience, literature, biologic plausibility, and clinical reasoning.

BOX 39-2 Percutaneous Tube Site Care

- Cleanse site with tap water and gentle soap, rinse, let dry
- A cotton-tipped applicator may be necessary to clean under an external bumper or disk
- Rotate catheter 360 degrees daily.
- Flush with 30 ml tap water (3 to 5 ml in pediatrics):
  - Every 4 hours
  - During continuous feeding
  - Before and after intermittent feedings
- Flush with 5 ml tap water before and after medication administration, and after measuring residual volume
- Instill each medication separately

Within 2 days after insertion, the adhesion formation of the stomach to the abdominal wall occurs; the gastrocutaneous tract forms within 1 to 2 weeks (Timratana et al, 2012). During this window of time, it is imperative to prevent accidental tube dislodgement and to monitor closely for infection. Initially, daily site care should include gentle cleansing with sterile water (Simons and Remington, 2013). A sterile gauze dressing should be applied over the site and changed daily to protect the site from external contamination and infection during this period while the gastrocutaneous tract is forming. Long term, a dressing is not necessary over the tube site and tap water can be used to cleanse the exit site. If desired, a pH-neutral mild soap can be used but should also be rinsed off. A cotton-tipped applicator may be necessary to clean under an external bumper or disk. When drainage is present, a moisture barrier may be used after cleansing around the tube to prevent moisture-associated skin damage (MASD) as long as the cause of the drainage is addressed and corrected (e.g., bacterial or fungal infection, hypergranulation tissue, and excessive gastric acid production). Nonadhesive absorptive dressings can be applied over the external fixation portion of the percutaneous tube if drainage is present. Best practice regarding placement of dressings under the external bumper of the PEG tube is unclear. Dressings should not be applied under the external fixation disk or bumper that will trap moisture or exert excess tension on the internal bumper against the gastric mucosal surface (Box 39-3). Extrathin hydrocolloids, thin silicone border foam dressings, or the relatively new hydroactive gauze dressings are potential options (Rollins et al, 2013).

Daily assessments should include the condition of the peritubular site and proper positioning of the stabilization device. The insertion site and surrounding tissue should be monitored for signs and symptoms of infection (e.g., erythema, induration, pain). The external bumper should rest lightly against the skin. Superficial infections occur in as many as 18% of patients (Simons and Remington, 2013). Soft tissue infections should be managed with culture-based antibiotics (see Plate 72B).

Tube Stabilization

Common complications related to gastrostomy or jejunostomy placement are (1) leakage of gastric or jejunal contents around the tube onto the skin and (2) tube dislodgment, both of which are frequently attributed to inadequate tube stabilization. Therefore postplacement nursing management must include measures to stabilize the tube.

Adequate tube stabilization requires proper internal positioning and proper external (skin-level) positioning. To achieve proper internal positioning, a tube that has a balloon, bumper, mushroom, or disk tip is used. These devices are positioned lightly against the anterior wall of the stomach (Figure 39-13). When a balloon tip is used, it must be inflated with an adequate volume of sterile water or air (in accordance with the manufacturer's guidelines) (Lord, 1997). Although saline may be readily available, it should not be used for balloon inflation because saline can crystallize and cause the balloon to rupture. Because water and air will diffuse through the walls of the balloon, adequacy of inflation should be checked weekly and whenever peritubular leakage is noted. Tubes with balloon tips should not be used as jejunal tubes because an inflated balloon within the jejunum is sufficient to obstruct the jejunum.

Adequate skin-level stabilization of the tube is necessary to prevent (1) lateral movement in the tube at skin level and (2) tube migration (in-and-out movements). Lateral movement of the tube contributes to leakage of gastric or intestinal contents onto the skin by eroding the tissue along the tract. Inflammation of the site can also develop from the presence of this chronic irritant. A stabilized tube should not allow lateral movement (Lord, 1997).

To maintain proper tube positioning in the stomach or small bowel, migration of the tube in and out of the tract must be prevented. Nonstabilized tubes are subject to migration as a result of gastric and intestinal motility and abdominal wall motion. The tube can migrate and obstruct the gastric outlet (causing gastric distention, nausea, and vomiting) and compromise tube function.

Historically, sutures have been used to stabilize tubes. However, sutures can cause tearing of the skin, with subsequent inflammation and significant pain at the suture site. In

---

BOX 39-3 Site Care for Drainage Tubes

- Change dressing every day.
- Remove dressing from site.
- Use a clean washcloth to cleanse the area around the tube with gentle soap and water.
- Use a dry washcloth to pat dry skin around tube.
- If necessary, reposition tube so that it does not kink or twist sharply.
- Secure fresh, split wound care dressing around tube site and over the retention disk using tape.
- Covering the tube site is not necessary while showering. These steps can be done in the shower or after the shower.

Note: Never submerge the tube site under water. No tub baths or swimming is permitted.

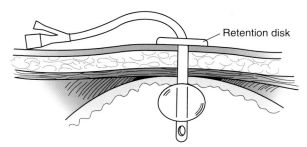

FIGURE 39-13 Proper stabilization of gastrostomy tube. Tube is secured between the anterior wall of the stomach and abdomen by a properly inflated internal balloon and externally with a tube stabilization device. Side-to-side mobility of the tube and tube migration are thus prevented.

FIGURE 39-14 Commercial external tube stabilization device.

FIGURE 39-15 Sample replacement gastrostomy tubes.

addition, sutures prevent tube migration, but they do not eliminate lateral tube movement. When sutures are used, an external tube stabilization device should be applied to provide more secure stabilization and comfort to the patient.

In the past, baby-bottle nipples have been used to secure gastrostomy tubes. Typically the nipple is cut along one edge, wrapped around the tube, and secured with tape where the tube exits from the nipple. This technique is not effective at preventing lateral movement or tube migration and should no longer be used.

Commercial external tube stabilization devices are readily available and should be used to secure percutaneous tubes (Figure 39-14). The commercial tube stabilization device is changed as needed; frequency is determined by the need to assess the tube site or provide site care. When frequent site care is required (as with newly placed tubes), a stabilization system that allows easy visualization of the site without removal of adhesives is desirable. The Hollister vertical drain/tube attachment device effectively holds tubes. The dressing is designed so that the tube comes straight out of the tract and is secured by the strap. Because the tube does not lie against the skin, there is no concern for development of a pressure ulcer along the tract. For smaller abdomens the tape ring can be removed. The vertical drain/tube attachment device can be left in place for 5 to 7 days.

Many tubes are being created specifically as gastrostomy tubes complete with stabilization features inherent in the design, thereby eliminating the need for commercial external stabilization devices. For example, the button has an internal dome, limited shaft length, and a flip-top cap to ensure stabilization of the tube. PEG tubes are designed with an internal bolster and an external bolster. The internal bolster can be a bumper, disk, or balloon that, when properly positioned, lies against the anterior stomach wall. Exteriorly, on the abdominal surface, the bolster is a bumper or disk that can be adjusted to lie snugly against the abdominal wall. This stabilization is critical to prevent dislodgment of the tube, mobility, obstruction, and peritubular leakage. A few Silastic catheter feeding tubes (with a balloon to secure the tube against the anterior stomach wall) have an adjustable external flange (Figure 39-15). Once the Silastic catheter is in position

and the balloon is inflated, the flange is slid down against the skin, stabilizing the catheter without the use of adhesives.

Regardless of the type of stabilization device or bolster used, adequate stabilization is critical to the success of the tubes. The devices secure the tube against the abdominal wall and against the anterior stomach wall. The tension between the internal and external securing devices should allow slight leeway from the skin to prevent erosion of the skin (i.e., device-related pressure ulcer) or gastric mucosa (known as buried bumper syndrome) (Lord, 1997; Simmons and Remington, 2013). This leeway should be monitored daily because changes in abdominal girth, as occurs with ascites, can develop, which exposes the patient to excess pressure under the external stabilization device. Modifications should be made as necessary.

Tube Patency

To maintain patency, all enteral feeding tubes require routine flushing (see Box 39-2). In adults, the tube should be flushed with 30 ml of water (3 to 5 ml in pediatrics) every 4 hours during continuous feeding, before and after intermittent feedings, after medication administration, and after measuring residual volume (Bankhead et al, 2009). It is also imperative that each medication be instilled separately and flushed with 5 ml of water before and after each. When the safety of tap water is questioned, sterile water should be used (Bankhead et al, 2009). Medications should be in liquid form or crushed and dissolved in tap water; enteric-coated, time-released, or sustained-release medications are not appropriate (Tong, 2010).

Occlusion of a feeding tube can result from administration of powdered or crushed medications in the feeding tube, viscous formulas, poor or inadequate flushing techniques, partially digested proteins, yeast, and aspiration of gastric or intestinal contents into the tube (Bankhead et al, 2009; Beyers, 2003). Instillation of 50 ml tepid water from a 60-ml syringe should be used initially to dislodge an occlusion allowing the water to dwell. This process can also assist in distinguishing a kinked tube from a clogged tube in that kinked tubes allow slow passage of water, whereas clogged tubes do not allow any passage of water. When irrigation with water fails, commercially available products have been reported. Clog Zapper, a powder containing a combination of enzymes (e.g., papain, cellulose, and alpha amylase) is reconstituted with water, instilled into the clogged tube, and allowed to dwell for 30 to 60 minutes. Two methods for the mechanical dislodgement of a clog include the Bionex Enteral Feeding Tube Declogger and the Bard PEG cleaning brush. Limited evidence is available in the use of these declogging strategies. The use of cranberry juice, chymotrypsin, carbonated drinks, and meat tenderizers is discouraged because they tend to precipitate in the feeding solution and cause adverse effects in patients with severe hepatic, renal, or coagulation abnormalities (Tong, 2010).

COMPLICATIONS

Complications associated with percutaneous tubes include local complications such as peristomal leakage, MASD, peristomal wound infection, and buried bumper syndrome. The wound specialist may see a patient with an intestinal tube for the first time when a skin complication develops. In addition to addressing the skin problem, investigation and correction of the underlying problem precipitating the skin irritation is essential.

Leakage

Leakage around the tube site warrants a thorough evaluation. Steps must be taken to correct any possible cause of the leakage. Replacing the tube with a larger size will not correct the problem. First check the adequacy of tube stabilization, appropriate balloon placement, adequate inflation of the balloon, and tube patency. The balloon should be deflated and reinflated with the amount of air or sterile water recommended by the manufacturer. Medications to reduce stomach acid may be warranted. Leakage may occur as a result of bolus feedings and may resolve with slower delivery or continuous delivery. When all attempts to halt the leakage fail, replacement of the tube may be necessary.

Moisture-Associated Skin Dermatitis

Moisture-associated skin dermatitis surrounding a tube most commonly results from chemical irritation (exposure to gastric or intestinal contents), the chronic presence of moisture, or fungal infection. If all attempts to halt leakage fail and tube replacement is not an option, methods to contain the drainage and protect the skin must be implemented. Hydrocolloids and absorbent dressings are often not appropriate because they will trap drainage and moisture against the skin, exacerbating MASD.

To contain drainage around a tube site, an ostomy pouch and catheter port can be applied. By attaching a catheter port to the pouch, the tube can exit the wall of the pouch through the port, which allows for feeding, suction, or gravity drainage to continue. The ostomy pouch then contains peritubular drainage (Figure 39-16). Such a pouching system is cost effective and allows collection, identification, and measurement of the drainage, as well as skin protection. Instructions for containing peritubular leakage are outlined in Box 39-4. The frequency of pouch changes is determined by the duration of the pouch seal, but on average the pouch is changed every 4 to 7 days. If a urinary pouch is selected, it may be necessary to "pop" the antireflux mechanism within the pouch, particularly when drainage is thick or contains particulate matter.

Fungal infections (e.g., candidiasis) can result when moisture is trapped at the insertion site. Corrective measures include protecting the skin from moisture with skin sealants or ointments, or containing the moisture with appropriate dressings. Antifungal medications (e.g., powders) may be necessary when extensive candidiasis is present.

Allergic contact dermatitis can occur when a patient's skin is sensitive to anchoring devices, tapes, soaps, or other commercial products. Medical adhesive–related skin injury (MARSI) in the form of mechanical trauma or folliculitis can also develop as a result of traumatic removal of adhesives used to anchor the tube (McNichol et al, 2013; O'Brien et al, 1999). These issues are discussed further in Chapter 5.

Peristomal Hyperplasia. An overgrowth of granulation tissue at the tube exit site can develop and is commonly referred to as *hyperplasia*. This overgrowth of granulation tissue occurs in response to chronic irritation of the tissue lining the tract. The source of the chronic irritation can be the type of tube material used (latex is more irritating than Silastic material), tube mobility (particularly in-and-out movements of the tube), and the chronic presence of excessive moisture.

FIGURE 39-16 Catheter access port attached to drainable ostomy pouch *(left)*. Two examples of a catheter access port *(right)*. (Courtesy NuHope and Hollister.)

BOX 39-4   Pouching Procedure for Leakage around Tube

1. Assemble pouch and catheter access device.
   a. Cut opening in barrier and pouch to accommodate tube site.
   b. Make small slit in anterior surface of pouch.
   c. Attach access device to anterior surface of the pouch.
   d. Tear paper backing on pouch or wafer but leave in place.
2. Prepare skin.
   a. Cleanse and dry skin.
   b. Treat any denuded skin (skin barrier powder to denuded area; skin sealant if needed).
   c. Apply thin layer of skin barrier paste to skin around insertion site, if needed.
3. Disconnect and plug tube.
4. Feed catheter through opening in pouch. Use water-soluble lubricant to pass tube, and use hemostat to pull tube through the pouch or barrier opening, anterior wall of the pouch, and access device.
5. Reconnect tube.
6. Ensure skin is dry. Remove paper backing from wafer and secure pouch to skin.
7. Secure tube to stabilization device with tape.

BOX 39-5   Instructions for Removal of Original PEG Tube

Equipment
- Nonsterile gloves
- Gauze (4 × 4)

Procedure
1. Obtain permission from physician.
2. Using dominant hand, grasp PEG tubing above bumper and rotate it 360 degrees. If it does not rotate freely, stop and call physician. If it rotates freely, wrap it around your hand to maintain a firm grip.
3. Use other hand to stabilize the patient's abdomen around the site.
4. While exerting moderate force, pull on PEG tube until inner bumper comes through skin opening. Slight bleeding may occur. If resistance is too great, stop and call physician.
5. Cover opening with gauze until ready to insert replacement gastrostomy tube. Insert tube immediately to prevent closure of the tract.

Note: Original PEG tube must be at least 2 weeks past time of insertion before nurse performs this procedure.

PEG, Percutaneous endoscopic gastrostomy.
Courtesy of Karen Huskey.

BOX 39-6   Instructions for Removal of Balloon Replacement Gastrostomy Tube

Equipment
- 20-ml Luer-Lok syringe
- Gauze (4 × 4)
- Nonsterile gloves

Procedure
1. Connect 20-ml syringe to balloon port of tube and aspirate all water out of balloon. (*Note:* Less than 20 ml may be present as a result of evaporation.)
2. Slowly withdraw tube from abdominal site.
3. Cover opening with gauze until ready to reinsert replacement tube. Insert tube immediately to prevent closure of the tract.

Hyperplasia may or may not be uncomfortable. However, when hyperplasia is allowed to persist, seepage from the overgrowth will develop and compromise the integrity of the external stabilization and skin integrity. Treatment should address the underlying causative factor. If chronic moisture is present, medications to reduce gastric reflux may be warranted. Adequacy of tube stabilization should be reevaluated. Once the cause is corrected, the hyperplasia should resolve. Occasionally debridement and cautery with silver nitrate sticks are warranted. Because it can be painful for the patient, cautery with silver nitrate sticks should be done infrequently and only by an experienced care provider.

TUBE REMOVAL

Enteral tubes are removed when the patient is able to resume adequate oral nutrition and may need to be removed when they are hopelessly occluded, kinked, or malpositioned. The method of removal will depend on the type of tube, the technique used to insert the tube, and the type of tube tip (Boxes 39-5 to 39-7). Percutaneous endoscopic gastrostomy tubes can be removed by external traction, endoscopy, or "cut and push" (Kejariwal et al, 2009). With the "cut and push" method, the outer bumper is loosened, the tube is rotated and advanced slightly into the stomach (to ensure the internal bumper is mobile and not attached to the gastric mucosa), and, while external traction is applied on the tube, the tube is severed at skin level. The internal portion of the tube will be expelled in the stool. A dressing is applied over the percutaneous tube site and replaced daily. Patients are NPO for 6 hours before the procedure and for 2 hours after the procedure. Performance of these PEG tube removals should be reserved for nurses who have successfully completed a formal competency check, such as nutritional therapist nurses and interventional radiology nurses.

PATIENT EDUCATION

Patient education is a key nursing responsibility and is absolutely critical to the patient with a gastrostomy or jejunostomy tube. Because the hospitalization period after tube placement may be brief to nonexistent, detailed caregiver education is essential, and outpatient follow-up care is imperative. In some situations, percutaneous tube placement may be performed strictly on an outpatient basis. In either case, home health care will be important to facilitate patient and caregiver independence in the process, safety with the procedure, and monitoring for complications. Key content areas to be included in a patient teaching plan are listed in Box 39-8.

BOX 39-7   Instructions for Insertion of Balloon Replacement Gastrostomy

Equipment

- Replacement gastrostomy tube of correct size
- 60-ml syringe with male tip
- Lubricant (e.g., K-Y jelly)
- Stethoscope
- Nonsterile gloves
- 20-ml Luer-Lok syringe
- 20 ml of sterile water

Procedure

1. Choose replacement gastrostomy tube that is the same size as the previously used tube unless otherwise indicated.
2. Draw up 20 ml of sterile water into syringe. Do not use saline.
3. Insert syringe into balloon port; fill balloon to ensure proper inflation.
4. Withdraw water out of balloon and lubricate distal end of gastrostomy tube.
5. Gently insert gastrostomy tube into existing opening in abdomen. Tube should go in without resistance. If resistance is detected, pull back and attempt to insert again at a slightly different angle. If resistance is met again, stop and call physician.
6. Once gastrostomy tube is inserted into existing tract, gastric contents should return into the tube. To confirm proper placement, instill 30 ml of air into gastrostomy tube and auscultate for sound, which should be heard in the stomach (not the abdomen).
7. Once placement is confirmed, fill balloon with 20-ml water-filled syringe. (Check balloon port to determine exact amount of water needed to fill balloon.)
8. After balloon is inflated, gently pull back on tube until resistance is felt, then slide down external bumper or disk until it rests lightly on the skin.
9. Rotate the catheter 360 degrees to confirm that tube has free rotation.
10. Cleanse skin around tube with soap and water; no dressing is necessary.

Courtesy of Karen Huskey.

BOX 39-8   Key Content for Patient Education

1. Name of procedure
2. Purpose for tube insertion
3. Characteristics of normal tube function
4. Type of tube placed
5. Size of balloon (if present)
6. Tube stabilization (why it is important, how it is achieved)
7. Routine site care (daily)
8. Weekly balloon inflation checks (if present)
9. Signs and symptoms of complications and appropriate response
10. Tube feeding schedule and procedure (when applicable)
11. Name of person to call with questions or problems
12. What to do if tube falls out

MISCELLANEOUS DRAIN TUBES

A drainage tube can be placed to drain an abscess or fluid collection that will not resolve on its own and antibiotics are ineffective. Although surgery may be performed to manage a fluid collection, surgery may not be appropriate due to local inflammation, the severity or location of the abscess, or the patient's comorbidities. With the assistance of computed tomography or fluoroscopy, a catheter can be placed anywhere in the body where pus accumulates. Once the drain is in place, the abscess may require a few weeks to a few months to resolve. The drain tube will facilitate resolution of inflammation so that a patient who does require surgical intervention will be in a more stable overall condition and therefore at decreased risk for complications associated with surgery. Each drain tube should be labeled so that documentation is clear and consistent among the physicians, nurses, and interventional radiologists. Drain tubes should be irrigated only when the provider who inserted the catheter gives specific instructions. Orders to irrigate the drainage tube should specify use of sterile saline, the amount of solution to use, and the frequency of irrigations. Slight force is used to irrigate the drain tube so that debris that has lodged in the lateral holes of the catheter can be dislodged.

CLINICAL CONSULT

A: Referral received to consult with an older adult patient admitted from a long-term care setting who had a PEG tube placed recently. Nurses report they have to change the gauze dressings around the site 4 or 5 times a day due to leakage around the site. Upon examination, the silastic bumper is not secure against the skin and gauze is taped to the peritubular site. The peritubular skin is erythematous with shallow islands of denudation.

D: Ineffective securement of PEG tube; peritubular MASD secondary to leakage of gastric contents.

P: Instruct nurses on proper technique for securing PEG. Manage skin denudement.

I: (1) Check balloon for proper inflation. (2) Cleanse skin with tap water and dab dry. (3) Dust skin barrier powder over denuded skin and apply thin silicone adhesive border foam with large center cut out to position over skin and around PEG site. (4) Position silastic bumper against thin silicone adhesive border foam dressing. (5) Cleanse site daily with tap water and cotton-tipped applicator.

E: Remove foam dressing after 7 days and discontinue; secure silicone bumper against skin. Reconsult if peritubular drainage resumes.

SUMMARY

Percutaneous tubes contribute to both quantity and quality of life for many patients. Regardless of who inserts the tube or the purpose of the tube, all percutaneous tubes require stabilization, and should be monitored for patency and complications. It should not be assumed that nursing staff are familiar with the appropriate care of percutaneous tubes. Furthermore, initial patient and caregiver instructions, as well as ongoing follow-up, is critical.

REFERENCES

Bankhead R, Rolandelli R: Access to gastrointestinal tract. In Rolandelli RH, editor: *Enteral and tube feeding*, Philadelphia, 2005, Elsevier Saunders.

Bankhead R, Boullata J, Brantley S, et al: A.S.P.E.N. Enteral nutrition practice recommendations, *JPEN J Parenter Enteral Nutr* 33(2):122–167, 2009.

Beyers PL: Complications of enteral nutrition. In DeChicco LE, Matarese MM, editors: *Nutrition support practice: a clinical guide*, Philadelphia, 2003, Saunders.

Bloch AS, Mueller C: Enteral and parenteral nutrition support. In Mahan LK, Escott-Stump S, editors: *Krause's food, nutrition, and diet therapy*, ed 11, Philadelphia, 2004, Elsevier.

Coates NE, MacFadyen BV Jr: Laparoscopic placement of enteral feeding tubes. In Latifi R, Dudrick SJ, editors: *Medical intelligence unit: current surgical nutrition*, Austin, TX, 1996, RG Landes.

DeChicco RS, Matarese MM: Determining the nutrition support regimen. In DeChicco LE, Matarese MM, editors: *Nutrition support practice: a clinical guide*, Philadelphia, 2003, Saunders.

Duh QY, McQuaid K: Flexible endoscopy and enteral access. In Eubanks WS, et al, editors: *Mastery of endoscopic and laparoscopic surgery*, Philadelphia, 2000, Lippincott Williams & Wilkins.

Foutch PG, Talbert GA, Gaines JA, et al: The gastrostomy button: a prospective assessment of safety, success and spectrum of use, *Gastrointest Endosc* 35(1):41–44, 1989.

Gauderer MWL, Olsen MM, Stellato TA, et al: Feeding gastrostomy button: experience and recommendations, *J Pediatr Surg* 23(1):24–28, 1988.

Gauderer MWL, Ponsky JL, Izant RF Jr: Gastrostomy without laparotomy: a percutaneous technique, *J Pediatr Surg* 15:872–875, 1980.

Gauderer MWL, Stellato TA: Gastrostomies: evolution, techniques, indications and implications, *Curr Probl Surg* 23:657–719, 1986.

Georgeson KE: Laparoscopic versus open procedures for long-term enteral access, *Nutr Clin Pract* 12(Suppl 1):S7–S8, 1997.

Georgeson KE: Laparoscopic gastrostomy. In Bax NMA, et al, editors: *Endoscopic surgery in children*, New York, 1999, Springer.

Gincherman Y, Torosian M: Enteral nutrition: indications, methods of delivery and complications. In Latifi R, Dudrick SJ, editors: *Current surgical nutrition*, New York, 1996, Chapman and Hall.

Gorman RC, Morris JB: Minimally invasive access to the gastrointestinal tract. In Rombeau JL, Rolandelli RH, et al: *Clinical nutrition: enteral and tube feeding*, ed 3, Philadelphia, 1997, Saunders.

Gorman RC, et al: Enteral feeding techniques. In Torosian MH, editor: *Nutrition for the hospitalized patient: basic science and principles of practice*, New York, 1995, Marcel Dekker.

Hanlon MD: Preplacement marking for optional gastrointestinal and jejunostomy tube site locations to decrease complications and promote self-care, *Nutr Clin Pract* 13:167, 1998.

Harbison SP: Intubation of the stomach and small intestine. In Yeo CJ, et al: *Shackelford's surgery of the alimentary tract*, ed 6, Philadelphia, 2007, Saunders.

Jung SH, Dong SH, Lee JY, et al: Percutaneous endoscopic gastrostomy prevents gastroesophageal reflux in patients with nasogastric tube feeding: a prospective study with 24 hour pH monitoring, *Gut Liver* 5(3):288–292, 2011.

Kejariwal D, Bromley D, Miao Y: The "cut and push" method of percutaneous endoscopic gastrostomy tube removal in adult patients: the Ipswich experience, *Nutr Clin Pract* 24(2):281–283, 2009.

Lord LM: Enteral access devices, *Nurs Clin North Am* 32(4): 685–704, 1997.

Lysen L: Enteral equipment. In DeChicco LE, Matarese MM, editors: *Nutrition support practice: a clinical guide*, Philadelphia, 2003, Saunders.

McNichol L: Medical adhesives and patient safety: state of the science: consensus statements for the assessment, prevention, and treatment of adhesive-related skin injuries, *J Wound Ostomy Continence Nurs* 40(4):365–380, 2013.

Naik RP, Joshipura VP, Patel NR: Complications of PEG – prevention and management, *Internet J Gastroenterol* 8(1):8, 2009.

O'Brien B, Davis S, Erwin-Toth P: G-tube site care: a practical guide, *RN* 62(2):52–56, 1999.

Patterson RS: Enteral nutrition delivery systems. In Grant JA, Kennedy-Caldwell C, editors: *Nutritional support nursing*, Philadelphia, 1988, Grune & Stratton.

Rollins H, Nathwani N, Morrison D: Optimising wound care in a child with an infected gastrostomy exit site, *Br J Nurs* 22(22):1275–1279, 2013.

Rombeau JL, Rolandelli RH: *Clinical nutrition: enteral and tube feeding*, ed 3, Philadelphia, 1997, Saunders.

Senadhi V, Emuron D, Singh R, et al: PEG tube placement in morbidly obese patients, *Endoscopy* 44:E53, 2012.

Simons S, Remington R: The percutaneous endoscopic gastrostomy tube: a nurse's guide to PEG tubes, *Medsurg Nurs* 22(2):77–83, 2013.

Timratana P, El-Hayek K, Shimizu H, et al: Percutaneous endoscopic gastrostomy (PEG) with T-fasteners obviates the need for emergent replacement after early tube dislodgement, *Surg Endosc* 26:3541–3547, 2012.

Tong A: Pancreatic enzyme products update, *Cleveland Clin Pharmacother Update* 13(6), 2010. http://www.clevelandclinic-meded.com/medicalpubs/pharmacy/pdf/Pharmacotherapy_XIII-6.pdf. Accessed August 19, 2015.

Wu JS, Soper NJ: Gastrostomy and jejunostomy. In Jones DB, et al, editors: *Laparoscopic surgery: principles and procedures*, ed 2, New York, 2004, Marcel Dekker.

Yarmus L, Gilbert C, Lechtzin N, et al: Safety and feasibility of interventional pulmonologists performing bedside percutaneous endoscopic gastrostomy tube placement, *Chest* 114(2):436–440, 2013.

Examples of Tools Used to Support Skin and Wound Care

AMERICAN COLLEGE PHYSICIANS EVIDENCE FOR PRESSURE ULCER RISK ASSESSMENT TOOLS

Characteristic	Quality of Evidence	Data
Braden scale		
Overall diagnostic accuracy	Moderate	Median sensitivity, 0.74 (range, 0.33 to 1.00); median specificity, 0.68 (range, 0.34 to 0.86) (cutoff ≤ 18); 1 poor-quality, 7 fair-quality, and 8 good-quality studies
Across settings	Low	No clear difference across settings (cutoff ≤ 15 to 18); 10 good-quality, 16 fair-quality, and 2 poor-quality studies
Optimal cutoff in different settings	Low	Lower optimal cutoff in acute care setting (sensitivity, 0.55; specificity, 0.94) (cutoff, ≤ 15) compared with long-term care setting (sensitivity, 0.57; specificity, 0.61) (cutoff, ≤ 18); statistical significance not reported; 1 good quality study
Difference according to race	Low	No clear differences between black and white patients; 1 fair-quality study (50)
Differences according to baseline pressure ulcer risk	Moderate	No clear differences; 1 good-quality and 2 fair-quality studies
Cubbin and Jackson scale		
Overall diagnostic accuracy	Moderate	Median sensitivity, 0.89 (range, 0.83 to 0.95); medium specificity, 0.61 (range, 0.42 to 0.82) (cutoff, ≤ 24 to 29); 1 good-quality and 2 fair-quality studies
Intensive care unit setting	Low	Similar diagnostic accuracy in intensive care unit patients compared with Braden and Waterlow scales; 1 good-quality and 1 fair-quality study
Norton scale		
Diagnostic accuracy	Moderate	Median sensitivity, 0.75 (range, 0.00 to 0.89); median specificity, 0.68 (range, 0.59 to 0.95) (cutoff, ≤14); 1 good-quality and 4 fair-quality studies
Waterlow scale		
Pressure ulcer incidence or severity (vs. clinical judgement)	Low	No difference compared with nurses' clinical judgment alone: RR, 1.40 (95% CI, 0.82 to 2.40); 1 good-quality study
Diagnostic accuracy	Moderate	Sensitivities, 0.88 and 1.00; specificities, 0.13 and 0.29 (cutoff, ≥ 10); 2 fair-quality studies
Diagnostic accuracy: direct comparisons among risk assessment scales	Moderate	No clear differences among scales; 2 good-quality and 4 fair-quality studies

RR, Relative risk.
Adapted from Qaseem A, Mir TP, Starkey M, et al: Risk assessment and prevention of pressure ulcers: a clinical practice guideline from the American College of Physicians, *Ann Intern Med* 162:359–369, 2015.

POLICY AND PROCEDURE: PREVENTION OF PRESSURE ULCERS

Policy:

All patients will have a skin inspection and be assessed for risk of pressure ulcers on admission (as soon as possible but at least within 8 hours), daily, and with significant change in condition. Appropriate preventive interventions will be implemented.

Risk Assessment Procedure:

Risk assessment includes determining a person's risk for pressure ulcer development using the appropriate Braden scale. Pressure ulcer preventive interventions will target risk factors as determined by the pressure ulcer risk assessment. For patients older than 16 years, the Braden scale will be used. For patients younger than 16 years, the Braden Q scale will be used.

Note: Braden Scale for Predicting Pressure Score Risk (Braden scale) is a standardized tool for determining level of risk for pressure ulcer development in adult patients. Level of risk scores are shown below; *however*, care plan development must be designed to decrease or eliminate each individual risk factor, as well as risk of skin breakdown from medical devices.

15 to 18 = Mild risk
13 to 14 = Moderate risk
10 to 12 = High risk
≤ 9 = Very high risk

Skin Inspection:

A head-to-toe skin inspection, including around and under medical devices, between all skin folds, and back of head. During inspection, pressure points are examined and palpated closely for any of the following conditions:

- Alteration in skin moisture
- Change in texture, turgor
- Change in temperature compared to surrounding skin (warmer or cooler)
- Color changes (e.g., red, blue, purplish hues)
- Nonblanchable erythema
- Consistency (e.g., bogginess [soft] or induration [hard])
- Edema
- Open areas, blisters, rash, drainage
- Pain

Note: Blanching erythema is an early indicator of the need to redistribute pressure. Nonblanching erythema is suggestive that tissue damage has already occurred or is imminent. Indurated or boggy skin is a sign that tissue damage may have occurred.

Preventive Interventions

1. Minimize or Eliminate Friction and Shear

   One or more of the following interventions and observations will be used to minimize or eliminate shear if it is identified as a risk factor:
   - Lift rather than drag patient's body when moving patient up in bed or chair.
   - Avoid elevating head of the bed more than 30 degrees unless contraindicated.
   - Decrease shear/friction by having patient sit in chair at 90-degree angle rather than reclining.
   - Use transfer methods that minimize sliding (e.g. mechanical lifts, HoverMatt, trapeze, surgical slip sheets).
   - Place a pad or pillow between skin surfaces that may rub together.
   - Apply heel and elbow pads to reduce friction (they do not reduce pressure).
   - Apply creams or lotions frequently to lower surface tension on skin and reduce friction.
   - Apply transparent film dressing, hydrocolloid dressing, or skin sealant to bony prominences (e.g., elbows) to decrease friction.
   - Keep skin well hydrated and moisturized.
   - Lubricate bedpan with incontinence care lotion or ointment before placing under patient. Position bedpan by rolling patient on and off rather than pushing and pulling bedpan in and out.
   - Apply skin protectants and ointments to protect skin from moisture. Excessive moisture weakens dermal integrity and destroys the outer lipid layer, so less mechanical force is needed to wound the skin and cause a physical opening.

2. Minimize Pressure

   Immobility is the most significant risk factor for pressure ulcer development. Patients who have any degree of immobility should be closely monitored for pressure ulcer development. One or more of the following interventions will be used if immobility is identified as a risk factor:

   Patients in Bed
   - Make frequent, small position changes.
   - Use pillows or wedges to reduce pressure on bony prominences.
   - Turn patient a minimum of every 2 hours.
   - Do not position patient lying on side directly on trochanter (hip).
   - Use pressure redistribution mattresses/surfaces.
   - Free-float heels by placing a pillow under calf muscle and keeping heels off all surfaces.
   - Avoid elevating head of the bed more than 30 degrees unless contraindicated.

   Patients in Chair
   - Encourage patient to shift weight every 15 minutes (e.g., perform chair pushups if able to reposition self; stand and reseat self if able; make small shift changes, such as elevating legs).
   - Reposition patient every hour if he or she is unable to reposition self.
   - Use chair cushions for pressure redistribution.

3. Minimize/Eliminate Pressure from Medical Devices
   - Follow manufacturer's instructions for appropriate use of medical devices (e.g., oxygen masks and tubing, catheters, cervical collars, casts, intravenous tubing, restraints).

- Routinely remove or reposition devices as needed for skin inspection, pressure relief, and pressure redistribution.
4. Manage Moisture

   Management of moisture from perspiration, wound drainage, and incontinence is an important aspect of pressure ulcer prevention. Moisture from incontinence may be a precursor to pressure ulcer development because of skin maceration and increased friction. Fecal incontinence is a greater risk factor than urinary incontinence for pressure ulcer development because the stool contains bacteria and enzymes that are caustic to the skin. In the presence of both urinary and fecal incontinence, fecal enzymes convert urea to ammonia, raising the skin pH. With a more alkaline skin pH, the skin becomes more permeable to other irritants. One or more of the following interventions will be used to minimize or eliminate moisture when it is identified as a risk factor:
   - Contain wound drainage.
   - Keep skin folds dry.
   - Evaluate type of incontinence (urinary, fecal, or both).
   - Implement toileting schedule or bowel/bladder program as appropriate.
   - Check for incontinence a minimum of every 2 hours and as needed.
   - Cleanse skin gently with pH-balanced cleanser at each soiling. Avoid excessive friction and scrubbing, which can further traumatize the skin. Cleansers with nonionic surfactants are gentler on the skin than are anionic surfactants in typical soaps.
   - Use incontinence skin barriers (e.g., creams, ointments, pastes, film-forming skin protectants) as needed to protect and maintain intact skin or to treat nonintact skin.
   - Consider use of stool containment devices. Rectal tubes not approved by the U.S. Food and Drug Administration will not be used.
   - Assess for candidiasis and treat as appropriate.

5. Maintain Adequate Nutrition/Hydration

   The patient who is malnourished and/or dehydrated is at increased risk for pressure ulcer development. One or more of the following interventions will be used when nutrition is identified as a risk factor:
   - Provide nutrition compatible with individual's wishes or condition.
   - Encourage hydration, as well as high-protein and high-calorie supplements, for the patient with multiple risk factors for pressure ulcer development.

6. Address Sustainability of Plan of Care and Goals

   The patient's ability to participate in pressure ulcer prevention interventions may be affected by physical and behavioral factors. Noncompliance may be related to inability to participate, lifestyle issues, cultural differences, medical condition, physical condition, lack of trust, or knowledge gaps. Possible activities to address include the following:
   - Provide education that increases patient/family knowledge of pressure ulcer risk and appropriate interventions.
   - Identify barriers to patient participation and develop strategies to address those barriers.

7. Documentation
   - All assessments and skin inspection findings will be documented within 24 hours of admission. A plan of care for prevention of skin breakdown, patient response to interventions, and informed refusals will be described and documented.

8. Patient/Family Education

   The patient, family, and/or caregivers will be educated on risk assessment and skin inspection technique. They will be informed of current status of risk assessment and skin inspection findings and will be involved in planning interventions.

POLICY AND PROCEDURE: WOUND ASSESSMENT, DOCUMENTATION, AND QUALITY TRACKING

Policy:

All wounds will be assessed upon admission or occurrence, weekly, within 24 hours of discharge, and with significant changes.

Procedure:

The following parameters will be documented:

A. Anatomic location of skin breakdown

B. Etiology (type) of skin breakdown

C. Classification of skin breakdown
   - Pressure ulcers will be classified according to the National Pressure Ulcer Advisory Panel (NPUAP) staging system.
   - All other wounds will be classified as either "partial thickness" or "full thickness."
     - *Partial thickness:* Wounds extend through the first layer of skin (the epidermis) and into, but not through, the second layer of skin (the dermis).
     - *Full thickness:* Wounds extend through both the epidermis and dermis and may involve subcutaneous tissue, muscle, and possibly bone.
     - *Approximated incisions:* Staples, sutures, or Steri-strips are present.

D. Wound measurements in centimeters

   Length and width: To ensure consistency, use the clock method for wound measurement. Visualize the wound as if it were the face of a clock. The top of the wound (12 o'clock position) is always toward the patient's head. Conversely, the bottom of the wound (6 o'clock position) is in the direction of the patient's feet. Therefore length will be measured from the 12 o'clock to the 6 o'clock position, using the head and feet as guides. Width will be measured from side to side, or from the 3 o'clock to the 9 o'clock position.

   Depth: The depth of the wound can be described as the distance from the visible surface to the deepest point in the wound, perpendicular to the skin surface. To measure the depth of the wound, use a sterile, flexible, cotton-tipped applicator.
   - Put on gloves and gently insert the applicator into the deepest portion of the wound.

- Grasp the applicator with the thumb and forefinger at the point level to the skin surface.
- Withdraw the applicator while maintaining the position of the thumb and forefinger.
- Measure (with a ruler marked in centimeters) from the tip of the applicator to that position.

Tunneling (also known as *sinus tracts*): This is a passageway under the surface of the skin that is generally open at the skin level. However, most of the tunneling is not visible.

- Put on gloves and gently insert the sterile cotton-tipped applicator into the deepest extent of the tunnel.
- Pinch the applicator at the point where it meets the wound edge.
- Hold the pinched length of the applicator next to a centimeter ruler to determine the depth of tunneling.
- Document the length and location of the tunnel using the clock method.

Undermining: Tissue destruction underlies intact skin. Both the direction and extent of undermining should be documented.

- Put on gloves and gently insert the sterile cotton-tipped applicator into the sites where undermining occurs.
- View the wound as though it were the face of a clock (as previously described). The 12 o'clock position corresponds to the wound edge that aligns toward the patient's head.
- Progressing in a clockwise direction, gently probe to determine the extent of undermining (e.g., 2 o'clock to 5 o'clock position).
- Insert the cotton-tipped applicator into the deepest area of the undermining. Grasp the applicator with thumb and forefinger at the point where it is level to the skin surface.
- Withdraw the applicator while maintaining the position of thumb and forefinger. Measure (using a ruler marked in centimeters) from the tip of the applicator to that position.
- Document the extent and deepest measurement of undermining in a manner similar to the following

example: "Undermining from 2 o'clock to 5 o'clock position. Deepest point is 2.5 cm at 3 o'clock position."

E. Wound bed appearance (type and percentage of tissue in the wound bed)
F. Exudate/drainage
   - Color
   - Amount (percentage saturating dressing and type of dressing)
G. Periwound
   - *All wounds:* Assess and document condition of periwound skin condition (maceration, induration, erythema)
   - *Lower extremity wounds:* Assess and document edema and dorsalis pedis and posterior tibial pulses and sensation
H. Presence or absence of local signs of infection/overcolonization
   - New/increased slough
   - Drainage excess, change in color/consistency
   - Poor granulation tissue (friable, bright red, exuberant)
   - Redness, warmth, induration around wound
   - Suddenly high glucose level in patient with diabetes
   - Pain or tenderness
   - Unusual odor
   - Lack of improvement after 2 weeks of optimal management (including elimination or reduction of pressure ulcer risk factors as well as cofactors to impaired wound healing)
I. Pain
   - Assess pain using a visual analogue scale or a faces rating scale
J. Patient/family education
   - Signs and symptoms of infection
   - Status or assessment of wound
K. Pressure ulcer reporting
   - Pressure ulcers that are present on admission will be reported to the physician/provider for evaluation and documentation in the physician's notes.
   - Facility acquired pressure ulcers will be reported to the physician/provider, and a quality tracking report will be sent to quality management for possible root-cause analysis.

POLICY AND PROCEDURE: WOUND MANAGEMENT

Policy:

A wound treatment plan will be initiated for a patient at the time of admission or upon development of a wound. The patient's treatment plan will be evaluated at least every week thereafter and revised as necessary. The treatment plan will be based on the principles outlined next.

Procedure:

A. Establish realistic goals related to wound management in collaboration with the patient, family, caregivers, and physician.
   - If wound healing is *not* a realistic goal, create a plan of care that will minimize pain, odor, and infection while optimizing quality of life.
   - If wound healing *is* a realistic goal, the following interventions should be incorporated into the care plan.

B. Control/eliminate causative factors.
C. Optimize nutrition.
   - Complete a nutritional screening on admission per nutritional assessment policy and procedure.
   - Consult registered dietician (RD) per nutritional assessment policy and procedure.
   - Reassess and consider RD consult if wound does not improve within 1 week of optimal wound management.
D. Assess, prevent, or manage pain.
E. Remove devitalized tissue when appropriate.
   - In the presence of adequate perfusion, remove devitalized tissue through mechanical, autolytic, or enzymatic debridement.
   - Heel ulcers with dry eschar need not be debrided if no signs of infection are present.

- Sharp debridement by a qualified professional should be conducted when indicated.
F. Cleanse wound.
  - Cleanse wound initially and at each dressing change.
  - Use minimal mechanical force while cleaning a wound.
  - Avoid cleaning wounds using abrasive or antiseptic agents. (Normal saline is most often appropriate.)
G. Provide a physiologic wound environment with appropriate dressings.
  - If blood supply to the wound site is adequate, keep the wound bed moist.
  - If blood supply to wound site is *not* adequate, keep the wound clean and dry.
  - Keep periwound skin dry and intact.
  - Control exudate.
  - Consider caregiver time.
  - Eliminate dead space.
  - Avoid overpacking the wound.
H. Manage bacterial colonization and infection.
  - When treating multiple wounds on the same patient, attend to the most contaminated wound last.

- Clean technique may be used for chronic wounds and pressure ulcers.
- Perform cleansing and debridement of wounds as appropriate.
- Consider a 2-week trial of topical antimicrobials as a course of treatment of wounds that are not healing after 2 weeks of optimal care.
- Protect wounds from exogenous sources of contamination (e.g., feces).
- Immediately report signs of infection to the physician.
I. Provide patient/family education.
  The patient, family, and/or caregivers will be educated regarding the following:
- Signs and symptoms of infection
- Status or assessment of wound
- Skin inspection and preventive interventions for skin breakdown (see policy on prevention of skin breakdown)
- Pressure ulcer risk assessment findings (see policy on prevention of skin breakdown)
- Dressing changes (if applicable)

POLICY: NAIL CARE

Purpose:

To identify patients who need expert nail clipping from a certified or trained specialist after discharge.

Responsibility:

Provider (referral for expert nail care)
Nursing (basic nail trimming)

Policy:

- *Expert nail clipping* is required for patients with nail disorders and conditions with risk factors known to lead to significant infection, poor wound healing, excessive bleeding, or limb loss. Expert nail care is not within the scope of nursing and requires a provider referral upon discharge to a podiatrist or trained/certified professional.
- *Basic nail clipping* is considered part of patient hygiene and within the scope of nursing practice.

Process:

A. The need for nail clipping is identified by the patient, family, hospital personnel, or provider.
B. The MD evaluates risk factors and determines if patient requires any of the following:
  - *Basic nail trimming* by staff nurse as specified in the *Nursing Procedure Manual*

- *Expert nail clipping* by a trained expert due to nail disorders and conditions with risk factors known to lead to significant infection, poor wound healing, excessive bleeding, or limb loss. Examples include but are not limited to the following:
  1. Onychophosis (incurvated or involuted nails)
  2. Onychogryposis (deformed, hypertrophic nails)
  3. Diabetes
  4. Rheumatoid arthritis
  5. Pernicious anemia
  6. Peripheral vascular disease
  7. Conditions that require warfarin (Coumadin)
  8. Neutropenia (absolute neutrophil count <1000).
  9. Thrombocytopenia (platelet count ≤60,000).
C. The MD orders *basic* nail trimming by nurse or generates a podiatry referral upon discharge if *expert nail clipping* is indicated. (*Note*: Inpatient podiatry consultations remain available for acute needs such as surgical procedures and debridement.)

Related Resources

Howes-Trammel S et al: Foot and nail care. In Bryant R, Nix D: *Acute and chronic wounds: current management concepts*, ed 5, St. Louis, 2015, Mosby/Elsevier.
Itano JK, Taoka KN: *Oncology Nursing Society core curriculum for oncology nursing*, ed 4, St. Louis, 2005, Saunders/Elsevier.

POLICY: ANTIEMBOLISM STOCKINGS

Purpose:

To assist health care providers in the appropriate assessment and use of antiembolism stockings (AES) and to delineate patient care requirements to minimize/eliminate risks associated with AES use.

Policy:

Use of AES may be indicated in the immobile/bedridden patient as a mechanical means of deep vein thrombosis (DVT)/pulmonary embolus (PE) prophylaxis in a patient who is at risk.

Procedure:

Adherence to the following assessment, use, and maintenance requirements is required. By definition, AES are elastic stockings that provide between 18 and 25 mm Hg gradient pressure. Medical center use is limited to knee-high stockings.

A. Indications for use:
1. An order by a licensed independent practitioner
2. For DVT/PE prophylaxis in the immobile/bedridden patient
3. *Contraindications* for use:
   a. Arterial insufficiency (including symptoms of claudication, lower extremity pain with elevation)
   b. Absent peripheral pulses
   c. Anatomic abnormality
   d. Dermatitis
   e. Loss of skin integrity
   f. Massive edema of legs or pulmonary edema from congestive heart failure
   g. Suspected or actual acute DVT
   h. Lower extremity ischemia or gangrene
   i. Recent vein ligation
   j. Recent skin graft
   k. Ambulatory patient

B. Assessment, care, and maintenance:
1. Initial assessment as noted in A, nos. 1 through 3.
2. Provide patient education, emphasizing the stocking is to be used only while the patient is immobile or bedridden. Once he or she is ambulatory, the stocking should be discarded.
3. Measure the patient for knee-high AES only after he or she has been supine for at least 30 minutes.
4. Measure the extremity(ies) for the appropriate size according to the manufacturer's directions and brand being used. (The ankle is the most important measurement.)
5. Ensure the patient's leg is clean and completely dry prior to initial application of the stocking.
6. *Safety check:* Apply the stockings according to nursing procedure and complete a safety check, including the following:
   a. Heel is located in the center of the heel pocket.
   b. Toes are freely mobile and patient reports no cramping.
   c. Fit is smooth over sensitive areas (toes, heel, anterior foot, ankle).
   d. Knit change at the knee is just below popliteal fossa.
7. Reassess lower extremity circulation within 1 to 2 hours after initial application. If circulation is diminished (i.e., toes discolored, patient reports numbness, burning sensation), remove the stockings and notify the ordering practitioner.
8. Remove the stockings for 30 to 60 minutes every shift and conduct a reassessment. Particular at-risk areas include the patient's toes, heels, malleolus, anterior ankle, and top of stocking (possible tourniquet effect). Once daily, wash the lower extremities and lubricate the skin. Allow the lubricant to absorb before reapplying the stockings. Powder can be used if the extremity is thoroughly dried prior to application.
9. Discontinue and discard the stockings when the patient is ambulatory.

C. Documentation:
1. *Stocking note:* Document as a progress note the initial assessment (including peripheral pulse assessment), measurements, size applied, and education provided.
2. Ongoing q.s. removal, assessment, and hygiene are recorded on the treatment record. Discontinuation of AES is also recorded on the treatment record.
3. Additional progress notes are required only when stockings require discontinuation due to impaired circulation, potential loss of skin integrity, or patient intolerance. Such progress notes will include provider notification.
4. Skin breakdown associated with use of the stockings requires an incident report to be initiated.

D. Special notes:
1. Alternative interventions effective for prevention of DVT/PE:
   a. Dorsal and plantar flexion of the foot at least 10 times every hour while the patient is awake. Such interventions should be documented on the treatment sheet.
   b. Progressing patients to an ambulatory status as soon as clinically and physically indicated is one of the most effective measures for DVT/PE prevention.
   c. AES are not recommended for use with sequential compression devices (SCDs). Rather, absorbent cotton stockings or stockinette is recommended for use.
   d. Mechanical foot pumps or compression therapy increase lower extremity peripheral blood flow.
2. Pharmacologic agents effective for prevention of DVT/PE:
   a. Low-molecular-weight heparin
   b. Warfarin
   c. Subcutaneous heparin
3. Little-known facts:
   a. AES *are not* effective in treating lower extremity edema in the upright patient. Ambulatory compression stockings (e.g., Jobst) can be ordered for this purpose. A variety of gradient pressure models (range 20 to 50 mm Hg) are available from the prosthetics department.
   b. Treatment of orthostatic hypotension may include ambulatory compression stockings (Jobst).
   c. Ankle-brachial index (ABI) is a noninvasive test that measures the patency of lower extremity arteries. ABI <0.8 indicates arterial occlusion. Normal ABI is 1.0 to 1.2. Although no data suggest a critical level for not using AES stockings, vascular devices should not be used if ABI is <0.8, which is the level where critical limb ischemia becomes a serious concern.

E. Patient/family education: Describe the purpose of the stockings before application, and instruct the patient to notify the nurse immediately of any burning, tingling, numbness, or pain following application. In rare situations where patients are discharged with AES, provide a written handout and review application, maintenance, laundering, and problem reporting with the patient.

INTERDEPARTMENTAL HANDOFF

Fairview Southdale Hospital Communication Tool

Hospital Handoff Information

   Date:_____ Time:_____

   Discharge/Transport from:

_____

Patient Sticker Here

Primary Patient Problem(s):

Allergies: **None**   **See Arm Band**   **Latex**

Safety Risks:
- ☐ **Full CODE**
- ☐ **DNR/DNI**
- ☐ **Fall Risk: Mental Status (orientation/confusion):**
- ☐ **Fall Risk: Functional Status (indep/limited mobility):**
- ☐ **Infection Risk:**   **MRSA**   **VRE**   **Other:**
- ☐ **Pressure Ulcer Risk (Braden ≤18)** — See back of sheet for interventions (excluding OR)
  - ○ **Existing Pressure Ulcer**   **Location:** _____ See back for interventions (excluding OR)
- ☐ **Restraints**
- ☐ **Suicide or Elopement Precautions–72 Hours HOLD** (**Security w/Patient**)

    Special Alert Care Plan: _____

Sensory Risk(s):
- ☐ **HOH**   **(R)**   **(L)**   **Both**
- ☐ **Vision Aids:**_____
- ☐ **Speech/Language difficulties:**_____

- ☐ **Interpreter Needed:**   **Yes**   **No**
    Contacted:_____

Equipment & Special Needs:
- ☐ **Needs assistance to transfer X_____ people (more than 2, please send on cart)**
- ☐ **Only guidance needed**
- ☐ **Uses cane/walker/other:**_____
- ☐ **Special Needs:**

    Able to have water: Yes   No

RN Signature:_____   **Ext:**_____

Note Patient Belongings:
_____Glasses _____Dentures _____Hearing aid _____Clothing _____Other (list)
Sending Department: _____ Initial
Receiving Department: _____ Initial
Discharging Department: _____ Initial

Return from procedural department:

Test #1
Signature:_____ ext:_____

Test #2
Signature:_____ ext:_____

ATTENTION NURSING:_____
_____
_____

The chart should remain with patient whenever possible.
Completion of this form is expected for patient safety, employee safety, tracking of patient belongings, and communication between inpatient and procedural areas.
A new form is needed each day or anytime greater than two procedures have occurred in one day.
This is not a permanent chart copy.

Pressure Ulcer Prevention[1]
Algorithm

ALLINA Hospitals & Clinics

Admission

Skin assessment (including history)

Head to toe inspection: Is there skin injury or pressure ulcer?

Yes → Develop an individualized care plan for treating and preventing further skin breakdown[2-4] If patient has a pressure ulcer on admission: Notify admitting physician and document in LDA group "Pressure injury/ulcer"

No

Daily pressure ulcer risk assessment; use Braden Scale. Complete holistic review for risk factors

Is there risk for skin breakdown or pressure ulcer?

No — Braden score > 18

Yes — *Braden score ≤ 18 or other risk factors

If pressure injury/ulcer is hospital acquired, document in LDA group and submit PVSR

Skin inspection Q shift if Braden ≤ 12 ; otherwise daily

Daily:
• Skin Inspection
• Braden Scale
• Holistic review of risk factors

Place "iceberg" magnet on patient's door to identify risk*

Develop target interventions[2-4] to address each risk area and include in the individualized plan of care ("Pressure ulcer prevention" secondary care plan) Review outcomes of plan and interventions

Mobility Activity Deficit — Yes

Moisture/ Incontinence — Yes

Nutritional Deficit — Yes

Braden Scale Risk Stratification

*Braden Scores:
At Risk: 15-18
Moderate Risk: 13-14
High Risk: 10-12
Very High Risk: ≤ 9

SKIN Bundle[5]
S = Skin Inspection & Risk Assessment
K = Keep pressure off – minimize pressure, friction, shear
I = Incontinence/moisture skin protection
N = Nutrition is optimized

Automatic consult goes to Dietitians: Braden score ≤ 14 and nutrition subscore is 1-2 for 3 consecutive days → NIP policy/order set

Review outcomes of plan and interventions

[1]Adapted from Armstrong DG et al: New opportunities to improve pressure ulcer prevention and treatment, *Adv Skin Wound Care* 21(10):469-78, 2008.
[2] Monahan FD: *Phipps' medical-surgical nursing: health and illness perspective*, ed. 8, St. Louis, 2007, Mosby/Elsevier.
[3]Perry AG, Potter PA: *Clinical nursing skills & technique*, ed. 6, St. Louis, 2006, Mosby/Elsevier.
[4] Tucker SM et al: *Patient care standards: collaborative planning and nursing interventions*, ed. 7, St. Louis, 2007, Mosby/Elsevier.
[5]MN Hospital Association, 2/2007, Road Map to a Comprehensive Skin Safety Program

* Magnets optional on high-risk patient care areas

Courtesy of M. Zink and S. Sendelbach, Allina Hospitals & Clinics.

Skin Care Instructions

Patient identification

Pressure Ulcer Prevention

☐ Turn and position every 2 hours
☐ Pressure ulcer prevention mattress (i.e., group 1)
☐ Specialty mattress (i.e., low air loss)
☐ Float Heels/heels off bed
☐ Chair cushion
☐ HOB no more than 30°
☐ Other _____

Care of moisture-related skin issues (perineal, groin, buttocks, skin folds)

☐ Antifungal cream to affected area, twice a day and after incontinence
☐ Perineal cleanser and barrier paste BID and after incontinence
☐ Other _____

Care of pressure-related suspected deep tissue injury or Stage I pressure ulcer

☐ _____ Suspected deep tissue injury (intact pressure-related nonblanchable, dark discoloration or blood blister) keep clean, dry and free from pressure/injury, discoloration may resolve or slough to reveal extent of skin breakdown. No dressings needed as long as tissue is intact

☐ _____ Stage I pressure ulcer (intact pressure-related nonblanchable erythema) keep clean, dry, and free from pressure breakdown. No dressings needed as long as tissue is intact

☐ _____ Blister keep clean, dry, and free from pressure breakdown. No dressings needed as long as tissue is intact

☐ _____ ointment to shallow _____ wound twice daily

☐ Other _____
_____
_____
_____
_____

ALGINATE DRESSING CHANGE PROCEDURE

Purpose:

Promote autolysis of necrotic tissue and absorb exudate.

Wound Location: _____   Dressing Change Frequency: _____

Supplies: (Circle all that apply):

a. Calcium alginate
b. Normal saline or hospital-approved wound cleanser to clean wounds
c. Tape
d. Gauze to dry periwound skin

e. Secondary dressing (ABD transparent dressing, border gauze)
f. Barrier ointment (zinc, Vaseline) or skin sealant
g. Sterile cotton-tipped applicators (Q-tips)
h. Other: _____

Procedure:

1. Wash hands and apply gloves.
2. Remove and discard dressing. Remove gloves and wash hands thoroughly per handwashing policy. Apply new gloves and put on appropriate personal protective equipment.
3. Cleanse with normal saline or hospital-approved wound cleanser.
4. Apply skin barrier to protect periwound skin from exudate.
5. Apply calcium alginate. If the wound has depth, gently fill wound space with alginate.
6. Cover with secondary dressings and secure as needed.

GEL/OINTMENT/ENZYME DRESSING CHANGE PROCEDURE

Purpose:

Enzymes promote enzymatic debridement in a moist environment. Ointments and gels facilitate autolysis.

Wound Location: _____   Dressing Change Frequency: _____

Supplies (Circle all that apply):

a. Gel/ointment/enzyme as applicable. (*Note:* Most ointments and enzymes come from pharmacy.)
b. Normal saline or hospital-approved wound cleanser
c. Secondary dressing (4 × 4 cover sponge, ABD, border gauze)
d. Tape

e. Sterile gauze
f. Barrier ointment or skin sealant
g. Sterile cotton-tipped applicators (Q-tips)
h. Other: _____

Procedure:

1. Wash hands and apply gloves.
2. Remove and discard dressing per facility policy. Remove gloves, wash hands, apply new gloves, and put on appropriate personal protective equipment.
3. Cleanse with normal saline or wound cleanser.
4. If needed, apply skin barrier around wound to protect patient's surrounding intact periwound skin from moisture.
5. Apply thin layer of ointment to wound base or saturate into moist sterile gauze for packing into wounds with depth.
6. Cover with secondary dressings and secure as needed.
   Note: Most enzymes require a moist environment to be effective.

HYDROCOLLOID DRESSING CHANGE PROCEDURE

Indication:

Noninfected, minimally exudative wound

Purpose:

Promote autolysis of nonviable tissue and provide a moist wound-healing environment.

Wound Location: _____   Dressing Change Frequency: _____

Supplies (Circle all that apply):

- Hydrocolloid
- Normal saline or hospital-approved wound cleanser
- Gauze to dry around wound

Procedure:

1. Wash hands and apply gloves.
2. Carefully remove and discard dressing per facility policy. Carefully remove gloves, wash hands, apply new gloves, and put on appropriate personal protective equipment.
3. Cleanse with normal saline or hospital-approved wound cleanser.
4. Apply hydrocolloid to wound base. Allow 1 additional inch of product to cover and protect surrounding intact periwound skin.
5. Apply paper tape if needed to prevent dressing edges from rolling up.

HYDROGEL-SATURATED GAUZE DRESSING CHANGE PROCEDURE

Indication:

Dry to minimally exudative wound

Purpose:

Donate moisture to prevent tissue dehydration, promote autolysis of nonviable tissue, and provide a moist wound-healing environment.

Wound Location: _____   Dressing Change Frequency: _____

Supplies (Circle all that apply):

a. Hydrogel product
b. Normal saline or hospital-approved wound cleanser to clean wounds
c. Tape
d. Gauze to dry around wound

e. Secondary dressing (ABD, 4 × 4 cover sponge, foam, border gauze)
f. Barrier ointment or skin sealant
g. Sterile cotton-tipped applicators (Q-tips)
h. Other: _____

Procedure:

1. Wash hands and apply gloves.
2. Remove and discard dressing. Remove gloves, wash hands, apply new gloves, and put on appropriate personal protective equipment.
3. Cleanse with normal saline or wound cleanser.
4. Apply skin barrier to protect periwound skin from exudate.
5. Spread apart gel-impregnated sterile gauze and gently place or pack in wound base (or saturate gauze with hydrogel from a tube).
6. Follow with additional sterile gauze only if needed to fill depth of wound.
7. Cover with secondary dressing and secure as needed.

WOUND AND SKIN CARE COMPETENCIES

Learner Name:_____

Learner: It is your responsibility to get the individual competencies in front of your preceptor for observation, checking off, and signatures.

Preceptor: It is your responsibility to observe, initial, and date each item only if learner is deemed competent by meeting each criterion.

Pressure Ulcer Prevention Competency Criteria	**Preceptor's Signature/Date**
1. Performs head-to-toe skin inspection and palpation, including under medical devices and between skin folds	
2. Documents accurate pressure ulcer risk assessment (e.g., Braden score)	
3. Develops and documents skin safety care plan; links individual risk factors to specific interventions	
4. Places patient *and all tubes* in proper position	
5. Prevents shear injury by keeping head of bed at 30 degrees or less with slight activation of knee gatch (20 degree)	
6. Uses draw sheet and gets assistance to minimize dragging patient against mattress while moving in bed	
7. Floats heels off of bed with use of pillows under legs and identifies alternatives to offloading heels when pillows are not effective	
8. Shifts weight every hour while in the chair	
9. Describes strategies for managing moisture and incontinence; identifies and finds relevant supplies	

Wound Assessment Competency Criteria	**Preceptor's Signature/Date**
1. Identifies self and explains procedure to patient	
2. Washes hands	
3. Gathers necessary supplies *before* beginning the procedure (measuring guide, cotton-tipped applicators, method for recording measurements, and dressing change supplies)	
4. Follows infection control guidelines for discarding dressings into the red container	
5. Cleans wound prior to assessment using appropriate infection control technique	
6. Notes correct anatomic location of wound	
7. Measures the wound's (in centimeters) height, width, depth, tunneling, and undermining	
8. Notes tissue type (red, granular, yellow, necrotic)	
9. Notes condition of periwound skin	
10. Notes presence or absence of signs of infection	
11. Applies new dressing according to step-by-step instructions	
12. Documents accurate wound assessment	

Wound Care Competency Criteria	**Preceptor's Signature/Date**
1. Washes hands	
2. Reviews step-by-step instructions for dressing change	
3. Gathers necessary supplies *before* beginning the procedure	
4. Follows infection control guidelines for discarding dressings	
5. Washes hands again after removing the dressing and applies new gloves	
6. Follows step-by-step instructions during dressing change, including a strategy for protecting the periwound skin	
7. Places patient in proper position	

Pouch Change Competency Criteria	**Preceptor's Signature/Date**
1. Empties ostomy pouch when one-third full of gas or stool	
2. Changes pouch *immediately* if leaking occurs and verbalizes why leakage can and should be prevented	
3. Reviews step-by-step instructions for ostomy pouch change procedure	

4. Gathers necessary supplies

5. Follows infection control guidelines for discarding pouch

6. Positions patient flat (or ensures no abdominal wrinkles) during procedure

7. Dries the skin completely before applying a new pouch

8. Follows step-by-step instructions during pouch change

Support Surface Competency Criteria   **Preceptor's Signature/Date**

1. Demonstrates use of CPR controls on a low air-loss surface

2. Explains rationale for using the least amount of linen possible under the patient

3. Demonstrates use of max inflate button on a low air-loss surface

4. Explains why max inflate should be used during repositioning on a low air-loss surface

5. Demonstrates appropriate selection of under pads (air permeable for air beds only)

6. Identifies process for selecting and obtaining pressure redistribution support surfaces for
   beds, chairs, and heels

Negative Pressure Wound Therapy (NPWT) Competency Criteria   **Preceptor's Signature/Date**

1. Locates and views video in resource room

2. Reviews step-by-step instructions

3. Identifies self and explains procedure to patient

4. Washes hands

5. Gathers necessary supplies *before* beginning the procedure

6. Follows infection control guidelines for discarding dressings into the red container

7. Washes hands again after removing the dressing and applies new gloves

8. Cuts the sponge to fit the wound so that the sponge does not overlap onto intact skin

9. Ensures that tubing is positioned so that the patient does not lie or sit on the tubing

10. Applies transparent dressing/drape to ensure adequate seal

11. Verbalizes or demonstrates how to change the canister

12. Verbalizes or demonstrates ability to interpret alarms, ensure correct pressure, and operate
    machine

SAFE SKIN GAP ANALYSIS: OPERATING ROOM

SAFE SKIN Practice The following key strategies for preventing OR-related pressure ulcers have been implemented:	Gap? Y/N	If yes, strategies to meet this practice	Person Responsible	Timeline
1a) A thorough preoperative skin inspection is performed the day of the procedure prior to hand-off to the perioperative team.				
1b) Pressure ulcer risk and status is communicated to perioperative staff.				
1c) Perioperative staff assesses the patient's surgical risk factors for pressure ulcer development.				
1d) An OR table mattress pad with pressure redistributing properties greater than the standard OR mattress pad is used for patient's at high risk for pressure ulcer development.				
1e) Facilities have a policy addressing patient transfer processes to prevent shearing of patient's skin during transfers.				
1f) Patient's pressure ulcer risk, correct patient position, and related equipment are communicated to the full perioperative team through a preoperative briefing or other communication strategy.				
1g) Responsibility for positioning and repositioning the patient is assigned and well defined.				
1h) When patient is in a supine position, the patient's heels are suspended off the surface.				
1i) Perioperative staff is educated on areas of increased risk for pressure ulcers, based on patient position, and strategies for reducing pressure ulcer risk.				
1j) Patients with expected postoperative hemodynamic instability and medical contraindications to turning are placed on a Group II pressure redistribution surface for postoperative care.				
1k) The perioperative nurse communicates patient's position in the OR, existing pressure ulcers, and preoperative pressure ulcer risk to the postoperative nurse.				
1l) Patient's heels are suspended off the bed/surface during postoperative care.				
1m) Postop patients are repositioned to alternate position than OR position if not medically contraindicated.				

AULTMAN SURGICAL/PROCEDURAL POSITIONING COMMUNICATION TOOL

PATIENT LABEL

AULTMAN
Surgical/Procedural Positioning Communication Tool
**Note Surgery Length In Hours _____

Circle affected area. Designate with an "I" for intraoperative or "P" for postoperative assessment. Describe the area in the comments section.

☐ SUPINE

Occiput   Arms and   Lumbar   Sacrum   Heels
            elbows   area   and coccyx

Scapulae   Thoracic
                vertebrae

Comments: _____
_____

☐ PRONE

Forehead,   Anterior   Dorsum
eyes, ears, shoulders   Knees   of the
chin   feet

                                   Toes

Iliac   Genitalia   Shins
crests (men)

Breasts/chest

Comments: _____
_____

☐ PRONE (JACKKNIFE)

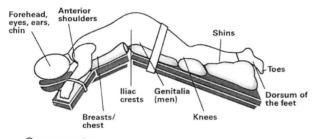

Forehead,   Anterior
eyes, ears, shoulders   Shins
chin

                              Toes

Iliac   Genitalia   Dorsum of
crests (men)   the feet

Breasts/   Knees
chest

Comments: _____
_____

☐ LATERAL

Arms   Ankles
                            and feet

                  Dependent hip   Legs   Dependent
Dependent side of Dependent   knee
the face and ear   shoulder
                   and axilla

Comments: _____
_____

☐ LITHOTOMY

Shoulders and
scapulae

                    Heels

                    Lateral
                    aspect of
                    the legs

                    Sacrum and
                    coccyx
Occiput   Hips

Comments: _____
_____

☐ SITTING

Scapulae

Ischial   Backs   Calcaneus
Tuberosities   of Knees

Comments: _____
_____

Form 202504 D: 02/10

SAFE SKIN GAP ANALYSIS: RESPIRATORY EQUIPMENT

SAFE SKIN Practice The following key strategies for preventing respiratory device-related pressure ulcers have been implemented:	Gap? Y/N	If yes, strategies to meet this practice	Person Responsible	Timeline
1a) Respiratory therapy is represented on the organization's pressure ulcer prevention team.				
1b) The skin beneath and around oxygen administration devices are thoroughly inspected at least every 8-12 hours.				
1c) Patients and caregivers are educated on the importance of frequent skin inspection beneath and around respiratory devices and of informing staff if they experience discomfort or pain beneath or around the devices.				
1d) Responsibility is clearly assigned (to a specific clinical discipline) for inspection and documentation of skin integrity around and under oxygen administration devices.				
1e) Abnormal skin integrity findings, site care, and interventions are documented in the patient's medical record in a location that is accessible to all relevant clinical disciplines.				
1f) Ear protectors are used on oxygen tubing as appropriate.				
1g) Strap tension and skin integrity beneath and around life sustaining CPAP and NPPV masks are checked at least every 4 hours, with oral intake, and with oral care.				
1h) During routine tracheostomy site care (at least every 8-12 hours) skin integrity and tension are checked under the straps, around and in back of the neck, around the stoma, and under the tracheostomy tube flange/faceplate.				
1i) Commercially available foam/collar type adjustable tracheostomy straps are used rather than ties or twill tape.				
1j) A standard procedure for management of tracheostomy sutures is in place.				
1k) The tension and skin integrity under and around ETTs and straps are checked every 2 hours with close attention to the neck, lips, and mouth.				
1l) When using commercial stabilizers, the position of the ETT (right, middle, left) is rotated at least every 2 hours.				

SAFE SKIN GAP ANALYSIS: CERVICAL COLLAR

SAFE SKIN Practice The following key strategies for preventing cervical collar-related pressure ulcers have been implemented:	Gap? Y/N	If yes, strategies to meet this practice	Person Responsible	Timeline
1a) Provider order, including frequency of use, is obtained for collar application.				
1b) Orthotist, or other trained provider, is consulted for appropriate collar fit.				
1c) Patients are removed from backboard on arrival in emergency department or as soon as possible.				
1d) Standardized processes are in place to achieve definitive care (e.g., collar removal, change to longer-term collar, within 24 hours or less).				
1e) If the patient condition permits, the skin is inspected and cleaned during change from transport collar to longer-term collar.				
1f) Staff is trained in proper technique for cervical collar placement.				
1g) A neurologic assessment is conducted after initial collar application, then every 8 hours (and as needed), or per provider orders.				
1h) Cervical collars are removed to cleanse, inspect, and palpate skin every 8-12 hours and removal of device and findings are documented.				
1i) Patient is log-rolled and repositioned every 2 hours (and as needed).				
1j) If collar has removable inner pads, pads are changed and washed every 24 hours (and as needed).				
1k) Staff is trained in proper technique for skin inspection and care of skin related to cervical collars.				
1l) Orthotists or other trained providers are available for staff questions or concerns.				
1m) Education provided to patients/family prior to discharge includes information on application, wearing and removal of collar, proper cervical alignment, skin care and inspection, and collar pad cleaning.				

SAFE SKIN ICU PLEDGE

Our ICU Safe Skin Team Pledge

We will:

1. **Keep our ICU patients moving** - Our team will develop a repositioning schedule for each patient (L-R-Center), based on the patient's condition, and will consistently follow the schedule to redistribute pressure for our patients.
2. **Float heels off the bed.**
3. **Immediately evaluate patients for the most appropriate surface** to redistribute pressure.
4. If a patient is not able to be adequately or routinely repositioned, our team will provide:
   - **Written confirmation** that patient cannot be repositioned from the physician with daily re-evaluation
   - At least **hourly mini shifts** off the tailbone
5. **Check our patients' skin beneath devices** - Every shift we will use opportunities such as oral care, vital sign checks, and respiratory treatments to look for skin issues.

PRESSURE ULCER PREVENTION PATIENT AND FAMILY EDUCATION

Preventing Pressure Ulcers (Bedsores)

A pressure ulcer, or bedsore, is a serious problem in the hospital and at home. Pressure ulcers can slow your recovery, causing pain, infections, and other problems.

What is a pressure ulcer?

A pressure ulcer is an injury to the skin and the tissue beneath it. It is caused by pressure on the skin.

Pressure ulcers tend to occur over bony body parts (elbow, heel, hip, etc.) that you sit or lie on for long periods of time. The pressure squeezes tiny blood vessels that supply the skin with nutrients and oxygen. When the skin goes without nutrients and oxygen for too long, a pressure ulcer forms. The area turns red at first. Unless treated quickly (changing your position, for example), the pressure can damage the skin and muscles.

Pressure ulcers are more likely to develop or worsen if you:
- slide down in a bed or chair.
- rub or create friction on the skin.
- cannot move or change positions.
- lose control of your bowel or bladder.
- don't get enough nutrients or fluids.
- have poor circulation or fragile skin.
- have problems thinking clearly.
- have problems feeling pressure or pain.

How can I prevent pressure ulcers?

- Limit pressure.
  - ▷ If you are in bed, change your position at least every 1 or 2 hours.
  - ▷ If you are in a chair and can shift your own weight, do so every 15 minutes. If you cannot shift your own weight, your caregiver should change your position at least every hour.

- Reduce friction.
  - ▷ When moving in bed, don't pull or drag yourself across the sheets. Also, don't push or pull with your heels.
  - ▷ Avoid repetitive movements. For example, don't scratch your foot by rubbing it on the sheets.

- Use padding carefully.
  - ▷ Avoid doughnut-shaped cushions. These can hurt the tissues under your skin.
  - ▷ Avoid using several layers (such as underpads, diapers and sheets) between you and your chair or bed.

- Protect your skin.
  - ▷ Have someone check your skin often. Tell your caregiver if anything looks unusual.
  - ▷ Clean your skin well after using a bedpan or soiling a diaper or pad.
  - ▷ Use moisturizer to prevent dry skin. Bathe every other day.
  - ▷ Don't rub or massage the skin over the bony parts of your body.
  - ▷ Make sure you are getting adequate nutrition, especially protein, as well as enough healthy liquids (e.g., water, milk and juice.)

If you have pain on your heels and buttocks, tell your caregiver. Pain may mean you have too much pressure on the skin.

If you must stay in bed for long periods of time:

- Try to keep the head of your bed as low as you can. If you need to raise it, raise it to the lowest point possible for as short a time as possible.

over

- Use pillows to keep your knees and ankles from touching each other.
- Avoid lying directly on your hipbone when on your side. Your care team may show you how to spread your weight more evenly.
- To keep your heels off the bed, place pillows under your legs from mid-calf to ankle. Never place pillows under the knee.
- Your caregiver may want to use a turning sheet to help you change position.
- If you cannot turn easily, ask your care team if you need a special mattress or mattress overlay to lessen the pressure.

If you have problems with bladder or bowel control:

- Only use pads made for incontinence (ones that pull moisture away from your skin).
- Clean the skin gently with a pH-balanced soap or cleansing product.
- Buy special cream or ointment to protect your skin from urine and stool. Ask your care team for suggestions.

If you have to wear stockings to prevent blood clots (antiembolism stockings):

- Your stockings should be removed at least twice a day to let your legs "breathe" and to check your skin for any redness or open sores.
- Once you can get up and move around freely, you no longer need to wear the stockings.

If you are in a chair or wheelchair:

- Remember that comfort and good posture are important.
- Change your position often. Spend time out of the chair several hours a day.
- Ask your care team if you need a special chair cushion.

If you wear oxygen tubing and/or a mask:

- Remember that these can cause pressure ulcers behind the ears, on the bridge of your nose, or even in your nostrils.
- These areas should be inspected by staff at least once a shift while you are in the hospital.
- Special pads may be used to protect these areas.
- Tell your caregiver if you are having pain or discomfort in these areas.

What else can I do?

Be active in your health care:

- Involve your family and caregivers.
- Ask questions. Be sure you know what is being done and why.
- Explain your needs, wants, and concerns.
- Learn what is best for you.

Knowing how to help your care team prevent pressure ulcers is an important part of your care.

Patient Safety | *Call to Action*

MEDICARE COVERAGE OF SUPPORT SURFACES

For all three support surface groups, patients should have a care plan established by their physician or home care nurse, which is documented in their medical records. This plan generally should include, among other things, education of the patient and regular assessment by a health care practitioner. Coverage for all three groups continues until the patient's pressure ulcer is healed. In addition to the previous common requirements, coverage for specific groups of support surfaces varies as follows:

GROUP 1 Support Surface

A group 1 support surface is generally designed to either replace a standard hospital or home mattress or as an overlay placed on top of a standard hospital or home mattress. Products in this category include mattresses, pressure pads, and mattress overlays (foam, air, water, or gel).

Coverage criteria (must meet one of the following):
- The patient is completely immobile.
	OR
- The patient is partially immobile with one of the following:
	- impaired nutritional status
	- incontinence
	- altered sensory perception
	- compromised circulatory status
- The patient has a pressure ulcer with one of the following:
	- impaired nutritional status
	- incontinence
	- altered sensory perception
	- compromised circulatory status

GROUP 2 Support Surface

A group 2 support surface is generally designed to either replace a standard hospital or home mattress or as an overlay placed on top of a standard hospital or home mattress. Products in this category include powered air flotation beds, powered pressure-reducing air mattresses, and nonpowered advanced pressure-reducing mattresses.

Coverage criteria (must meet one of the following):
- The patient has large or multiple Stage III or IV pressure sores on the trunk or pelvis
	OR
- The patient had a myocutaneous flap or skin graft for a pressure sore on the trunk or pelvis and has been on a group 2 or 3 support surface.
	OR
- The patient has a Stage II pressure sore located on the trunk or pelvis AND has been on a comprehensive pressure sore treatment program (which has included the use of an appropriate group 1 support surface for at least 1 month)

GROUP 3 Support Surface

A group 3 support surface is a complete bed system known as air fluidized.

Coverage criteria (must meet ALL of the following):
- The patient has a Stage III or Stage IV pressure ulcer AND
- Is bedridden or chair-bound AND
- Would be institutionalized without the use of the group 3 support surface AND
- Is under the close supervision of the patient's treating physician AND
- At least 1 month of conservative treatment has been administered (including the use of a group 2 support surface) AND
- A caregiver is available and willing to assist with patient care AND
- All other alternative equipment has been considered and ruled out.

Support Surface Examples Using CMS Criteria for Reimbursement	
Category, Description, and Medicare Codes	**Product Examples***
Group 1 Mattresses, pressure pads, and mattress overlays; foam, air, water, or gel Medicare Codes: E0181-E0189, E0196-E0199, A4640	EHOB-WAFFLE® Mattress Overlay Gaymar-Sof.Care II SpanAmerica-Geo Matt MAX KCI-TheraRest® SMS Hill-Rom Tempur-Pedic
Group 2 Powered air flotation beds, powered pressure-reducing air mattresses, and nonpowered advanced pressure-reducing mattresses Medicare Codes: E0193, E0277, E0371, E0372, E0373	Gaymar Plexus Air Express LAL Sizewise-Sunflower Pulse, True Low Air Loss SpanAmerica-Pressure Guard CFT KCI-First Step® HillRom-VersaCare Talley Medical Quattro Overlay™
Group 3 Complete bed systems known as air fluidized Medicare Code: E0194	Hilrom-Clinitron At·Home® AFT KCI-KCI's FluidAir® EliteTM

Reference: Centers for Medicare and Medicaid Services (CMS) Medicare Policy Regarding Pressure Reducing Support Surfaces Information for Medicare Fee for Services Health Care Professionals MLN Matters Number: SE1014 August 17, 2010. Available at https://www.cms.gov/MLNMattersArticles/downloads/SE1014.pdf. Accessed September 13, 2010.
*Note: product examples and group classification came from the manufacturer's website and are not inclusive. Websites accessed September 13, 2010.

SATISFACTION SURVEY

■   Wound, Ostomy, Continence, Foot Care Nursing Program   ●Riverwood
                                                                 HEALTHCARE CENTER

Recently, you have received services of our Wound, Ostomy, Continence, Foot Care Nursing Program. Please take a moment to give us your assessment of the program to aid us in evaluating our services.

Please indicate below the service you received (check only one)

☐ Wound Care   ☐ Ostomy Care   ☐ Continence Care   ☐ Foot & Nail Care

Please indicate the most recent date of service ....

Response Definition: P=Poor   F=Fair   G=Good   VG=Very Good   E=Excellent

	P	F	G	VG	E
1. Procedures, treatment and care practices were thoroughly explained by staff..............................	☐	☐	☐	☐	☐
2. Professionalism of staff	☐	☐	☐	☐	☐
3. Staff members were friendly and encouraging	☐	☐	☐	☐	☐
4. The space provided for care and education was adequate...	☐	☐	☐	☐	☐
5. Comfort and pain issues were addressed appropriately and in a timely manner.............................	☐	☐	☐	☐	☐
6. How would you rate the Wound, Ostomy, Continence, Foot Care Nursing Program?	☐	☐	☐	☐	☐

	Y	N
7. Were your questions regarding your condition answered to your satisfaction?	☐	☐
8. Have you continued with the home instructions regarding care and prevention?....................................	☐	☐
9. Has this program assisted you in changing your self-care habits?..	☐	☐
10. Were you provided with appropriate education regarding your condition?	☐	☐
11. Would you recommend the Wound, Ostomy, Continence, Foot Care Nursing program to others?.....................	☐	☐

Is there anything in the program that could be added or changed that would be helpful to you?

Please feel free to make any comments regarding the program inside the box below. Include your name and telephone if you would like someone to contact you regarding the services you received.

Please make no marks below this line

ACTIVITY LOG

WOUND/SKIN CARE SERVICES   Month _____

Daily Activity, Patient Case Mix, and Time Summary (1 unit = 15 minutes)

1. Pressure Ulcer (PU) nosocomial 2. PU-present on admission 3. Skin tear 4. Surgical wound 5. Incontinence 6. Venous 7. Arterial 8. Neuropathic 9. Mixed 10. Tube 11. Colostomy 12. Ileostomy 13. Urostomy 14. Committee work 15. Quality management 16. Staff education 17. Research/Trials 18. _____ 19. _____

Patient	Unit #	1	2	3	4	5	6	7	8	9	10	11	12	13	14	15	16	17	18	19	20	21	22	23	24	25	26	27	28	29	30

Self-Assessment Exercises

QUESTIONS

A. Principles of Assessment

1. Distinguish between assessment and evaluation of healing.

2. Which of the following methods is an example of categorizing a wound by classification?
   a. Linear measurements
   b. Photographs
   c. Staging
   d. Wound molds

3. A full-thickness wound is one that:
   a. involves the muscle layer
   b. extends into the dermis
   c. is limited to the epidermis
   d. contains necrotic tissue

4. List 10 indices of wound healing that should be assessed and recorded.

5. Eschar can be described as which of the following?
   a. Viable tissue
   b. Necrotic tissue
   c. Fibrin
   d. Granulation tissue

6. Describe eschar.

7. Describe slough.

8. List six factors known to damage the skin.

9. Which of the following is described as a lesion that is raised, solid, and less than 1 cm in diameter?
   a. Macule
   b. Papule
   c. Pustule
   d. Nodule

10. A blister that measures 1.5 cm in diameter may also be called which of the following?
    a. Bulla
    b. Pustule
    c. Vesicle
    d. Wheal

11. Which of the following statements about erosion is *true*?
    a. Erosion involves the loss of epidermis and dermis.
    b. Erosion heals by scar formation.
    c. Erosion involves partial loss of epidermis.
    d. Erosion extends into subcutaneous tissue.

12. Which of the following accurately characterizes chemical skin irritation?
    a. Erythema with satellite lesions
    b. Erythema and erosion of skin
    c. Ulcerations with necrotic tissue in wound bed
    d. Ulcerations with pustules

13. Which of the following characterizes varicella-zoster virus?
    a. It requires prior exposure to genital herpes.
    b. It is reactivated by mechanical trauma.
    c. It consists of a bilateral vesicular rash.
    d. It develops along one or two dermatomes.

14. State the two phases of an allergic contact dermatitis.

15. Candidiasis can be described as which of the following?
    a. Pustular or macular papular rash with erythema
    b. Papular rash within the hair follicle
    c. Pustular rash in clusters
    d. Vesicular rash with plaque formation

16. Which of the following statements about herpes simplex virus is *true*?
    a. It initially develops as papules.
    b. Secondary lesions consist of necrotic plaques.
    c. Erythema signifies a secondary infection.
    d. Vesicles are uniformly shaped and grouped.

17. Which of the following is a usual result of severe traumatic injury with associated wounds?
    a. Increased metabolic rate for 10 to 14 days after injury
    b. Decreased metabolic rate to help conserve energy for the first 2 to 5 days after injury
    c. Decreased metabolic rate for 48 hours, then increased for the following 10 to 14 days
    d. Unknown metabolic consequences (cannot be determined without more information)

18. An 82-year-old man describes his situation to you as you obtain a history. Which of the following indicates risk of malnutrition?
    a. Eating alone
    b. Inability to prepare his own food
    c. Low income
    d. All of the above

19. Mrs. France is a 60-year-old African American woman who is admitted to the hospital after an automobile accident that resulted in a penetrating chest wound and a ruptured spleen. You see her for her wounds 2 weeks after surgery and are concerned whether she is experiencing acute injury–related malnutrition because her:
    a. albumin is 2.4 g/dl, prealbumin is 28 mg/dl, and her CRP is 1.8 mg/L
    b. albumin is 2.8 g/dl, prealbumin is 12 mg/dl, and her CRP <0.8 mg/L
    c. albumin is 3.6 g/dl, prealbumin is 0.6 mg/dl, and CRP is 2.5 mg/L
    d. none of the above

20. The nutritional status of a 5-foot-tall, 54-year-old woman with a venous leg ulcer of 18 months is being evaluated. Which of the following leads to the definitive diagnosis of disease-related malnutrition?
    a. Weight loss of 10 pounds in 1 year
    b. Body mass index of 16 kg/m²
    c. Albumin level of 3.4 g/dl
    d. Petechiae

21. Nutritional screening (versus nutritional assessment) is characterized by:
    a. being performed by a WOC nurse; results in a diagnosis, done on all patients
    b. being performed by a dietitian; results in a diagnosis; performed only on patients who are at risk, obese, or have a wound
    c. being performed by the bedside nurse; results in identification of nutritional risk; performed on all patients
    d. being performed by the bedside nurse; results in diagnosis of malnutrition/no malnutrition; performed only on patients who are at risk, obese, or have a wound

22. Mr. Zabo is a 75-year-old man who is retired and lives alone. He is healthy except for a painful arterial ulcer on his right leg that has been present for nearly 2 years, and he needs a "water pill for his high blood pressure." He eats one meal a day, usually at the local coffee shop. Most often, that meal is usually lunch. Over the past 3 months he has lost 15 pounds and first noticed the weight loss because his pants were loose on him. Your initial suspicion is that he has which of the following?
    a. Starvation-related malnutrition
    b. Disease-related malnutrition
    c. Acute or injury-related malnutrition
    d. None of the above

23. Mr. Eddie is a 57-year-old man with type 1 diabetes that you have been seeing because he is receiving NPWT for a lower extremity nonhealing left stump wound. He is hemodynamically stable, but you note he looks more edematous than when you saw him 3 days ago and his NPWT output has increased, although his weight has increased 2 kg. He is on an appropriate diabetic diet. His oral intake is recorded as good for 1 day and not recorded for the other 2 days since you last saw him. Review of his blood work shows he is stable, including his glucose of 101 g/dl and creatinine of 1.9, but his albumin has dropped from 4.8 gm/l to 1.9 g/dl in the past 3 days. He says he is tired and refuses to get up in the chair. Based on his change in condition and his blood work, you question whether he is:
    a. hyperglycemic
    b. hypoglycemic
    c. overhydrated
    d. underhydrated

24. In patients with a wound, zinc supplementation should be ordered on:
    a. everyone
    b. those with a chronic wound
    c. those with established zinc deficiency
    d. those with a BMI <18.5 or >30 kg/m²

25. Which of the following sentences most accurately describes patients' protein needs for repair after injury?
    a. They increase to provide energy for basal functions.
    b. They increase to support anabolism.
    c. They decrease because of reduced basal metabolic rate.
    d. They decrease to conserve losses.

26. The most ideal way to feed a person with a healing wound is:
    a. enterally with a nasogastric tube because it is the least time consuming
    b. parenterally, as it is associated with a low infection rate and reduced risk of aspiration
    c. orally because it maintains gut function and enhances independence
    d. it doesn't matter—there is no ideal way to feed a person with a wound.

27. Which of the following best describes the pain associated with conservative sharp debridement?
    a. Noncyclic acute wound pain
    b. Cyclic acute wound pain
    c. Chronic wound pain
    d. All of the above

28. Which of the following pain assessment scales would be most appropriate for a nonverbal nursing home resident with severe Alzheimer disease and a Stage IV sacral pressure ulcer?
    a. McGill Pain Questionnaire
    b. Pain Assessment in Advanced Dementia (PAINAD) scale
    c. Visual analogue scale
    d. Wong-Baker faces scale

29. Explain why wounds confined to the epidermal and dermal layers heal by regeneration, whereas wounds that extend through the dermal layer into the subcutaneous tissue or fascia or muscle layer must heal by scar formation.

30. Explain what is meant by primary-, secondary-, and tertiary-intention wound healing.

31. Identify the major components of partial-thickness repair.

32. Explain why epidermal resurfacing and dermal repair proceed more rapidly when the wound surface is kept moist.

33. Summarize the activities that occur in the three key phases of repair for full-thickness wounds healing by primary intention (in order).

34. Which of the following cells are responsible for collagen synthesis?
    a. Macrophages
    b. Neutrophils
    c. Fibroblasts
    d. Platelets

35. The process of contraction is important for wound healing in which of the following?
    a. Wounds healing by primary intention
    b. Wounds healing by secondary intention
    c. Superficial abrasions
    d. Partial-thickness wounds

36. Explain why large wounds healing by secondary intention may require skin grafting, whereas large, partial-thickness wounds will epithelialize.

37. Summarize the differences between acute and chronic wound healing.

38. List at least six factors that affect wound healing.

39. Which of the following characterizes the molecular environment of a chronic wound?
    a. High levels of growth factors
    b. Increased levels of proteases (matrix metalloproteinases)
    c. Increased levels of protease inhibitors (tissue inhibitors of metalloproteinase)
    d. Excessive collagen synthesis

40. Which of the following is true about darkly pigmented skin compared to lighter skin?
    a. Darker skin has less functional integrity.
    b. Darkly pigmented skin can mask erythema or redness seen with pressure ulcers or dermatitis.
    c. Light skin has a higher prevalence of keloids.
    d. All of the above

41. Standard interventions to enhance tissue perfusion for wound healing include:
    a. application of cooling blanket
    b. fluid restriction to control edema
    c. management of pain and anxiety
    d. raise the head of the bed

42. Which of the following factors affect both perfusion and oxygenation?
    a. Smoking and obesity
    b. Pain and anxiety
    c. CHF and diabetes
    d. Obesity and cancer

43. Which of the following explains why obesity is a risk factor for poor healing?
    a. Adipose tissue is less perfused than lean tissue.
    b. Many obese people are dehydrated.
    c. Obese persons often are hypotensive.
    d. Skin is pulled tight by obesity.

B. Principles of Wound Management

1. What are the three principles of wound management?
    a. Debridement, control of infection, and exudate management
    b. Establishment of a treatment goal, wound cleansing, and physiologic local wound care
    c. Assessment of the host, debridement, and physiologic local wound care
    d. Address the wound etiology, support the host, and maintain a physiologic local wound environment

2. Which of the following interventions indicates an attempt to control or eliminate the etiology of a venous ulcer?
    a. Resizing of shoe to include orthotics
    b. Applying an alginate and foam cover dressing
    c. Monitoring blood glucose levels
    d. Encouraging elevation of the leg three times daily

3. Which of the following statements about semiocclusive dressings is true?
   a. They are occlusive to liquids and gases.
   b. They are occlusive to liquids but transmit moisture vapor and gases.
   c. They are occlusive to gases and vapors but transmit liquids.
   d. They are inconsistent in their nonocclusive properties.

4. In the patient with a new approximated surgical wound, the primary wound care objective is:
   a. autolysis
   b. hydration
   c. cleansing
   d. protection

5. Dressing selection is primarily based on which of the following?
   a. Forms of the dressing
   b. Characteristics of the wound
   c. Product availability and cost
   d. Number of dressing changes required daily

6. In the patient with a highly exudative pressure ulcer, which category of dressings should be considered?
   a. Hydrocolloids
   b. Collagens
   c. Transparent dressings
   d. Alginates

7. Which of the following statements about wound care products is *true*?
   a. Hydrocolloids absorb more exudate than alginate dressings.
   b. Transparent dressings are contraindicated for Stage II pressure ulcers.
   c. Wound fillers can be used to fill undermining and tunnels.
   d. Silver-impregnated dressings are indicated when critical colonization is suspected.

8. List seven objectives for local wound management.

9. Which of the following methods of debridement is nonselective?
   a. Autolysis
   b. High-pressure irrigation
   c. Enzymatic
   d. Surgical sharp

10. High-pressure wound irrigation requires which of the following?
    a. Bulb syringe
    b. Daily dressing changes
    c. Personal protective gear
    d. Expensive equipment

11. List three considerations in the use of enzymatic debridement.

12. Selection of debridement approach is guided by all of the following *except:*
    a. patient's age
    b. presence of wound infection
    c. extent and type of necrotic tissue
    d. clinician experience

13. The risk of transient bacteremia is associated with which of the following debridement techniques?
    a. Autolysis
    b. Conservative sharp
    c. Enzymes
    d. Wet-to-dry dressings

14. The most accurate means of obtaining data on planktonic phenotype organisms in a chronic wound is:
    a. blood work - increased WBCs
    b. blood work - increased C-reactive protein
    c. wound culture - swab culture
    d. wound culture - tissue biopsy

15. Wound infection is present when which of the following cluster of signs/symptoms is seen:
    a. Wound size is bigger; wound is red and bleeding
    b. Wound is malodorous; wound size has not decreased in 3 weeks
    c. Body temperature is increased; exudate present is increased
    d. Slough is present; wound size has not changed in 4 weeks

16. Current thinking about quantitative wound cultures is that $>10^5$ CFU:
    a. accurately evaluates wound bioburden
    b. overestimates wound bioburden
    c. underestimates wound bioburden
    d. none of the above

17. Mr. Z has had his chronic sacral pressure ulcer debrided. It now is clean and 5×7 and about 1 cm deep. You anticipate the new treatment will be:
    a. topical antiseptic, e.g., silver dressing
    b. topical antibiotic, e.g., gentamicin
    c. systemic antibiotic, e.g., Keflex
    d. systemic antibiotic, e.g., honey

18. Systemic antibiotics are appropriate treatment during what phase of the continuum of bioburden?
    a. Contamination
    b. Colonization
    c. Critical colonization/biofilm
    d. Infection

19. To get the most accurate culture, it is important that the specimen be taken from:
    a. healthy wound tissue
    b. pus
    c. necrotic tissue
    d. exudate
    e. slough

20. Quantum sensing in biofilm allows organisms to communicate in order to:
    a. module genes
    b. reduce metabolism
    c. live in a hypoxic environment
    d. all of the above

21. You are treating 10 patients with various chronic wounds. About how many do you expect will have biofilm present?
    a. 1 in 10
    b. 3 in 10
    c. 6 in 10
    d. 9 in 10
    e. All 10 patients

22. Which of the following must be included in the comprehensive wound treatment of a 47-year-old patient with an open wound of the abdomen secondary to a retroperitoneal abscess?
    a. Wet-to-dry dressings
    b. Pain control
    c. Debridement of granulation tissue
    d. Treatment for depression

23. Which of the following is *not a primary* mechanism of action of negative pressure wound therapy (NPWT)?
    a. Wound edge contraction
    b. Wound environment stabilization
    c. Reduction of bioburden
    d. Wound surface microdeformations

24. Bioburden reduction with use of NPWT is believed to occur through which of the following?
    a. Removal of growth factors
    b. Increased perfusion
    c. Irrigation daily with normal saline
    d. Creation of hypoxic environment for bacteria with suction

25. Which of the following describes appropriate use of NPWT in the care of enteric fistulas?
    a. It can only be used after exploration of the enteric fistula.
    b. It is only used to contain effluent.
    c. It is never indicated with enteric fistulas.
    d. The wound should be covered with a wound liner instead of porous foam filler dressing.

26. Serious complications associated with NPWT, including death, are related to which of the following?
    a. Hemorrhage
    b. Retrograde migration of bacteria from canister to wound surface
    c. Fluid and electrolyte depletion
    d. Excess wound moisture

27. Contraindications to NPWT include which of the following?
    a. Patient taking anticoagulants
    b. Treated osteomyelitis
    c. Nonenteric or unexplored fistulas
    d. Postsurgical dehiscence

28. Which of the following statements about hyperoxygenation that occurs with hyperbaric treatment is *true*?
    a. Hyperoxygenation occurs because the hemoglobin molecule is saturated with oxygen molecules.
    b. Hyperoxygenation results from increasing the oxygen-carrying capacity of the plasma.
    c. Several treatments are needed to achieve hyperoxygenation.
    d. Hyperoxygenation may be sustained for 8 to 10 hours after exposure.

29. All of the following personal care items are contraindicated during hyperbaric treatment *except*:
    a. hairspray
    b. hearing aids
    c. contact lenses
    d. perfume

30. True or False: Wound care dressings with a petrolatum base should be removed during hyperbaric treatment.

31. True or False: Hyperbaric oxygen is a definitive treatment of hard-to-heal wounds.

32. List three types of adhesion molecules or adhesion receptors that participate in inflammation.

33. True or False: Growth factors are proteases.

34. All of the following growth factors have shown significant benefit in healing acute or chronic wounds in clinical trials *except*:
    a. fibroblast growth factor
    b. epidermal growth factor
    c. transforming growth factor-β
    d. insulinlike growth factor

35. Which of the following statements about cellular- and tissue-based products (CTPs) is TRUE?
    a. All CTPs provide an extracellular matrix (ECM).
    b. All CTPs provide growth factors.
    c. All CTPs are derived from animal sources.
    d. All CTPs mimic native tissues to promote healing.

36. Acellular CTPs are designed to:
    a. deliver living cells to the wound bed
    b. replace the need for a split-thickness skin graft
    c. function as an extracellular matrix (ECM) scaffold
    d. provide a dermal and epidermal covering

37. Describe the sources of CTP components.

38. Name an epidermal, dermal, and bilayer product available in the United States.

39. Living bilayered CTPs provide:
    a. keratinocytes and fibroblasts
    b. blood vessels and fibroblasts
    c. melanocytes and keratinocytes
    d. macrophages and blood vessels

40. True or False: Allogeneic cell-based CTPs are temporary and biodegradable.

41. List at least three essential steps to using CTPs successfully.

42. Debridement is contraindicated in which of the following wounds?
    a. A pressure ulcer that is covered with 75% yellow slough
    b. A noninfected heel ulcer that is 100% covered with dry eschar in a patient with arterial disease
    c. An infected wound with eschar that is separating from the surrounding skin
    d. A pressure ulcer with slough and eschar in a terminally ill patient

43. Which of the following frequently causes procedural wound pain?
    a. Adhesive dressings
    b. Wet-to-moist gauze
    c. Debridement
    d. All of the above

44. Which of the following is included among best practices for managing wound pain?
    a. Assuming that the pain is bearable
    b. Medicating for pain after the procedure
    c. Using a combination of strategies
    d. Addressing nonprocedural pain before procedural pain

45. True or False: Decreasing swelling by compression in patients with a venous ulcer has been shown in several studies to reduce venous ulcer pain.

46. List five interventions for pain reduction during dressing changes.

47. An incision healing without complication becomes impermeable to bacteria within:
    a. 24 hours
    b. 2 to 3 days
    c. 1 week
    d. none of the above

48. In the patient with a new approximated surgical wound, the primary wound care objective is:
    a. autolysis
    b. hydration
    c. cleansing
    d. protection

49. Which of the following is *not* appropriate for a sutured postoperative incision?
    a. Keep moist with a topical antibiotic ointment.
    b. Maintain original postoperative dressing for 48 to 72 hours.
    c. Begin showering 48 to 72 hours postoperatively.
    d. Protect surgical incision from exposure to sun.

C. Pressure Ulcers

1. Define pressure ulcer.

2. What is the role of muscle in preventing pressure ulcers?
   a. Muscle redistributes pressure load.
   b. Muscle provides the blood supply to the skin.
   c. Muscle enables blood vessels to resist shear injury.
   d. Muscle concentrates pressure over the bony prominence.

3. Describe how intensity of pressure and duration of pressure affect tissue ischemia.

4. Which of the following are major factors that contribute to pressure ulcer development?
   a. Shear, smoking, and friction
   b. Age, smoking, and blood pressure
   c. Nutrition and stress
   d. Shear, friction, and nutritional debilitation

5. Which of the following statements about blanching erythema is *false*?
   a. It resolves once pressure is removed.
   b. It indicates deep tissue damage.
   c. It is an area of erythema that turns white when compressed.
   d. It implies that pressure is not adequately relieved or reduced.

6. The undermining that is commonly observed with pressure ulcers may be the result of which of the following?
   a. Shear
   b. Friction
   c. Maceration
   d. Advanced age

7. Nonblanchable erythema of intact skin describes which classification of pressure ulcer?
   a. Suspected deep tissue injury
   b. Stage I
   c. Stage II
   d. Stage III

8. Exposed tendon describes which classification of pressure ulcer?
   a. Stage III
   b. Stage IV
   c. Unstageable
   d. Partial thickness

9. A brown, dry wound base on the right trochanter describes which classification of pressure ulcer?
   a. Suspected deep tissue injury
   b. Stage III
   c. Stage IV
   d. Unstageable

10. A blood-filled blister on the heel describes which classification of pressure ulcer?
    a. Suspected deep tissue injury
    b. Stage I
    c. Unstageable
    d. Iatrogenic

11. Intact, nonblanchable, persistent purple discoloration over the coccyx describes which classification of pressure ulcer?
    a. Suspected deep tissue injury
    b. Stage I
    c. Unstageable
    d. None of the above

12. An intact, serous-filled blister on the heel describes which classification of pressure ulcer?
    a. Suspected deep tissue injury
    b. Stage I
    c. Stage II
    d. Stage III

13. Application of a skin barrier ointment to the perineal skin addresses which pressure ulcer risk factor?
    a. Impaired mobility
    b. Impaired activity
    c. Moisture
    d. Nutrition

14. Keeping the head of the bed less than 30 degrees addresses which pressure ulcer risk factor?
    a. Impaired mobility
    b. Friction/shear
    c. Moisture
    d. Nutrition

15. Repositioning the patient every 2 hours helps to address which pressure ulcer risk factor?
    a. Impaired mobility
    b. Nutrition
    c. Altered sensory perception
    d. Both a and c

16. Which is the best rationale for obtaining a pressure redistribution mattress?
    a. The patient has a pressure ulcer on both trochanters and sacrum.
    b. A nurse requests a lateral rotation low air-loss bed because he does not have enough time to turn his patient every 2 hours.
    c. The patient is on a ventilator.
    d. Both a and c.

17. Which of the following is the most appropriate intervention for a Stage II ischial tuberosity pressure ulcer?
    a. Pressure redistribution mattress
    b. Pressure redistribution chair cushion
    c. Bed rest
    d. Wound culture

18. Which of the following is an appropriate treatment option for the adult to prevent chemical skin irritation due to acute diarrheal consistency fecal incontinence?
    a. Apply moisturizer twice per day.
    b. Remove all skin barrier ointment when cleansing perianal area after incontinent stool.
    c. Apply moisture barrier ointment or paste.
    d. Apply transparent dressing over perianal skin.

19. The most effective pressure ulcer prevention plan uses:
    a. protocols for total risk assessment scores
    b. strategies to minimize individual pressure ulcer risk factors
    c. turning teams
    d. bundles

20. Friction damage to the skin is characterized by which of the following statements?
    a. It is commonly seen in the periwound field under adhesives.
    b. It results from prolonged elevation of the head of bed.
    c. Tissue necrosis can be present.
    d. Injury typically is very shallow and limited to epidermis.

21. Prolonged moisture on the skin due to urinary incontinence has which of the following effects?
    a. Thickening and strengthening of collagen bonds
    b. Decreased resistance to mechanical trauma
    c. Ulceration due to caustic nature of urine
    d. Stabilization of skin's normal flora

D. Lower Extremity Ulcers

1. Rest pain is indicative of which of the following?
   a. Mild occlusive disease, as occurs with 25% occlusion
   b. Moderate occlusive disease, as occurs with 50% occlusion
   c. Advanced occlusive disease, as occurs with 90% occlusion
   d. Need for amputation

2. Risk factors for lower extremity arterial disease include which of the following?
   a. Alcoholism
   b. Hypertension
   c. Elevated high-density lipoprotein levels
   d. Diabetes insipidus

3. What type of pain is claudication?
   a. Pain that exists without precipitating activity
   b. Pain that develops when the patient elevates the legs
   c. Pain that is triggered by moderate-to-heavy activity
   d. Pain that worsens with rest

4. Which of the following ankle-brachial index (ABI) values is indicative of calcification of the vessel wall in a person with diabetes?
   a. 0.95 to 1.1
   b. 0.5 to 0.95
   c. 0.5
   d. >1.3

5. Which of the following descriptions is classic for an arterial ulcer?
   a. Highly exudative
   b. Presence of red granulation tissue
   c. Common location above medial malleolus
   d. Dry wound bed

6. Which of the following describes the situation in which maintenance of an eschar-covered arterial ulcer is preferred?
   a. The involved limb can be revascularized.
   b. The $TcPO_2$ is 20 mm Hg.
   c. The wound is infected.
   d. Indications of infection are absent and potential for healing is limited.

7. Describe how a competent venous system and the calf muscle pump work together to prevent venous hypertension.

8. Which of the following levels of pressure would be considered therapeutic for graduated compression when a patient has an ABI of 0.95 in the lower extremity?
   a. 20 mm Hg compression at the ankle
   b. 25 mm Hg compression at the ankle
   c. 30 mm Hg compression at the ankle
   d. 50 mm Hg compression at the ankle

9. Which of the following management options would be *best* for the patient with a venous ulcer complicated by arterial disease, as evidenced by an ABI of 0.5?
   a. Use leg elevation to control edema and 20 mm Hg graduated compression wrap.
   b. Use pneumatic compression or graduated compression to provide pressures in the 25 to 30 mm Hg range.
   c. Recommend Trental (pentoxifylline) as an alternative to compression.
   d. Delay any treatment until patient undergoes revascularization.

10. Distinguish between elastic and nonelastic static compression products, and explain which is best for the sedentary patient.

11. Which of the following symptoms would indicate venous dermatitis instead of cellulitis?
    a. Erythema, elevated temperature
    b. Erythema, crusting, and itching
    c. Pain, fever, and bullae
    d. Inflammation, pain, and exudate

12. Venous contact dermatitis can be best managed with which of the following treatments?
    a. Antibiotic cream daily
    b. Lanolin cream twice a day
    c. Topical corticosteroid daily for 1 week
    d. Antifungal powder twice per day

13. Instructions to the patient being fitted for compression stockings for venous insufficiency include which of the following?
    a. Apply stockings first thing in the morning.
    b. Do not remove stockings at bedtime, only when bathing.
    c. Launder the stockings once per week.
    d. Do not perform ankle exercises while wearing the stockings.

14. Lipedema occurs:
    a. in both sexes equally
    b. in the feet and the legs
    c. in both legs
    d. often in conjunction with cellulitis

15. Which of the following is the gold standard for diagnosing lymphedema?
    a. Isotopic lymphoscintigraphy
    b. Magnetic resonance imaging
    c. Computed tomographic scan
    d. Lymphangiogram

16. Comorbid conditions associated with lymphedema may include which of the following?
    a. Venous ulcer disease
    b. Obesity
    c. Hepatic disease
    d. All of the above

17. The Kaposi-Stemmer's sign is the ability to pinch the skin:
    a. at the base of the second and third toes
    b. on the dorsal surface of the foot
    c. between the third and fourth fingers
    d. of the great toe

18. Identify the types of neuropathy and the effects of each on skin integrity.

19. Which of the following is the primary cause of diabetic foot ulcers?
    a. Peripheral neuropathy
    b. Infection
    c. Edema
    d. Peripheral arterial disease

20. Which of the following findings is suggestive of osteomyelitis in the patient with a diabetic foot ulcer?
    a. Abnormal bone scan
    b. Nonhealing ulcer
    c. Abnormal x-ray study findings
    d. All of the above

21. Identify factors other than topical therapy that must be addressed in the management plan of a patient with a diabetic foot ulcer.

22. Identify routine precautions that should be included in the teaching of the patient with lower extremity neuropathic disease.

23. Which of the following is *not* important information in gathering the patient's pertinent health history?
    a. Arthritis status
    b. Smoking habits
    c. Vision problems
    d. Nasal polyps

24. In assessing the anatomic level in the lower extremity at which arterial insufficiency becomes apparent, which of the following is diagnostically most useful?
    a. Segmental pressures
    b. Femoral bruit
    c. Venous refill time
    d. Ankle-brachial index

25. When instructing the patient and caregiver on proper shoe fit, which of the following is important to emphasize?
    a. Shoes should be selected based on the printed shoe size provided by the manufacturer.
    b. Shoes should be tested for fit early in the morning before the patient is too fatigued to adequately assess how it feels.
    c. Shoes should be fitted while the patient is sitting with the foot elevated on a slanted shoe-fitting stool.
    d. Shoes with heavy rubber soles that curl over the top of the toe area should be avoided.

26. Which of the following is *not* recommended when treating warts on the foot, particularly in younger individuals?
    a. Electrocautery
    b. Liquid nitrogen (cryotherapy)
    c. Salicylic acid
    d. Capsaicin ointment

27. Onychomycosis is:
    a. a bacterial infection
    b. commonly painful
    c. a fungal infection
    d. treatable with bleach solution soakings in persons with weak or frail skin

28. Options for toenail debridement should include the use of all of the following *except:*
    a. manual nippers
    b. mechanical rotary tools fitted with tungsten carbide burs
    c. salicylate solutions
    d. personal protective equipment to reduce exposure to dust

29. Which of the following causes foot odor?
    a. Fungi
    b. Isovaleric acid
    c. Foot powders
    d. Acetic acid

30. Natural, age-specific changes of the foot include which of the following?
    a. Bunions
    b. Narrowing of the foot
    c. Thickening of fat pad over calcaneous
    d. Decreased range of motion

31. The patient should notify his or her physician when any of the following develop *except:*
    a. foot pain that persists for more than 72 hours
    b. foot pain that increases with elevation of the legs
    c. swelling of one leg or foot that persists less than 8 hours
    d. any sudden progression of a foot deformity

32. What causes maceration between the toes?
    a. Inflammation
    b. Allergy
    c. Excessively dry skin
    d. Excessively moist skin

E. Other Types of Wounds

1. Which of the following descriptions is representative of a skin tear classified as category III using the Payne-Martin scale?
   a. Partial-thickness wound with epidermal flap that can be approximated
   b. Both epidermis and dermis are pulled apart as if incisions were made
   c. Partial-thickness wound with no epidermal flap
   d. Full-thickness wound that occurs in skin wrinkle

2. Which of the following terms refers to a tinea infection of the nails?
   a. Tinea pedis
   b. Tinea cruris
   c. Tinea corporis
   d. Onychomycosis

3. Suggestions to prevent tinea infections include which of the following?
   a. Wash hair daily.
   b. Avoid wearing socks.
   c. Wear flip-flops or sandals in public places instead of going barefoot.
   d. Use antideodorant rather than antiperspirant.

4. Which of the following medication histories places the patient with fecal or urinary incontinence at risk for candidiasis?
   a. Prophylactic use of an antifungal agent
   b. Recent antibiotic use
   c. Current use of anticoagulants
   d. Current use of antiseizure medications

5. Which of the following characteristics is distinctive for perianal herpes simplex?
   a. Common location is inner thighs or groin
   b. Associated with history of moisture and antibiotics
   c. Initial manifestations are painful clusters of vesicles
   d. Commonly has a pathergy response

6. Which of the following is *not* appropriate for a sutured postoperative incision?
   a. Keep moist with a topical antibiotic ointment.
   b. Maintain original postoperative dressing for 48 to 72 hours.
   c. Begin showering 48 to 72 hours postoperatively.
   d. Protect surgical incision from exposure to sun.

7. Which of the following hygiene practices is *not* recommended in the presence of radiation skin damage?
   a. Warm showers
   b. Antimicrobial soap to prevent infection
   c. Washing hair with baby shampoo
   d. Shaving with a straight-edge razor

8. Which of the following interventions to promote comfort is *not* recommended in the presence of radiation skin damage?
   a. Gently apply (do not rub) a petrolatum-based product to dry, irritated skin.
   b. Use aloe vera to soothe and cool the skin.
   c. For burning and itching, apply normal saline compresses as needed.
   d. Wear loose, soft, breathable, nonbinding clothing that protects skin from sun and wind.

9. The surgical procedure used to relieve compartment syndrome and nerve damage from tissue edema is known as:
   a. grafting
   b. fasciotomy
   c. escharotomy
   d. incision and drain

10. Which of the following interventions is recommended when the traumatic wound is heavily colonized?
    a. Surgically debride daily.
    b. Pack with Silvadene-coated gauze dressings twice daily.
    c. Surgically close the wound by approximation of wound edges within 36 hours.
    d. Pack the wound with one-quarter strength Dakin solution twice daily temporarily.

11. The wound that undergoes malignant transformation is known as a:
    a. Marjolin ulcer
    b. fungating wound
    c. fistula
    d. draining wound

12. Odor control in a malignant cutaneous wound includes applying:
    a. TNF (tumor necrosis factor) topically every day
    b. gentamycin powder topically every day
    c. metronidazole powder topically with every dressing change
    d. either b or c to the wound every day

13. A condition in which the skin develops superficial blistering and a sandpaper feel and exfoliates after exposure to bacterial toxins is known as:
    a. toxic epidermis necrosis (TEN)
    b. epidermolysis bullosa
    c. staphylococcal scalded skin syndrome (SSSS)
    d. calciphylaxis

14. General signs and symptoms of vasculitis include which of the following?
    a. Sandpaper feel to skin
    b. Severe pruritus
    c. Fever and arthralgias
    d. Mental confusion and imbalance

15. The extent of irreversible tissue damage due to frostbite is primarily influenced by which of the following?
    a. Lowest tissue temperature achieved
    b. Rewarming process
    c. Body part that is involved
    d. Speed with which skin froze

16. Which of the following factors are known to contribute to bowel fistula formation?
    a. Hypotension, tension on the suture line, distal bowel obstruction
    b. Diabetes mellitus, anemia, hematoma formation at site of anastomosis
    c. Compromised blood flow to area of anastomosis, distal bowel obstruction, presence of foreign body close to suture line
    d. Hypoalbuminemia, electrolyte imbalance, tension at the suture line

17. Radiation-induced endarteritis can be expected to develop:
    a. During the first month after irradiation
    b. Between 1 and 3 years following irradiation
    c. Up to 5 years following irradiation
    d. At any time after irradiation

18. Define the involved structures for the following fistulas:
    a. Enterocutaneous
    b. Colocutaneous
    c. Vesicovaginal
    d. Rectovaginal
    e. Colovesical
    f. Atmospheric enterocutaneous fistula

19. Which of the following is the major cause of death in the patient with a fistula?
    a. Malnutrition
    b. Sepsis
    c. Fluid and electrolyte imbalance
    d. Hypotension

20. Which of the following fistulas in an adult would be appropriately managed with a pouching system?
    a. Output during the past 4 hours required four dressing changes and skin is inflamed.
    b. Output during past 24 hours was 50 ml and nonodorous.
    c. Output is noncorrosive and skin is intact.
    d. Output is nonodorous, contained with dressings, and skin is intact.

21. Skin barrier ring or paste used when pouching a fistula achieves which of the following objectives?
    a. Absorb moisture from denuded skin.
    b. Increase tack of pouch adhesive.
    c. Level irregular skin surfaces.
    d. Protect the skin from adhesives.

22. A percutaneous tube that is placed to relieve a high ureteral obstruction is a:
    a. Jackson Pratt drain
    b. gastrostomy tube
    c. Penrose drain
    d. nephrostomy tube

23. The purpose of stabilizing a percutaneous tube is to:
    a. minimize exit site erosion
    b. enhance gastric peristalsis
    c. allow the tube to move with peristalsis and respirations
    d. reduce the length of time the tube will be needed

24. Which of the following is an appropriate initial first step in managing leakage from a gastrostomy site?
    a. Inflate an additional 2 ml of air or saline into the balloon.
    b. Apply an ostomy pouch to contain the drainage and protect the skin.
    c. Cauterize the tract with silver nitrate.
    d. Determine the cause for the leakage.

25. To clean the jejunostomy tube site, the nurse should do which of the following?
    a. Use a cotton-tipped applicator and warm water once daily.
    b. Use a skin cleanser three times daily.
    c. Apply bacitracin ointment once daily.
    d. Dab with diluted hydrogen peroxide once daily.

ANSWERS

A. Principles of Assessment

1. Assessment includes verification and interpretation of observations made. Evaluation of healing involves monitoring and assessment documented over time to reveal patterns and trends that indicate improvement or deterioration in the wound. (Chapter 6)

2. c (Chapter 6)

3. a (Chapter 4)

4. Indices of wound healing (Chapter 6)
   - Etiology/type of skin damage
   - Factors that impede healing
   - Duration of wound
   - Anatomic location of wound
   - Extent of tissue loss (stage)
   - Characteristics of wound base
   - Type of tissue
   - Percentage of wound containing each type of tissue observed
   - Dimensions of wound in centimeters (length, width, tunneling, undermining)
   - Exudate (amount, type, odor)
   - Wound edges
   - Periwound skin
   - Presence or absence of signs of infection
   - Pain

5. b (Chapter 6)

6. Eschar is necrotic (devitalized) tissue. Appearance is leathery (black or brown). Eschar can be soft, firm, adherent, or loose. (Chapter 6)

7. Slough is soft, moist, avascular (necrotic/devitalized) tissue; it may be white, yellow, or tan; it may be loose or firmly adherent. (Chapter 6)

8. Factors known to damage the skin include mechanical, chemical, vascular, allergic, infectious, immunologic, burn, and disease-related types. (Chapter 5)

9. b (Chapter 5)

10. a (Chapter 5)

11. c (Chapter 5)

12. b (Chapter 5)

13. d (Chapter 5)

14. The two phases of an allergic contact dermatitis are the sensitization phase and the elicitation phase. (Chapter 5)

15. a (Chapter 5)

16. d (Chapter 5)

17. a (Chapter 27)

18. d (Chapter 27)

19. b (Chapter 27)

20. b (Chapter 27)

21. c (Chapter 27)

22. a (Chapter 27)

23. c (Chapter 27)

24. c (Chapter 27)

25. b (Chapter 27)

26. c (Chapter 27)

27. a (Chapter 25)

28. b (Chapter 25)

29. Wounds involving only the epidermis and dermis heal relatively quickly because epithelial, endothelial, and connective tissue can be reproduced. Wounds extending through the dermis and involving deeper structures must heal by scar formation because the deep dermal structures, subcutaneous tissue, and muscle do not regenerate. (Chapter 4)

30. Wounds that are well approximated with minimal tissue defect are said to heal by primary intention. Wounds that are left open and allowed to heal by production of granulation tissue are said to heal by secondary intention. Wounds are described as healing by tertiary intention when there is a delay between injury and reapproximation of the wound edges. (Chapter 4)

31. The major components of partial-thickness repair are inflammatory response, epithelial proliferation and migration, and reestablishment and differentiation of epidermal layers. If dermis is involved, connective tissue repair proceeds concurrently with reepithelialization. (Chapter 4)

32. A moist wound surface facilitates epidermal migration because epidermal cells can migrate only across a moist surface. In a dry wound, epidermal cells must tunnel down to a moist level and secrete collagenase to lift the scab away from the wound surface in order to migrate. Connective tissue repair begins earlier when the wound surface is kept moist because new connective tissue forms only in the presence of suitable exudate. (Chapter 4)

33. Inflammatory phase: hemostasis and inflammation. Proliferative phase: neoangiogenesis, matrix deposition/collagen synthesis, epithelialization, and, when a full-thickness wound is left to heal by secondary intention, contraction of wound edges. Maturation phase: matrix deposition and collagen lysis. (Chapter 4)

34. c (Chapter 4)

35. b (Chapter 4)

36. There is a limit to epidermal cell migration. In full-thickness wounds, epidermal cells are present only at the wound margins. In partial-thickness wounds, epidermal cells are present in the lining of hair follicles and sweat glands, as well as at the wound periphery. (Chapter 4)

37. Chronic wounds are likely to begin with circulatory compromise as opposed to injury. Injury initiates hemostasis, which triggers the wound-healing cascade; circulatory compromise does not trigger the wound-healing cascade. Chronic wounds contain higher levels of proteases (i.e., neutrophil elastase and matrix metalloproteases ([MMPs]), resulting in the prolonged presence and increased volume of proinflammatory cells (cytokines). (Chapter 4)

38. Factors that affect wound healing include tissue perfusion and oxygenation, nutritional status, infection, diabetes mellitus, corticosteroid administration, immunosuppression, and aging. Systemic factors include renal or hepatic disease, malignancy, sepsis, hematopoietic abnormalities, and stress. (Chapter 4)

39. b (Chapter 4)

40. b (Chapter 3)

41. c (Chapter 28)

42. a (Chapter 28)

43. a (Chapter 35)

B. Principles of Wound Management

1. d (Chapter 18)

2. d (Chapter 12)

3. b (Chapter 18)

4. d (Chapter 18)

5. b (Chapter 18)

6. d (Chapter 18)

7. d (Chapter 18)

8. Objectives for local wound management are to prevent and manage infection, cleanse the wound, remove nonviable tissue (debridement), maintain an appropriate level of moisture, eliminate dead space, control odor, eliminate or minimize pain, and protect the wound and periwound skin. (Chapter 18)

9. d (Chapter 17)

10. c (Chapter 17)

11. Considerations in the use of enzymatic debridement include the following (Chapter 17):
    - Enzymes are inactivated by heavy metal ions (chlorine, silver, mercury).
    - Enzymes may be used to debride an infected wound.
    - Enzymatic debridement necessitates dressing changes at least daily.
    - Selection of debriding enzyme is primarily based on clinician preference, cost, availability, and ease of use.

12. a (Chapter 17)

13. b (Chapter 17)

14. d (Chapter 16)

15. c (Chapter 16)

16. c (Chapter 16)

17. a (Chapter 16)

18. d (Chapter 16)

19. a (Chapter 16)

20. d (Chapter 16)

21. c (Chapter 16)

22. b (Chapter 16)

23. c (Chapter 21)

24. b (Chapter 21)

25. a (Chapter 21)

26. a (Chapter 21)

27. c (Chapter 21)

28. b (Chapter 22)

29. c (Chapter 22)

30. True (Chapter 22)

31. False (Chapter 22)

32. Selectins, integrins, cell adhesion molecules (Chapter 20)

33. False (Chapter 20)

34. d (Chapter 20)

35. d. All CTPs mimic native tissues to promote healing. (Chapter 19)

36. c. Function as an extracellular matrix (ECM) scaffold. (Chapter 19)

37. Sources for the components of CTPs include autologous (derived from the patient's own body), allogeneic (derived from humans other than the patient; also called *homografts*), xenographic (derived from nonhuman sources, e.g., porcine, bovine, equine, avian, etc.; also called *heterografts*), biosynthetic (biologic and manufactured materials), and synthetic (manufactured materials). (Chapter 19)

38. Epicel, Dermagraft, Apligraf (Chapter 19)

39. a. Keratinocytes and fibroblasts (Chapter 19)

40. True. Although autologous cellular CTPs (i.e., skin grafts) will survive (referred to as *take*), the allogeneic CTPs are temporary and biodegradable. Allogeneic fibroblasts survive from 3 to 8 weeks in the patient, and allogeneic keratinocytes survive only 2 to 3 weeks. (Chapter 19)

41. (1) Address underlying pathology; (2) Correct systemic factors interfering with wound healing; (3) Identify and treat clinical infection prior to application; (4) Debride all necrotic tissue and excess granulation tissue, fibrinous slough, and surrounding callus prior to application; (5) Ensure complete contact and stabilization of CTP in wound bed by using bolster dressings, NPWT, or sutures to secure CTP in place; (6) Prevent accumulation of fluid under CTP by fenestrating product prior to application; (7) Keep CTP without synthetic backing moist; (8) Follow package insert for directions specific to individual products. (Chapter 19)

42. b (Chapter 16)

43. d (Chapter 26)

44. c (Chapter 26)

45. True (Chapter 26)

46. Minimize the degree of sensory stimulus (e.g., drafts from open windows, or prodding and poking); allow patient to perform his or her own dressing change; allow time-outs during painful procedures; schedule dressing changes when the patient is feeling best; give an analgesic and then schedule the dressing change when its peak effect occurs; soak dried dressings before removal; avoid use of cytotoxic cleansers; avoid aggressive packing; minimize number of dressing changes; prevent periwound trauma; position and support wounded area for comfort; consider using low-adhesive or nonadhesive dressings; and offer and use distraction techniques (e.g., headphones, television, music, warm blanket). (Chapter 26)

47. b (Chapter 34)

48. d (Chapter 34)

49. a (Chapter 34)

C. Pressure Ulcers

1. A pressure ulcer is localized injury to the skin and/or underlying tissue, usually over a bony prominence, as a result of pressure or pressure in combination with shear. (Chapter 7)

2. a (Chapter 7)

3. Amount and duration of pressure share an inverse relationship in producing tissue ischemia. A long time is needed for low pressure to create ischemia, whereas a short time is needed for high pressure to cause tissue ischemia. (Chapter 7)

4. d (Chapter 8)

5. b (Chapter 7)

6. a (Chapters 7 and 8)

7. b (Chapter 7)

8. b (Chapter 7)

9. d (Chapter 7)

10. a (Chapter 7)

11. a (Chapter 7)

12. c (Chapter 7)

13. c (Chapter 8)

14. b (Chapter 8)

15. d (Chapter 8)

16. a (Chapter 9)

17. b (Chapter 9)

18. c (Chapter 5)

19. b (Chapter 5)

20. d (Chapter 5)

21. b (Chapter 5)

D. Lower Extremity Ulcers

1. c (Chapter 11)

2. b (Chapter 11)

3. c (Chapter 11)

4. d (Chapter 11)

5. d (Chapter 11)

6. d (Chapter 11)

7. A competent venous system includes deep veins, superficial veins, and perforator veins. The perforator veins (communicating veins) connect the deep and superficial veins to transport blood. Veins function by one-way valves to prevent backflow. The calf muscle pump and one-way valves work together to propel venous blood back to the heart. During ambulation, the calf muscle contracts and pumps the blood out of the deep veins, and the one-way valves in the perforator system close to prevent backflow into superficial veins. When the calf muscle relaxes, the valves in the perforator veins open to permit blood flow into the deep veins. (Chapter 12)

8. c (Chapter 12). 30 to 40 mm Hg is considered a therapeutic level. 20 to 25 mm Hg compression is considered a light compression, whereas 50 mm Hg is a very high compression usually indicated for lymphedema.

9. d (Chapter 12). An ABI of 0.5 indicates ischemia, and any additional compression to a leg with compromised arterial circulation could increase claudication and put the patient at risk for ischemic damage. In addition, the wound will not heal unless revascularization is performed.

10. Elastic compression devices deliver a sustained pressure, regardless of the patient's activity level. Nonelastic compression devices compress the calf muscle during ambulation. The constant compression increases interstitial tissue pressure to reduce leakage of fluid from capillaries. The sedentary patient should be managed with elastic compression devices because he or she has decreased calf muscle pump action. (Chapter 12)

11. b (Chapter 12)

12. c (Chapter 12). Lanolin skin products and topical antibiotic creams should not be used because of sensitivities to topical creams/lotions that develop in the patient with chronic venous insufficiency.

13. a (Chapter 12). Compression stockings need to be applied in the morning before the patient gets out of bed to prevent the return of ankle edema, which can occur as soon as the patient dangles the foot over the edge of the bed. Ankle exercises can be performed while the stockings are worn.

14. c (Chapter 13)

15. a (Chapter 13)

16. d (Chapter 13)

17. a (Chapter 13)

18. Autonomic: Results in decreased sweating and oil production, loss of skin temperature regulation, and abnormal blood flow in the soles of the feet. Resultant xerosis can precipitate fissures, cracks, callus, and finally ulceration. Sensory: Loss of protective sensation leads to lack of awareness of pain and temperature change, resulting in increased susceptibility to injury. Minor trauma caused by poor-fitting shoes or an acute injury can precipitate a chronic ulcer. Motor: Affects the muscles required for normal foot movement and can result in muscle atrophy, resulting in collapse of the arch, cocked-up or claw toes, hammertoes, and weight redistribution from the toes to the metatarsal heads, which leads to increased pressures and subsequent ulceration. (Chapter 14)

19. a (Chapter 14)

20. d (Chapter 14)

21. Glycemic control, offloading, callus management, pain control, education (Chapter 14)

22. Routine precautions in the teaching of the patient with lower extremity neuropathic disease include the following (Chapter 14):
   - Wash feet daily; dry carefully, including between the toes.
   - Test the water with hands or elbow.
   - Do not soak feet.
   - Apply moisturizing cream to feet, but not between toes.
   - Do not use heating pad or hot water bottle to warm feet.
   - Do not use chemical corn or callus removers or corn pads.
   - File away calluses with pumice stone.
   - Do not walk barefoot; wear slippers with rubber sole; no open toes or heels; avoid pointed-toe shoes or boots; do not wear sandals with strap between toes.
   - Buy shoes later in the day when feet are their largest.
   - Inspect shoes for objects inside before putting them on.
   - Wear clean socks every day; avoid nylon socks; no tight elastic or seams.
   - Do not smoke; exercise regularly.

23. d (Chapter 15)

24. a (Chapter 15)

25. d (Chapter 15)

26. d (Chapter 15)

27. c (Chapter 15)

28. c (Chapter 15)

29. b (Chapter 15)

30. d (Chapter 15)

31. c (Chapter 15)

32. d (Chapter 15)

E. Other Types of Wounds, Tubes, and Fistulas

1. c (Chapter 5)

2. d (Chapter 15)

3. c (Chapter 15)

4. b (Chapter 5)

5. c (Chapter 5)

6. a (Chapter 34)

7. d (Chapter 5)

8. a (Chapter 5)

9. b (Chapters 31 and 32)

10. d (Chapter 31)

11. a (Chapter 37)

12. c (Chapter 37)

13. c (Chapter 30)

14. c (Chapter 30)

15. b (Chapter 30)

16. c. (Chapter 38)

17. d. (Chapter 38)

18. a. An enterocutaneous fistula is between the small bowel and the skin.
    b. A colocutaneous fistula is between the colon and the skin.
    c. A vesicovaginal fistula is between the bladder and the vagina.
    d. A rectovaginal fistula is between the rectum and the vagina.
    e. A colovesical fistula is between the colon and the bladder.
    f. An atmospheric enterocutaneous fistula is between the small bowel and the open abdominal wound bed.

19. b (Chapter 38)

20. a (Chapter 38)

21. c (Chapter 38)

22. d (Chapter 39)

23. b (Chapter 39)

24. d (Chapter 39)

25. a (Chapter 39)

A

Abdominal incisions, 64
Abscess, 494, 577
Absorbent dressings, 535–536
Accreditation, 2
Acellular extracellular matrix
    scaffolds, 329, 330–331t
Acetic acid, 290–291t
Ace-type bandages, 218
Achilles tendon
    description of, 264
    reflex testing of, 268
Achilles tendonitis, 278
Acid burns, 477
Acquired lymphedema, 228
Active support surfaces, 167–170,
    168–169t
Acute fecal incontinence, 89
Acute limb ischemia, 187
Acute lymphedema, 228
Acute pain, 389
Acute phase response, 411–412
Acute wounds
    characteristics of, 64
    cleanup, 67
    description of, 490
    healing of, 68
    molecular imbalances in, 346b
    negative pressure wound therapy
        for, 352
Adherence, 428
Adherens junctions, 339
Adhesion molecules, 338–341, 338f,
    339f
    cadherins, 339
    cell, 339
    integrins, 338
    selectins, 338–339
Adhesive dressings, 85
Adjunctive interventions, 105–106
Adolescents, 51
Adult learning, principles of, 432b
Advance beneficiary notice, 25
Advance practice nurse, physician
    services provided by, 34
Advanced trauma life support
    (ATLS), 464–465
Advancement flaps, 492
Affordable Care Act (ACA), 30–31
Age
    foot changes associated with,
        263, 276
    pressure ulcer and, 131
    skin changes related to, 51–56
Air, as surface support, 166
Air-fluidized support surfaces,
    168–169t, 171
Albumin, 412
Alginate dressings, 309, 536
Alkali burns, 477
Allergens, 58–59
Allergic contact dermatitis, 48–49,
    101, 575

AlloDerm, 329, 330–331t
Allogeneic ECM scaffolds, 329–332
Allograft, 483
Alternating current, 370t
Alternating-pressure support
    surfaces, 167–170
Ambulatory payment classification,
    30b, 33
Ambulatory venous hypertension,
    205–207
American Burn Association, 479t,
    486
American Society for Metabolic
    and Bariatric Surgery, obesity
    definition, 508
Amorphous hydrogels, 315
Amperage, 370t
Amplitude charge, 370t
Amputations
    economic burden of, 240
    foot ulcer as cause of, 252–253
    infection as cause of, 251–252
    lower extremity arterial disease,
        200–201
    peripheral arterial disease as risk
        factor for, 243
    prevention program of, 246t
    traumatic wounds, 471
Anabolic steroids, 416–417
Analgesics, 199
Ancillary staff, 28
Androgens, 416–417
Anesthetic risk, 490
Angiogenesis, 44
Anhidrosis, 271
Ankle
    circumference of, 179
    flexibility testing of, 268
    range of motion, 180, 267f
Ankle flare, 178
Ankle joint equinus, 243
Ankle pumps, 212
Ankle-brachial index, 193–194,
    194b, 209–210
Anterior tibial artery, 265
Antiarmor devices, 463–464
Antibacterial, 284b
Antibiotics, 284b
    beads, 469
    diarrhea associated with, 90
Antidepressants, 405
Antiembolism stockings, 218
Antiepileptics, 405
Antiinflammatory cytokines, 341t
Antimicrobials, 284b
    burn wound management using,
        482–483
    topical, 290–291t
    for wound odor, 537
Antioxidants, 57
Antiplatelet agents, 198
Antiseptic, 284b
    topical, 289

Anxiety, 433–434
AP-1 nuclear transcription
    complex, 56–57
Apligraf, 328t, 333
Apnea, sleep, obesity and, 512
Apocrine glands, 50, 52–53t, 265
Arch, 274
Arginine, 414–415
Arm muscle circumference, 411
Aromatherapy, 235
Arterial insufficiency, 211–212
Arterial perfusion, 209–210
Arterial ulcers, 186–203, 201b
    antiplatelet agents for, 198
    assessment of, 191–193
    atherosclerosis as cause of,
        187–188
    bypass grafts for, 197–198, 197f
    characteristics of, 184–185t
    dressings for, 200
    endovascular procedures for, 198
    epidemiology of, 186–187
    etiology of, 187–188
    history of patient with, 191–192
    hyperbaric oxygen therapy for,
        199
    intermittent pneumatic
        compression for, 199
    management of, 197–200
    measures to improve perfusion,
        197
    mixed arterial-venous disease,
        199
    noninvasive testing for, 193–196
        ankle-brachial index, 193–194,
            194b
        computed tomographic
            angiography, 196
        Doppler waveform studies,
            193f, 195, 196f
        duplex angiography, 196
        exercise stress testing, 195
        magnetic resonance
            angiography, 196
        pulse volume recordings, 195
        segmental limb pressure
            measurements, 195–196
        skin perfusion pressure, 195
        toe-brachial index, 194–195
        transcutaneous oxygen
            pressure (TcPO2), 195
    pathology of, 191
    pharmacologic therapy for,
        198–199
    sickle cell disease as cause of,
        188
    surgical options of, 197–198
    topical therapy for, 200, 200b
    vasculitis as cause of, 188
Arteries, lower extremity, 183f
Arteriography, 196–197
ASEPSIS scoring tool, 500–501,
    501b

Assessments, 109–118
    burn injuries, 480
    fistula, 548–549, 548b
    focused physical, 112–113, 112b
    lower extremity. see Lower
        extremity assessment
    lower extremity neuropathic
        disease. see Lower extremity
        arterial disease (LEAD),
        assessment of
    nutritional status. see Nutritional
        status assessment
    skin. see Skin assessment
    venous ulcers, 209–212
    wound. see Wound assessment
Association of Women's Health,
    Obstetric and Neonatal
    Nurses (AWHONN), on
    diaper dermatitis, 521
Atherosclerosis, 187–188
Athlete's foot, 96
At-risk population, 15
Atrophie blanche lesions, 178, 210
Attention deficit hyperactivity
    disorder, 485
Aural barotrauma, 366
Autografts. see Skin grafts
Autolysis, 296–297
Autonomic nervous system, 420
Autonomic neuropathy, 241
Avlosulfon. see Dapsone
    (Avlosulfon)
Axial flaps, 492
Axonotmesis, 466

B

Bacitracin/neomycin/polymyxin,
    483
Bacteria
    colonization, 284, 284b
    contamination, 284, 284b
    on skin, 47
Bacterial bioburden
    biofilm, 284b, 285
    burn injuries, 482
    colonization, 284, 284b, 285b
    contamination, 284, 284b
    continuum of, 284–288, 284b
    critical colonization, 284b, 285
    management of, 288–292
    negative pressure wound therapy
        reduction of, 350
    topical wound management
        affected by, 321
Bacterial biofilms, 47–48
Bacterial infections
    cellulitis, 97
    erysipelas, 97
    erythrasma, 98
    folliculitis, 98
    impetigo, 98–99
Balanced Budget Act of 1997
    (BBA), 31

Ballistic injuries, 463
Banding, 381
Bariatric bed, 508–509, 510t
Bariatric task force, 513
Bariatric treatment chair, 29
Bariatrics, 508
Baromedical Nurses Association, 364
Barotrauma, aural, 366
Basal cell carcinoma (BCC), 458
Basal cells, 42
Basal keratinocytes, 42
Basement membrane zone, 44
Bates-Jensen Wound Assessment Tool, 121
Behavioral Risk Factor Surveillance System, 239
Benzopyrones, 236
BGC Matrix, 483
Bilayer Matrix Wound Dressing, 333
Bilayered cellular- and tissue-based products, 333–334
Billing. see also Reimbursement
   acronym related to, 30b
   hospital-based clinic vs. freestanding clinic, 22
   incident to, 34
Bioactive molecules, 74–75
Biobrane, 330–331t, 332, 483
Bioburden
   bacterial
      biofilm, 284b, 285
      burn injuries, 482
      colonization, 284, 284b, 285b
      contamination, 284, 284b
      continuum of, 284–288, 284b
      critical colonization, 284b, 285
      infection secondary to. see Wound infection
      management of, 288–292
      negative pressure wound therapy reduction of, 350
      topical wound management affected by, 321
   definition of, 284b
Bioelectrical impedance analysis, 232
Biofilm matrix, 283
Biofilm phenotype, 283
Biofilms, 47–48, 284b, 285, 289–292
Bioimpedance spectroscopy, 232
Biosynthetic extracellular matrix scaffolds, 330–331t, 332–333
Biothesiometer, 246f, 247b
Biovance, 330–331t
Biphasic PC electrical stimulation, 372
Blanching erythema, 132–133
Blast injuries, 463
Bleeding control, 464–465, 536
Blood dyscrasias, 458–459, 459t
Blood flow, 182, 371
Blood pressure, 131
Body composition, 414
Body mass index (BMI), 411, 508, 508b

Body temperature, pressure ulcer risks, 132
Bone biopsy, 292
"Bottoming out," 163–164
Bounding land mines, 463
Boyle's gas law, 361–362, 364
Braden Q scale, 518–520, 519t
Braden Scale, 144–147, 145t
Bridging technique, 557, 557f, 558b
Brown recluse spider, 443
Bruise, 136
Bruit, 182
Buerger disease, 188
Bullet wounds, 462–463
Bullous impetigo, 98
Bullous pyoderma gangrenosum, 444
Bunionette, 277t
Bunions, 242t
Burn centers
   referral to, 476b, 479
   school reentry programs, 486
Burn injuries, 487b
   American Burn Association categories of, 479, 479t, 486
   assessment of, 480
   care, phases of, 480–486
      acute/wound care, 481–485
      autograft closure, 483–484
      bioburden management, 482–483
      cellular- and/or tissue-based products, 483
      emergent, 480–481
      escharotomy, 481
      fasciotomy, 481
      fluid resuscitation, 480
      hydrotherapy, 482
      rehabilitation, 485–486
      surgical excision, 483–484
      topical antimicrobials, 482–483
   chemical, 477
   contact, 476
   contractures, 485–486
   deep circumferential, 481
   discharge planning for, 486
   edema caused by, 480
   electrical, 476
   emotional support for, 481
   enteral nutritional support for, 480
   epidemiology of, 475
   evaluation of, 477–479
   flame, 475–476
   fluid and electrolyte-imbalance caused by, 479
   hypermetabolic response to, 479–480
   infection in, 482
   inflammatory mediators, 479
   inhaled hot air, 476
   itching secondary to, 485–486
   Lund-Browder chart for estimating, 477–479, 478f
   major, 479t
   minor, 479t

Burn injuries (Continued)
   moderate, 479t
   outpatient management of, 486–487
   pain control for, 481
   pathophysiology of, 479–480
   pediatrics, 484–485, 484b, 524
   rehabilitation for, 485–486
   scald, 476
   scarring in, 485–486
   severity of, 477, 478f
   skin integrity loss caused by, 479
   thermal, 475–476
   tissue damage zones, 477
   total body surface area of, 475, 477–479
   types of, 475–477
   wound
      fungal infection of, 482
      infection of, 482
      stabilization of, 480–481
      sunscreen protection, 487
Burow's solution, 96
Business plan, 21, 22b
Bypass grafts, 197–198, 197f

C

C fibers, 388
Cadaveric human skin, 334
Cadexomer iodine, 289, 290–291t
Cadherins, 339
Calcaneus, 264
Calcific uremic arteriolopathy, 448
Calciphylaxis, 136, 448, 493
Calcitriol, 50–51
Calcium alginate, 310–312t
Calf circumference, 179
Calf muscle pump, 205
   dysfunction of, 208–209, 209b
   exercise for, 212
Callus, 248, 270t, 276f
Calories, 414
Candida albicans, 87
Candidiasis, 95–96
Capillary closing pressure, 128, 163b
Capillary occlusion, 132–134, 134f
Capillary pressure, 128, 128f
Capillary refill, 182, 182b
Capillary wall, 134
Carbohydrates, 58, 415
Carboxymethylcellulose, 314
Care transitions, 436
Caregiver, 429
Carotene, 43
Carotenoids, 43
Catastrophizing, 388
Catecholamines, 420
Catenins, 339
Cathode, 369
CDS, 328t
Cell adhesion molecules (CAMs), 339
Cell therapy, 334
CellSpray XP, 328t

Cellular- and tissue-based products, for wounds, 325–336, 327b, 335b
Cellulitis, 97
   characteristics of, 237
   compression bandaging for, 237
   dermatitis vs., 211t
Centers for Disease Control (CDC), on surgical site infections, criteria for, 501–502, 502t
Centers for Medicare & Medicaid Services (CMS), 15-16. see also Medicaid; Medicare
   national coverage determinations, 35–36, 35b
   responsibilities of, 30
Centre for Evidence-Based Medicine (CEBM), 7
Certifications, 2
   eligibility criteria, 2
   hyperbaric oxygen therapy, 364
   value of, 2b
Certified wound, ostomy, and continence nurse (CWOCN), 11–12
Certified wound care nurse, 11
Certified wound care specialist, 12
Certifying organizations
   accreditation, 2
   comparing of, 2, 2b
   eligibility criteria, 2
Chair cushions, 167
Change agent, 4, 4b
Charcoal dressings, 537, 558
Charcot arthropathy, 242t, 277
   description of, 243
   treatment of, 255
Charcot foot, 243, 256t
Charcot restraint orthotic walker, 254–255, 255f
Charge, 370t
Chart audits, 17
Charts
   documentation needed for, 26, 26t
   preparation, storage, and electronic medical records, 24
Chemical burns, 477
Chemical cauterization, 297
Chemokine, 341
Chilblain, 456t
Child abuse, 485, 485b
Child neglect, 485, 485b
Children. see also Pediatrics; Premature infants
   dressings for, 526–527
   FLACC pain scale for, 393–394, 393t
   gastrostomy tubes for, 522
   pressure ulcers in, 518–520, 519t, 520b
Chlorhexidine, 51–55, 290–291t
Chloromycetin, 537
Chromophore, 301
Chronic limb ischemia, 187
Chronic lymphedema, 228

Chronic pain, 387
Chronic venous disease, 204, 205–209
  classification of, 207
  risk factors for, 208–209
  valvular dysfunction associated with, 208b
  venous ulcers. see Venous ulcers
Chronic venous insufficiency, 204, 209b. see also Venous ulcers
  arterial insufficiency evaluations, 211–212
  arterial perfusion associated with, 209–210
  assessment of, 209–212
  diagnostic evaluation of, 211–212
  duplex ultrasound evaluations, 212
  edema associated with, 210
  hemosiderosis associated with, 210
  lipodermatosclerosis associated with, 210
  obesity and, 212
Chronic Wound Pain Experience model, 394–395, 394f, 395f
Chronic wounds, 284
  bacterial bioburden in, 284–288
  characteristics of, 73–74, 73b, 73f
  denervation, 74
  growth factors in, 74
  healing of, 64
  infection, databased paradigms of, 286t
  inflammatory substances, 73
  miscellaneous host conditions, 74
  molecular imbalances in, 346b
  negative pressure wound therapy for, 352–353
  pathology of, 73
Circulation, 49
Claw toes, 241, 242t, 277t
Clinic
  benefits of, to organization, 22b
  billing differences, 22
  clinical consult, 38b
  continuous quality improvement plan, 30
  equipment necessary for, 28
  financial viability, 22–24
  hospital-based. see Hospital-based clinic
  management, 21–22, 23t
  outpatient, 38b
  physical space, 22
  policies, procedures, and guidelines, 29, 29b
  referral network, 28
  room equipment, 28–29
  space and supply needs for, 23b
  staff. see Staff
  structure of, 22–24, 23b
  wound care supplies, 29
Clinic operations, 24–30
  chart preparation, storage, and electronic medical records, 24

Clinic operations (Continued)
  compliance program, 24–27
  consents, 24
  hours of operation, 24
  scheduling, 24
Clinical consult, 18b
Clinical decision-making, 3
Clinical signs and symptoms checklist, 287
Clinician, 429
Clonidine, 405
Closed suction system, for fistula effluent, 553
Closed-cell foam, 165
Clostridial myonecrosis, 363
Clostridium difficile, 90
Clostridium difficile-associated diarrhea, 90
Clostridium perfringens, 494
Clostridium tetani, 465–466
Clot formation, 67
Coccyx, 114f
Coder, insurance and billing, 27–28
Codes/Coding
  Current Procedural Terminology, 37
  Distinct Procedural Service, 37
  medical condition, 36
  National Correct Coding Initiative, 25t, 37
  procedure, 36
  services and supplies, 32b, 36–38
  supply, 36–37
Cognitive ability, 433
Cold injury, 456t
Collagen, 44, 46, 415
  aging and, 55–56
  synthesis of, 70–71
Collagen dressing, 309–313
Collagenase, 297, 341
Collar, 154t
Colonization, 284, 284b
  criteria for, 285b
Communication, 51
Community program, 17
Community-associated methicillin-resistant Staphylococcus aureus, 97
Compartment syndrome, 467–468
Compensatory antiinflammatory response syndrome (CARS), 467, 467t
Complete decongestive physiotherapy, 234–235
Compliance program, 24–27
  insurance authorization, 25
  objectives, 24
  treatment orders, 25–26
Composite dressing, 313
Compression garments, 218–219
Compression stockings, 218, 219b, 219f
  lymphedema managed with, 235
Compression therapy, 213–216, 214t, 220f
  contraindications, 213, 216
  devices for, 213–214

Compression therapy (Continued)
  features of, 214–216
  inelastic, 215
  intermittent pneumatic compression, 213–214, 219–220
  negative pressure wound therapy vs., 351–352
  suggestion for, 215b
  types of, 215t
  wraps, 215, 216–218, 217f
    application technique for, 216–217
    long-stretch reusable, 218
    multilayer, 217–218
    paste, 217–218, 217b
    reusable inelastic device, 219, 219f
    single-layer reusable, 218
Computed tomographic angiography, 196
Concordance, 428
Congenital lymphedema, 228
Connective tissue disorders, 446–448
Connective tissue growth factor, 340t, 344–345
Consents, 24
Conservative instrumental debridement, 299, 299b
Conservative sharp wound debridement, 299–300
  policy and procedure, 300b
Constitutive synthesis, 43
Consultant, 3, 4b
Contact burns, 476
Contact dermatitis, 101
  allergic, 101
Contact inhibition, 65
Contact layers, 313, 537
Containment devices, 91–93
Contamination, 284, 284b
Continued maintenance debridement, 289
Continuing medical education, 17
Continuous Assessment Record and Evaluation (CARE), 119
Continuous lateral rotation, 170
Continuous quality improvement plan, 30
Contractor audit, 26–27
Contractures, 485–486, 494
Coordination testing, 269
Copper, 415–416
Corns, 270t, 276f
Corporate compliance, 24
Corticosteroids, 446t
  tensile strength affected by, 70–71
  tinea managed with, 96
  venous dermatitis symptoms managed with, 211
Cortisol, 131–132
Cost effectiveness, 16–17
Creatinine, 413
Crest pads, 275t
CRIES pain scale, 393–394, 393t

Critical closing pressure, 128
Critical colonization, 284b, 285, 289–292
Critical limb ischemia, 187
Cues to action, 430t, 431
Cultural competence, 436
  steps to improve, 436b
Culture- and tissue-based products, 325–326
Cumulative incidence, 13b, 14
Cuneiform bones, 264, 265f
Curette, 272
Current, 370t
Current Procedural Terminology, 30b, 34t, 37
Custom-molded shoe, 255f
Cyclosporine, topical, 445, 446t
Cymetra, 329, 330–331t
Cytokines, 341–342
  antiinflammatory, 341t
  biologic roles of, 337–338
  definition of, 337
  inflammatory cell, 340–341
  macrophage secretion of, 340
  production of, 341
  proinflammatory, 341t
  in wound healing, 341t

D
Dakin's solution, 290–291t
Dapsone (Avlosulfon), 443
Darkly pigmented skin
  assessment of, 111–112, 112b
  characteristics of, 41b
  dermatologic disorders associated with, 43–44
  erythema detection in, 112
  pressure ulcer staging in, 135
  ultraviolet radiation protections, 48
  vitamin D levels on, 50–51
Debridement
  nail, 271, 272b
  wound. see Wound debridement
Debulking procedures, 236
Decision support tools, 9
Decubitus ulcer, 127. see also Pressure ulcer(s)
Deep incision infection, 502
Defensins, 47–48
Degree of activity, 146
Dendrocytes, 49
Deodorizers, 536–537, 555
Dependent rubor, 181
Depression, 433–434
Dermagraft, 328t, 329
Dermal and bilayered cellular- and tissue-based products, 334
Dermal and bilayered culture- and tissue-based products, 327–329, 328t
Dermal fibrosis, 210–211
Dermal papillae, 45
Dermal proteins, 46
Dermal thermometry, 182
Dermal-epidermal junction, 44, 52–53t, 86

DermaMatrix, 330–331t
Dermatitis, 178
    allergic contact, 48–49, 575
    chemical, 87–88
    contact, 101
    diaper, 87–88, 520–522
    incontinence-associated, 88,
        510–511
    intertrigo, 90–91
    perineal, 87–88
    radiation, 102t, 105b
Dermatoheliosis, 55, 56
Dermatomes, 100f
Dermatophytes, 96, 276–277
Dermis, 41f, 44–46, 52–53t
    cells in, 46
    development of, 51
    eccrine glands, 49–50
    fibroblasts in, 44–45
    papillary, 45, 45f, 49
    proteins in, 44
    repair of, in partial-thickness
        wound, 65–66
    reticular, 46
    vasculature in, 44, 52–53t
DESIGN R tool, 121
DESIGN tool, 121
Desmosomal proteins, 42
Desmosome, 42
Desquamation, 103
Diabetes mellitus
    ankle joint equinus associated
        with, 243
    Charcot foot associated with, 243
    economic burden of, 240
    lower extremity arterial disease
        risks, 190
    peripheral arterial disease in,
        243–244
    prevalence of, 239
    substance P, 69
    wound healing affected by,
        78–79t
Diabetic foot infections, 251, 252t
Diabetic foot ulcers, 258b
    callus, 242–243
    characteristics of, 250
    classification of, 250–251, 250t
    early intervention, 252–253
    economic burden of, 240
    evaluation of, 249–252
    ischemic, 250
    lower extremity amputations
        secondary to, 239–240
    with lower extremity arterial
        disease, 250
    management of, 252–258
        early intervention, 249b,
            252–253
        felted foam dressing, 254
        glycemic control, 253
        multidisciplinary approach
            to, 252
        offloading, 253–255
        total-contact cast, 253–254,
            253f
    pathogenesis of, 240–244

Diabetic foot ulcers (Continued)
    prevalence of, 239
    prevention of, 252–253
    risk classification of, 245t
    risk factors for, 244b
        classification of, 244
        motor neuropathy, 241
        musculoskeletal
            abnormalities, 241–243,
            242t
        neuropathy, 252
        peripheral neuropathy,
            240–241
    sensory neuropathy as risk factor
        for, 241
    size classification system, 251t
    topical therapy, 257
    University of Texas classification
        system, 250–251, 251t
    vascular status, 247–248
    Wagner foot wound classification
        system, 250, 250t
    wound
        debridement, 256
        management of, 255–257
        topical care of, 257
Diabetic neuropathy
    autonomic, 241
    glycemic control and, 253
    vasa nervosum associated with,
        252
Diagnosis code, 30
Diagnostic studies, level of
    evidence for, 9t
Diapedesis, 68
Diaper dermatitis, 87–88, 520–522
Diaper rash. see Incontinence-
    associated dermatitis (IAD)
Diarrhea
    antibiotic-associated, 90
    Clostridium difficile-associated,
        90
Diazepam, 403t
Dietitian, 13
Diffuse neuropathy, 241
Diffusion of Innovations Theory,
    4, 5t
Direct current, 370t
Directed percutaneous endoscopic
    jejunostomy, 568
Disease-related malnutrition, 409,
    413t
Disinfectant, 284b
Dismounted IED injury pattern,
    463
Documentation
    for chart, 26, 26t
    contractor audit, 26–27, 27b
    payer audit, 26–27, 27b
    reimbursement, 26
    wound debridement, 26
Dominant dystrophic
    epidermolysis bullosa
    (DDEB), 450b
Doppler waveform studies, 193f,
    195, 196f
Dorsalis pedis, 265

Dorsalis pedis pulse, 265
Drainage tubes, 577
Draining wounds
    definition of, 542
    management of, 541–561
Dressings, 105
    absorbent, 535–536
    alginate, 309, 536
    application of, 318–319
    for arterial ulcers, 200
    atraumatic changes or removal
        of, 318, 535–536
    caregiver considerations, 321
    changing of, 317–319, 400b
    charcoal, 537, 558
    collagen, 309–313
    compatibility issues for, 320
    composite, 313
    contact layers, 313, 537
    exudate volume and, 117–118
    fiber gelling, 309
    fistula effluent containment
        using, 550
    foam, 313–314
    formulary for, 310–312t
    gauze, 316–317
    hemostatic, 465t
    hydrocolloid, 314
    hydrogel, 314–315, 537
    infection control of, 317–318
    ingredients in, 309
    inspection of, 110
    moisture-retentive, 400
    negative pressure wound therapy
        and, 354–355, 469
    pain management during
        removal of, 355b, 400b
    pediatric, 526–527
    securing of, 319
    selection of, 319–321, 319b
    semiocclusive, 307t
    silver antimicrobial, 482
    specialty absorptive, 316
    surgical, 504
    topical antimicrobials for, 321
    transparent film, 316
    wet-to-dry, 298, 316–317, 469
    wound location consideration, 321
    wound odor affected by, 118
Droperidol, 403t
Drug-induced vasculitis, 448
Dry gangrene, 494
Duplex angiography, 196
Duplex ultrasound, 212
Durable medical equipment, home
    use of, Medicare guidelines
    for, 37b
Durable medical equipment,
    prosthetics, orthotics, and
    supplies (DMEOS), 30b, 31
Dysesthesia, 403t
Dyslipidemia, lower extremity
    arterial disease risks, 190

E
Early-delayed fascial closure, 471
Eccrine glands, 49–50, 52–53t, 265

Edema
    chronic venous insufficiency, 210
    control of, 399–400
    definition of, 178–179
    distribution of, 179
    extent of, 179
    grading scale for, 180b
    hyperbaric oxygenation for, 362
    lower extremity, 178–179
    negative pressure wound therapy
        for, 350–351
    pattern of, 179
    pitting, 179, 179f
    reduction of, and wound fluid
        removal, 350–351
    types of, 180t
    venous, 180t
Education
    of patient. see Patient education
    staff, 29
    as wound specialist, 1–2
Educational assessment, 432b
Educator, 3–4, 4b
Elastic foam, 165
Elastin, 44, 46, 71
Elastosis, 46
Elderly, 86. see also Older adults
Electrical burns, 476
Electrical stimulation, 369–376, 374b
    antibacterial effects of, 371
    blood flow effects of, 371
    contraindications, 371–372, 372b
    definition of, 369
    device for, 369, 370f
    effects of, 369–371
    fibroblast effects, 370
    galvanotaxic effects, 369–370
    indications for, 371–372
    payment coverage for, 373–374
    PC (pulsed current), 372–373, 374t
    terminology associated with,
        370t
    tissue oxygen, 371
    types of, 372–373
    waveforms used in, 373f
Electrolytes, 416
    replacement, 544
Electronic medical records, 9, 24
Elephantiasis, 229–230
Emergency centers, mattresses used
    in, 166–167
Endothelial cells, 69–70
Endotoxins, 283–284
Endotracheal tube, 154t
Endovenous laser ablation, 223
Enteral feeding
    description of, 562
    gastrostomy button for, 571, 571f
    gastrostomy tube for. see
        Gastrostomy tubes
    jejunostomy tube for. see
        Jejunostomy tubes
Enteric fistulas, 353, 547
Enteric tubes, nursing management
    of, 572–575
Enteroatmospheric fistula (EAF),
    542

Enterocutaneous fistulas, 541–542, 542f, 547
Envelopment, 163–164
Enzymatic debridement, 297
Epibole, 73
Epicel, 327, 328t
Epidermal appendages, description of, 40
Epidermal culture- and tissue-based products, 327, 328t
Epidermal growth factor (EGF), 66, 340t, 343–344
Epidermal-dermal junction, 52–53t, 55
Epidermis, 40–44, 41f, 52–53t
  in adolescents, 55
  resurfacing, 65
  stratum basale, 41f, 42–44
  stratum corneum, 41
  stratum germinativum, 42–44
  stratum granulosum, 41f, 42
  stratum lucidum, 41–42, 41f
  stratum spinosum, 41f, 42
Epidermolysis bullosa, 450–452, 450b, 451t
  anemia and, 451
Epidermolysis bullosa simplex (EBS), 450b
Epinephrine, 402
Epithelial resurfacing, 65–66, 66f
Epithelialization
  delayed in, 73, 73f
  of full-thickness wounds, 69
Eponychium, 266, 266b
Erysipelas, 97
Erythema, 112
  blanching, 132–133
  nonblanching, 133
Erythema multiforme (EM), 454b
Erythrasma, 98
Eschar, debridement of, 295–296
Escharotomy, 481
Estrogen, 416–417
Ethylenediamine tetraacetic acid (EDTA), 290–291t
Eutectic mixture of local anesthetics (EMLA)
  cream, 402b
  for pediatric patients, 525–526, 527t
Evaluation and management (E&M) service code, 30b, 36
Evidence, research, rating of, 8t
Evidence-based care, 5–7
Exercise, 212
Exercise stress testing, 195
Exostectomy, 255
Exotoxins, 283–284
Explosive munitions, 463–464
Extracellular matrix, 75
  abnormalities, 74
  degradation of, 76
  factors affecting the formation of, 69
  fibroblasts in, 76
  provisional, 69–71
  wound healing functions of, 73

Extracellular matrix scaffolds, 483
  acellular, 329, 330–331t
  biosynthetic, 330–331t, 332–333
  checklist for using, 326b
  classification of, 326–333
  synthetic, 333
  xenographic, 332
Extravasation, 452–454
  assessment, 453
  intervention, 453–454
  in pediatric patients, 524–525, 524b
  prevention, 453
  risk factors for, 453b
  wound care specialist role in, 452
Exudate
  description of, 117–118, 319–320
  malignant cutaneous wounds, 537–538
  pouches for collection of, 537–538
E-Z Derm, 330–331t, 332

F

Facilitator, of evidence-based practice and quality improvement, 4b, 5–9
Facility reputation, 142
Facultative synthesis, 43
Falls, 172
Fasciocutaneous flaps, 492
Fasciotomy, 467–468, 481
Fat-free compartment, 414
Fats, 414, 415
Fat stores, measurement of, 411
Fecal impaction, 89
Felted foam dressing, 254, 254f, 275t
Fentanyl, 403t
Fetus
  skin of, 51, 55b
  wound healing in, 63–64, 75–76
Fiber gelling dressing, 309
Fibrin, 337
Fibrin cuff theory, 209
Fibrin sealants, 546
Fibroblast(s)
  in dermis, 44–45
  electrical stimulation effects on, 370
  in extracellular matrix, 69–71
  growth factor secreted by, 340t, 345
  matrix metalloproteinase secretion by, 339–340
  myofibroblasts differentiation of, 72
  ultrasound effects on, 380
  in wound bed, 70–71
Fibroblast growth factor, 340t, 345
Fibronectin, 44
Field blockade, 402
Filaggrin, 42
Filariasis, 229–230
Film dressings, 316
Financial outcomes, 16–17
Financial viability, 22–24

Fiscal intermediaries, 25t, 35
Fissures, of feet, 271
Fistulas
  algorithm for selecting, 550f
  assessment of, 548–549, 548b
  classification of, 542–543, 543b, 544t
  closure of, 544
  complex, 543b, 543f
  complications associated with, 542
  conservative management of, 546
  cutaneous opening, 554
  definition of, 542
  effluent from
    accurate measurement of, 559
    characteristics of, 548, 549t
    closed suction systems for, 553
    dressing for, 550
    nonpouching options for, 552–553
  enteric, 353, 547
  enterocutaneous, 541–542, 542f, 547
  epidemiology of, 541–542
  etiology of, 541–542
  external, 543
  fluid and electrolyte replacement for, 544
  gastrointestinal, 541
  high-output, 543, 545t
  internal, 543
  low-output, 543
  management of, 541–561, 560b
  manifestations of, 544
  medical conditions associated with, 541–542
  medical management of, 544–547
  negative pressure wound therapy for, 553
  nonsurgical treatment of, 544–546
  nursing management of, 547–560
    abdominal topography, 548–549
    assessment, 548–549, 548b
    evaluation of, 560
    goals of, 547–548, 547b, 560
    planning and implementation, 549–560
  nutritional recommendations for patients with, 546t
  nutritional support for, 545–546
  output control, 544–545
  perifistula skin, 549
  pouches for
    adaptations to, 556–557
    adhesive sheets to enlarge pouch adhesive surface, 556, 556b
    adhesive skin barrier surface, 554–555
    bridging technique, 557, 557f, 558b

Fistulas (Continued)
  capacity of, 555
  catheter ports, 557–558
  change procedure, 553b
  cost containment, 560
  ease of use, 559, 559b
  effluent measurement, 559
  examples of, 555f
  film, 555
  odor control, 558
  options and features of, 553–555, 554b
  outlet, 555, 555f, 556b
  patient comfort, 558–559
  patient mobility, 559
  saddlebagging, 556–557, 556f, 557b
  silicone molding, 557, 558b
  temporary, 556b
  tips for, 554b
  trough procedure, 557–558, 559b, 559f
  wound access, 555
  risk factors for, 541–542
  sepsis caused by, 542, 544
  simple, 543, 543b
  skin barrier products for, 550, 551f, 551t
  skin breakdown, 550
  somatostatin for, 545
  spontaneous, 542
  spontaneous closure of, 544, 546, 547b
  surgical treatment of, 546–547
  terminology, 542–543, 543t
  vaginal, 552–553, 552f
Fistula tract, 546
5-aminosalicylic acid (5-ASA), topical, 446t
FLACC pain scale, 393–394, 393t
Flame burns, 475–476
Flaps and grafts, 353
Flash freeze, 456t, 457
Floating heels, 150
Flow sheets, 9
Fluid, as support surfaces, 165–166
Fluid replacement, 544
Foam dressings, 313–314, 319t
Foam overlay, 165f
Foam sclerotherapy, 223
Foam support surfaces, 164–165, 168–169t
Focal neuropathy, 241
Focused physical assessment, 112–113, 112b
Folliculitis, 95, 98
Foot. see also Legs; Lower extremity
  age-related changes, 263
  anatomic structures of, 264f
    dorsal view, 265f
  arteries of, 183f
  care of, 263–282
  cutaneous components of, 265–266
  flexibility exercises of, 268t
  functional ability, 268–269
  functions of, 263–264

Foot (Continued)
  hygiene for, 269–271, 270t
  maceration of, 269
  muscular components of, 264
  musculoskeletal function of, 267–268
  neurovascular of, 264–265
  physical assessment of, 266–269, 267b, 270t
  range of motion, 267f
  skeletal components of, 264, 264f
  structure of, 263–266
  subcutaneous components of, 265–266
  ulcers of. see Diabetic foot ulcers
Foot diseases and disorders
  caregiver education, 280
  chronic, 263
  family education, 280, 280b
  fungal infections, 276–277
  home remedies for, 280–281
  malformations, 277t
  offloading techniques, 274–276, 275t
  padding for, 274–276
  patient education, 280, 280b
  prevention of, 270t
  quality-of-life effects, 263
  referral for, 280
  types of, 263
  ulceration and amputation risk, 269
Foot imprints, 248–249
Foot infections
  assessment of, 270t
  diabetic, 251, 252t
Foot odor, 270–271
Foot ulcers. see Diabetic foot ulcers
Footprint, 274f
Footwear, 248–249, 248b, 273–274, 273b, 274f
Forefoot
  anatomy of, 264f
  malformations of, 277–279, 277t
Forefoot test, 249, 249f
Formulary
  dressings, 310–312t
  pressure ulcer prevention program, 156–157
  wound care, 29
Fournier's gangrene, 136
Freestanding clinic
  billing differences, 22
  financial stability, 23–24
  regulatory issues, 22
Frequency, 370t
Friction, 85, 130, 145t, 147, 164
Frostbite, 456–458
  classification of skin injury, 457
  injury, classification system, 457t
  management of, 457–458
  rapid rewarming, 457
  risk factors for, 456, 456b
  standard protocol for, 458b
Frostnip, 456t
Full-thickness skin grafts, 484

Full-thickness wounds, 113–114
  characteristics of, 64, 64f
  "cleanup" of, 67
  epithelialization of, 69
  granulation tissue formation, 69–71, 70f
  healing of, 64
  primary intention healing of, 64f, 66, 67f, 72t
    hemostasis, 67, 72t
    inflammation, 67–69
    maturation, 71, 72t
    proliferation, 69–71
    remodeling, 71
  repair of, 66–71, 67f
  secondary intention healing of, 64f, 71–73, 72t
Functional-sensory status assessment, 179–181
Fundamentals of Hyperbaric Medicine, 361
Fungal infections
  burn wounds, 482
  candidiasis, 95–96
  enteric feeding tube, 575
  foot, 276–277
  home remedies for, 280–281
  nail, 279
Fungating malignant wound, 534

G

Gabapentin, 403–404
Galvanotaxis, 369–370
GammaGraft, 328t, 334
Gangrene, 494
Gastrointestinal (GI) fistulas, 541
Gastrostomy
  definition of, 562
  Janeway, 564, 564f
  percutaneous endoscopic, 566, 567f, 568f, 576b
  Stamm, 563–564, 564f
  Witzel, 564, 564f
Gastrostomy button, 571, 571f
Gastrostomy tubes, 563
  for children, 522
  complications of, 575–576
  conversion of, to gastrostomy-jejunostomy tube, 569–570
  feeding tube features, 570–571
    material composition, 570
    ports, 570–571
    tip configurations, 570, 571f
    tube diameter, 570
  leakage around, 93, 573b, 575
  moisture-associated skin dermatitis, 575–576
  nursing management of, 572–575
  occlusion of, 574–575
  ostomy pouch for drainage containment, 575, 575f
  patency of, 574–575
  patient education, 576, 577b
  peristomal hyperplasia, 575–576
  placement of, 563–570
    algorithm for, 563f

Gastrostomy tubes (Continued)
  complications of, 575–576
  endoscopic approach, 566–568, 567f, 568f, 572
  interventional radiologic approach, 569
  "over the wire" (Sachs-Vine) technique, 566, 568f
  "pull" (Ponsky) technique, 566, 567f
  "push" (Russel) technique, 566
  removal of, 576, 576b
  replacement of, 574f, 576b, 577b
  site
    care of, 572–573, 572b
    selection of, 572
    stabilization of, 573–574, 573f, 574f
  surgical approaches, 563–565, 564f, 572
    laparoscopic, 565
    open, 563–565
Gastrostomy-jejunostomy tube, 569–570
Gauze dressings, 316–317, 317b, 317t
  continuously moist saline gauze, 317
  disadvantages of, 317t
  guide to appropriate use of, 317b
  hypertonic saline-impregnated gauze, 317
Gel support surfaces, 165
General neuropathic pain, 403t
Genodermatoses, 40
Glamorgan scale, for pressure ulcers, 518–520, 519t
Glucocorticoids, 131–132
Glucose, 415
Glutamine, 415
Gluteus maximus muscle flap, 496
Glycemic control, 253, 503
Glycosaminoglycans, 44
Goniometer, 180, 268f
Goose bumps, 49
GraftJacket, 329, 330–331t
GraftJacket Xpress, 329–332, 330–331t
Graft-*versus*-host disease, 455–456
Gram stain, 287
Grants, 17
Granulation tissue
  factors affecting the formation of, 71
  formation of, in proliferative phase of wound healing, 69–71, 72t
  healthy, signs of, 72, 115
Great toe, 264
Greater trochanteric ulcers, 495–496, 496f
Ground substance, 44
Group health plans, 32–33
Growth factors, 337, 348b
  autocrine action of, 342, 342f
  biologic roles of, 337–338
  in chronic wound, 74

Growth factors (Continued)
  clinical practice use of, 345–348
  cloning of, 342
  connective tissue, 340t, 344–345
  discovery of, 342
  epidermal, 340t, 343–344
  families of, 343–345
  fibroblast, 340t, 345
  inflammatory cell, 340–341
  insulinlike, 66, 345
  keratinocyte, 340–341
  keratinocyte proliferation affected by, 66
  low levels of, 74
  macrophage secretion of, 68
  in neoangiogenesis, 69–70
  paracrine action, 342
  platelet-derived, 66, 344
  purification of, 342
  radiation ulcer healing, 105
  receptors for, 342–343, 342f, 343f
  transforming growth factor-β, 340t
  vascular endothelial, 44, 69
Gunshot wounds, 466

H

Hair, 49, 52–53t
Hallux rigidus, 277t
Hallux valgus, 242t, 277t
Hammer toes, 241, 242f, 242t, 277t
Handoffs, 155–156
Harris mat, 248–249, 249f
Harris-Benedict equation, 414
Head circumference, 411
Head-of-bed elevation, 149
Health belief model, 429–436
  concepts and application of, 430t
Health education materials, 434t
Health Insurance Portability and Accountability Act (HIPAA)
  compliance with, 24–25
  Privacy Rule, 24–25, 25t
Healthcare Common Procedure Coding System (HCPCS), 30b, 34t, 35
Healthy tissue, characteristics of, 468t
Heel
  eschar of, 493
  pressure ulcers of, 150
Heel pain, 278
Heel spur, 242t, 278, 278f
Hematoma, 136, 501
Hemidesmosomes, 44
Hemoglobin A_{1c}, 253
Hemorrhage control, 465
Hemorrhagic shock, 464–465
Hemosiderin staining
  chronic venous insufficiency, 210
  lower extremity venous disease, 178
Hemosiderosis, 210
Hemostasis
  agents for, 465t
  in full-thickness wound repair, 67, 72t

Henry's law, 361–362
Heparin-binding epidermal growth factor, 344
Herpes simplex virus, 99–100
  nursing care for, 100
Herpes zoster, 100–101
Heterotopic ossification, 471–472
High-frequency ultrasound, 379–381
Hindfoot
  anatomy of, 264f
  malformations of, 277
HIPAA. see Health Insurance Portability and Accountability Act (HIPAA)
Histamine, 48–49
Homocystinemia, lower extremity arterial disease risks, 190–191
Honey, 290–291t, 291
Horizontal spray land mines, 463
Horse chestnut seed extract, 213
Hospice care, 531–532
Hospital outpatient facility settings, 33
Hospital-based clinic, 22, 33
  billing differences, 22
  referrals, 22–23
  regulatory issues for, 24
Hours of operation, for clinic, 24
House fires, 476
Hyaff-11, 333
Hyalomatrix PA, 330–331t, 333
Hyaluronan, 44
Hyaluronic acid, 51
Hydration, 57
  laboratory measures of, 412t
Hydrocolloid dressings, 105, 314, 319t
Hydrofera blue, 290–291t
Hydrogel dressings, 314–315, 319t, 537
Hydrogel sheets, 315
Hydrogen peroxide, 290–291t
Hydrosurgical water knife, 301
Hydrotherapy, 298, 482
Hydroxylation, 70–71
Hygiene, foot, 269–271, 270t
Hyperactive deep tendon reflexes, 268
Hyperalgesia, 405
Hyperbaric oxygenation, 361–368, 367b, 423
  application of, 364–366
  aural barotrauma associated with, 366
  breath holding during, 366
  chambers used in, 364–365, 365f, 366b
  claustrophobia associated with, 366
  clostridial myonecrosis treated with, 363
  contraindications of, 364, 364b
  definition of, 361
  edema management with, 362
  effects of, 362t
  history of, 361

Hyperbaric oxygenation (Continued)
  indications for, 362–364, 362b, 363t
  investigational uses of, 364b
  mechanism of, 362t
  necrotizing fasciitis treated with, 363
  patient preparation and safety, 365–366
  physiologic effects of, 361–362
  pressurized high-oxygen environment, 365–366
  protocols for, 364–366
  seizure activity during, 366
  side effects of, 366
  situations for, 364b
  staff education and certification, 364
  visual acuity changes during, 366
  wound healing effects, 362t
  wound-related indications of, 363t
Hyperglycemia, 253, 502
Hyperkeratotic callus, 256
Hyperkeratotic lesions, 276, 276f
Hyperproliferative scarring, 76, 77t
Hypertension
  ambulatory venous, 205–207
  lower extremity arterial disease risks, 190
Hypertonic saline-impregnated gauze, 317
Hypertrophic scars, 76, 485
Hypoactive deep tendon reflexes, 268
Hypodermis, 45f, 46
Hyponychium, 266, 266b
Hypothermia, 308, 420–421
Hypothermia-induced vasoconstriction, 420
Hypoventilation syndrome, obesity and, 512
Hypoxia
  angiogenesis and, 69–70
  fibroblast affected by, 71
  wound bed, 65–66
  wound healing affected by, 78–79t
  wound tissue, 419–420

I
ICD-10, 25t, 30b, 36
Immersion, 163–164
Immune reactions, 454–456
Immunization, 465–466
Immunosuppression, 78–79t
Impetigo, 98–99
Incidence, 13–14
  cumulative, 13b, 14
  definition of, 13–14
  pressure ulcer, 125
Incidence density, 13b, 14
Incident-to-physician services, 34–35
Incision
  dehiscence, 512
  topical care of, 503–505, 504b

Incontinence-associated dermatitis (IAD), 88, 510–511
  conditions associated with, 89–90
  in pediatric patients, 520–522
Indentation force deflection (IFD), 165
Infancy, definition of, 516, 517t
Infection, 284b, 286–288, 292
  bacterial. see Bacterial infections
  criteria for, 285b
  diabetic foot, 251, 252t
  fungal. see Fungal infections
  lower extremity arterial disease risks, 191
  osteomyelitis, 256, 292
  prevention of, in arterial ulcers, 199–200
  skin. see Skin infections
  surgical site, 501–502, 502t, 503t
  wound. see Wound infection
Infectious Diseases Society of America (IDSA), 292
Inflammation
  acute phase response to, 412t
  adhesion molecules and receptors, 338–341
  cell proteases, 339–340
  control of, 399–400
  duration of, 68–69
  extracellular matrix effects on, 68–69
  lower extremity arterial disease risks, 191
  neutrophils in, 339–340
Inflammatory response
  contributing factors, 75–76
  in partial-thickness wounds, 65
Informed refusal, 437–438
Infrastructure, maintenance of, 11b
Ingrown nail, 279, 280f
Inhaled hot air burns, 476
Injury-related malnutrition, 409–410, 413t
Innovation, 4, 5t
Insulinlike growth factor, 66, 340t, 345
Insurance and billing coder, 27–28
Integra, 330–331t
Integra Bilayer Matrix Wound Dressing (BMWD), 333
Integra Dermal Regeneration Template (IDRT), 332–333
Integra Flowable Wound Matrix, 333
Integra Matrix Wound Dressing, 333
Integrated bed systems, 167
Integrins, 338
Interdigit neuroma, 277t
Interdisciplinary team, 9–10, 10t, 27–28, 27t
Interface tissue pressures, 162, 163b
Interleukin, 341
Interleukin-1β, 340, 341–342

Intermittent pneumatic compression
  arterial ulcers managed by, 199
  lymphedema managed with, 235
  venous ulcers managed by, 219–220
International Skin Tear Advisory Panel (ISTAP), 85
International Working Group on the Diabetic Foot, 244, 245b
Internet, 6, 7t
Interpulse interval, 370t
Intertrigo, obesity and, 509
Intertrigo dermatitis, 90–91, 95
Intervention studies, level of evidence, 8t
Interventional radiologic approach, 569–570
Intervention-based research, 8t
Intestinal bypass, 547
Ionizing radiation, 102
Iron, 415–416
Irritant contact dermatitis, 48–49
Irritants, 58–59
Ischemic pain, 181, 192b
Ischemic ulcers. see Arterial ulcers
Ischial ulcers, 496, 496f
ISTAP. see International Skin Tear Advisory Panel (ISTAP)

J
Janeway gastrostomy, 564, 564f
Jejunostomy
  definition of, 562
  needle catheter, 565, 565f
  percutaneous endoscopic, 566–568, 568f
  Witzel, 564–565
Jejunostomy tubes
  complications of, 575–576
  feeding tube features, 570–571
    material composition, 570
    ports, 570–571
    tip configurations, 570, 571f
    tube diameter, 570
  leakage around, 573b, 575
  moisture-associated skin dermatitis, 575–576
  nursing management of, 572–575
  occlusion of, 574–575
  ostomy pouch for drainage containment, 575, 575f
  patency of, 574–575
  patient education, 576, 577b
  peristomal hyperplasia, 575–576
  placement of, 563–570
    complications of, 575–576
    interventional radiologic approach, 569
    laparoscopic surgical approach, 565, 566f, 572
    percutaneous endoscopic, 566–568, 572
  removal of, 576, 576b
  site
    care of, 572–573, 572b
    selection of, 572

Jejunostomy tubes (Continued)
  stabilization of, 573–574, 573f, 574f
  surgical approaches of, 563–565
    laparoscopic, 565
    open, 563–565
Jock itch, 96
Junctional epidermolysis bullosa (JEB), 450b

K

Kaposi-Stemmer sign, 232
Keloids, 43–44, 76, 485
  expansion of, 76
  sites of, 76
Keragraf, 328t
Keratin, 41
Keratinocyte growth factor, 345
Keratinocytes, 41, 65
  growth factors that affect, 66
  in partial-thickness wounds, 65
Kidney disease, lower extremity arterial disease risks, 191
Kinase domain, 342
Kinesio taping, 235

L

Lacerations, 85–87
Lactoferrin, 290–291t, 291
Lamellipodia, 65
Laminin, 44
Land mines, types of, 463
Langerhans cells, 48–49
Laparoscopy
  gastrostomy, 565
  jejunostomy, 565, 566f
Laplace's law of physics, 216, 216b
Laser debridement, 301
Laser surgery. see Endovenous laser ablation
Laserskin, 328t
Late preterm infant, definition of, 517t
Lateral shear, 149
Lean body mass, 414
Legs. see also Foot; Lower extremity
  arteries of, 183f
  assessment of. see Lower extremity assessment
  general appearance of, 177–179
  skin temperature of, 182
  trophic changes, 177
  veins of, 177–178
Leukocytes
  chemotactic attraction of, to wound, 338
  margination of, 68
Levine technique, for wound culture collection, 288, 288b
Lidocaine, liposomal, for children, 526
Limb elevation, 212
Limb ischemia, chronic vs. acute, 187
Limb-threatening infections, 256–257
Lipedema, 180t, 230–231, 231t

Lipodermatosclerosis, 178, 210
Lipopolysaccharide, 65–66
Liposomal lidocaine, for children, 526
Litigation avoidance, 142
Local coverage determinations, 30b, 35–36, 173
Local warming, 422
Long-stretch reusable wraps, 218
Lorazepam, 403t
Loricrin, 42
Low air-loss support surfaces, 171
Lower extremity. see also Foot; Legs
  arteries of, 183f
  veins of, 205
Lower extremity amputations
  diabetes mellitus as cause of, 240
  economic burden of, 240
  foot ulcers as cause of, 252–253
  infection as cause of, 251–252
  peripheral arterial disease as risk factor for, 243
  prevention program for, 246t
Lower extremity arterial disease (LEAD), 186. see also Arterial ulcers
  amputations for, 200–201
  assessment of, 192b
  invasive testing for, 178b, 196–197
  limb preservation strategies, 200b
  lower extremity assessments for, 193
  noninvasive testing for, 178b, 193–196, 194t
    ankle-brachial index, 193–194, 194b
    computed tomographic angiography, 196
    Doppler waveform studies, 193f, 195
    duplex angiography, 196
    exercise stress testing, 195
    magnetic resonance angiography, 196
    pulse volume recordings, 195
    segmental limb pressure measurements, 195–196
    skin perfusion pressure, 195
    toe-brachial index, 194–195
    transcutaneous oxygen pressure (TcPO2), 195
  obesity and, 511
  pain history, 192–193
  patient education, 200–201
  pharmacologic therapy for, 198–199
  purpura and petechiae associated with, 178
  risk factors for, 188–191, 189b
    diabetes mellitus, 190
    dyslipidemia, 190
    emerging types of, 190–191
    homocystinemia, 190–191
    hypertension, 190
    infection, 191
    inflammation, 191

Lower extremity arterial disease (Continued)
    kidney disease, 191
    modifiable, 189–190, 189t, 198
    predisposing, 190
    smoking, 189
Lower extremity assessment, 177–185, 178b, 184b
  arterial ulcers, 193
  blood flow, 182
  capillary refill, 182, 182b
  dependent rubor, 181
  diagnostic testing, 178b, 182–184
  edema, 178–179
  elevational pallor, 181, 181b
  functional-sensory status, 179–181
  general appearance of limb, 177–179
  lower extremity arterial disease, 177, 193
  pain management, 181
  perfusion, 181–182
  pulse, 182, 182b
  skin color, shape, and integrity, 178
  skin temperature, 182
  trophic changes, 177
  veins, 177–178
Lower Extremity Assessment Project (LEAP), 471
Lower extremity neuropathic disease (LEND), 182
  assessment of, 244–252
    footwear, 248–249, 248b
    lower extremity and foot physical examination, 245–248
    patient history, 244
    risk factors, 244
    skin and nail condition, 248
    wound sites, 250t
  description of, 239
  epidemiology of, 239–240
  management of, 252–258
    early intervention, 252–253
    glycemic control, 253
    multidisciplinary approach to, 252
    offloading, 253–255
  nail assessment, 248
  skin assessment, 248
  wound sites, 250t
Lower extremity ulcers
  arterial. see Arterial ulcers
  characteristics of, 181t
  neuropathic, 181t
  pain management, 181, 181t
  venous, 181t. see also Venous ulcers
Lower extremity venous disease (LEVD), 204. see also Venous ulcers
  assessment of, 209–211, 209b
  atrophie blanche lesions associated with, 178, 210
  classification for, 208t

Lower extremity venous disease (Continued)
  hemosiderin staining for, 178
  obesity and, 511
  venous dermatitis associated with, 210–211, 211t
Lund-Browder chart, 477–479, 478f
Lymphangitis, 236
Lymphatic system
  anatomy of, 229f
  capillaries, 228
  drainage, 227
  function of, 227–228
Lymphedema, 227–238, 237b
  acquired, 228–230
  acute, 228
  adjunctive therapy, 235
  assessment of, 232–233
  benzopyrones for, 236
  in cancer patient, 227
  cellulitis associated with, 237
  characteristics of, 180t
  chronic, 228
  clinical presentation of, 227
  complete decongestive physiotherapy for, 234–235
  complications of, 236–237
  diagnostic tests for, 231–232
  epidemiology of, 227
  idiopathic, 228
  incidence of, 227
  Kinesio taping for, 235
  limb protection, 233
  limb size measurements, 232–233
  lipedema vs., 231t
  lymphatic flow promotion, 233
  management of, 234–236
  pathophysiology of, 227–228
  pharmacology, 236
  physical assessment, 232–233
  prevention of, 233
  primary, 228
  pruritus associated with, 233
  resources for, 237b
  secondary, 228–230
  selenium therapy for, 235
  skin care for, 233
  stages of, 230, 230t
  surgery for, 235–236
  teaching points for, 233b
  treatment of, 234t
  types of, 228–230
Lymphedema praecox, 228
Lymphedema tarda, 228
Lymphokine, 341
Lymphoscintigraphy, 231

M

Maceration, 95, 269, 320, 536
Macrodeformation, using negative pressure wound therapy, 351
Macrophages, 49
  cytokines secreted by, 340–341
  growth factors secreted by, 68
Mafenide acetate, 482–483
Maggots, 298

Magnetic resonance angiography, 196
Magnetic resonance imaging (MRI), for osteomyelitis, 292
Malignancy-related wounds
    atraumatic dressing changes, 535–536
    bleeding control or prevention in, 536
    care objectives for, 534–538
    cutaneous wounds, 534
    description of, 534
    exudate from, 537–538
    fungating, 534
    Marjolin ulcer, 534
    odor control in, 536–537
    pain control for, 534–535
    periwound skin management in, 536
    pruritus associated with, 534–535
Malignant cutaneous wounds, 534
Mallet toe, 247, 277t
Malnutrition, 408–410
    acute disease-related, 409–410
    criteria for, 413t
    diagnosis of, 413
    disease-related, 409, 413t
    injury-related, 409–410, 413t
    in obese patients, 513
    pressure ulcers in patient with, 493
    risk factors for, 409b
    screening for possible, 410
    starvation-related, 409, 413t
Malnutrition Universal Screening Tool (MUST), 410
Marjolin ulcer, 458, 534
Marketing, 15–18
Martorell hypertensive ischemic leg ulcer, 448–450, 449t
Mast cells, 49
MatriDerm, 330–331t
MatriStem, 330–331t, 332
Matrix metalloproteinases (MMPs)
    in chronic wounds, 73
    extracellular matrix degradation, 76
    inflammation affected by, 339–340
    in partial-thickness wound repair, 65–66
    remodeling control by, 71
Mattress overlays, 166
Mattresses
    replacement, 166
    support surfaces use of, 166–167
McGill Pain Questionnaire, 390
Meaningful use, 24
Mechanical rotary tool, 272b, 273
Mechanical stretch, 351–352
Mechanotransduction, 351
Medicaid, 32. see also Centers for Medicare & Medicaid Services (CMS)
    billing rate, 22
    eligibility requirements, 32

Medical adhesive-related skin injury (MARSI), 93–94, 522
    assessment, prevention and treatment for, 94b
Medical-grade honey, 315–316
Medicare, 31-32. see also Centers for Medicare & Medicaid Services (CMS)
    authorization, 25
    definition of, 31
    fiscal intermediaries, 35
    local coverage determinations, 35–36
    managed care plan, 33–34
    national coverage determinations, 35–36
    nurse practitioner reimbursement, 34b
    Part A, 31
    Part B, 31
    support surface reimbursement by, 172–173
Medicare administrative contractors, 25t, 30b, 35
Medicare Advantage plan, 31–32
Medicare Coordination of Benefits, 33
Medicare Physician's Fee Schedule (MPFS), 33
Medicare Secondary Payer Program, 32–33
Medigap, 33
Mediskin, 332
Meige disease, 228
Meissner corpuscles, 50
Melanin, 43
Melanocortin-1 receptor (MC1R), 43
Melanocytes, 43
Melanoma, 57
Melanosomes, 43
Meperidine, 403t
Merkel cells, 50
Metabolism, 50–51, 54t
Metatarsophalangeal (MTP) joint, 264, 265f
Methicillin-resistant Staphylococcus aureus (MRSA), 97, 257, 317
Methicillin-resistant Staphylococcus epidermidis, 97
Methodology, 14–15
Metronidazole, 90, 537
Microdeformation, negative pressure wound therapy, 351–352
Micronized purified flavonoid fraction, 213
Microvascular tissue perfusion, 244
Midazolam, 403t
Midfoot
    anatomy of, 264f
    malformations of, 277
Mid-upper arm circumference, 411
Minerals, 415–416
Mini Nutritional Assessment (MNA), 410

Mini Nutritional Assessment (MNA)-Short Form, 410
Mixed nociceptive/neuropathic, 389–390
Mobility
    definition of, 146
    fistula pouch and, 559
Moisture
    in Braden Scale for the Prediction of Pressure Ulcer Risk, 145t, 146
    pressure ulcer caused by, 130
    skin damage associated with, 509, 509t
    wound environment, 307–308
Moisture vapor transmission rate (MVTR), 307–308
Moisture-associated skin damage (MASD), 87–89, 520
    prevention and treatment for, 91–93, 92t
    types and interventions, 91b
Moisture-retentive dressings, 400
Monokine, 341
Morbid obesity, definition of, 508
Morphine, 403t
Morton neuroma, 277t
Motor neuropathy, 241
Multidisciplinary team, 9–10, 10t
Multiorgan dysfunction syndrome (MODS), 467, 467t
Mupirocin, 290–291t
Muscle strength reflexes, 268
Muscle wasting, 414
Muscular pain, 403t
Musculoskeletal abnormalities, 241–243, 242t
Myocutaneous flaps, 492
Myofibroblasts, 71

N

Nail(s)
    anatomy of, 266b
    care of, 263–282
        clinical consult, 281b
        summary, 281
    debridement of, 271
    growth of, 266
    lower extremity neuropathic disease and, 248
    structure of, 266, 266f
    trimming of, 271, 272b
Nail bed, 266, 266b
Nail disorders, 279–280
    onychatrophia, 279t
    onychocryptosis, 279, 279t, 280f
    onychogryposis, 279t
    onychomycosis, 279t
    onychophosis, 279t
    paronychia, 248, 279t, 280, 280f
Nail file, 272
Nail plate, 266, 266b
Nail rasp, 272
Nail root, 266, 266b
Nasal oxygen, 154t
Nasogastric tube, 154t

National Correct Coding Initiative, 25t, 37
National Database of Nursing Quality Indicators (NDNQI), 14
National Patient Safety Goals, 24
National Pressure Ulcer Advisory Panel (NPUAP), 85
    classification system, 135b
Necrotic tissue, 295
Necrotic wound
    management of, 200
    topical therapy for, 200b
Necrotizing fasciitis, 363, 442–443, 468, 494
Needle aspiration, for wound culture collection, 288
Needle catheter jejunostomy, 565, 565f
Negative acute phase reactants, 411–412
Negative pressure wound therapy (NPWT), 350–360, 358b, 442–443
    adjunctive interventions for, 355
    application of, 354–358
    compression therapy and, comparisons between, 351–352
    contraindications, 353, 353b
    debridement before, 354
    definition of, 350
    devices, in palliative wound care, 538
    dressings used with, 355, 469
    edema reduction using, 350–351
    factors to consider before discharge, 358b
    fluid removal using, 350–351
    hemorrhage considerations, 354
    history of, 350
    indications for, 352–353
    intermittent versus continuous, 355
    macrodeformation using, 351
    mechanical stretch using, 351–352
    mechanism of action, 350–352
    microdeformation using, 351–352
    pain management, 354–355
    patient discharge/transfer of care, 357–358
    for pediatric patients, 527, 527t
    precautions for, 353–354, 353b
    procedure components of, 355–357, 356b, 357f, 358f
    product selection, 355
    skin grafts and, 497
    systems, 351t
    transitioning, from inpatient to home, 358b
    uses of, 352–353
    wound bed preparation using, 495
    wound contraction using, 351
Neoangiogenesis, 69–70

Neoepithelium, 69
Neonatal Skin Condition Scale, for pressure ulcers, 519t, 520b
Neonates, 393–394, 393t
  bathing and moisturizing of, 516–517
  definition of, 516, 517t
  eutectic mixture of local anesthetics (EMLA) for, 525–526, 527t
  skin characteristics of, 516–518
Nerve block, 402
Neuromas, 242t
Neuropathic pain, 389
  assessment of, 245
  management of, 389, 403t
  pharmacologic interventions for, 403t
  somatic, 389
  visceral, 389
Neuropathic ulcers, 181t
  characteristics of, 184–185t
Neuropathy
  peripheral, 240–241
  sensory, 241
Neuroplasticity, 389
Neuropraxia, 466
Neurotmesis, 466
Neutrophils, 284, 339–340
  at wound space, 68
Nippers, 271
Nitrogen balance, 413
Nociception, 388
Nociceptive pain, 389
Nonadherent dressings, 105
Nonblanching erythema, 133
Nonbullous impetigo, 98–99
Noncompliance
  complicated regimens, 433
  definition of, 428
  eliminating, 428–440, 438b
    goal setting, 429
    significance, 428–429
    modifying variables, 432–436
      activity and mobility, 434–435, 435b
      care transitions, 436
      cognitive ability, 434
      cultural factors, 436
      depression, anxiety, and pain, 433–434
      dexterity, 434
      education and knowledge, 432–433
      finances and available resources, 435
      potential or actual side effects, 435–436
Noncontact low-frequency ultrasound, 381–382, 381f
Nonfacility/freestanding sites, 33
Nonphysician practitioners, 34
Nonsteroidal antiinflammatory drugs, 402–403
Nonuremic calciphylaxis, 448
Nurse, 3t, 12
Nurse coordinator, 27

Nurse practitioner, 34b
Nutrition, 58, 408
  deficiencies in, 411t
  malnutrition, 408–410, 413t
  overnutrition, 408
  pressure ulcer risks, 130–131, 147
  skin integrity affected by, 58
  starvation, 409, 413t
  undernutrition, 408
  wound healing and, 414–416, 415t
Nutritional status assessment, 410–413, 417b
  anthropometric measures, 411, 411t
  clinical signs, 410–411, 411t
  dietary intake, 413
  functional, 413
  history and clinical diagnosis, 410
  laboratory data, 411–413
  physical examination, 410–411, 411t
  screening and, 410–413
  systematic approach, 410
Nutritional support, 416–417. see also Enteral feeding
  fistula management with, 545–546
  goals of, 416
  preferred route of, 417
  sequence of events for, 416b
Nutritionist, 13

O

Oasis Matrix, 330–331t, 332
Obesity, 58
  altered skin function in, 508, 509t
  chronic venous insufficiency and, 212
  comorbidities associated with, 507
  criteria-based protocols for, 513
  definition of, 508
  dry skin and, 508
  economic impact of, 507
  hypoventilation syndrome and, 512
  incisions and sutured wounds on, 512
  incontinence-associated dermatitis and, 510–511
  malnutrition and, 513
  morbid, 508
  nutritional considerations in, 513
  oxygenation affected by, 421
  physical environment on, accommodations in, 511b
  pressure management in, 508–509
  pressure ulcers and, 508
  prevalence of, 507
  quality improvement for, 513–514, 514b
  skin fold management in, 509–510
  skin integrity and, 512
  sleep apnea and, 512

Obesity (Continued)
  surgical considerations in, 511–513
  surgical site infection risks, 421, 503
  tracheostomy care and, 513
  unique needs in, 508–511
  wound complications and, 512
  wound healing affected by, 78–79t, 421
Occupational therapist, 12
Odor
  fistulas pouch, 558
  foot, 270–271
  wound. see Wound odor
Offloading, 274–276
  diabetic foot ulcers managed with, 253
  pressure ulcers managed with, 148–153
  repetitive stress, 275t
Older adults
  pressure ulcers in, 126
  protein deficiency in, 414
  skin in, 52–53t
Omega-3 fatty acids, 415
Omega-6 fatty acids, 415
Onychatrophia, 279t
Onychocryptosis, 279, 279t, 280f
Onychogryposis, 279t
Onychomycosis, 279, 279t
Open abdomen closure, 470–471
Open-cell foam, 165, 313–314
Open fractures, 466
Open laparotomy, 563
Operating room
  mattresses used in, 166–167
  support surfaces used in, 166–167, 167b
Operations report, 15b, 17–18
Opioids
  addiction to, 405
  sedation concerns with, 404, 404t
  side effects of, 405
  wound pain managed with, 401b, 403–404
OrCel, 328t, 334
Organic compounds burns, 477
Osteoarthritis, 276
Osteomyelitis, 252, 284b, 292, 363, 469
  sensitivity and specificity of tests for, 292t
Ostomy, for pediatric patients, 523
  online resources, 523b
Outcome and Assessment Information Set (OASIS), 119
Outcomes report, 15b, 17–18
Outreach programs, 17
"Over the wire" (Sachs-Vine) technique, 566, 568f
Oxandrin. see Oxandrolone (Oxandrin)
Oxandrolone (Oxandrin), 416–417
Oxygen
  supplemental, 422–423
  wound healing role of, 419–420

Oxygen mask, 154t
Oxygen therapy
  hyperbaric, 105
    for arterial ulcers, 199
    gangrene treated with, 494
    necrotizing fasciitis treated with, 494
  topical, 366–367
Oxygenation, 419–427, 425b
  factors that alter, 420–421
  interventions to improve, 422–424, 422t
  obesity effects on, 421
  response to, 424–425
  smoking effects on, 421

P

Pain, 433-434. see also Wound pain
  burn injury, 481, 484
  causes of, 389f
  classifications of, 388–390
  heel, 278–279
  history-taking, 390
  intensity scales, 390, 391f, 393t
  ischemic, 181
  lower extremity ulcer, 181, 181t
  malignant wound, 534–535
  mixed nociceptive/neuropathic, 389–390
  neuropathic, 181
  nociceptive, 389
  patterns of response to, 387
  perceptions about, 386–387
  perfusion and oxygenation, 420
  physiology of, 387–388
  pressure ulcers, 387
  site of occlusion and location of, 192t
  venous ulcers, 389–390
Pain Assessment in Advanced Dementia, 391, 391–392t
Palliative care
  definition of, 531–532
  description of, 531
Palliative wound care, 532, 538b
  comorbidities, 532
  definition of, 532
  indications for, 532
  interventions for, 535t
  maceration prevention, 536
  malignancy-related wounds
    atraumatic dressing changes, 535–536
    bleeding control or prevention in, 536
    care objectives for, 534–538
    cutaneous wounds, 534
    description of, 534
    exudate from, 537–538
    fungating, 534
    Marjolin ulcer, 534
    odor control in, 536–537
    pain control for, 534–535
    periwound skin management in, 536–537
    pruritus associated with, 534–535

Palliative wound care (Continued)
negative pressure wound therapy devices in, 538
nonmalignancy-related wounds, 532–534
pressure ulcer, 533–534
wound types, 532
Pallor, elevational, 181, 181b
Papillary dermis, 45, 45f, 49
Para-aminobenzoic acid, 101
Paresthesia, 403t
Paronychia, 248, 279t, 280, 280f
Partial-thickness wound, 113–114
characteristics of, 64, 64f, 65–66
definition of, 65
dermal repair in, 66
epidermal repair, 65–66
regulatory factors in, 66
healing of, 64, 65t
inflammatory response in, 65
repair of, 65–66, 65t
Patch tests, 101–102, 102b
Pathergy, 444
Pathogens, 46–48
Patient education
enteral feeding tube, 576, 577b
foot diseases and disorders, 280, 280b
health education materials, 434t
Joint Commission statements for, 432b
lymphedema, 233b
pressure ulcers, 153–155
printed materials, 433, 434t
Patient goal setting, 429
Patient handoffs, 155–156
Patient perceptions, 429–436
Patient refusal algorithm, 437f
Patient trust, 142
Patient-controlled analgesia (PCA), 481
Payer audits, 26–27
Pediatrics. see also Children; Premature infants
antimicrobial agents on, 517, 517t
anxiety and discomfort in, addressing, 525–526, 526t
bathing and moisturizing for, 516–517
burn/thermal injury in, 524
diaper dermatitis in, 520–522
dressing selection for, 526–527
extravasation injury in, 524–525, 524b
gastrostomy tubes for, 522
incontinence-associated dermatitis in, 520–522
medical adhesive-related skin injury (MARSI) in, 522
negative pressure wound therapy for, 527, 527t
nutritional support for, 525
organic, natural, and herbal products on, 517–518
ostomy for, creation of, 523
pouching in, 523–524, 523b

Pediatrics (Continued)
pressure ulcers in, 516–518
Braden Q scale, 518–520, 519t
Glamorgan scale, 518–520, 519t
risk assessment in, 518
skin care needs of, 516–530, 527b
skin characteristics of, 516–518
skin inspection in, 518
topical antiseptics on, 516–518, 517t
Pentoxifylline, 105, 213
Perceived barriers, 430, 430t
Perceived benefits, 430, 430t
Perceived severity/susceptibility, 429–430
Perceived threat, 429–430
Percutaneous endoscopic gastrostomy (PEG), 566, 567f, 568f, 576b
Percutaneous endoscopic jejunostomy, 566–568, 568f
Percutaneous tube
aspiration risk, 563b
gastrostomy. see Gastrostomy tubes
jejunostomy. see Jejunostomy tubes
nursing management of, 562, 577b
Perforator veins, 205
Perfusion, 419–427, 425b
assessment of, 181
factors that alter, 420–421
interventions to improve, 422–424, 422t
oxygen levels, 419
skin flaps, 492
wound healing role of, 419–420
Periderm, 52–53t
Perifistula skin, 549
Perineal dermatitis, 87–88, 520
differential diagnosis of, 89t
Perionychium, 266, 266b
Perioperative recommendations, for pressure ulcer prevention, 152t
Peripheral arterial disease, 186
lower extremity amputation risks, 243
Peripheral neuropathy, 240–241
Peripheral vascular disease, 186
Perirectal abscess, 136
Peristomal hyperplasia, 575–576
Periungual, 266b
Periwound skin, 118
care of, 399
cleansing and protection, 318
condition of, 320
palliative wound care for, 536
pathology common features, 118t
protection, 319–320
Perometer, 179
Pes cavus, 242t
Pes covus, 242t
Petechiae, 178

pH, skin, 47
Phalanges, 264
Pharmaceuticals, 29
Pheomelanin, 43
Phosphatases, 343
Photoaging, 55, 56
Photographic Wound Assessment Tool, 121
Photography, 121–122, 121b
Physical assessment, focused, 112–113, 112b
Physical therapist, 12
Physician, incident-to services for, 34–35
PICOT, 5, 6b
Pilosebaceous unit, 47
Pitting edema, 179, 179f
Planktonic bacteria, 47–48, 284b
Planktonic phenotype, 283
Plantar fasciitis, 242t, 278
Plantar warts, 276
Platelet-derived growth factors, 66, 340t, 344
Platelets
adhesion of, 339
degranulation of, 339
Polarity, 370t
Polyarteritis nodosa (PAN), 447t
Polyhexamethylene biguanide (PHMB), 290–291t, 291
Polymethylmethacrylate (PMMA), 469
Polyurethane foam dressings, 313
Ponsky ("pull") technique, 566, 567f
Popliteal artery, 265
Positive acute phase reactants, 411–412
Posterior tibial artery, 265
Postherpetic neuralgia, 101
Postinflammatory hypopigmentation, 43–44
Pouch, fistula
adaptations to, 556–557
adhesive sheets to enlarge pouch adhesive surface, 556, 556b
adhesive skin barrier surface, 554–555
algorithm for selecting, 550f
capacity of, 555
catheter ports, 557–558
change procedure, 553b
cost containment, 560
ease of use, 559, 559b
effluent, accurate measurement of, 559
examples of, 555f
exudate collection with, 538
film, 555
odor control, 558
options and features, 553–555, 554b
outlet, 555, 555f, 556b
patient comfort, 558–559
patient mobility, 559
saddlebagging, 556–557, 556f, 557b

Pouch, fistula (Continued)
silicone molding, 557, 558b
temporary, 556b
tips for, 554b
trough procedure, 557–558, 559b, 559f
wound access, 555
Pouching, for stomas, in pediatric patients, 523–524, 523b
Povidone-iodine, 290–291t
Prealbumin, 412
Premature infants, skin of, 51, 52–53t, 54t
Preprocessed information sources, 6t
Pressure
capillary, 128, 128f
capillary occlusion caused by, 132–134
cellular response, 133f
differential diagnosis, 136b
intensity of, 128–129
Pressure mapping, 162, 163f
Pressure redistribution
pressure ulcers prevention program use of, 148–153
support surfaces, 162, 168–169t
Pressure ulcer(s), 124–139, 136–137b
at-risk patient populations, 129–130
Braden Scale for the Prediction of Pressure Ulcer Risk, 143
capillary occlusion-related ischemia, 132–134
causative factors, 127–132
age, 131
blood pressure, 131
body temperature, 132
duration of pressure, 128f, 129–130, 129f
friction, 130
intensity of pressure, 128–129, 128f
miscellaneous factors, 132
moisture, 130
nutritional debilitation, 130–131
shear, 130
smoking, 132
stress, 131–132
tissue tolerance, 129–132
classification of, 135–137
contributing factors, 128f
on darkly pigmented skin, 112b, 135
definition of, 124
differential diagnosis of, 136b
duration of life, 126
economic effects, 125–126
family education about, 153–155
floating heels for, 150
frequency of, 127f
friction, 85, 145t, 147
greater trochanteric, 495–496, 496f
heels, 150

Pressure ulcer(s) (Continued)
high-frequency ultrasound for, 380
incidence of, 125
ischial, 496, 496f
lymphatic function impairment associated with, 134–135
in malnourished patients, 493
medical device-related, 151–153, 153b, 154t
monitoring, assessment and evaluation of, 119b
mucosal, 136
multiple, 496
obesity and, 508
palliative care for, 533–534
patient education about, 153–155
patient populations vulnerable to, 126–127
in pediatric patients, 518–520
Braden Q scale for, 518–520, 519t
Glamorgan scale for, 518–520, 519t
Neonatal skin condition scale for, 519t, 520b
risk factors for, 518
prevalence of, 125
quality of life, 126
recurrence of, 497
reperfusion injury associated with, 134
repositioning frequency to prevent, 148
repositioning techniques to prevent, 148–151
reverse staging of, 136–137
risk assessment for, 144b
risk factor for
assessment of, 143–147
intraoperative, 151b
sacral, 495, 495f
screening for, 143–147
seated position and, 150–151
shear, 84, 145t, 147
sites for, 127f
skin safety interventions based on risk factors, 146t
spinal cord injury patients, 126
stages of, 135b
surgical management, 491, 496
terminology associated with, 127
visual inspection of, 112
wound bed assessments, 135–136
Pressure ulcer prevention program (PUPP), 140–161, 158b
best-practice audit prevention, 142b
best-practice bundle for, 143–155
hydration, 147
nutrition, 147
offloading, 148–153
pressure redistribution, 148–153
risk assessment and screening, 143–147

Pressure ulcer prevention program (Continued)
skin health, 147, 147b
skin inspection and assessment, 143
components of, 143
decision-making tools, 156–157
documentation, 155, 156b
effectiveness of, 140
emergency centers, 151
family education, 153–155
formularies, 156–157
infrastructure for, 155–158, 156b
justification of, 140–142
medical device-related pressure ulcer, 151–153, 154t
national priority, 140–141
operating room, 151
outcome measure, 158
palliative care, 532–533
patient education, 153–154
patient handoffs, 155–156
quality tracking and evaluation of, 157–158
reimbursement for, 141, 141b
staff
accountability, 157, 158b
education and competence of, 157
team members, 155
technology to support, 157
unavoidable pressure ulcer identified, 141–142
Pressure Ulcer Scale for Healing, 120–121
Pressure/shear factor, 85, 147
Preterm infant, definition of, 517t
Prevalence, 13
definition of, 13
formula for, 13b
Primary intention wound healing, 64, 64f, 66, 72t
Primary malignant wound, 458
Primary wound closure, 499
PriMatrix, 330–331t, 332
Privacy, 24
Procedural hospital settings, 151–153
Productivity tracking, 16–17
Profilaggrin, 42
Prognostic studies, level of evidence for, 9t
Program coordinator, 4b, 9–13
Proinflammatory cytokines, 341t
Propionibacterium acnes, 47–48
Proprioception, 269
Prospective payment system (PPS), 33
Prostacyclins, 252
Protection, 46–49, 54t
against pathogens, 46–48
against ultraviolet radiation, 48
Protein(s)
dermal, 46
matrix, 75
wound healing requirements, 414

Protein deficiency, 130–131
Protein kinase C-beta, 252
Proteoglycans, 44
Prothrombin, 67
Pruritus
epidermolysis bullosa and, 452
lymphedema and, 233
malignancy-related wounds, 534–535
Pseudofolliculitis, 46
Pseudomonas aeruginosa, 47–48, 283
biofilms, 289
Pulsatile lavage, 298–299
Pulsating pressure, 167–170
Pulse, 182, 182b
Pulse duration, 370t
Pulse volume recordings, 195
Pulsed current (PC) electrical stimulation, 372–373, 374t
Purpura, 178
Pyoderma gangrenosum, 443–446, 493
bullous, 444
data in workup, 445b
diagnosis of, 444–445, 444b
diagnostic criteria, 445b
manifestations of, 444
systemic diseases associated with, 444b
treatment of, 445, 446t
ulcerative lesion, characteristics, 444
vegetative, 444

Q
Quality improvement, 7–9
for obese patients, 513–514
wound specialist role, 5
Quality of life
chronic pain effects on, 387–388, 388b
foot diseases effect on, 263
pressure ulcers effect on, 126
wound pain effects on, 387–388

R
Radiation recall, 103
Radiation therapy
for hyperproliferative scarring, 77t
skin care during, 103–106, 104t, 105b
skin damage caused by, 102–106
Radiation-induced endarteritis, 542
Random flaps, 492
Randomized clinical trial (RCT), 7
Rapid thrombelastography (r-TEG), 464–465
Reactive hyperemia, 132–133
Reactive oxygen species, 56–57, 68–69, 339–340
Reactive support surface, 168–169t, 170–171
Recertification requirements, 2
Recessive dystrophic epidermolysis bullosa (RDEB), 450b

Rectal pouches, 91–93
Referrals, 28
Refusal, informed, 437–438
Regional block, 402
Reimbursement. see also Billing
documentation for, 26
factors that influence, 33–36
fiscal intermediaries, 35
group health plans, 32–33
incident-to services, 34
Medicaid. see Medicaid
Medicare. see Medicare
nonphysician practitioners, 34
support surfaces, 172–173
wound management, 321–322, 322b
Remodeling phase, of wound healing, 71, 341
Removable cast walkers, 253
Reperfusion injury, 134
Replacement mattresses, 166
Research, 5
utilization, 5–6
Resources, 16
efficient use of, 16
Results
benchmarks, 14
generalizability, 14
Rete pegs, 41f, 42
Reticular dermis, 46
Reticular veins, 178
Retinol-binding protein, 412
Revenue generation, 16–17
Rewarming, 457
Rheumatoid arthritis, 447t
Risk scale, 143–144
RNA transcription factor, 342–343
Romberg test, 269, 269b
Room equipment, 28–29
Rotation flaps, 492
Rubor, dependent, 181
Rule of nines, 477–479, 478f
Russel ("push") technique, 566

S
Sacrum
anatomy of, 114f
pressure ulcers of, 495, 495f
Saddlebagging, 556–557, 556f, 557b
Saline, 382
Satellite lesions, 95
Scab, 65
Scald burns, 476
Scale, 29
Scar formation, wound healing through, 63
Scarring
excessive, 76, 77t
hyperproliferative, 76, 77t
Scleroderma, 46
Seated position, 150–151
Sebaceous gland, 47, 52–53t
Sebum, 47
Secondary healing, 491
Secondary lymphedema, 228
Secondary-intention wound healing, 64, 64f, 72, 72t

Sedation, 403t, 404, 404t
Segmental limb pressure, 195–196
Selectins, 338–339
Selective blockade, 402
Selenium, 235
Self-efficacy, 430–431, 430t
Semiocclusive dressings, 307–308, 307t
Semmes-Weinstein monofilament test, 245, 247b, 247f
Sensation, 50, 54t
Sensitivity, 143–144
Sensory neuropathy, 241
Sensory perception, 146
Sepsis, 467t, 542
Serial abdominal closure, 470–471
Seroma, in surgical wounds, 501
Serum proteins, 411–412
Sesamoid bone, 264
Severe Cutaneous Adverse Reaction (SCAR) classification system, 454, 454b
Sharp debridement, 299–301
Shear, 84–85, 85f
    description of, 130
    repositioning techniques for, 148–151
    transferring without lateral, 149
Shear strain, 164
Shear stress, 164
Shivering, 49, 421
Short Nutritional Assessment Questionnaire (SNAQ), 410
Sickle cell anemia, 459t
Sickle cell disease, 188
Silicone molding, 557, 558b
Silver, 290–291t, 291
Silver antimicrobial dressings, 482
Silver sulfadiazine, 482
Single-layer reusable compression wraps, 216, 218
Skin, 40–62
    in adolescents, 51
    age-related changes in, 51
    bacterial species on, 47
    basement membrane zone, 44
    clinical consult, 59b
    color of, 40, 41b
    communication functions of, 51
    dark. see Darkly pigmented skin
    dermis. see Dermis
    description of, 40
    elasticity of, 55–56
    epidermis. see Epidermis
    factors altering, 51–59
        age, 51–56
        hydration, 57
        medication, 58
        nutrition, 58
        smoking, 58
        soaps, 57–58
        sun exposure, 56–57
    fetal, 51, 55b
    flora on, 47
    formulary for, 271t
    functions of, 46–51
    hydration of, 57

Skin (Continued)
    hypodermis, 46
    immune system, 48–49
    inspection of, 110, 110t
        pressure ulcers, 143
    layers of, 40–46
        basement membrane zone, 44
        dermis, 44–46, 45f, 52–53t
        epidermis, 40–44, 45f, 52–53t
    lower extremity, 178
    metabolic functions of, 50–51
    monitoring of, 110
    in newborn, 52–53t, 54t
    in older adults, 52–53t, 54t
    photoaging effects on, 56, 56b
    in premature infants, 51, 52–53t, 54t
    protective functions of, 46–49
    sensation functions of, 50
    thermoregulatory functions of, 49–50
    thickness of, 52–53t
    vitamin D synthesis in, 50–51
Skin adhesives, 500
Skin assessment, 82, 110–112
    dark skin, 111–112
    documentation of, 109
    lighting necessary for, 110–111
    parameters of, 111t
    in pressure ulcer prevention program, 143
    significance of, 109
Skin barrier products, 550, 551f, 551t
Skin care, 103–106, 104t
    barrier products, 550, 551f, 551t
    lymphedema prevention with, 233
    during radiation therapy, 103–106, 104t, 105b
Skin cleansers, 91
Skin damage
    allergic factors that cause, 101–102
    assessment of, 82
    chemical irritants, 88–89
    classification of, 84b
    etiology of, 102
    mechanical forces that cause, 82–87
        friction, 85
        lacerations, 85–87
        shear, 84–85, 85f
        skin stripping, 85–87
    moisture-associated with, 87–89
    pathophysiologic characteristics, 102–103
    pathophysiologic process, 88
    risk factors of, 103
    types of, 82–108, 106b
    vascular, 94–95
Skin diseases, 40
Skin flaps, 85–86, 497–498
Skin folds
    inspection of, 110
    management, in obese patient, 509–510

Skin grafts, 491, 497
Skin immune system, 46, 48–49
Skin infections, 95
    bacterial, 97–99
    cellulitis, 97
    dermatophyte, 96
    erysipelas, 97
    erythrasma, 98
    folliculitis, 95, 98
    fungal, 95–96
    herpes simplex virus, 99–100
    impetigo, 98–99
    varicella-zoster virus, 100–101
    viral, 99–101
Skin injury, classification of, 457
Skin integrity, mechanical threats to, obesity and, 512
Skin lesions, 83t
Skin perfusion pressure, 195
Skin phototype system (SPT), 48
Skin pigmentation, 43–44
    characteristics of, 41b
    dark
        assessment of, 111–112
        characteristics of, 41b
        dermatologic disorders associated with, 43–44
        erythema detection in, 112
        vitamin D levels on, 50–51
    demographics of, 40
    sun exposure effects on, 48
Skin safety committees, 9–13
    certification in wound care, 10–12
    dietitian or nutritionist, 13
    director, 12
    membership of, 10
    nursing, 12
    occupational therapy, 12
    physical therapy, 12
    potential members of, 11b
    responsibilities of, 10, 11b
    social services, 13
    speech therapy, 12–13
    unit-based skin champions, 12
    utilization review, 13
Skin sealant, 87, 92t
Skin stripping, 85–87
    prevention of, 87b
Skin substitutes, 327
    bilayered, 333–334
    burn injuries managed with, 483
    checklist for using, 326b
    classification of, 326–333
    dermal, 327–329, 328t
    epidermal, 327, 328t
    wound closure using, 491–492
Skin tears
    care plan for, 86–87, 86b
    classification system, 86t
    ISTAP classification system for, 85–86
    prevention of, 86
    risk factors for, 86
Skin temperature, 182
Skinfold measures, 411
Sleep apnea, obesity and, 512

Slough, 295
Slow movement/incremental turns, 149
Smoking, 58
    lower extremity arterial disease risks, 189
    oxygenation affected by, 421
    skin health affected by, 132
    wound healing affected by, 78–79t, 421
Soaps, 57–58
Social Security Amendments, 31
Social services, 13
Social worker, 13
Sodium cromoglycate, 446t
Sodium hypochlorite, 290–291t
Sodium thiosulfate, 448
Soft silicone contact layers, 313
Somatic pain, 389
Somatostatin, 545
Spasms, 494
Specialty absorptive dressings, 316
Specialty beds, 16
Specificity, 143–144
Speech therapist, 12–13
Spider bites, 443
Spider veins, 178
Spinal cord injury, pressure ulcer risks, 126
Splint, 154t
Split-thickness skin grafts, 483–484, 491, 497
Staff, 27–28
    ancillary, 28
    clinic director, 27
    education of, 29
    insurance and billing coder, 27–28
    interdisciplinary team, 27t
    nurse coordinator, 27
    orientation program, 3
    retention, 17
    satisfaction, 17
Stakeholders, 3
Stamm gastrostomy, 563–564, 564f
Standing wave, 381
Staphylococcal scalded skin syndrome, 441–442
Staphylococcus aureus, 283, 441
    biofilms, 289
    methicillin-resistant, 97, 257, 317
Staples, for surgical wounds, 499–500
Starkid Skin Scale, for pressure ulcers, 519t
Starvation-related malnutrition, 409, 413t
Static land mines, 463
Statins, 199
Status indicator, 37
Stem cells, epidermal, 42, 49
Stemmer sign, 179, 232
Steri-Strips, 500
Stevens-Johnson syndrome, 454, 454b
Stoma, pouching for, in pediatric patients, 523–524, 523b

Stratum basale, 41f, 42–44
Stratum corneum, 41, 41f
Stratum germinativum, 41f, 42–44
Stratum granulosum, 41f, 42
Stratum lucidum, 41–42, 41f
Stratum spinosum, 41f, 42
Stress, 420
  autonomic nervous system
    response to, 420
  pressure ulcer risks, 131–132
Styloid process, 264
Subcutaneous, 52–53t
Subfascial endoscopic perforator
  vein surgery, 221–223
Substance P, 69
Subungual, 266b
Sucrose, for pain management, in
  infants, 525
Suction-assisted lipectomy, 236
Sun exposure, 48, 56–57
Sunburn, 57
Sunscreens, 57
Superficial venous system, 205
Supervised walking programs, 198
Support surfaces, 16, 162–176, 175b
  active (alternating pressure),
    167–170, 168–169t
  air fluidized, 168–169t, 171
  care setting-specific formulary,
    172–175
  categories of, 162, 166–171,
    168–169t
  chair cushions, 167
  continuous lateral rotation,
    168–169t, 170
  definition of, 162
  effectiveness evaluation, 173b
  emergency room, 166–167
  entrapment risks, 172
  fall risks, 172
  fatigue of, 162–163
  features of, 166–171, 168–169t
  fluids as, 165–166
  foam, 164–165, 168–169t
  gel, 165
  guidance for, 163b
  inspection of, 175b
  integrated bed system, 167
  interface tissue pressure, 162
  life expectancy of, 162–163
  low air loss, 168–169t, 170–171
  maintenance of, 174
  mattress overlays, 166
  mattresses, 166–167
  Medicare reimbursement, 173
  medium used in, 164, 164f
  microclimate control, 164
  moisture control considerations,
    164
  nonpowered static air, 164f
  operating room, 162, 167b
  patient need, 171–172
  physical concepts, 162–164
  pressure redistribution, 163–164,
    168–169t
  purchasing, 173
  reactive, 164f, 170–171

Support surfaces (Continued)
  reimbursement for, 172–173
  renting of, 173, 174t
  safety of, 174
  selection criteria for, 171–175
  size of patient considerations,
    172
  therapeutic functions of,
    162–164
  weight of patient considerations,
    172
Suprathel, 330–331t
Surgery
  abscess treated with, 494
  decision making, 490–491
  fistula management with, 546
  gangrene treated with, 494
  gastrostomy tube placement
    during, 563
  history of, 490
  lymphedema treated with, 235
  necrotizing fasciitis treated
    with, 494
  nonoperative conditions, 493
  in obese patients, 511–513
  patient assessment before, 490
  preoperative management,
    494–495
  pressure ulcers treated with,
    491, 496
  radiation-induced wounds
    treated with, 105
  reconstructive, 490–498, 491f,
    498b
  reducing cofactors, 494–495
  traumatic wounds treated with,
    493–494
  wound assessment before,
    490–491
  wound bed preparation for, 495
Surgical debridement, 289,
  300–301
Surgical site infection (SSI),
  501–502, 502t, 503t
Surgical wounds, 499–506, 505b
  ASEPSIS scoring tool for,
    500–501, 501b
  assessment of, 500–503
  closure of, 499–500
  description of, 499
  healing of, impediments to,
    500b, 501–503
  infections of, 501–502
  skin adhesives for, 500
  staples for, 499–500
  sutures for, 499–500
  systemic conditions on, 502–503
  topical incision care, 503–505,
    504b
Sutures
  for surgical wounds, 499–500
  tube stabilization using, 573–574
Swab technique, for wound culture
  collection, 288, 288b
Sweat glands, 49–50
Sweating, 49–50
Systemic circulation, 206f

Systemic inflammatory response
  syndrome (SIRS), 467, 467t
Systemic lupus erythematosus
  (SLE), 447t

T

T lymphocytes, 68
Tagliacozzi flap, 490
Tarsals, 264, 264f, 265f
Tarsometatarsal (TMT) joints, 264
Team model terms, 10t
Telangiectasias, 103, 178
Tendo-Achilles lengthening, 255
Tertiary-intention wound healing,
  64, 64f
Testing standards, 2
Tetanus, 465–466
Thalassemia, 459t
Thermal burns, 475–476
Thermal injuries, 463
  in pediatric patients, 524
Thermoregulation, 49–50, 54t
Thrill, 182
Thrombin, 67
Thromboangiitis obliterans, 188
Thyroxin-binding prealbumin, 412
Tinea, 96, 96b, 276–277, 279t
Tinea incognito, 96
Tissue
  healthy, characteristics of, 468t
  nonviable, 115
  type of, 115
  viable, 115
Tissue anoxia, 128
Tissue biopsy, 288
Tissue expansion, for wound
  closure, 492–493
Tissue flaps, 492, 492b
Tissue hypoxia
  smoking as cause of, 132
  wound, 419–420
Tissue inhibitors of
  metalloproteinases, 75, 340
Tissue macrophages, 49
Tissue oxygen, 371
Tissue tolerance, 129–132
Tobacco cessation, 190b
Toe-brachial index, 194–195
Topical antimicrobials, 289,
  290–291t
Topical incision care, 503–505,
  504b
Topical medications, 400–402
Topical nitrogen mustard, 446t
Topical oxygen therapy, 366–367
Topical wound care, 454
Total body surface area (TBSA),
  475, 477–479
Total contact cast (TCC), 253–254,
  275t
Total thigh flap, 496
Touch, 50
Tourniquet, 465
Toxic epidermal necrolysis (TEN),
  441, 454–456, 455t
  "with spots," 454b
  "without spots," 454b

Toxic shock syndrome, 442
Tracheostomy care, obesity and,
  513
Tracheostomy straps, 154t
Traditional high-frequency
  ultrasound, 379–381
Transcutaneous oximetry (TcPO2),
  248
Transcutaneous oxygen pressure
  (TcPO2), 195
Transcutaneous oxygen tension,
  424, 424f
Transdisciplinary, 9–10, 10t
Transducer, 379–380, 379f
Transepidermal water loss (TEWL),
  44, 51
  neonatal skin and, 516
Transferrin, 412
Transforming growth factor-β,
  340t, 344
Transgastric jejunal tube, 569f
Transient amplifying cells, 42
Transient bacteremia, 300
Transparent film dressings,
  316, 319t
Transposition flaps, 492
Transpyloric percutaneous
  endoscopic jejunostomy,
  567–568, 568f
Transthyretin, 412
Traumatic wounds, 462–474, 472b
  acute management of, 464–468
  advanced trauma life support
    for, 464–465
  amputation of, 471
  antibiotic beads for, 469
  assessment of, 466
  ballistic injuries, 463
  blast injuries, 463
  bleeding control, 464–465
  bone exposure, 468
  bullet wounds, 462–463
  care, components of, 463b
  debridement of, 467
  description of, 462
  dressings for, 469
  explosive munitions, 463–464
  gunshot wounds, 466
  heterotopic ossification, 471–472
  immunization, 465–466
  irrigation of, 466
  negative pressure wound therapy
    for, 469
  nerve injury repair, 466–467
  open abdomen closure, 470–471
  with open fractures, 469
  subacute management of,
    468–472
    serial irrigation and
      debridement, 468–469,
      468t
  surgery for, 493–494
  thermal injuries, 463
  vehicle crashes, 464
  war wounds, 462–464
Treatment orders, 25–26
Trophic changes, 177

Tropocollagen, 46
Trough procedure, 557–558, 559b, 559f
Trovafloxacin, 257
Tuberosity of fifth metatarsal, 264
Tubes. *see* Drainage tubes; Gastrostomy tubes; Jejunostomy tubes
Tubular sleeve, 218
Tumor, 534
Tumor necrosis factor-α
  in inflammatory phase, 68–69, 340
  wound healing role of, 341t
Tunneling, 116–117, 117f
Turning patients in bed, 148–149, 148f, 157f
24-hour urine creatinine, 413

U

Ulcers. *see* Arterial ulcers; Diabetic foot ulcers; Pressure ulcer(s); Venous ulcers
Ultrasonic debridement, 382
Ultrasonic low-frequency debridement, 382–383, 383t
Ultrasound, 379–383, 379f, 383b
  definition of, 379
  device for, 379f
  high-frequency, 379–381
  low-intensity, 380
  noncontact low-frequency, 381–382
Ultrasound mist, 299
Ultraviolet light, 377–385, 378f, 383b
  bacteriocidal effects, 378
  conditions exacerbated by, 379b
  contraindications, 378–379, 379b
  equipment for administering, 378f
  indications for, 378
  physiologic effects of, 380
  precautions for, 378–379, 379b
  use of, 378
  UV-A, 377
  UV-B, 377
  UV-C, 377
Ultraviolet radiation exposure
  protection against, 48
  skin effects, 50–51
Unavoidable pressure ulcer, 141–142, 142b
Undersea Medical Society, 361
Ungual, 266b
Unite Biomatrix, 332
Universal precautions, 317–318
University of Texas classification system, 250–251, 251t
Unprocessed resources, 6, 7t
Urocanic acid, 42
Utilization review (UR) specialist, 13

V

Vacuum-assisted closure, 351t
Vaginal fistula, 552–553, 552f
Validity, 143–144

Vancomycin-resistant *Staphylococcus aureus*, 257
Varicella-zoster virus, 100–101
Varicose veins, 177–178, 210
Vasa nervosum, 252
Vascular damage, 94–95
Vascular endothelial growth factor, 44, 69, 344, 420
Vasculitis, 188, 446–448, 447t
Vasculogenesis, 44
Vegetative pyoderma gangrenosum, 444
Vehicle crashes, 464
Veins
  appearance of, 177–178
  lower extremity, structure and function, 205, 207f
  perforating, 207f
  valvular dysfunction, 208
  varicose, 177–178, 210
Velcro wraps, 219
Venous dermatitis, 210–211, 211t
Venous edema, 180t
Venous ulcers, 112–113, 204–226, 224b. *see also* Chronic venous insufficiency
  ablation procedures for, 223
  adjunct therapies for, 221
  arterial perfusion associated with, 209–210
  assessment of, 209–212
  characteristics of, 184–185t, 211
  diagnostic evaluation of, 211–212
  epidemiology of, 204–205
  follow-up for, 223–224
  history of patients, 208t, 209
  lifelong maintenance for, 223–224
  lipodermatosclerosis associated with, 210
  management of, 212–213
    compression therapy, 213–216
    exercise, 212
    failure to progress, 220–221
    horse chestnut seed extract, 213
    limb elevation, 212
    local wound care, 220–221, 222f
    micronized purified flavonoid fraction, 213
    pentoxifylline, 213
    pharmacologic therapy, 212–213
    weight control, 212
  mixed arterial-venous disease, 199
  pain associated with, 389–390
  pathology of, 209
  prevalence of, 204
  protease levels in, 346f
  recurrence rates, 223
  surgical interventions, 221–223
  surgical treatments for, 223t
  trapping theory of, 209
  varicosities associated with, 210

Venous ulcers (*Continued*)
  white blood cell activation theory of, 209
Venous valves, 207f
Ventral hernia, 470
Vesicants, 452, 452t
Viral infections, 99
Visceral pain, 389
Viscoelastic foam, 165
Viscoelastic gel, 165
Viscous fluid, as support surface, 166
Visual analog scale, 391f
Vitamin A, 131, 415
Vitamin C, 131, 415
Vitamin D, 50–51
Vitamin E, 131
Vitamins, 415
  deficiency of, 131
Voltage, 370t
Volume support, 423–424
V-Y advancement flap, 496

W

Wagner foot wound classification system, 250, 250t
War wounds, etiology of, 462–464
Warming, 422
Warts, 276
Water, as support surface, 166
Waveform, 370t
Weibel-Palade bodies, 339
Weight, 411
Werner syndrome, 46
Wet gangrene, 494
Wet to dry dressings, 469
Wet-to-dry gauze debridement, 298
Wind chill temperature, 456
Witzel gastrostomy, 564, 564f
Witzel jejunostomy, 564–565
World Health Organization Pain Clinical Ladder, 400, 401b, 401f
World Wide Web, 6
Wound
  acute. *see* Acute wounds
  anatomic location of, 113
  bioburden effects on, 283
  burn
    fungal infection of, 482
    infection of, 482
    stabilization of, 480–481
    sunscreen protection, 487
  cellular- and tissue-based products for, 325–336, 327b, 335b
  chronic. *see* Chronic wounds
  classification systems for, 114
  cleansing of, 318, 399, 536
  culture of, 287
  depth measurements, 116, 117f, 320
  drainage of, 538
  duration of, 113
  filling of, 319
  financial impact of, 435
  full-thickness. *see* Full-thickness wounds

Wound (*Continued*)
  ischemic, 493
  length measurements, 116, 117f
  malignancy-related. *see* Malignancy-related wounds
  measurement of, 115–116, 116t
  packing, 319
  partial-thickness. *see* Partial-thickness wound
  preventable, reduction of, 16
  senescence and, 321
  shape of, 117
  size of, 115–117
  surgical. *see* Surgical wounds
  traumatic. *see* Traumatic wounds
  tunneling, of 320
  uncommon, 441–461, 459b
  undermining of, 320
  width measurements, 116, 117f
Wound assessment, 113–118, 122b
  anatomic location of, 113
  bacterial burden, 118
  classification systems for, 114
  depth measurements, 116, 117f
  edge, 118
  etiology and differential diagnosis, 112–113
  exudate, 117–118
  length measurements, 116, 117f
  parameters of, 113b
  periwound skin, 118
  regulatory documentation tools, 119
  shape of, 117
  before surgery, 490–491
  tissue involvement, 113–114
  tissue type in, 113–114
  tunneling, 116–117, 117f
  undermining, 116–117, 117f
  width measurements, 116, 117f
Wound-Associated Pain Model, 395f
Wound base
  tissue color in, 115
  tissue types in, 115, 320
Wound bed
  descriptors of, 115t
  fibroblasts in, 70–71
  hypoxia, 65–66
  preparation of, 346, 495
  pressure ulcer staging after assessment of, 135–136
  principles of, 347t
  tissue in
    color of, 115
    type of, 115
Wound care
  costs of, 16
  supplies for, 29
  venous ulcers, 220–221, 222f
Wound care orders, 322
Wound care practice
  factors that affect the success of, 1
  stakeholders in, 3
Wound care program, 1
  policies and procedures, 9

Wound clinic. *see* Clinic
Wound closure
    methods for, 491–493
    secondary healing, 491
    skin graft for, 491
    skin substitutes for, 491–492
    surgical, 499–500
    tissue expansion for, 492–493
    tissue flaps for, 492, 492b
Wound contraction
    negative pressure wound therapy
        for, 351
    in secondary-intention wound
        healing, 64f, 72
Wound conversion, 477
Wound debridement, 295–305, 303b
    algorithm for, 301f
    clinician experience and
        competence, 302
    condition and goals for the
        patient, 302
    conservative instrumental, 299
    conservative sharp, 299–300,
        299b, 399
    continued maintenance, 289
    definition of, 299
    diabetic foot ulcers, 256
    documentation of, 26
    maintenance of, 302–303
    methods of, 296–301
        autolysis, 296–297
        biosurgical, 298
        chemical, 297–298
        enzymatic, 297
        hydrosurgical water knife, 301
        hydrotherapy, 298
        laser, 301
        maggots, 298
        mechanical, 298–299
        pulsatile lavage, 298–299
        selective *versus* nonselective,
            296b
        sharp, 299–301, 402
        ultrasonic mist, 299
        wet-to-dry gauze, 298
        wound irrigation, 298–299
        wound status, 302
    necrotic tissue, 295
    before negative wound therapy,
        354
    odor control with, 537
    pain management during, 399
    progression of, 302–303
    purpose of, 295
    selection of, 301–303, 301f
    supplies for, 29
    traumatic wounds, 467
    ultrasonic, 382–383
    wound irrigation, 298–299
    wound status, 302

Wound edge, 118
Wound environment
    characteristics of, 306–308
    moisture level in, 307–308
    normal temperature, 308
    objectives for, 307t
    pH, 308
Wound exudate, 117–118
    description of, 319–320
    malignant cutaneous wounds,
        537–538
    pouches for collection of,
        537–538
Wound filler, 317
    examples of wound
        characteristics matched
        with, 354t
Wound fluid, removal of, 350–351
Wound healing, 79b
    acute wounds, 64
    assessment of cofactors, 113t
    assessment of instruments, 120b
    chronic wounds, 64
    cytokines in, 341t
    delayed, 283
    effect of perfusion in, 419–420
    environment, 64–65
    factors that affect, 78–79t, 494
    faster rates, 16
    full-thickness wounds, 64, 66,
        71–73
    goal of, 429
    imbalance molecular
        environments of, 347f
    inflammatory phase of, 68, 72t
    maturation of, 71, 72t
    mechanism of, 63–64
    mediators of, 74–75
    nutrient needs for, 414–416
    obesity effects on, 421
    oxygen in
        effect of, 419–420
        important roles of, 420t
    partial-thickness wounds, 64,
        65–66, 65t
    phases of, 337–338
    potential for, 429
    predicting, 119–120
    primary intention, 64, 64f, 504
    process of, 64–73
        cascade of events, 67f
    reassessment of, 119–122
    remodeling phase of, 71, 341
    role of nutrients, 415t
    scar formation as form of, 63
    scarless
        characteristics of, 75b
        in fetus, 63–64
    secondary, 64, 64f, 72t
    smoking effects on, 78–79t, 421

Wound healing (*Continued*)
    surgical, impediments to, 500b,
        501–503
    systemic support for, 199–200
    tertiary, 64, 64f
    tools for documentation and
        evaluation of, 120–121
    topical oxygen therapy, 366–367
Wound infection
    chronic wound, 287
    clinical consult, 293b
    conservative sharp debridement,
        299
    cultures for, 287–288
    evaluation of, 292–293
    laboratory tests for, 287–288
    manifestations of, 286–287
    risk factors for, 287b
    signs and symptoms of, 287
    surgical, 501–502
Wound irrigation, 298–299, 318, 466
Wound management
    costs of, 16
    documentation of, 321–322, 322b
    principles of, 306–308, 307b
    reimbursement for, 321–322,
        322b
    topical, 306–324, 322b, 445–446
        bacterial bioburden, 321
        extravasation wounds, 454
    wound environment
        characteristics, 306–308
Wound management plan
    barriers to, 431t
    care transitions, 436
    mistrust, 435–436
    noncompliance with. *see*
        Noncompliance
    skepticism, 435–436
Wound Matrix, 332
Wound odor, 118
    assessment of, 321
    charcoal dressings for, 537
    control of, 536–537
    debridement for, 537
    deodorizers for, 536–537
    topical antimicrobials for, 537
Wound Ostomy and Continence
    Nurses Society, 371
Wound pain, 386–398, 396b.
        see also Pain
    acute, 389
    assessment of, 390–394
    care models, 394–395, 394f, 395f
    causes of, 389f
    chronic, 404b
    classification of, 388–390
    consequences of, 387–388
    debridement, 302, 390, 399
    goals for, 390

Wound pain (*Continued*)
    history-taking, 390
    intensity scales, 390, 391f, 393t
    management of, 399–407, 406b
        addiction concerns, 405–406
        complications of, 404–405
        dressings, 400
        injectable medications for, 402
        nonpharmacologic pain
            control, 399–400
        opioids, 401b, 402–403, 403t
        pharmacologic, 400–406
        systemic medications for,
            402–404
        topical medications for,
            400–402
    mixed nociceptive/neuropathic,
        389–390
    neuropathic, 389
    nociceptive, 389
    physiology of, 388
    quality of life effects, 387–388
Wound Pain Management model,
    394f, 395
Wound specialist
    educational preparation, 1–2
    factors that affect the success
        of, 1
    functions of, 2–13
    responsibilities of, 2–13
    roles of, 2–13, 3t, 4b
        benefits of, 15
        change agent, 4
        consultant, 3
        educator, 3–4
        facilitator of evidence-based
            practice and quality
            improvement, 5–9
        marketing of, 15–18
        program coordinator, 9–13
Wound tissue hypoxia, 419–420
Wound treatment associate
    (WTA), 12

X

Xelma, 330–331t
Xenograft, 483
Xenographic extracellular matrix
    scaffolds, 332
Xerosis, 271
Xylitol, 290–291t, 291

Z

Zinc, 415–416
Zone of coagulation, 477
Zone of hyperemia, 477
Zone of stasis, 477
Z technique, 288